PATHOLOGY
FOR THE
HEALTH
SCIENCES

For my students

PATHOLOGY FOR THE HEALTH SCIENCES

Written and illustrated by

NICHOLAS J. VARDAXIS

Department of Medical Laboratory Science
Royal Melbourne Institute of Technology

CHURCHILL LIVINGSTONE
EDINBURGH   HONG KONG   LONDON   MADRID   MELBOURNE
NEW YORK AND TOKYO 1995

CHURCHILL LIVINGSTONE
Medical Division of Longman Group Limited

Distributed in the United States of America by Churchill
Livingstone Inc., 650 Avenue of the Americas, New York,
N.Y. 10011, and by associated companies, branches and
representatives throughout the world.

First edition 1994: Macmillan Education Australia Pty Ltd
UK edition 1995: Longman Group Ltd.

ISBN 0 443 05324 3

British Library Cataloguing in Publication Data
A catalogue record for this book is available from the
British Library.

Library of Congress Cataloging in Publication Data
A catalog record for this book is available from the Library
of Congress.

Typeset in Times
by Superskill Graphics, Singapore

Printed in Hong Kong

Contents

Preface

This text was written with the students of the health sciences in mind and presents an introduction to the subject of pathology. The material has been arranged in a such a way that the essentials of the subject are covered in Part I, on general pathology, and then in Part II, on systemic pathology, each organ system of the body is covered in greater detail. The student may at any time, of course, refer to Part II for more detail about a disease process affecting a particular organ system, but the topics have been arranged in a logical order, such that each chapter follows on from the next and the information is slowly built up on the previous chapter's foundation. At the end of each chapter a section of questions that examine the understanding of the material and case studies illustrating the information presented in that chapter has been included. It is suggested that the student tackle these questions and case studies before proceeding to the next chapter. In addition, lists of relevant further reading material are provided for the interested student who wishes to pursue a topic further.

In its modern definition pathology is taken to be 'the study of disease by scientific methods, elucidating its causes and effects'. It nowadays has input from several specialized areas: **morbid anatomy** (or gross pathology); **histopathology and cytology**; **biochemistry** (clinical pathology); **haematology**; **medical microbiology**; **immunology**; and **genetics**. Each of these branches is a very specialized area but in any given disease process specialists in these different fields may be called upon to help in the diagnosis of disease and also help in the clarification of the cause of disease. A rather more specialized branch of the subject is **forensic pathology**, and in this discipline pathology shows an overlap with the law as often a forensic pathologist will be called upon as a specialist witness in a court of law in order to provide vital information about the cause of death of a person. As students you may have been introduced already to the methods and means of study of disease in some of these fields. However, this text focuses on the areas of theoretical pathology and morbid anatomy which are interrelated disciplines and an understanding of which is essential in the study of disease.

Pathology laboratories undertake a very wide variety of scientific tests which may be required for the diagnosis of many diseases. At a time when our lives are becoming increasingly intertwined with science and technology, primary health practitioners have come to depend more and more on laboratory tests for accurate diagnosis, since it is only on this basis that proper treatment may be undertaken. You will be introduced to some of the important and commonly encountered tests as far as diagnosis of disease is concerned in the fields of pathology, morbid anatomy and clinical pathology. You will observe the intimate relationship between disease as it manifests itself in the body and disease as it is evident at the cellular, tissue and organ levels.

This pathology text is by no means an exhaustive treatise on pathology, nor does it delve too deeply into the molecular causation of disease; however, it aims to solve many of the problems that face students who are embarking on the study of disease. These are, firstly, the difficulty in coping with the extensive terminology and nomenclature of pathology; secondly, the difficulty in relating changes to or aberrations from normal structure and function to the more overt manifestations of disease such as signs and symptoms; thirdly, the interpretation of pathological changes evident in tissues or organs. This text aims to solve these problems by stressing the dynamic nature of disease and repair processes and by encouraging observation of structural changes in disease and discussion of the underlying mechanisms. This depends on considerable practical experience in analysis of pathological material and therefore sessions in the laboratory are seen to be an essential experience which should be undertaken in conjunction with a course in theoretical pathology. Studying pathology improves one's powers of **observation** and **deduction**, both fundamental to study in any branch of medicine or science. The understanding of general principles of pathological processes is an important objective.

An adequate knowledge of anatomy and physiology is essential and is presupposed as both of these subjects are prerequisites for the study of pathology. This text will help you in coping with the extensive work load that must be covered in your course of pathology.

Nicholas J. Vardaxis
Melbourne, November 1992

Part I

General Pathology

1

Introduction to the Study of Disease

The World Health Organization has defined health as a condition of complete physical, mental and social well-being. This is an idealistic definition and compromises often have to be made as the state defined by the World Health Organization is very hard to attain in the real world. To be 'healthy' is often erroneously equated in the minds of many people as being free of disease and this is because the presence of disease is such an obvious and uncomfortable feature of people's lives. Disease has always plagued and fascinated humans, its causation having been a subject of endless speculation, philosophical discussions, scientific hypotheses and experimentation.

In the past, pathology was regarded as the study of dead bodies, mainly as a means of establishing the cause of death. In its modern guise pathology is the scientific study of disease and its causation. The history of pathology is an interesting field of study as it overlaps in many cases with other fields of intellectual activity, such as religion, philosophy and science. The concept of disease and its causation has progressed through the centuries from an essentially spiritual concept to a physical, scientifically explicable state that may be studied in a similar manner to any other branch of science.

Modern-day pathologists have many resources available to them with which they are able to study disease and its causation. However, it is not surprising that even today the causes of many diseases are still unknown. Although we may diagnose such diseases, describe them accurately and sometimes treat them more or less effectively, we still know little about their causes and hence we are powerless to prevent their occurrence. It is only when we study a disease and its causation that we are able to deal with it effectively, not only treating it when it arises but also being able to prevent it.

History of Pathology

Primitive and ancient people knew little about the causes and processes of disease, although they were able to see the outward signs of disease and knew how it felt to be sick. Primitive people regarded disease as a divine punishment for wrongdoing and various evil spirits and demons were held responsible for bringing about the disease. The witchdoctors of these cultures tried to treat disease by exorcizing the demons out of the body. The ancient Mesopotamians and Egyptians (*c*. 2500 BC) also held demons responsible for many ailments but often they also took a more practical, empirical approach to the treatment of disease. Ancient Egyptian papyri mention several identifiable diseases and their treatments, which were often vegetable, animal and mineral preparations, or even simple surgical procedures. Even though the Egyptians embalmed the bodies of their dead, the priest-doctors knew surprisingly little of the normal anatomy and function of the human body as it was the slaves and not the doctors that carried out the mummification process.

The contagious nature of certain diseases was known in Biblical times, hence the sufferers of leprosy were said to be 'unclean' and kept apart from the community. Ancient China and other Eastern civilizations were also aware of the nature of contagion, smallpox being a typical infectious disease that the ancient Chinese physician knew a lot about and did much to try and confer immunity to. Ideas about disease in most of these civilizations were a complex philosophical and spiritual *mélange*. Many herbal preparations were prescribed and some age-old Eastern treatments for disease, including acupuncture and tactile therapies, are still popular and in use today throughout the world.

The ancient Greeks contributed significantly to the study of medicine. Hippocrates (*c*. 400 BC) believed that disease could be caused by external factors, not evil demons. He described accurately many diseases and treated diseases in a common-sense manner, stating that nature was the greatest healer. Some quite complex surgical operations were carried out by the ancient Greeks with a great deal of success. On the other hand, some other ancient Greek thinkers took a more philosophical view of disease and explained it by postulating the existence of four essential body humours (body fluids) that corresponded to the four 'elements', earth, fire, air and water. Figure 1.1 illustrates the basis of the **humoral aetiology of disease** as was propounded by the ancient Greek philosophers.

Such ideas were initiated by Empedocles, Pythagoras, Anaximenes and Heraclitus of Ephesus amongst others. The four humours were **phlegm**, **blood**, **yellow bile** and **black bile**. Disease was due to imbalances of these four humours caused by improper drainage or production of the humours. **Dyscrasia** is a term meaning 'improper mixing' and refers to this improper mixing of the humours to cause disease. This term is still used nowadays to describe some conditions of the blood. It was maintained that a **phlegmatic** person tended to be flaccid and obese with thin hair, narrow blood vessels and white pasty skin. They were said to be slow in movement and intelligence, even-tempered and not given much to gastric or venereal pleasures. A **plethoric** person had an excess of blood, and, although

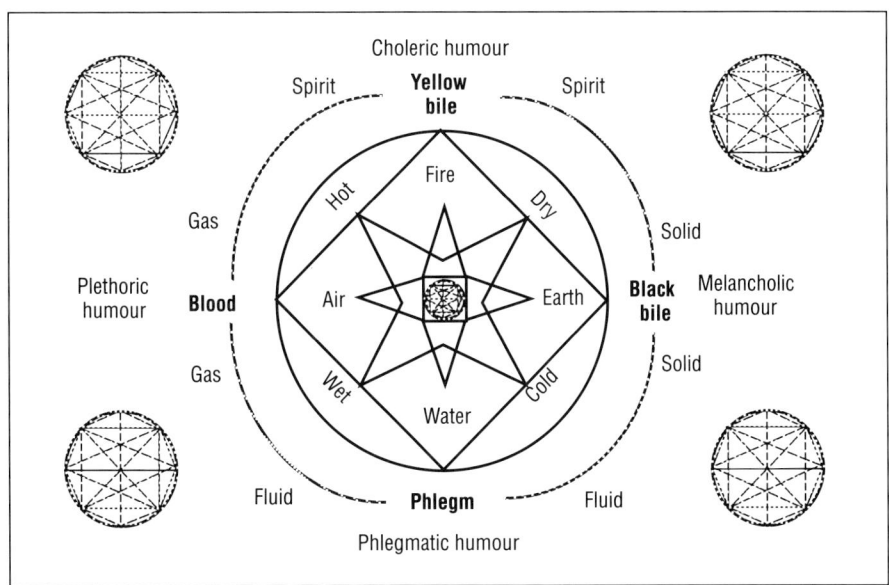

Figure 1.1 *The humoral aetiology of disease as propounded by the ancient Greek philosophers*

obese, tended to be robust and active, moderately hypersexed with a good appetite and a full strong pulse. A **choleric** person tended to be thin, energetic, with a strong inclination to sexual pleasure, fastidious of food, a strong rapid pulse and good blood vessels. The **melancholic** type was typically dark and hairy, with narrow blood vessels, slow pulse, large appetite and inclined towards sexual activity.

The importance of this humoral system of pathology cannot be stressed enough. It was the predominant ancient theory of disease causation and it was adopted widely in the ancient world. With some variations, the humoral system persisted until the end of the 18th century, only slightly affected by the discoveries of the 16th and 17th centuries. Traces of this system are still in evidence today, especially in the alternative medicine areas of naturopathy, traditional Chinese medicine, homoeopathy and so on. The excessive use of bleeding, purgation, sweating and other, often detrimental, modes of therapy over the centuries was a direct outcome of this system of regarding disease.

The Romans continued the Greek tradition and Celsus, a Roman, wrote a book on medicine in 30 AD. Galen, a Greek who lived and practised in Rome, performed dissections and also found various drugs (about 500) which could be used in treatment of disease, and some of which are still used today in the same form. Galen, however, performed most of his studies on pigs because of the ban on dissecting human cadavers, and therefore was responsible for the dissemination of much inaccurate information, which persisted for centuries after his death (see Figure 1.2).

During the Middle Ages very little new material became known about the nature of disease and superstition reigned supreme. Many ancient writings (often those of a fanciful or superstitious nature) were accepted blindly as the truth and medical people did not do any new work. In many cases such ancient writings contained serious errors and fallacies, and even if a perspicacious observer saw such errors he dared not contradict. Some progress in the study of disease occurred in the East during the Middle Ages, in the Arabian world, where great hospitals were founded and the ancient Greek and Roman knowledge and traditions were maintained. The humoral system of pathology was widely adhered to and was used in the diagnosis and treatment of all diseases. Avicenna, the great Persian physician, wrote many important works on medicine and his 'Canon' was a standard text in the mediaeval world. The Byzantine empire also had very proficient physicians and the church with its many monasteries was often involved in the running of hospitals and looking after the sick.

It was not until the Renaissance that dissections were carried out more scientifically and many discoveries were made about the anatomy and function of the human body, but also the changes in disease were studied. The Swiss physician Paracelsus (alias Aureolus Theophrastus Bombastus von Hohenheim) was a controversial figure who advanced chemotherapy by preparing and prescribing many compounds of iron, antimony, zinc and mercury. Paracelsus was also the first to make a partial break from tradition in that he refuted aspects of the humoral pathology system. The Belgian anatomist Andreas Vesalius (*c.* 1550) performed painstaking dissections on human cadavers and pointed out the errors propounded by Galen's writings, correcting approximately 200 anatomical errors of Galen. Giovanni Battista Morgagni, an Italian (1682–1771), pioneered the autopsy examination and anatomical pathology, and Bonet at about the same time compiled all previous dissections and pointed out differences between normal and diseased organs. In the 18th century the Englishman John Hunter (1728–1793)

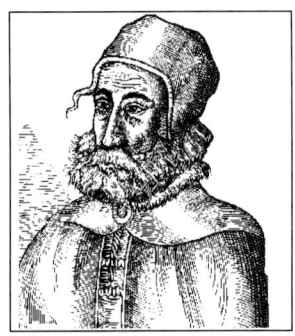

Claudius Galen 131–201 AD

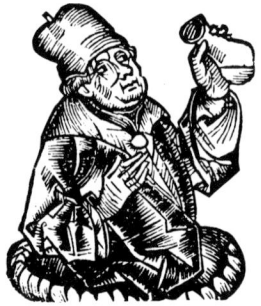

Ibn Sina Avicenna 980–1037 AD

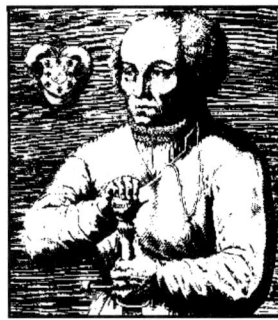

Paracelsus 1493–1541 AD

Figure 1.2   *Some famous physicians of the past*

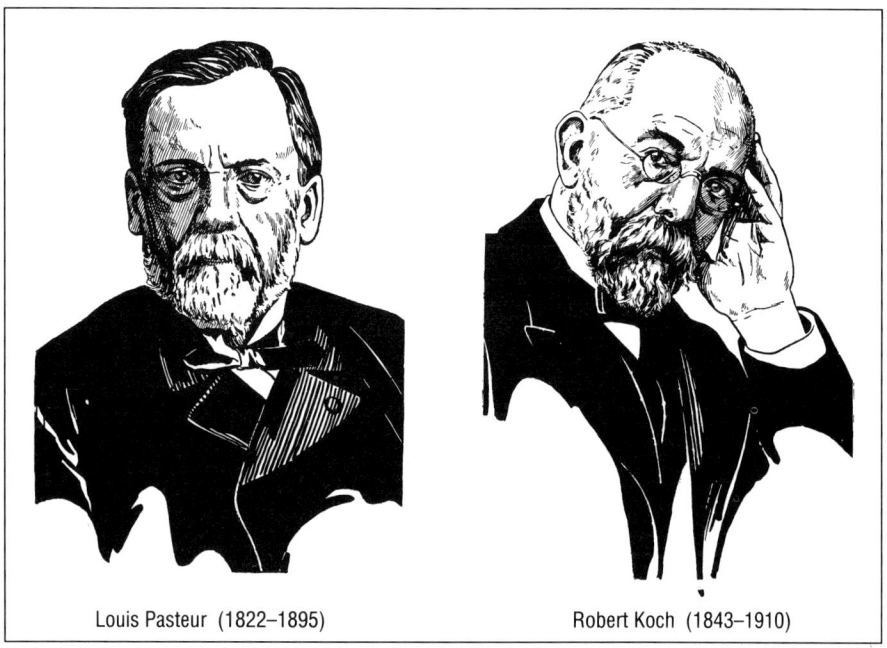

Louis Pasteur (1822–1895) Robert Koch (1843–1910)

Figure 1.3 *The two most famous microbiologists of the 19th century*

first began experimental pathology (using himself as a subject in his studies on venereal diseases!).

During the 19th century many advances were made in the study of disease and its causes. Louis Pasteur (France) and Robert Koch (Germany) discovered the micro-organisms which caused some serious diseases and helped develop vaccines to prevent diseases (refer to Figure 1.3). Also, at the end of the 19th century, advances were made in cellular pathology and immunology. Carl Rokitansky (1804–1878), the Bohemian pathologist, wrote an extensive treatise on diseases of the arteries and performed over 30 000 autopsies, publishing his findings. Rudolf Virchow (1821–1902) is considered to be the 'father' of cellular pathology and some of his work is still valid today. Virchow was the first pathologist who looked for the causes of disease at a cellular level and tried to understand the nature of injury as it affected cells.

Clinical pathology began in hospital ward 'side rooms' where very simple tests were performed to help diagnose disease. As the number of tests which could be performed increased, the pathology laboratory came into being. In the 20th century, with the advent of electron microscopy and better technology, disease can be studied at the ultrastructural and molecular level. Pathology laboratory investigations now utilize many different departments and specialities, which are described below.

Histopathology and cytology are specialities in which tissues and cells are examined for abnormalities under the microscope. The structure of the tissue and the relationship between one cell and another cell may give valuable information about the nature of disease. Rudolf Virchow was the first pathologist to stress the importance of cellular changes in disease. The examination of cellular changes is often the only conclusive method of diagnosing a particular disease. Diseases such as tumours are conclusively diagnosed by these specialities. Very often, pieces of tissue removed from the body during life (tissue biopsies) are sent to the histopathology laboratory in order to diagnose disease (refer to Figure 1.4).

Biochemistry is often referred to as 'clinical pathology' and examines body fluids. Blood, serum, urine and cerebrospinal fluid may be examined for abnormal components and metabolic studies may be carried out. Usually when most people return from their doctor's surgery and say that they have had a 'blood test' done, they have had blood taken for some biochemical examination to be carried out. Diseases of metabolism such as diabetes, alkalosis or phenylketonuria rely on this discipline for diagnosis. Detecting the level of cholesterol and other lipoproteins as an indicator of cardiac disease risk is another common test that is carried out by this department.

Microbiology is the specialized area in which in-

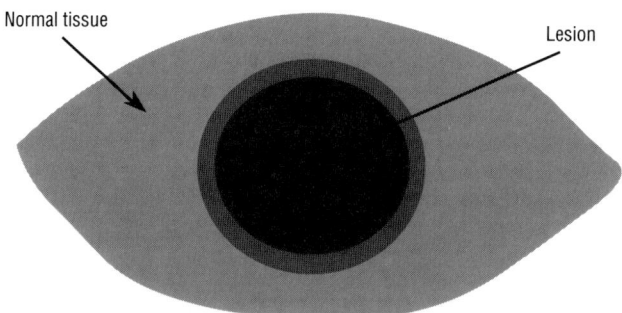

A small, 1.5 cm diameter, well-circumscribed lesion excised for biopsy. Note that a sleeve of normal tissue around the lesion has also been removed and the zone of interaction between the normal tissue and the lesion is also included. This zone of interaction may provide important clues about the nature of the disease process.

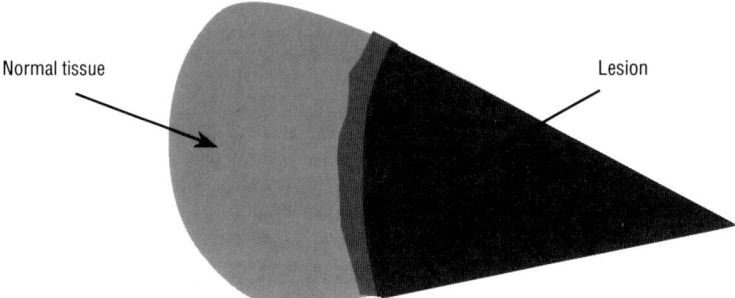

Excision biopsy from a larger, 6 cm diameter lesion including once again a portion of normal tissue, a portion of the lesion and the zone of interaction between the two regions.

Figure 1.4   *Excision biopsies of lesions of different sizes may give important clues as to the aetiology of the disease process active in the diseased tissue*

fectious diseases are studied. Specimens from a case of suspected infectious disease are sent to the laboratory which is responsible for identification of microorganisms causing many diseases. Bacterial, viral, fungal, protozoal and parasitic diseases may be diagnosed, for example diphtheria, urinary tract infections, influenza, thrush, worm infestations.

Haematology examines the blood and blood cells to identify any blood abnormalities and clotting defects. A blood sample is taken and diseases such as leukaemia, anaemia and haemophilia may be diagnosed in this department.

Immunology and serology are two specialities which have grown very rapidly over the past twenty years as our knowledge of the body's immune system has increased dramatically. Such departments now identify abnormalities in the body's immune system, diagnose allergies and hypersensitivity states and autoimmune diseases. Serological reactions also con-

firm the diagnosis of many infectious diseases (especially viral ones) by using very specific antigen–antibody reactions. A disease such as AIDS would be diagnosed by this speciality.

Medical genetics examines the genetic material of cells for detection of genetic defects. A very important part of the work carried out here is the construction of pedigrees for families where a certain disease is very prevalent and the subsequent genetic counselling of prospective parents. Prenatal diagnosis of genetic defects is also carried out. Diseases such as Down's syndrome, Tay-Sachs disease and anatomical defects are diagnosed by this speciality.

In any disease the importance of these specialized fields and the many tests performed is variable. Currently, the diagnosis of a disease does not just depend on recognition of signs and symptoms but also on the results of special tests which may either confirm or rule out suspected diseases, thus enabling a differential diagnosis. For example, if diabetes mellitus is suspected from the clinical presentation, biochemical tests are required (sugar levels in blood or urine). In the case of a lump being palpated, a tumour is suspected and histological tests are required. Tissue is examined under the microscope to see whether a tumour is benign or malignant and what type of tumour it is.

It should be noted that in disease, tissue may be taken by **biopsy**, that is, removal of tissue from the living body to examine its structure, biochemistry, etc., or **autopsy** (= necropsy, post mortem), where dissection of the cadaver is carried out to examine the viscera for disease processes. Examination of the cadaver for pathology is an important learning exercise and the serious study of pathology is unthinkable without the examination of post mortem material. **Pathology museums** house specimens of gross pathology and are a great aid to the students of pathology.

In almost every speciality listed above new developments and rapidly expanding technology have meant that electronic equipment and mechanical techniques are being relied upon more and more for the diagnosis of disease. The **X-ray machine, computerized tomography scanner, nuclear magnetic resonance machine, ultrasound machine** and many more such instruments are being utilized more and more for looking at diseased tissues in non-invasive ways and aiding in rapid diagnosis. In the laboratories, **electronic cell sorters and counters** are being used to analyse blood, a host of electronic **analysers** will very rapidly and accurately measure concentrations of chemicals in body fluids and **computerized systems** are now standard in many microbiology laboratories and are being used in identification of bacteria from clinical specimens. Many more such technological gadgetry is being added to the diagnosticians' armamentarium, helping to make diagnosis of disease more accurate, more effective and quicker.

Nature of Disease and Aetiology

Disease may be described using a framework of four areas of information:

Topography (T) — site of occurrence
Morphology (M) — changes caused in the tissues
Aetiology (AE) — cause, if known
Function (F) — functional manifestations of disease.

This is the basis of the Systematized Nomenclature Of Pathology (SNOP) system of classification of disease, an internationally recognized system. By using a stand-ard system of numbers to classify disease according to the four variables above, a consistent, uniform method of disease classification may be arrived at: for example M4001 Bronchopneumonia T28, AE1600 (T28 = lung; M4001 = patchy pneumonia; AE1600 = due to infection with *Staphylococcus aureus*). This system allows for any disease to be accurately and reproducibly classified using coded numbers and information sent to or received from overseas to be accurately interpreted. However, routinely, a useful way to classify disease is by its aetiology. Broadly, diseases are either **genetically determined** or **acquired** (see Figure 1.6).

Genetically Determined Disease

There are four major groups of disorders which are genetically determined and in these the disease arises because of some defect in the DNA of the cell, either abnormalities in the information stored in the DNA or a defect in the way in which that information is read and interpreted by the cellular machinery (i.e. gene defects or anomalies of gene expression).

Cytogenetic Disorders

This implies that abnormal numbers of chromosomes are present in cells, or alternatively that the chromosomes are damaged in some gross way (e.g. arms of chromosomes may break off and either be lost or attach to inappropriate places on other chromosomes). Such disorders can be readily detected by looking at dividing cells of the individual under a microscope and counting the chromosomes or observing them for abnormalities. The medical genetics laboratory is involved in this, taking photographs of dividing cells and then cutting and pasting the chromosome pairs on a chart to construct a **karyotype** of that individual. Examples of these disorders and their abnormal karyotypes are: Down's Syndrome (trisomy 21, 47 chromosomes in each cell — refer to the chapter on central nervous system disorders); Turner's syndrome (45, X0 chromosomes in each cell); Klinefelter's syndrome (47, XXY chromosomes in each cell); and the so-called 'super males' (47, XYY chromosomes in each cell — these are phenotypically normal males, although they may be slightly taller than average, and it is said that they are more likely to exhibit antisocial behaviour).

Let us look at the profile of a typical cytogenetic disorder, **Klinefelter's syndrome**. This disorder is the commonest cytogenetic disorder affecting the sex chromosomes. The affected individual usually has 47 chromosomes in each of his cells, the extra chromosome being an additional X, such that his genotype is XXY. Rarely, extra X and Y chromosomes are present also, or the patients may be **mosaics**, some of their cells being 46, XY cells and some of their cells being 47, XXY cells (Figure 1.5). The abnormality results from the non-disjunction of the sex chromosomes during

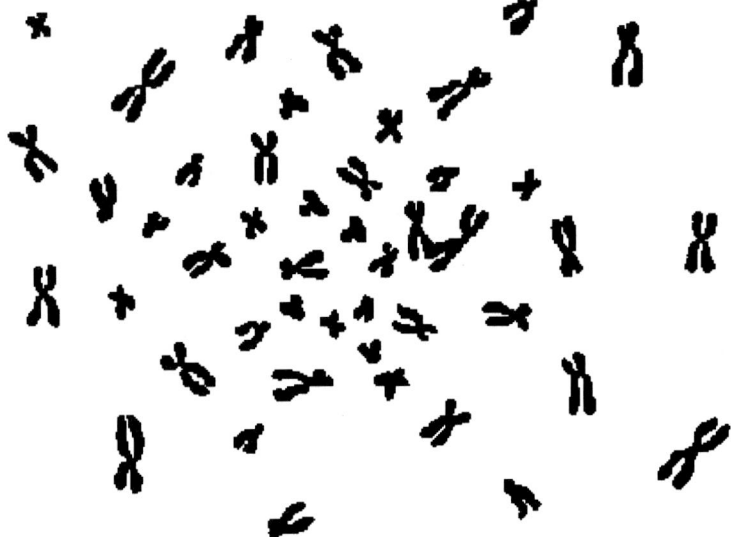

Chromosome spread from a dividing cell ready to be sorted for karyotyping (are these from a normal individual?). The chromosomes are cut out and pasted out as below into the A, B, C, D, E, F, G and sex chromosome groups.

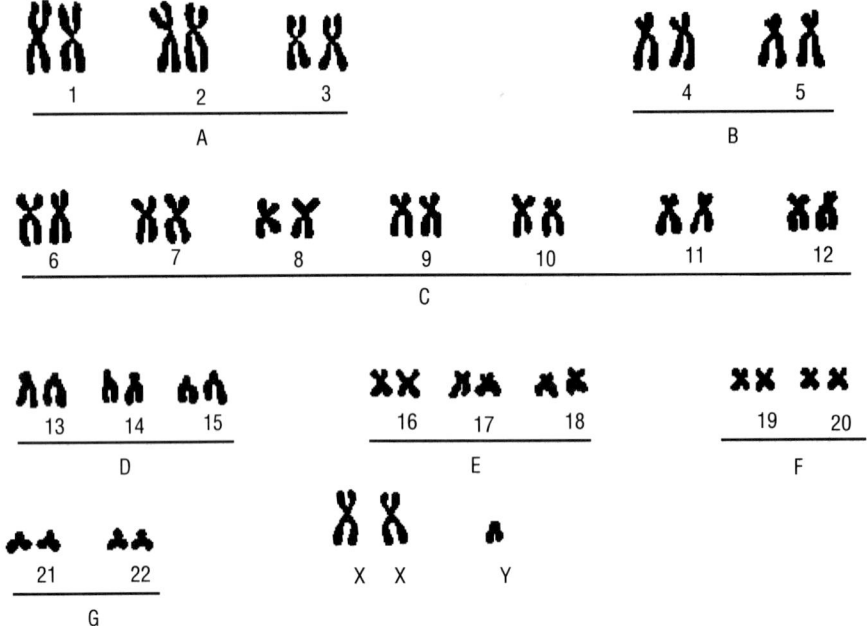

Karyotyped chromosomes from an individual with Klinefelter's syndrome, karyotype 47, XXY.

Figure 1.5   *The karyotyping procedure, used for identifying cytogenetic disorders*

meiosis and the extra X chromosome may be inherited from the mother's ovum or the father's sperm cell. It is thought to arise because of irradiation of the ovaries or testes, or it may occur if the mother is of advanced age.

A wide range of presentations of Klinefelter's syndrome is noted clinically because of the variation of genotypes that are seen. Typically, patients have a **hypogonadism**, where the testes are poorly developed and atrophic, **gynaecomastia** (enlarged breasts) and reduced body hair. These changes are consistent with low levels of testosterone in the blood and raised urinary gonadotropin levels. Most patients with Klinefelter's syndrome are sterile as a result of the abnormalities in hormonal levels and the testicular maldevelopment, but occasionally patients who exhibit mosaic forms of the disease will be fertile. The patients with this disorder appear to be tall because of their very long legs and there may be a degree of mental retardation relating usually to the number of extra X chromosomes that are present. A patient with an XXY sex genotype may be only slightly retarded or, in some cases, of normal intelligence. It should be noted that cytogenetic disorders of up to 49, XXXXY are compatible with life, although there is profound mental deficiency and severe physical abnormalities in these people.

Mendelian Defects

These are gene defects, resulting from **mutation** of DNA and are inherited in a similar fashion to other genetic characteristics, such as eye colour. The defects may be **autosomal** (i.e. carried on any chromosome except the X chromosome) or **sex-linked** (i.e. carried on the X chromosome). They may be **dominant** or **recessive**. Examples include: familial hypercholesterolaemia (autosomal dominant, prevalence 1 in 500); haemophilia (sex-linked recessive, prevalence 1 in 10 000); phenylketonuria (autosomal recessive, prevalence 1 in 12 000); polycystic kidney disease (autosomal dominant, prevalence 1 in 10 000); cystic fibrosis (autosomal recessive, prevalence 1 in 2000).

Let us look at the profile of a typical Mendelian defect, phenylketonuria (PKU). This disorder occurs in a variety of forms but classical PKU is seen to occur commonly in people of Scandinavian origin and is rare in blacks and Jews. The affected people have a defect in phenylalanine metabolism due to a lack of the enzyme phenylalanine hydroxylase that normally converts phenylalanine to tyrosine. The amino acid phenylalanine accumulates in the body of affected babies from the time of birth, reaching toxic levels within a few months. Although the babies appear nor-

mal at birth, when the phenylalanine reaches toxic levels there is stunting of growth, brain damage and mental retardation. The individuals suffer from seizures and other neurological anomalies and there is depigmentation of the hair and skin with an eczematous rash apparent throughout the body. Because the phenylalanine reaches very high levels, minor metabolic pathways develop and the excess amino acid is partially metabolized into phenylpyruvic acid, phenylacetic acid and o-hydroxyphenylacetic acid that are excreted in large quantities in the urine and sweat. It is these excreted metabolites that impart a strong 'mousy' or musty odour to the affected infants.

Classical PKU may be prevented by dietary means early on in life and dietary restrictions are enforced as soon as the condition is diagnosed and continued throughout life. A number of screening tests may be used in the postnatal period to diagnose PKU and these include the **Guthrie Inhibition Assay** involving a test with bacteria requiring phenylalanine for growth. In this test some serum taken from the infant to be tested is incubated with these bacteria and if phenylalanine is present the bacteria grow adequately; if phenylalanine concentrations are low the bacteria do not grow. Other tests on blood from the newborn may also be performed and in this respect recombinant DNA technology is proving to be a very powerful technique in the diagnosis of many of the Mendelian disorders. As this technique may be used with as few as 10 to 100 cells (through utilization of the polymerase chain reaction) very small volumes of blood are needed and the technique may also be performed on dried blood.

Multifactorial Inheritance Disorders

In these disorders a particular set of genes or a certain genetic assortment of an individual (the presence of many distinct genes in a certain pattern) make that individual more likely to develop a disease. It should be realized that this is a rather simple way of regarding these diseases as the influence of external, environmental factors (e.g. diet) may be very important in determining whether or not the disease will develop or how severely the individual may be affected. Typical diseases which develop within such frameworks are certain forms of diabetes mellitus and hypertension.

Congenital Malformation

In these disorders, complex non-Mendelian/polygenic causes are involved and the mechanism is poorly understood, generally because we know so little about normal development and differentiation. It is suspected that such disease may often be caused by aberrant gene expression leading to abnormal differentiation during histogenesis and organogenesis. The results of such aberrations of gene expression are gross anatomical defects. There are many examples of these disorders ranging from the innocuous (harelip), to the serious (many types of heart defects), to the fatal (absence of an organ, e.g. anencephaly, congenital absence of the brain).

Acquired Disease

Most diseases are acquired and are due to the effects of some external environmental factor. The genetic make-up of an individual may influence the susceptibility to external disease-causing agents. Hence in the development of acquired disease there are various factors to be considered in order to understand the disease fully.

The **causative agents** (aetiologies derived from the environment, e.g. bacteria which are inhaled into the respiratory tract) are the primary and most important determinant in the development of an acquired disease. **Predisposing factors** may be genetic or environmental and make the disease more likely to develop in those individuals who are so predisposed (e.g. inherited immune deficiencies or cigarette smoking, making someone more likely to contract respiratory infections). **Contributory factors** make the disease progress more rapidly or make the disease more severe (e.g. malnutrition, alcoholism, causing a disease to be more severe in the individuals affected).

There are many causative agents and types of injury in the group of acquired disorders and these include physical and chemical agents, micro-organisms, immune factors, deficiencies and various other causes relating to the mental state of the patient. The ways of dealing with disease by our medical care givers may also contribute to the development of disease instead

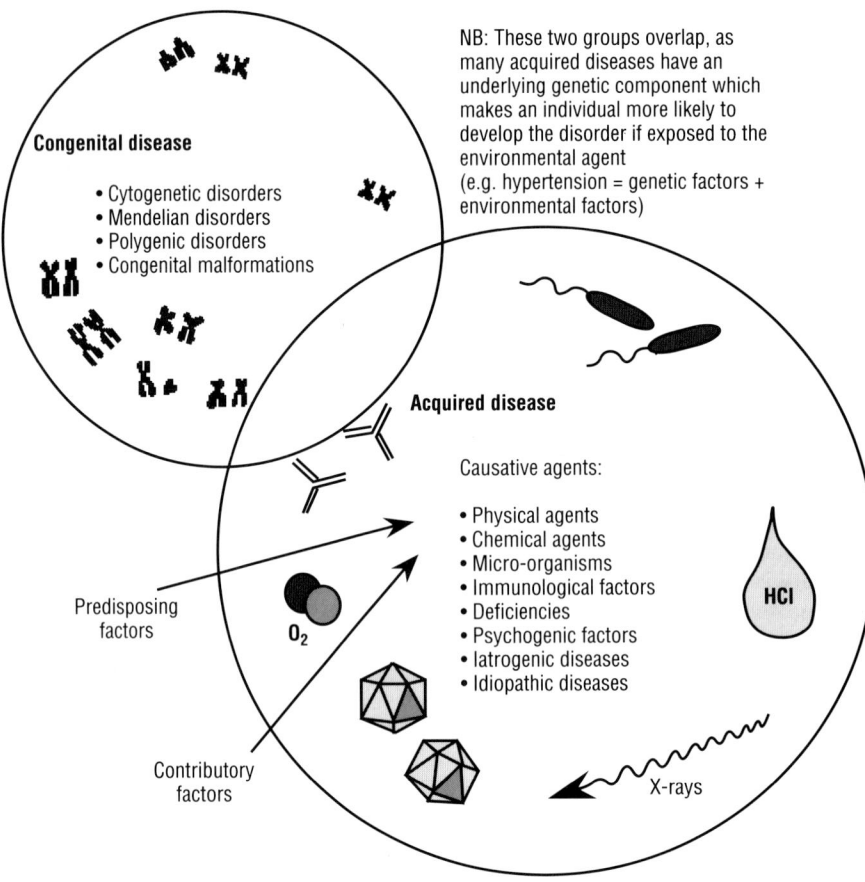

Figure 1.6   *The aetiology of disease subdivided into congenital and acquired groups*

of curing it, and some diseases are a direct effect of inappropriate treatment by the care givers. It should also be noted that within this group of acquired diseases are included some diseases that have an unknown aetiology.

Physical Agents

A very large group of agents interacting with the tissues can cause direct damage: cold, heat, mechanical trauma (laceration, rupture, fracture, etc.); X-rays, γ rays, UV light and other radiation; products of radioactive decay (e.g. neutrons, α, β rays). Generally, these agents will cause direct damage to cells by destroying the cell's macromolecules, the genetic material being especially prone to damage by the various forms of electromagnetic radiation, while heat, cold and trauma will cause disruption to the cell's integrity, thus seriously compromising its function.

Chemical Agents

Almost any chemical substance may be toxic or cause injury if it is given at the appropriate dosage (e.g. consider oxygen toxicity which develops if pure oxygen is breathed for a length of time). Generally, most chemical injuries are caused by corrosive or highly toxic substances small doses of which have deleterious effects. These chemicals may be naturally occurring or synthetic, organic or inorganic, for example arsenic, phosphorus, lead, mercury, hydrochloric acid, DDT, alkaloids, toxins. A considerable amount of research has been carried out in relation to particularly active chemical substances known as **free radicals**. These are highly reactive atoms or molecules that have free, single electrons that may combine with the first available reagent that they encounter. If free radicals form in cells, they will combine with cellular macromolecules, leading to abnormalities in cellular functioning. Free radical injury is now known to be important in many diseases and the formation of free radicals may seriously contribute to the pathogenesis of many disorders whose primary aetiology is due to another agent, rather than a chemical.

Organisms

Other animate agents may interact adversely with the tissues of the body, causing infections and infestations. Bacteria, viruses, fungi, protozoa, helminths and other parasites cause the infectious diseases, many of which are very serious or fatal if left untreated. Before the days of vaccination, antibiotics and chemotherapy, infections were the major cause of death, especially in childhood. Examples of such infectious diseases are diphtheria (caused by a bacterium called *Corynebacterium diphtheriae*); ' 'flu' (caused by the influenza virus); athlete's foot (caused by fungi, e.g. *Epidermophyton*); amoebic dysentery (caused by a protozoon, *Entamoeba histolytica*) and roundworm infestation (caused by a parasitic worm called *Ascaris lumbricoides*). Effective chemotherapy of most of the infectious diseases has reduced the death rate due to these aetiological agents; however, even today some infectious diseases still exact a fatal toll (e.g. AIDS caused by the *Human Immunodeficiency Virus*). In developing countries infectious disease is still very prevalent and some easily curable infections remain a scourge as there is inadequate medical care and major socioeconomic problems prevent people from seeking medical treatment.

Immune Diseases

The immune system protects the body from invasion by foreign, non-self material. However, the immune system has been aptly described as the 'two-edged sword' as sometimes it can mediate very serious disease. Allergies, hypersensitivities (e.g. hay fever) and autoimmune diseases such as rheumatoid arthritis fall within this group. Immune deficiency states arise if the immune system fails to develop normally (e.g. Bruton disease) or if it is crippled in some way (e.g. AIDS). Diseases due to anomalies of immune system function are a prime example of disorders that span the two major groups of aetiologies — genetic and acquired. It is known, for example, that genetic factors are very important in determining normal immune responses and the presence of certain inherited factors will interfere with normal immunity or predispose to the development of hypersensitivity or autoimmune disease. Immune disease is also grouped together with the acquired diseases as some external environmental stimuli (i.e. exposure to a substance foreign to the body or encountering a micro-organism in an infection) will bring about the manifestations of the abnormal immune response.

Deficiencies

Most people equate these disorders with nutritional deficiencies arising out of inadequate dietary intake or unbalanced dietary intake, for example **Kwashiorkor**, a severe protein deficiency commonly seen in Third World countries and avitaminoses such as **beriberi**. However, a deficiency which is a very common cause of injury in tissues is oxygen deficiency which is seen when the blood supply to an organ is interrupted for a length of time. Such a deficiency is the commonest cause of death in developed societies such as ours, in the guise of heart attacks and strokes. It should be noted that this oxygen deficiency is intimately linked with disorders of the vascular system and there is a complex aetiology to these diseases of vessels, with many important factors predisposing and contributing to the development of lesions.

Psychogenic Factors in Disease

It is known that psychological factors such as stress, anxiety and personality type contribute to the development of disease, or in fact may be the prime cause of some diseases. For example, it is known that psychogenic factors are important in the development of chronic peptic ulcers. Hypertension and other vascular diseases are often aggravated by anxiety, as evidenced by the 'relaxation response' where some patients with high blood pressure can lower it by taking up yoga or meditation. In these disorders, which depend on the mental state of the patient, a patient may literally think themselves into a disease state (something which the witch doctor knows and which his victim knows when the former points the 'bone of death' at the latter, who promptly dies, so absolute being the belief in the power of the witch doctor!). Anxiety and stress can interact with the immune system and a lowering of immunity is seen when a person is experiencing such states, thereby increasing the susceptibility to infection (something that students become very aware of around the time of the examinations!). Often, psychogenic factors are very important contributory or predisposing factors to the development of a disease if not the primary aetiological factor associated with a particular disease.

Iatrogenic Diseases

These disorders develop as a result of medical intervention for the treatment of a disease. The health professional may be guilty of overtreatment of a disease (too enthusiastic?) or undertreatment or maltreatment of disease (not knowing enough pathology?). The wrong medication may be administered, the wrong dosage may be calculated, or a disease may be misdiagnosed and the treatment decided upon may be totally inappropriate. Often the side effects of drugs may be overlooked, especially in the paediatric, gerontological or frail patient, and these side effects may be more serious than the disease for which the drugs were administered. An example of such a disease is the administration of penicillin to a patient who is allergic to this antibiotic. The administration of the drug will initiate a series of hypersensitivity reactions that may have a fatal outcome.

Idiopathic Diseases

The precise cause of these diseases is unknown but they may be well characterized clinically. Alternative names that may be used for idiopathic disease are 'primary' disease or 'essential' disease. Typical examples are: sarcoidosis, a chronic inflammatory disease; most brain tumours; primary hypertension. Often diseases that have a known pathogenesis will have an unknown aetiology and a typical example of such a disorder is rheumatoid arthritis (RA). It is known that RA is an autoimmune disease and the mechanism of the development of the lesions has been elucidated. Much is known about the genetic predisposition to the disease and many of the other predisposing and contributory factors around RA have been documented. However, the precise aetiological agent that functions as the trigger for the series of autoimmune reactions that lead to RA is unknown. The prevention and treatment of these idiopathic disorders may be difficult or often impossible.

Introduction to Key Terms in Pathology

Before beginning a course of pathology it is necessary to be aware of some common terms used routinely in the subject and to introduce some simple underlying concepts. As in the study of a foreign language, we need to be familiar with a simple vocabulary before we begin to utter meaningful sentences.

Pathology is the scientific study of disease, elucidating its causes and effects. The word pathology is derived from two Greek words: πάθος (*pathos*), 'suffering or distress', and λόγος (*logos*), a 'treatise' or 'study'. **Disease** is an abnormal variation in the structure and/or function of any part of the body; literally, a state of departure from ease. It should be noted that conditions that the layperson may not consider to be 'disease' may be disease to a pathologist. For example, a six-digit hand causes no suffering or distress, is compatible with life and is not considered as a disease by a non-pathologist. A pathologist sees this as disease, however, because it represents an abnormal variant of the structure of the body.

Morphology is the appearance of the diseased or injured tissue both macroscopically and microscopically. Different diseases may be recognized by their characteristic morphologies. It should be noted that the same disease in different sites may show a similar or identical appearance. For example, tuberculosis shows an identical appearance whether it occurs in the lungs, liver, spleen, bone or kidney.

Topography is the site of the body in which the disease manifests itself. Some diseases characteristically occur in only one site of the body, for example cirrhosis of the liver or dust inhalation diseases of the lungs. Other diseases may be seen in many body sites, the same aetiology being responsible.

Aetiology is the term given to the cause of disease. A typical example of an aetiology of a disease is infection with a specific bacterium. *Staphylococcus aureus* is a bacterium which when introduced into tissues will cause an abscess (a boil or a pimple). Hence, this bacterium is the aetiology of the abscess. When the cause of a disease is unknown we refer to it as an **idiopathic** disease. Pathology involves not only the scientific study of the disease process itself but also the aetiology (causes) of disease. Once the aetiology is known, methods of prevention and cure can be discovered. Other terms commonly used for diseases whose aetiology is unknown, synonymous with idiopathic, are **primary** and **essential**.

Pathogenesis is the mechanism by which a disease is produced once initiated by its causative agent. Going back to the example of *Staphylococcus aureus* causing an abscess, clearly the bacterium is the aetiology but the pathogenesis is the complex way in which the bacterium is introduced in the tissue and all of its subsequent biological activities that induce damage in the tissue with the typical response of the body to that damage, manifesting as an abscess. The complex of aetiology/pathogenesis associated with a characteristic disease produces signs and symptoms in the patient that we identify as a specific disease presentation.

Diagnosis is the procedure whereby a disease is identified by its unique characteristics: aetiology, morphology and functional aberrations which give rise to symptoms and signs. The **symptoms** of a disease are what the patient perceives as being wrong with him- or herself and often are what force the patient to seek medical advice, while the **signs** are what the examining health professional perceives as being abnormal and these signs may not necessarily be obvious to the patient. Appropriate laboratory investigations can then be carried out in order to help in the definitive diagnosis of the disease. This involves a series of tests to help differentiate the disease in question from other related, similar diseases.

Differential diagnosis refers to the process where a group of pathological states of similar characteristics are considered as likely candidates for the disorder that the patient is presenting with. The process of differential diagnosis is a very important one as it is here that the expert knowledge of the diagnostician or the pathologist is tested in the 'real world'. A presenting patient will exhibit a variety of symptoms and signs and it is up to the pathologist to correlate these with any other changes or deviations from the normal that are apparent in tissues or in the results of the various tests that have been carried out, arriving logically at a 'short list' of possibilities. Further investigations may then be required to arrive at a more precise diagnosis.

Presumptive diagnosis is the initial diagnosis which is arrived at by the examiner and is based on the presenting features of the case, i.e. morphology, signs and symptoms, natural history. There may be several such presumptive diagnoses, all part of the differential diagnosis of the disease. **Definitive diagnosis** is the final diagnosis which is arrived at by the examiner and is based not only on the presenting features of the case, i.e. morphology, signs and symptoms, natural history but also on the results of more specific examinations and tests which are carried out in order to rule out similar disease processes.

Complications are new and/or different pathological entities which may occur as the disease progresses. These may involve more of the tissue or organ than the initial lesion involved, or the disease may spread to involve more distant sites or the whole body. Important complications are often metabolic and biochemical in origin, indicating the disordered function of the diseased part. A **sequela** is any 'sequel' of a disease process, i.e. a complication, a resolution or any outcome of the disease process. The **natural history** of a disease is the way the disease evolves if it is left untreated.

Treatment is the method whereby medical workers may alter or arrest the natural history of the disease in order to minimize symptoms and stop or reverse damage. Treatments may be many and varied depending on the disease and the medical practitioner involved. Treatment may consist of drug administration, diet changes, radiation, surgery, psychotherapy, physiotherapy, etc., or a combination of different types of treatment.

Prognosis is the probable outcome of the disease whether treated or untreated. The prognosis is usually based on statistical data gained through collation of information on those who have suffered from the same disease. It may be expressed as percentage survival for a set time (usually 5 years) as in the case of cancer: for example, the number of patients with lung cancer who survive for 5 years following diagnosis of their condition is 7–10%. From the statistics available for a specific disease it is possible to express prognosis as **excellent** or **good** if minimal residual change will occur in the patient; **guarded** if the outcome is uncertain but may cause some alteration to normal physiology; and **poor** or **grave** if the patient will be permanently debilitated or if death is the likely outcome.

Acute disease is one which is expected to run its course over a fairly short time, hours to days. A typical example of an acute disease is a mild thermal burn on a finger. It lasts for only a few hours and complete healing has occurred within a day or so. **Subacute** disease is less well defined but takes a longer course, weeks to months. A wound is an example of a subacute disease. Healing takes a few weeks to occur. **Chronic** disease may take months to years or perhaps the lifetime of an individual to run its course.

Severe disease is one which is likely to produce many effects on the patient, with often an unpleasant outcome resulting in permanent disability or death. Severe diseases may be very difficult or impossible to treat effectively. An example of a severe disease is that of a malignant brain tumour, which is usually fatal within a few weeks from diagnosis. **Moderate** disease is one that is less likely to produce much tissue damage and injury, and usually responds well to treatment. Adult onset diabetes mellitus is an example of a moderate disease. **Mild** disease is one which usually lasts

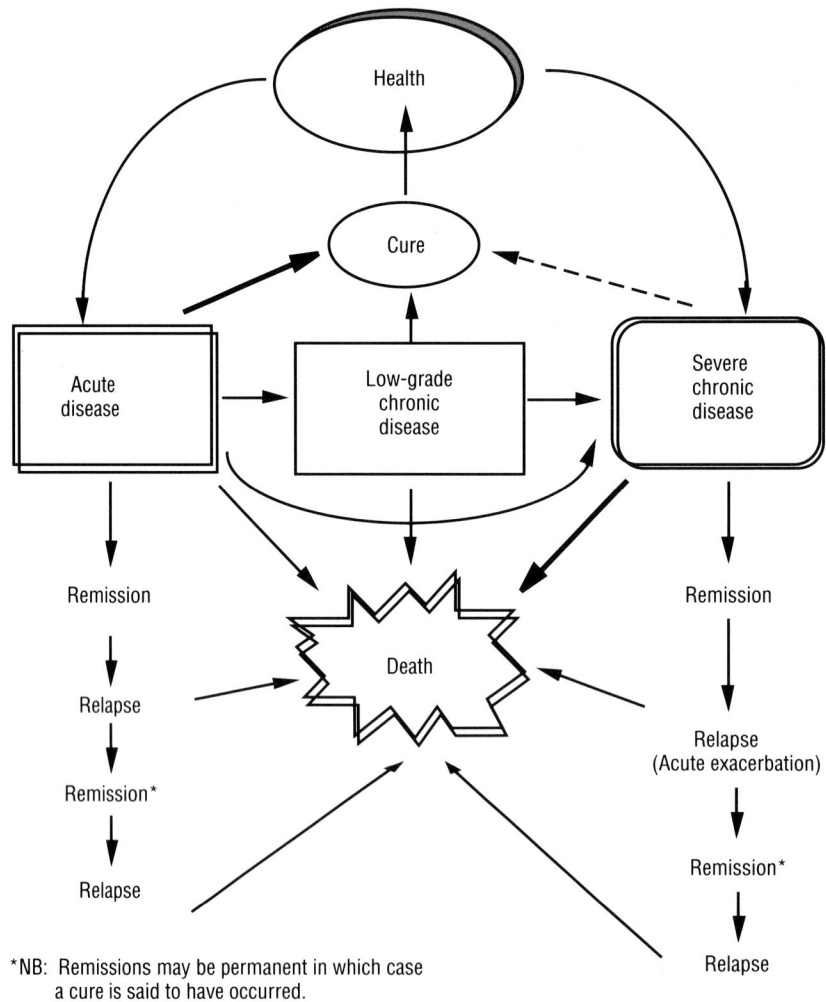

*NB: Remissions may be permanent in which case a cure is said to have occurred.

Figure 1.7 *Natural history of disease with possible outcomes*

for a short period of time and is treated easily and completely, not leading to serious complications or to death. Mild disease examples are the common cold (upper respiratory tract infection due to a rhinovirus), fibroids of the uterus (a common, benign tumour of women) and a mild thermal burn.

Lesion refers to the region of tissue directly affected by the disease process and may be readily seen when the tissue is examined with the naked eye or viewed under the microscope. Usually, when the disease process is described the size of individual lesions is stated in centimetres or millimetres. An example of a lesion is a localized region of infection as is seen in the case of an abscess (a boil or a pimple).

Localized disease is one which is confined to a small area of tissue. An abscess is a localized disease. **Widespread** disease is one involving extensively much tissue or whole organs. Acne is widespread disease as infection occurs in many regions throughout the skin of the affected individual, the face, trunk and back being usually involved severely. **Systemic** disease is one which involves many systems in the body and usually its manifestations are evident in almost every tissue in the body. Diabetes mellitus is a systemic disease in which most tissues of the body are affected.

Remission of a disease refers to the state where injury to the tissue is temporarily halted, the symptoms and signs of the disease disappear, and the patient begins to feel better. If a remission is permanent, a cure is said to have been effected. Remissions may be spontaneous or achieved by treatment. **Relapse** of a disease is a state of renewed tissue injury and damage with signs and symptoms becoming apparent again. It occurs after a remission. **Exacerbation** is a state of increased tissue injury and damage occurring in an established disease or a low grade, mild disease, making the disease more severe (see Figure 1.7).

Revision Questions

1. What do you understand by the term 'pathology'?
2. What does the humoral aetiology of disease purport? Is this of any relevance to pathology today?
3. Match the famous physician with the contribution he made to the study of disease:

   (a) Paracelsus   (i)   Famous French 19th century microbiologist

   (b) Robert Koch   (ii)   Roman medical encyclopaedist (1st century AD)

   (c) Claudius Galen   (iii)   Belgian anatomist of the 16th century

   (d) Ibn Sina Avicenna   (iv)   German pathologist of the 19th century

   (e) Cornelius Celsus   (v)   Ancient Greek physician, famous for his 'oath'

   (f) Karl Rokitansky   (vi)   Persian physician who wrote the 'Canon'

   (g) Andreas Vesalius   (vii)   Pioneer of the autopsy examination

   (h) John Hunter   (viii)   Graeco-Roman physician (2nd century AD)

   (j) Hippocrates   (ix)   German microbiologist of the 19th century

   (k) Giovanni Battista Morgagni   (x)   English experimental pathologist (18th century)

   (l) Louis Pasteur   (xi)   Swiss physician interested in chemotherapy

   (m) Rudolf Virchow   (xii)   Bohemian pathologist of the 19th century

4. Explain the difference between a cytological examination of tissue and a histopathological examination of tissue.
5. What is the difference between a biopsy and an autopsy?
6. Of what use is the autopsy examination?
7. Explain briefly the SNOP system of nomenclature of disease. Why is this useful?
8. Differentiate between cytogenetic and Mendelian disorders, giving an example of each one.
9. What are 'free radicals'?
10. Distinguish between the two related terms 'aetiology' and 'pathogenesis'.
11. What is a 'lesion'?
12. Give an example of an acquired disease. State what its aetiology is and also what contributory and predisposing factors are important in its development.
13. What is meant by the term 'prognosis' in pathology?
14. Distinguish between 'presumptive diagnosis' and 'definitive diagnosis'.

Introductory Crossword

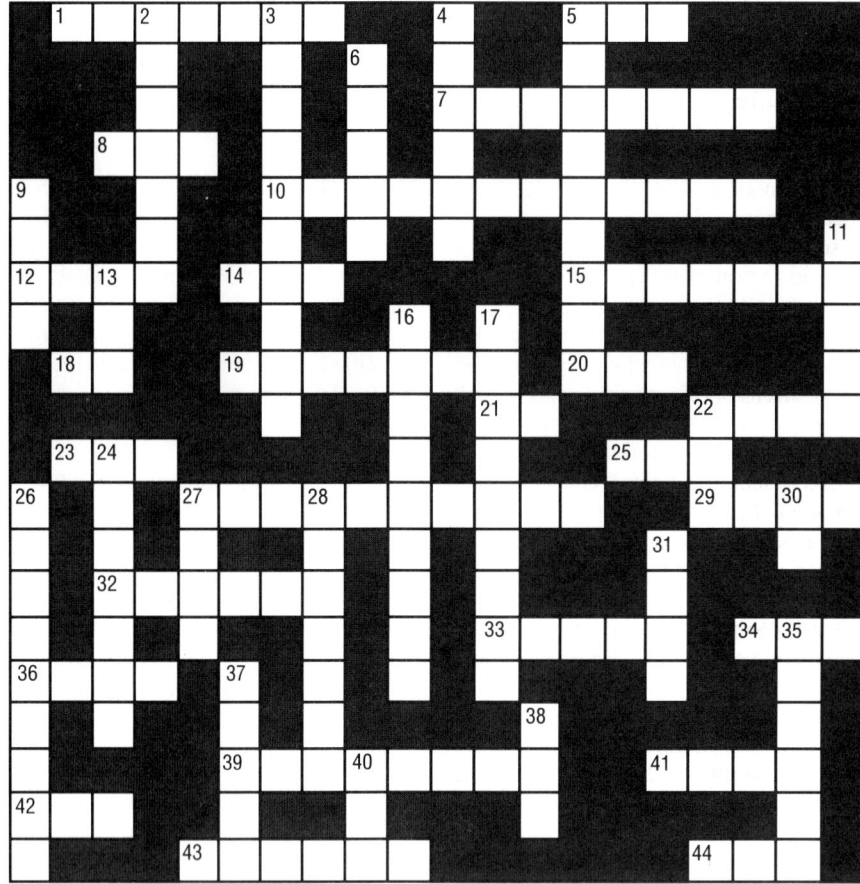

CLUES

ACROSS

1. A long-lasting process, present for months to years (7).
5. The genetic material of the nucleus (3).
7. This process lasts for days to weeks (8).
8. The _ _ _ smear test is an example of a cytological diagnostic technique (3).
10. The mechanism by which an aetiological agent causes the disease process (12).
12. The complete eradication of a disease with return to wellness and health (4).
14. The energy molecule of the cell (3).
15. Any conclusion or complication of a disease (7).
18. An element found in bone (2).
19. Any abnormality in structure and/or function of a tissue or organ (7).
20. The metabolism of fat occurs in this organelle (1, 1, 1).
21. A disease caused by *Mycobacterium tuberculosis* (2).
22. The commonest symptom patients present with (4).
23. The gametes of the female (3).
25. A Mendelian disorder where there is abnormality in the metabolism of phenylalanine (3).
27. The characteristic appearance of a disease process (10).
29. When damaged tissue is removed from the body this is left behind as evidence of healing (4).
32. A famous Roman physician who wrote the first medical encyclopaedia (6).
33. The lesion of tertiary syphilis (5).

34. A system of blood groups (1, 1, 1).
36. The longest cytoplasmic process arising from a neurone (4).
39. A famous Italian physician, the first to perform autopsies (8).
41. This substance is formed in fat necrosis of the pancreas when free fatty acids combine with calcium (4).
42. A charged atom or molecule (3).
43. A stress placed upon a tissue causing disruption to its structure and function (6).
44. Karyotype associated with Klinefelter's syndrome (3).

DOWN

2. A new phase of disease activity after a remission (7).
3. A disease due to an unknown aetiology (10).
4. The part of a tissue seen to be affected directly by the disease process (6).
5. The procedure leading to the identification of a particular disease (9).
6. A disease process lasting for hours to days (5).
9. A German microbiologist of the 19th century (4).
11. A Graeco-Roman ancient physician who lived between 131–201 AD (5).
13. The genetic material found in ribosomes (3).
16. The scientific study of disease (9).
17. The cause of a disease (9).
22. A thick, yellowish fluid formed in areas of inflammation (3).
24. A German pathologist of the 19th century (7).
26. The lack of blood in tissue (9).
27. A disease which is not severe, easily overcome (4).
28. A French microbiologist of the 19th century (7).

30. A chemical element, often used for poisoning (2).
31. A form of physical injury (4).
35. The removal of living tissue from the body as an aid in diagnosis (6).
37. *Homo sapiens* (5).
38. The cause of AIDS (1, 1, 1).
40. This is the site of protein synthesis in the cell (1, 1, 1).

Further Reading

Antonarakis SE. 'Diagnosis of Genetic Disorders at the DNA Level.' *N Engl J Med* 1989; **320**: 153.

Gordon R. *Great Medical Mysteries*. Book Club Associates, London, 1984.

Hamlyn Publishing Group. *Medical People and Practices*. Life, Love and Family Health Series, Marshall Cavendish Ltd, London, 1970.

Hamlyn Publishing Group. *The Fringes of Medicine*. Life, Love and Family Health Series, Marshall Cavendish Ltd, London, 1970.

Leavesley JH. *Medical By-Ways — Famous Diseases and Diseases of the Famous*. ABC Enterprises and W Collins, Sydney, 1985.

Lechevalier H. *Three Centuries of Microbiology*. McGraw-Hill, New York, 1965.

Long ER. *A History of Pathology*. Dover Publications, New York, 1965.

Sandison AT. 'Diseases in the Ancient World.' *Rec Adv Histopathol* 1981; **11**: 1.

Starobinski J. *A History of Medicine*. Prentice-Hall International, London, 1965.

Upton AC. 'Environmental Medicine. Introduction and Overview.' *Med Clin N Am* 1990; **74**: 235.

Woo SLC. 'Molecular Basis and Population Genetics of Phenylketonuria.' *Biochem* 1989; **28**: 1.

2

Injury and the Response of the Body to Injury

The normal cell is a dynamic system of constantly changing chemical and structural entities. A typical human cell comprises a plasma membrane, endoplasmic reticulum, ribosomes, Golgi apparatus, lysosomes, vacuoles, mitochondria, cytoplasmic fluid, nuclear membrane, nuclear protein and nucleic acids (condensed into chromosomes at cell division) and nucleolus (see Figure 2.1). Some cells are considerably more specialized and may contain a variety of other structural elements. All cells have the ability to ingest fluid by pinocytosis and solid particles by phagocytosis. Cell division occurs in somatic cells by mitosis and in this process the chromosome number is preserved, such that the mother cell gives rise to two identical daughter cells the same as itself. In the gonads, the germ cells are capable of mitotic division but also of meiosis, in which the mother cell divides to give rise to two identical cells but with each daughter cell having half the number of chromosomes of the mother cell, and this forms the gametes (ova and sperm). Some specialized cells in the adult have lost their ability to divide (e.g. neurones) and thus once they are injured and die they will not be replaced by similar cells.

The appearance and specialization of cells of the body vary considerably depending on the function of the cell, tissue or organ. For example, some cells are ciliated (respiratory tract epithelium), others have a phagocytic function (white blood cells). Although the cells of the body vary widely in their appearance, their function and structure, they all respond similarly to stresses that damage their constituents.

Rudolf Virchow, the famous German pathologist of the 19th century, was the first to describe the responses of cells to injury. Cellular responses to injury are the cornerstone of pathology and they must be completely understood if a complete comprehension of any disease is to be achieved.

Cellular Response to Injury

Cellular Reactions in Disease

At the cellular level, disease can be visualized as an

adaptation to a noxious stimulus, or an injury. **Injury** is a stress which is placed upon cells and tissues in the body causing a variation in their structure and function. This results in a pathological process operating, leading to macroscopical changes, symptoms and signs, clinical evidence of disease. **Trauma** is a more specific term. It is injury caused by a mechanical or physical agent (e.g. bacterial infection causes injury to tissues while a car accident results in trauma).

The causes of injury have been discussed previously, for example oxygen lack, physical agents, chemical agents, biological agents, immunological

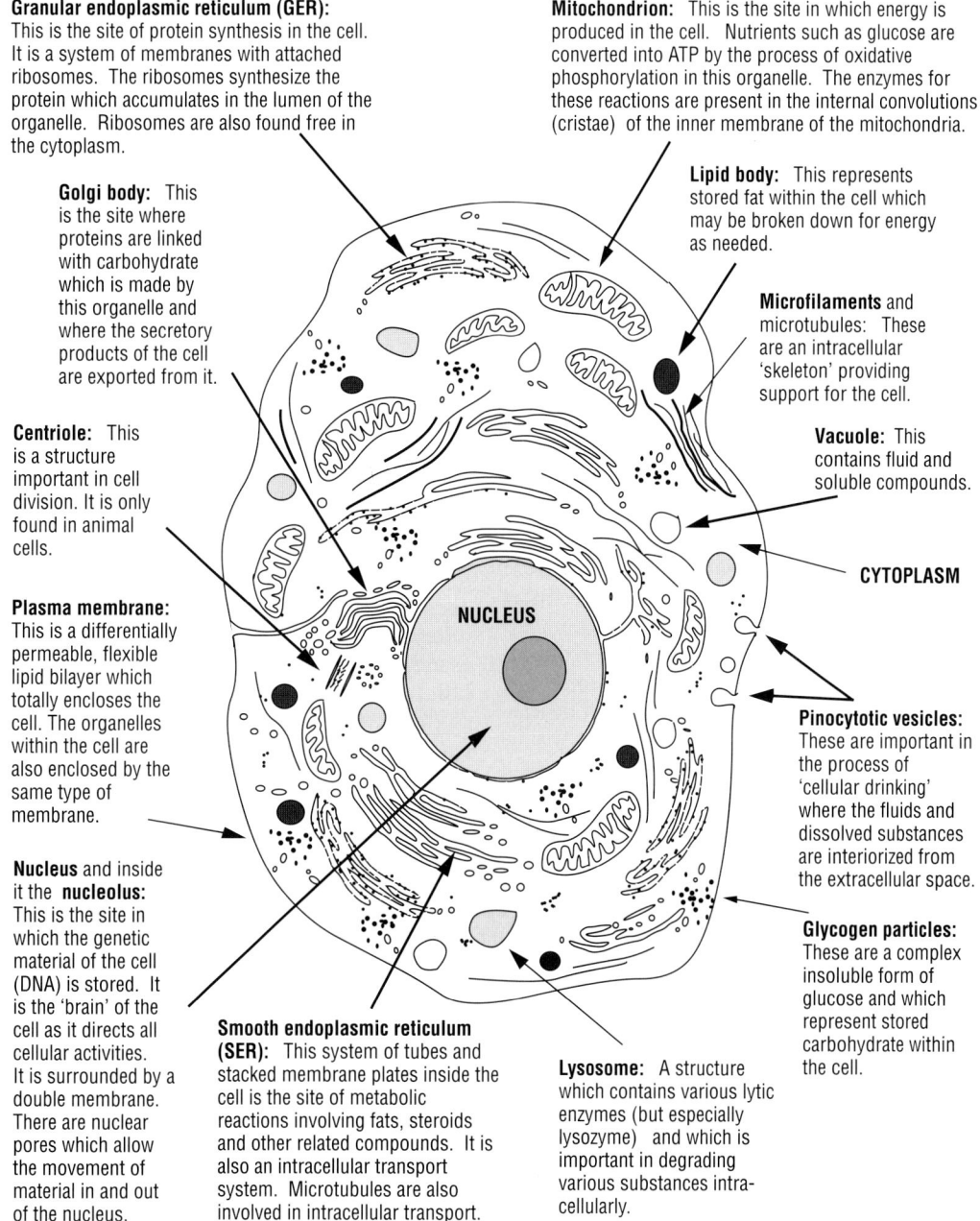

Granular endoplasmic reticulum (GER): This is the site of protein synthesis in the cell. It is a system of membranes with attached ribosomes. The ribosomes synthesize the protein which accumulates in the lumen of the organelle. Ribosomes are also found free in the cytoplasm.

Golgi body: This is the site where proteins are linked with carbohydrate which is made by this organelle and where the secretory products of the cell are exported from it.

Centriole: This is a structure important in cell division. It is only found in animal cells.

Plasma membrane: This is a differentially permeable, flexible lipid bilayer which totally encloses the cell. The organelles within the cell are also enclosed by the same type of membrane.

Nucleus and inside it the **nucleolus:** This is the site in which the genetic material of the cell (DNA) is stored. It is the 'brain' of the cell as it directs all cellular activities. It is surrounded by a double membrane. There are nuclear pores which allow the movement of material in and out of the nucleus.

Smooth endoplasmic reticulum (SER): This system of tubes and stacked membrane plates inside the cell is the site of metabolic reactions involving fats, steroids and other related compounds. It is also an intracellular transport system. Microtubules are also involved in intracellular transport.

Mitochondrion: This is the site in which energy is produced in the cell. Nutrients such as glucose are converted into ATP by the process of oxidative phosphorylation in this organelle. The enzymes for these reactions are present in the internal convolutions (cristae) of the inner membrane of the mitochondria.

Lipid body: This represents stored fat within the cell which may be broken down for energy as needed.

Microfilaments and microtubules: These are an intracellular 'skeleton' providing support for the cell.

Vacuole: This contains fluid and soluble compounds.

CYTOPLASM

Pinocytotic vesicles: These are important in the process of 'cellular drinking' where the fluids and dissolved substances are interiorized from the extracellular space.

Glycogen particles: These are a complex insoluble form of glucose and which represent stored carbohydrate within the cell.

Lysosome: A structure which contains various lytic enzymes (but especially lysozyme) and which is important in degrading various substances intracellularly.

NUCLEUS

Figure 2.1   *Structure and function of a typical animal cell*

mechanisms. Not all of these types of injury will lead to immediate cell death. Removal of the noxious stimulus may lead to partial or complete recovery. If compensatory mechanisms fail, the stimulus can lead to cellular changes which result in:

- **lethal injury**, i.e. **necrosis** or death of cells, while still part of the living body;
- **acute or chronic sublethal injury** — reactive changes and inflammation, which may be followed by recovery or by necrosis;
- **alterations in growth and/or differentiation**.

Lethal cellular injury may lead to organ/tissue disease which is clinically acute or chronic, depending on the number of cells killed and the ability of surviving cells to compensate. Acute, lethal cellular injury involving small numbers of cells at widely spaced intervals of time may cause chronic disease (e.g. alcoholic cirrhosis of the liver). In addition to the severity of the injury, another factor which determines what the cellular response will be is the nature of the cells themselves. Cells of the body are conveniently divided into two groups: **parenchymal cells**, which are the specialized cells in every organ responsible for carrying out that organ's function, and **connective tissue cells**, which are the supporting cells, comprising fibroblasts, glial cells, blood vessels and phagocytes. Although there are many different types of injury the body has only limited ways of responding. The parenchymal cells of the tissue or organ are said to undergo the **cellular response to injury**, while the connective tissue undergoes the change known as **inflammation** or the **inflammatory response**. It should be kept in mind that when a tissue is injured the response that will be seen is dependent not only on the **type** of tissue that is injured (i.e. whether it is a parenchymal tissue or a connective tissue), but also, very importantly, on the **severity** of the injury (refer to Figure 2.2).

Cell Injury

Cell injury is the central problem in pathology. Since the body may be regarded as an organized system of cells, the basis of disease may ultimately be traced to disturbances of cellular structure and function. This principle of **cellular pathology** was put forward by the German pathologist Rudolf Virchow in 1858. The normal cell is in a **homeostatic steady state** in which energy is required to maintain its internal environment (refer to Figure 2.3). Cell injury results when a homeostatic stress is placed upon the cell, altering its steady state. The injury may be reversible (e.g. fatty change) or it may be irreversible, resulting in cell death.

Abnormalities in cell division may also be seen. **Amitosis** is the process of cell division in which the injured cell divides but does so without preparation and duplication of chromosomes, thus giving rise to two cells with unequal numbers of chromosomes (e.g. 20 in one cell and 26 in the other). This form of abnormal cell division is followed by the rapid degeneration and death of both of these abnormal cells. Amitosis may be seen in skin cells that have been exposed to radiation or in other tissue cells exposed to sublethal concentrations of certain chemicals.

Ischaemia, a state in which blood supply is inadequate for tissue needs, is probably the most common cause of cell injury. Cells subjected to ischaemia pass through a sequence of changes, culminating in necrosis. Different cell types reach the point of **biochemically irreversible injury** (the biochemical definition of cell death) at different rates: at 37°C **neurones** undergo necrosis in 3 to 5 minutes, **myocardium** in 30 to 40 minutes (most other body cells resemble myocardium in this respect) and **fibroblasts** after many hours.

Beyond this 'point of no return', cells continue to undergo spontaneous degenerative changes: **autolysis**, indicating degradation of cellular components by the cell's own lytic enzymes, and **coagulation**, whereby the cellular proteins are denatured and coagulate. After some hours, these processes result in changes in the morphology of the cell that can be recognized microscopically as **histological necrosis**. Similar sequences of changes occur in many other forms of injury to cells. Consequently, ischaemia is often used as a model for cell injury in general. In ischaemia, the fall in available oxygen prevents the process of oxidative phosphorylation and the mitochondria become condensed. Anaerobic glycolysis provides an alternative mode of ATP generation. This results in the breakdown of glycogen and the accumulation of lactate and hydrogen ions. This fall in pH causes peripheral clumping of nuclear chromatin which is a reversible change.

With continuing ischaemia, ATP production by anaerobic glycolysis begins to fail. The deficiency in ATP causes the failure of the membrane ion pumps. Na^+, K^+ and Ca^{2+} diffuse along their concentration gradients, resulting in a net influx of water and swelling of the ER. The cytoskeleton is also disrupted. These are still reversible changes and the cell will return to normal if oxygen is readmitted to the area. If the ischaemia continues, damage to mitochondrial membranes leads to high-amplitude swelling of these organelles. Flocculent densities appear in the mitochondrial matrix due to protein denaturation. This change indicates that the cell has reached the 'point of no return' and this signifies an **irreversible change**, the cell having reached **biochemical death**. The remaining cellular changes will develop even if oxygen supply is re-established.

Autolysis begins to occur. The destruction of cellular macromolecules is accelerated by the release of lysosomal enzymes. The breakdown of nucleic acids leads to a loss of ribosomes and dissolution of the nucleus (karyolysis). Some of the products of autolysis are soluble and escape from the cell, leading to a reduction of cell weight. There is also progressive **coagulation** of cell proteins, an effect opposite to that of autolysis and this has been illustrated graphically in Figure 2.4.

Cell death is easily recognized under the microscope (Figure 2.5). A rather featureless, ghost-like outline of the cell remains. Nuclear breakdown is complete. The cytoplasm appears eosinophilic due to protein denaturation and loss of DNA and RNA, which are basophilic. Intracellular membranes form multilamellar stacks and it is almost impossible to recognize organelles.

Less severe injury, for example a partial, chronic ischaemia, leads to a delay in the biochemical necrosis of the cells subject to the injurious stimulus. The cells nevertheless react to the injury and undergo the well-characterized **reactive changes** to injury before un-

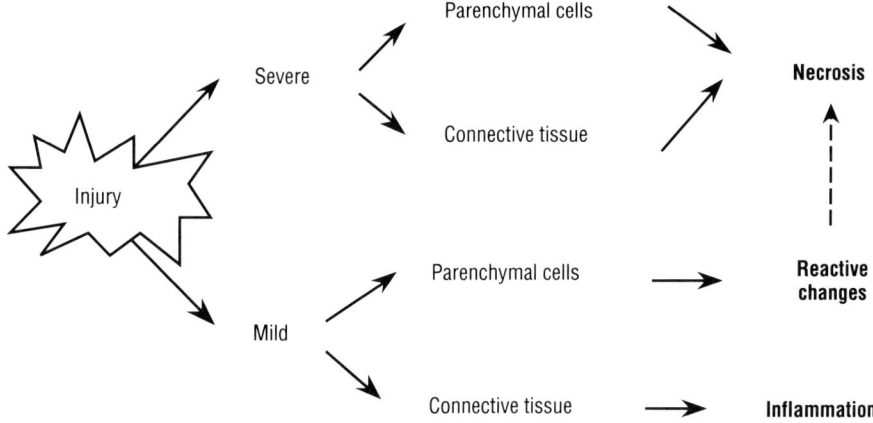

Figure 2.2   *The response of cells to injury depends to a large extent on the severity of the injury and the type of cell that is injured*

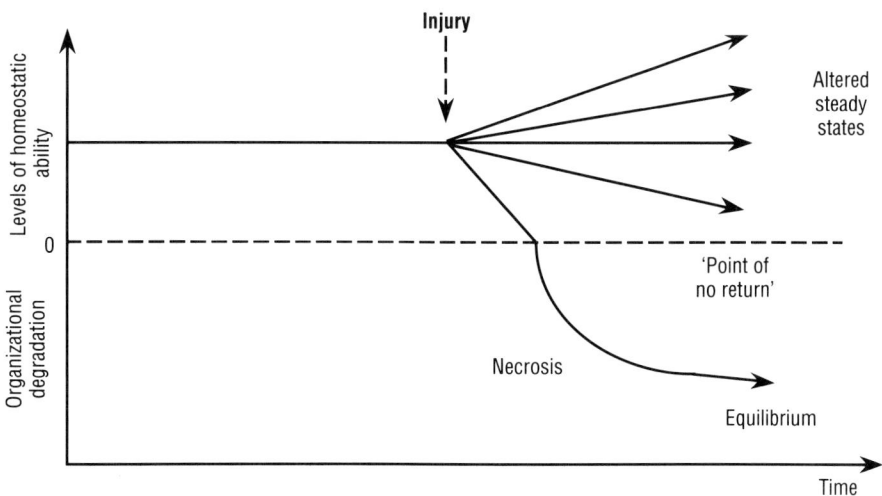

Figure 2.3   *The response of cells to injury may reflect ability or inability to cope with the injurious agent*

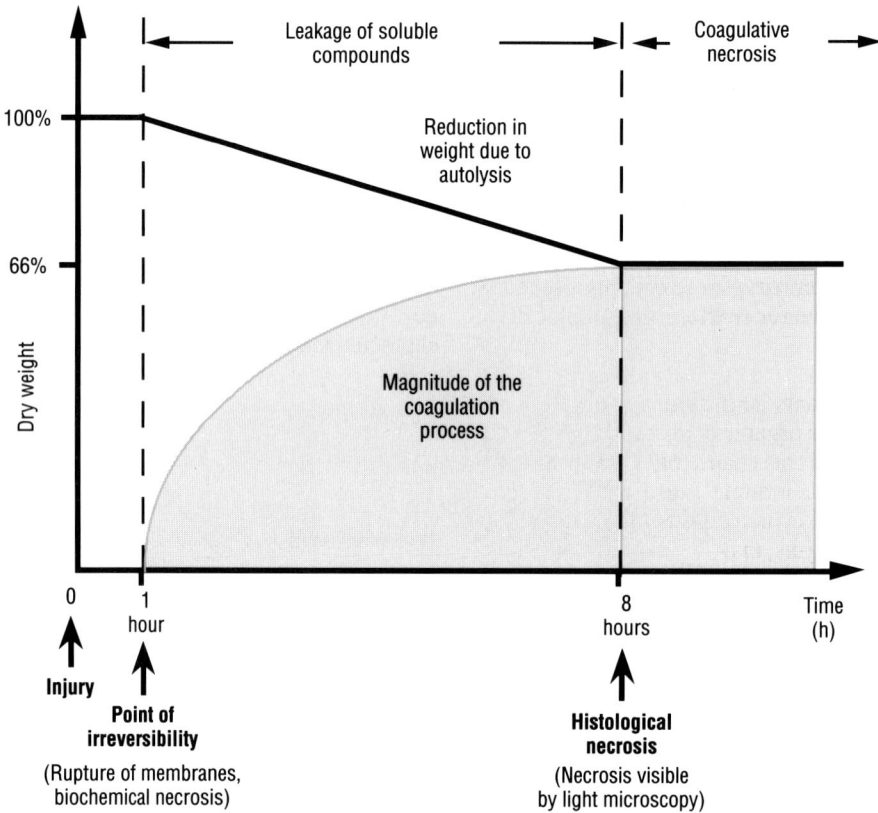

Figure 2.4   *The process of coagulative necrosis, as it may occur in a region of ischaemia, illustrated graphically*

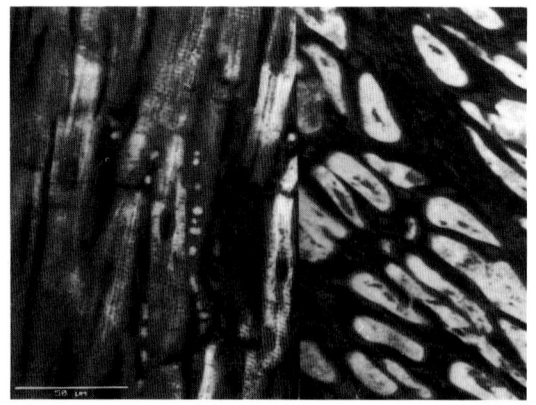

Figure 2.5   *Coagulative necrosis of myocardium (right) compared to normal myocardium (left). Note shrinkage of cells, loss of nuclei and striations (scale bar is 50 μm)*

dergoing necrosis. A characteristic feature of these reactive changes is that in their early stages at least, they are **reversible**.

Necrosis

Necrosis means death of cells or tissues while still part of the living body. It may occur suddenly or it may be preceded by gradual and potentially reversible damage. A more severe form of injury will lead to more rapid necrosis. The types of injury or aetiologies of disease discussed previously may lead to necrosis of cells or tissues if severe. Some common causes of necrosis are discussed below.

Anoxia
Anoxia (oxygen deficiency) is most commonly due to impairment of blood supply. If an end-artery (i.e. one

without adequate collateral supply) is obstructed, the blood supply to the tissue of that vascular bed is suddenly cut off, the tissue becomes **ischaemic** and dies. A region of **ischaemic necrosis** is termed an **infarct**. It should be noted that anoxia may be seen in tissue that is not ischaemic. That is, although it is well supplied with blood it may be anoxic. This occurs typically in carbon monoxide poisoning.

Different cells can tolerate **ischaemia** (impaired blood flow, and hence anoxia) to different degrees. Nerve cells die after only a few minutes, while fibroblasts can survive for hours.

Toxins and Infection
Certain bacteria, plants and animals (e.g. spiders, snakes) produce toxic organic compounds which even in very small quantities may cause cell damage amounting to necrosis. The bacterium *Clostridium perfringens* produces a lecithinase which digests the lipoprotein of cell membranes. Toxins may be distributed via the blood stream and injure cells remote from the infection site. Some toxins accompanying bacterial infection cause inflammation and **thrombosis** (intravascular clotting of the blood during life) thus producing ischaemic necrosis of cells of vascular endothelium.

Immunological Injury
Many infections produce T-cell-mediated immunological damage, for example *Mycobacterium tuberculosis* evokes an immune reaction (hypersensitivity) which leads to necrosis of cells in the vicinity of the bacterium. In many allergic reactions, the immune response instead of protecting the body will harm tissues and kill normal body cells. In the large group of autoimmune diseases, the immune system fails to recognize the host's tissues as 'self' and mounts an immune response against self components, with much tissue damage and necrosis.

Intracellular Infection
Viruses proliferate within cells and in so doing may kill the infected cells (cytopathic effects, CPE, refer to changes in the virus-infected cells which may be seen with the light microscope and which may be characteristic of specific viruses). Certain types of bacteria will also cause intracellular infections with a similar result, for example, *Rickettsia* spp., *Chlamydia* spp., *Listeria monocytogenes*.

Chemical Poisons
Certain chemicals injure cells, especially those in the organs of excretion and metabolism where their concentration is probably greatest. Thus many drugs or chemical poisons will kill cells of the kidney (acute

tubular necrosis) or liver (centrilobular necrosis). Very frequently in cases of poisoning, renal or hepatic failure is the ultimate cause of death.

Physical Agents
Cells exposed to heat die rapidly at temperatures above 55°C. Cold is less harmful and many cells or even small animals may survive freezing and thawing under controlled conditions. Necrosis occurs in frost-bite because of damage to capillaries leading to thrombosis. Radiation such as X-rays and gamma rays destroys the genetic material of cells and may destroy other macromolecules in the cell, leading to necrosis. Trauma will directly damage cells and vessels, causing their death.

Types of Necrosis

Necrosis produces distinct microscopic and macroscopic changes in tissues which may be seen some hours after the cells die. Both microscopically and macroscopically appearances of necrotic tissue may vary. The type of necrosis depends on the cause, the tissue affected and whether or not superimposed infection is present.

Coagulative Necrosis

Coagulative necrosis is most commonly seen in solid tissues and commonly seen in infarcts, for example heart, kidney, spleen and lung infarcts.

Macroscopically the necrotic area may become swollen, firm, lustreless and is pale unless it contains much blood. Histologically, the outlines of dead cells are usually visible but intracellular detail is lost and the cell looks structureless (like coagulated protein; see Figure 2.5).

Colliquative or Liquefactive Necrosis

Necrotic cells in the brain become softened due to their lipid nature and ultimately turn into a turbid fluid. This 'liquid' form of necrosis is termed colliquative or liquefactive necrosis. Colliquative necrosis of this type is known as **autolysis** because the cells essentially lyse themselves through the action of their own intracellular lytic enzymes in their lysosomes (Figure 2.6).

Another type of colliquative necrosis is **suppuration** (or sometimes referred to as suppurative necrosis) which occurs in lesions where large numbers of polymorphonuclear neutrophils have collected in an inflammatory response. This suppuration forms a vis-

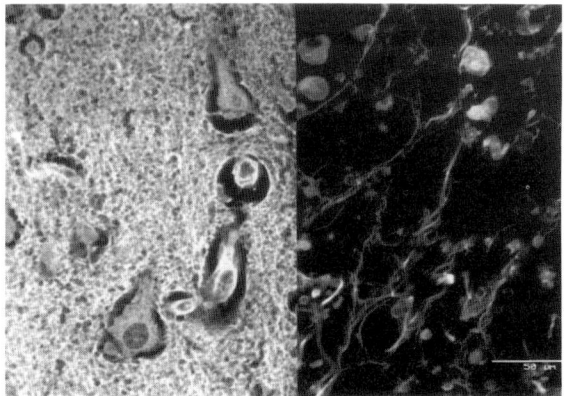

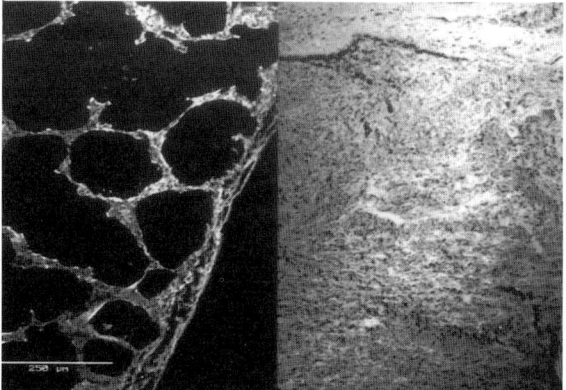

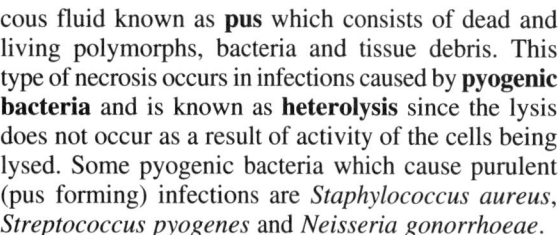

Figure 2.6   *Colliquative necrosis of the brain (right) compared to normal brain (left). Note loss of neurones as the tissue almost completely liquefies (scale bar is 50 μm)*

Figure 2.7   *Caseous necrosis of the lung (right) compared to normal lung (left). Note the conversion of the tissue into a solid, cheese-like mass (scale bar is 250 μm).*

cous fluid known as **pus** which consists of dead and living polymorphs, bacteria and tissue debris. This type of necrosis occurs in infections caused by **pyogenic bacteria** and is known as **heterolysis** since the lysis does not occur as a result of activity of the cells being lysed. Some pyogenic bacteria which cause purulent (pus forming) infections are *Staphylococcus aureus*, *Streptococcus pyogenes* and *Neisseria gonorrhoeae*.

Some authors prefer to distinguish between autolytic and heterolytic necrosis by calling the former colliquative and the latter liquefactive.

Caseous Necrosis

Caseous necrosis is so named because of its cheese-like consistency. This form of necrosis occurs in tuberculosis and has a dry, friable (crumbly) appearance. The necrotic tissues lose all structure and bear no resemblance to normal tissues macroscopically or microscopically. This type of necrosis occurs because of special biochemical attributes of the bacterium *Mycobacterium tuberculosis* but also very important are factors relating to the immune system and the nature of the response that the body mounts against this organism specifically. Almost any tissue in the body may be affected by tuberculosis and caseous necrosis may thus be seen anywhere in the body (Figure 2.7).

Gangrenous Necrosis

Necrotic lesions affecting skin or mucosal surfaces

(e.g. bowel) are frequently infected by bacteria which causes putrefaction (the production of foul-smelling gas with brown, green or black tissue discolouration). This putrefactive form of necrosis is called **gangrene** (or gas-gangrene if gas is produced in the tissues). The main causative bacterium is *Clostridium perfringens* but other bacteria such as *Peptostreptococcus* spp. and *Bacteroides* spp. may also be involved.

Gummatous Necrosis

Gummatous necrosis is a variant of coagulative necrosis and differs from it in appearance in that the necrotic tissue is slightly yellower in colour and has a more rubbery consistency than the tissue which has undergone coagulative necrosis. It characteristically occurs in the tertiary stages of syphilis (infection with *Treponema pallidum*), where **gummata** form in tissues. This stage of syphilis may be seen many decades after the primary infection and gummata may be found in any organ of the body, but especially in the heart, blood vessels and brain.

Fat Necrosis

In acute pancreatitis there is release of many digestive enzymes into the pancreatic and surrounding tissues. Liberated lipases act on surrounding adipose tissue, for example the omentum, and cause fat necrosis, as is shown in Figure 2.8. The fatty acids released through

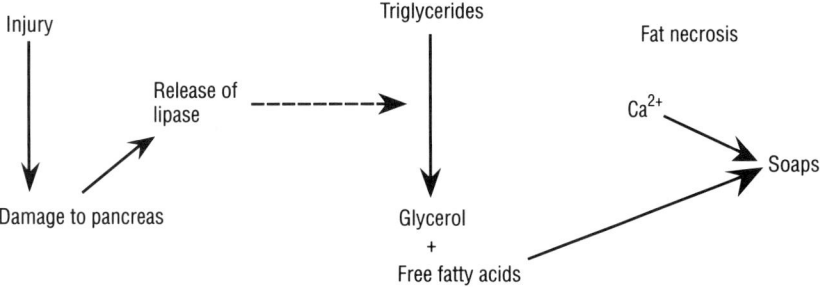

Figure 2.8 *The mechanism of pancreatic fat necrosis*

the digestive action of lipase combine with calcium ions to form 'soaps' (a soap being the salt of a fatty acid). This gives the necrotic adipose tissue a pale blue (basophilic) appearance histologically. The process is known as 'saponification' (Figure 2.9). The necrotic tissue may later calcify leaving hard gritty masses.

Alternatively, fat necrosis may follow traumatic injury to adipose tissue, for example after a blow to the breasts. The adipose cells are destroyed and release their fats. These fats are degraded and the tissue undergoes necrosis, fibrosis and calcification, forming an area that is felt as a hard lump within the tissue.

Fibrinoid/Hyaline Necrosis

Small arteries and arterioles in hypertension (high blood pressure) undergo degeneration in their walls known as hyaline degeneration and fibrinoid necrosis. This is seen most prominently in hypertensive kidney disease. Hyaline degeneration is so named because of the glassy, eosinophilic (smooth pink) appearance of the affected wall of an arteriole or small artery. Fibrinoid necrosis, affecting arteriolar walls, is so named because of the resemblance to fibrin in the necrotic wall, appearing bright pink and smudgy histologically. This form of necrosis is a variant of coagulative necrosis.

Reaction to Dead Tissue

Necrotic tissue excites an inflammatory response in the tissue around it and ultimately the mass of necrotic cells is removed by the inflammatory process. The compounds released by the breakdown of the necrotic cells during autolysis are what stimulate the inflammatory response in the living tissue surrounding the necrotic area and many phagocytic cells enter the area of necrosis from adjacent inflamed vessels. These phagocytes break down and remove the necrotic debris. Where possible necrotic tissue is replaced by the same kind of tissue by multiplication (regeneration) of surrounding healthy tissue cells. Often, however, this cannot be accomplished and repair occurs by connective tissue and a **scar** is left behind.

Sometimes dead tissue becomes calcified as it attracts calcium salts, and it cannot be removed. This is especially the case where large areas of necrotic tissue are present. Such a result is termed **pathological calcification**. This is the process whereby calcium salts are deposited in the soft tissues. The type of calcium salts deposited are similar to those within bone, i.e. hydroxyapatite, a basic, complex calcium phosphate. Small amounts of iron and magnesium salts may be deposited in association with the calcium. There are two different types of pathological calcification, dystrophic calcification and metastatic calcification.

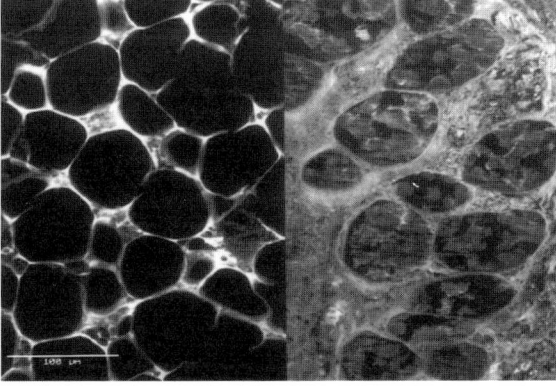

Figure 2.9 *Fat necrosis in the omentum associated with pancreatitis (right) compared to normal adipose tissue (left). There is saponification as the freed fatty acids combine with calcium (scale bar is 100 μm)*

Dystrophic Calcification

This occurs despite normal levels of plasma calcium and in the absence of derangements in calcium metabolism. Dystrophic calcification occurs in areas of necrosis as dead and dying tissue has an affinity for calcium salts. Calcium is deposited in regions of coagulative, caseous and fat necrosis especially. The larger the area of necrosis and the longer it persists in the body, the more chance there is of calcification occurring. Regions of coagulative necrosis may become calcified. The lungs in cases of tuberculosis frequently show large regions of calcification of the caseous necrosis, and damaged heart valves and the walls of arteries may show deposits of calcium which binds onto the necrotic tissue. If skeletal muscle is damaged, in certain situations it will attract calcium salts and a region of calcification and inflammation in the muscle gives rise to the condition of **myositis ossificans**. Certain tumours which have necrotic centres also show calcification (Figure 2.10).

Under the microscope, the regions of calcification show basophilic, amorphous, granular or clumped deposits of calcium within the tissue. These deposits may be palpated in the fresh tissue as hard, gritty deposits.

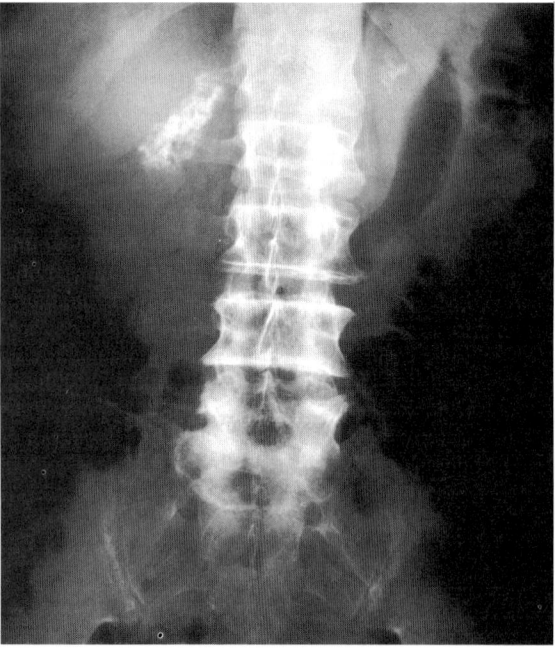

Figure 2.10 *Abdominal X-ray showing dystrophic calcification of the adrenal gland (courtesy of Dr Thomas Molyneux, RMIT)*

It is not unusual in some cases to see massive calcium deposits as occurs, for example, in a tuberculous lymph node, where the whole node is converted to a pebble of calcium salts. In the course of time, the focus of dystrophic calcification may be converted to **heterotopic bone**. This term implies bone formed in exotic sites, distant from the skeleton. In this particular case, mesenchymal cells are brought to the site of calcification via the bloodstream, they differentiate into osteogenic cells, begin to lay down bone and eventually the area of calcification is converted into a region of bone, some such bony areas even containing a marrow cavity with blood-forming cells.

On occasion, dystrophic calcification will occur in very small areas of necrosis which involves only single cells or small groups of them. Such calcified cells act as foci of crystallization and they attract more calcium salts which are laid down in layers around the 'seed crystal' of original calcified cells. The result of this process is multiple small grains of calcification within the tissue. These lamellated grains of calcification are termed **psammoma bodies** (i.e. 'sand grains') and are a feature of some brain tumours.

Metastatic Calcification

In this type of pathological calcification the deposition of calcium occurs even in normal, living tissues and it is always the result of some derangement of calcium metabolism, which is reflected by raised plasma calcium levels, **hypercalcaemia**. There are many causes of hypercalcaemia, including abnormal hyperactivity of the parathyroid glands (**hyperparathyroidism**), vitamin D intoxication, systemic sarcoidosis and increased mobilization of calcium from bones due to a variety of causes. It should be noted that if necrotic tissue is present in an individual with hypercalcaemia, the calcium deposition is greatly enhanced and accelerated. Metastatic calcification may occur in a variety of tissues around the body but is most commonly seen in the walls of blood vessels, the kidneys, lungs and gastric mucosa. Metastatic calcification deposits tend to be more delicate than those encountered in dystrophic calcification and thus rarely give rise to large concretions or calculi.

In both cases of pathological calcification, the deposits of calcium cause no clinical dysfunction but on occasion, massive involvement of the lungs compromises respiration, large deposits in the kidneys cause renal damage and deposition in the wall of blood vessels may hamper their function causing interference in the blood supply to the tissues that they irrigate.

Sublethal Injury — Reactive Changes

Reactive changes tend to occur in response to mild injury, for example low toxin concentrations or short exposure to heat or partial oxygen lack (**partial chronic anoxia** as occurs in arterial disease). Without sufficient oxygen, oxidative phosphorylation fails. Certain toxins may also interfere directly with the oxidative phosphorylation processes occurring in the mitochondria. Interference with this leads to inhibition of mitochondrial activity resulting in depressed ATP in the cell. The first system to fail in the cell due to lack of ATP is the Na^+/K^+ pump which serves to maintain physiological cation distributions about the cell membrane and in so doing controls the electrical potential of the cell and the influx of water. The osmotic pressure inside the cell is normally high and so water tends to constantly flood into the cell along its concentration gradient, hence the need for the ion pump in the cell membrane. When the Na^+/K^+ pump fails, water floods into the cytoplasm from the extracellular compartment or other intracellular compartments, for example nuclear sap. This results in cellular or subcellular swelling with shrinkage of some other compartment as water redistributes. This accumulation of water is known as **hydropic change**. In addition, anoxia leads to increased anaerobic metabolism as a compensatory mechanism. Increasing levels of toxic metabolites lead to denaturation and clumping of proteins in the cytoplasm and nucleus. This may be seen under the microscope as staining irregularities in the cells.

In some cells (e.g. liver cells, kidney tubule cells and heart muscle cells) lipids may also accumulate within the cell due to impaired lipid metabolism. This lipid accumulation is known as **fatty change** and may still be a reversible process if the cell recovers. The lipid is seen in vacuoles which may become very large such that the cell may resemble an adipose cell (Figure 2.11). Such fatty change is seen in the liver of alcoholics, who through the constant consumption of alcohol (a toxin), injure their liver cells (the major site of alcohol detoxification in the body). The whole of the liver becomes enlarged, pale and full of fats within the cytoplasm of the cells. Even at this stage the fatty change in the liver is reversible and if alcohol is no longer consumed, the liver will go back to normal. If alcohol consumption is continued, the liver cells will die. Reactive changes will become **degenerative changes** if the injurious stimulus continues to act, thus causing more damage to the cellular components. In this case the damage to the cells becomes too great and these changes are **irreversible**, eventually leading to necrosis (refer to Figure 2.12).

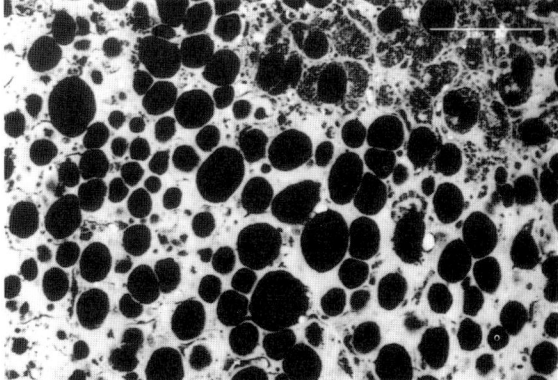

Figure 2.11 *Fatty change of the liver associated with chronic alcohol abuse. Note the resemblance of the injured liver cells to adipocytes (scale bar is 50 μm)*

Swelling of intracellular structures and cytoplasm leads to stretching and finally rupture of their bounding and internal membranes. If lysosomal membranes rupture, release of digestive enzymes occurs which aids in the destruction and digestion/dissolution of cell contents (**autophagy**). Nuclear changes such as shrinkage (**pyknosis**) and nuclear fragmentation (**karyorrhexis**) may occur. If the nucleus is dissolved by this process **karyolysis** is said to occur. Membrane rupture is usually a late phenomenon, but may occur early in such diseases as gout, haemochromatosis and the pneumoconioses.

The redistribution of water leads to swelling of some compartments, for example the cytoplasm and mitochondria, and shrinkage of other compartments, for example the nucleus. Increased acidity and altered fluid volume lead to precipitation and denaturation of proteins including essential enzymes. Another change which occurs with degenerative changes is that calcium ions may flood into the cytoplasm and precipitate intermediary metabolites as sparingly soluble calcium salts and calcium soaps.

Light Microscopic Appearances of the Above Stages

In the **early reversible stage**, cell swelling ('cloudy swelling' or **hydropic change**) and **fatty change** occur. These changes are seen as characteristic microscopic features in a section prepared by conventional histopathological techniques. Very characteristic of fatty change is liver tissue which has been injured by alcohol (seen, for example, in a dedicated drinker!).

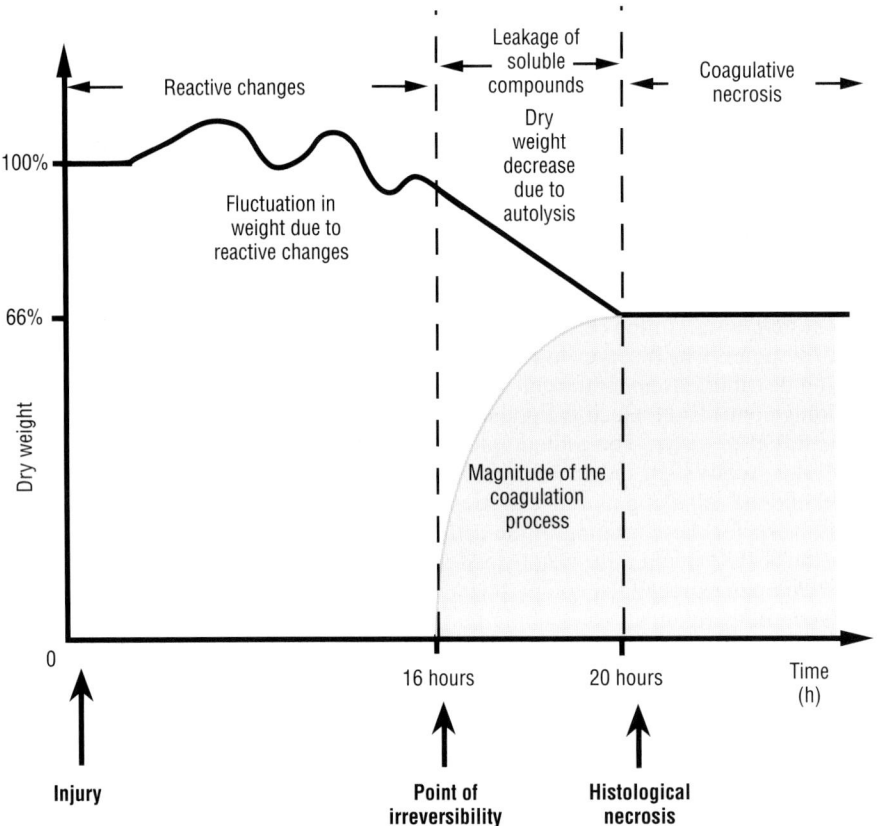

Figure 2.12 *The response of parenchymal cells to sublethal injury, as may be seen in a region of oligaemia, involves reactive changes of the cells before they undergo necrosis*

Similarly, hydropic change will be seen in cases of chemical poisoning in the cells of the kidney tubules or once again in the liver (after inhalation or ingestion of carbon tetrachloride liver cells undergo hydropic and fatty change). Changes in staining characteristics of the cell may occur: loss of the cytoplasmic basophilia (bluish mauve colour) may be noticed and the cells may appear excessively stained with eosin. This reflects abnormalities in protein metabolism. In some cells **loss of glycogen** may be a prominent feature of cell injury (special stains are available for staining intracellular glycogen).

In the **irreversible stage**, necrosis (cell death) occurs, encompassing coagulation of cytoplasm, loss of cell outline, cell shrinking, dystrophic calcification, nuclear changes (pyknosis, karyorrhexis, karyolysis) and intense eosinophilic staining. Changes seen in necrosis include clumping of denatured nucleoprotein about the nuclear membrane, making the nucleus look empty with a broken up, irregular membrane (karyorrhexis: nuclear fragmentation). If chromatin clumping is associated with nuclear shrinkage the nucleus appears like a tiny dark blue mass (pyknosis: nuclear condensation). If lysosomal enzymes digest the nucleus then the nucleus dissolves (karyolysis: loss of nucleus).

Degenerative Changes seen in Cells in Disease

When cells are damaged but not killed, they may recover function but tend to accumulate metabolic products whose intermediary metabolism is disturbed. The commonest accumulation is with fat (fatty change), especially in the liver or kidney as described previously. Other products that can accumulate include filaments and glycogen (hyaline degeneration) and in some cases pigments accumulate from breakdown of haemoglobin or melanin.

In damaged cells lysosomes tend to accumulate and fuse with damaged organelles, as a mopping up of damaged structures gets under way. Some components of the damaged cell cannot be broken down by the lysosomal enzymes and these inert indigestible remains are stored in the cell for the rest of its life as **lipofuscin**, which is a brownish pigment. When very abundant, lipofuscin colours cells brown. The same may be seen if cells are starved of nutrients, for example diminished nutrients in blood or tissue fluids causes them to derive their energy by digesting their own protein and constituents. This results in **atrophy** (shrinking of the cells). Such atrophic cells are usually packed with lysosomes and breakdown products. The brown shrunken appearance of the heart in old age is aptly called brown atrophy.

Cell shrinkage may lead to cell disappearance. In such cases the missing cells may be replaced by fat cells or fibroblasts (connective tissue). Atrophy may be a normal process such as involution of embryonic remnants, for example the umbilical vessels, or the general shrinkage of tissues with ageing or disuse. This change is due to a type of cell death known as **apoptosis** and examples of it may be seen in the invo-lution of the uterus, breast or thymus. Apoptosis is a 'physiological' process of cell death and is thought to be programmed into certain cells, developing at a certain stage in their life cycle. The information for apoptotic cell death is in the DNA and the process develops when such genetic information is activated.

In apoptosis the cell begins to lose water and begins to shrink. The nucleus shrinks and eventually undergoes pyknosis and karyorrhexis. The cell continues to shrink and the organelles begin to group together, forming membrane-bound bodies (called apoptotic bodies) within the cell cytoplasm. Eventually the cell breaks up and releases the membrane-bound fragments containing dense cytoplasmic contents and condensed organelle remnants. The surrounding, surviving parenchymal cells then phagocytose the cell fragments and degrade them using the components as nutrients (Figure 2.13). This type of cell death occurs in isolated cells or small groups of cells within the tissue at any one time and is not accompanied by inflammation or other degenerative changes. It causes (over a period of time) a shrinkage of the tissue in which it is occurring and is sometimes termed **shrinkage necrosis**.

Injury to cells may be reflected in the connective

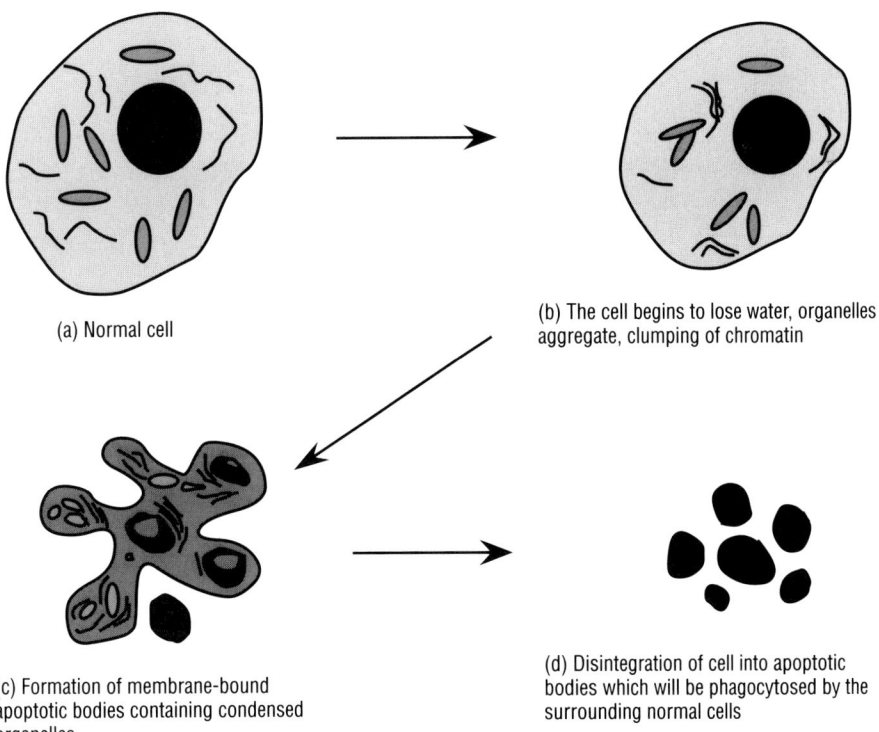

(a) Normal cell

(b) The cell begins to lose water, organelles aggregate, clumping of chromatin

(c) Formation of membrane-bound apoptotic bodies containing condensed organelles

(d) Disintegration of cell into apoptotic bodies which will be phagocytosed by the surrounding normal cells

Figure 2.13   *The process of apoptosis ('shrinkage necrosis')*

tissue matrix they lie in. There may be changes in the amount of collagen in the matrix or calcification of the matrix, or deposition of pigments or carbohydrate/protein-rich material (amyloid) in the matrix. This amyloid material consists of immunoprotein (as seen in multiple myeloma or rheumatoid arthritis). The accumulation of amyloid is irreversible and is usually seen in those disorders which are associated with abnormal immune function.

Summary of Parenchymal Cell Response to Injury

Severe injury to all types of cells in the body leads to immediate death or **necrosis** of cells.

Mild injury to tissue such as partial chronic anoxia or toxic action of alcohol on liver cells will evoke a different response:

1. Some cells, severely affected, will die quickly, undergoing necrosis (refer to Figure 2.14).
2. Some cells will survive for many hours undergoing various **reactive changes** then may later die. Reactive changes seen histologically include:
    *   Fatty change
    *   Loss of glycogen stores, abnormal mitochondria
    *   Loss of cytoplasmic basophilia (staining characteristic)
    *   Hydropic change
    *   Vacuolation, coagulation, and
    *   Nuclear changes (irreversible)

When cells undergo reactive changes, the point of irreversibility is delayed for some hours before the cell undergoes necrosis. The reactive changes, which are reversible in the early stages, occur during the delay phase. If the injury is removed before the point of irreversibility is reached then the cell may recover, but usually its life span is shortened (refer to Table 2.1).

Connective tissue in the region responds by undergoing the series of changes known as acute inflammation.

3. Some cells will appear unaffected, however, their lifespan may be shortened.
4. Those cells sufficiently far removed from the injury will not be affected.

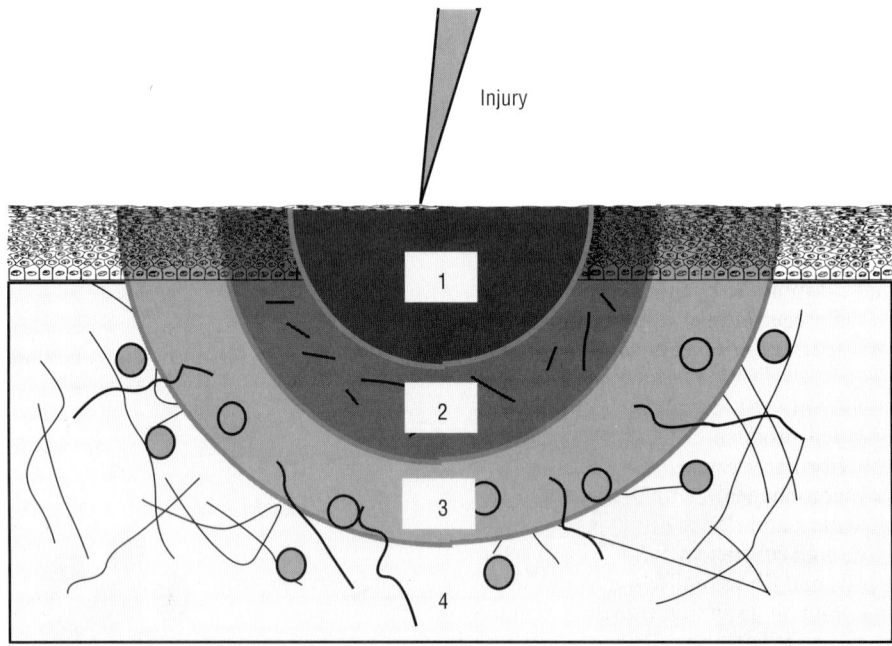

Zone 1: Necrosis
Zone 2: Reactive changes
Zone 3: Minimal effects
Zone 4: No injurious effects

Figure 2.14   *Summary of responses of parenchymal cells to injury*

Table 2.1 *Summary of reactive changes of parenchymal cells to sublethal injury*

Organelle involved	Substance involved	Microscopic appearance	Functional significance
Membranes, smooth ER	Electrolytes and Water	Hydropic change Swelling	Failure of ATP production
Mitochondria	Carbohydrate	Decreased glycogen Mitochondria abnormal	ATP production decreased
Ribosomes, granular ER	Protein	Loss of cytoplasm basophilia	Inhibition of protein synthesis
Endoplasmic reticulum	Fat	Fatty change	Infiltration by fat, impaired metabolism, serious effects
Lysosomes	Enzymes	Autophagy Vacuolation Autolysis	Destruction of cell components, organelles
Nucleus	Nucleic acids	Pyknosis Karyorrhexis Karyolysis	End-stage effects (Moribund cells)

Inflammation

An injury to tissue results in both a parenchymal cell response and a connective tissue response. Inflammation is the way in which connective tissue responds to sublethal injury. If injury to connective tissue is severe then necrosis will occur in its various components just as necrosis will occur in the parenchymal cells of an organ.

The components of connective tissue are: **fibroblasts**, which produce collagen and other connective tissue fibrillar proteins; **phagocytes** (polymorphs and macrophages), which wander through the tissue, ingesting and destroying particles and debris; **matrix** (ground substance), which fills the spaces between the cells and fibres; and **blood vessels**, which supply tissues with nutrients and oxygen, removing metabolites and carbon dioxide. **Lymphatic vessels** are also present, draining excess tissue fluid and returning it to the circulation.

In the inflammatory response certain characteristics may be observed:

- The reaction to injury is mostly the same even with widely differing types of injury.
- The response is not a single process but several interrelated responses.
- The inflammatory response is generally beneficial as part of the body's defence system. However, it can at times be harmful or even lethal if mounted inappropriately.

Inflammation in an organ is designated by the organ name plus the suffix **-itis**, for example tonsillitis, appendicitis, conjunctivitis, peritonitis, hepatitis. Some exceptions are pleurisy and pneumonia.

Inflammation may be either acute or chronic. Chronic inflammation is discussed in the section at the end of this chapter.

Acute Inflammation

Acute inflammation may be briefly defined as 'the reaction that begins in a tissue after sublethal injury and ends with complete healing'.

Celsus described the **cardinal signs** of inflammation in the first century AD. They are:

Calor — **heat**

Rubor — **redness**
Dolor — **pain**
Tumor — **swelling**
Functio laesa — **loss of function**, was added by
Virchow many centuries later

These five cardinal signs of acute inflammation may
easily be observed in mild thermal injury (burns) to the
skin. There is redness, heat when touched, swelling
and pain. The skin affected will not carry out normal
functions such as perspiration, temperature regulation,
tissue barrier, etc. Loss of function may not occur in
all cases of acute inflammation, however.

Examination of the injured area histologically was
first carried out by Julius Cohnheim, a German pathologist, in 1882, and he found that the examination
of living inflamed tissue under the microscope explains the cardinal signs. Cohnheim observed that in
acute inflammation there is:

- sustained **vasodilatation** (dilated blood vessels);
- **hyperaemia** (increased blood flow in vessels);
- **increased vascular permeability** (more fluid enters the tissue spaces from the vessels);
- **inflammatory exudate formation**;
- **slowing of blood flow** or **stasis** (complete stoppage
  of flow);
- **margination** and **diapedesis** of leukocytes (white
  cells move to sides of vessels and 'stick' there, then
  actively move through endothelial cell junctions);
- **leukocytic chemotaxis** and **emigration** (white cells
  move to damaged areas).

If an area which is acutely inflamed is examined
under the light microscope Cohnheim's observations
may be verified. Taking a simple, mild thermal burn in
the skin as the typical acute inflammatory lesion we
may see the following changes occurring. Immediately following the injury, there is a transient **vasoconstriction** of the arterioles. This does not always
occur with burns but is a prominent feature of other
types of injury (mainly traumatic injury) and is seen
with the naked eye as a **blanching** of the area. The
next stage involves a **vasodilatation** of the arterioles
and venules in the injured area and the opening up of
many vascular channels which had previously been
carrying little or no blood. Blood flow through the area
may increase up to tenfold.

This is the **hyperaemia** of inflammation and is what
makes the area appear red to the naked eye. Initially,
for the first one or two hours after the injury, the blood
flow is extremely rapid. The blood cells become packed
in the central part of the blood vessel, with plasma
being in contact with the vascular wall. This is an
exaggeration of the **axial flow** which is seen in normal

vessels. The vast increase in the blood flowing through
the area gives it its red, hot, inflamed look and feel.
Accompanying the increase in blood flow is a great
swelling of the area, the **oedema**, of the acute inflammatory response. This fluid is derived from blood
plasma and it escapes the vessels because their walls
show **increased vascular permeability**, thus allowing
more blood and protein to escape the circulation with
greater ease than normal. The fluid which collects in
the tissue spaces as a result of this process is called
inflammatory exudate and its protein concentration
is higher than that of normal tissue fluid. The proteins
in it are plasma proteins, which points out its derivation from blood plasma.

Gradually, the blood flow through the inflamed vessels decreases and may even stop in some vessels, the
latter situation called **stasis** of the blood. This stasis
may persist and result in the death and disintegration
of the affected vessels and the tissue which they supply with blood. However, in most cases flow begins
again and eventually will return to normal. As the flow
slows down the blood cells begin colliding with the
vascular wall, rolling along it and it is observed that
neutrophilic leukocytes from the blood stream start to
adhere to the surface of the endothelial cells lining the
vessels. Progressively more and more neutrophils adhere to the endothelial surface, until the whole luminal
surface of the vessel becomes covered with leukocytes;
this is the **margination** or 'pavementing' of the
leukocytes.

The next stage involves the active amoeboid movement of the neutrophils through the vascular wall to
the extravascular spaces. Each cell insinuates its way
between the endothelial cells, pushing apart the closed
junctions of the cells and squeezing through into the
tissue spaces. This process is called **diapedesis**. Once
the neutrophils are in the tissue spaces they emigrate to
sites adjacent to the vessels, being attracted to those
sites by chemical targets, for example groups of necrotic
cells releasing products of autolysis or groups of bacteria releasing metabolites and toxins. The movement
of the leukocytes in response to a chemical gradient is
known as **chemotaxis**. The neutrophils will then
phagocytose particulate matter.

Formation of Inflammatory Exudate

Normal Vessels and Transudate Formation

The **endothelium** of small blood vessels is the single
layer of cells that line the internal aspect of vessels and
is composed of very flattened, elongated cells which
adhere to the connective tissue underneath, fitting to-

gether like the cobblestones in a pavement. With the electron microscope, the capillary and venule endothelium is distinguished into three distinct classes (Figure 2.15).

In **continuous endothelium vessels** the lumen of the vessel is surrounded by a continuous cylinder of endothelium 0.2–0.3 µm thick composed of a single endothelial cell bent over itself much like a brandy snap. The cytoplasm of the cell contains all the usual organelles found in other cells. This is the commonest type of vessel found in the body and such vessels are found in skin, muscle and nervous system (Figure 2.16).

Fenestrated endothelium vessels resemble the continuous vessels but the endothelium shows multiple perforations in the cytoplasm of the endothelial cells, making them look rather like sieves. These openings are called fenestrae and are covered by a thin, differentially permeable diaphragm, thinner than a single plasma membrane. This type of vessel is found in the mucosae of the gastrointestinal tract, in the kidney and glandular organs (Figures 2.17 and 2.18).

Sinusoidal endothelium vessels are lined by endothelium which shows large open pores in the cytoplasm of the cells. These are wide open gaps, not covered by a diaphragm. These vessels are found in the liver, spleen and bone marrow.

The structure of the vascular endothelium is important in the exchanges that occur between the interior of the vessel and the extracellular fluid that surrounds the vessel. The endothelial cell cytoplasm is the barrier across which such exchanges occur. Normally the passage of substances across the vascular endothelium occurs according to pressure and concentration gradients. The diffusion of small molecules and gases (e.g. K^+, Na^+, Cl^-, sugars, CO_2, O_2) occurs through the closed cell to cell junctions and is governed by simple passive diffusion gradients. The molecules are small enough to pass through the narrow passage between the cell junctions. Bulk movement of water occurs through the wall of the vessels and is due to chemical and osmotic

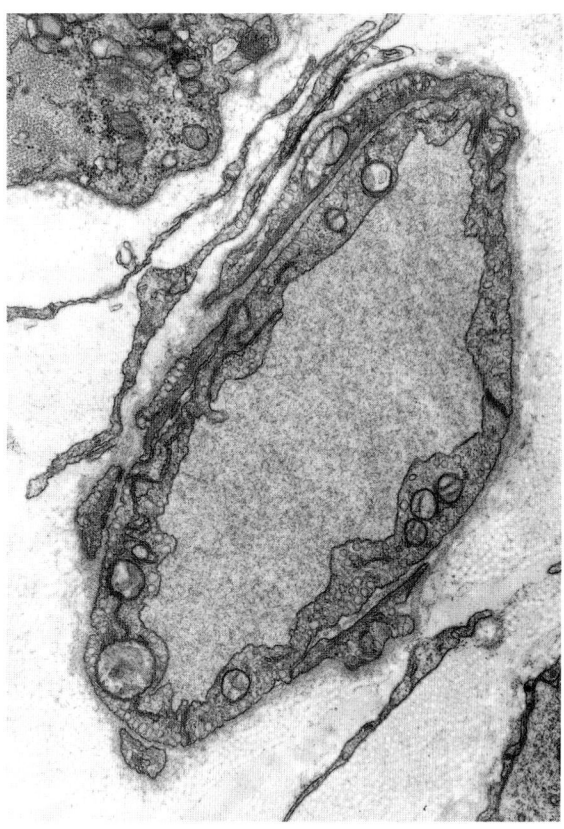

Figure 2.16   *A continuous endothelium capillary of skeletal muscle (×28 000)*

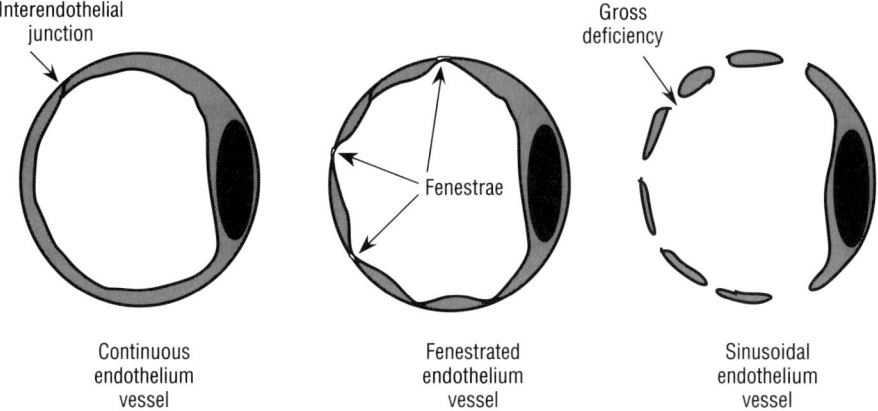

Figure 2.15   *Types of vascular endothelium in the body*

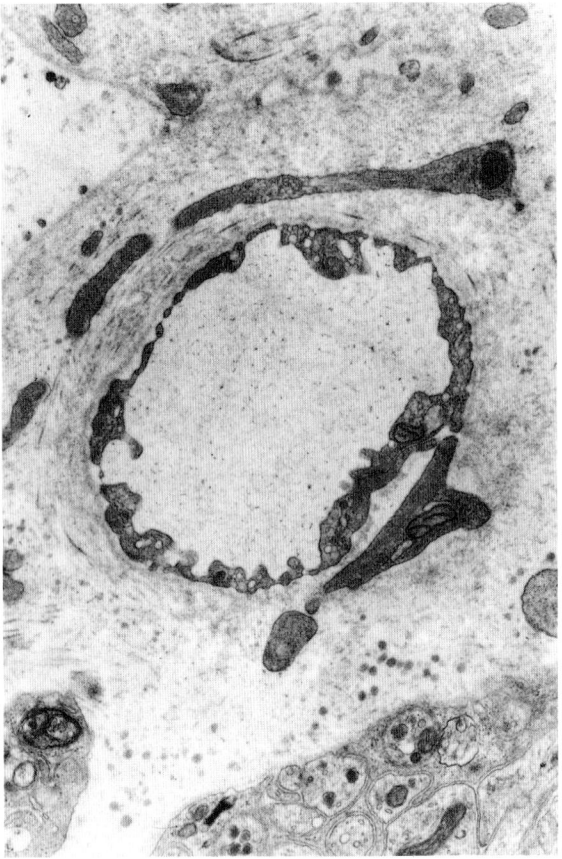

Figure 2.17 *A fenestrated endothelium capillary of stomach mucosa (×20 000)*

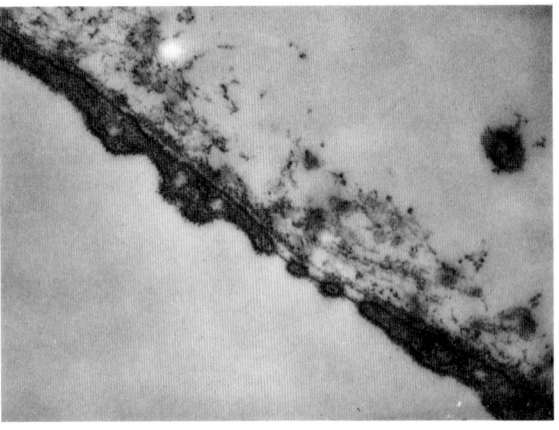

Figure 2.18 *Detail of the fenestrae of a fenestrated endothelium capillary of stomach mucosa (×110 000)*

forces. This was first described by the physiologist Starling for normal vessels and these forces are known as **Starling forces** (Figure 2.19). The hydrostatic pressure within the arteriolar end of the capillary bed is higher than the colloid oncotic pressure outside the vessel such that there is a movement of water out of the vessel into the tissue space at the arteriolar end. Conversely, the hydrostatic pressure within the venular end of the capillary bed is lower than the colloid oncotic pressure outside it and hence water tends to move into the vessel from the tissue fluid at the venular end. The net effect is that almost as much water leaves the vessel as it enters it. An examination of the pressures shows that there is slight loss of fluid from the vessel into the extravascular spaces, and this is what forms the tissue fluid. A small amount of **plasma protein** also leaves the vessels together with the water. This escaped protein cannot re-enter the vessel because of chemical and osmotic considerations. Excess tissue fluid and protein are collected by the **lymphatic vessels**. These are blind-ending, thin vessels within the tissues, one function of which is to take up the protein and excess fluid and through a system of larger and larger vessels return that fluid and protein to the circulation via the thoracic duct. The walls of the lymphatics are permeable to protein only from outside in and they also possess valves, making protein and lymph flow one way.

The measure of lymph flow and protein content of the lymph from any tissue is an indication of the protein leakage from the blood vessels into the tissue fluid of that area. In an area where the capillaries and venules are lined by continuous endothelium, for example the skin, there is little lymph volume and the protein content of the lymph is low normally. Where the capillaries of the tissue are lined by fenestrated endothelium, for example the intestine, there is a higher outflow volume of lymph which contains a higher amount of protein. In tissues where there are sinusoidal vessels, for example the liver, there is a very large volume of lymphatic outflow which is very high in its protein content. These findings are not surprising when we consider the structure of the endothelium in the three types of vessels. It is obvious that the protein leakage from sinusoidal and fenestrated vessels occurs through the pores and fenestrae, but it may be asked, how does the protein escape the continuous endothelium vessels? Three theories have been put forward:

1. Via pinocytotic vesicles (i.e. through exocytosis).
2. Slow seepage through closed junctions (just as fluid and small solutes escape).
3. Escape through momentary openings of the endothelial junctions.

In order to determine which theory best explains the behaviour of vessels, inflamed vessels were examined at the first stages of inflammation where large volumes of fluid and much protein escaped the circu- lation. It was found that following injury to tissue, anaerobic metabolites and other substances build up in the injured area. These substances stimulate **mast cells** (basophil polymorphonuclear leukocytes not in circu-

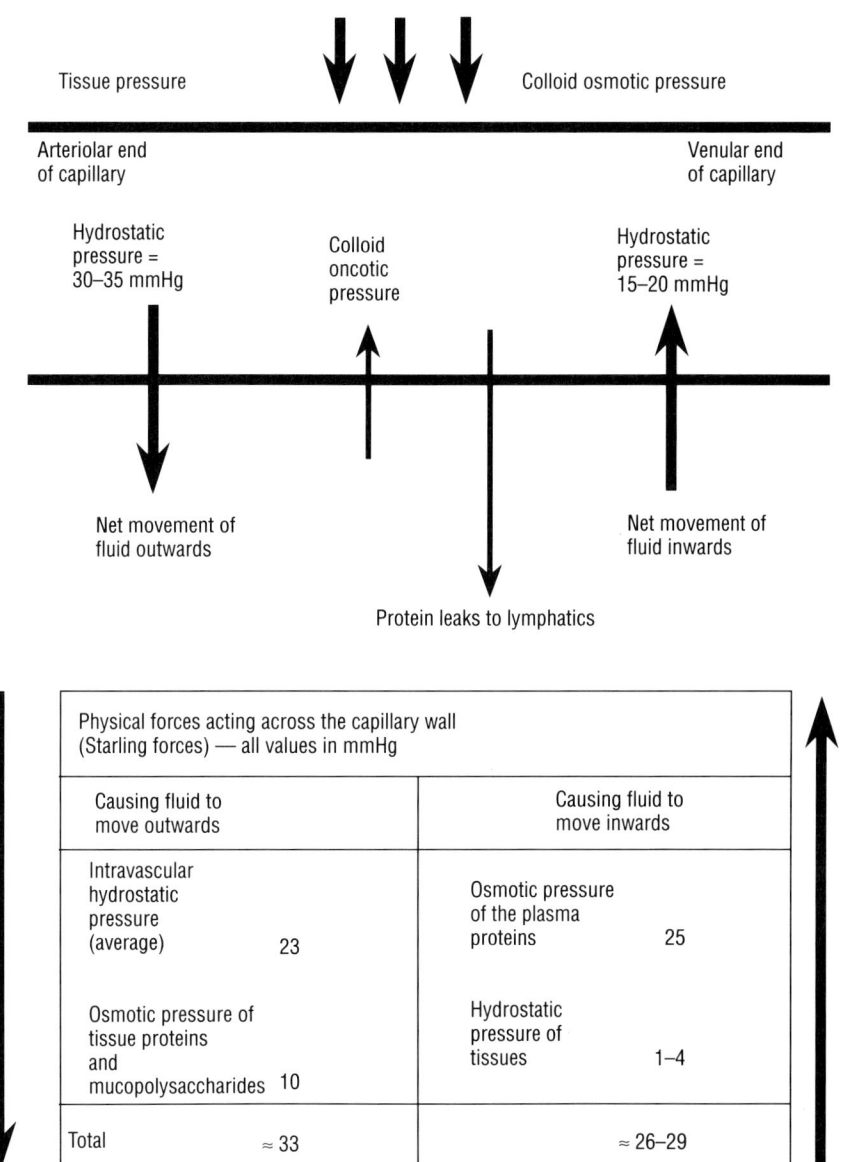

Figure 2.19 *Starling forces — as a result of the discrepancy of forces acting to force fluid in and out of small vessels, the net effect is that some fluid escapes the circulation, becoming the interstitial fluid that bathes the cells. Some protein also escapes with this fluid. Fluid and protein are returned to the circulation via the lymphatics*

lation but residing in connective tissue) to degranulate and release pharmacologically active substances such as histamine, kinins, prostaglandins and many others. These substances have a direct effect on blood vessels. The initial stimulant is **histamine** which causes dilatation of venules and increased vascular permeability, following a brief arteriolar constriction. The leakage of fluid and protein following release of histamine lasts for approximately 15 to 20 minutes. It has been shown by many studies that release of histamine and other such **permeability factors (mediators of inflammation)** induce the formation of openings or gaps in vessels by causing the endothelial cellular junctions to separate. These mediators are derived from a variety of sources in the inflamed tissues. Important sources are damaged tissues, the complement cascade, the kinin enzyme system and arachidonic acid metabolites (see Figure 2.20). When the permeability factors cease to act, the junctions of the cells reclose and the vessels stop leaking fluid and protein. Do gaps of this type occur in all kinds of vessels? Are gaps a feature of the inflammatory response only or are they seen in physiological situations also? Are permeability factors the only causes of gap formation? To answer these questions, the technique of **vascular labelling** was developed.

Vascular Labelling and its Importance in Inflammation

Vascular labelling is a technique used in experimental animals and involves the intravenous injection of a particulate marker substance in colloidal suspension (Figure 2.21). Something like Indian ink or a dye such as Monastral blue is used. What happens normally is that the marker particles circulate for some time and are eventually taken up by phagocytic cells such as Kupffer cells in the liver. If following the Indian ink injection an intradermal histamine injection is given, the vessels in the region start to leak fluid and protein since the histamine has induced gaps in their walls. Together with the protein, there is leakage of the carbon particles of the Indian ink. The carbon particles are too large to move past the basement membrane which surrounds the vessel and so are trapped as deposits beneath the open endothelial cell junction which is leaking protein and carbon. When the junction recloses, a deposit of carbon or dye particles are left trapped between the endothelium and basement membrane thus 'labelling' the vessel that was leaking carbon (and therefore also leaking fluid and protein). This marker particle deposit is readily seen under the microscope — and even to the naked eye the area appears grey (Figures 2.22 and 2.23).

With this technique it was found that histamine affects only the small venules and arterioles, causing gaps to form in their endothelial cell junctions. Histamine did not cause gaps to form in the endothelial cell junctions of capillaries. It was also found by using vascular labelling in physiological situations (i.e. in vessels that were not exposed to histamine, not inflamed) that in normal continuous vessels there were some deposits of marker particles beneath closed junctions. This indicated that momentary openings of cell junctions occurred even in non-inflamed vessels. How-

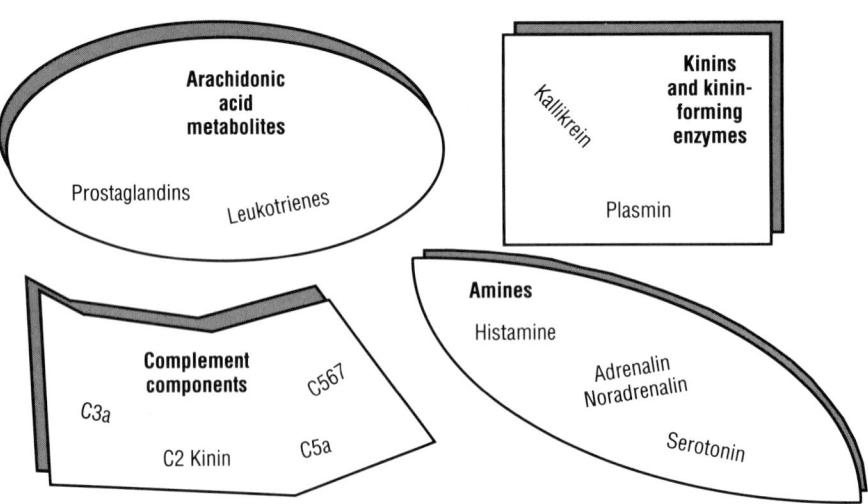

Figure 2.20 *Chemical mediators of the acute inflammatory response*

ever, this occurred rarely and a considerable proportion of the protein has been shown to leak via exocytosis (carbon particles are also found in vesicles within endothelial cells in vascular labelling studies). Generally the opening of intercellular endothelial junctions is a hallmark of the inflammatory response. It has been shown to occur in all types of vessels and it is triggered by many endogenous mediators of inflammation (e.g. histamine, bradykinin).

The mechanism through which gaps form in vessels has also been elucidated and is due to the presence of the contractile proteins **actin** and **myosin** which occur in many types of cells, including endothelium. There is good evidence that mediators of inflammation such as histamine cause the activation of actin/myosin system in venules and arterioles, the result being a contraction of the endothelial cell, causing the opening of the endothelial cell junction. However, this is a short-lived reaction as the effects of histamine are over within 15–20 minutes. How then may we explain the different patterns of inflammatory oedema which are sometimes seen to occur for long periods of time (such

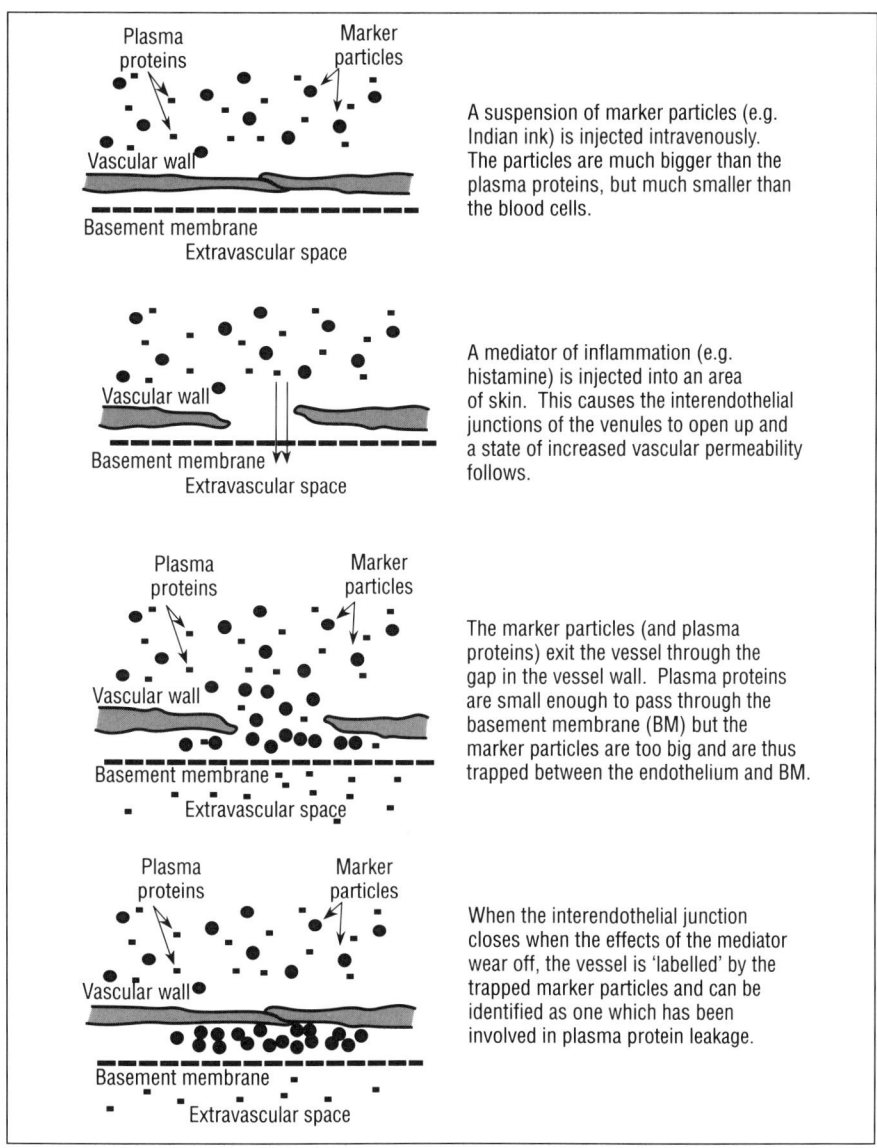

Figure 2.21 *The vascular labelling technique*

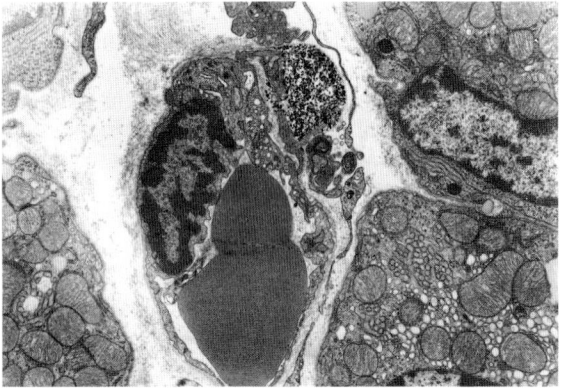

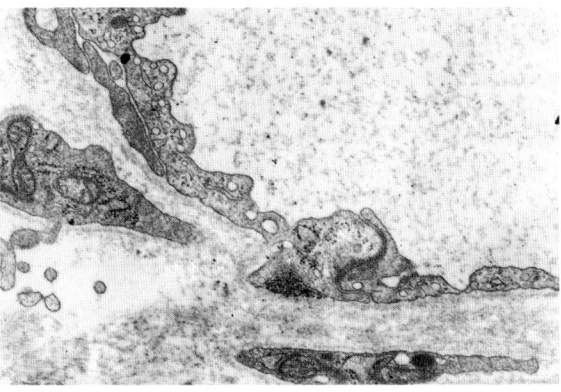

Figure 2.22 *Vascular labelling of a fenestrated endothelium capillary of stomach mucosa after injury through application of ethyl alcohol. Note the carbon marker particles trapped between a closed interendothelial junction and the basement membrane. Two erythrocytes are within the lumen of the vessel (×19 000)*

Figure 2.23 *Detail of vascular labelling deposit in a fenestrated endothelium capillary of stomach mucosa after injury through application of ethyl alcohol. The marker particles (ferritin) are trapped between a closed interendothelial junction and the basement membrane (×52 000)*

as in severe burns) or those that are seen after considerable time following the injury (such as in sunburn, where leakage occurs several hours after exposure to the sun)? In order to answer this question we need to consider the severity of the injury and the effect this injury has on the tissue and vessels.

We may divide injuries into three major types: mild, moderate and severe. With **mild injury** (such as mild thermal burn) there is only minor tissue damage and the vessels are largely intact. Vascular leakage is mainly a function of histamine release from mast cells and is seen to occur early in the sequence of events following the injury and lasts for a relatively short time. With **moderate injury** (such as sunburn or a more severe burn) the damage to tissue is greater and the vessels have also been injured. There is once again release of histamine which causes the initial swelling of the area. The gaps in the vessels reclose when the effects of histamine wear off. However, since the vessels have been injured they undergo reactive changes to injury and eventually, some endothelial cells will undergo necrosis. This will cause the formation of large gaps in the vessels several hours following the injury and associated with this will be a marked swelling of the area due to the accumulation of considerable quantities of inflammatory exudate. With **severe injury** (such as severe burns) there is considerable injury to tissue and also immediate injury and necrosis of the endothelium of vessels. This has the effect of causing large deficiencies to form in vessels due to stripping of their endothelium, thus allowing large quantities of fluid

and protein to escape for considerable periods of time following the injury. Eventually leakage will be checked by repair mechanisms operating in the area. It is evident that in addition to gaps forming in endothelium in response to mediators of increased permeability, gaps also form in response to direct injury of endothelium. The type of gap that forms in a particular situation will depend on the nature of the injurious agent as well as the severity of the injury (Figure 2.24).

Nature of Inflammatory Exudate

It was mentioned earlier that one of the features observed by Cohnheim in inflamed sites was hyperaemia, that is, an increase in the blood flow to the damaged area, sometimes by as much as a factor of ten. Fluid then leaves the microcirculation as a result of venular dilatation and increased capillary permeability. Venules and capillaries form gaps between their endothelial cells either in response to mediators of increased permeability or as a result of direct injury to endothelial cells. The fluid which normally bathes the cells is a **transudate** (S.G. < 1.012), a fluid low in protein which has been filtered out of vessels. In inflammation, the fluid which accumulates is an **exudate**, rich in protein as vascular permeability changes lead to increased protein leakage (S.G. > 1.018). This exudate causes swelling in the tissue. However, this inflammatory exudate, although having considerably more protein than tissue fluid, is found to have about half the plasma concentration of proteins. If inflammatory exudate forms from plasma which comes out of sizeable gaps in vessels, why is not the concentration of proteins in exudate the same as the plasma concentration of proteins? This is because essentially two processes contribute to the formation of inflammatory exudate: (a) escape of plasma into the extravascular spaces via gaps in the endothelium of vessels, and (b) disruption of the Starling forces; that is, the colloid oncotic pressure in the inflamed vessel will be the same as before but the vasodilatation and hyperaemia will cause an increase in the amount of water leaving the vessels by **ultrafiltration** at the arteriolar and venular ends of the microcirculatory bed that is inflamed. Thus the exu-

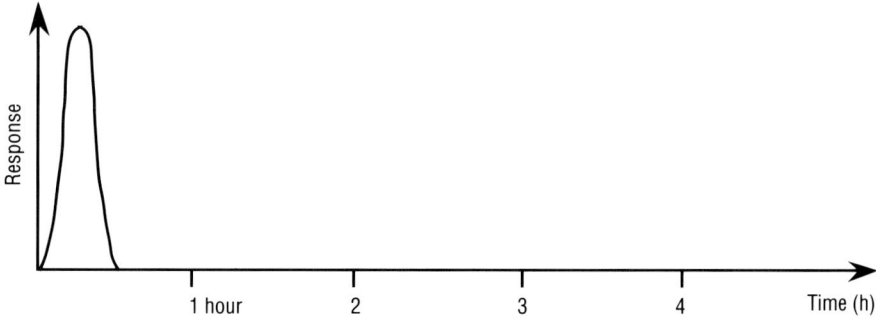

(a) Histamine-type response: short lived but intense

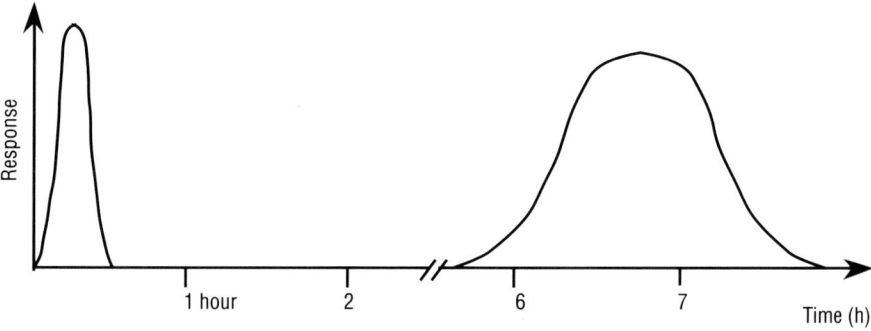

(b) Mild direct injury response: biphasic. Short lived, intense initially, followed by a long-lived intense response many hours later

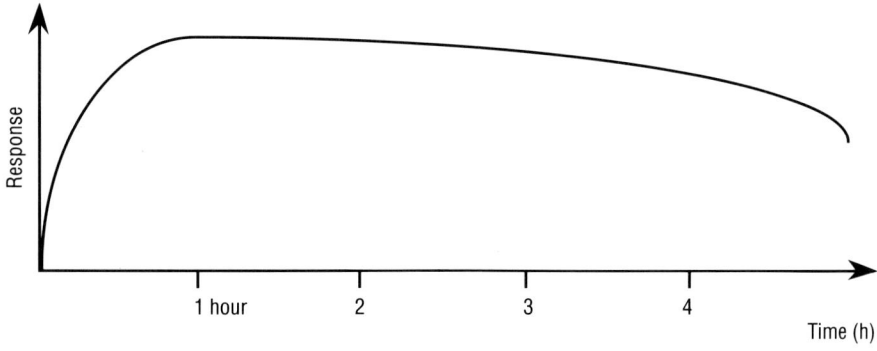

(c) Severe direct injury response: long lived and intense

Figure 2.24 *The severity of vascular injury related to exudate formation*

date is diluted by this water lost from the circulation through a magnification of the normal process of tissue fluid formation.

In acute inflammation the character of the exudate is descriptive of the inflammation:

1. **Serous inflammatory reaction** — in response to mild injuries, such as a minor burn, there is usually formation of a watery exudate low in protein, perhaps forming a skin blister. This is seen to occur in mild burns, sunburn, some hypersensitivity (allergy) reactions and chemical injury. Serous fluid may also accumulate in body cavities, for example within the pericardium, pleura and peritoneal cavity.

2. **Fibrinous exudate** — in more severe types of injury the fluid is an exudate rich in fibrinogen so that fibrin forms in the tissues. The gaps which form in vessels are large enough to allow large protein molecules to escape (Figure 2.25); for example in uraemia there is a fibrinous pericarditis. This causes adhesion of the two layers of the pericardium and a characteristic sound is auscultated, the 'friction rub'. A similar situation occurs in the pleura.

3. **Suppuration** — in severe types of injury (especially in infections caused by pyogenic bacteria) the infiltrate contains large numbers of neutrophils resulting in a purulent or suppurative inflammation, for example suppurative appendicitis. The exudate is known as pus and the localized collection of pus is called an abscess or an empyema (see Figure 2.30).

4. **Haemorrhagic inflammatory reactions** — these occur when injury has caused rupture or necrosis of vessel walls, for example haemorrhagic infections such as meningococcaemia (septicaemia caused by *Neisseria meningitidis*).

Early in inflammation the principal reactive site is the venule. Exudation and white cell emigration begins there. Later, and with more severe injury, the capillaries also play their role. The formation of the exudate (a fluid rich in protein) in the extravascular tissues gives inflammatory swelling (**tumor**) or oedema. The increased blood flow to the area (hyperaemia) cause the redness (**rubor**) and the heat (**calor**). The increased tissue pressure and accumulation of tissue breakdown products and pharmacologically active substances stimulate nerve endings at the site, causing pain (**dolor**). Movement increases tissue pressure in the damaged area and so reflex muscle spasm about the injured site produces further irritation resulting in loss of function (**functio laesa**).

Eventually in all inflamed sites, exudate formation is controlled and the visible swelling diminishes. This is because of several controlling factors operating, tending to limit the effects of inflammation. Firstly, blood platelets will migrate to the area of endothelial cell damage and denudation and will adhere to the exposed subendothelial connective tissue, 'plugging up' the leaking vessel. This is especially noticeable in severe injury with extensive endothelial cell damage. Secondly, the arterioles will gradually constrict, returning to their normal diameter. The blood flow will return to normal, less blood will enter the area and the Starling forces will return to normal. Thirdly, the effects of endogenous mediators of increased permeability will wear off and any gaps caused by these will close. Lastly, the distensibility of the tissue, which is limited, and the rise in pressure in the extravascular fluid will tend to prevent more inflammatory exudate from forming. Eventually, the lymphatics will remove most of the inflammatory exudate and the swelling in the area will disappear.

Cellular Aspects of Acute Inflammation

When we look at a piece of tissue which is acutely inflamed under the microscope, the most obvious and characteristic feature seen is in most cases the large accumulation of leukocytes present in the extravascular spaces. These cells comprise the **inflammatory infiltrate**, as distinct from the inflammatory exudate, the latter term referring to the fluid portion of the inflammatory response. As Cohnheim noticed after the inflammatory exudate had formed, the blood flow in the inflamed area slowed considerably or even stopped altogether (**stasis**). This disrupts the axial flow of the

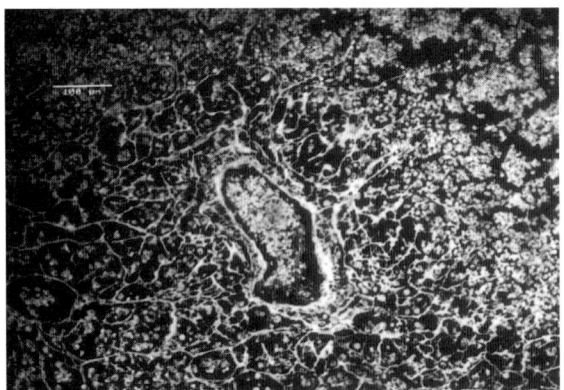

Figure 2.25 *Strands of fibrin being deposited around an inflamed venule in bacterial meningitis (scale bar is 100 μm)*

blood in the vessel and allows interaction of the blood cells with the endothelium of the vessel. A very notable feature of this interaction is the adherence of neutrophils to the endothelium of inflamed vessels such that they form a layer of cells resembling a pavement (**margination** or **pavementing**; Figure 2.26).

It is apparent that some change has occurred in the vascular endothelium making it 'stickier', allowing the neutrophils to adhere to its surface. Experimental work on this aspect of the inflammatory response has revealed that the injured endothelium in inflammation is not metabolizing normally and that there is a dearth of certain metabolites in the immediate area of such damaged endothelial cells. Notably, prostaglandin production is decreased and it has been shown experimentally that it is the lack of the prostaglandin PGI_2 that allows the adherence of neutrophils to the endothelium. The intact, healthy endothelium produces this substance and thus prevents the adherence of neutrophils and also of platelets. This change in the metabolism of the endothelial cells is not a non-specific feature of all increased permeability states, it is only seen in certain situations. For example, if histamine is injected intradermally, there is hardly any leukocytic adherence to the endothelium of leaking vessels. If, however, there is bacterial infection of the skin or skin damage caused by a burn, there is quite considerable leukocytic adherence to the inflamed endothelium. It should also be remembered that leukocytic adherence occurs after inflammatory exudate formation and most of the gaps in the endothelium would be reclosed.

Once the leukocytes have marginated and are firmly stuck to the endothelium, they form pseudopodia and begin to actively crawl through the vessel wall, searching for the closed interendothelial cell junctions. They insert their pseudopodia in the junction, prize it apart and crawl through the closed junction, actively pushing it apart as they go through it. Individual cells take about 2–12 minutes to pass through the vascular wall and into the extravascular spaces. Very little plasma is lost when the cells go through and the basement membrane is degraded by the neutrophils as they go through it. This process of leukocytic emigration through the vascular wall is termed **diapedesis** (Figure 2.27). Later, the basement membrane is reconstituted. That inflammatory exudate formation and diapedesis are separable events is demonstrated by the experiment where some serum is injected subcutaneously in the rat. There is an almost immediate increase in vascular permeability of the area caused by gap formation in vessels. In this phase no leukocytes escape the circulation. Four hours later, vascular leakage has stopped, the gaps have closed, but diapedesis is at its peak, many

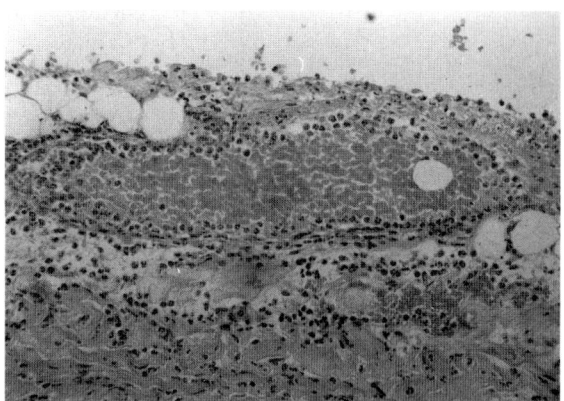

Figure 2.26 *An inflamed venule in pericardium showing the process of pavementing. Numerous neutrophils have adhered to the inner aspect of vascular endothelium in preparation for diapedesis (×100)*

neutrophils escaping the vessel with little loss of fluid or protein.

The typical cell accumulating in areas of acute inflammation is the **polymorphonuclear neutrophilic leukocyte** (abbreviated forms are 'neutrophil', 'polymorph' or 'pus cell'). Neutrophils originate in the bone marrow and move into the circulation where they comprise approximately 60% of all white cells, their life span being about a week. If they leave the bloodstream and go into the tissues their life span is approximately 48 hours. They are cells with a highly characteristic appearance, having a multilobed nucleus (two to five lobes), and a pale cytoplasm containing numerous granules. These granules are lysosomes which contain lytic enzymes, mainly **lysozyme**. The function of the neutrophil is **phagocytosis**. Phagocytosis is the process whereby cells take up particulate matter and break it down ('cellular eating'). Neutrophils ingest and destroy bacteria and other microbes and are very important in controlling infection in the body. They may also ingest and destroy necrotic tissue and other debris, fibrin and other particulate matter. Often, where there are many bacteria present or where there are large accumulations of necrotic debris, neutrophils will migrate to the area and release their cellular contents, 'exploding' in the process, destroying themselves but also a lot of the surrounding debris in 'kamikaze' style. Neutrophils have also been shown to have a secretory function, being able to secrete various substances important in inflammation. They release some substances which cause fever (**endogenous pyrogens**),

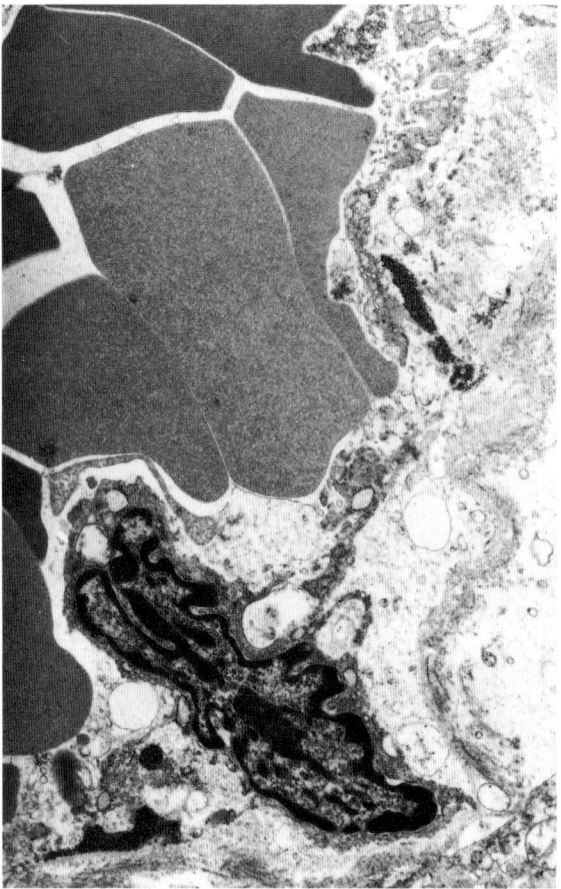

Figure 2.27 *A neutrophil in the process of diapedesis through the interendothelial junction of a fenestrated endothelium capillary of stomach mucosa after injury through direct application of ethyl alcohol (×50 000)*

some substances able to attract other neutrophils (**chemotactic factors**) and also **vasodilators** that increase blood vessel diameter.

Once the neutrophils are in the extravascular spaces they show ordered motion, moving towards targets like groups of bacteria, necrotic cells or debris. They do so in response to chemical substances that attract them and they respond to the concentration gradient of these substances, going from areas of low concentration to areas of high concentration. Such a response to chemical attraction is called **chemotaxis**, and neutrophils have considerable chemotactic ability, allowing them to 'home in' on regions where they are needed. Obviously if bacteria have entered the tissue and are the cause of injury and inflammation, neutrophils are

required at that site to phagocytose the bacteria and rid the tissue of the injurious agents. Hence the neutrophils come out of the vessels and move chemotactically towards the bacteria in response to the metabolites and toxins elaborated by the micro-organisms.

A day or so following neutrophil margination and diapedesis, when the neutrophils have destroyed most of the microbes or have lysed the necrotic debris, monocytes from the bloodstream enter the tissues becoming the **mononuclear phagocyte** more commonly called **macrophage** or **histiocyte**. Macrophages are large, oval cells with a large oval nucleus and a finely granular cytoplasm. Their life span in the tissues varies from weeks to many months or even years. They are also phagocytic cells but they are larger and more sluggish than the neutrophils. Their function is to clear the last remaining debris in the area and generally to 'mop up the battlefield'. They almost never release their lysosomal enzymes and, rather, break down particulate matter by phagocytosis. They also have a very important secretory function, producing and releasing substances which have a modulatory role in the inflammatory and immune response (Figure 2.28).

When macrophages have finished cleaning up areas of inflammation they remain in the tissue as wandering phagocytic cells or they proceed to the lymph nodes which drain the area and remain there as cells important in the immune response and capable of interacting with lymphocytes in future immune responses. In many organs of the body there are large numbers of resident macrophages, permanently residing there and whose function is to phagocytose debris and particulate matter. These macrophages are known collectively as the **reticuloendothelial system** or as the **mononuclear phagocytic system**. Examples of such cells are the Kupffer cells in the liver, sinusoid lining cells of the spleen and subcapsular sinus cells in the lymph nodes. The process of phagocytosis as an important defence mechanism to infection was pointed out by Elie Metchnikoff in the 19th century (see Figure 2.29).

Sequelae of Acute Inflammation

Following an injury the acute inflammatory response may progress in different ways. The **sequelae** (a **sequela** is any possible result, complication or conclusion of a pathological process) of acute inflammation depend on many factors: the causative agent, the extent of damage, the tissue involved, the magnitude of the inflammatory response and the possible persistence of the causative agent. The possible sequelae of acute inflammation are:

- Resolution
- Suppuration
- Repair
- Chronic inflammation

Resolution

Resolution means a complete restoration of normal structure and function. It is the most favourable outcome of acute inflammation but unfortunately is often not the most likely. Resolution can only occur when injury to the tissues is slight and/or the tissues have a high regenerative capacity. It also occurs where the products of the acute inflammatory response (exudate) can be spontaneously eliminated. Lobar pneumonia (an infection of the lungs) is the best example of resolution. Lobar pneumonia is caused by *Streptococcus pneumoniae* which stimulates a rapid acute inflammatory response within the alveolar spaces.

Initially the vessels in the alveolar walls become hyperaemic or **congested** with the extra blood flow. Exudate rich in fibrin then collects in the alveoli as the vessels leak fluid. Many red blood cells also become

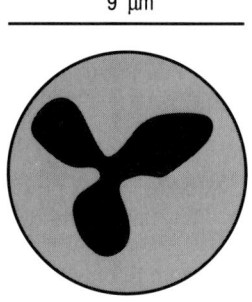

9 μm

A polymorphonuclear neutrophilic leukocyte: 'neutrophil', 'polymorph', 'pus cell'

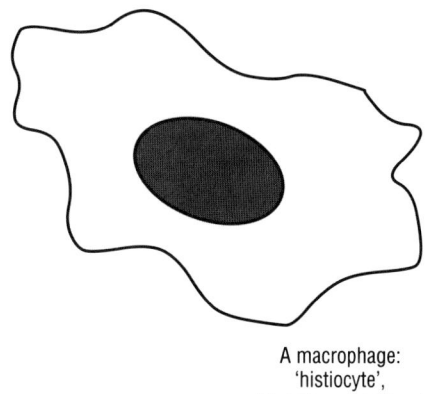

A macrophage: 'histiocyte', 'Kuppfer cell of liver'

Figure 2.28 *The cells involved in acute inflammatory responses*

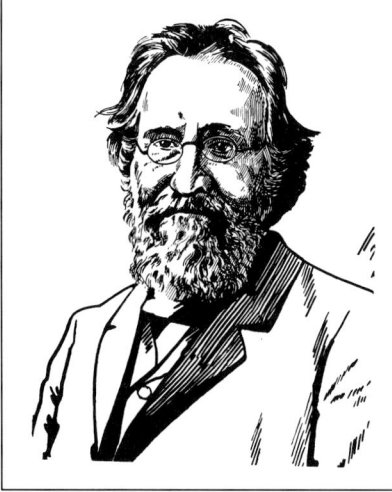

Metchnikoff was a Russian biologist who did a great deal of work on the process of phagocytosis. He showed with a series of elegant experiments that inflammatory cells played a major defensive role in the body.

The development of this theory took up 20 years of his life and was put forward in his book *Defence Mechanisms Against Infectious Disease* (1901).

Metchnikoff's views were violently opposed by many fellow scientists who believed that the primary defence mechanism against injurious agents was a humoral response, a concept stimulated by Buchner's observations on the bactericidal power of normal serum.

Figure 2.29 *Elie Metchnikoff (1845–1916)*

forced out of vessels and collect in the alveolar spaces giving a **consolidated** (solid) appearance to the portion of the lung involved. The lung macroscopically resembles red liver tissue, so this phase of lobar pneumonia is known as **red hepatization**. As well as abundant exudate, fibrin and red blood cells, neutrophils then leave the vessels by diapedesis and accumulate within the alveoli. These white blood cells fill the alveoli giving the affected lobe a solid, grey appearance. This phase of pneumonia is known as **grey hepatization**.

If the patient overcomes this infection the exudate and infiltrate are quickly removed. The fibrin, red blood cells and dead polymorphs are phagocytosed and digested by macrophages present in the alveoli or recruited from the circulation. These macrophages are often stained with haemosiderin (a breakdown product of haemoglobin from red blood cells) when seen histologically. The exudate is made more liquid by the action of digestive enzymes from leukocytes and much is coughed up by the patient and removed or may be removed via the lymphatics. Thus the alveoli are undamaged and cleared of all inflammatory exudate within days. Alveoli refill with air so that normal structure and function are restored. Resolution is said to have occurred.

If, however, exudate is not removed promptly or if alveolar walls, etc. have been damaged then **organization** of the exudate will occur, so fibrosis or scarring follows. Resolution has not occurred in this case and there is permanent damage. Bronchopneumonia does not resolve, the exudate becomes organized and scarring follows. This is repair rather than resolution.

Suppuration

In some acute inflammations, for example in infections by **pyogenic** (pus-forming) bacteria, there is substantial exudate and infiltrate. Large numbers of neutrophils being present may then lead to necrotic tissue with dead and living neutrophils, dead and living bacteria. This inflammatory fluid is known as **pus** and the process as **suppuration**. The pus may become walled off initially by fibrin and then by granulation (repair) tissue around it. Such a localized collection of pus is known as an **abscess**. This may grow if the bacteria persist and the tissue forms more pus. The pressure inside the abscess increases causing it to expand outwards along regions of least resistance. This is known as 'pointing' (Figure 2.30).

Usually it expands or points towards the closest epithelial surface via which the abscess will burst and empty the contents of the abscess cavity, thus dis-charging and eliminating its contents. If the abscess is in the skin, the pointing and discharge of pus is advantageous since the bacteria are eliminated. However, if the abscess is in an internal organ and if it discharges inside the body, this may have serious consequences as the bacteria in the pus may infect other organs and cause more abscesses to form. The residual collapsed region of the abscess heals by organization and fibrosis, forming a scar.

Regeneration and Repair

Following acute inflammation, especially when there has been necrosis of the parenchymal cells of the tissue, there must be a restoration or replacement of tissue which has been lost. This restoration is known as regeneration or repair.

Restoration by Parenchymal Cell Division — Regeneration

Not all cells of the body are capable of division and differentiation allowing replacement of lost cells with identical cells. There are three groups: labile cells, stable cells and permanent cells.

Labile cells continue to multiply throughout life. They include cells of epithelial surfaces and lymphoid and haemopoietic cells. Multiplication of these labile cells replenishes cells that are being continually lost by shedding or wearing out. The lining of the small intestine is being replaced totally every few days. Similarly, skin cells are constantly replaced as they slough off and bone marrow constantly replenishes old blood cells that are destroyed in the spleen.

Stable cells retain the capacity to regenerate but do so only when stimulated as a result of acute cell loss since their normal survival is long term. The viscera of the body fall into this category. They do not normally engage in mitotic activity but have the potential to do so (e.g. it is possible experimentally in animals to remove up to two-thirds of the liver and within weeks the liver has returned to normal weight and cell number). The regeneration which occurs may not reconstitute an organ of entirely normal microscopic anatomy but the numbers of cells have been replaced and function may be normal.

Mesenchymal cells also fall into this category, for example fibroblasts retain great regenerative capacity and the ability to differentiate along various lines (multipotential cells). In injuries involving bone fibroblasts may divide and differentiate to form chondroblasts or osteoblasts.

Permanent cells are so differentiated and specialized that they have lost the ability to divide, for example the nerve cells and striated muscle cells (skeletal and cardiac muscle cells). Smooth muscle cells may be capable of division. Regeneration of permanent cells is impossible so when lost they must be replaced by connective tissue, forming a scar to replace lost bulk.

Remaining cells may undergo hypertrophy (enlargement in size).

The regeneration of tissue following injury depends not only on the type of tissue destroyed, but also on the preservation of the normal architectural framework. For example, in kidney disease if a portion of tubular epithelium is destroyed by a toxic substance but the

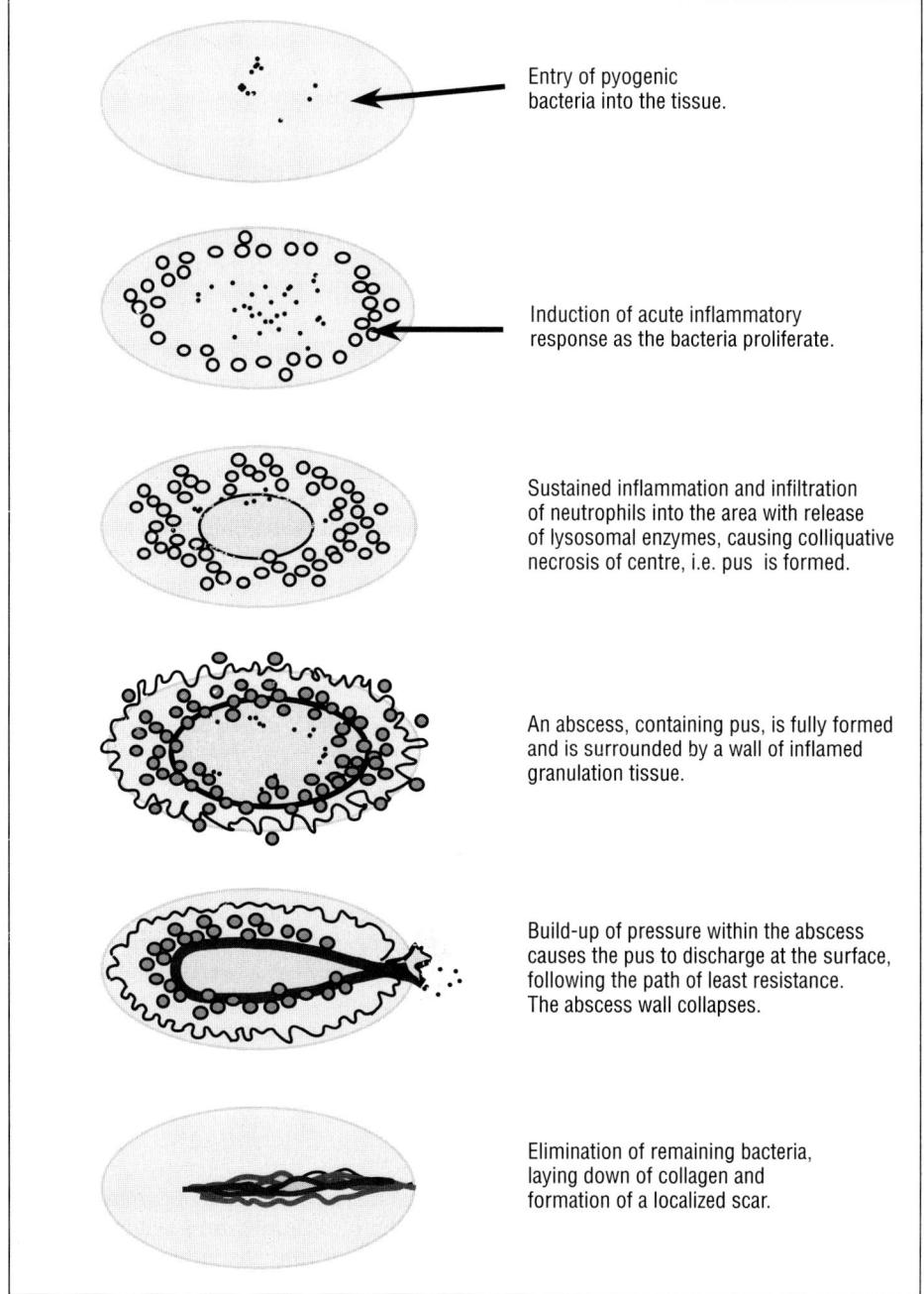

Entry of pyogenic bacteria into the tissue.

Induction of acute inflammatory response as the bacteria proliferate.

Sustained inflammation and infiltration of neutrophils into the area with release of lysosomal enzymes, causing colliquative necrosis of centre, i.e. pus is formed.

An abscess, containing pus, is fully formed and is surrounded by a wall of inflamed granulation tissue.

Build-up of pressure within the abscess causes the pus to discharge at the surface, following the path of least resistance. The abscess wall collapses.

Elimination of remaining bacteria, laying down of collagen and formation of a localized scar.

Figure 2.30 *The formation and fate of an abscess*

more resistant stroma (supporting tissue) is preserved, the remaining viable epithelial cells will divide and reline the tubules restoring function. However, if the stromal architecture is destroyed as in a renal infarct, regeneration cannot take place and scarring ensues.

Repair by Connective Tissue — Organization

This is the usual consequence of most tissue damage. It is an efficient method of closing and repairing tissue defects but it results in replacement of special tissue by **collagen**. This localized loss of organ parenchyma thus results in some loss of function.

The process of healing an injured area by granulation tissue and replacement with connective tissue is known as **organization**. The process of repair of connective tissue will be discussed in detail later when describing wound and fracture healing.

Briefly, following acute traumatic loss of tissue the 'gap' is filled by blood coagulum (fibrin mesh with trapped blood cells). Following a more gradual process after necrosis, the defect is filled initially by inflammatory exudate and infiltrate. All dead tissue and inflammatory debris must be removed by action of macrophages and it is only then that **granulation tissue** begins to fill the area (Figure 2.31). This consists of fibroblasts producing collagen and 'budding' (proliferating) capillaries. The fibroblasts divide and migrate into the area, along with the budding capillary

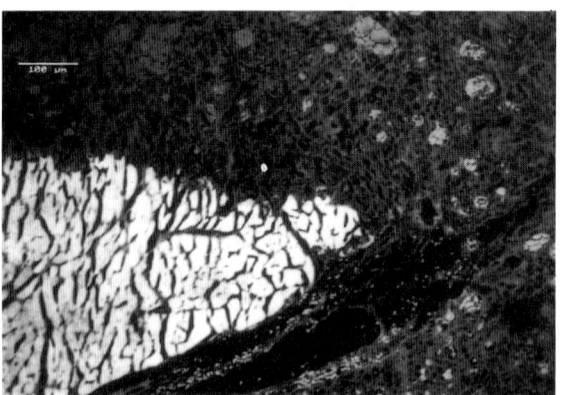

Figure 2.31 *Granulation tissue forming around a region of myocardial coagulative necrosis (pale, wedge-shaped region). The new vascular channels formed in the granulation tissue provide nutrients and cells important in the resorption of the necrotic area and its replacement by scar (scale bar is 100 μm)*

loops. The collagen produced initially in granulation tissue is rather wispy and immature but later thickens giving the scar more tensile strength. Granulation tissue migrates inwards towards the centre of an injured area, from the undamaged margins.

This granulation tissue matures into **scar tissue** as time progresses. Mature scar tissue has few fibrocytes, is avascular as vessels are no longer required once active proliferation has ceased, and consists largely of mature collagen. As it matures scar tissue contracts leaving a smaller area of connective tissue to replace the lost tissue.

Chronic Inflammation

Finally, acute inflammation may progress to chronic inflammation. If the injury or stimulus which produced acute inflammation has not been removed then the inflammatory response will continue at the same time as repair or healing is taking place. Thus the inflammation has entered a chronic phase.

Chronic inflammation is defined as 'the prolonged phase in which destruction of tissue and inflammation are proceeding at the same time as attempts at healing'. For example, in chronic pyelonephritis there may be recurrent acute infections in the kidney over a long period of time (usually years), and the kidney shows evidence of chronic inflammation and repeated acute inflammations when examined histologically. Chronic inflammation is discussed in detail at the end of this chapter.

Function of the Acute Inflammatory Process

Acute inflammation was defined as the process which commenced with sublethal injury and finished with complete healing. Its function therefore is to effect healing in tissues and repair the damage that has been caused by the various injurious stimuli that act in the tissue. All components of the inflammatory process are important in this respect and they all have beneficial effects.

Exudate Formation

The increased volume of extracellular fluid caused by influx of **inflammatory exudate**, serves to dilute and help flush away toxins and metabolites which may be present at the site of injury. This diminishes tissue damage due to toxic injury of cells.

Fibrinogen is one of the proteins in the exudate which forms strands of fibrin once in the tissues. The fibrin meshwork so formed may help to limit movement of bacteria by providing a mechanical barrier which helps to wall off infection from the rest of the body. Fibrin is also very sticky and helps to 'glue' together damaged or torn tissues. Protein components of plasma called **immunoglobulins (antibodies)** neutralize toxins and kill bacteria. Another complex series of plasma proteins called **complement** have important effects and enhance the inflammatory response. Finally, the **drainage** of the inflammatory exudate to the regional lymph nodes carries fragments of bacteria and other microbes to the reactive cells of the immune system present in the lymph nodes and hence stimulates immunity. Thus, the tissues are protected from future infections with the same microbes.

Infiltrate Formation

The infiltration of large numbers of **neutrophils** at the sites of acute inflammation is extremely important as these cells are active in the process of phagocytosis and degranulation. The neutrophils will ingest and destroy micro-organisms in the area thus guarding against widespread infection. These inflammatory cells are also very important in the breakdown of necrotic tissue, denatured proteins and other debris. Hence these are the prime cells which 'clean up' the area which has been injured and the prime cells in preventing infection spreading extensively to involve more tissue.

Macrophages also are important in the phagocytic process and they serve as the cells which 'mop up' any debris left behind in the tissue after the neutrophils have been active. However, the macrophages are also extremely important in immune system reactions and their phagocytic action is accompanied by stimulation and activation of lymphocytes in the specific phase of the immune response.

Granulation Tissue Formation

Granulation tissue forms in areas that have been acutely inflamed whenever there is need for repair and healing by scar tissue formation (Figures 2.32 and 2.33). It comprises newly formed capillaries that 'bud off' existing blood vessels, proliferating fibroblasts that lay down collagen and some inflammatory cells, predominantly macrophages, that phagocytose debris. The function of granulation tissue is to provide blood and nutrients to the area being repaired and to provide a source for inflammatory cells and new blood vessels to the damaged area. Very important in repair are the **fibroblasts** which are found in granulation tissue. These cells divide and lay down collagen and matrix components which on maturation will become the fibrous scar that is seen in repair reactions. **Myofibroblasts** are specialized fibroblasts which contain many bun-

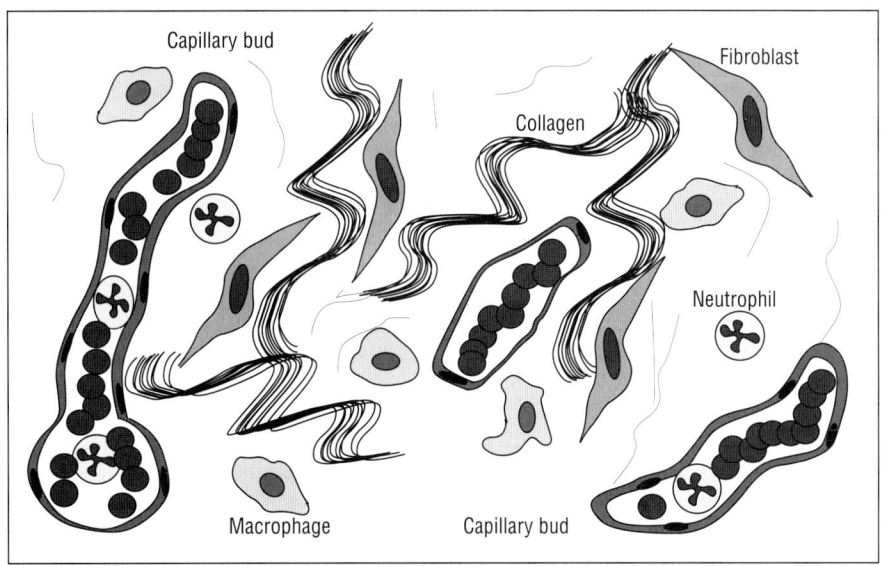

Figure 2.32 *The structure of granulation tissue*

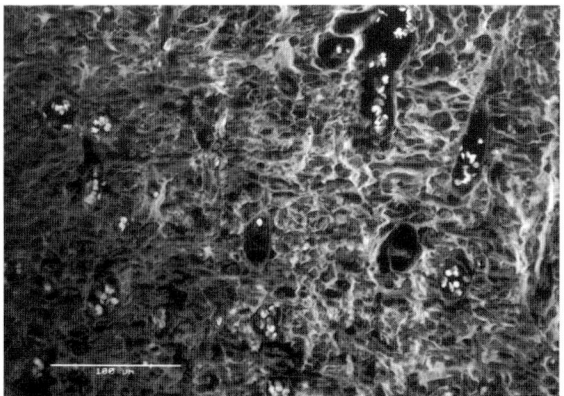

Figure 2.33 *Granulation tissue forming around a 12-day wound in rat skin. Collagen is being laid down by fibroblasts around the vascular sprouts (scale bar is 100 μm)*

dles of actin and myosin filaments and are capable of prolonged contractile actions. It is these cells that are important in the process of wound contraction (see the section on wound healing and repair).

Wound Healing — Tissue Repair

A **wound** may be defined as any disruption of the tissues or organs of the body caused by injury. The healing of wounds is a situation in which the acute inflammatory response plays a very important role and in most cases is an example of healing, which is the main reason why the inflammatory response occurs. As previously discussed, the healing of wounds may be through **regeneration** (replacement of lost tissue by parenchymal cells) and/or **repair** (fibrous scar tissue replacement). Regeneration can occur only in labile or stable cells and not with permanent cells which are unable to undergo mitosis. There are many different types of wounds, the most common of which are caused by injury to the tissues by physical or mechanical agents, **trauma**, therefore, being the commonest aetiology of wounds.

A **contusion** is the common 'bruise' and is most often caused by injury with a blunt instrument. The skin above the contusion remains unbroken, but there may be extensive injury beneath it with damage to blood vessels, leading to haemorrhage. Contusions are most often seen on the face and torso.

An **abrasion** is an open surface wound, very superficial and involving only the epidermis and upper dermis

('scrape' or 'graze'). It is caused by friction injury and occurs usually on exposed areas of the skin.

An **avulsion** is usually a large, open wound where the extensive tissue loss prevents approximation of the wound margins. It is caused by cutting, gouging or tearing of tissue. It is commonly found on the face, hands and legs. An X-ray of the wound may be required in order to rule out bone damage.

Surgical wounds are usually clean-cut wounds which are planned to minimize damage and injury, and in which minimal tissue loss occurs. Usually their margins are approximated, so that the wound heals quickly and with minimum amount of scar tissue formation. They are commonly found on the thorax and abdomen.

A **puncture** is typically a small wound that may involve deep tissues and results from injuries with sharp pointed objects. It may occur anywhere in the body but occurs frequently on the chest or abdomen. It may be required to X-ray or CT-scan the wound, in order to rule out retention of injuring object, presence of haematoma and deep tissue and bone damage.

Lacerations are usually open, large, ragged wounds which extend deeply into the subcutaneous tissues. They result after injury with sharp or blunt instruments, usually after considerable force has been applied, such that the tissue is penetrated, crushed and torn. Much necrotic debris and blood clot is to be found in such wounds and there may be retention of external material (glass and wood fragments, gravel, debris, etc.). These wounds may occur anywhere in the body and X-rays may be taken to rule out deeper tissue and bone damage.

Missile wounds are the result of high-velocity tissue penetration such as occurs with gunshot wounds. There may be two wounds, at the missile entry and exit sites, or alternatively there may be a single wound with the missile lodging in the tissues. Considerable haemorrhage may occur and the patient may be in shock.

When discussing the healing of wounds it is usual to consider the course of events following a wound to the skin and subcutaneous tissues. However, connective tissue repair is similar in most tissues following injury and tissue loss. Whatever the nature of the wound, the healing mechanisms that operate are similar resulting in repair of the damage, and any differences that may be seen are usually quantitative rather than qualitative; that is, the amount of scar tissue finally formed varies, depending on the tissue that was lost and had to be replaced. When an **avulsion wound** is inflicted to skin and subcutaneous tissues the sequence of events in repair or healing of the wound is as follows (refer to Figure 2.34):

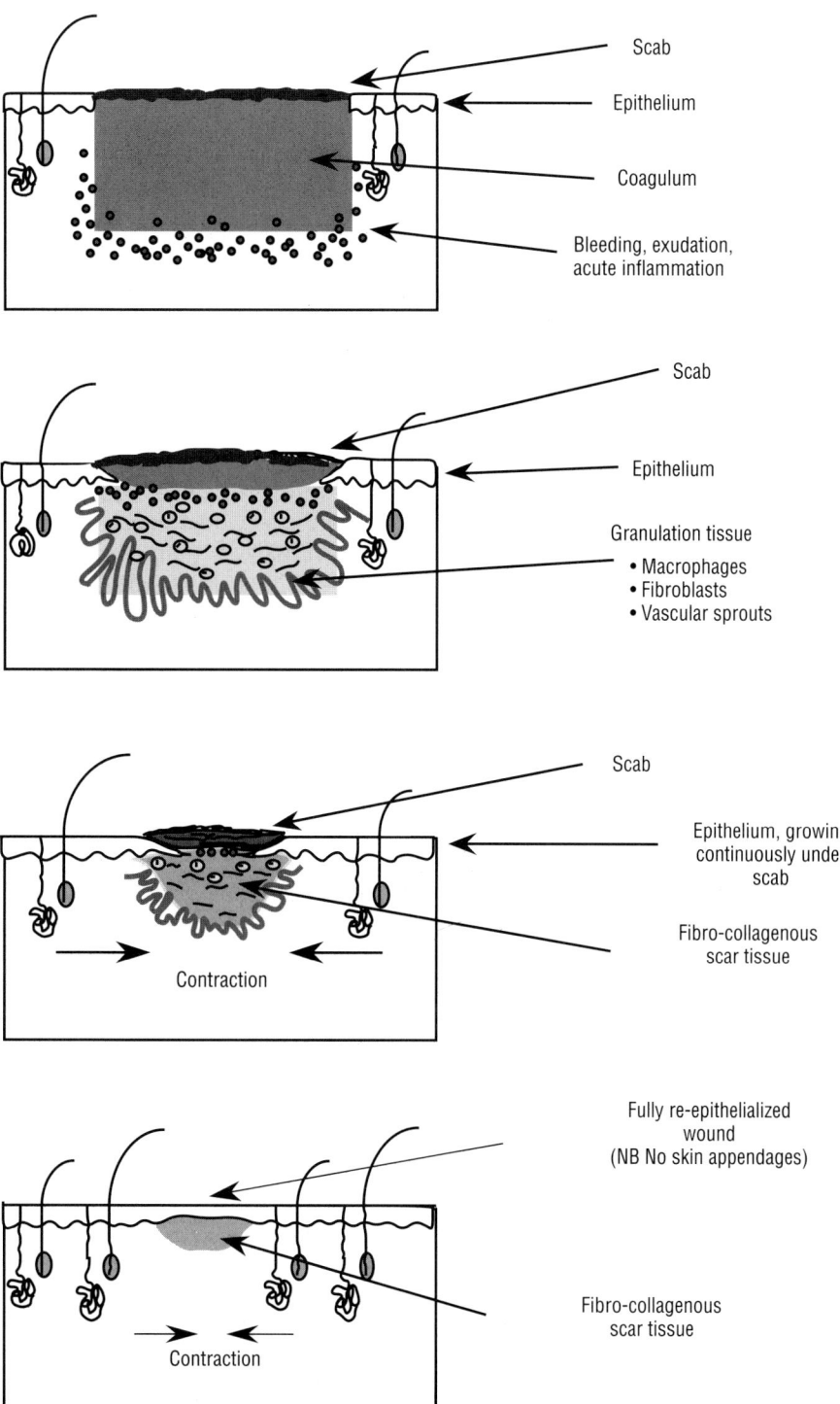

Figure 2.34   *Wound healing by secondary intention*

Closure of the Defect ('filling the gap', 0–2 hours)
There is immediate **haemorrhage** into the wound so that the epithelial discontinuity is covered by a **coagulum** (blood clot). This coagulum forms as the fibrinogen becomes **fibrin** once out of the vessels and forms a mesh trapping blood cells within it. This blood clot then desiccates (dries out) forming a hard protective **scab**.

Removal of Debris (2–24 hours)
In response to the injury there is an acute inflammatory response at the wound margins with exudation and infiltration and emigration of leukocytes. Ultimately all the dead tissue and debris in the wound beneath the scab is removed by the action of neutrophils and macrophages.

Formation of Granulation Tissue (24–36 hours)
At the wound margins (base and sides) the capillaries proliferate forming capillary buds or loops which invade the blood clot, using the supporting scaffold of the fibrin mesh of the clot. Fibroblasts in the normal tissue surrounding the wound are stimulated at the same time to divide and migrate into the clot, along with the capillary buds. This highly vascular tissue rich in young fibroblasts and newly formed capillaries is called **granulation tissue** (so named for its finely granular appearance when viewed with the scab removed). Fibroblastic proliferation and migration and capillary budding proceed inward from the wound margin at a rate of up to 0.1 mm/hour, while the inflammatory response is still active in the centre of the injured area. Phagocytosis of debris continues.

Epithelial Regeneration (36–72 hours)
As the granulation tissue matures and moves into the wound gap another process begins at the margins of the wound: the surrounding epithelial cells (basal cells of the skin) divide. As the epithelium proliferates it covers over the wound beneath the scab, from the margins toward the centre. This regenerating epithelium uses the granulation tissue beneath the scab as a base upon which to grow. Thus, this process of **re-epithelialization**, like granulation, proceeds inwards from the edges of the defect. The time required to fill the wound depends on the size of the wound, but for most medium-sized wounds the process is complete within 7–14 days.

Scar Formation — Synthesis of Collagen (3–7 days)
Collagen is synthesized and secreted by the fibroblasts in the granulation tissue; initially in soluble form the collagen is deposited extracellularly. After deposition of collagen, chemical changes occur in the immature collagen and there is cross-linking between adjacent collagen fibres. Hence this early, wispy collagen becomes thicker with time. There is also a breakdown of newly formed collagen by enzymatic action of macrophages and the laying down of new collagen by fibroblasts. Hence, macrophages and fibroblasts perform a **remodelling** of the early scar and ultimately fibres remain orientated in such a way as to be parallel to the wound, thus providing the scar and tissue with maximum tensile strength.

Scar Contraction (7–8 days)
Fibroblasts are capable when active of developing longitudinal contractile myofilaments so that they resemble smooth muscle cells. These specialized cells are known as **myofibroblasts**. It is known that myofibroblasts contract in a healing wound and this serves to draw the edges of the wound together, reducing the size of the tissue defect and resulting in shrinkage of the scar. Collagen fibres also shrink somewhat as the scar ages. In addition, in the early phase of wound healing there is marked contraction as the coagulum and scab dehydrate. The result is a wound much smaller in area than that initially. Experiments in the skin of rabbits have shown that a wound originally 40 cm^2 in area is reduced in about 5 weeks to a wound 3–4 cm^2 in area. This represents a reduction of approximately 90%.

Scar Maturation ('blanching of the scar', 3–4 weeks)
Early scar tissue is highly vascularized with granulation tissue and appears quite red. By progressive proliferation of fibroblasts and laying down of collagen and contraction of the scar it loses its vascularity. The pressure of increasing collagen fibres laid down compresses the capillaries, which are no longer required. Thus the scar 'blanches' (becomes white) and gains strength over the course of months. Ultimately the scar is converted into a line composed almost entirely of collagen fibres and is avascular. Hence the wound has healed, with scar tissue closing the defect and regeneration of epithelium growing across the wound under the scab, which eventually drops off leaving a complete layer of epithelium covering the wound. Skin appendages such as hair follicles and sweat glands are unable to regenerate and so this scarred area will not contain such specialized structures. The process of repair by connective tissue or scarring is also known as **organization** or **fibrosis**.

The type of wound healing just described, where a fairly large defect is involved, is also known as '**healing by second intention**'. A neat surgical wound, where an incision is made and the defect is later closed or apposed by suturing, is known as '**healing by first intention**'. In this latter case the defect left by the wound is small and heals more quickly, requiring less scar tissue formation. Hence it is a common procedure to **approximate** wound margins, bringing them closer together and stitching them in order to diminish the time required for wound healing and also to minimize scar tissue formation. As the scar matures and contracts tensile strength is gained. One week after surgery 50% of the previous tensile strength is attained. After two weeks 70% of tensile strength is gained and sutures are usually removed at about this time (depending on the size of the wound and the area of the body involved).

Aberrations of Wound Healing

In some individuals, the laying down of excessive amounts of collagen forms a protruding, tumorous growth of scar tissue known as **keloid**. This tends to occur more commonly in people with dark skin pigmentation, being rare in Nordic type Caucasians and redheads. Instead of contracting and settling down, as most scars do, keloid scars may continue growing, producing large protruding masses. This bulging scar is disfiguring and unsightly but often removal of the keloid simply leads to further keloid scar formation. Laser therapy may be employed in this case.

Another deviation is the formation of excessive amounts of granulation tissue which protrudes from the wound above the level of the surrounding skin and may block re-epithelialization. This **exuberant granulation** is sometimes referred to as 'proud flesh' because of its pouting, bright-pink appearance. It sometimes requires surgical removal to permit restoration of epithelial continuity. Another term frequently used for this condition is **pyogenic granuloma**, but this is an unfortunate misnomer as the described changes are neither suppurating nor granulomatous.

Factors which Impair Wound Healing

These are many and may be divided into the localized and generalized factors. By far, the most commonly encountered are those of a localized nature, in particular, infection, poor blood supply, excessive movement and widely separated wound margins.

Localized Factors

Lack of adequate immobilization. If the wound is in constant motion, epithelium and granulation tissue are jarred out of place with bleeding, death of cells and great delay in the healing process because the granu-

lation tissue has to be reformed and the debris removed. Hence it is important to keep a healing wound as immobile as is practicable.

Lack of adequate blood supply/oxygenation. It is essential that a healing wound has an adequate blood supply. Oxygen is important in formation of the granulation tissue and also in preventing wound infection and necrosis. If a wound is in an area which has a poor blood supply it will heal slowly and has a greater risk of becoming infected. Surgical incisions are planned in a way that will allow rapid vascularization of the wound margins and hence effective granulation of the wound. In people with vascular diseases, wounds in the extremities, especially the feet, may turn into nasty, spreading ulcers which persist for long periods, may become infected and lead to gangrene, necessitating amputation of the limb.

Infection. This is by far the most common and most important factor delaying wound healing. If the wound becomes 'septic', that is, infected by micro-organisms, wound healing will be considerably more difficult. Bacteria present will cause damage to tissue and so scar tissue will not be able to form well. Wound infection may occur owing to an injury under dirty conditions and with dirty objects, for example working in soil or on farms, surgery (especially bowel surgery), or even post-surgical hospital infection. Dirty wounds are those that contain foreign material such as soil, dust, splinters of wood and glass, gravel, or alternatively wounds containing large amounts of necrotic tissue and blood clot. The presence of the debris acts as the source of the infection and also shelters the micro-organisms from the inflammatory and phagocytic process. As more bacteria multiply in the wound, toxins and metabolites are produced, destroying more and more tissue and protracting the inflammatory response. Wound healing will not progress normally until all bacteria are eliminated. The body responds by accumulating more neutrophils in the area such that **pus** is formed. It is essential that all wounds be properly cleaned, with excessive blood clot, necrotic tissue and foreign debris removed. This is a process known as **débridement**. It is best to leave dirty wounds open after cleaning them until granulation tissue has started to form as this tissue is very resistant to infection. Then the wound may be sewn up without fear of infection.

A normally healing, healthy wound looks pink, the exudate is watery and present in low volumes. The tissue around the wound is pinkish and not very painful or swollen. The bluish edge of the ingrowing epithelial margins may be discerned just under the edge of the scab. On the other hand, an infected wound looks very red, is swollen and quite painful. The exudate is copious and may be purulent and no epithelium is to be seen growing around the wound margins.

Wound separation. As previously discussed, wound healing is much quicker in a small wound, especially when the edges of the defect can be surgically apposed.

Generalized Factors

Nutrition. Deficiencies in such substances as vitamin C (ascorbic acid), vitamin A and protein will seriously interfere with wound healing as these factors are essential in repair by connective tissue formation and regeneration. Hence malnourished or starving individuals will show impaired wound healing (alcoholics, the elderly, mentally deficient people, Third World country inhabitants, Aborigines). Vitamin C in particular is essential in the formation of normal collagen and granulation tissue. In **scurvy**, wounds heal extremely poorly with bleeding and further tissue damage occurring.

Age. Wound healing is impaired in the elderly. There may be many factors involved. It generally takes much longer for a wound to heal in the elderly and vascular disease, hence a poor blood supply to the healing wound, malnutrition as well as ageing of connective tissue cells and less efficient inflammatory response may be involved. In the very young wounds heal much more quickly and usually with minimal scarring.

Drugs/hormones. Certain drugs and hormones will impair wound healing by suppressing the inflammatory response, immune response and scar formation. For example, people on **corticosteroid therapy** or people with tumours of the adrenals which produce excessive levels of glucocorticosteroids. These hormones have a direct anti-inflammatory effect, also depressing protein and polysaccharide synthesis and inhibiting wound contraction.

Generalized diseases. People with generalized vascular disease, as, for example, elderly people with atherosclerosis or diabetes, heal wounds poorly especially when these wounds are in the extremities (toes, feet, legs). Slowed or diminished wound healing is a feature of vitamin C deficiency (scurvy), ischaemic areas such as in peripheral vascular disease or varicose ulcers and in people suffering from diabetes. Patients with generalized malignancies, widespread cancers or leukaemia will also show greatly delayed or absent wound healing.

Healing in Specialized Tissues

Central Nervous System

The central nervous system (CNS) possesses no fibroblasts except those in the meninges and those around blood vessels. The supporting cells in the CNS are the glial cells, and it is these cells that are involved in tissue repair. If an area of brain is damaged, colliquative necrosis will occur and acute inflammation will follow. The number of neutrophils in the area is low, the majority of inflammatory cells being macrophages derived from circulating monocytes and resident microglial cells. Macrophages will phagocytose the lipid-rich fluid and they will appear under the microscope as very large, rounded cells with an abundant foamy cytoplasm. Such cells are termed **gitter cells** or **compound granular cells**.

As granulation tissue forms around the region of damage the glial cells, mainly astrocytes, begin to proliferate and they form a dense aggregate around the damaged region. The astrocytes are cells with many cytoplasmic processes full of fibrils and it is these processes that will form a dense meshwork of fibres that will surround the region of injury. The end result of this process is a glial scar and the region is an area of **gliosis**, the CNS equivalent of fibrosis elsewhere in the body. If the area of injury is large, a fluid-filled cavity often remains and the gliosis surrounds the area, giving an appearance very much like a cyst; this is the so-called **apoplectic cyst** that may be seen after ischaemic necrosis of the brain.

If the injury in the CNS involves the meninges and vessels, healing will occur in these areas in the normal way, with fibrosis and collagenous scarring. At the junction between the regions of gliosis and fibrosis, the astrocytic processes attach to the collagen fibres.

Peripheral Nerves

If a peripheral nerve is injured, damaged or severed, the axons distal to the site of injury will degenerate. The nerve axons become beaded with the myelin breaking up into fatty droplets. The axon breaks up into irregular segments so that within three weeks there is no trace of the damaged nerve remaining. Macrophages will take up and digest the lipids and the fragments of damaged tissue. Meanwhile, the Schwann cells around the damaged axon will swell up and divide, forming a column of cells that marks the course of the lost axon.

The severed ends of axons at the proximal end of the nerve that has been damaged will become bulbous. Fibrils in the cytoplasm of the axon begin to elongate and cytoplasmic outgrowths begin to grow into the Schwann cell masses randomly. If an axonal sprout finds a mass of Schwann cells it will grow into it at a rate of 2 to 5 mm a day. Once the regenerating axonal processes reach the end organ they will reinnervate it, and in many cases normal function is restored. However, this is not always the case, as often the regenerating axon will not encounter the proliferated Schwann cell masses. In this event the regenerating axonal sprouts will form a useless tangled mass of processes.

Muscle

Both striated and smooth muscle will under most circumstances scar if they are damaged, but in special cases will regenerate. Prolonged ischaemia of striated muscle will result in necrosis of tissue and scarring will be the result. Trauma will also result in scarring as the traumatic inflammatory response seen after the injury will bring about the removal of damaged and necrotic fibres and their replacement by scarring. At the junction of the damaged striated muscle and the normal muscle the muscle cells that have been severed will form bulbous ends and these will elongate slightly into the scar tissue in an abortive attempt at regeneration. However, there is no nuclear division and the process of cytoplasmic elongation stops very soon after the injury.

The best example of striated muscle regeneration occurs after Zenker's toxic degeneration of muscle. This occurs when there is toxic damage to muscle as seen in association with typhoid fever and other serious infections. The surviving muscle fibres extend into the endomysial tissue, eventually reoccupying the spaces that the original fibres occupied. There is no scarring in this instance. It appears that there may be some nuclear division involved in this process.

Smooth muscle cells in most cases respond to injury by undergoing replacement fibrosis. In some cases, the smooth muscle cells proliferate but the stimuli that cause this are poorly understood. It appears that smooth muscle cell proliferation may be inappropriate in some cases, as occurs, for example, in lung infarct healing, where smooth muscle cells divide randomly amongst the scar tissue.

Cartilage

Slight injury to cartilage is able to be repaired through regeneration. However, this only occurs with minimal injury which does not interfere too much with the nutrition of the tissue. Under most circumstances injury to the tissue is quite severe and the cartilage will degenerate, followed by granulation tissue formation around the damaged cartilage, leading to fibrosis. Frequently, damaged cartilage will ossify.

Solid Organs

The liver is a stable tissue containing cells that retain their ability to divide in the adult. Minor liver injury will usually result in little or no scarring. If more substantial liver injury occurs, scarring is more widespread, but at the same time the surviving liver cells are stimulated to divide. This effect is seen best with **cirrhosis** of the liver where chronic damage to liver (commonly due to chemical agents such as alcohol) results in regeneration of liver cells. The regenerative nodules of liver cells in the organ consist of normal hepatocytes, but usually some compromise in function of the organ is observed, as the architecture of the tissue is disrupted.

In experimental animals, such as rats, if two-thirds of the liver are removed surgically, the remaining hepatocytes will begin to undergo mitosis by the middle of the second day after surgery and the liver will have reached approximately its original mass by the end of the second week after the operation. Little fibrosis accompanies this regeneration. Experimental models for human cirrhosis have been developed in laboratory animals such as rats. Usually a toxic chemical such as carbon tetrachloride is administered and the injury to the liver that results stimulates the same response as is seen in humans: fibrosis and regenerative nodule formation.

Kidney tissue responds to injury largely by fibrosis. Specialized structures such as the nephron will not regenerate and no new glomeruli are formed. However, in some cases, especially after toxic injury to tubules, it is possible to observe mitosis in the surviving epithelium lining damaged tubules. If there is damage to the specialized part of the nephron, regeneration of the tubule will not alter the fact that the affected nephron will not function normally as far as excretion is concerned.

Pancreas and other glandular tissues usually show marked regenerative ability. Experimental studies involving resection of pancreas have shown that the surviving duct cells will rapidly divide and form branching sprouts. At the ends of these new growths acinar cells will form and in their cytoplasm zymogen granules are found. It is suspected that regeneration of other glands, both endocrine and exocrine, commonly occurs in many situations around the body after injurious stimuli.

Bone Fracture Healing — Tissue Regeneration

Bone fracture is any discontinuity of bone resulting after mechanical forces act on a bone. It includes bone breaks, cracks and crushing injuries. Fracture may occur in two ways: direct application of force to the bone or force transmitted indirectly along the line of the bone (e.g. fracture of the radius due to falling on an outstretched hand). There are many types of fractures, some of which are illustrated in Figure 2.35. The various types of fractures in specific body sites involving a particular bone are often named after the famous physician or surgeon who first described them, but this nomenclature (an example of **eponymic** nomenclature) is rapidly become obsolete in favour of a more general type:

Avulsion fracture: the separation of a small piece of bone cortex at the site of attachment of a ligament or tendon.

Comminuted fracture: the bone is divided into three or more parts (the bone is crushed and splintered, usually into many small fragments).

Complete fracture: the whole cross-section of the bone is involved. Complete fractures may have fracture lines that are **transverse**, **oblique** or **spiral**.

Compound fracture: the skin or mucosal surface is pierced by the ends of a fractured bone, such that the bone protrudes into the external environment. Usually extensive soft tissue trauma and necrosis is also seen in this type of fracture and the risk of infection is great.

Compression fracture: a fracture produced by compression of bone and is commonly seen in the vertebrae.

Dislocation fracture: occurs near an articulation with a consequent dislocation of the joint, as, for example, occurs with the fracture of the femoral head.

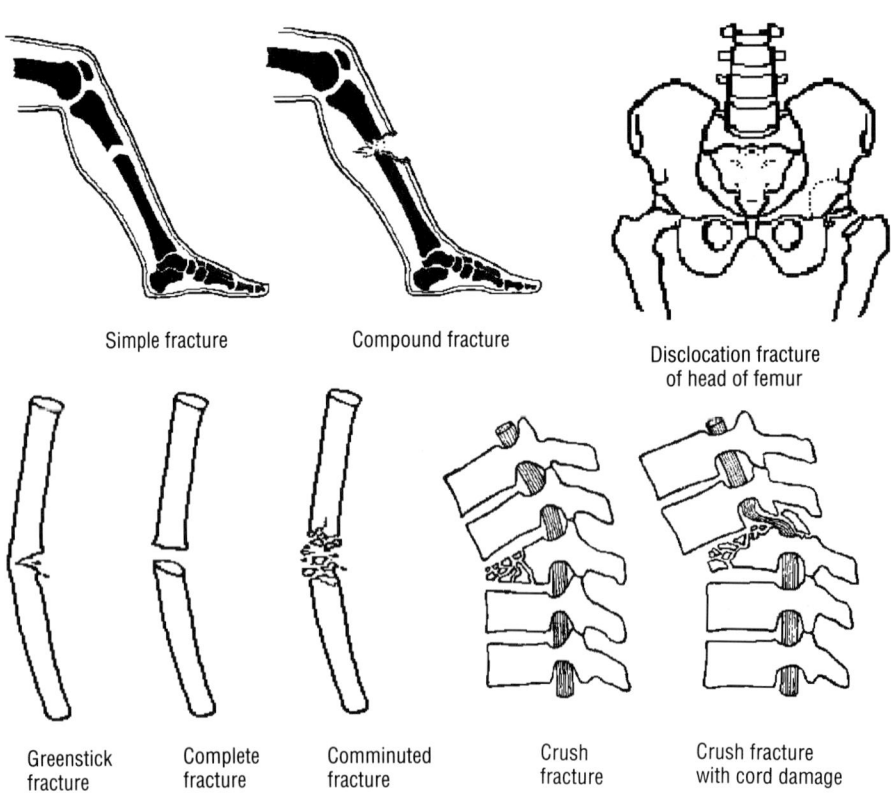

Simple fracture   Compound fracture

Dislocation fracture
of head of femur

Greenstick   Complete   Comminuted   Crush   Crush fracture
fracture   fracture   fracture   fracture   with cord damage

Figure 2.35 *Some types of bone fracture*

Double fracture: where the bone breaks cleanly in two places.

Fissure fracture: there is an incomplete fracture in the bone which does not involve the whole cross-section, i.e. a crack through the bone.

Greenstick fracture: this is a fissure fracture, with bending of the bone on its convex side only. This is seen commonly in children's bones which are more elastic or may be seen in the elderly with osteomalacia, a bone-softening disease.

Impacted fracture: one bone fragment becomes firmly wedged or 'telescopes' into the other fragment, as, for example, may occur with fractures of the lower limb bones.

Incomplete fracture: an alternative name for a fissure fracture.

Indirect fracture: the bone in this case fractures at a point distal to the point where the maximal force was applied.

Simple fracture: the bone is divided into two parts only and the overlying soft tissues are intact, without protrusion of the broken ends into the exterior of the body.

Stress fracture: this occurs where there is excessive overuse of a bone, for example the 'march fracture' seen in the metatarsals of army recruits after they have been marching continuously. Often the fracture line is difficult to detect on X-ray until new bone has formed at the site.

Spiral fracture: the line of breakage in the cross-sections of the bone forms a spiral that twists around the bone.

Spontaneous fracture: a sudden violent or unexpected movement, or unaccustomed and exaggerated repetition of movements places unaccustomed stress upon a normal bone and may result in fracture. Hence, electroconvulsive therapy (ECT) for psychiatric illness without anaesthesia or muscle relaxation therapy leads to spontaneous fracture in up to 20% of cases. '**March fracture**' of the metatarsal is another example of spontaneous fracture. Also, people who do excessive weight-training and muscle-building programmes may suffer spontaneous fractures. In some cases of tetanus, the extremely forceful contractions induced in opposing pairs of muscles by the tetanus toxin causes bones to fracture spontaneously.

Some common sites of bone fracture are associated with certain types of occupation, recreational activity or a special form of stress that is applied to a bone. The rugby or football player involved in an awkward tackle very often breaks his clavicle. Skiing accidents, especially involving novices to the slopes, frequently cause fractures of the tibia. Hockey players regularly sustain fractures of the humerus (often just above the level of the elbow), radius or ulna. Trampolinists and other athletes who land awkwardly after jumps risk breaking their ankles with a subsequent 12-week period of immobility prescribed. Fractures caused by a fall most often involve the bones of the wrist as the natural reaction when falling is to outstretch the hands in order to protect oneself. The elderly very frequently break the neck of the femora, even with minimal stressing forces.

Normal bone is very strong and has tensile and crushing strengths that are about the same, between 9 and 16 kg/mm^2, thus being nearly as resistant to bending and twisting as cast iron! Therefore, great force must be applied in order to break a normal bone, and this usually implies that a lot of trauma to the soft tissues will be seen with most fractures. It should be kept in mind that children's bones are much more pliable than adults' and also, in old age, the bones tend to become more brittle. This explains why an infant who falls out of a first-story window may not sustain any fractures, while an elderly woman crossing the road, who in her hurry trips over the kerb and falls only a short distance, may break the neck of the femur, a fracture that may require many months to heal. Alternatively, very commonly, patients with fractures present with **pathological fracture**, that is, a fracture which occurs in bone which is already diseased, thus requiring only minimal force in order to break it owing to bone weakening. Pre-existing bone diseases, such as tumours, genetic disorders, osteoporosis and osteomalacia, should always be considered and excluded when dealing with a bone fracture.

The process of fracture healing is similar to the process of wound healing, which has already been described, with the exception that instead of connective tissue scar formation there must be formation of new bone and remodelling of bone. Thus, this represents **regeneration** rather than repair of the broken bone. Incomplete, simple fractures heal the most quickly but another important factor is age of the patient, bone regeneration being perfect and relatively rapid the younger the patient is.

There are three principles that are used in order to treat fractured bones. Firstly, any displacement in the bone must be corrected and the broken bony ends must be aligned in the anatomically correct position. This is called **reducing a fracture**. Secondly, the bony parts must be immobilized for a sufficiently long time so as to allow healing to occur. Various types of splinting have been devised in order to keep the bone immobile, most commonly plaster of Paris impregnated bandages being used. The splinting may be used in conjunction with **traction** (a pulling force across the break), which will help align the bone. Thirdly, damage to the soft tissues must also be treated in order to avoid excessive scar tissue formation and to avoid prolonged rehabilitation. Following these three precautions, the body's own healing processes are allowed to act and the bone regenerates. The process of bone fracture healing is outlined in Figure 2.36.

Haematoma Formation ('Blood Clot', 0–24 hours)

At the time of injury, bleeding occurs from severed and damaged vessels at the fracture site. A periosteal tear may result in blood seeping into surrounding tissues, including muscle. This intramuscular haemorrhage may be sometimes subsequently organized, and

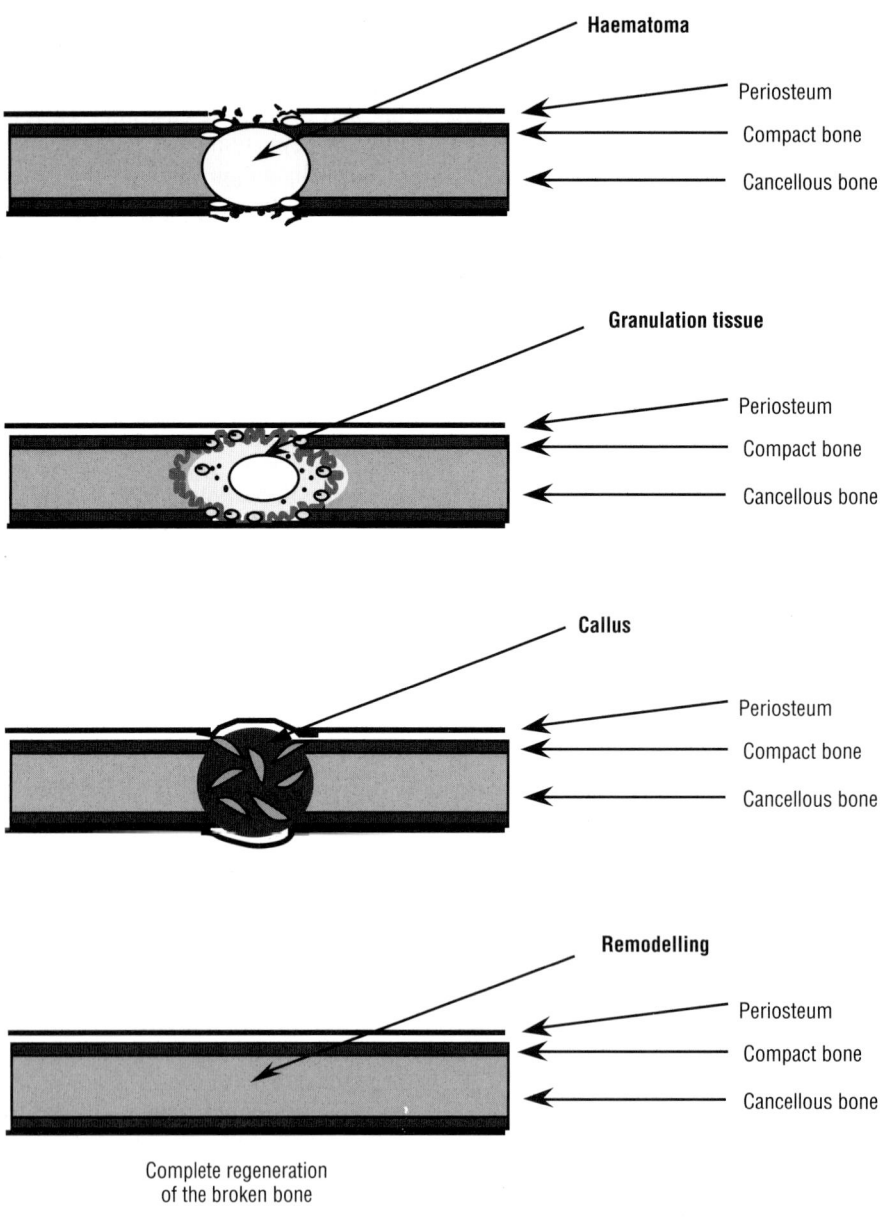

Figure 2.36 *Bone fracture healing; bone regeneration*

dystrophic calcification with subsequent **ossification** (bone formation) may occur in the surrounding muscle, resulting in the condition of **myositis ossificans**. The blood clot and fibrin strands that form inside the fracture cavity are the first attempt by the body to unite the broken bone ends and the fibrin 'glue' forms a wide bridge joining the bone fragments together and acts as a scaffold for future tissue repairing mechanisms.

Traumatic Inflammatory Response (1–3 days)

Inflammation occurs in response to the tissue injury as tissue breakdown products are released by autolysis. The inflammation proceeds with typical formation of exudate and polymorph infiltration. The exudate fluid causes distension of the periosteum, so that the haematoma assumes a fusiform (spindle) shape. Usually, in simple fractures not many neutrophils accumulate in the area as there is no infection and little tissue debris that they phagocytose.

'Demolition' (2–7 days)

The inflammatory response continues with macrophages infiltrating the clot removing fibrin, red blood cells, inflammatory exudate and debris. **Osteoclasts** are activated and begin to lyse bone on either side of the broken bone, such that in an X-ray of the fracture, decalcification of the bony ends will be seen around the fracture cavity. This increases the calcium concentration locally and also allows the new osteoid formed to merge with the pre-existing osteoid. Dislodged bone fragments undergo necrosis as their blood supply has been cut off, and are broken down and removed by macrophages and osteoclasts.

Formation of Granulation Tissue (3–8 days)

Capillary loops and fibroblasts derived from periosteum and endosteum grow into the clot. Fibroblasts are multipotential mesenchymal cells, and are capable of differentiating into osteoblasts or chondroblasts. Granulation tissue is highly vascular and the periosteum is vital in supplying the necessary blood and nutrients. In a fracture of the neck of the femur, the vessels which supply the periosteum are sometimes damaged, cutting off blood supply to the head of the femur and resulting in avascular necrosis of the bone. In cases such as this the necrotic broken bone fragment will not regenerate.

Formation of Provisional Fracture Callus (7–25 days)

Mesenchymal cells differentiate into chondroblasts and osteoblasts and they migrate into the fracture cavity. They then begin to form both the collagen fibres and the osseomucin ground substance in which the fibres are embedded. This is **osteoid tissue**, which is formed during the maturation of granulation tissue. The collagen fibres are laid down in a random fashion. As in the repair of ordinary connective tissue, progressive devascularization now occurs. The osteoblasts then secrete **alkaline phosphatase**, and the phosphate concentration rises.

Meanwhile, lysis of bone fragments has resulted in a high local concentration of calcium and thus all the ingredients are present for the formation of bone mineral. Calcification of the osteoid now occurs about the randomly distributed fibres, forming a loose 'woven bone' which unites the fractured bone ends. This mass of young, irregular bone spicules forming across the fracture gap is called the **provisional callus** and depending on its position is further specified as external, intermediate and internal. The provisional callus is the second attempt at union of the fractured bone ends.

In fracture healing, the formation of woven bone is dependent on adequate immobilization of the fracture site. If immobilization is inadequate, then repeated disorganization and injury to the granulation tissue mass occurs and the fibroblasts may differentiate only to chondroblasts instead of osteoblasts, and thus cartilage is laid down instead of bone. If no differentiation of fibroblasts occurs, then fibrous tissue (scar) is formed instead of bone. If cartilage is produced, this splints the fracture and diminishes movement and in some cases subsequent ossification of the cartilage may occur. Ossification of fibrous tissue is, however, exceedingly rare, if it occurs at all.

Formation of Definitive Fracture Callus (1–3 months)

The cartilage or woven bone is infiltrated by capillaries, osteoclasts and a second wave of fibroblasts. The original disordered bone spicules of the provisional callus are demolished and new bone is now laid down about the capillaries using the blood vessels as the centre of concentric layers of bone, resulting in the formation of Haversian systems of lamellar bone. This ordered, lamellar bone which forms across the fracture gap is called the **definitive callus** and represents the third and strongest attempt at union of the broken bony ends. New bone is also laid down from the periosteum inwards, forming a wide sleeve of newly laid down cortical bone around the fracture region.

Remodelling (3–12 months)

Continued laying down and removal of bone (osteoblast/osteoclast activity) results in remodelling of the new bone to form a structure very similar to the original. External callus is removed, intermediate callus is remodelled into compact bone containing Haversian systems and the internal callus becomes hollow, continuous with and invaded by cells of the marrow cavity. The remodelling of the bone is directed by the muscle and weight-bearing stresses that are placed upon the bone. If the bone has been well aligned ('well set'), perfect reconstruction of the bone occurs and when the process has been completed there will be no radiological evidence of the previous bone fracture; that is, fracture healing is now complete and bone regeneration has occurred.

It should be kept in mind that a fracture heals clinically well before it heals radiologically and therefore use of the broken bone will occur before the X-rays reveal a completely regenerated bone. It is essential when bone remodelling is occurring to begin to use the limb lightly in order to place the normal stresses on the bone thus directing bone deposition along the normal lines of stress. One disadvantage of keeping healing bone fractures immobile for any length of time is the atrophy observed in the muscles around the fracture site and the stiffness of the joints involved. It should be noted that the healing time for fractures will depend very much on the age of the patient, the site fractured, the severity of the fracture, the blood supply of the bone involved, the adequacy of the treatment and whether there is pre-existing bone disease present. A rough guide for the otherwise healthy young adult is six weeks for a spiral fracture of the upper limb and twelve weeks for a transverse one. Double these times are required for fractures of the lower limbs. However, children's bones heal twice as fast, while the bones of the elderly may take twice as long, or longer, to heal. Certain diseases of bones will prevent the natural healing mechanism from operating at all. For example, if a malignant tumour is present in the bone and this has been the cause of a fracture, it is unlikely that the fracture will heal unless the tumour is first eradicated.

Aberrations of Bone Fracture Healing

The final success of healing of the fracture depends on good alignment of the broken bone ends, adequate blood supply to the newly forming bone, on the amount of bone tissue that needs to be replaced, on the degree of immobilization of the fracture site, and the path of differentiation of the fibroblasts. If immobilization is adequate, fibroblasts differentiate to form osteoblasts and bone is formed. If immobilization is not complete, fibroblasts form into chondroblasts and cartilage is laid down which may later ossify. When there is little or no immobilization, fibroblasts lay down collagen only, forming scar tissue. If scar joins the bone ends, that is, a **fibrous union**, little or no further change occurs. The fracture is permanently unstable and healing is unsatisfactory. When this occurs a 'false joint' is said to be present in the bone — the condition known as **pseudoarthrosis**. This is is especially common in highly mobile sites, for example fractures of the ribs.

Non-union, that is, complete lack of union of bone, results if soft tissues become interposed between the fractured bone ends. A uniting haematoma is not formed and union of any sort may not possible. Sometimes there may be attempts at healing by fibrous tissue formation, the two bony ends being joined quite firmly by strands of collagenous fibrous tissue and a pseudoarthrosis once again results.

If the fracture has not been aligned well and there is anatomical malalignment, the bone will not heal straight and in that case there may be **deformity**, **angulation** and **displacement** of the healed bone fracture. If this occurs in a straight, long bone the deformity is particularly marked and there may be compromise of function of the affected limb. Once this has occurred, the only remedy is to re-break the bone and set it correctly.

If the bone fracture is a comminuted one and a large volume of bone has undergone necrosis and is removed, there will be a large fracture cavity between the broken bone ends. If the bone ends are apposed (brought closer together) and bone healing occurs, the resulting healed bone will be considerably shorter than the original bone. This will lead to deformity and compromise in function of the limb. In order to prevent this, an orthopaedic surgeon must insert pins which will keep the bony ends the required distance apart and allow the regenerating bone to fill in the gap. This procedure generally increases the time taken for the fracture to heal, but is of benefit since no deformity will result. The metals used for fixing broken bones are stainless steel, vitallium or titanium, as these metals resist corrosion by the body fluids and do not cause irritation or injury to the living tissue. In **inlay fixation**, a pin or a nail is inserted along the long axis of the bone, whereas in **onlay fixation** a metal plate is fixed to the surface of a bone, overlapping with the two ends of the fracture (Figure 2.37). One example of the inlay technique is the **Kuntscher nail** used for the fixation of a broken femur. The ends of the broken bone are exposed by the orthopaedic surgeon and a shaft is drilled in each direction into the broken bone ends. A guide wire is inserted until it emerges at the buttock through the skin. The nail is then hammered from above, along the guide wire, across the fracture line and into the lower bone fragment. The wire is then withdrawn, the pin being left in place within the drilled cavities of the bone.

It must be stressed that dead bone will not regenerate and this is particularly important in certain situations in the body that are notorious for their poor blood supply: the carpal scaphoid bone, the shaft of the tibia and the neck of the femur. Fractures of the neck of the femur, in particular, are a big problem, especially in the elderly, where there may be associated dislocation. The femoral head in this case undergoes necrosis and needs to be replaced by a **prosthesis** (artificial joint) in a surgical procedure known as an **arthroplasty**. This procedure is very commonly carried out in the elderly after fractures and is also carried out to replace severely arthritic joints.

Factors which Impair Bone Fracture Healing

Union will take longer than normal to occur if adverse influences are present after the establishment of a uniting haematoma. If these adverse influences are severe, fibrous union may occur. Such adverse influences are many and, as was the case with the healing of soft tissue wounds, they may be divided into the localized and generalized.

Localized Factors

Lack of adequate immobilization. Movement causes damage to the granulation tissue resulting in re-bleeding and disorganization. In clinical practice fracture movement is minimized by splinting the fracture. Externally plaster casts are used, or internally, rods (nails and pins), plates, screws or fixateurs may be used.

Infection. Infection prolongs the acute inflammatory phase and bacteria or their toxins disorganize the clot and cause necrosis. Under these conditions, delayed union, mal-union or non-union may result. Infection is more common in a compound fracture where the bone has pierced the skin. In this situation it is essential to have ensured that infection is not present before closing up the wound and setting the bone. A mass of necrotic tissue, blood clot or dead bone fragments are the perfect environment for bacterial multiplication. When the wound is infected and the fracture is involved there may be suppuration, **osteomyelitis** (infection of the surrounding bone and marrow cavity), tetanus or gangrene.

Poor blood supply. While complete loss of blood supply leads to necrosis of the bone, poor blood supply leads to poor granulation tissue formation, anoxia, diminished nutrients and increased metabolites in the area, therefore a great delay in healing. In peripheral vascular disease, diabetes or regions of anatomically poor blood supply (fractured neck of femur, scaphoid fracture) there will be delayed healing. Under these circumstances, adequate immobilization is of the utmost importance.

Localized bone disease. Pre-exisiting disease, such as a malignant tumour in the immediate area of the frac-

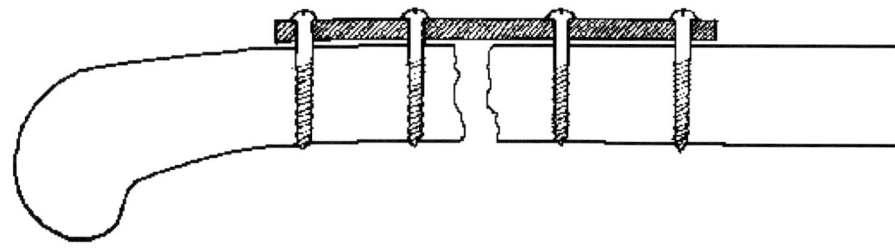

Figure 2.37 *Onlay fixation of a fracture in which quite a lot of bone has been lost across the fracture gap. The broken bony ends need to be pinned in a way such that the healing reconstitutes the bone that was lost, preventing a shortening of the healed bone*

ture (possibly the cause of a pathological fracture), greatly delays or even totally hampers the process of fracture healing.

Generalized Factors

Poor nutrition. Malnutrition affects fracture healing as it does wound healing. Essential nutrients include vitamin C, vitamin A, vitamin D, proteins and calcium. In the malnourished individual bone fracture healing will be greatly delayed but will still proceed even if it is at the expense of other tissues in the body. Thus, existing bone may be resorbed to provide the necessary calcium to heal the fractured bone, the injured taking priority over the healthy tissue. Vitamin C is essential in collagen formation and in scurvy, bone fractures heal very poorly. Vitamin D is essential in calcium metabolism and is needed if the fractured bone is to heal normally.

Generalized vascular disease. Atherosclerosis is the major factor of importance here as in this disorder the lumen of arteries is narrowed thus allowing less blood to flow into the tissues, therefore inducing in the tissues a state of chronic, partial ischaemia. Fewer nutrients and less oxygen reach the tissues, and more tissue metabolites accumulate in the tissue fluids. There is decreased blood supply to bone in these patients and therefore bone fracture healing is greatly delayed.

Generalized bone disease. A lesion or disease which weakens bone may lead to fracture with even minimal strain. This may occur in **hyperparathyroidism** (osteitis fibrosa cystica), in **osteogenesis imperfecta**, in benign **tumours** and cysts of bone (e.g. hydatid cyst, or giant cell tumour of bone) or malignant tumours of bone, both primary or secondary. Indeed, pathological fracture through a metastasis (secondary tumour) may be the first presentation of **cancer** (malignant tumour). **Paget's disease** of bone is another example of a bone disease which may cause pathological fractures. If such a disease pre-exists in a fractured bone, healing may be greatly delayed or even absent, as pathological processes are active at the site preventing the normal body healing response from taking place.

Other generalized disease. When a patient is very debilitated due to widespread disease in other parts of the body, bone fracture healing will be greatly delayed as the body's resources are depleted and normal healing processes are diminished. Examples of such diseases are **diabetes mellitus**, **advanced carcinomatosis** (widespread cancer in many tissues), **leukaemia** and **severe systemic infections**.

Ageing. As with wound healing, fracture healing tends to be less efficient in old age, the major reasons for this being a complex interaction of various factors. Many elderly people have a poor diet lacking in protein, vitamins and calcium. Widespread atherosclerosis of great severity is also found in the elderly and this accounts for the ischaemia seen in sites of tissue repair. Cell mobility and metabolism are decreased in the elderly, an effect of generalized body atrophy, hormonal changes and ischaemia. The elderly also suffer from many debilitating disorders such as diabetes, cancers and generalized bone diseases such as **osteoporosis** and **osteomalacia**. The changes seen in bone with these conditions are illustrated in Figure 2.38. All of the above factors interact and decrease the efficiency and completeness of bone regeneration in the elderly patient.

Review of the Body's Response to Injury

The pathways of the various reparative and healing mechanisms occurring in the body after injury are summarized in Figure 2.39. It can be seen that depending on the severity of the injury and the nature of the tissue that is injured the body will respond in slightly different ways. Lethal injury in both parenchymal and connective tissues is followed by necrosis. Sublethal injury in parenchymal tissue is followed by reactive changes whereas in connective tissue sublethal injury will induce acute inflammation. Reactive changes may be overcome if the tissue is not severely injured and the tissue may go back to normal.

Necrotic tissues may become infected or they may calcify. They will excite inflammatory responses and depending on the degree of tissue damage and the regenerative capability of the tissue, resolution may follow, or scarring, or regeneration or any combination of these. Specific examples of tissue responses to injury have been covered and different outcomes in various tissues have been exemplified.

Chronic Inflammation

Chronic means long-lasting. As was mentioned earlier the typical acute inflammatory response lasts for up to a few days. Chronic inflammation implies a process that persists for a long period of time, lingering on for

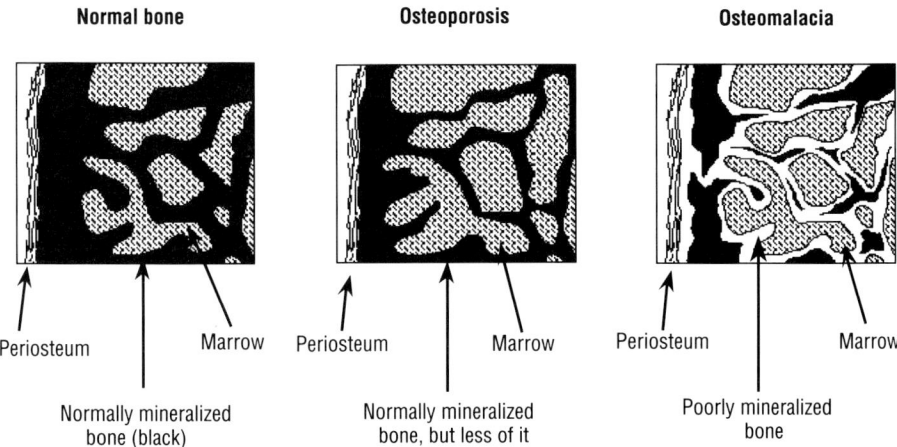

Figure 2.38 *Osteoporosis and osteomalacia predispose to pathological fractures and healing of the broken bone will be greatly delayed or prevented in patients with these conditions*

weeks or many months. Acute and chronic inflammation are related processes but there are good clinical and biological reasons for distinguishing between them. Chronic inflammation may be defined as the prolonged process in which destruction of tissue and inflammation are proceeding at the same time as attempts at healing. Chronic inflammation results and persists because of a persistent irritant stimulus, which the body cannot remove or destroy, or owing to the nature (the physical or biochemical features) of the causative agent which favours its persistence, or because of factors relating to the immune system, which because of the presence of the persistent injury is in a state of constant activation. All of these factors may operate together and are in many cases interrelated.

Chronic inflammation is of two main types and the responses are distinguished on the basis of their origin. The first type of response is the **sequela** to unresolved acute inflammation and the second type is chronic inflammation *ab initio* (i.e. a typical chronic inflammatory response from the beginning, without a pre-existing acute phase). It may be odd to talk about a *chronic* inflammatory condition which arises as such immediately, but in this case the inflammation varies so much from the typical acute inflammatory response that it is considered to be a different entity altogether.

Characteristics of Chronic Inflammation

Whereas acute inflammation is mainly exudative, chronic inflammation is largely cellular (productive or proliferative). The predominant cells present are not usually neutrophils as in acute inflammation but rather **lymphocytes**, **plasma cells**, **macrophages** (and their derivatives) and **fibroblasts**. The presence of lymphocytes and plasma cells indicates that immunological mechanisms are involved. The presence of fibroblasts indicates that the processes of repair are occurring concurrently with the inflammation. Thus the chronic inflammatory response is said to be **pleomorphic** since a large variety of different cells are present in the inflamed tissues simultaneously. When the tissue undergoes necrosis, there may develop different types of tissue necrosis, such as suppurative, caseous, gummatous, coagulative or fibrinoid.

The histological appearance of the inflamed tissue is in the majority of cases **non-specific**, that is, the same cellular reaction may be seen in response to many different agents and the cellular picture gives no indication of the cause of the inflammation. It should be kept in mind, however, that transition from acute to chronic inflammation may occur when the injury persists, and also that acute inflammation may supervene in chronically inflamed tissues, so it is not uncommon to see a 'mixed picture' histologically.

Chronic inflammation developing as a sequela to acute inflammation occurs in cases where the agent that causes acute inflammation cannot be eradicated and the reaction continues. For example, in staphylococcal osteomyelitis there is an initial acute inflammation and bone necrosis. Bacteria can survive in this dead bone (sequestrum) and are inaccessible to the body's defences. Hence chronic inflammation ensues. The same situation may be seen in a typical chronic

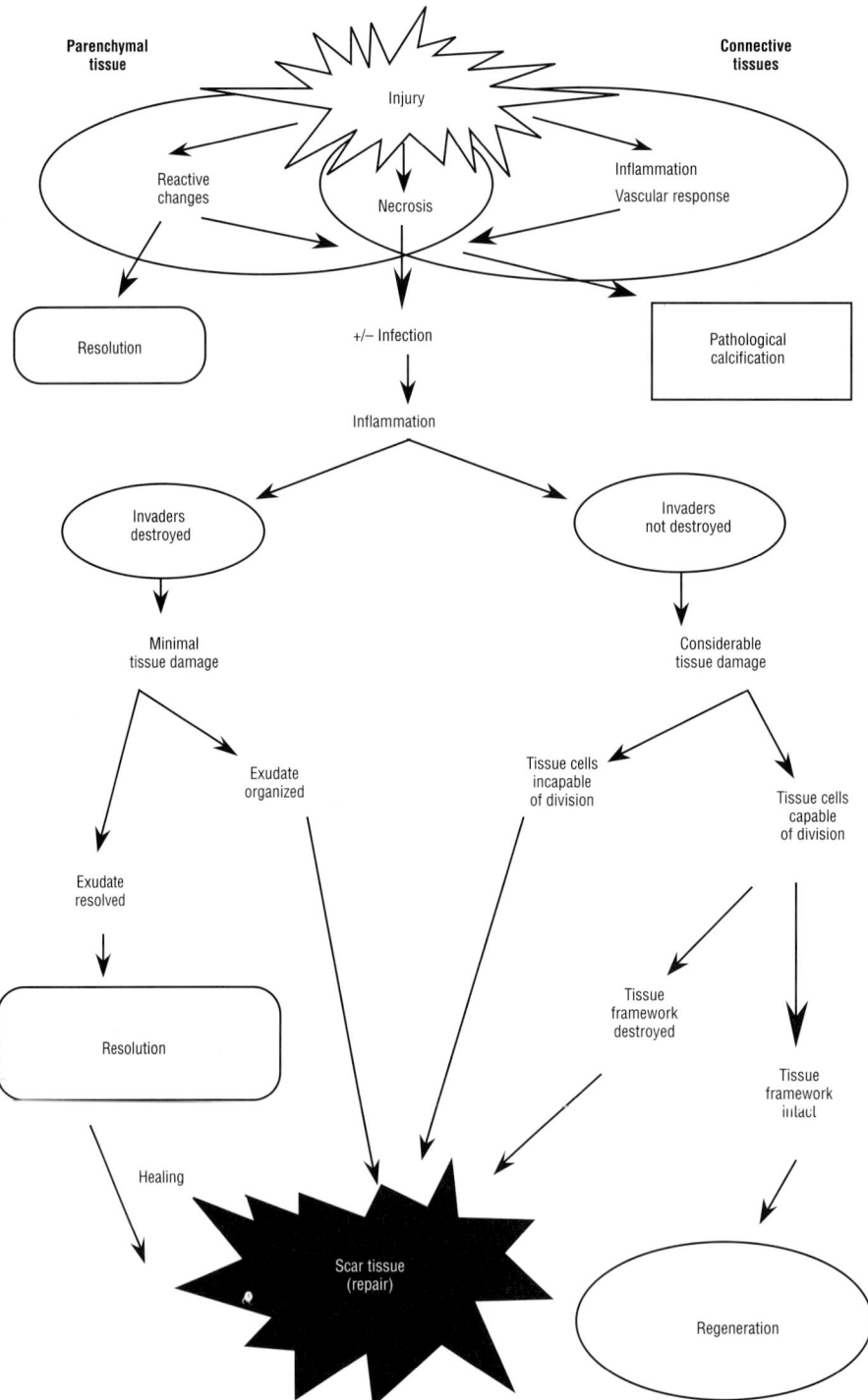

Figure 2.39   *The spectrum of the body's response to injury*

abscess as considered earlier. In this case the bacteria causing the abscess cannot be eliminated from the tissues and therefore the suppuration, tissue damage and necrosis persist for a long time. Granulation tissue which forms around the abscess cavity may be considered to be an attempt at healing as the body is trying to 'wall off' the lesion, preventing the spread of bacteria and the damage of more tissue. A chronic peptic ulcer is another example of this inflammation. Acid damages stomach or duodenal mucosa, acute inflammation begins, and fibrous scar repairs the damage. The inflammation becomes chronic as the acid constantly damages the tissue, and the body constantly repairs the damage by fibrosis. Certain immunological reactions and autoimmune disease may also be considered to be of this type of response, for example rheumatoid arthritis, beginning with a typical acute inflammatory response, but persisting and being converted into a chronic inflammation in which tissue destruction constantly proceeds in association with scarring. In all of the above examples the nature of the inflammation may be considered to be an essentially typical acute inflammatory response (histologically) in that neutrophils and macrophages with granulation tissue formation are the predominant features. The only reason the reaction is termed 'chronic inflammation' is because it persists for a long time. Perhaps it may be better to consider these states as a 'protracted acute inflammation'. Some pathologists prefer to give this protracted acute inflammation the name of **subacute inflammation**.

Chronic inflammation *ab initio* (with no acute phase) is caused by injurious agents that do not provoke an acute inflammatory response; that is, we will not see the typical cardinal signs of acute inflammation when the injurious agents enter the tissue. For example, sterile foreign bodies such as catgut, talc, asbestos fibres, silica particles and some micro-organisms, when entering the tissues, will induce the typical pleomorphic, productive cellular response of chronic inflammation, without hyperaemia, exudation, etc. Some of the micro-organisms inducing chronic inflammation *ab initio* are *Mycobacterium tuberculosis,* the cause of TB, *Mycobacterium leprae*, causing Hansen's disease (leprosy), *Treponema pallidum*, causing syphilis, and *Actinomyces* spp., causing madura foot. In addition, there are some idiopathic diseases which fall into this group, the prime example being **sarcoidosis**.

Forms of the Chronic Inflammatory Response

The chronic inflammatory response may vary depend-

ing on the site involved and the causative agent. Also, one or another component of the response may predominate thus leading to several histological and clinical presentations. These different types of response may be either sequelae of acute inflammation or alternatively chronic inflammation *ab initio*.

Chronic Fibrous Inflammation

In this form, there is marked **fibrosis** (laying down of fibrocollagenous tissue), i.e. scarring, for example rheumatoid arthritis of advanced standing showing fibrosis of the joints involved (pannus formation and **ankylosis** — fused joint surfaces). Another example is chronic inflammation of a duct or viscus, which will show marked deposition of fibrous tissue around the wall, leading to **stenosis**, reduction of luminal diameter and obstruction.

Chronic Serous Inflammation

Serous exudate formation is a marked feature of this type of response. Serous inflammation occurs commonly on serous membranes such as pleura, pericardium, synovium and peritoneum. In the early stages of rheumatoid arthritis, for example, chronic synovitis with serous effusion into the joint space is seen. Other examples are tuberculous pericarditis and tuberculous peritonitis, where large volumes of serous fluid accumulate. Chronic bursitis in joints due to mechanical injury may also take this form. It should be noted that the fluid which accumulates is not an exudate but rather an increased quantity of the **serous transudate** which is normally found in these areas.

Chronic Suppurative Inflammation

This occurs in chronic inflammation when pus formation is a feature, and is characteristically a reaction where chronic inflammation is a sequela of acute inflammation, for example a chronic abscess such as a **carbuncle** or a **furuncle**. **Sinus formation** may be a feature in such reactions where the abscess cavity forms a channel which continuously empties the pus formed to the exterior of the body, through skin or a mucosal surface.

Chronic Ulcerative Inflammation

An **ulcer** is a localized excavation of tissue usually on

the skin or mucosal surface and it involves deeper tissues, such as the dermis, submucosa or parenchyma of organs. Some bacterial infections may produce chronic ulcers, for example *Mycobacterium ulcerans* infection, causing the tropical ulcers seen in the skin of people living in the tropics. Ulceration may result from physical or chemical injury, the latter exemplified in **chronic peptic ulcers**. Immune damage of a chronic nature also produces ulcerations, for example **ulcerative colitis**.

Chronic Granulomatous Inflammation

This is a very typical form of chronic inflammation characterized by the formation of one or more **granulomata**. A granuloma is a grain-like lump in the inflamed tissue and is composed of masses of chronic inflammatory cells aggregated in characteristic deposits. A granuloma should not be confused with granulation tissue, which is an entity associated with healing, whereas in most cases granulomata are associated with

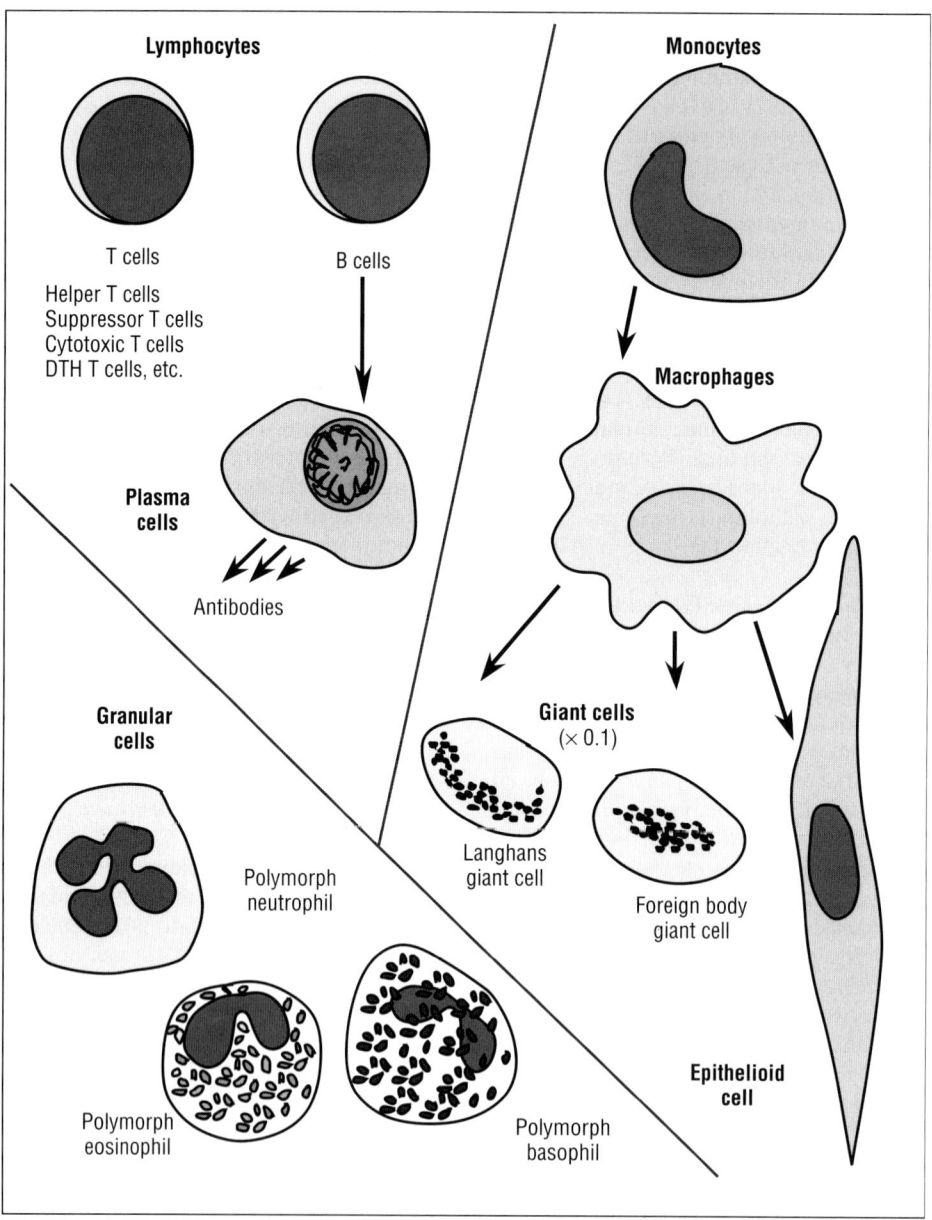

Figure 2.40   *The various types of cells that may be found in sites that are chronically inflamed*

tissue damage and destruction. Granuloma formation is linked with important immune system manifestations of altered function and it may be said that granulomata form whenever the immune system is trying to cope with a particularly difficult or uncharacteristic situation. Some authors suggest that all granulomata are manifestations of **hypersensitivity**, that is, an inappropriate immune response which causes damage to tissues instead of protecting them. The nature of the initiating injurious stimulus in granuloma formation is certainly unusual and it may be the main factor in initiating the formation of such structures. A typical example of granuloma formation in tissues is tuberculosis. The infecting micro-organism in this case is *Mycobacterium tuberculosis*, which is a specialized bacterium in that it possesses a very thick cell wall rich in **mycolic acid**, a waxy substance, which renders the bacterium resistant to the destructive effects of lysozyme inside phagocytic cells. Thus when these bacteria enter the tissues, they are ingested by macrophages but are able to survive intracytoplasmically, stimulating the macrophage to initiate immune responses which may lead to hypersensitivity and granuloma formation. Since chronic granulomatous inflammation and tuberculosis are very important processes and characteristic chronic inflammatory states they will be discussed in detail.

Granulomatous Inflammation

Cellular Aspects of Granulomatous Inflammation

Certain noxious agents excite chronic granulomatous inflammation which is characterized by the formation of granulomata, aggregates of chronic inflammatory cells. The types of cells present in all granulomata are constant, such that granulomata due to different causes are very similar, although not exactly alike. For example, the granuloma that forms in tuberculosis is almost identical to the granuloma that forms in sarcoidosis, the only difference being that the granuloma of TB contains a central region of caseous necrosis. The characteristic cell types in a granuloma are the **mononuclear phagocytes** (**macrophages**) and their many derivatives as can be seen in Figure 2.40. Macrophages in tissues are derived from blood monocytes and are important cells in phagocytosis and immunity. They retain their capability of division and differentiation once in the tissues and they have a long life span, of months or years. The macrophage undergoes two transformations in regions of chronic inflammation, forming epithelioid cells and giant cells.

Epithelioid cells were so named because they resemble certain epithelial cells. They are flattened and elongated in shape with an oval, vesicular nucleus, pale-staining eosinophilic (pink) cytoplasm and an indistinct cell membrane. These cells are modified macrophages which have lost their ability to phagocytose particulate matter. Apparently they have a secretory role and it is thought that they secrete **monokines**, substances essential in stimulating and prolonging the immune response in localized areas. Epithelioid cells are a characteristic feature of many types of granulomata, for example those of tuberculosis, sarcoidosis and leprosy.

Giant cells are very large cells, 40 to 100 μm in diameter, and they are a multinucleate syncytium containing 50 or more nuclei. When the nuclei are clustered about the periphery of the cell in a 'horse-shoe' or circular pattern the cell is called a **Langhan's giant cell** (Figure 2.41). If the nuclei are scattered about the cytoplasm in a random fashion, more centrally, the cell is known as a **foreign body giant cell** (Figure 2.42). The essential difference seems to be that if previous immunological sensitization of the macrophages has occurred, Langhan's giant cells tend to form, as in TB. However, both types of giant cells may be seen together. Giant cells form whenever there is material in the tissue that the macrophages have difficulty in phagocytosing or destroying, such as *Mycobacterium* spp., talc granules, asbestos, surgical silk or wood splinters. Many macrophages attempt to phagocytose the same particles together and in the process fuse together to form the giant cell (Figure 2.43). There may be subsequent nuclear division without cellular division of the giant cell, giving rise to the large syncytia. It is now quite clear that giant cells do

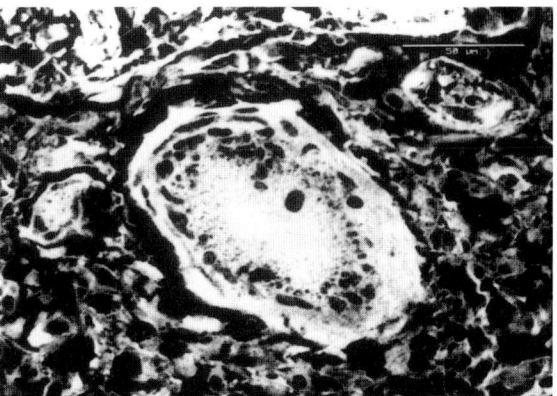

Figure 2.41 *A Langhan's giant cell in a tubercle. Note the horseshoe arrangement of the many nuclei of the syncytium (scale bar is 50 μm)*

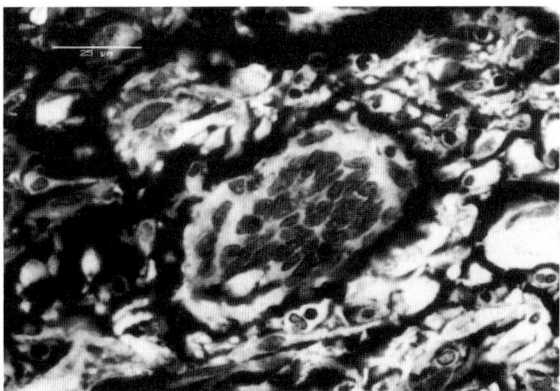

Figure 2.42 *A foreign body giant cell in a granuloma of sarcoidosis (scale bar is 25 μm)*

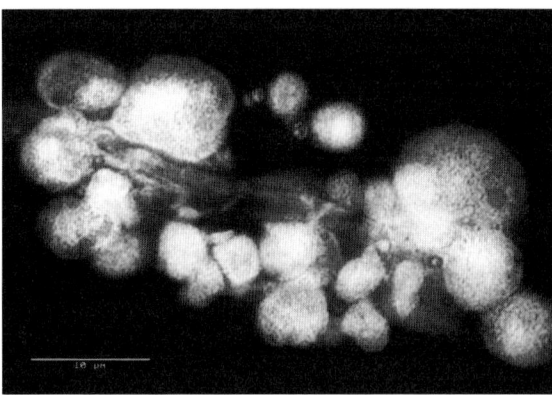

Figure 2.43 *Living macrophages in cell culture aggregating around a cellulose fibre. Giant cells are forming as the macrophages attempt to phagocytose the offending foreign particle (scale bar is 10 μm)*

not have an improved phagocytic capability; in fact the contrary is true — they are sluggish, sessile cells that do not seem to do much once they have formed. It is thought that they arise in tissues as a result of a biological accident rather than as a result of a specific adaptive manifestation of macrophage function in sites of chronic inflammation.

Lymphocytes or, as they may be sometimes described in histopathology, 'small round cells' are the immunological effector cells and both T cells and B cells may be found in granulomata although the T cells predominate. The presence of many lymphocytes in granulomata underlines the importance of immune mechanisms in the formation of these structures. They represent an attempt by the immune sys-

tem to cope with the injurious agent, largely through the cell-mediated immune response. The presence of delayed-type hypersensitivity T cells and secretion of lymphokines in areas of chronic inflammation are thought to be of importance in the chronicity of the immune response where granulomata form.

Plasma cells are differentiated B lymphocytes and are the cells involved in antibody production. These are not a prominent feature of granulomata, indicating that the humoral immune response is not as active in these structures. However, they may be found in very large numbers in other sites of chronic inflammation such as the synovium in rheumatoid arthritis, where production of **auto-antibodies** may be a very important step in the pathogenesis of the disease (Figure 2.44).

Granulocytes (neutrophils, eosinophils and basophils) may occasionally be found in sites that are chronically inflamed but are generally not numerous nor prominent cells. In the case of typical granulomata, these cells are absent. In the case where an **active chronic inflammatory response** is evident, neutrophils may be seen in large numbers in association with many chronic inflammatory cells. In these responses a site which is already chronically inflamed is injured or damaged and a phase of acute inflammation is seen on top of the pre-existing chronic inflammation. A typical example is the active chronic synovitis of rheumatoid arthritis, where episodes of acute inflammation punctuate the long-lasting chronic inflammation. In these situations a very complex histological appearance may be seen. Eosinophils may be prominent in some conditions, for example **parasitic infestations**, where the eosinophil count of the blood may be considerably raised as well as large numbers of these cells accumu-

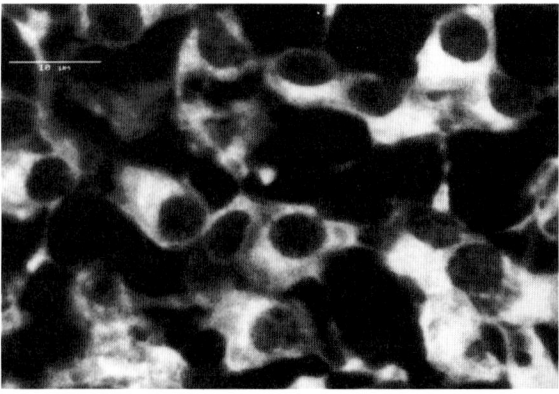

Figure 2.44 *Plasma cells secreting antibody. From an inflamed synovial membrane of a patient with rheumatoid arthritis (scale bar is 10 μm)*

lating in the region of parasitic invasion and damage. Another case where numerous eosinophils may be found is in **allergic conditions**, such as asthma, where nasal polypi may form containing very large numbers of eosinophils.

Fibroblasts are the collagen-producing cells and may be found in the periphery of granulomata, attempting to wall off the lesions, or may in fact be the prime component of the granuloma, as occurs in **silicosis** in the lung where the granulomata form in response to silica particle inhalation. In the case where constant damage to tissue characterizes the chronic inflammation, fibroblast proliferation and fibrosis may be a prominent feature of the body's attempts at healing, for example a chronic peptic ulcer.

Histological Structure of the Granuloma

The chronic inflammatory reaction is focal in its distribution, each focus being called a granuloma. Where the aetiological agent that has caused their formation is known, these granulomata are called **specific**. For example, in the case of tuberculosis the specific granulomata are known as **tubercles**. Other specific granulomata are those of leprosy, talc and histoplasmosis. In the cases where the aetiological agent that causes the granulomata is not known, they are called **non-specific**, as is the case with those of **sarcoidosis** or **Crohn's disease** (see Table 2.2).

If we examine a typical specific granuloma, the tubercle, it will be evident that the granuloma is mainly a collection of the pleomorphic infiltrate of chronic inflammation, with varying degrees of degeneration and necrosis. The structure of this typical granuloma is shown in Figure 2.45. The way in which these lesions develop is as follows. As soon as the *Mycobacterium tuberculosis* bacteria enter the tissues they stimulate a non-specific inflammatory response in which macrophages enter the tissues and start to phagocytose the bacteria. The macrophages cannot digest the bacteria, they secrete monokines which attract more macrophages and lymphocytes. Macrophages differentiate into epithelioid cells and giant cells and tissue damage occurs both through the direct toxic effects of the bacterial multiplication, and through the immune response harming the tissue. This has as an effect the creation of a central mass of **caseous necrosis**. In other types of granulomata, there may be coagulative necrosis (as in sarcoidosis) or fibrinoid necrosis (as in rheumatoid nodules). The central region of necrosis is surrounded by an area of epithelioid cells and macrophages, with occasional giant cells among them (mostly Langhan's giant cells in tubercles). Towards the periphery is a large zone of lymphocytes, some plasma cells (not many in TB), macrophages and finally a region of fibroblasts and collagen around them. As the infection progresses and more tissue is damaged, the granuloma may grow and coalesce with other

Table 2.2 *The causes of granulomatous inflammations*

Infectious	Non-infectious	Unknown cause
Mycobacterial infection • Tuberculosis • Atypical mycobacterioses • Leprosy • Other mycobacterioses Mycotic infection • Blastomycosis • Cryptococcosis • Coccidioidomycosis • Histoplasmosis Treponemal infection • Syphilis • Yaws Parasitic infections • Schistosomiasis	Chemical causes • Berylliosis • Talc granuloma Autoimmunity • Rheumatoid nodule • Granuloma of Crohn's disease	• Cat scratch disease • Sarcoidosis • Granuloma of Crohn's disease • Rheumatoid nodule

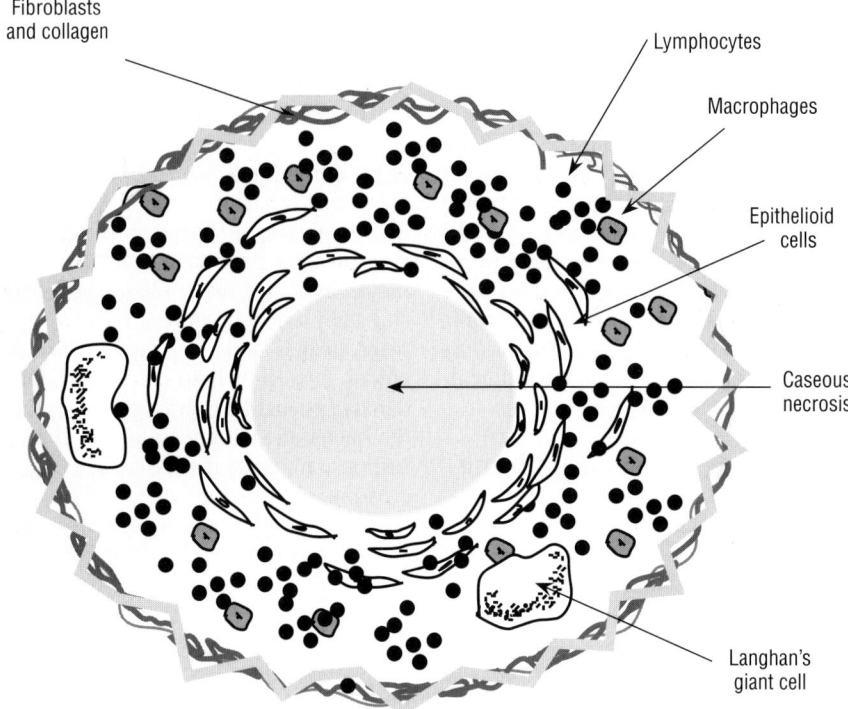

Figure 2.45 *This is a typical, specific, granuloma of chronic inflammation, the tubercle. It is specifically caused by infection with* Mycobacterium tuberculosis. *The hallmark of the tubercle is a central region of caseous necrosis, not found in other types of chronic inflammatory granulomata*

granulomata around it to form quite large lesions filled with extensive degenerating necrotic areas. Occasionally, the presence of the caseous material or other debris may stimulate an acute inflammatory response in which case there will be many neutrophils accumulating in the area, and even suppuration may be seen. The same will occur if secondary bacterial infections develop.

Pulmonary Tuberculosis

Tuberculosis is an infectious disease caused by a bacterium known as *Mycobacterium tuberculosis*. Rarely it may also be caused by atypical mycobacteria, such as *Mycobacterium bovis* (seen in cattle) or *Mycobacterium scrofulaceum*. The tubercle bacillus is a slender, acid-fast rod which stains by the Ziehl-Neelsen method. The cell wall contains complex lipid (mycolic acid) which elicits an immune response, a hypersensitivity, and may also have a role in production of caseous necrosis (caseation) seen in TB. The

disease is usually droplet-spread, where the infective droplets are inhaled via the airways. *M. bovis,* in the past, had been spread via the gastrointestinal tract through infected milk, but this is now rare due to cattle immunization and pasteurization of milk. There are two distinct phases in the development of tuberculosis: primary and post-primary (secondary) TB.

Primary Tuberculosis

Following exposure to the tubercle bacilli, usually from a person who already has the disease, in 95% of cases an asymptomatic primary infection will develop while 5% of cases will develop symptomatic infection and very few will develop a fulminating miliary TB (blood-spread of the organisms with involvement of many organs). Severe infection in this primary stage usually occurs in the very young, those with lowered resistance to infection, or those who have received a high infective dose of bacteria.

The site where the acid-fast bacilli lodge is the

alveoli, usually subpleurally in the mid-zone of the lung. Initially, neutrophils may ingest the bacilli but macrophages are recruited in larger numbers and after a few hours only macrophages will be found in the area. An inflammatory reaction ensues, and tubercle bacilli are ingested by macrophages but not killed. Few lymphocytes are involved at this stage as there is no immunity at first. A **Mantoux test** given at this time will be negative.

Over the next 2–3 weeks a tubercle develops at this primary site, with epithelioid cells, giant cells and lymphocytes. This primary lesion which is single and 1–2 cm in size is called the **Ghon focus**. Caseation is present and the tubercle enlarges gradually. The mycobacteria, in macrophages, spread to the local hilar lymph nodes in which tubercles and caseation also form. These caseous masses may be quite large. The combination of the Ghon focus and caseous lymph nodes is known as the **Ghon complex** or primary complex. The Ghon complex will most often heal by fibrosis and often calcify, becoming easily visible on a chest X-ray.

Occasionally the outcome is less favourable and the infection may progress and spread along the airways, giving rise to **tuberculous bronchopneumonia** ('galloping consumption'), or spread via the bloodstream, giving rise to **miliary TB**. In both these cases the infection is rapidly fatal.

In the usual case, with a healed Ghon complex the individual has now become sensitized to the tubercle bacilli and a challenge with the Mantoux test will be positive. It should be noted that viable mycobacteria may remain dormant in such lesions for many years and upon suitable circumstances may be reactivated to give rise to post-primary TB.

Post-primary (Secondary or 'Re-infection') Tuberculosis

Post-primary or re-infection tuberculosis occurs when there is already some immunity to the tubercle bacilli, either from prior primary infection or from BCG vaccination (a live vaccine using attenuated *M. bovis* named after its French discoverers as Bacille Calmette et Guérin). It may result from further inhalation of mycobacteria or it may be a reactivation of a dormant primary lesion, especially in cases of malnutrition, alcoholism or an illness which is debilitating.

It is in fact the immune response to *M. tuberculosis* which causes the damage to tissue, not the action of the bacteria themselves. The person infected with tubercle bacilli becomes sensitized to the bacteria, displaying a hypersensitivity which is cell-mediated

(T lymphocytes) and cytotoxic (causing tissue necrosis). It is a delayed hypersensitivity response (Type IV). In this response, the T lymphocytes which are sensitized will produce lymphokines to activate and stimulate macrophages which will then be more able to kill the tubercle bacilli. In the post-primary or re-infection phase of TB the lesion formed is usually in the apex of the lung which is well ventilated (*M. tuberculosis* is strictly aerobic and requires oxygen for growth). The right lung is often involved. In this case the lymph nodes are not usually involved but the lesion may consist of several tubercles which caseate and coalesce to form larger lesions. The progress of this phase is slower because of the partial immunity of the individual which means that the body is immune against the organisms and is attempting to resist the infection. The large caseous lesion may eventually liquefy (due to enzymatic action) and the liquid contents, containing living bacilli, may then be spread via bronchi or blood. A person is most infective when a discharging tuberculous cavity is present.

Miliary Tuberculosis

Spread of tubercle bacilli may occur via the bloodstream by erosion of a tubercle as it enlarges into the wall of a blood vessel. This causes a discharge of bacilli directly into the bloodstream, or by lymphatic spread into the thoracic ducts and into the venous blood. Miliary tuberculosis is so named because of the appearance of numerous tiny tubercles (which result from such widespread dissemination simultaneously) resembling tiny 'millet seeds' scattered throughout the tissues. Miliary TB is 100% fatal without antibiotics, most deaths being from tuberculous meningitis (Figures 2.46 and 2.47).

Tuberculous Bronchopneumonia

When the tubercles enlarge and erode an airway, the spread of tubercle bacilli along bronchi and bronchioles causes tuberculous bronchopneumonia which is also rapidly fatal without treatment. This used to be known as 'galloping consumption' because of the rapid death of the patient.

Other Complications

TB may be disseminated almost anywhere in the body: kidneys, brain, spine, bone, gastrointestinal tract and even skin. There may also be a direct involvement of

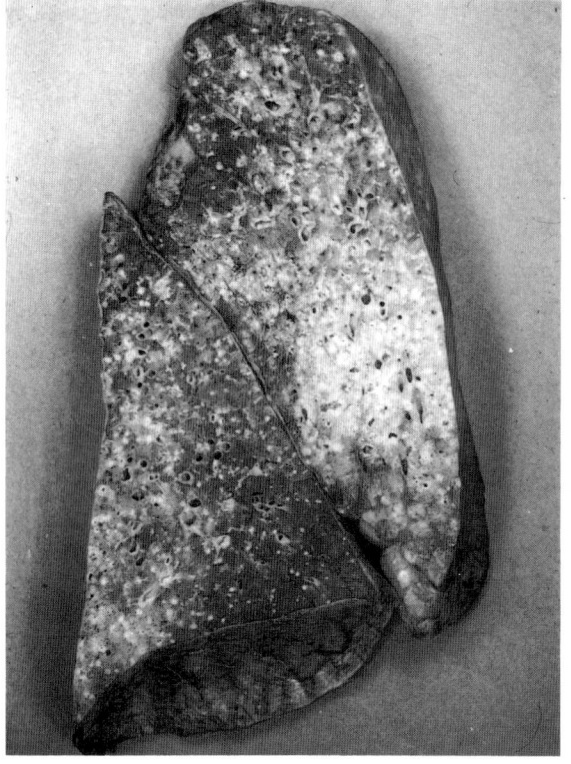

Figure 2.46   *Miliary tuberculosis of the lungs in a debilitated 70-year-old male*

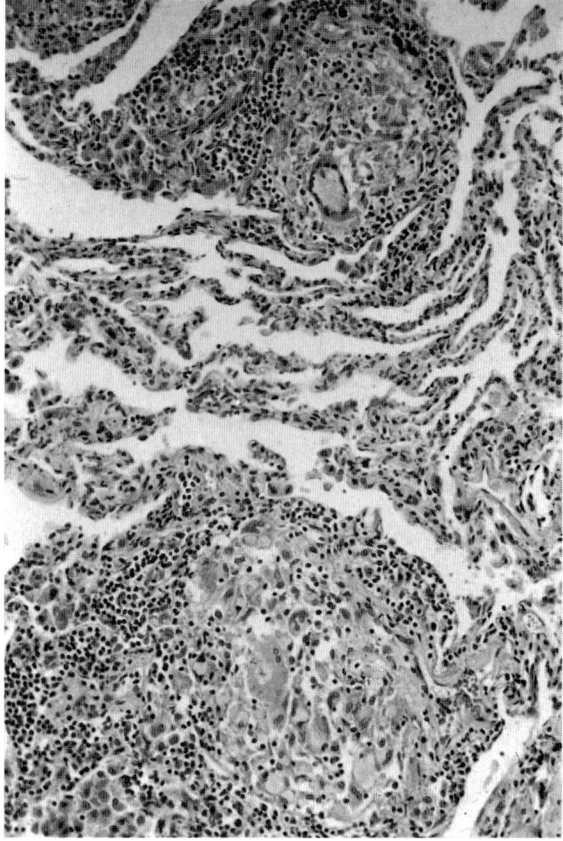

Figure 2.47   *Two tubercles in the lungs of a patient with a history of tuberculosis*

adjacent structures. Tuberculous pleurisy may be present which usually produces a serous effusion, and also the pericardium may be involved (tuberculous pericarditis). Even following treatment and 'healing' of tuberculosis it is possible for reactivation of the disease to occur. Reactivation appears to be associated with altered immunity. It is predisposed to by diabetes, chronic alcoholism, malignant disease (especially lymphosarcoma), steroid therapy, stress of various kinds.

Revision Questions and Case Studies

Injury and Necrosis

1. Write brief notes on the following:
   (a) Reactive changes of cells to mild injury
   (b) Pathological calcification
   (c) The body's reaction to dead tissue
2. Discuss the response of parenchymal cells to severe, lethal injury.

3. What different types of necrosis may occur in the body? Discuss the characteristic features of each of these types of necrosis and give an example of each one.
4. What is meant by the term 'biochemical necrosis' when it is applied to a cell responding to injury?
5. Differentiate between the following terms and give examples of these processes:
   (a) Fatty change
   (b) Fat necrosis
6. What occurs in the process of reactive changes to injury? Outline these processes if they occur as a result of ischaemia in the myocardium. Differentiate between the various forms of reactive changes and give examples of other types of injury that may cause such changes in various tissues.
7. List the various genetically determined forms of disease and give two diseases as an example of each aetiology.
8. List the various causes of acquired disease and give two disorders as an example of each cause.

9. Outline the process of necrosis as it occurs in a region of the myocardium.
10. Differentiate between dystrophic calcification and metastatic calcification and give an example of a disease in which each one occurs.
11. What is an iatrogenic disease? Give three examples of such disease.
12. Differentiate between the following factors in the causation of disease:
    (a) Causative agent
    (b) Predisposing factor
    (c) Contributory factor
13. State the characteristic type of necrosis that would be associated with the following disorders:
    (a) A region of anoxic necrosis in the myocardium
    (b) A region of anoxic necrosis in the spleen
    (c) A region of necrosis in the omentum in association with pancreatic damage
    (d) Infection of tissue with *Mycobacterium tuberculosis*
    (e) Infection of tissue with *Treponema pallidum*
    (f) Infection of tissue with *Clostridium perfringens*
    (g) Infection of tissue with *Staphylococcus aureus*
    (h) A region of anoxic necrosis in the brain
    (i) The wall of a small arteriole in the kidney of a patient with hypertension
    (j) A region of anoxic necrosis in the wall of a vein
14. What is meant by the term 'differential diagnosis'?
15. Distinguish between the following terms:
    (a) Remission
    (b) Relapse
    (c) Cure
    (d) Exacerbation

16. Which departments or specialities of pathology would be important in the diagnosis of the following diseases?
    (a) Diabetes mellitus (a disease characterized by raised levels of blood sugar)
    (b) Breast cancer (a disease in which abnormal cells are found in the breast tissue)
    (c) Down's syndrome (a disease where there is an abnormal chromosome number in all cells of the body)
    (d) Lobar pneumonia (a bacterial infection of the lungs)
    (e) Di-George syndrome (a disease where there is abnormal immune function)
    (f) Iron deficiency anaemia
    (g) Leukaemia (a disease where there are increased numbers of abnormal white cells in the circulation)
    (h) Cancer of the cervix (a disease where abnormal cells are proliferating on the lining of the uterine cervix)
    (i) Phenylketonuria (a genetic disease where increased levels of abnormal metabolites are found in the blood and urine)
    (j) Tuberculosis of the lungs (a bacterial infection of the lungs)
17. Define the following terms:
    (a) Autolysis
    (b) Heterolysis
    (c) Autophagy
    (d) Karyorrhexis
18. Differentiate between biochemical necrosis and histological necrosis.

Case study 1. Below is a photograph of a chromosome spread prepared from dividing bone marrow cells de-

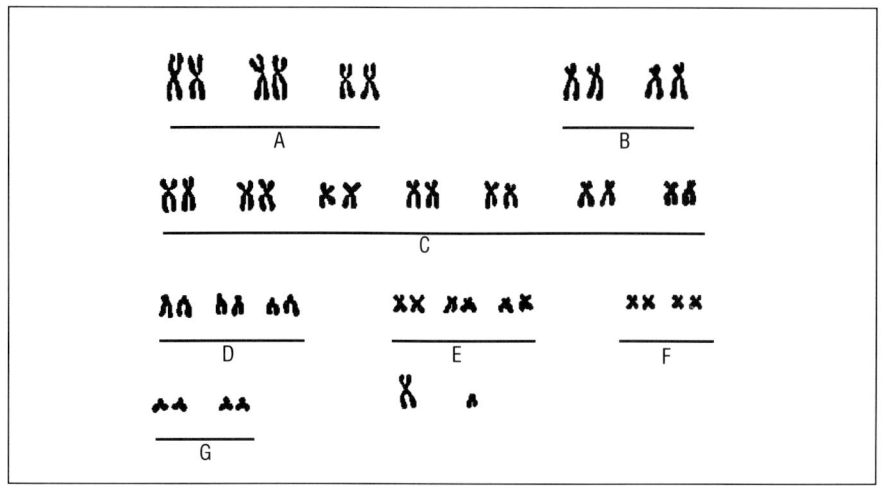

rived from a 9-month-old Caucasian male, rather pale, with blue eyes and sandy-coloured hair, who shows evidence of failure to thrive, increased myotonus, dermatitis and mental retardation (delayed development, behaving as 4 month old). The baby was delivered on a sheep station by the boy's father and there were no obstetric complications, the father having been a male nurse in the past. The parents of the baby are both normal. Biochemical tests have been ordered on the baby's urine and blood.

(a) Give the karyotype and identify the abnormality, if any, in the chromosome spread.
(b) What is the differential diagnosis?
(c) What is the most likely diagnosis?
(d) What is the incidence of this disorder?
(e) How is this disorder normally diagnosed?

Case study 2. A 51-year-old Aboriginal male is admitted to hospital with a presumptive clinical diagnosis of 'taboparesis'. The patient was exposed to *Treponema pallidum* 25 years ago and serological tests are positive for syphilis and hepatitis B. A sample of cerebrospinal fluid reveals the following results after biochemical and microscopic analysis: protein, 95 mg/100ml (N = 15–45); glucose, 70 mg/100ml (N = 50–80); chloride, 715 mg/100ml (N = 710–750); cells, 67 lymphocytes/ml (N = up to 5/ml); organisms, nil cultured.

The patient has a staggering gait, impaired postural adjustment, and Charcot's joints in the knee and hip, with gross swelling with effusion in the joint. X-ray examination reveals articular cartilage destruction and osteophyte formation, with calcification of the capsular tissues. While in hospital the patient commits suicide by jumping off a fourth floor balcony. An autopsy is carried out and examination of the brain reveals thickened and opaque meninges firmly adherent to an atrophic, small brain with wide sulci and shrunken gyri. When sectioned the brain shows a loss of the normal distinct line of demarcation between the thinned grey matter and the white matter. In the spinal cord there is marked decrease in the size of the dorsal columns, maximal in the lumbar region, with atrophy of the posterior roots and thickening of the meningeal membranes, more so posteriorly.

(a) Is the presumptive clinical diagnosis correct?
(b) What is the causative agent and what is the stage of the disease?
(c) What is the characteristic necrosis that is associated with this disorder? Describe an area of this necrotic tissue as it would appear to the naked eye.

(d) Why were there no organisms isolated from the cerebrospinal fluid?

Acute Inflammation

1. What is inflammation? Discuss the process of acute inflammation with special reference to characterizing features, forms of presentation, cellular aspects and macroscopic appearance of inflamed sites.
2. Discuss the formation of an abscess after the introduction of bacteria into the liver and indicate the possible sequelae of this disorder.
3. Discuss the process of acute inflammation and indicate its characteristics, various forms, macroscopical and microscopical features. Outline the steps in the formation of exudate and infiltrate and the possible sequelae of the inflammation. Ensure that you cover thoroughly the clinical manifestations of the acute inflammatory response and also that you explain the purpose and advantageous effects of this process.
4. Describe all the possible sequelae that may occur in tissue after completion of the acute phase of inflammation, and give examples of each.
5. Discuss the mechanism of formation of inflammatory exudate in acute inflammation.
6. Of what significance is the technique of vascular labelling in studies of acute inflammation?
7. Explain the sequence of events leading to the formation of inflammatory exudate in a typical biphasic response (e.g. sunburn). Ensure that you explain why two peaks are observed in the formation of inflammatory exudate with this type of response.
8. Distinguish between the various types of inflammatory exudate and give a situation in the body and condition as an example of each one:
    (a) Serous exudate
    (b) Fibrinous exudate
    (c) Suppurative exudate
    (d) Haemorrhagic exudate
9. Outline in detail the various functions and beneficial effects of the acute inflammatory response.
10. What is the role of complement in the acute inflammatory response?
11. How are prostaglandins involved in acute inflammation?
12. Explain briefly the way in which normal Starling forces are instrumental in the formation of interstitial fluid.
13. Why does a fever often accompany an acute inflammatory response?

14. What are the effects of histamine on blood vessels in acute inflammation?
15. What is the function of the macrophage?
16. What is meant by the term 'diapedesis' and which are the first cells that take part in this process in acute inflammation?
17. What are the five cardinal signs of acute inflammation? What processes occurring in the microvasculature account for these changes that are seen with the naked eye in the tissues?
18. What determines whether regeneration or repair will occur in a tissue that has been injured and inflamed?

Wound and Bone Fracture Healing

1. It has been said that the healing of wounds in the soft tissues resembles very much the healing of a fractured bone. Discuss, comparing and contrasting the two types of healing.
2. Describe the appearance of the margin of an uncomplicated healing wound (at 4 days) as it appears microscopically and indicate the significance of the structures present.
3. What is a myofibroblast? Where is it found and what is its function?
4. What are some of the factors delaying wound healing and which one of these is the most commonly encountered?
5. What is a pseudoarthrosis and what is a common way in which it may form in a bone?
6. Describe the structure of granulation tissue and indicate its function by noting what its result is.
7. What is a callus and what is its function?
8. When is a bone fracture called a 'pathological fracture'? Give three examples of pathological fractures.
9. Distinguish wound healing by primary intention and wound healing by secondary intention.
10. What is keloid and under what circumstances is it likely to form?
11. Discuss the factors that are important in delaying or impairing bone fracture healing.
12. Define the following terms:
    (a) Avulsion wound
    (b) Avulsion fracture
    (c) Contusion
    (d) Laceration
13. What is meant by the term 'arthroplasty' and when is it necessary to resort to such a procedure?
14. What are some of the factors that contribute to the delay in wound and fracture healing that is seen in old age?

15. What is meant by the term 'débridement'? Why is this important in wound healing?
16. What is meant by the term 'simplification' of a wound?

Case study 1. A 74-year-old Caucasian woman has undergone treatment in the past 2 years for breast cancer (including mastectomy, chemotherapy and radiotherapy). She has now been admitted to hospital after what has seemed to be a spontaneous, compression fracture of one of her lumbar vertebrae.

(a) What possible explanations can you offer as to why the normal stresses of daily life on the bone in this case should have been enough to fracture it?
(b) What treatment is available in cases such as this?
(c) Will the bone fracture heal in this particular instance?

Case study 2. A 19-year-old Caucasian male motorcyclist sustains the following injuries in an traffic accident: a comminuted, compound fracture of the right femur, bilateral simple and complete radial neck fractures with a partial fracture of the right clavicle. By the time he is examined in casualty the thigh injury has been in contact with dirt and gravel for more than 6 hours.

(a) Which of the above fractures is likely to heal the most quickly and how long would this take (approximately)?
(b) What is the usual form of treatment for fractures of the neck of the radius?
(c) What are the possible complications that may occur in the fracture of the femur as described above?

Case study 3. While walking down the street you see an elderly woman in front of you trip, slip and fall gently a short distance along the footpath. Despite what has seemed to you to be a 'soft fall' the woman complains of excruciating pain in her left hip and on examining it you suspect the possibility of a fracture of the head of the femur. Assuming that your diagnosis is correct:

(a) Why has the minimal stress on the bone in this case been enough to fracture it?
(b) What would you do to help the woman?
(c) Would this woman be a likely candidate for arthroplasty of the hip? Why/why not?

Case study 4. A 43-year-old Caucasian female presents at a clinic with a burn wound on her right forearm which she sustained while cooking 6 days ago. She informs you that she treated it herself by washing it immediately with cold water and then by bandaging it for a couple of days. You examine the wound and observe: an irregular, 4 cm in diameter, very red wound which is markedly swollen. The exudate on the surface is thick and copious and in the depth of the wound you see some pus. The edges of the wound are red and swollen and the surrounding skin is also inflamed. Palpating the left axillary lymph nodes you find them enlarged and tender. You see signs of lymphangitis on the forearm.

(a) What is the presumptive diagnosis?
(b) What steps are to be taken in definitive diagnosis and treatment?

Chronic Inflammation

1. Compare and contrast the processes of acute and chronic inflammation. Mention macroscopic and microscopic appearance, characteristics of the cellular response, various presentations in different tissues and the sequelae of these processes.
2. Describe the histological criteria distinguishing acute and chronic inflammation. Discuss briefly some of the factors which may contribute to the chronicity of the response.
3. Is the chronic inflammatory response of benefit to the body? (*Hint:* Think of the cell types that are involved in this process.)
4. Describe briefly the various forms of the chronic inflammatory response.
5. Describe the appearance of a typical granuloma as seen with the naked eye and as it appears under the microscope.
6. Distinguish between specific and non-specific granulomata and give two examples of each of these types of granuloma.
7. What is the function of epithelioid cells?
8. Discuss the active chronic inflammatory response and give examples of such a reaction in tissues.
9. How does tuberculosis develop in human tissue? Differentiate between primary and secondary tuberculosis and explain what a Ghon focus is in your answer.
10. Define the following terms:
    (a) Ankylosis
    (b) Stenosis
    (c) Furuncle
    (d) Carbuncle
    (e) Ulcer
11. Differentiate between tuberculous bronchopneumonia and miliary tuberculosis.
12. What is meant by the term 'pleomorphic, productive response' when used to describe the chronic inflammatory response.
13. What is the function of the lymphocyte?
14. Differentiate between the following granulomata, stating whether they are infectious or non-infectious and specific or non-specific:
    (a) Tubercle
    (b) Sarcoid granuloma
    (c) Leproma
    (d) Talc granuloma
    (e) Granuloma of Crohn's disease
    (f) Syphiloma
    (g) Granuloma of berylliosis
15. What evidence is there that immune factors are important when the body mounts a chronic inflammatory response?
16. In a chronic abscess, surrounding the central region of pus there are many plasma cells in the granulation tissue. What is the function of these cells in this instance?

Case study. A 28-year-old Indian male is admitted to hospital with a presumptive diagnosis of 'gangrene' in the index and middle fingers of the right hand. Upon examination he is found to have anaesthesia of the affected digits but also of the ring finger of the right hand, of the digits of the other hand and of the toes on both feet. The two affected digits are severely damaged by repeated trauma which the patient has not felt. There is considerable damage to these digits and there is infection, considerable blackening and a foetid smell. The patient migrated to Australia 15 years ago from Calcutta to join his sister who was already living in Melbourne. He is married with one 4-year-old child. The right index and middle fingers are surgically amputated and laboratory investigation indicates the presence of acid-fast bacilli, free in the tissue and within macrophages.

(a) What is the diagnosis?
(b) What is the characteristic microscopical lesion associated with this disorder?
(c) Is this a curable disease? What is the treatment?

Response to Injury Crossword

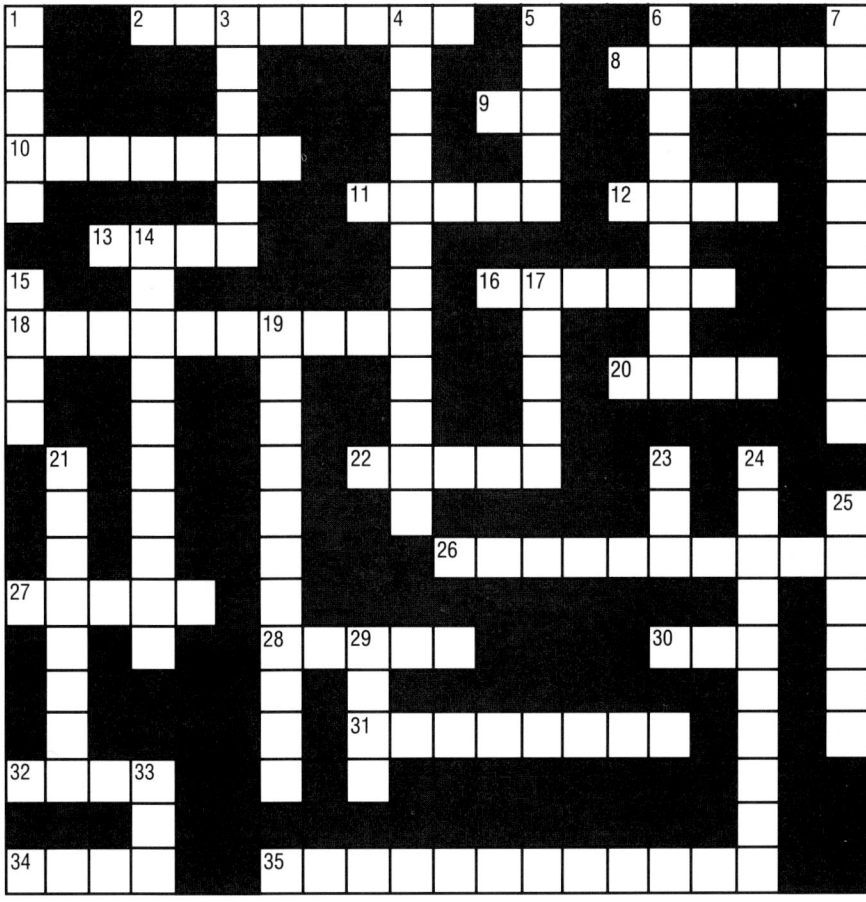

CLUES

ACROSS

2. A German pathologist of the 19th century who described the miscroscopic changes occurring in inflammation (8).
8. The solid network-like protein that forms when plasma proteins leak out of vessels in inflammation (6).
9. A disease that causes tubercles to form in tissues (2).
10. The fluid part of the acute inflammatory response is called thus (7).
11. One of the cardinal signs of acute inflammation, due to vasodilatation (5).
12. If this powder enters tissue a granuloma will form (4).
13. The end result of the fibrous form of the chronic inflammatory response (4).
16. The complete stoppage of blood flow in an acutely inflamed tissue (6).
18. Increased blood flow through a tissue during acute inflammation (10).
20. This cardinal sign of acute inflammation is only observed in inflamed skin (4).
22. Raised tissue pressure due to swelling and direct effects of mediators and tissue breakdown products cause this cardinal sign of acute inflammation (5).
26. This cell gives rise to the epithelioid cells and giant cells in the granulomata of chronic inflammation (10)

27. He described the triple response of acute inflammation (5).
28. Excess tissue fluid and inflammatory exudate will eventually be absorbed and form this fluid (5).
30. A factor causing delay in wound and fracture healing (3).
31. He described the forces (bearing his name) that are acting on small blood vessels and which are important in the formation of tissue fluid (8).
32. A tropical disease, similar to syphilis, causing granulomata in tissues, caused by *Treponema pertenue* (4).
34. The dried coagulum that covers the surface of a healing wound is called thus (4).
35. The process whereby cells take up particles into their cytoplasm in order to destroy and digest them (12).

DOWN

1. Higher than normal body temperature (5).
3. An 18th century English pathologist who stated that inflammation was a salutary process (6).
4. Response of connective tissues to sublethal injury (12).
5. One of the cardinal signs of acute inflammation (5).
6. An inflammatory mediator causing vasodilatation, hyperaemia and increased vascular permeability (9).
7. The cellular parts of the inflammatory response (10).
14. The ordered movement of cells, in response to a chemical gradient (9).
15. The _ _ _ _ focus is the first site affected in pulmonary tuberculosis (4).
17. The swelling that is seen as a cardinal sign in acute inflammation (5).
19. This cell type lines all blood vessels in all parts of the body (11).
21. A small, window-like pore that is found in some types of endothelium in the body (8).
23. Histamine induces the formation of a _ _ _ in the endothelial cell junction (3).
24. Passage of cells through junctions of endothelium (10).
25. Healing through the formation of scar (6).
29. The _ _ _ _ cell secretes histamine (4).
33. _ _ _ acute inflammation is one lasting for days to weeks (3).

Further Reading

Injury and Necrosis

Arends MJ, Wyllie AH. 'Apoptosis: Mechanisms and Roles in Pathology.' *Int Rev Exp Pathol* 1991; **32**: 223.

Arstila AU, Hirsimäki P, Trump BF. 'Studies on the Subcellular Pathophysiology of Sublethal Chronic Cell Injury.' *Beitr Pathol* 1974; **152**: 211.

Cheung JY, Bonventre JV, Malis CD, Leaf A. 'Calcium and Ischemic Injury.' *N Eng J Med* 1986; **314**: 1670.

Connor JM, Ferguson-Smith MA. *Essential Medical Genetics*, third edition, 1991; Blackwell Scientific Publications Ltd, Oxford.

Duvall E, Wyllie AH. 'Death and the Cell.' *Immunol Today* 1986; **7**: 115.

Emery AEH, Rimoin DL. *The Principles and Practice of Medical Genetics*, second edition, 1990; Churchill Livingstone, Edinburgh.

Holloway M. 'Fetal Law. Experimental Surgery May Feed Ethical Debates.' *Sci Am* 1990; September: 17.

Searle J, Kerr JFR, Bishop CJ. 'Necrosis and Apoptosis.' *Pathol Annu* 1982; **17**(2): 229.

Trump BF, Laiho KA, Mergner J, Arstila AU. 'Studies on the Subcellular Pathophysiology of Acute Lethal Cell Injury.' *Beitr Pathol* 1974; **152**: 243.

Walker NI, *et al.* 'Patterns of Cell Death.' *Meth Arch Exp Pathol* 1988; **13**: 18.

Wyllie AH. 'Commentary: What is Apoptosis?' *Histopathology* 1986; **10**: 995.

Acute Inflammation

Cohnheim J. *Lectures in General Pathology*, Translated by McKee AD, 1889; New Sydenham Society, London.

Colditz IG. 'The Margination and Emigration of Leukocytes.' *Surv Synth Pathol Res* 1985; **4**: 44.

Finlay-Jones J, Kenny P, Hart P, Nulsen M, McDonald P. 'Abscesses.' *Today's Life Sci* 1990; **2**(7): 38.

Hurley JV. *Acute Inflammation*, second edition, 1983; Churchill Livingstone, Edinburgh.

Issekutz AC. 'Role of the Polymorphonuclear Leukocytes in the Vascular Responses of Acute Inflammation.' *Lab Invest* 1984; **50**: 605.

Majno G, Palade GE. 'Studies on Inflammation I. The Effect of Histamine and Serotonin on Vascular Permeability: An Electron Microscopic Study.' *J Biophys Biochem Cytol* 1961; **11**: 571.

Majno G, *et al.* 'Studies on Inflammation II. Effects of Histamine and Serotonin Along the Vascular Tree: A Topographic Study.' *J Biophys Biochem Cytol* 1961; **11**: 607.

Movat HZ (ed.). *The Inflammatory Reaction*, 1986; Elsevier, Amsterdam.

Parish C, Willenborg D, Cowden W. 'Novel Inhibitors of Inflammation.' *Today's Life Sci* 1990: **2**(7): 20.

Ryan GB, Majno G. 'Acute Inflammation.' *Am J Pathol* 1977; **86**: 183.

Smith W, Matthias L, Gamble J, Vadas M. 'Endothelial Cells and the Regulation of Inflammation.' *Today's Life Sci* 1989; **1**(5): 26.

Stossel TP. 'Phagocytosis.' *Semin Haematol* 1975; **12**: 83.

Wound and Bone Fracture Healing

Clark RAF, Henson PM (eds). *The Molecular and Cellular Biology of Wound Repair*, 1988; Plenum Press, New York.

Gabbiani G, Ryan GB, Majno G. 'Presence of Modified Fibroblasts in Granulation Tissue and their Possible Role in Wound Contraction.' *Experientia* 1971; **27**: 549.

Hamlyn Publishing Group. *Surgery Today*, 1969; Life, Love and Family Health Series, Marshall Cavendish Ltd, London.

Heughan C, Hunt TK. 'Some Aspects of Wound Healing Research.' *Can J Surg* 1975; **18**: 118.

Ingber DE, Folkman J. 'How Does Extracellular Matrix Control Capillary Morphogenesis?' *Cell* 1989; **58**: 803.

Ketchum LD, Cohen IK, Masters FW. 'Hypertrophic Scars and Keloids.' *Plast Reconstr Surg* 1974; **53**: 140.

Knapp TR, Daniels JR, Kaplan EN. 'Pathologic Scar Formation.' *Am J Pathol* 1977; **86**: 47.

Majno G. 'The Story of the Myofibroblasts.' *Am J Surg Pathol* 1979; **3**: 535.

McKibbin B. 'The Biology of Fracture Healing in Long Bones.' *J Bone Joint Surg* 1978; **60**(B): 150.

Montandon D, D'Andrian G, Gabbiani G. 'The Mechanism of Wound Contraction and Epithelialization.' *Clin Plast Surg* 1977; **4**: 325.

Sevitt E (ed.). *Bone Repair and Fracture Healing in Man*, 1981; Churchill Livingstone, Edinburgh.

Shosham S. 'Wound Healing.' *Int Rev Conn Tiss Res* 1981; **9**: 1.

Smith R. 'Recovery and Tissue Repair.' *Br Med Bull* 1985; **41**: 295.

Sporn MB, Roberts AB. 'Peptide Growth Factors and Inflammation, Tissue Repair and Cancer.' *J Clin Invest* 1986; **78**: 329.

Chronic Inflammation

Beutler B, Cerami A. 'The Biology of Cachectin/TNF-α.' *Ann Rev Immunol* 1989; **7**: 625.

Boros DL. 'Granulomatous Inflammations.' *Prog Allergy* 1978; **24**: 13.

Epstein WL. 'Granuloma Formation in Man.' *Pathobiol Annu* 1977; **7**: 1.

Kunkel SL, *et al.* 'Cellular and Molecular Aspects of Granulomatous Inflammation.' *Am J Resp Cell Mol Biol* 1989; **1**: 439.

Lucas SB. 'Histopathology of Leprosy and Tuberculosis — An Overview.' *Br Med Bull* 1988; **44**: 584.

Nathan CF. 'Secretory Products of Macrophages.' *J Clin Invest* 1987; **79**: 319.

Sheffield EA. 'Editorial: The Granulomatous Inflammatory Response.' *J Path* 1990; **160**: 1.

Smith KA. 'Interleukin-2.' *Sci Am* 1990; March: 26.

Sutton JS, Weiss L. 'Transformation of Monocytes in Tissue Culture into Macrophages, Epithelioid Cells and Multinucleated Giant Cells: An Electron Microscopic Study.' *J Cell Biol* 1966; **28**: 303.

Unanue ER. 'Co-operation between Mononuclear Phagocytes and Lymphocytes in Immunity.' *N Eng J Med* 1980; **303**: 977.

3

Fluid Disturbances, Blood and Vascular Disorders

Disturbances in the body fluids and vessels are a very important group of disorders as they are extremely common in incidence and may be sufficiently severe to cause death. As blood vessels and body fluids are found in all parts of the body, diseases affecting these two elements affect any tissue of the body, or, as occurs frequently, the whole body may show evidence of the effects of such diseases.

Arterial disorders and their complications are directly responsible for approximately half of all deaths in the Western world. Atherosclerosis and its complications in the form of thrombosis, embolism and infarction are the prime cause of 'heart attacks' and 'strokes'. Hypertension (high blood pressure) is commonly associated with many of these disorders.

One disorder in the group of these body fluid and vascular disorders may directly cause another, or it may be so intimately linked with it that it is only a matter of time before one disorder will bring about the other as a sequela. Hypertension, for example, is a major risk factor in atherosclerosis and people with high blood pressure will develop atherosclerosis more rapidly and more severely than the person with normal blood pressure. Once atherosclerosis has developed in a vessel, thrombosis (clotting of blood inside the vessel) will supervene and this will bring about infarction (ischaemic necrosis).

Oedema

Oedema is the abnormal accumulation of fluid in the intercellular tissue spaces or in the body cavities. It should not be confused with swelling which may be due to an intracellular accumulation of fluid. When something is swollen it may or may not be oedematous. The intracellular increase in fluid is a reactive change of cells to injury and is called hydropic change and is due to a disturbance of the sodium/potassium pump in the cell membrane. Oedema is due to accumulation of fluid in the extracellular spaces and is almost always due to disruption of the normal Starling forces acting across vessel walls. The difference between oedema and hydropic change is shown in Figure 3.1.

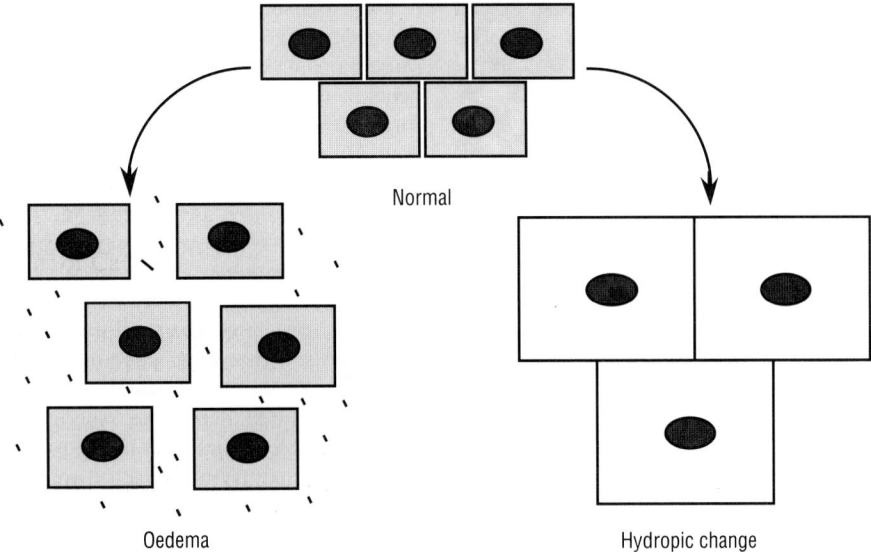

Normal

Oedema

Hydropic change

Figure 3.1 *Oedema compared to hydropic change*

Oedema may occur as a localized process, for example seen only in one organ or one limb, or it may be systemic (or generalized) where it causes diffuse swelling of all tissues and organs of the body, becoming very obvious in the subcutaneous tissues. In this latter case it is often referred to as **anasarca**. Collection of oedema fluid in the peritoneal cavity is called **ascites** and may cause gross swelling of the abdomen. Oedema in the pleural cavity is called **hydrothorax** and in the pericardium **hydropericardium**. The older terms hydrops and dropsy which also refer to generalized oedema are rarely used nowadays.

Non-inflammatory oedema fluids which have a low protein content are known as transudates while the protein-rich fluids forming in areas which are acutely inflamed are called exudates. The determination of protein content of the oedema fluid in a patient may be used to find out if the patient has, say, an uncomplicated heart failure and a pleural transudate or whether there is a superimposed infection in the lungs, yielding an exudate.

Localized Oedema

Localized oedema is seen most commonly in sites which are inflamed and where there is a localized increase in the vascular permeability. **Inflammatory oedema** and the factors which lead to its development were mentioned earlier: active hyperaemia of the region, increased osmotic pressure of the interstitial fluid, increased hydrostatic pressure in the capillaries and increased vascular permeability. In this case the localized oedema is a protein-rich exudate and is most usually quite quickly resorbed. It must be kept in mind that active hyperaemia may occur under physiological situations also, for example in exercising muscle where there may be transient formation of a transudate leading to a short-lived local oedema. The prominence of the muscles in an exercising athlete are a typical example of this process of physiological oedema due to increased blood flow.

Localized oedema is also a feature of many **allergic** or **hypersensitivity reactions**, for example hay fever, hives and the Arthus reaction. These reactions are all inflammatory in nature and the oedema is due to the accumulation of exudate which persists as long as the cause of the allergy persists.

Another cause of local oedema is the **obstruction of lymphatics**. The cause of obstruction may be a tumour, trauma and injury, inflammation and scarring, radiotherapy, or protozoan infestations such as filariasis which block the lymphatics. Under normal conditions the lymphatics constantly drain small amounts of fluid from the interstitial spaces. When the lymphatics are blocked the tissue fluid increases in volume causing swelling and concurrently increasing tissue pressure causing more fibrous tissue to be laid down, leading to gross thickening of the tissue. In long-standing cases the skin swells and thickens so much that it resembles the skin of elephants. The deformed oedematous and thickened limbs of such people are shaped like those of elephants hence the term **elephantiasis** to describe this condition.

Impaired venous drainage of an area, whatever its cause, can sufficiently raise the capillary pressure, leading to the formation of local oedema in an area. Phlebothromboses (blood clotting in the veins), especially seen in the leg veins, or with incompetent venous valves commonly encountered in varicose veins and compression of the veins by external pressures (e.g. garters!) may cause localized oedema.

Even in the normal individual, the legs remaining immobile for long periods of time (sitting or standing for many hours) may cause oedema of the legs and feet. This is due to the lack of leg muscle movement which normally aids the drainage of blood from the leg veins. Venous return of blood depends much on muscular movement and if the legs are immobile there is a pooling of blood in the veins with a rise in venous blood pressure, resulting in oedema.

Generalized Oedema

In the human, generalized oedema is not detectable unless an extra five kilograms of water is retained in the tissues. It first becomes noticeable in the extremi-

ties and is usually called **pitting oedema** since when the oedematous region is depressed with the finger a pit remains when the finger is withdrawn. Generalized oedema is seen in many diseases, including various forms of heart disease, renal disease, liver disease and endocrine disorders.

Right heart failure. In this case the right heart is not pumping blood fast enough, leading to a generalized increase in the venous pressure which causes an increased hydrostatic pressure within the capillaries and the formation of extra tissue fluid. However, this is not enough to cause oedema since the lymphatics are able to cope with the excess fluid, removing it from the area. Underlying endocrine pathogenic mechanisms are responsible as outlined in Figure 3.2.

The major contributing factor important in this case as well as in many other cases of generalized oedema is that the reduced blood flow through the kidney causes it to secrete increased amounts of renin. This stimulates the adrenal cortex to secrete more aldosterone. The resulting hyperaldosteronism has the effect of increased sodium retention by the kidney which causes the pituitary gland to secrete antidiuretic hormone, the overall result being that more water is retained by the body contributing to the oedema caused by the right heart failure. The importance of water and sodium retention in the causation of this type of oedema

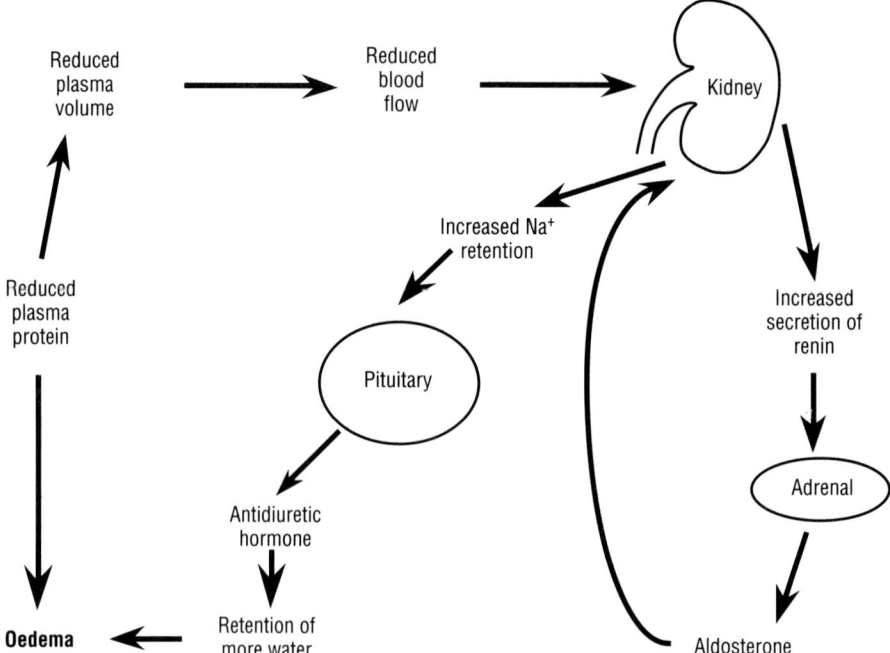

Figure 3.2 *Mechanism underlying the pathogenesis of generalized oedema*

is shown by the benefits of drugs which promote water and sodium excretion, leading to control of the oedema (these drugs are termed **diuretics**).

Renal disease. Diseases such as glomerulonephritis, acute renal failure and others which cause the loss of much protein in the urine may cause oedema. This is because the plasma protein level goes down as protein is lost from the kidney in the urine and the lowered plasma proteins interfere with the normal Starling forces, with the formation of oedema. Once again the reduced plasma volume activates the aldosterone, anti-diuretic hormone system which retains more sodium and water in the body. As more water is retained the plasma is further diluted and a vicious cycle is created.

Cirrhosis of the liver. This is sometimes the cause of generalized oedema and in particular, often leads to ascites. Two major mechanisms are involved: (1) injury to the liver with loss of the synthesis of plasma albumin; and (2) the development of portal hypertension which is due to the widespread scarring within the liver. As much as 5 or 10 litres of fluid may accumulate and again a mechanism of sodium retention is thought to act and to contribute to the formation of the oedema.

Malnutrition. This may cause oedema as is exemplified by the disease kwashiorkor, which is a form of dietary deficiency of protein. The level of plasma proteins decreases as an effect of the lack of proteins in the diet and the decreased osmotic pressure in the plasma leads to the formation of oedema.

Other clinical states. Oedema can be caused by certain other conditions such as protein loss from the intestine, normal pregnancy, toxaemia in pregnancy, idiopathic cyclic oedema in women and the ingestion of certain drugs, the prime example being oestrogen. The pathogenesis of the disease varies from one to the other of these disease states but the oedema seen with them is rarely as severe as that encountered with the causes mentioned above. Oestrogen causes oedema by acting to stimulate sodium and water retention. The mild cyclic oedema which is seen in many normal women of child-bearing age is a response to fluctuating oestrogen levels during the menstrual cycle.

Oedema of the brain and lungs is the most life threatening form of abnormal fluid retention. Oedema in the brain is important since any increase in the volume of fluid within the cranium will cause an increase in intracranial pressure as the fluid accumulates within a confined space. In the lungs accumulation of fluid within the alveoli will seriously affect respiration, resulting in a water-logged lung which may result in the 'drowning' of the patient.

Brain oedema is encountered with brain trauma, infections, hypertensive crises and obstruction to the venous outflow. The oedematous brain is heavier than normal, the sulci are narrowed and the swollen gyri are flattened where they press against the skull. The ventricles are compressed and on section the white matter may appear soft and gelatinous. The grey matter may appear widened. There is much accumulation of fluid within the actual brain substance and swelling of the neurones and glial cells is also present (Figure 3.3).

Swelling of the brain leads to increased intracranial pressure with resultant headaches, vomiting and convulsive seizures. Herniation of the brain stem or cerebellar tonsils into the foramen magnum may precipitate death. Cerebral oedema may develop within hours of brain injury, requiring immediate corrective steps to save the patient's life.

Pulmonary oedema is a very common clinical problem and is seen in left ventricular failure, renal disease, shock, infections and allergies within the lungs. The oedema is usually confined to or more marked in the lower lobes. In long-standing conditions, however, all lobes may become affected. The lungs assume a rubbery, gelatinous consistency and if they are cut a frothy, blood-stained fluid escapes. Under the microscope there may be seen widening of the alveolar walls, but most evident is the precipitation of a granular pink, protein-poor coagulum in the alveoli.

When present for protracted time intervals this fluid is prone to infections, producing a pneumonia which in this case is called a **hypostatic pneumonia**. Pulmonary oedema is important since it impedes the normal

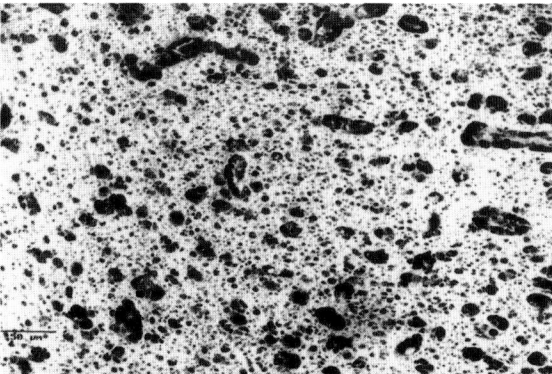

Figure 3.3 *Oedema of the cerebrum after head trauma. The neurones have liquefied and much oedema fluid may be seen around the blood vessels (scale bar is 50 μm)*

ventilatory function of the lungs. Characteristically as the respired air bubbles through the fluid within the alveoli, a variety of abnormal air sounds, called **rales**, are produced. In extremely advanced cases there are extremely loud rales, popularly called the 'death rattle'.

Haemostasis and Haemorrhage

Haemorrhage, or 'bleeding', may be defined as the escape of blood from the circulation. This may be due to: **trauma** causing rupture of vessels; **disease** of the vascular wall, for example atheroma, which weakens the wall, leading to rupture of the vessel; or **blood clotting failure** so that even slight damage to vessels cannot be 'plugged up' to prevent blood loss.

Haemostasis

Before discussing haemorrhage it is important to understand haemostasis, which is the process of preventing blood loss from the circulation. Whenever a blood vessel is severed or ruptured haemostasis ensures that vascular changes, coagulation of blood and subsequent repair mechanisms stop the loss of blood from the circulation. In order to preserve normal blood circulation it is important that:

1. blood stays fluid in normal vessels;
2. if blood is escaping from vessels it must coagulate; and
3. there must be a clot-lysing system.

The coagulation system of the blood has evolved to fulfil these prerequisites.

Haemostatic Mechanism

There are three components to the haemostatic mechanism and also a system for lysing the clot that forms as a result of haemostasis. Following damage to a vessel the first component to come into operation is **vasoconstriction**. Once the injury has been inflicted, constriction of smooth muscle in the walls of the small vessels is an important mechanism in reducing blood flow through them and hence limiting blood loss. Another effect, that of **vascular spasm**, is initiated in the smooth muscle of the damaged larger arteries, causing reduction of blood flow into the injured area — thus minimizing loss of blood from the ruptured vessels. Vascular spasm may be a local myogenic effect or neurogenic and involving the autonomic nervous system via a sympathetic reflex. The extent of vaso-

constriction depends on the nature of the injury: when the damage to vessels is a smooth cut or a clean incision (e.g. a paper cut or a sharp razor incision), spasm and constriction is likely to be minimal, and the bleeding is generally quite severe. When the injury to the tissue involves crushing or mangling with a great deal of disruption to the vessels, the spasm may be so intense as to cause almost a complete stoppage of blood flow.

The second component of the haemostatic mechanism is **adhesion** and **aggregation of platelets**, forming a haemostatic plug. Platelets are cell fragments of the giant bone marrow cell, the megakaryocyte, and are present in the normal bloodstream in numbers of approximately 250 000 per μL of blood. Minor trauma to small vessels occurs in everyday life. These tears are immediately plugged by platelets, which are attracted to the exposed collagen of the basement membrane and subendothelial connective tissues. Platelets contribute both to vascular function (by plugging microscopic haemorrhages) and to clot formation, by supplying essential clotting factors.

The third component of the haemostatic mechanism is **blood clot formation** (fibrin clot). Fibrinogen is a soluble plasma protein, the function of which is to be converted under certain circumstances to the insoluble, strand-like protein **fibrin**. Both the damage to the vascular wall and the aggregation and degranulation of platelets set in motion the blood clotting mechanism, the final effect of which is the conversion of fibrinogen to fibrin. The fibrin networks thus formed are incorporated into the platelet plug, the whole structure being referred to as the **haemostatic plug**. Within 3 to 6 minutes, the entire cross-section of the injured vessel is filled with the clotted blood, composed of blood platelets, cells and fibrin strands. In this way the loss of blood from the damaged vessel has been stopped.

The clot lysing system in the bloodstream, which breaks down the insoluble fibrin networks to soluble products, is called the **fibrinolytic mechanism**. It is composed of four elements: plasminogen, plasmin, activators and inhibitors. Plasmin is the fibrin-dissolving enzyme. This mechanism is important in the dissolution of any fibrin clots which have formed spontaneously in the circulation and also in the dissolution of haemostatic plugs which are no longer needed in the injured vessel which has been repaired.

Fibrin Formation

Endothelial cells line the vessels and promote a smooth flow of blood by:

• discouraging platelet adhesion (production of prostacyclin, PGI_2);

- secreting substances which lead to fibrin dissolution (fibrinolysis);
- releasing heparin secreted by neighbouring mast cells.

Blood flow is regulated by smooth muscle fibres of the terminal arterioles which respond to neurogenic stimuli or blood-borne vasodilators and constrictors.

When there is damage to a vessel, platelets become activated and react in the following way. They **adhere** to damaged endothelium and exposed collagen by becoming 'sticky'. There is release of **vasoconstrictors**, especially 5-hydroxytryptamine (5HT = serotonin), from damaged endothelial and tissue cells to produce a local vasospasm. The platelets **aggregate** to seal the site of injury, thus forming a platelet plug. Platelets then **release** platelet factor 3 (PF_3), which initiates blood clotting, and release other factors that attract more platelets to the area and also contribute to the formation of fibrin in the clotting process. The clotting process results from an interaction of plasma proteins at the site of blood loss giving rise to a controlled production of **fibrin**. Fibrinogen, which is a soluble blood protein, in the presence of thrombin is converted to fibrin — an insoluble strand-like protein. This forms a mesh, trapping blood cells and sealing the site and provides the basis for permanent healing. **Retraction** of the platelet–fibrin clot to form a firm mass, which is attached to the damaged wall and totally plugs up any damage, is the result of haemostasis.

Blood coagulation passes through four stages: (1) initiation; (2) generation of prothrombinase; (3) generation of thrombin; (4) fibrin formation. There are two closely linked systems of blood coagulation as shown in Figure 3.4 and these comprise the intrinsic system and the extrinsic system. The **intrinsic system** (= blood thromboplastin system) is so called because all required factors are present in the normal circulating blood, thus giving rise to spontaneous clotting of shed blood. This is illustrated if some blood is placed in a clean glass tube and allowed to stand. The blood will clot in approximately 10 minutes, totally as a result of the action of the intrinsic system. The **extrinsic system** (= tissue thromboplastin system) is so called because an external source of tissue extract takes part. This is illustrated by adding some minced tissue to freshly drawn whole blood within the glass tube. Under these conditions the blood will clot in 10 seconds instead of 10 minutes.

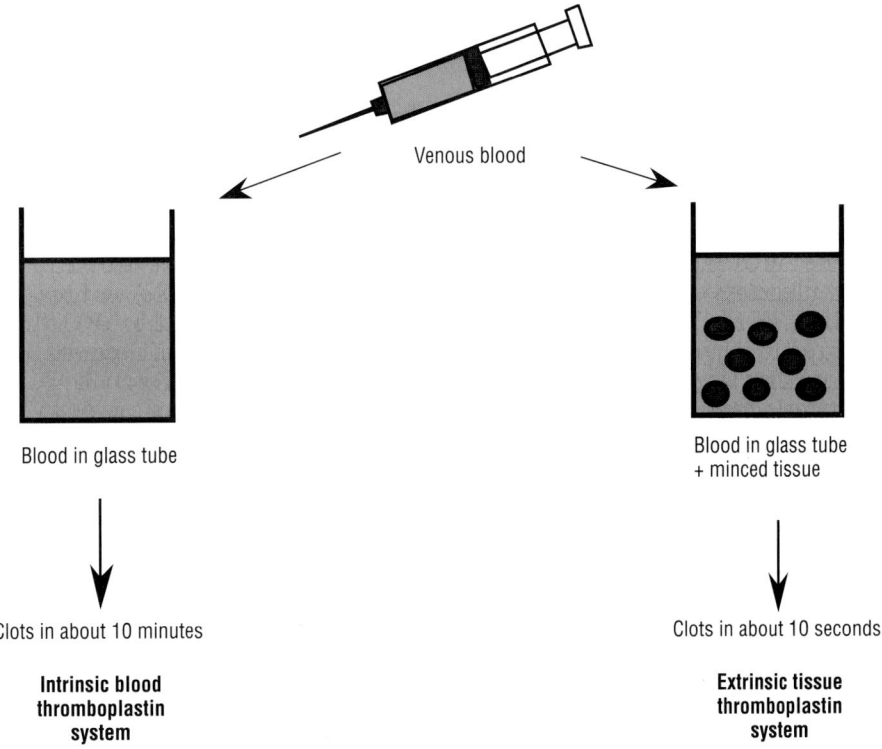

Venous blood

Blood in glass tube

Clots in about 10 minutes

Intrinsic blood thromboplastin system

Blood in glass tube + minced tissue

Clots in about 10 seconds

Extrinsic tissue thromboplastin system

Figure 3.4 *Mechanisms of fibrin formation*

Both intrinsic and extrinsic pathways lead to the final common pathway of thrombin activation converting fibrinogen to fibrin. In fact, tissue injury and vascular damage usually occur together. The extrinsic system generates thrombin, which aggregates platelets causing them to initiate the intrinsic system, so there is an interaction of the two systems (Figure 3.5).

It should be noted that many substances will interfere with the blood clotting cascade and many of these substances are used *in vivo* clinically, or *in vitro* in the laboratory. For example, **heparin** is a naturally occurring anticoagulant found in many cells (e.g. mast cells). Its inhibitory effects are derived from its activity as a potentiator of antithrombins, which act on thrombin, inactivating it and making it unable to mediate fibrin formation. **Aspirin** also inhibits blood clotting by interfering with platelet function, its effects lasting for 7–10 days if sufficiently high doses are ingested. A number of substances are used in the laboratory to prevent the spontaneous clotting of blood samples

withdrawn from the circulation; for example **citrate** or **oxalate** ions interfere with the clotting process by binding calcium, thus forming insoluble precipitates. Calcium ions are an essential component in the blood coagulation cascade (Ca^{2+} = factor IV) acting as a cofactor. Usually citrate- or oxalate-treated tubes are available in the haematology clinic for blood sample collection.

Fibrinolysis

Having prevented blood loss from a damaged vessel by formation of a blood clot, it is important that this clot may also be lysed in order to re-establish normal blood flow through the vessel and also to limit or localize clot formation to the damaged area. Hence there is a balanced system of blood clotting and clot dissolution or fibrinolysis. There is a paired system of (1) clotting proteins and inhibitors of coagulation and (2) fibrinolysis and its inhibitors.

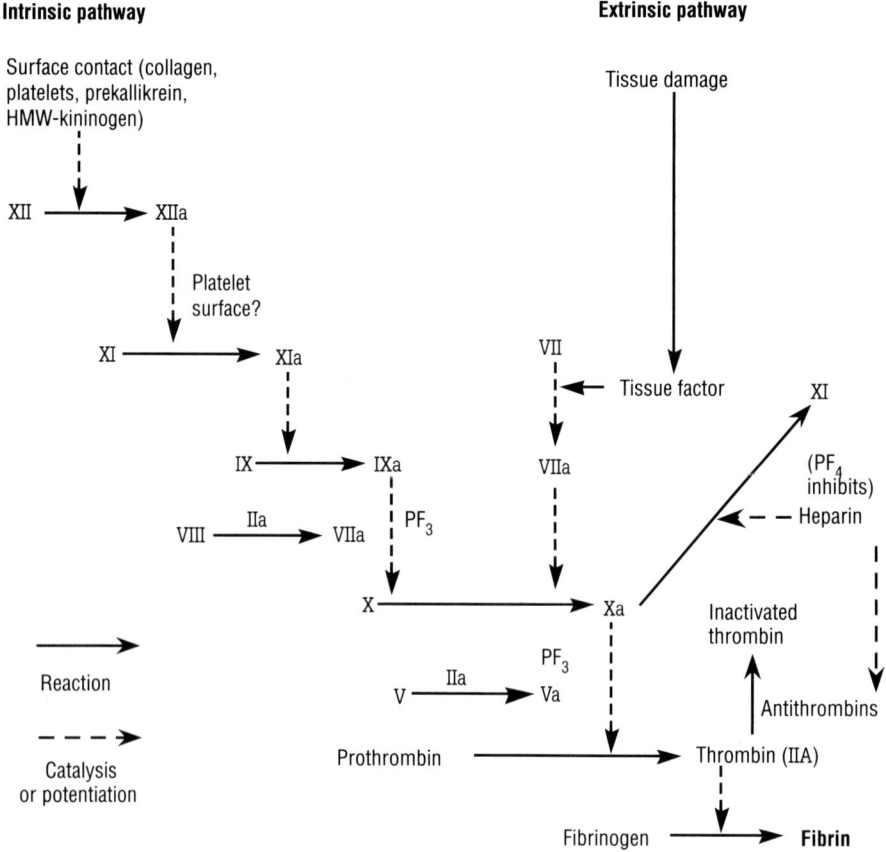

Figure 3.5 *The two pathways in the clotting cascade that may result in fibrin formation*

In fibrinolysis the effective agent is **plasmin**, which destroys fibrin, releasing fibrin degradation products (FDP) which also inhibit thrombin, thus preventing clotting. Plasmin also acts on fibrinogen and other blood clotting factors and so must be in the inactive form in the blood. The inactive protein is **plasminogen**. Normally plasminogen is laid down with fibrin in the clot and plasmin is slowly released to produce autodigestion of the clot, due to intrinsic and extrinsic activators. Hence there is a self-limiting mechanism in blood coagulation.

The balance between blood clotting and fibrinolysis or clot dissolution is very important and deficiencies in either of these systems may lead to either haemorrhagic disease; (lack of blood clotting) or to excessive thrombosis (blood clot formation), both of which are potentially fatal.

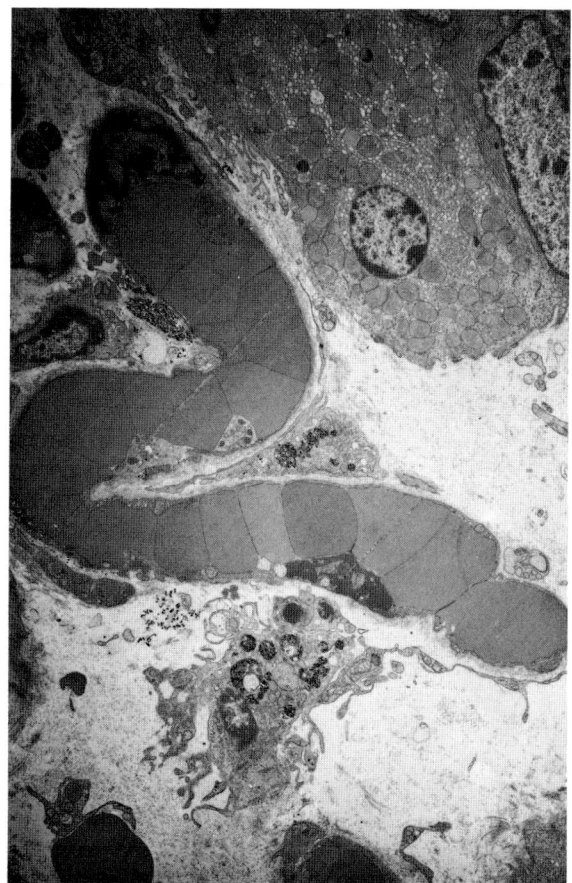

Figure 3.6 *A congested capillary in stomach mucosa after injury through application of ethyl alcohol (×52 000)*

Haemorrhage

There are many reasons why blood loss from the circulation may occur: trauma, damaged vessels, vascular disease, inflammatory and neoplastic erosion of vessels and also hypertension (high blood pressure) causing rupture of blood vessels, for example in the brain (CVA — cerebrovascular accident). Under many circumstances the normal homeostatic mechanisms which prevent blood loss from the circulation will not be adequate to prevent haemorrhage occurring (Figures 3.6 and 3.7).

Haemorrhage may be either external or internal. **External haemorrhage** (exsanguination) is where blood is lost from the body. In this case the blood may be lost directly into the environment, as through a penetrating wound in the skin, or it may be lost indirectly, when there is chronic bleeding into the gastrointestinal system, as, for example, from a colonic cancer. **Internal haemorrhage** is blood loss into the tissues. This is known as **haematoma** formation (blood clot in the tissues). Internal blood loss or haemorrhage may occur into a body cavity also, for example haemothorax, haemoperitoneum or haemopericardium. When minute haemorrhages occur into the skin, mucous membranes or serosal surfaces, they are known as **petechiae** (= petechial haemorrhage). If the haemorrhages are slightly larger they are known as **purpura**.

A subcutaneous haematoma (larger than 1–2 cm) is known as an **ecchymosis** (= bruise) When an ecchymosis occurs due to haemorrhage in the skin it is readily visible and the colour changes seen in a bruise as time passes give an indication of what happens to the blood once lost into the tissues.

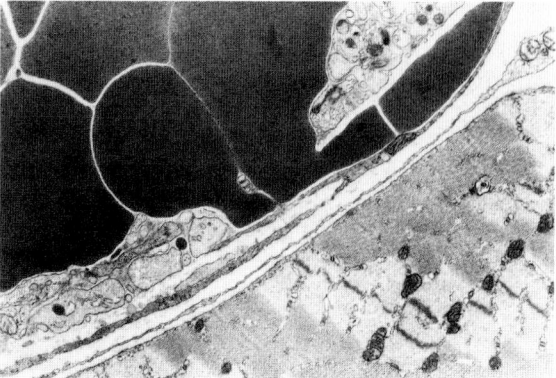

Figure 3.7 *Passive diapedesis of erythrocytes through an open interendothelial junction in an inflamed venule in skeletal muscle (×8000)*

Course of a Haemorrhage

Haemorrhage into the tissues results in an inflammatory response and eventual removal of blood by macrophages with organization and repair. As the red blood cells are degraded by macrophages colour changes in the bruise are seen. Immediately the blood escapes from an artery it is bright red in colour indicating oxygenated haemoglobin. Within seconds the colour changes to a cherry-red due to removal of oxygen by the surrounding tissue cells. The bruise is thus initially a deep red colour caused by the freshly escaped red blood cells with release of **haemoglobin**. As the haemoglobin degrades the colour alters. The bruise becomes green-blue as haemoglobin is converted to **biliverdin**, then green-yellow as it degrades to **bilirubin**, and finally becomes a brown-orange colour as **haemosiderin**, an insoluble pigment, is produced. As degraded red blood cells are removed by macrophages the haemosiderin pigment is seen as large granules inside these macrophages.

In hypoxic tissues (low oxygen tension) with haemorrhage, for example in a haemorrhagic infarct, **haematoidin** pigment may be seen as a brown, crystalline substance which is derived from bilirubin. When there are many macrophages containing these break-down products of haemoglobin this may be an indication of an old haemorrhage in the tissue. Sometimes jaundice may follow a major haemorrhage due to the excessive release of bilirubin which accumulates in the skin.

Clinical Implications of Haemorrhage

The clinical implications of haemorrhage depend on:

- **volume** of blood loss;
- **rate** of blood loss;
- **site** of haemorrhage.

For example, a slow loss of up to 30% of blood volume may have no serious clinical effect. **Anaemia** may result but there will be regeneration of blood by the bone marrow. However, rapid loss of 20% of blood volume, or loss of just 50 ml or less in a strategic area such as the brainstem may result in **death** (see Figure 3.8). Also, external haemorrhage may **deplete iron stores** (iron is present in the haem portion of haemoglobin). Internal haemorrhages permit the reabsorption and re-utilization of iron. It is possible to survive a loss of up to 20% blood volume without adverse effects. This is due to the homeostatic mechanisms which help to maintain normal circulation following loss of blood.

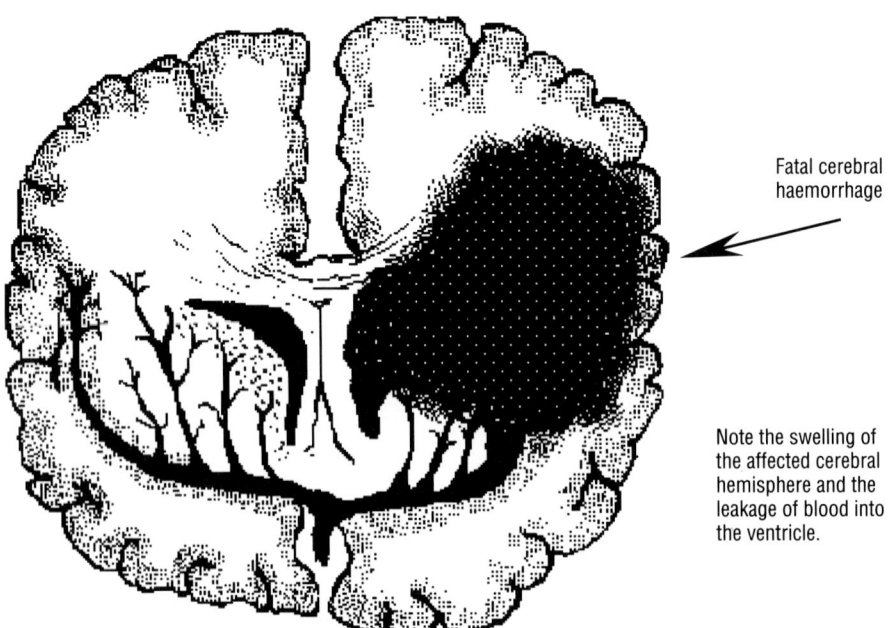

Fatal cerebral haemorrhage

Note the swelling of the affected cerebral hemisphere and the leakage of blood into the ventricle.

Figure 3.8 *Situation of a haemorrhage has important clinical effects as is seen with this cerebral haemorrhage (one type of 'cerebrovascular accident' or CVA)*

Haemorrhage leads to a lowered blood volume or **hypovolaemia**. This leads to a lowered cardiac output and lowered blood pressure which in turn could lead to brain and heart damage owing to diminished oxygen and ultimately could cause death.

Haemorrhage into certain sites of the body may be rapidly fatal because of anatomical or functional considerations. Bleeding into the brain may cause rapid death as the blood is escaping inside the cranial cavity, within a non-expandable bony 'box'. Thus, the soft nervous tissue is compressed and damage to neurones occurs. Unless these patients are treated as surgical emergencies they most often die rapidly. Another sensitive site is the pericardium. If bleeding occurs into the pericardium there may be excessive pressure put on the myocardium and prevention of normal cardiac function. Such a situation is also rapidly fatal, especially if a large volume of blood enters the pericardial cavity in a short time, as may occur, for example, following a myocardial infarct (heart attack), with rupture of the necrotic region of myocardium and release of a massive volume of blood into the pericardial sac.

Homeostatic Mechanisms

In order to minimize the effects of blood loss the following mechanisms occur:

- **Vasoconstriction**. Blood vessel constriction causes an increased peripheral resistance, and thus an increased blood pressure.
- **Aldosterone production by the kidney**. Aldosterone increases water conservation (preventing fluid loss via the kidneys), thus increasing the blood volume and in turn increasing the blood pressure.
- **Tachycardia**. The heart beats more rapidly, thus decreasing circulation time which helps increase oxygen delivery to the tissues.

However, these mechanisms fail if blood is lost too quickly or if a very large volume is lost all at once. Also, if the haemorrhage is situated in a vital organ such as the brain these homeostatic mechanisms are of little benefit.

Haemorrhagic Diatheses

In certain people there is an increased tendency to haemorrhage. There are many reasons for this increased bleeding tendency and the bleeding disorders are collectively known as **haemorrhagic diatheses**. The main cause of this abnormal haemorrhage is failure of blood coagulation and numerous coagulation defects are known. In the patients suffering from these disorders, even insignificant trauma (e.g. a shaving cut) may lead to serious or life threatening haemorrhage. The haemostatic plug formed is very fragile and easily disrupted, such that after the initial vasoconstriction following the injury is over, the rush of the blood back into the dilated vessel will cause breakdown of the plug and bleeding from the vessel will begin again. There are many genetic and acquired disorders affecting the coagulation cascade.

A failure in blood clotting can occur due to faulty fibrin formation and there are a number of disorders in which the prime defect is associated with fibrin formation. Many factors in the clotting cascade may be affected and may be either totally absent in the body or, alternatively, defective in their function.

Genetic Defects of Clotting Factors

Haemophilia A. This is an X-linked recessive defect (therefore mainly affecting males, the females being most usually carriers of the trait), characterized by a life-long tendency to haemorrhage, due to a prolonged coagulation time. There is a deficiency of factor VIII in the blood and the first indication of the disorder occurs at the age of 2–3 years when slight trauma is followed by excessive bleeding. Haematemesis, haematuria and melaena may occur and when investigated they will show no local cause. **Haemarthroses** are common and since they are recurrent, inflammation and organization in the joint will lead to ankylosis. Large haematomata may form in the soft tissues and if not resorbed may lead to the formation of large hardened masses surrounded by fibrous tissue, the so-called 'pseudotumours'.

Treatment of haemophiliacs is by correction of the factor VIII deficiency through injection of factor concentrates derived from purified human blood. The injections are performed by the patients themselves and generally patients are also educated about avoidance of activity likely to cause trauma to tissues. All daughters of known haemophiliacs will be carriers and they will go on to transmit the disease to 50% of their sons and the carrier trait to 50% of their daughters. Intermarriage in the royal families of Europe in the 19th century ensured that the haemophiliac trait was transmitted to many offspring. Queen Victoria was a famous carrier and Alexis, the czarevich of Russia, son of Nicholas II, the last Czar, was a haemophiliac. The incidence of haemophilia A is 12 cases per 100 000 males in the population.

Christmas disease (Haemophilia B). This is another X-linked recessive defect, which is clinically identical to haemophilia but the deficiency is one of factor IX. It was named Christmas disease in 1952 as this was the name of the first patient in which the disorder was described. Some of the female carriers of this disorder show a minor tendency to bleed, but otherwise the disease is very similar to haemophilia. The incidence of haemophilia B is about one case per 100 000 males in the population.

Von Willebrand's disease (pseudohaemophilia). This is an autosomal dominant deficiency of factor VIII, leading to prolonged bleeding time and a normal coagulation time, platelet count and prothrombin time. The disorder manifests itself early in childhood, some babies bleeding from the umbilical stump after delivery, with the tendency to haemorrhage continuing throughout life. However, with increasing age the bleeding tendency becomes less severe and it is only rarely that life-threatening haemorrhages occur. The most common presentations of these patients are: bruising, multiple haemorrhages in mucous membranes, excessive bleeding following tooth extractions, haematemesis and haematuria. Women with the disorder may present with menorrhagia or there may be excessive postpartum haemorrhage. The disease is controlled by factor VIII supplementation.

Haemophilia C. This is a bleeding disorder due to factor XI deficiency. It is inherited as an autosomal dominant trait, very prevalent in some ethnic groups, especially Jews. It is a rather rare disorder with an approximate incidence of one case per 500 000 population. The disease is less severe than haemophilia A and bleeding episodes are more easily controlled with disabling haemarthroses developing very rarely.

Afibrinogenaemia. This is an exceedingly rare disorder where there is a congenital deficiency of normal fibrinogen in the blood, making it virtually incoagulable. It is an autosomal dominant defect and transfusions of plasma or fibrinogen extracts prepared by cryoprecipitation are required for treatment.

Acquired Defects of Clotting Factors

Combined clotting factor deficiencies, deficiencies of a combination of factors, for example factors II, VII, IX, X, are seen in a variety of clinical cases where patients present with a haemorrhagic diathesis. It should be noted, however, that such disorders are acquired and are secondary developments of other diseases in the body. Deficiencies of clotting factors may be seen in **malnutrition** or **malabsorption syndromes** as occur, for example, in chronic obstructive jaundice. In this case, there is a deficiency of the raw materials from which the clotting factors are manufactured, especially vitamin K, which is essential in the synthesis of factors II, VII and XI.

Liver disease very often leads to clotting factor deficiencies as the liver is the site for synthesis of many clotting factors (fibrinogen = factor I; prothrombin = factor II; factors V, IX, X). A common condition leading to a haemorrhagic diathesis is **cirrhosis of the liver**.

Premature birth, where the liver is not fully functional, will often be accompanied by a bleeding tendency; this, however, is only transient and disappears as soon as the liver begins to produce its full quota of clotting factors.

Acquired afibrinogenaemia may be found in cases of very severe liver disease and the clinical presentation of these patients resembles that of patients with congenital afibrinogenaemia.

Acquired factor IX deficiency is seen in kidney disease (nephrosis) and is due to unknown causes and it may also be seen in vitamin K deficiency.

High levels of circulating anticoagulants may cause a bleeding tendency due to the fact that these substances will directly interfere with the coagulation cascade. Excessive therapeutic levels of aspirin or heparin will cause this. Also, some patients with liver disease, tuberculosis, systemic lupus erythematosus and macroglobulinaemia have abnormally high levels of plasma globulins. This hyperglobulinaemia has an anticoagulant effect.

Purpura

Purpura means purple in Latin and refers to multiple purplish bruises on the skin or mucosal surfaces, resulting from capillary haemorrhages. The haemorrhages are usually small and called **petechial haemorrhages.** They are distributed over large areas of the skin or mucosae, but occasionally larger haemorrhages may occur. Purpura may be seen for various reasons and there are many aetiological factors which predispose to or lead to purpuric haemorrhages. The causes can be subdivided into various groups depending on whether they are due to platelet abnormalities or whether they are due to small vessel disorders.

Thrombocytopenic Purpura

Thrombocytopenia (deficiency of platelets) is said to occur when the platelet count of blood is less than

100 000 platelets per μL. Platelets are extremely important in the process of blood clotting and thrombosis. The structure of these small cell fragments is quite complex (see Figure 3.9). Lowered blood platelet numbers result from a variety of causes and once thrombocytopenia is present, spontaneous bleeding will occur. The mechanism is not clear but it is not simply a matter of defective haemostatic plug formation. It appears that normal platelet numbers are essential in the maintenance of the normal structure and function of capillary walls. It may be that secretion of platelet-derived growth factor (PDGF) in the microvasculature is essential for the maintenance of capillary endothelium. Thrombocytopenic purpura results from a variety of diseases that will destroy platelets, leading to a reduction in their circulating number.

Reduced platelet production from bone marrow. Decreased megakaryocyte numbers in the bone marrow will lead to decreased platelet production and is caused by marrow-depressing drugs (e.g. cytotoxic drugs), poisons (e.g. nitrogen mustard gas), leukaemia and idiopathic marrow hypoplasia. An idiopathic form of this disorder is seen in children and young adults. The disease is usually self-limiting, often disappearing spontaneously shortly after onset. Occasionally, chronic relapsing forms occur.

Reduced megakaryocyte maturation. This occurs in association with infections especially some viral ones such as infectious mononucleosis, measles and chicken pox.

Destruction of circulating platelets. **Hypersplenism** (enlarged spleen) as caused by a variety of disorders (e.g. portal hypertension, lymphomata, thalassaemia, Gaucher's disease) will be overdestructive for platelets and other blood cells. The spleen normally removes old red blood cells, platelets and particulate matter from the bloodstream. It is a major site for antibody synthesis, especially in response to circulating antigens, and it also synthesizes many lymphocytes. It acts as a reservoir for red blood cells but this function is not as important in the human as it is in the lower animals where the spleen may release many red blood cells into the circulation when there is an acute demand for them (e.g. following haemorrhage).

Antibodies against platelets. In some disorders (e.g. systemic lupus erythematosus — SLE) the immune system may produce antibodies against platelets. These specific antibodies will combine with the platelets, mediating their breakdown and destruction. In other autoimmune manifestations of antibody-mediated destruction of platelets, drugs such as quinine, sedormid or sulphamethazine combine with platelets. In hypersensitive individuals antibodies to these drug–platelet complexes form and bind to the platelets and the platelets are destroyed.

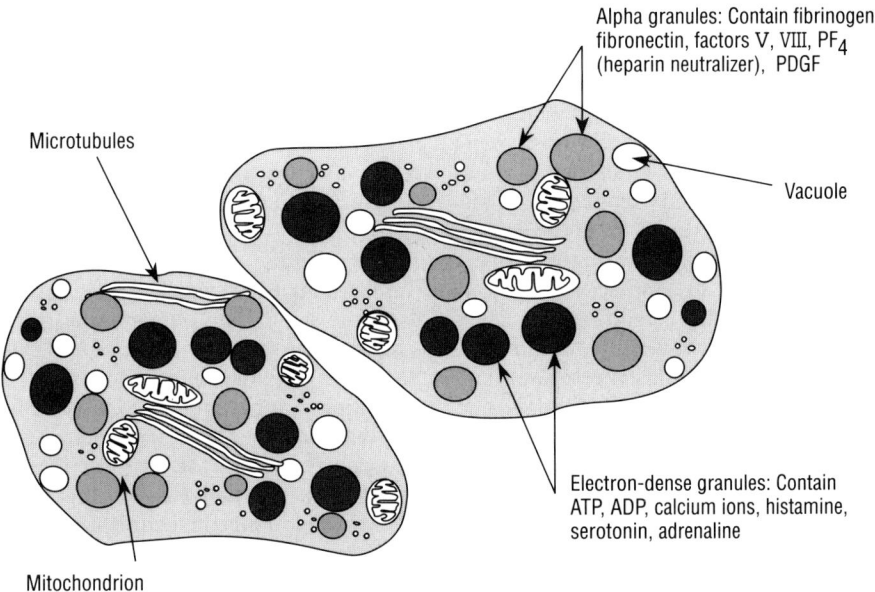

Alpha granules: Contain fibrinogen, fibronectin, factors V, VIII, PF_4 (heparin neutralizer), PDGF

Microtubules

Vacuole

Electron-dense granules: Contain ATP, ADP, calcium ions, histamine, serotonin, adrenaline

Mitochondrion

Figure 3.9 *Blood platelets or 'thrombocytes'*

Paradoxical consumption thrombocytopenia. In this case the platelets initially are normal in both structure and function. The thrombocytopenic state results after platelets are used up in vast numbers in a short period of time. A condition where this occurs is **disseminated intravascular coagulation** (DIC), which may be triggered off by septicaemia or alternatively by amniotic fluid embolism as a complication of childbirth. Vast numbers of platelets are used up in the circulation as clots form in vessels, leading subsequently to thrombocytopenia and haemorrhage. Hence it is paradoxical as clotting and haemorrhage occur to excess in the same patient.

Non-thrombocytopenic Purpura

When the platelet count is normal ($\approx$ 250 000 per μL) and platelet function is normal, purpura may result from vascular defects. **Congenital vascular defects** are rare and autosomally inherited. The small blood vessels (mainly capillaries) are very thin walled and excessively fragile, thus tending spontaneously to rupture and bleed. Some examples of these disorders are: **hereditary haemorrhagic telangiectasia**, where microvascular dilatations make the capillaries balloon outwards and rupture; **hereditary capillary fragility**, where the capillary endothelium is congenitally weak and liable to rupture; **connective tissue disorders**, where the supporting perivascular connective tissues are weak and provide little support for the vessels.

Purpura may result from **acquired vascular defects**. **Henoch-Schönlein purpura** follows infections, especially streptococcal, where the vascular basement membrane has been damaged by immune complex deposition. This type of purpura is seen especially in children. **Infections** may cause direct damage to capillaries. This is true particularly of Gram negative organism infections as occurs with septicaemias and meningococcal infections. Severe scarlet fever and haemorrhagic smallpox may also cause this toxic damage. **Drug-induced damage** to capillaries is seen in numerous hypersensitivities which manifest themselves as 'drug rashes', commonly following administration of sulphonamides and corticosteroids. Vessel weakening is also seen in **debility**, **protein starvation**, **scurvy** and **old age**. **Toxic capillary damage** may occur when there are high circulating levels of toxic substances, for example excessive levels of urea in uraemia.

Qualitative Platelet Abnormality Purpura

This is the condition described as **thrombasthenia**. In this case platelet count is normal or above normal but platelets are abnormal in their function. They cannot take part in the haemostatic mechanism and purpura results. This tends to be a fairly rare condition in the congenital form, as occurs, for example, in Von Willebrand's disease which also affects platelet function. Acquired platelet defects occur with administration of certain drugs, for example drugs of cytotoxic therapy, anticoagulants and anti-inflammatory drugs (especially aspirin). Other conditions such as uraemia, diabetes and scurvy also interfere with platelet function.

Laboratory Tests for Coagulation Defects

Laboratory tests for coagulation are indicated if a patient presents with a history of haemorrhages which are purpuric or ecchymotic in nature. Alternatively, the patient may present with difficulty in stanching a wound, prolonged bleeding from minor trauma sites or an iron deficiency anaemia (in the last case, an internal haemorrhage may be the cause, and the patient may not be aware that he or she is losing blood). There are many different tests in use and each of these has a specific function and may give an indication of where the problem lies. Some of the more important ones are outlined below. See also Figure 3.10.

Full Blood Examination
A sample of the patient's peripheral blood is collected and sent to the laboratory. A blood smear is made, the number and morphology of the formed elements of the blood being examined. This procedure checks for quantitative and morphological abnormalities in the platelets (thrombocytopenia and thrombasthenia). Normal platelet numbers are from 150 000 to 400 000 per μL of blood. A low platelet number may indicate that the cause of the bleeding is thrombocytopenic purpura.

Bleeding Time
This particular test checks gross vascular status and also platelet function. A controlled puncture incision is made in the free hanging ear lobe (Duke method) or the volar aspect of the forearm (Ivy method). A piece of blotting paper is applied to the bleeding drop (with care that the paper does not touch the skin) every 30 seconds. The length of time for bleeding to stop is recorded, the normal value being between 3 and 7 minutes. A prolonged bleeding time may be indicative of thrombocytopenia or thrombasthenia. It should be noted that aspirin ingestion can interfere with bleeding time results, giving prolonged bleeding times for anything up to 7 days after ingestion.

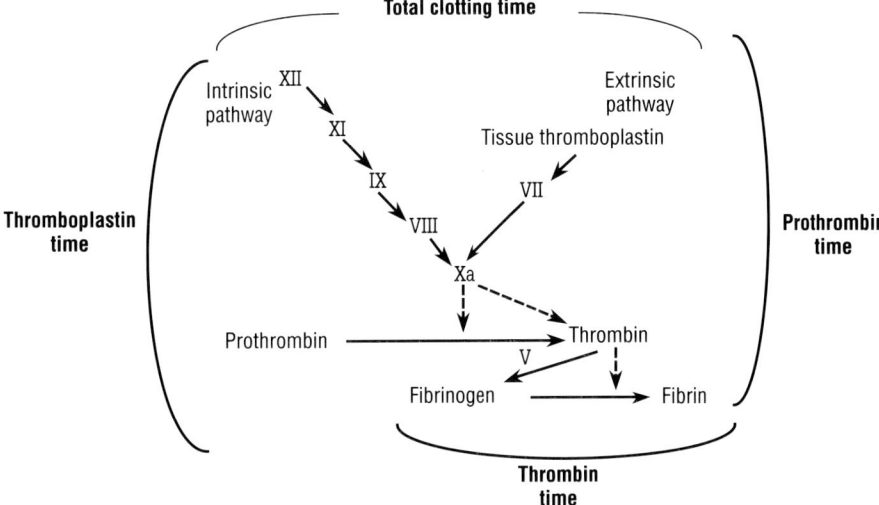

Figure 3.10 *Laboratory tests for blood clotting function*

Prothrombin Time

This test checks the functioning of the extrinsic pathway of blood coagulation and tests for the normal functioning of the following factors: factor I (fibrinogen), factor II (prothrombin), factor V (prothrombin accelerator), factor VII (proconvertin), factor X (Stuart-Prower factor). An aliquot of the patient's citrated blood is mixed with phospholipid and tissue thromboplastin (derived from brain tissue). As the calcium ions have been removed by the citrate, clotting does not occur. Calcium ions are then added in excess and the clotting time is recorded, the normal being 11–13 seconds. Prolongation of prothrombin time shows abnormalities in the clotting factors listed above, and indicates that further testing may be needed to check for normal liver function and for vitamin K deficiency.

Activated Partial Thromboplastin Time

This is the single most useful test for coagulation defects as it tests for the intrinsic coagulation pathway and checks for deficiencies in the following: factor I (fibrinogen), factor II (prothrombin), factor V (prothrombin accelerator), factor VIII (antihaemophilic globulin), factor IX (Christmas factor), factor X (Stuart-Prower factor), factor XI (plasma thromboplastin antecedent) and factor XII (Hageman factor). The principle of the test is to activate factors XI and XII in citrated plasma by incubating the test system with kaolin (a contact activating agent which greatly enhances reproducibility of results) and then adding a platelet substitute such as chloroform extract of brain tissue and recalcifying. The clot should form in 26 to 42 seconds

normally. Abnormalities in this test indicate that one or more of the factors listed above are defective.

Thrombin Time

The patient's citrated plasma and an exogenous aliquot of thrombin are mixed, the clotting time measured, normal values being 10–13 seconds. This test indicates abnormalities in fibrinogen polymerization or low levels of fibrinogen.

Whole Blood Coagulation Time

This is the oldest and simplest test but it is not always a reliable indicator of clotting disorders as it may be normal when coagulation is defective. A sample of blood is removed from the patient by venepuncture and a millilitre is placed in a clean glass tube, 12 cm by 1 cm, and the tube is inverted every 30 seconds until the clotted blood can support its own weight. The normal coagulation time is 4–10 minutes and tests are run in duplicate. If whole blood coagulation times are prolonged, then blood coagulation is very abnormal (refer to Figure 3.10).

Tourniquet Test (Hess's Test)

A sphygmomanometer cuff is placed around the upper arm and inflated until the pressure is at a point midway between the diastolic and systolic pressures. The pressure is thus maintained for 5 minutes. When the cuff is removed the antecubital fossa is inspected for petechial haemorrhages. Normally there are none to, at the most, four in an area covered by a 3 cm diameter circle (the size of a 50 cent piece).

It should be noted that with any of the above tests performed, a clear history from the patient should be obtained, with details of a personal as well of a familial nature being taken. Particular care should be taken in enquiring about the severity of haemorrhages following operative procedures, dental extractions, menstrual blood, etc. The time course of the current problem should be ascertained and the patient examined for evidence of cutaneous and mucous membrane haemorrhages. A large variety of drugs has been implicated in the causation of haemorrhagic diatheses and the patients should be questioned as to the types of medication they are on and also if they have been exposed to any toxic chemicals or substances in their workplace. Some patients may be self-administering large doses of analgesic preparations which contain aspirin and this may cause haemorrhage. Some may have been given heparin therapeutically, and heparin enhances the neutralizing effects of antithrombin III on factors IXa, Xa, XIa and plasmin, therefore prolonging prothrombin time, partial thromboplastin time and thrombin time.

Shock

Shock is not a specific disease but rather a clinical syndrome with many presentations. The clinical state of shock results from reduction of the effective circulating blood volume. This circulatory insufficiency leads to an imbalance between the metabolic needs of the tissues and the blood available to them. There will be lowered oxygen and nutrients available to cells and an increase of metabolites. This in turn may lead to cell damage, reactive changes and necrosis. Depending on the severity of the syndrome, shock may be either reversible or irreversible. Two major clinical syndromes are distinguished: primary shock and secondary shock.

Primary shock develops very quickly after injury, pain or emotional reactions; and it is a transient response (unless accompanied by extensive trauma or severe haemorrhage). Fluid balance is not usually affected. It is a neurovascular reaction accompanied by extensive peripheral vasodilatation which results in **syncope** (fainting). This form of shock occurs only in humans and may be seen at first as sighing respiration, yawning, nausea and vomiting and eventually loss of consciousness and lowered blood pressure. A reduction of cerebral blood flow leads to the loss of consciousness. It is possible that fainting helps divert blood to the brain by causing the patient to fall to the ground. When the horizontal position is assumed, recovery soon occurs, as the blood rushes back to the brain.

Primary shock also occurs when blood is lost very quickly. This type of shock is followed by a redistribution of the remaining blood. The less evolved animals are able to literally 'wring out' their spleen, thus forcing the erythrocytes which were sequestered there into the circulation to replenish those that were lost. This response also occurs in humans, but is of limited usefulness. It should be noted that primary shock may progress to secondary shock, as may occur, for example, after a car accident where a person may go into primary shock as a result of fright and pain of his injuries and then following this the blood loss sustained may give rise to the fluid imbalances which characterize secondary shock.

Secondary or **delayed shock** is a disturbance of fluid balance which results in reduced peripheral circulation. It is manifested by lowered blood volume (hypovolaemia), reduced blood flow, haemoconcentration and renal functional deficiency. Secondary shock manifests itself with a variety of signs and symptoms:

* the patient appears ill (nauseated, pallid, sweating) and complains of **weakness**;
* systolic arterial pressure is low (**decreased BP**);
* **pulse rate is rapid** and **feeble**;
* respiration rate increases (**tachypnoea**);
* **tachycardia** follows;
* skin is **cold** and **clammy**;
* **confusion** and apathy may be present;
* there is **depression of general metabolic activity**;
* there may be peripheral **cyanosis**;
* **oliguria** (lowered urinary output) and even **anuria** (no urine) may follow.

It should be kept in mind that these symptoms and signs are important in diagnosis as secondary shock is essentially a clinical syndrome and not a distinct pathological entity. Different patients will present with a different assortment of the above symptoms and signs and the clinical presentation may vary depending on the precipitating aetiological factors.

Aetiological Factors in Shock

Hypovolaemic shock is caused most commonly by haemorrhage, but may also be due to loss of plasma or loss of salt and water (e.g. burns, dehydration). In **cardiogenic shock** there is no effective cardiopulmonary pumping action and this type of shock is seen in myocardial impairments, pulmonary emboli, etc. **Septic shock** (= endotoxic shock) is caused by widespread vasodilatation of blood vessels in bacterial sepsis, while **neurogenic shock** is caused by reflex nervous effects of prolonged, severe pain dilating capillaries and veins throughout the peripheral circulation. The causes of these different types of shock are discussed in greater detail below.

Hypovolaemia

Haemorrhage is the commonest type of cause precipitating hypovolaemia. The severity of the shock state that results will depend very much on the amount of blood that is lost and the speed with which the loss occurs. A rapid, severe loss has always important effects which may be fatal. Losses of 20% or less of the blood volume are tolerated well; sudden losses of 35% of the blood volume may be fatal. However, if the bleeding is slow (extending over 24 hours), losses of up to 50% of the blood volume may be tolerated. Losses above 50% of the blood volume are always life threatening. With the fall in blood volume, there is lowered venous return to the heart, lowered systemic blood pressure, tachycardia (increased heart rate), reduced stroke volume, lowered cardiac output and drop in peripheral blood pressure.

There is in response to these generalized effects a reflex sympathetic vasoconstriction which results in increased peripheral resistance but not constriction to either cerebral or coronary arteries. In fact there is vasodilatation of cerebral and coronary arteries so that blood is shunted to the vital organs. The sympathetic vasoconstriction is supported by release of adrenal catecholamines, aldosterone, antidiuretic hormone and the activation of the renin–angiotensin system. All of these act to conserve fluid and support the falling blood volume and blood pressure. However, while the heart and brain are protected, the vasoconstriction increases lack of perfusion of peripheral tissues, causing tissue anoxia which leads to metabolic acidosis with anaerobic glycolysis releasing pyruvate and lactate into the circulation. The fall in blood pressure, and impairment of renal function, leading to oliguria and even anuria are both important problems in shock as they may have serious or fatal consequences.

As well as haemorrhage, extensive body burns can cause massive loss of fluids and electrolytes. For example, if a leg is involved in a burn over its total surface, up to 6 litres of fluid can escape in a short time. This is equivalent to a severe haemorrhage. Other causes of hypovolaemia include other forms of body fluid loss such as induced by vomiting, diarrhoea, dehydration and electrolyte depletion.

Cardiogenic Shock

This represents a circulatory collapse resulting from a suddenly developing insufficiency of the heart. It is most commonly seen in myocardial infarction, serious cardiac arrhythmias, massive pulmonary embolism, rupture of cardiac valves or of the papillary muscles. This type of shock may lead to rapid death, especially if the primary cardiac condition precipitating it is not diagnosed or treated immediately. The importance of cardiogenic shock as a cause of death in people who have had a myocardial infarct (heart attack) has been pointed out, as 20% of such people die before reaching hospital, usually 4 hours after the ischaemia has affected the heart.

Septic Shock

In endotoxic shock, many bacteria (especially implicated are the Gram-negative bacteria, e.g. *Pseudomonas aeruginosa*) multiply within the bloodstream, causing an overwhelming infection. Breakdown products of the bacterial cell wall (= endotoxins) are released into the circulation through the action of phagocytes, and these cell wall fragments have a pyrogenic effect and are also directly toxic to capillary endothelium. Endotoxins are important in the release of vasoactive substances which cause numerous microcirculatory derangements.

Microcirculatory Derangements

These refer to a variety of changes in the peripheral circulation which cause profound disturbances in homeostasis. There is pooling of blood in the peripheral circulation, disseminated intravascular coagulation and abnormal permeability of capillaries with loss of plasma, water and a subsequent decrease in blood volume. These mechanisms may underlie the shock seen in patients with sepsis, endotoxaemia and also contribute to cardiogenic shock. Endotoxins may trigger release of vasoactive substances causing peripheral pooling. Hypoxic injury to autonomic control centres and release of such substances as histamine, bradykinin and acetylcholine cause loss of peripheral resistance and expansion of the microcirculation with increased permeability and transudation of large volumes of fluid. Released lysosomal enzymes may contribute directly to such microcirculatory injury. In the individual patient several mechanisms may act at the same time to bring about the reactions seen in shock.

Whatever the aetiology of shock, the end result is very similar — a low perfusion hypoxic injury to cells and an ever widening circle of metabolic imbalances leading to cellular effects that are similar in mechanism to those already discussed in cellular injury. Changes in tissues of the body are:

1. **Liver**: fatty change of the hepatocytes, with usually no or minimal functional implications. If the shock state resolves, the hepatocytes will return to normality.
2. **Lungs**: congestion and oedema leading to respiratory embarrassment. The changes in respiration seen in shock patients are a combination of neurogenic effects on the lungs and local effects caused by the decreased surface area available for gas exchanges.
3. **Brain**: loss of consciousness may be followed by permanent damage due to anoxic oedema, raised intracranial pressure and neuronal necrosis, with regions of cerebral softening developing. Permanent brain damage may follow protracted shock.
4. **Kidneys**: acute renal tubular necrosis with oliguria or anuria. This is an effect of grossly diminished blood flow to the renal parenchyma, the patient often going into renal failure.
5. **Heart**: fatty change and hydropic change of the myocardial cells will be seen. If the shock state persists for any length of time, these reactive changes may progress to necrosis, which may have important functional implications.

By far, the best prognosis for patients is seen in hypovolaemic and neurogenic shock. If such patients are promptly treated, the pathological changes developing are minimal and the tissues return to normal after suffering only reactive changes. However, in cardiogenic and septic shock, the prognosis is much graver, even with treatment; mortality rates in these cases is often as high as 70–80%.

Thrombosis

Thrombosis is the process resulting in the formation of a solid or semi-solid mass from the constituents of the blood, within the vascular system, during life. The resulting mass is called a **thrombus** and varies in composition depending on the conditions and situations under which the thrombus forms. Thrombosis (thrombus formation) must be distinguished from post-mortem clot formation which is simply the passive clotting of blood after death due to cessation of blood circulation. A post-mortem clot is dark red, shiny, wet,

non-adherent and moulds to the shape of the blood vessel. It has two distinct layers: an upper layer of clotted plasma (so-called 'chicken fat jelly') and a lower layer of sedimented red blood cells (like 'redcurrant jelly'). Thrombosis is also different from the process of haematoma formation as the thrombi form within vessels, unlike haematomata, which form in the tissues. A thrombus is often a **laminated** structure. It appears firm, friable, has a granular surface and is adherent to the vessel wall. The laminated appearance is due to successive deposition of platelets and fibrin (appearing pale) and layers of red and white cells and fibrin (appearing red). These layers when viewed in cross-section are known as the **lines of Zahn**. In thrombosis, platelets initially stick to the endothelial surface of the vessel, aggregate and disintegrate. Platelet damage leads to accumulation of clotting factors, causing fibrin deposition. The fibrin mesh traps red and white cells, and is followed by further deposition of aggregated platelets.

The three components of the normal haemostatic mechanism (namely, endothelial cells, platelets and the coagulation cascade) interact in many ways and are in an equilibrium in the normal circulation. There are factors that inhibit and factors that enhance intravascular coagulation of blood.

Endothelial Cells

Factors inhibiting thrombosis. Intact endothelium insulates blood and coagulation factors in the circulation from the highly **thrombogenic** subendothelial components. Endothelial cell membranes repel platelets, inhibiting their adherence, an effect mediated by synthesis of prostacyclin (PGI_2) by the normal endothelium. In addition, endothelial cells actively degrade ADP, which is a potent platelet aggregating agent. **Thrombomodulin** is a substance on the surface of the endothelial cell and this binds thrombin, reducing the clotting activity of the latter. The thrombomodulin–thrombin complex activates protein C which lyses factors V and VIII. Endothelial cells also possess **heparan sulphate**, which binds onto **antithrombin III**, greatly enhancing its anticoagulant properties (i.e. inactivation of factors IXa and Xa).

Factors favouring thrombosis. Damage or injury to the endothelium promotes platelet adhesion and clotting of blood. Denudation of the endothelium exposes the basement membrane collagen which is highly thrombogenic. **Von Willebrand factor**, which is synthesized by endothelial cells, is essential for the adherence of platelets to the subendothelium. **Tissue factor** is released by damaged endothelial cells and this activates the clotting cascade via the extrinsic pathway. Injured endothelium also binds factors IX and X, thereby enhancing their activity greatly.

Platelets

Factors favouring thrombosis. Platelets possess two types of granules in their cytoplasm and these contain substances favouring thrombosis and coagulation of blood.

Alpha granules, containing:	**Electron-dense granules,** containing:
Fibrinogen	ATP, ADP
Fibronectin	Calcium ions
Factors V, VIII	Histamine
Platelet factor 4	Serotonin
(a heparin neutralizer)	Adrenaline
Platelet-derived growth factor (PDGF)	

Once platelets come into contact with the collagen of the basement membrane, they are activated and three reactions take place:

- **adhesion** of platelets to basement membrane;
- **secretion** of granule components;
- **aggregation** of more platelets, with manufacture of PF_3, enhancing clotting.

Coagulation Cascade

Factors favouring thrombosis. The coagulation cascade involves a series of pro-enzymes that, once activated, will culminate in the formation of **thrombin**, which is an enzyme converting the soluble plasma protein **fibrinogen** to an insoluble, fibrillar protein, **fibrin**. The coagulation cascade may be activated by the **intrinsic** or the **extrinsic** pathways, the intrinsic mechanism being more important in thrombosis.

Factors inhibiting thrombosis. Once the coagulation cascade has been initiated it is controlled lest the clotting involve all of the blood in the vasculature. The **fibrinolytic system** is the main controlling mechanism. **Plasminogen** is present in plasma and may be activated by **tissue plasminogen activator** (secreted by most tissue cells and endothelium) to form **plasmin**. Plasmin breaks down fibrin, fibrinogen and clotting factors VIII and V.

General Factors Predisposing to Thrombosis

These factors are referred to as **Virchow's Triad** since it was Rudolf Virchow who first formulated them. All thrombi have formed in response to these factors either acting alone or in various combinations. Vascular diseases in particular are likely to give rise to all three factors in Virchow's Triad. Thrombosis is predisposed to by:

- changes in the vessel wall;
- changes in blood flow;
- changes in blood constituents.

Changes in the Vessel Wall

Any change to the smooth endothelial surface of a vessel wall predisposes to platelet deposition. Intact vascular endothelium produces prostaglandins which inhibit thrombosis. When endothelium is injured it no longer produces these antithrombotic substances and thrombosis is enhanced.

Damage to the endothelium may be caused by a wide variety of processes:

- Atherosclerosis is very important in this context (mainly abdominal aorta, coronary arteries).
- Cardiac infarction (thrombosis in the left ventricle overlying an area of infarction).
- Infection.
- Toxic injury, for example endotoxin.
- Poisons, chemicals, for example derivatives of cigarette smoke.
- Cholesterol (in hyperlipidaemia).
- Immune mechanisms.

Changes in Blood Flow

Stasis of flow is a very important factor, for example venous stasis in congestive heart failure, dehydration, prolonged bed rest (leg vein thrombosis post-operatively). Also, in very long operations when the patient is anaesthetized venous stasis is a prominent feature, especially in the leg veins. **Turbulence** of flow is also important and may occur with distortion of the vessel lumen due to narrowing or dilatation, for example rigid valves, aneurysms. Disruption to the normal laminar flow of the blood is thus caused by both stasis and turbulence.

Changes in blood flow have the following effects. They:

- may cause damage to the intima;
- bring platelets into prolonged contact with the endothelium;
- prevent dilution and clearance of clotting factors;
- allow the build-up of thrombi and prevent their removal.

Alteration in the Blood Constituents

Excessive normal components and abnormal components within the blood may constitute a **thrombotic diathesis**, that is, a predisposition to thrombosis or clotting. Conditions include:

- **Thrombocythaemia**: an increased number of platelets promotes clotting of blood causing hypercoagulability; this occurs post-operatively, post-partum, post-haemorrhage, but also following splenectomy and in polycythaemia rubra vera.
- **Polycythaemia**: increases in red blood cell numbers that occur in this condition also involve increased platelet count. The blood has increased viscosity, flow is reduced and red cell clumping occurs, which contributes to an increased thrombotic tendency.
- **Plasma proteins**: in such conditions as **macroglobulinaemia** (high globulin levels in the blood) increased blood viscosity promotes stasis and thrombosis.
- **Hyperlipidaemia**: increased blood lipids are very important in this context as they increase the coagulability of the blood.
- **Hypercoagulability of the blood**: this is due to excessive clotting factors produced by the liver and by excessive platelet numbers.
- **Hyperoestrinism**: excessive oestrogen levels, either endogenous or administered therapeutically, will make thrombosis more likely.

Clinical Risk Factors of Thrombosis

The above-mentioned generalized risk factors of thrombosis are considered when a patient is admitted to hospital and the clinical risk of thrombosis developing after, say, an operative procedure may be estimated. The following risk factors are considered to be important clinically and predispose to thrombosis:

- **Age**: generally, the older the patient, the greater the risk.
- **Health status**: the presence of other disease predisposing to thrombosis; e.g. atherosclerosis, hyperlipidaemia, diabetes, obesity, varicose veins, cancer (especially lung, genitourinary tract or gastrointestinal tract cancers), ulcerative colitis.
- **Heart condition**: cardiac infarction, cardiac failure, rheumatic heart disease, arrhythmias.
- **History**: patients with previous thrombotic episodes.
- **Blood disorders**: hypercoagulability of blood, thrombotic diathesis, platelet disorders, thrombocytosis (increased platelet production or decreased destruction, e.g. splenectomy).
- **Immobility**: patients in a coma or patients with paralysed limbs, patients to be operated upon and undergoing generalized anaesthesia. Also diminished mobility in old age, bed confinement, aeroplane trips.
- **Post-operative risk:** especially 10 days after abdominal and pelvic surgery.
- **Pregnancy and childbirth**: in the early post-partum period thrombosis is a major complication. During pregnancy raised levels of coagulation factors occur.
- **Hormonal**: high levels of oestrogens as in oral contraceptives and hormonal dysfunctions are a high risk. The risk of disseminated vascular thrombosis and CVA (stroke) is 5–6 times higher in women using high-dose oestrogen pills.
- **Cigarette smoking**: components of tobacco smoke enter the circulation and are thrombogenic.
- **Septicaemia**: the presence of bacteria in the blood often causes thrombosis (DIC, see below).

Types of Thrombi

Thrombi may be classified according to many different criteria as outlined in Figure 3.11.

Arterial thrombi form at sites of endothelial damage. They consist of layers of platelets interspersed with fibrin. Venous thrombi can develop in the absence of endothelial damage, they are predisposed to by stasis. They are gelatinous, moist and dark and often consist of trapped blood cells in a meshwork of fibrin filaments. Cardiac thrombi form in the cavities of the heart most commonly in association with myocardial infarction (heart attack). Capillary thrombosis occurs especially with septicaemias (some types of thrombi are illustrated in Figure 3.12).

A **platelet thrombus** is composed almost entirely of platelets. It forms the initial portion of a coralline thrombus and also the endocardial vegetations (on heart valves). These thrombi may be known as platelet 'plugs' which seal small areas of damage in vessels (Figure 3.13). A **coralline thrombus** is the typical laminated thrombus which may become occlusive, for example in a coronary artery or deep leg vein thrombosis.

A **propagating thrombus** is one in which progressive extension of the thrombus occurs following thrombotic occlusion in the venous system. This type has a more gelatinous, moist, deep red appearance, consisting mostly of blood cells trapped in a fibrin meshwork.

A **mural thrombus** is a thrombus adherent to one aspect of the wall of a large vessel or heart chamber which does not completely occlude the lumen, for example, a thrombus overlying a myocardial infarct.

A **ball thrombus** is an unattached, spherical, cardiac thrombus within the cavity of the atrium or ventricle, too large to pass through the valve orifices, and which may cause intermittent valve obstruction.

A **septic thrombus** may form as a result of infection, or a previously bland thrombus may become secondarily infected, as, for example, in thrombophlebitis.

Site of occurrence:	**Appearance:**
• Arterial (arteriothromboses)	• White (conglutination)
• Cardiac — atrial	• Red (coagulation)
— ventricular	• Mixed (laminated)
— valvular (vegetations)	**Microbiology:**
• Venous (phlebothromboses)	• Bland (not infected)
(thrombophlebitis)	• Septic (infected)
• Capillary	
Type:	**Aetiology:**
• Mural (lumen not obstructed totally)	• Atherosclerosis
• Occlusive (lumen obstructed totally)	• Thrombotic diathesis
• Propagating (growing, enlarging)	• Post-operative
• Coralline (irregular, branching)	• Hormonal/oestrogen
• Vegetations (thrombi on heart valves)	• Toxic
• Ball (unattached to wall, in heart esp.)	• Other

Figure 3.11 *Classification of thrombi*

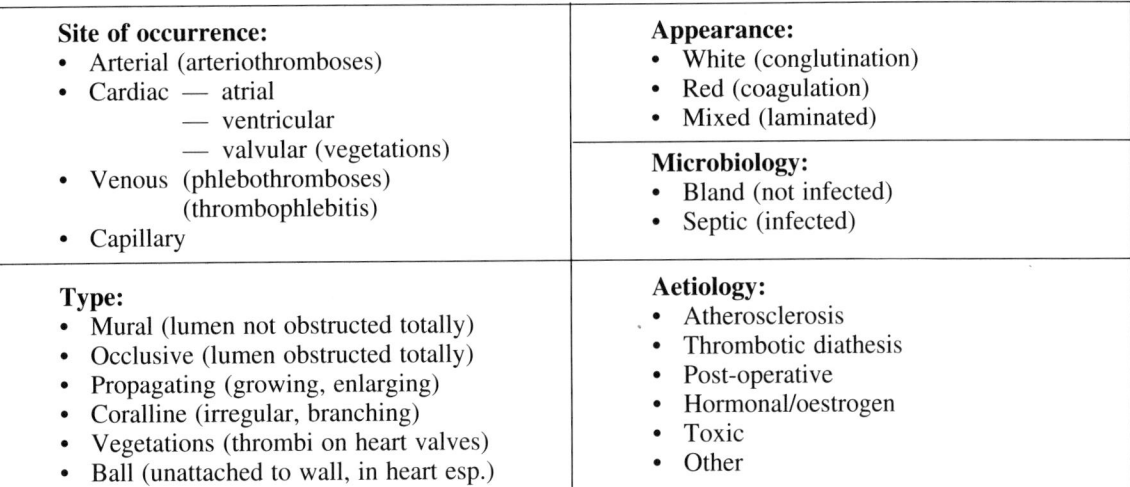

A mural, mixed thrombus

An occlusive mixed thrombus

A mural, platelet thrombus

An occlusive red thrombus

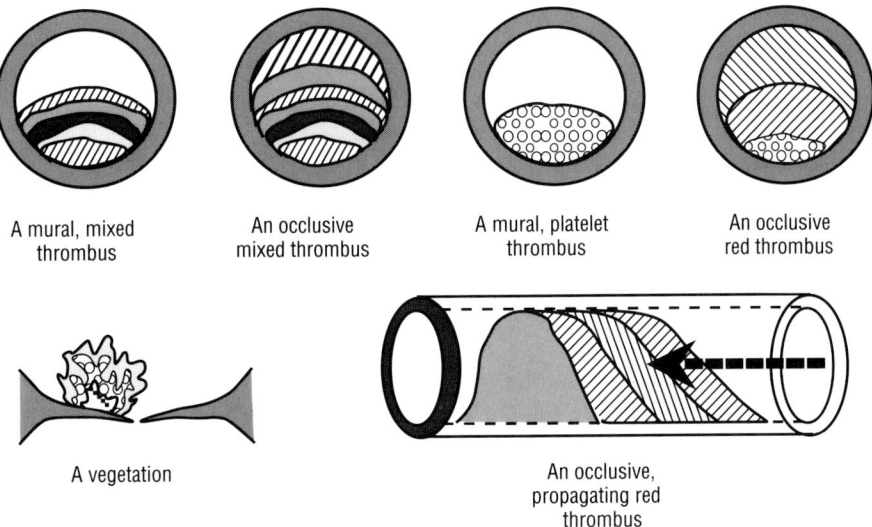

A vegetation

An occlusive, propagating red thrombus

Figure 3.12 *Some types of thrombi*

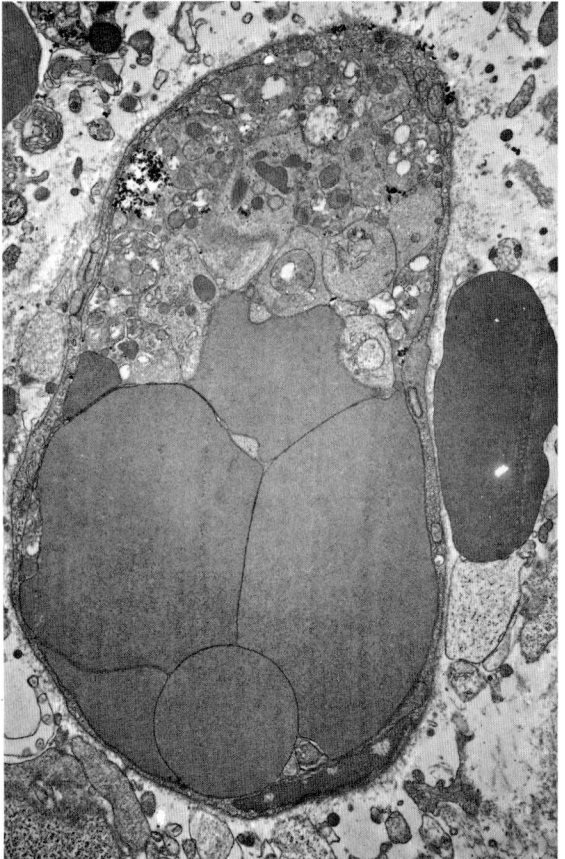

Figure 3.13　*A platelet plug forming in response to a region of damage in a capillary in stomach mucosa after injury through application of ethyl alcohol (×11 000)*

Propagation and Fates of Thrombi

When a thrombus forms and occludes the lumen of a vessel, there is cessation of blood flow. Stasis of flow leads to further propagation of the thrombus up to the next branches where flow is occurring. This process generally continues until a point of bifurcation of the vessel, whereby the blood is diverted and no further thrombus may then form. The thrombus that has arisen from this additive process from the initial thrombus is termed a **propagating thrombus**.

The sequelae of thrombosis are many and which sequela occurs depends on the site where the thrombus has formed, its size and the health of the patient.

Lysis. Thrombi can be rapidly dissolved by enzymatic action (plasmin) and the previously occluded lumen of the vessel may become patent once again. This is the most favourable outcome. Spontaneous small thrombi form often in every healthy person's blood stream but the lytic action of the plasmin system ensures that this type of thrombosis is symptomless.

Retraction and recanalization. Retraction of the thrombus first occurs as the clot matures and the fibrin strands consolidate with the platelets. This tends to decrease the size of the thrombus unevenly and cracks appear in the substance of the coagulum. In an occlusive thrombus this process may also allow some blood to start flowing past the obstruction. The second episode of retraction occurs as a result of the acute inflammatory process which is initiated at the site. Neutrophils from the bloodstream and also from inflamed vasa vasorum move into the thrombus and actively begin to resorb the necrotic thrombotic material. The organization process then begins as macrophages and granulation tissue moves into the thrombus. Fibroblasts begin to lay down collagen and endothelial cells around the thrombus divide, begin to cover the surface of the thrombus and also grow inwards to line the cracks in the centre of the thrombus. This leaves space within the vessel lumen allowing blood flow to be partially re-established (Figure 3.14).

Granulation tissue capillaries communicate through the clot, enlarging and resulting in perforation of the clot by many small vessels. This allows blood flow to be re-established. The process whereby new vascular

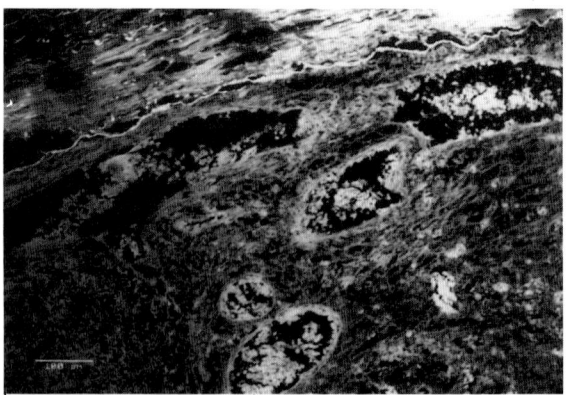

Figure 3.14　*Organizing thrombus in a vein. Recanalization has progressed to the stage where new vascular channels are forming in the granulation tissue that is infiltrating the thrombus. The wavy line of the elastic laminae of the vascular wall is seen at the upper edge of the micrograph (scale bar is 100 μm)*

channels form through an organized and scarred thrombus is termed **recanalization of the thrombus** (see Figure 3.15).

Calcification. The clot may be very large, such that the process of organization and recanalization may not

progress to completion. The partially organized clot (within a vein usually) will subsequently undergo dystrophic calcification forming a **phlebolith**.

Detachment, embolism. Small fragments of the thrombus can break off and lodge downstream, form-

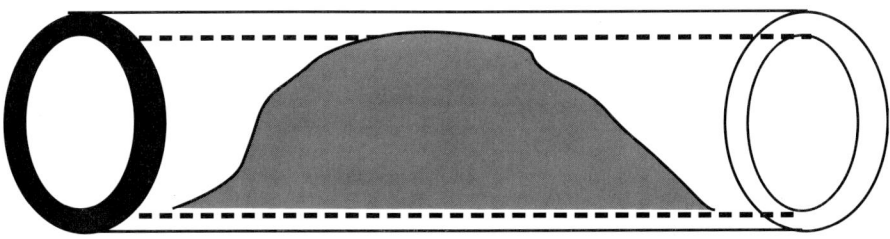

Occlusive thrombus forms in a vessel

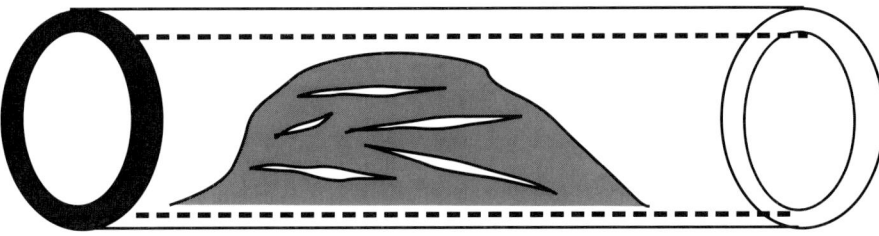

Retraction of thrombus with 'cracks' forming in it

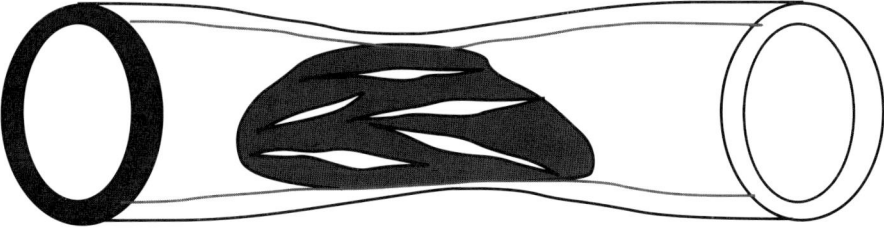

Inflammation, organization, re-endothelialization

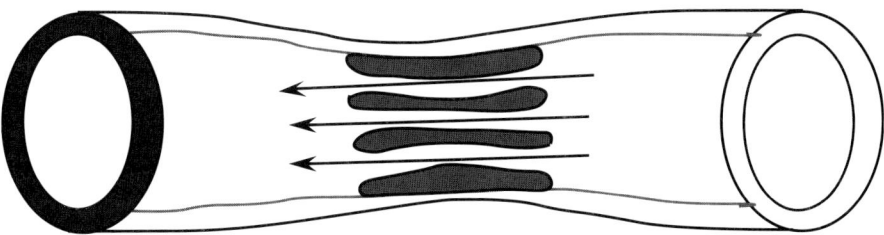

Recanalized thrombus

Figure 3.15 *The process of thrombus organization and recanalization*

ing emboli. For example, pulmonary embolism from deep vein leg or pelvic thrombosis may lead to sudden death or pulmonary ischaemic necrosis. A propagating thrombus may detach when it reaches the junction with a larger vein. The process of detachment of thrombi which lodge elsewhere is termed **thromboembolism**.

Infection. An infected thrombus is softened by proteolytic bacterial products so that portions may detach and produce septic infarction, pyaemic abscesses or mycotic aneurysms, Osler's nodes in the skin.

Thrombotic Conditions

Cardiac thrombosis follows myocardial infarction, valve prostheses, cardiac aneurysm, bacterial endocarditis and atrial fibrillation. If present in the left side of the heart it leads to systemic thromboembolism. Frequently, cerebral infarction (stroke) follows on from this condition.

Arterial thrombosis results from atherosclerosis or aneurysmal dilatation. The effects are **occlusion** and **embolism**. The condition is seen most frequently in the abdominal aorta, the coronary arteries, common carotids, renal arteries and cerebral arteries.

Venous thrombosis is also termed **phlebo-thrombosis** if it is not complicated. It usually results from stasis, especially if the blood is hypercoagulable. Venous thrombosis can also occur with inflammation of veins by irritant substances (e.g. IV catheters, drug abuse). It is very easy for infection to occur in these thrombi and the site becomes red, swollen, painful and hot. This symptomatic venous thrombosis is termed **thrombophlebitis**. Infected thrombi can lead to **pyaemia** (carriage of pyogenic organisms in the blood and formation of abscesses at distant sites). Non-infected thrombi in veins can also cause local tenderness and distant embolism.

Cavernous sinus thrombosis arises as an infection with suppuration in the sinuses or skin of the upper half of the face with thrombosis of the associated vessels. The infection is usually unilateral but spreads rapidly to the other side via the circular sinus. Patients are acutely ill and febrile, with severe retro-orbital pain and protruding eyes. There is oedema of conjunctivae and eyelids, with paralysis of extra-ocular muscles and paraesthesia of the trigeminal nerve. Complications include blindness, cerebral oedema, cerebral abscess and death. If diagnosed early, the condition responds to aggressive therapy with intravenous antibiotics.

Migratory thrombosis is characterized by the formation of thrombi in many different veins at different times but situated close together. It is an uncommon but significant manifestation of cancer, especially pancreatic cancer.

Disseminated intravascular coagulation (DIC) occurs when there is widespread triggering of coagulation and fibrinolysis within the circulation. It is diagnosed by laboratory findings of decreased circulating fibrinogen and platelets and increased circulating fibrin degradation products. The condition is caused by introduction into the circulation of foreign substances, and by burns, trauma, surgery, infections, amniotic fluid embolism, incompatible blood transfusion, snakebite, septicaemia (especially with Gram-negative bacteria), cancer of the prostate, lung and pancreas.

In most of these conditions cellular fragments or toxins are widely disseminated and cause widespread deposition of minute amounts of fibrin in the circulation, with consumption of clotting factors and platelets. Activation of plasmin occurs with dissolution of clots.

Effects of DIC include impaired renal blood flow which can cause acute renal tubular necrosis. Consumption of platelets and clotting factors leads to excessive haemorrhage from sites of trauma and shock develops. Treatment, paradoxically, is with heparin and infusion of platelets and clotting factors.

Embolism

Embolism is defined as the transfer of abnormal material by the bloodstream and its subsequent impaction in the vascular system. The solid or insoluble material is called an **embolus** and the commonest type of embolus is a **thromboembolus** which is derived from a dislodged thrombus elsewhere in the vascular system. The site at which the embolus lodges depends very much on the site at which it has arisen, as the diameter of the embolus and the diameter of blood vessels further downstream is what will determine impaction.

Types of Embolism

Thromboembolism (Thrombotic emboli)

Thromboemboli are due to dislodged thrombi originating in arteries, veins or in the heart. Thromboemboli arise very commonly from veins. In **pulmonary embolism** emboli arise mostly from the deep leg veins (95% of venous emboli are from these veins) or veins in the pelvis, and may be very large. The thrombus becomes detached, passes through the right atrium and ventricle of the heart and passes into the pulmonary arteries, impacting in the lungs where the vessels become progressively narrower. If a large embolus lodges in the lung arteries (e.g. a **saddle embolus** which lodges astride the bifurcation of the pulmonary vessels), the patient may die very quickly as there will be serious compromise of the blood flow through the lungs, leading to systemic hypoxia and a massive strain on the right heart.

When the emboli are smaller they are less likely to cause death as they travel to more peripheral areas of the lungs where they impact and cause infarcts. These patients may present with severe dyspnoea, pleuritic chest pain, cyanosis, loss of consciousness and sometimes they may die as more lung areas become involved in the inflammatory process generated by the necrosis and exudate that fills the lung tissue. Treatment is often unsuccessful, hence the most important factor is prevention of leg vein thrombosis in patients at risk.

Minor pulmonary emboli, unless multiple, have little detectable effect in healthy lungs. Pulmonary infarction may sometimes occur. If deep vein thrombosis is discovered early, treatment is with **anticoagulants** (e.g. intravenous heparin at first, then oral warfarin) to prevent propagation of the thrombus.

Arterial emboli are usually thrombotic debris originating on atherosclerotic plaques. Their effects depend on their location. Showers of emboli thrown up from the carotid arteries produce transient ischaemic attacks (TIA) in the brain which may manifest themselves as dizziness, loss of vision, paraesthesiae or loss of consciousness. If large emboli lodge in the brain vessels then a cerebrovascular accident (CVA) or 'stroke' occurs. Thrombi arising in the aorta or iliac vessels may impact in the popliteal or smaller arteries and cause occlusion leading to arterial insufficiency in the distal portion of the leg which may resolve or progress to loss of the limb.

Cardiac emboli usually arise from a mural thrombus in the atrium in atrial fibrillation or are attached to the ventricle in myocardial infarction. They may also arise from infected heart valves (vegetations) in bacterial endocarditis. If infected, these emboli can cause septic infarcts when they block an end-artery (for example in the kidney), or may cause multiple metastatic abscesses.

Fat Embolism

Fat emboli are emboli of fat globules which arise mostly from bone marrow following severe fractures, usually through the tibia and femur which have fatty marrow. Fat embolism may also occur in burns severe

enough to involve subcutaneous adipose tissue. They also arise as a result of rupture of atheromatous plaque which releases the lipid material inside the plaque. Usually only minute globules of fat escape but if large amounts of fat are released into the circulation the consequences are severe: cerebral insufficiency, pulmonary infarction or oedema and haemorrhage, and possibly death. Onset may be after a symptom-free period, with symptoms of cerebral disturbances such as restlessness, confusion, aggression, drowsiness or coma, associated with dyspnoea (difficulty in breathing) and tachypnoea (rapid breathing). A petechial rash may be seen. If the patient can be tided over the dangerous period of hypoxia, fat embolism is spontaneously reversible, although high levels of oxygen may be necessary in resuscitation.

Gas Embolism

Gas which enters the bloodstream acts as a 'solid' physical mass unless it is small enough such that it can dissolve quickly.

Air embolism
A large bubble of air admitted into a vessel does not dissolve quickly and may cause obstruction. If the jugular vein is opened air can be sucked into the right ventricle of the heart. If the volume of air is large enough (> 100 ml of gas), the pumping action of the heart causes severe foaming or frothiness, impeding the circulation and leading to loss of cardiac output and possible death. Smaller bubbles of air are dissolved and eliminated through the lungs. The risks are even greater with open-heart surgery or if bubbles of air enter the pulmonary veins (e.g. with pleurocentesis). In this case systemic embolism may block a coronary or cerebral vessel and lead to ischaemia, necrosis or death.

Major risks are:

- incision of large neck veins (surgery, homicide or suicide attempts);
- faulty intravenous therapy technique;
- injection of air or gas (pneumoperitoneum, pneumothorax, Fallopian tube inflation, other diagnostic and surgical procedures);
- separation of placenta during contractions of the uterus in childbirth with rise in intra-uterine pressure if the foetal head is engaged;
- chest injuries affecting the lungs — air is forced into vessels in the negative pressure phase of respiration;
- cerebral surgery (open veins, venous sinuses);
- open-heart surgery.

Nitrogen Embolism (Caisson Disease)

This may also be known as 'decompression disease', 'nitrogen narcosis' or 'the bends' (note that the term 'nitrogen narcosis' refers to an intoxicating effect that high levels of nitrogen have on nervous tissue and not an effect of nitrogen embolism). Nitrogen embolism occurs when deep-sea divers are decompressed too rapidly (ascending to the water surface too rapidly). Deep in the sea, pressures are much greater than atmospheric pressure. At greater pressure there is an increased amount of dissolved gases in the blood. Tiny bubbles of nitrogen form as gases come out of solution when the return to lower pressures is too rapid. Oxygen and carbon dioxide gas are quickly absorbed but the inert nitrogen gas remains in the tissues with a special affinity for fat, as in subcutaneous tissue and nervous tissue.

The 'bends' occur as bubbles of nitrogen lodge in muscles, bones and joints, causing severe pain, and the patient bends over as a response to this pain. Larger bubbles may occlude pulmonary capillaries or vessels in the central nervous system. Nitrogen bubbles lodging in the brain result in mental disturbance or coma. Nitrogen bubbles in the lungs cause 'the chokes', that is, dyspnoea, difficulty in breathing. Spinal cord damage may also occur, resulting in paraplegia. Treatment is by recompression in a pressure chamber followed by slow decompression to reabsorb the nitrogen.

Tumour Embolism

Malignant tumours, especially sarcomata, may spread via the bloodstream, producing disseminated secondary deposits. These tumour emboli are usually tiny but occasionally large fragments of tumour may break off and impact in blood vessels.

Tissue Fragments

Tissue fragments may dislodge and produce emboli. Occasionally atheromatous plaque fragments, biopsy material and traumatized tissue may form emboli.

Foreign Bodies

Catheter tips, fragments of disintegrating heart valves and insoluble matter used to contaminate drugs used by addicts may form emboli with serious consequences. Parasites may also act as emboli as occurs, for example, in cerebral malaria (the protozoön causing malaria known as *Plasmodium* has phases in the bloodstream).

Helminth parasites or their products may also lodge in vessels (e.g. microfilaria worms).

Amniotic Fluid Embolism

This is a rare complication of childbirth (approximately one in 50 000 to 80 000 deliveries). When it does occur it is totally unpredictable, mostly unpreventable and often fatal. It occurs typically in older multiparous women with difficult deliveries. The symptoms are sudden dyspnoea, cyanosis, collapse, haemorrhage, convulsions and coma, occurring during or shortly after delivery. Death occurs in 85–90% of patients.

At autopsy foetal squames (keratin), fat, mucin and lanugo (hair) are found in the pulmonary arterioles and capillaries of the dead woman. Disseminated intravascular coagulation is a frequent accompaniment of this condition as amniotic fluid is rich in a thromboplastin-like substance and hence highly thrombogenic.

The pathogenesis of the condition is that the foetal head (or presenting part) wedges into the lower uterine segment, and the force of the uterine contractions causes partial tearing of the uterine wall, exposing and opening branches of the uterine veins. Under this increased pressure during contractions, amniotic fluid containing shed foetal products is forced into the maternal veins (sometimes maternal placental vessels) and this infusion is carried to the lungs and causes DIC. This may deplete fibrinogen in the blood, causing bleeding tendencies.

Emergency caesarean section rescues up to 40% of babies whose mothers have died during labour in this tragic way.

Results of Embolism

The results of embolism depend on:

- the site of origin (whether arteries or veins);
- the site of impaction;
- the presence of collateral circulation;
- infection (whether septic or aseptic emboli are involved).

Death may occur suddenly due most commonly to pulmonary embolism, usually from deep vein thrombosis. Alternatively death may result from cerebral embolism causing a cerebrovascular accident, or more rarely due to coronary artery embolism causing a fatal heart attack.

Embolic occlusion of a vessel supplying a part or the whole of an organ with poor collateral blood supply leads to ischaemic tissue necrosis, or **infarction**.

Infarcts in vital organs such as the heart or brain may be fatal.

Embolism may result in obstruction of the femoral artery (or even brachial artery). The affected limb then becomes cold, pale and numb with no pulse. If the collateral supply is adequate there may be recovery of blood supply to the limb. When the collateral supply is inadequate **gangrene** may result.

Infarction

Infarction is an area of anoxic (usually ischaemic) necrosis produced by an acute interruption of blood supply. This is usually due to thrombosis and/or embolism. Infarction may be due to obstruction of arterial blood supply or obstruction of venous drainage from the organ. Infarction occurs where collateral blood supply is inadequate to allow survival of the tissues. Hence, organs which are highly vascular, such as skin, thyroid and liver, are rarely sites of infarction. Infarction occurs more commonly in tissues with end-arteries, such as kidney, spleen, heart and brain.

Types of Infarcts

Pale or anaemic infarcts occur, for example, in kidney, heart, spleen and brain tissue after occlusion of end-arteries, implying that no more blood may enter that region of tissue. The blood already in the infarcted region is drained away by the veins and this gives the infarct a very pale appearance, an effect enhanced by the coagulation of protein (refer to Figure 3.16).

Red or haemorrhagic infarcts occur, for example, in lung and intestine, which have a dual blood supply. Alternatively, red infarcts may result if a vein is occluded (usually by formation of thrombus *in situ*) or when an occluded artery readmits blood to the infarcted tissue (i.e. if a thromboembolus in the artery is broken down *after* the tissue has undergone necrosis). Interruption of arterial blood supply produces anoxic necrosis more certainly than does venous occlusion as veins can produce bypass channels more readily than arteries. **Mixed infarcts** occur, for example, in the heart where there is partial readmission of the blood into the infarcted area after the tissue has undergone necrosis.

A **bland infarct**, the most usual type, is one which has not been infected and occurs, for example, in the heart, while a **septic infarct** is one which has secondarily become infected and occurs, for example, in the gut or in the lungs.

In **recent infarcts**, there is still evidence of the necrosis and the organization process is still new. **Organized infarcts** show little evidence of necrotic tissue, most of it being replaced by scar. This represents the most usual outcome of infarction and is the healing response of the body to the injury which has created the region of ischaemic necrosis.

In **calcified infarcts** the necrotic tissue tends to undergo dystrophic calcification and very large infarcts may calcify.

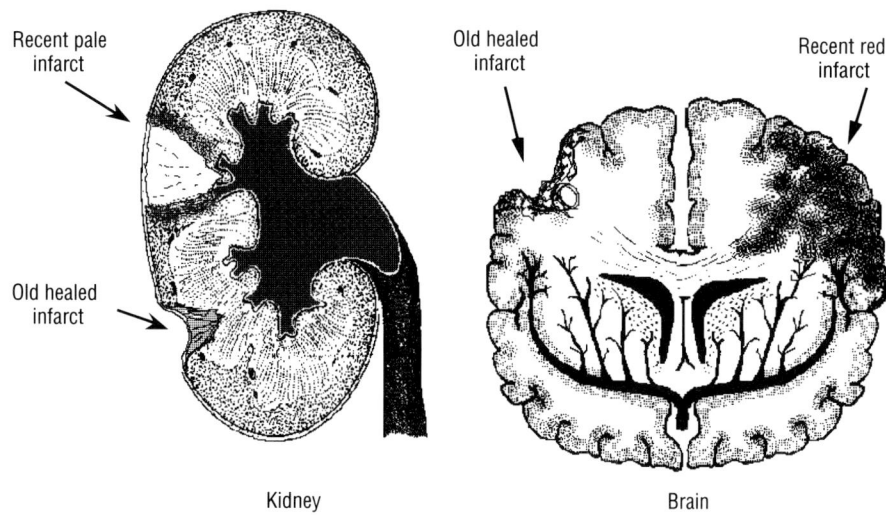

Kidney · Brain

Figure 3.16 *Some types of infarcts illustrated*

Appearance and Nature of Infarcts

All infarcts appear red eventually as blood passes into the area with the initiation of the inflammatory response and formation of the granulation tissue, which will grow into the infarcted region bringing with it cells of inflammation and repair. In solid organs, large infarcts are areas of coagulative necrosis and when the blood is drained by the venous system, few red blood cells remain in the area which appears pale. Large infarcts may remain pale as the inflammatory response is inadequate to remove totally all of the necrotic tissue and such large infarcts are more likely to calcify (Figure 3.17)

Most infarcts result from thromboembolic occlusion of nutrient arteries to various organs, the most commonly involved being heart, brain and kidneys. The thromboembolus is usually derived from a thrombus which has formed on atheromatous plaques in arteries (arterial thromboemboli) or damaged heart muscle regions (cardiac thromboemboli seen in association with necrotic muscle in the heart; a stroke very commonly may follow a heart attack). Infarction due to venous occlusion almost always follows *in situ* formation of thrombi in the vein occluded. Venous thromboemboli will lodge in the pulmonary arteries with resulting pulmonary infarction. This is because the pulmonary vessels are of decreasing diameter down to the level of the alveolar capillaries and this means that all thromboemboli arising in the peripheral venous system (most usually thrombi form in the leg veins) will be arrested in the lungs.

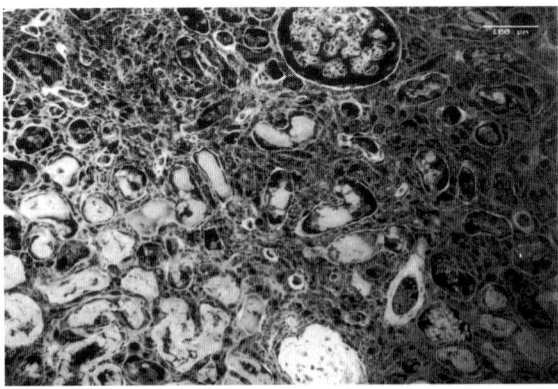

Figure 3.17 *A renal infarct. The edge of the necrotic region is seen to traverse the upper left corner of the micrograph through to the right bottom corner. A normal glomerulus is at the top of the micrograph while a necrotic one below shows coagulation (scale bar is 100 μm)*

Occlusion to a vessel may also occur as a result of large **atheromatous plaques** growing and gradually occluding the lumen of a vessel, as may occur in branches of the coronary artery (the interrelationship of some common vascular disorders is seen in Figure 3.18) A growing **tumour** may compress a vessel and compromise blood supply distally (many rapidly growing malignant tumours very often have central infarcted regions where they have compressed their own blood supply). **Torsion** (twisting) of the pedicles of mobile viscera (e.g. gut) or solid organs (e.g. ovary, testis) will twist the blood vessels in the pedicle, causing thrombosis and infarction. Usually in this last example a red infarct results as the veins are more readily compressible than arteries and the testis and ovaries have no venous by-pass mechanisms. Lastly, fibrocollagenous tissue adhesions in tissues may cause compression of vessels trapped in the collagenous scar, resulting in infarction (e.g. intestinal adhesions following surgery).

Infarcts tend to be conical (wedge-shaped in section), involving the peripheral part of an organ, reflecting the occluded vascular tree, with the apex of the cone at the point of focus of occlusion, the external aspect of the organ forming the base of the cone. In the affected areas pressure drops following vascular obstruction so blood from surrounding tissue suffuses into the infarcted area in the early stages. There is a hyperaemic border around the infarct due to the inflammatory response, so in the early stages the infarct most usually appears pale with a red border.

Microscopically, for a few hours the infarct margin is stuffed with blood, then after approximately 24 hours necrosis becomes visible, usually coagulative. Red blood cells lyse and haemosiderin is seen, often inside macrophages. The inflammatory response at the border which later extends into the centre of the infarct enables phagocytic removal of necrotic debris. Finally there is organization of the infarct or repair by fibrocollagenous connective tissue replacement, which grows in from the margins. Eventually, all that remains is a depressed scar (**fibrosis**).

The time course of a typical pale infarct in tissue resulting from arterial occlusion is given below:

- **0–6 hours**: the infarcted tissue is slightly paler than the surrounding tissue, its margins poorly defined.
- **8–10 hours**: the infarct is very pale and the margin between it and the normal tissue is well defined.
- **10–30 hours**: there is a very hyperaemic border around the infarcted region as the inflammatory response commences in reaction to the breakdown products of cells released at the site.

- **30–72 hours**: the hyperaemic border is wider and more pronounced around the infarcted region and granulation tissue forms, which begins to resorb the necrotic tissue. The infarcted area is very pale, dense and shrunken.
- **72 hours–14 days**: the infarcted tissue is gradually replaced by fibrocollagenous scar tissue as the granulation tissue infiltrates the necrotic tissue. Macroscopically the infarct will appear redder and redder as the granulation tissue vessels grow into it.

Infarcts of the central nervous system undergo colliquative (liquefactive) necrosis, leaving a cystic space filled with turbid fluid. **Gliosis** (not fibrosis) occurs in the brain so the cyst may be criss-crossed by strands of glial cells, lined by glial cells and filled with fluid. Such a structure occurring in brains of survivors of cerebral infarction are termed **apoplectic cysts** as the old term for a stroke was apoplexy.

Septic infarction may occur when an infarct has superimposed infection, causing colliquative necrosis and abscess formation or alternatively gangrene. This may be caused by an infected or septic embolus (such as valve vegetations in bacterial endocarditis breaking off) or by secondary infection of an established infarct, for example in the bowel or in the lungs.

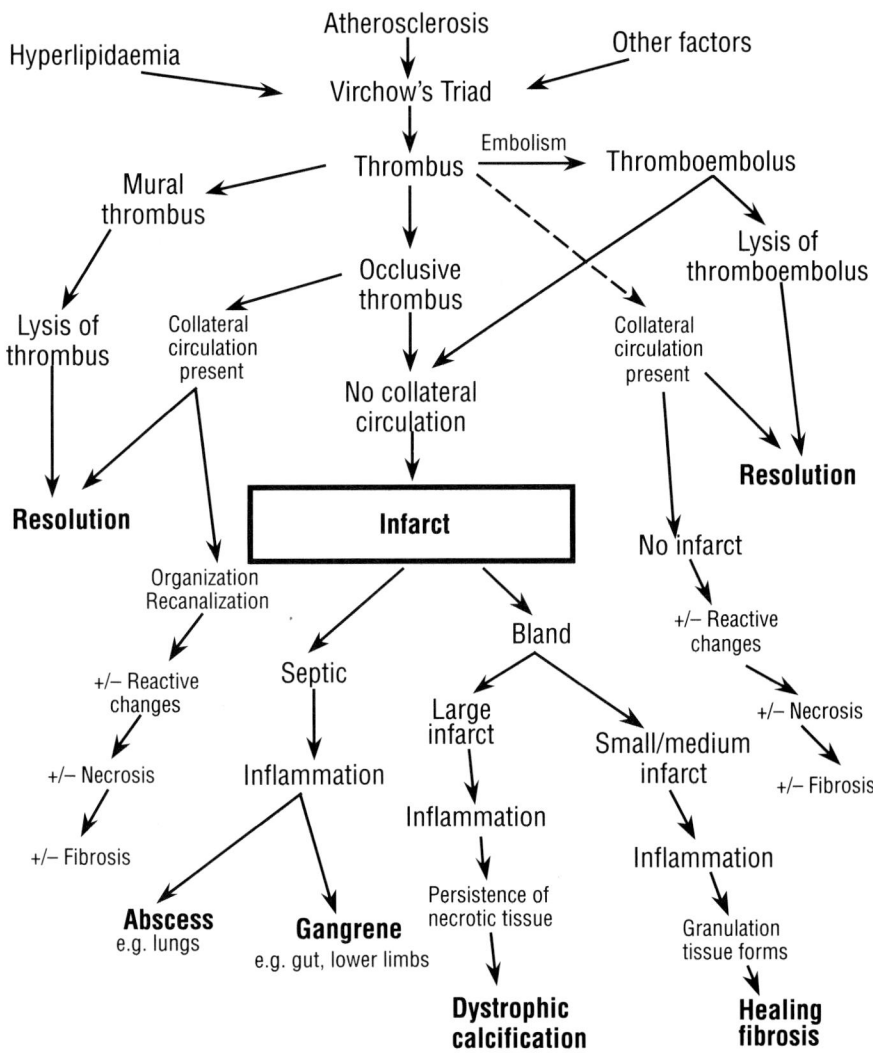

Figure 3.18 *Interrelationship of some common vascular disorders*

Hypertension

Hypertension is a persistent rise in blood pressure. Blood pressure fluctuates considerably under emotional and other stresses and also increases with age, and hence there is no universally accepted numerical value for a 'raised blood pressure'. It is the diastolic pressure which is most important in hypertension and if the diastolic pressure is greater than 95 mmHg it is regarded with suspicion. Persistent blood pressure at 140/95 mmHg is considered to be hypertension (i.e. systolic 140 mmHg/diastolic 95 mmHg). Hypertension is very common, affecting approximately one-third of the population. Its effects are often lethal and yet it remains asymptomatic until late in its course, by which time irreversible damage has already occurred.

Hypertension is an important risk factor in coronary heart disease and in cerebrovascular accident ('stroke'), and may also lead to renal failure and to left ventricular failure ('heart failure'). The detrimental effects of blood pressure elevation increase continuously as the pressure increases. There is a correlation between high salt intake and hypertension in people who are genetically predisposed. The prevalence of hypertension increases with age. If it is present in young adults it tends to be severe, and there is more frequently an underlying cause. Overall, women are more commonly affected than men but this is mostly in older age groups. Males under 50 years of age are more commonly affected.

Measuring Blood Pressure Correctly

When taking a blood pressure measurement the patient's arm must be horizontal at the level of the fourth intercostal space. Otherwise, hydrostatic pressure effects may cause an error of as much as 10 mmHg in either the systolic or diastolic pressure. The cuff should be placed snugly on the upper arm, it should be of a suitable width and the deflation should be at the proper rate. Ensure that the patient is relaxed, comfortable and in pleasant surroundings as emotional state may greatly influence the blood pressure.

Be aware of the **auscultatory gap**, which is a zone of silence in the Korotkoff sounds starting 10–30 mmHg below the true systolic pressure and continuing downwards for 20–30 mmHg towards the diastolic pressure (refer to Figure 3.19). You may be misled if you randomly inflate the cuff to the silence of the gap. If you then deflate the cuff, the reappearance of the sounds will be mistaken for the systolic pressure reading. To avoid this, always take blood pressure by the palpatory method. Put your finger or stethoscope on the radial pulse and inflate the cuff until the pulse disappears. When you then deflate, you can be certain that the first reading will not be in the auscultatory gap.

Blood Pressure Curve Analysis

A typical blood pressure curve is shown in Figure 3.20. The **systolic blood pressure** is indicated by the

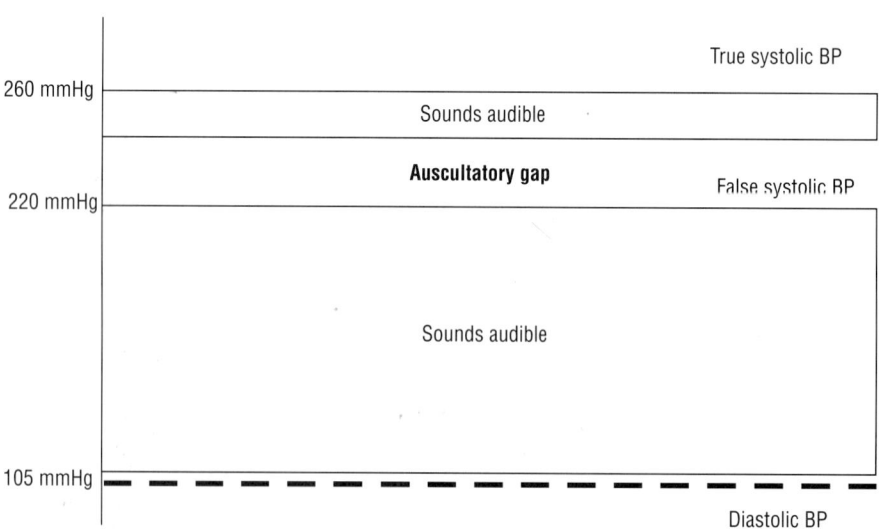

Figure 3.19 *The presence of an auscultatory gap while taking blood pressure measurements of some patients*

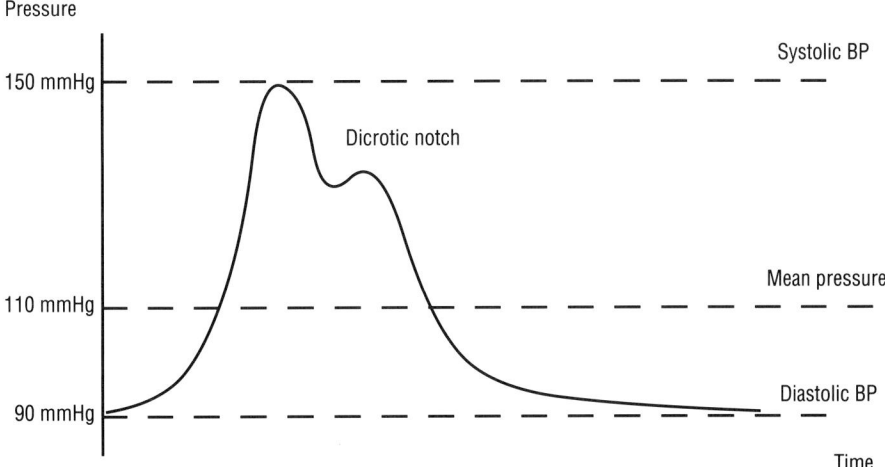

Figure 3.20 *A typical blood pressure curve*

crest of the blood pressure curve and represents the maximal pressure generated within the vascular tree coincident with the peak of ventricular systole. The **diastolic blood pressure** is indicated by the trough of the blood pressure curve and represents the minimal pressure within the vascular tree coincident with the end of ventricular diastole. The major single determinant of diastolic pressure is **arterial resistance**. An important factor in the development of hypertension is increases in arterial resistance of the peripheral arterioles. The **pulse pressure** is the difference between systolic and diastolic blood pressure. It is mainly a function of the volume of blood ejected by the heart during systole. The **mean pressure** is the average blood pressure within the vascular tree throughout the cardiac cycle. For clinical purposes a good approximation for this value is worked out by adding a third of the pulse pressure to the diastolic pressure:

Mean pressure = 1/3 Pulse pressure + Diastolic pressure

i.e. for the curve in Figure 3.14:

MP = 20 + 90 = 110 mmHg

Remember that blood pressure is a function of cardiac output (which is the product of heart rate by stroke volume) and peripheral resistance. Therefore, changes in blood pressure may have either cardiac causes or peripheral circulatory causes, or both. In viewing the blood pressure curve in Figure 3.20 it is evident that the length of diastole is longer than the length of systole and therefore the arterial pressure during most of the cardiac cycle is closer to diastolic than systolic pressure. It thus becomes apparent why diastolic pressure increases are more important in hypertension than systolic pressure increases.

Types of Hypertension

Ninety per cent of hypertension is **idiopathic** (**primary** or **essential** hypertension) Of the remaining 10%, the majority is due to renal disease, but also may be due to endocrine disease. Where the cause of the raised blood pressure is known, the condition is known as **secondary** hypertension.

Both primary and secondary hypertension may also be divided into **benign hypertension**, which follows a slowly progressive course compatible with long life, or **malignant hypertension**, in which there is a fulminant severe increase in blood pressure. It should be noted that these are clinical divisions. Benign hypertension is associated with a long course, developing over a period of many years or decades and is generally compatible with a long life, unless a myocardial infarct or cerebral infarct supervenes. The disorder shows some important lesions in the kidneys.

Malignant hypertension runs an accelerated course and may kill the patient in several months. It is associated with some characteristic and specific signs, a diastolic pressure above 120 mmHg, renal failure, hypertensive retinopathy, bilateral retinal haemorrhages and exudates with or without papilloedema. Unless treated, the majority of patients with malignant hypertension are dead within one year. Malignant hypertension may develop in previously normotensive individuals *de novo*, or may be superimposed on previously existing benign hypertension. It tends to occur more commonly in the younger age group, generally in people aged between 30 and 40 years.

Both forms of hypertension affect many tissues in the body and thus the disorders must be considered as systemic diseases with prime effects on the vascular system, kidney and spleen. Both forms increase the risk of developing other vascular diseases such as arteriosclerosis.

Causes of death in hypertension are:

• cerebral haemorrhage;
• renal failure (uraemia);
• congestive heart failure;
• coronary occlusion (coronary heart disease).

The following clinical findings are common in hypertension:

• Retinal changes: sclerosis, haemorrhage, oedema — all of which may lead to blindness.
• Renal changes: arteriolosclerosis, infarcts, scarring, hyalinization of glomeruli.
• Vascular changes: predisposition to atherosclerosis, predisposition to aneurysm formation, predisposition to aneurysm rupture.

Malignant Hypertension

This is a disorder which is less commonly seen than benign hypertension but is important as it may cause death in a very short period of time. Very high blood pressures may be seen, the patients presenting with readings of up to 280/180 mmHg. It may arise *de novo*, or it may supervene on pre-existing benign hypertension. There are very important and characteristic pathological features in the kidney: initially there is damage to arterioles mediated by the effects of age, genetics, inflammatory processes in the wall and direct effects of the high blood pressure. There is hyperplasia of the smooth muscle in the wall of the arterioles and plasma proteins (but especially fibrinogen) infiltrate into the arterial wall and fibrin is formed intramurally. The clotting mechanism is then activated and microthrombi form on the luminal aspect of the damaged vessel. Fibrinoid necrosis of the vessel wall develops as a result of the high pressure, the inflammation and ischaemia. The changes in the arterial walls are described as a **necrotizing arteriolitis** and this term describes both the necrosis and inflammation that are features of the disease.

As the blood attempts to pass through the obstructed

lumen of these vessels there is damage to the erythrocytes, more thrombosis, fibrin deposition and a vicious cycle begins. The tissue becomes progressively more ischaemic and the kidney is stimulated to produce renin which causes aldosterone to be secreted, causing a further elevation of the blood pressure. The vascular changes develop in the arterioles of other tissues in a similar way to that already described for the kidney vessels. Thus, **malignant arteriolosclerosis** develops markedly in the kidney, spleen, brain and extremities.

Changes in the kidney which are particularly marked are referred to as malignant nephrosclerosis and necrotizing arteriolitis (refer to Figures 3.21, 3.22 and 3.23). Macroscopically the kidney looks normal or slightly shrunken with small, petechial haemorrhages in the cortex giving it a 'flea-bitten' appearance. The arterioles show fibrinoid necrosis of the wall, and the so-called 'onion-skinning' refers to the concentric hyperplastic and degenerating layers of the arterial wall resembling the cut surface of an onion.

The glomeruli are involved in the ischaemia and undergo various pathological processes including thrombosis and haemorrhage, finally undergoing fibrinoid necrosis, showing **hyalinization** (a 'glass-like' appearance — a descriptive term to indicate the uniform, eosinophilic appearance of the necrotic glomeruli which look like pink glass). Approximately 20% of glomeruli are involved in this disease process (Figure 3.24).

At the same time, the tubules show non-specific reactive and degenerative changes of ischaemia and may often contain clumps of coagulated plasma pro-

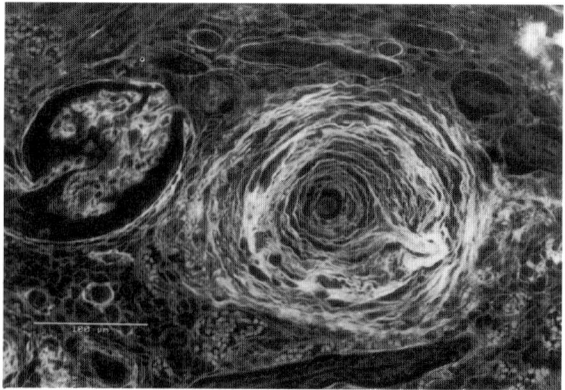

Figure 3.21 *Malignant arteriosclerosis showing characteristic 'onion skinning' of the vascular wall (scale bar is 100 μm)*

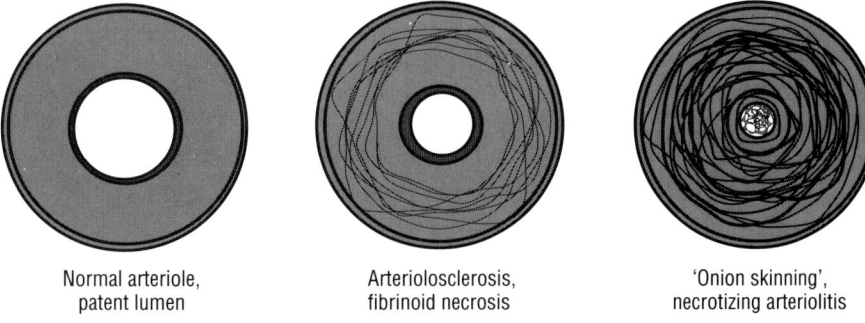

| Normal arteriole, patent lumen | Arteriolosclerosis, fibrinoid necrosis | 'Onion skinning', necrotizing arteriolitis |

Figure 3.22 *The arteriolar changes seen in malignant hypertension*

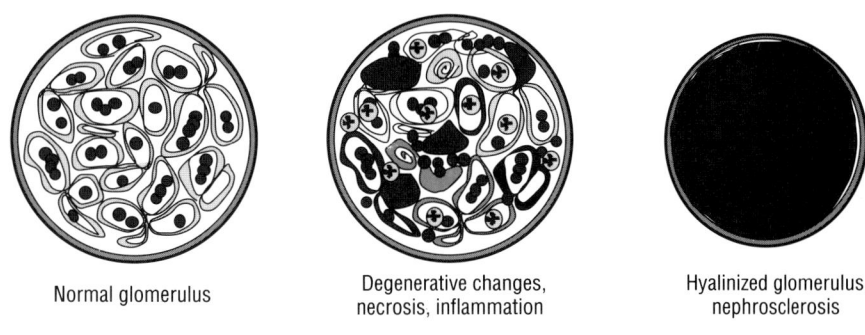

| Normal glomerulus | Degenerative changes, necrosis, inflammation | Hyalinized glomerulus, nephrosclerosis |

Figure 3.23 *Glomerular changes seen with malignant hypertension*

tein which has escaped through the damaged glomeruli. These clumps of coagulated protein in the tubules look amorphous and eosinophilic and are called **protein casts** as they assume the shape of the tubular lumen like a plaster cast would. These protein casts are excreted in the urine and may be detected by microscopy (Figure 3.25).

Eventually, all these rapidly developing changes in the kidney lead to renal failure. The patient may notice **haematuria** (blood in the urine), and **proteinuria** (protein in the urine) may be detected. Damage to arterioles in other tissues may cause sudden onset of cerebral manifestations of disease such as headaches, nausea, vomiting, loss of consciousness, convulsions. Arterioles in the eye are also affected very severely in malignant hypertension and various changes in the retinal disc will cause visual derangements. There is **papilloedema** (oedema of the optic disc = papilla), due to congestion of retinal veins, haemorrhages in the retina, microthrombosis in the arterioles and degenerative changes in the arteriolar wall. Blindness may result in longstanding untreated cases.

The effects of malignant hypertension on the patient

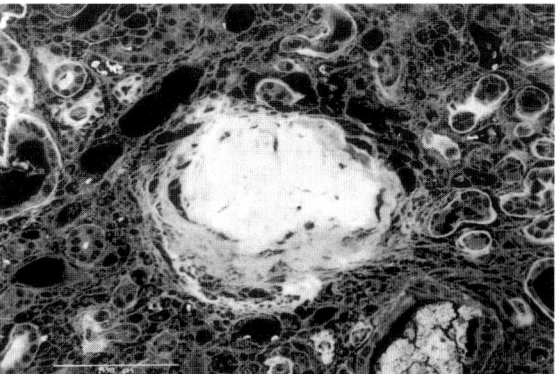

Figure 3.24 *Malignant nephrosclerosis where a glomerulus has been completely hyalinized, the capillaries now being a mass of fibrinoid necrosis (scale bar is 100 μm)*

are due to the arteriolosclerosis with considerable tissue damage, especially in the kidney. The patients show **left-sided hypertrophy** of the heart (thickening

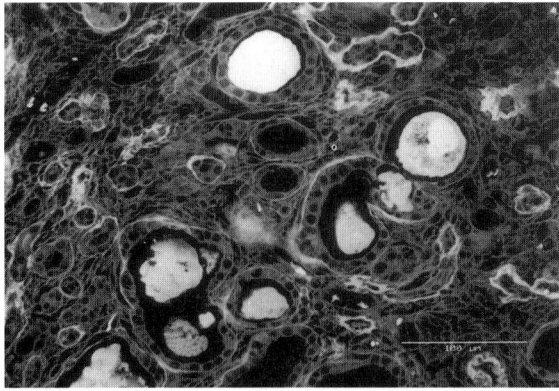

Figure 3.25 *Tubules in a kidney from a patient with hypertension showing characteristic protein casts in the tubular lumen (scale bar is 100 μm)*

of the left ventricular wall in response to the increased work load on the heart) and this may progress to **congestive heart failure** as the coronary arteries may be unable to supply the heart muscle with its demands for increased blood supply.

Prognosis for patients with malignant hypertension is generally poor, even with treatment. If untreated, most patients will die within one year of diagnosis, usually of **renal failure** and uraemia. Occasionally, patients may die of cerebrovascular accidents or cardiac failure. Treatment of patients is with antihypertensive drugs (α-adrenoceptor and β-adrenoceptor blockers usually). The percentage of patients surviving for 2 years with treatment is 75% and for 5 years with treatment is 50%. The long-term survival of the patient depends on how early in the course of the disease treatment commenced, the extent of renal damage sustained by the patient, the severity of arteriosclerosis and the ease of control of other disease processes coexisting with or causing the hypertension.

Benign Hypertension

This is the commonest form of hypertension (95% of cases) and is one which is slowly progressive and more easily controlled with treatment. It may however, be totally asymptomatic for many years. Characteristically, in these patients changes known as **benign nephrosclerosis** develop in the kidneys. Some degree of such kidney changes is seen at autopsy of most people over the age of 60 years. In the younger age groups severity and frequency of lesions are aggravated by the coexistence of diabetes mellitus.

The basic anatomical lesion of benign hypertension is hyaline arteriolosclerosis, which develops in many vessels throughout the body but is especially marked in renal arteries and arterioles. The arterial wall first becomes thickened with reduplication of elastic layers as more collagenous tissue is laid down with splitting of the elastic fibres, a change known as **elastosis**. There is subsequently degeneration of, deposition of plasma proteins in, and fibrinoid necrosis of the arteriolar wall. Lipids are deposited in the wall and the lumen is greatly decreased in size causing marked ischaemia of the glomeruli and other tissues supplied by these vessels. The glomeruli show axial thickening, fibrosis and hyalinization, all of these changes becoming more marked as the disease progresses over many years. There is diffuse tubular atrophy, tubular cast formation and interstitial fibrosis of the kidney (see Figures 3.26 and 3.27).

Patients with benign hypertension may have few or no signs and symptoms for many years as the blood pressure rises slowly over time. There may be mild proteinuria and haematuria. Ischaemia of many tissues may lead to manifestations such as poorly healing wounds in the lower limbs and other peripheral tissues and there may be gangrene. Generally these changes develop much more quickly and severely if the patient with hypertension is also a diabetic. Hypertension is a prime risk factor in the development of **atherosclerosis**, the prime degenerative disease of importance in the arterial system. Hypertensive hypertrophy of the left ventricle is a major complication of the disease and most patients with advanced hypertension die of myocardial insufficiency, congestive heart failure and myocardial infarcts. Cerebrovascular accidents are also an important cause of death. The renal lesions progress slowly and generally there is enough renal substance left for the kidneys to carry out their function; rarely do patients with benign nephrosclerosis develop renal failure.

The prognosis of benign hypertension is much better than that of malignant hypertension as it is easier to treat and control the disorder. Patients may live for many years, even with untreated benign hypertension — in fact, many patients with benign hypertension have few symptoms or signs and their condition may remain undiagnosed. Drug or alternative treatments are quite successful in lowering the blood pressure. Changes in lifestyle, diet review, sensible exercise are all additional means of dealing with hypertension and may be important in determining the progression of the disease. It should be noted that benign hypertension may suddenly progress to malignant hypertension, thereafter following the course of that disorder.

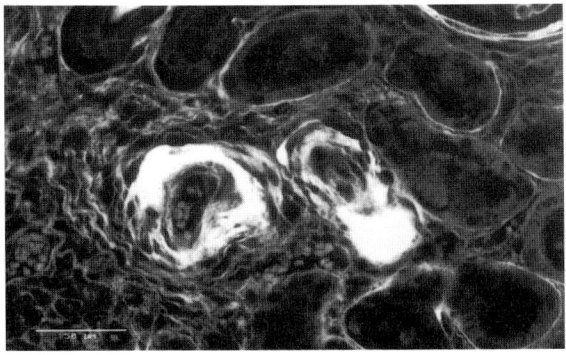

Figure 3.26 *A section from the kidney of a patient with benign hypertension showing arterioles with fibrinoid necrosis (very bright acellular regions) in their walls (scale bar is 50 μm)*

Hence, all patients with benign hypertension should be carefully monitored regularly.

Aetiology and Pathogenesis of Hypertension

Primary Hypertension

It has already been said earlier that most cases of hypertension (90%) are **idiopathic**, that is, we do not know the causes. Hypertension is believed to arise as a result of an interaction of complex, polygenic genetic causes and environmental factors. Many studies have shown evidence for the genetic factors as there is a high degree of concordance in twins, siblings and families. The control of blood pressure normally is a complex homeostatic mechanism depending on neu-ral, hormonal and haemodynamic controls (see Figure 3.28).

Environmental influences affect to a great degree the development of the hypertension and also its severity. Numerous epidemiological studies have shown that external factors may be more important than genetic factors in certain situations. For example, Chinese living in China have a low incidence of hypertension, but once they migrate to a Western country the incidence of the disease approaches that of the native population. Studies have indicated that important external factors involved in determining the development of the disease include: stress and lifestyle, personality type, obesity, inactivity, smoking of cigarettes and oral contraceptive use. The external factor which has generated the greatest interest by far is common salt (NaCl) ingestion. Some researchers maintain that high salt intake is the greatest risk factor and point to data collected from cases of hypertension developing in certain racial groups living in different geographical areas: natives living in the highlands of New Guinea, remote inland areas of Africa and Brazil traditionally have a low sodium diet and the incidence of primary hypertension in these people is very low. If these natives migrate to the coastal areas, their dietary intake of sodium increases and so does their incidence of hypertension. The daily consumption of salt increases in these people from virtually nil to 8 grams or more per day and correlates well with the very low incidence of hypertension in the remote areas to the high incidence of 8 to 25% of the population in the coastal areas. Despite data like these, it is now believed that elevated NaCl intake is not a prime factor in hypertension and in most human cases genetic factors are more important. This is supported by the fact that many people remain normotensive despite consuming large quantities of salt daily. Experimental studies in rats also support this suggestion.

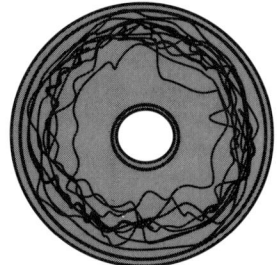

Hyaline arteriolosclerosis,
fibrinoid necrosis

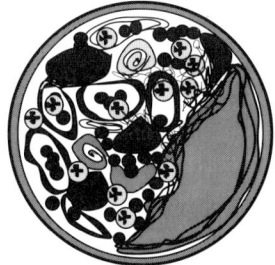

Degenerative changes,
benign nephrosclerosis

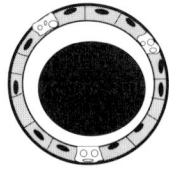

Tubular atrophy,
protein cast formation

Figure 3.27 *The changes in arterioles and renal tissue seen in benign hypertension*

Females tend to be affected more than males in primary hypertension, usually showing first signs of the disorder in their fourth or fifth decade (refer to Figure 3.29). The incidence of the disease rises with age and as much as 50% of the population over the age of 50 years may have a degree of hypertension. Note, however, that the disease is mild and slowly progressive (i.e. benign hypertension), thus frequently remains undiagnosed and subclinical.

Secondary Hypertension

This is defined as hypertension which occurs secondarily to other conditions. This accounts for only 10% of cases of high blood pressure. There are many known causes of secondary hypertension but by far the most important cause is renal disease, while other causes are endocrine disorders and some hormone-secreting tumours, the most important one being the rare **phaeo-**

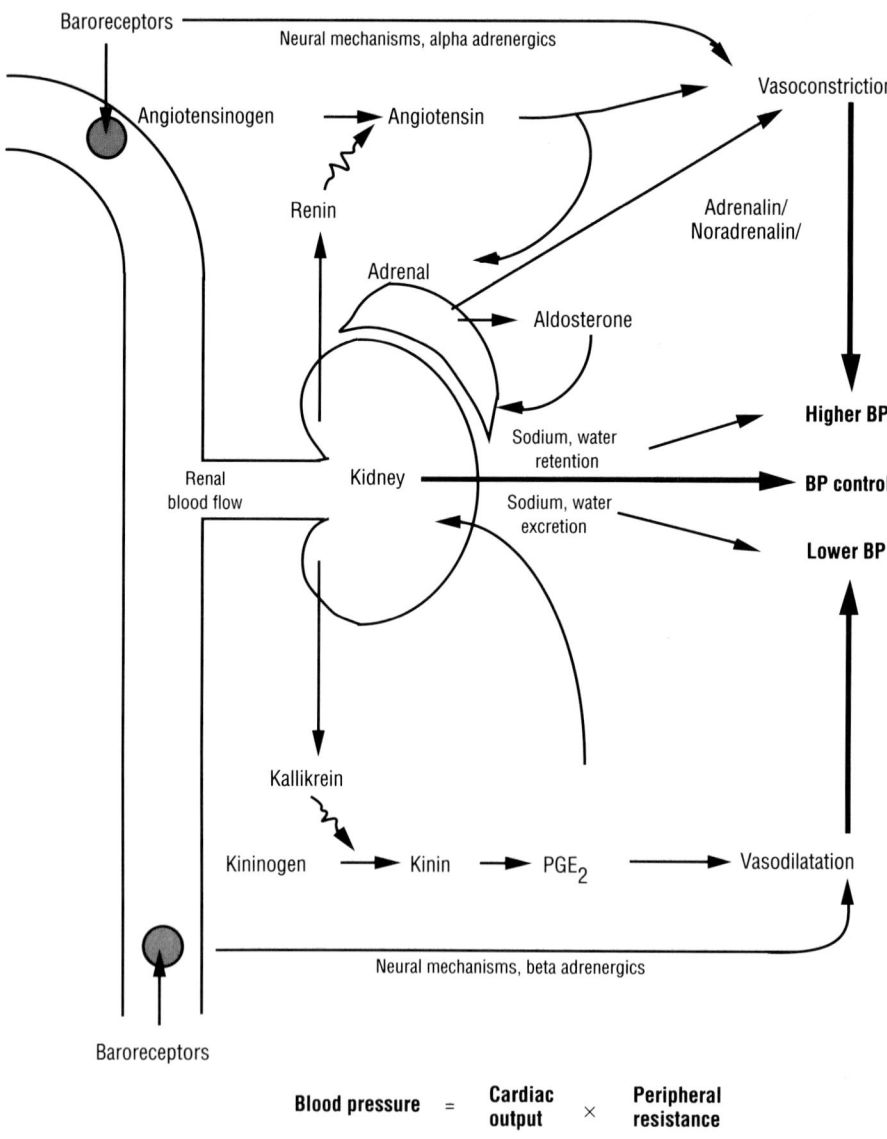

Figure 3.28 *The control of blood pressure*

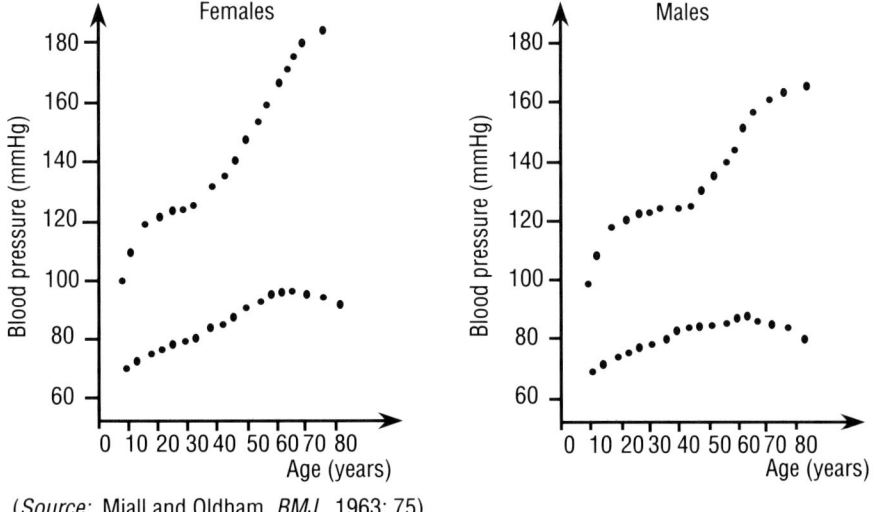

(*Source:* Miall and Oldham, *BMJ* 1963; 75)

Figure 3.29 *Mean systolic and diastolic blood pressures in a population in New South Wales*

chromocytoma. A small number of cases of secondary hypertension have neurological causes.

Renal Causes

Renal ischaemia or diminished intrarenal arterial blood pressure is a potent stimulus for secretion of renin, an enzyme synthesized and stored in the cells of the juxtaglomerular apparatus. Renin splits off angiotensin I from a circulating α2 globulin, angiotensinogen, which is manufactured in the liver. Angiotensin I is then converted to angiotensin II. Angiotensin II acts on vascular smooth muscle to cause vasoconstriction, increasing peripheral resistance. Angiotensin II and angiotensin III stimulate release of adrenal aldosterone, which causes sodium and fluid retention. Thus renal hypertension is induced.

Causes of renal hypertension include **renal artery stenosis** by atheroma, fibromuscular hyperplasia or compression by external masses. This narrowing of the renal artery causes a reduced blood flow to the kidney, activating the mechanism mentioned above. **Renal diseases** are another cause. Renal hypertension may follow intrinsic diseases of the kidney such as **chronic glomerulonephritis**, **polycystic renal disease** and **chronic pyelonephritis**. It may also follow **hydronephrosis**. In Australia, **analgesic nephropathy** is an important cause. The diseased kidney secretes excessive renin which leads to systemic hypertension. Unilateral nephrectomy is curative, unless the other kidney is also damaged or diseased.

Endocrine Causes

Hyperaldosteronism, hypersecretion of steroid hormones from the adrenal cortex, in **Conn's syndrome** (primary hyperaldosteronism) and in **Cushing's syndrome** (secondary hyperaldosteronism due to excessive ACTH secretion by the pituitary), is an important cause of hypertension. A functioning **tumour of chromaffin tissue**, usually an adenoma of the adrenal medulla known as **phaeochromocytoma**, elaborates high circulating levels of catecholamines, particularly noradrenaline, which elevates blood pressure. In certain **lung tumours** excessive quantities of ACTH are secreted, which cause a Cushingoid syndrome with hypertension.

Hyperoestrinism, either endogenous (e.g. tumours of the ovary) or exogenous (e.g. contraceptive pill or therapeutic administration of **oestrogens**), produces a mild elevation of blood pressure. In the presence of oestrogen, increased quantities of angiotensinogen are elaborated by the liver, leading to increased levels of angiotensin and aldosterone in the body.

In **diabetes mellitus** (insulin deficiency) hypertension is common and there are associated kidney lesions (**Kimmelstiel-Wilson bodies**) which are seen in about 20–30% of diabetic kidneys.

Neurological Disorders

With conditions that cause increased intracranial pressure, lesions of the hypothalamus and lesions of the brainstem, hypertension may also occur due to effects on control mechanisms of blood pressure. Some cases of hypertension respond to changes in lifestyle and this is known as the **relaxation response**. Patients with hypertension who undertake meditation, yoga and other such stress reduction measures and effectively reduce their high blood pressure are few, but nevertheless this group shows the significance of autonomic nervous sytem mechanisms that are important in some cases of hypertension.

Arteriosclerosis

The diseases of arteries are a varied group and depend very much on the type and calibre of artery affected, as different disease processes affect different arteries. In order to understand the disease of the arteries, it is important to understand some of their distinctive, normal structural and functional characteristics (refer to Figure 3.30).

Arteries are divided into three major categories, depending on their size and a variety of histological features: **large and elastic arteries** including the aorta; **medium-sized muscular arteries**, also referred to as distributing arteries; and **small arteries**, less than 2 mm in diameter, that are for the most part within the substance of organs. Whatever the type of artery, the basic structure of the wall is the same, being divided into three major layers: the **tunica intima** (the layer closest to the lumen), the **tunica media** (the middle coat) and the **tunica adventitia** (the outermost layer). These layers are most easily distinguished in the larger vessels and generally become more and more indistinct as the vessels get smaller. At the level of the arterioles these layers are indistinguishable.

Large elastic arteries of the body include the aorta and its major branches. The *tunica intima* of these vessels is composed of a thin layer of endothelial cells, smooth and continuous, resting on a basement membrane. Below this is a layer of mucopolysaccharides and myointimal cells, the properties of which are intermediate of those of smooth muscle cells and fibroblasts. The outer limit of the intima is composed of a poorly defined zone of elastic fibres arranged longitudinally. The *tunica media* is a thick muscular layer, rich in elastic fibres. Muscle cells and elastic laminae are arranged in more or less alternate layers and the media is separated from the adventitia by a condensation of the elastic tissue, referred to as the external elastic membrane. The *tunica adventitia* is a loosely defined mass of connective tissue, surrounding the vessel, in which elastic and nerve fibres are dispersed and in which the small nutritive vessels of the arteries, the *vasa vasorum*, are found.

The great quantity of elastin in the wall of these vessels makes them very resilient and their rebound after systole helps the blood to move forward in the arterial system. In the ageing process, the elastic fibres are replaced by fibrocollagenous tissue as they deteriorate. The vessels lose their elasticity and the arteries stretch and elongate, becoming tortuous.

The **muscular arteries** have a wall in which the three layers described above are well defined. The intima is well separated from the media by a compact wavy, internal elastic membrane. The media is composed of many layers of smooth muscle, arranged in concentric circular and spiral rings. There are fine elastic fibres within the media also and it is well separated from the adventitia by the external elastic lamina. The adventitia resembles that of the elastic arteries, but contains more nerves, indicating the important role that autonomic control plays in the regulation of blood flow through these vessels.

In **small arteries** there is progressive loss of the external elastic membrane and then of the internal elastic membrane, such that there is virtual loss of definition between the three layers at the pre-arteriole level. In **arterioles** the wall is composed of the endothelial lining, which rests on scant connective tissue. Below this there is a muscular layer surrounded by a connective tissue adventitia. The thickness of the wall is about the same as the diameter of the lumen. The arterioles are well supplied by nerve endings of the autonomic nervous system, as it is they, together with the small arteries, that respond to nervous control of vascular flow.

The differentiation of these three types of arteries is important in pathology, as each class of vessel tends to have its own pattern of diseases and lesions. For example, atheroma occurs most commonly in the elastic and muscular arteries, while the small arteries and arterioles show more commonly fibromuscular tissue proliferation and hyalinization.

Veins are generally thin-walled vessels with relatively large lumina. The three separate coats seen in arteries are not as well defined in the veins as the elastic laminae are present in only the largest veins. Also, the media is much thinner and uneven in its distribution. The veins are thus predisposed to abnormal dilatations, compression and easy penetration by tumours and inflammatory processes.

Arteriosclerosis is not a specific pathological entity. It is a term that means 'hardening of the arteries'. This term is sometimes used vaguely and inaccurately. Arteriosclerosis describes a group of arterial disorders which have in common the features of thickening and loss of elasticity of artery walls. There are three major morphological and clinicopathological variants of arteriosclerosis which are very specific disease entities. These are:

- **atherosclerosis**, the most common and the most important;
- **Mönckeberg's medial calcific sclerosis**, common, less serious;
- **arteriolosclerosis**, important, commonly occurs in hypertension.

Atherosclerosis

This is the disease which is the greatest killer in the Western world. It is global in distribution and in the last few decades has reached epidemic proportions in the economically developed countries. It has a long

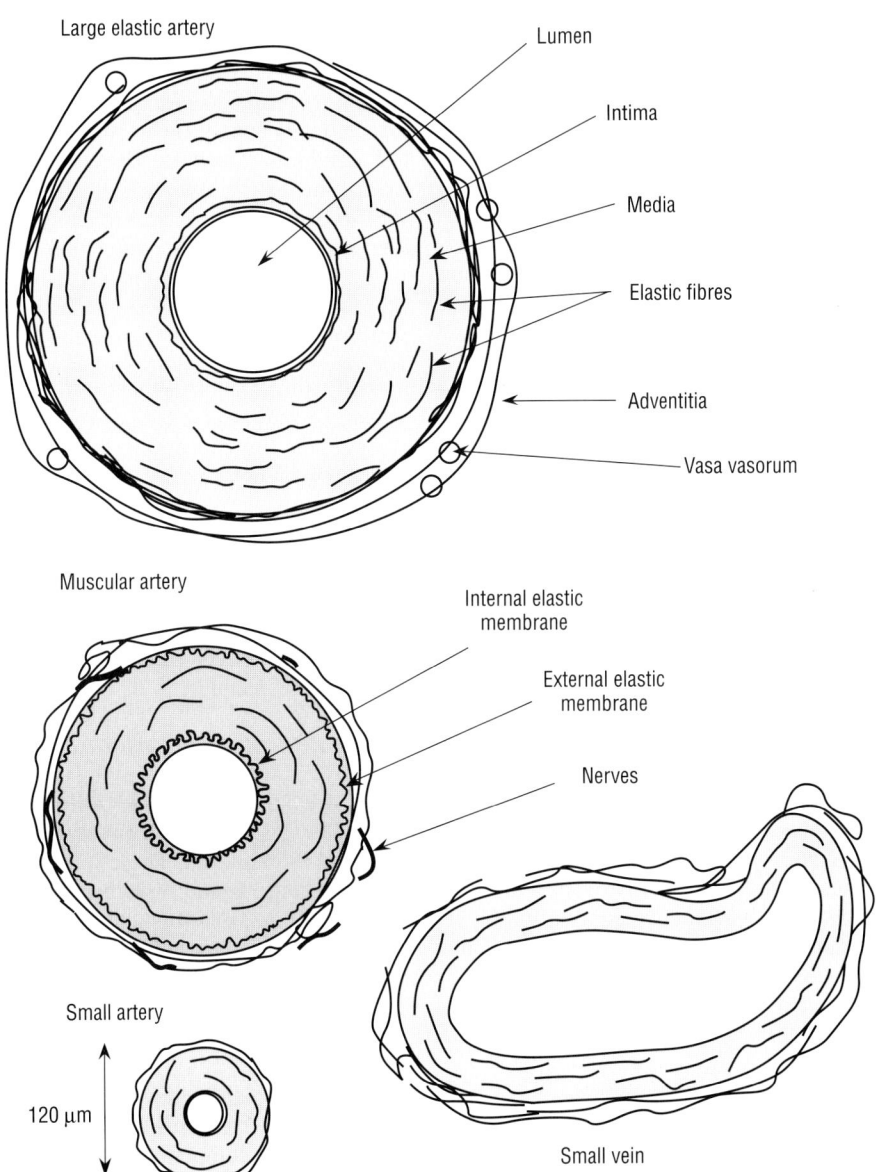

Figure 3.30 *The structure of normal blood vessels*

course and it only causes serious complications when it produces arterial insufficiency. Although any artery may be affected, the aorta, coronary and cerebral arteries are most commonly affected. This is why **myocardial infarcts** ('heart attacks') and **cerebral infarcts** ('strokes') are the two main consequences of this disease. Myocardial infarcts alone account for approximately 20% of all deaths in Western societies.

The disease itself is asymptomatic or 'silent', illness being the result of its complications, the incidence of which increases with age. Almost everyone is affected by old age. Before the age of 45 years males are affected twice as commonly as females (M:F = 2:1). Above the age of 45 years (post-menopausal) more women become affected and eventually women and men are affected equally (M:F = 1:1).

Its variable severity and incidence among nations and individuals, social and ethnic groups is evidence that atherosclerosis is not an inevitable consequence of life. Research in the field of atherosclerosis is looking for both the cause as well as the reason why some people have only mild disease while others are severely affected.

Atherosclerosis is a disease of large and medium size arteries. The coronary, carotids, abdominal aorta, iliac and femoral vessels are primarily affected. The basic lesion is called the **atheroma** or **fibro-fatty plaque**. This consists of a raised focal plaque within the intima of the vessel and in the plaque is a core of lipid, mostly cholesterol, which is usually complexed to proteins and esters. Covering the plaque is a fibrous cap. The term atherosclerosis is taken from the words *ather* (Greek: porridge, gruel) and *sclerosis* (Greek: hardening). At first, these atheromata are sparsely distributed, but as the disease advances, they become more and more numerous, often coalescing to cover the entire luminal aspect of the artery affected.

The disease has an insidious course and may progress for 20 to 40 years without producing any symptoms. Its very slow, progressive course and the fact that the lesions may not cause symptoms until a long time has passed often means that atherosclerosis may not be diagnosed during life, but is discovered as a finding at post-mortem examinations. During life, angiography may be used to detect atheroma, or in the case of advanced, calcified lesions, radiography may be of diagnostic importance.

Development of Atheromatous Plaques

The lesions of atherosclerosis have been divided into four types according to their morphology. These are discussed below.

Fatty Streaks

The fatty streak is important not because it causes any serious disturbance in the blood flow dynamics in the vessels, but because some researchers think it may be the precursor of the typical atheromatous plaque. There is no firm evidence which implicates fatty streaks as the precursors of atheroma. Fatty streaks occur in the aorta of children of all ages in all parts of the world, even in nutritionally deprived children in undeveloped nations where atherosclerosis is rare. These streaks are virtually always present by the age of 10 years and their extent increases with age — though they can regress. The fatty streaks are shallow, yellow intimal plaques, beginning as lesions less than 1 mm in diameter, and they soon grow to streaks 2 mm in width and 1–2 cm long. They are flattened or slightly raised lesions, lifting the endothelium slightly, and are often hard to distinguish macroscopically unless they have been stained with a lipophilic stain.

The hallmark of fatty streaks is lipid deposition in the intima and the lesions are composed predominantly of **lipophages** ('foam cells'), which are lipid laden macrophages, and smooth muscle cells. Lipid is also found extracellularly and proteoglycans, collagen and elastic fibres are present in variable amounts. Fatty streaks tend to occur more commonly in the thoracic aorta, at the aortic valve ring, in the abdominal aorta and later in the coronary arteries. As can be seen from their distribution, some of these locations are always involved by atherosclerosis (coronary arteries), while others are spared (thoracic aorta). In the third decade, fatty streaks begin to disappear and in sites where atherosclerosis develops they are replaced by typical atheromatous plaques.

Early Atheromatous Plaques

These are smooth, ovoid, yellow, slightly raised button-like lesions which involve the intima of the aorta and its branches. These lesions are often called **musculoelastic lesion** or **intimal cushion**. They represent small areas of thickening or plaque formation, often first developing at branch points in arteries or at the ostia of branches as they come off the larger arteries. At first there is a patchy distribution of the lesions in affected arteries with large unaffected areas in between.

These early plaques have been unequivocally associated with atherosclerosis and they are composed of essentially four components: **cells** (including vascular smooth muscle cells and macrophages); **connective tissue** fibres and matrix; **plasma proteins**; and **lipids** (usually very little lipid is found within them). These four components occur in varying proportions depending on the age of the lesion. There are smooth muscle cells (myointimal cells) and these together with collagen and elastin fibres form a fibrous plaque which thickens as the lesion ages. A small central mass of essentially low-density lipids and lipophages is seen, which gradually enlarges and is surrounded by proliferated myointimal cells and fibrous tissue (Figure 3.31).

Fully Developed Atheromatous Plaque

The fibrous cap forms and thickens considerably as the lesion enlarges. These plaques may coalesce as they enlarge. There is considerably more lipid contained in the centre of the plaque — often seen as cholesterol crystals or clefts (Figure 3.32) — and greater amounts of fibrous tissue and myointimal cells. Foam cells are still seen in large numbers and there is necrosis of the intima and degeneration of the media as the plaque encroaches on the media, causing its atrophy and thinning (see Figure 3.33).

Complicated Plaque

In complicated plaques there may be: **calcification** of the degenerate plaque which may be patchy or massive; **ulceration** of the overlying endothelium and cap — and rupture of the plaque with debris entering the bloodstream (cholesterol emboli); **thrombosis** occurring over the ulcerated plaque (Figure 3.34); **thromboembolism** often following thrombosis; **infarction** often seen in association with atherosclerosis and thrombosis; **haemorrhage** occurring into the plaque (from the

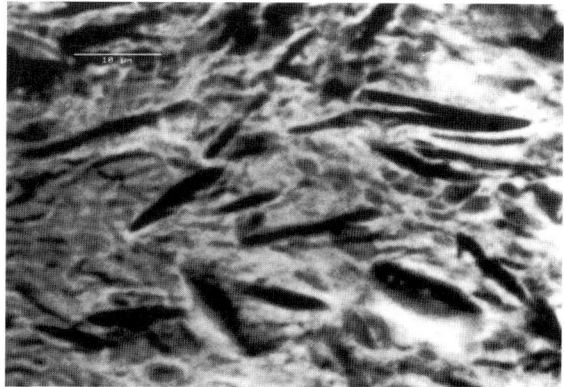

Figure 3.32 *Fibrofatty material at the centre of a typical atheromatous plaque showing the cholesterol clefts (dark spaces) occupied by needle-shaped crystals of cholesterol (scale bar is 10 μm)*

vascular lumen or from the branches of the vasa vasorum).

Risk Factors in Atherosclerosis

High blood lipid, serum lipoprotein and cholesterol levels. A raised level of serum low-density lipoprotein or raised levels of cholesterol (e.g. in hypothyroidism) increase the incidence of atherosclerosis and its complications. The ratio of low-density lipoproteins (LDL) to high-density lipoproteins (HDL) is important and appears to be mainly influenced by genetic factors but also by diet. The ratio is also raised in certain congenital conditions (e.g. familial xanthomatosis).

Blood pressure. The higher the blood pressure, the greater the risk, especially in patients over 45 years of age. Benign hypertension of long duration is particularly important in this context.

Cigarette smoking. It is not clear how tobacco raises the incidence of atherosclerosis, but epidemiological evidence indicates that smoking is a very important contributory factor. One mechanism may be the destruction of endothelial cells by tobacco smoke components which enter the circulation from the lung capillaries. The damage to the endothelium by these components initiates formation of the atheromatous plaque.

Diabetes mellitus. The incidence and extent of atherosclerosis is increased in diabetics due to altered fat metabolism and hyperlipidaemia (high blood lipids, high LDL/HDL ratio).

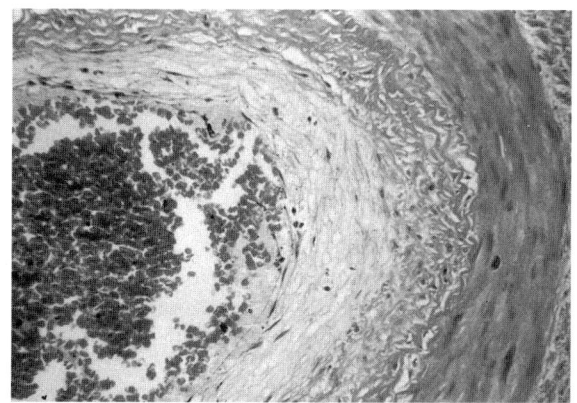

Figure 3.31 *A small artery showing an early atheromatous plaque in its intima (×100)*

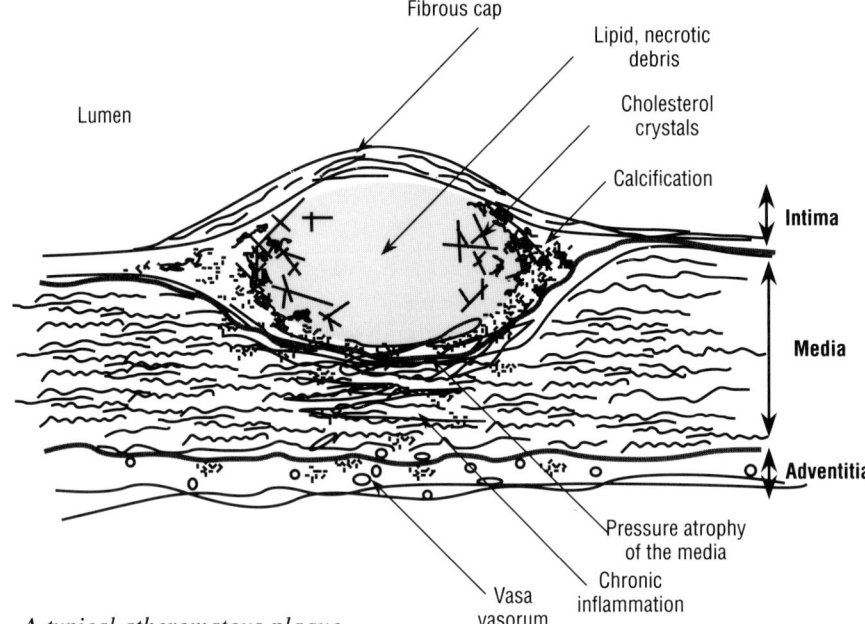

Figure 3.33 *A typical atheromatous plaque*

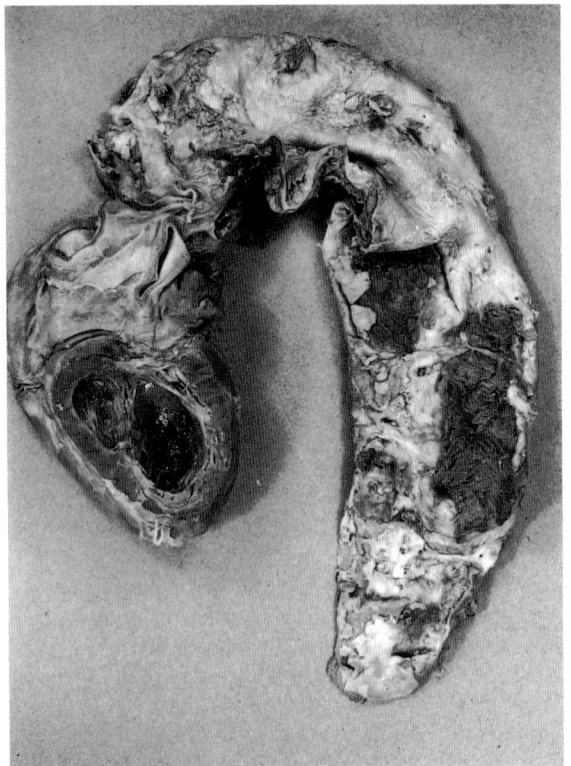

Figure 3.34 *Aorta from a 70-year-old male, showing extensive atheroma and complicating thrombosis*

Genetics (heredity). It is not clear how this factor operates but the risk of atherosclerosis and its complications appears to run in families. One mechanism is postulated to be the differences in the metabolism of fats by various individuals. It is suspected that some people have a better capacity to metabolize fats and also to incorporate these fats into HDL rather than LDL.

Hormonal factors. Women, until the age of menopause, are less likely to suffer the consequences of atherosclerosis than men. The risk is equal by the age of 65 to 70 years. The beneficial effects are linked with the high oestrogen levels which affect lipid metabolism, thus pre-menopausal women are protected by their female sex hormones.

Diet. There is evidence that reducing the content of cholesterol or reducing the saturated fatty acid/polyunsaturated fatty acid ratio (LDL/HDL) leads to decreased morbidity and mortality from atherosclerosis.

Other risks. Other factors may also contribute to a lesser extent to development of atherosclerosis. These include lack of exercise, obesity, stress and certain behaviour patterns (e.g. Type A personality).

Pathogenesis of Atherosclerosis

The initial lesion in atherosclerosis is said to be fatty streaks in patchy distribution, mostly in the aorta and large arteries. Over the years these may enlarge to form true atheromatous plaques which may occlude the lumen of large arteries. There are various factors involved in how these plaques develop, and many theories have been proposed to account for the development of the disease. These are discussed below.

Haemodynamic stress. Hypertension is contributory to atherosclerosis. Atherosclerosis develops in haemodynamically stressed arteries usually at or near sites of increased stress such as bifurcations. Atherosclerosis only affects pulmonary arteries when pulmonary hypertension is present. Haemodynamic stress such as turbulence and increased pressure of flow may damage the endothelial lining of arteries. It may stimulate intimal thickening and perhaps make the endothelium more permeable to lipids.

Lipid infiltration hypothesis. Hypercholesterolaemia or hyperlipidaemia is important in the pathogenesis of atherosclerosis but the mechanism is not well understood. Atheromatous plaques are rich in cholesterol, and high-cholesterol diets have been shown to cause atherosclerosis in experimental animals. Certainly there may be some direct insudation of lipids through the intima but more complex changes must be involved. In the presence of hypercholesterolaemia the endothelial lining is damaged. Once the lipids are inside the vessel wall, the smooth muscle cells are induced to proliferate and fibrosis occurs on the surface of the plaque in reaction to the damage. The alternative name of this theory is the **imbibition theory of Virchow** as it was first put forward by the great German pathologist in 1856.

Thrombogenic theory. Rokitansky, in 1852, put forward this theory and called it the **encrustation hypothesis**. It purports that when there is damaged endothelium in an artery, platelets aggregate at the sites of exposed subendothelial connective tissue. This platelet plug or thrombus may be microscopic, but there follows further thrombosis with the thrombus becoming organized and incorporated into the intima, which re-endothelializes. This lesion resembles early changes of atheromatous plaque as macrophages break down the thrombus leaving the lipids to accumulate. Hence this theory assumes that lipids in the plaque are generated from the breakdown of platelets.

Monoclonal theory. Benditt put forward this theory after his observations on the phenotype of smooth muscle cells in atheroma. It is known that in atherosclerosis, smooth muscle cells from the media migrate and proliferate in the intima. Fibrous connective tissue is also laid down in the intima. Platelets release factors which stimulate myointimal cell migration and proliferation. Fibrous tissue which forms the superficial subendothelial cap of the atheromatous plaque is possibly also provided by myointimal cells like myofibroblasts, which can lay down collagen and other connective tissue components.

Evidence suggests that all the myointimal cells derive from a single precursor cell (smooth muscle cell). In the normal population of smooth muscle cells there are two phenotypes: type A and type B. The phenotypic difference is a subtle one and revolves around whether the muscle cells have one or other form of a specific enzyme in their cytoplasm. This difference in phenotype may be detected by special tests. Benditt observed that smooth muscle cells in atheromatous plaques were all of a single type, type A or type B, unlike smooth muscle cells in normal arterial medias which are a mixed population, 50% type A and 50% type B. He suggested that atheromatous plaques were like a benign tumour of the arterial wall, the smooth muscle cells representing the neoplastic component.

To explain the lipid content of the plaque, the theory maintains that deep within the lipid-rich layer of the atheromatous plaque are regions of necrosis. These may be due to toxic effects of lipids and ischaemia, although the deeper part of the plaque is supplied by branches of the vasa vasorum which extend into the normally avascular intima of affected arteries. Since the atheromatous plaque has a distinct fibrous cap it is possible that lipid may insudate into the plaque from the vasa vasorum.

Response to injury theory. This theory was put forward by Ross and his co-workers and it is one which combines many elements of other theories outlined above. Essentially, Ross purports that the initiating stimulus in the pathogenesis of atherosclerosis is intimal injury. This injury may take the form of many guises: hyperlipidaemia, hypertension, metabolic imbalances, tobacco smoke components, autoimmunity and infection. Subsequently, there is insudation of lipid into the intima and thrombosis. There follows migration of smooth muscle cells from the media into the intima and their proliferation in that site in response to platelet factors which are released from the thrombus (e.g. PDGF), with, finally, organization of the thrombus and re-endothelialization. This sequence of events is repeated many times, leading eventually to the formation of the typical plaque.

This is the currently accepted theory and it explains many of the observed epidemiological, clinical and morphological data that have been amassed in relation to the disease. It should be noted that it is a combination of the features of many previous theories and as such it is highly successful in explaining many more observations than any single previous theory was able to do.

General Effects of Atherosclerosis

The plaque of atherosclerosis may cause narrowing of the lumen of an artery causing **ischaemia**. This is very often seen in the coronary arteries, leading to chronic ischaemia of the heart muscle, reactive changes and eventually necrosis of heart muscle bundles. The condition manifests itself clinically as **angina pectoris** a sharp chest pain upon exertion which radiates down the left arm. This represents the inability of the coronary arteries to cope with the increased demand for blood by the straining heart.

Thrombosis may occur over ulcerated plaque, causing total occlusion, and resulting in infarction or possbly in **embolism** which causes infarction at a distant site.

Rupture of plaque (rupture of the fibrous cap) may occur releasing showers of fatty debris into the blood as small emboli. **Haemorrhage** into the plaque may result in thrombosis in the wall and thickening which may occlude the vessel.

Damage of the media may result when the plaque causes a weakening of the vessel wall and its increase in size leads to medial damage predisposing to **aneurysm** formation (dilatation of the weakened area of wall) and rupture of the vessel.

Effects of Atherosclerosis at Different Sites

The majority of people reach old age with moderate or severe atherosclerosis and yet have no symptoms. When symptoms do occur they affect the following sites and lead to the sequelae outlined below (refer also to Figure 3.36):

- **Coronary arteries**: occlusion causes **ischaemic heart disease**, or **coronary heart disease**, **angina**, **myocardial infarction**, **arrhythmias**.
- **Cerebral arteries and carotid arteries**: gradual narrowing causes slow impairment of mental function. Acute obstruction causes **cerebral infarction** ('stroke'). Rupture causes cerebral or subarachnoid **haemorrhage** (cerebrovascular accident — CVA).
- **Vertebral arteries**: obstruction is an important cause of **cerebral ischaemia**.
- **Aorta**: atherosclerosis affects particularly the distal aorta. **Aneurysms** may form and rupture rapidly causing death. Emboli may obstruct leg arteries causing infarction of distal parts and **gangrene** of the toes. Ischaemia of the genitalia may cause **atrophy** and **impotence** in males.
- **Leg arteries**: increasing obstruction causes **intermittent claudication** and gangrene. (Intermittent claudication is caused by ischaemia to muscles: upon exertion, walking even short distances, the muscles are painful and the sufferer must rest and walking must be undertaken in short intervals).

Mönckeberg's Medial Sclerosis

This is a common disease affecting men and women equally over the age of 50 years. It affects small and medium-sized muscular arteries. The limb and genital arterial supplies are especially affected. Vessels quite commonly involved are: femoral, tibial, ulnar, radial and coronary arteries. Essentially this is an idiopathic disease but various experimental studies have suggested that it may be involved with prolonged muscular contraction and degeneration of arterial smooth muscle. Prolonged, increased levels of vasoconstrictors such as catecholamines and nicotine in experimental animals lead to vascular spasm which is followed by degeneration of muscle cells and calcification in the media. Mönckeberg's medial calcification may co-exist with atherosclerosis but is not related to it.

The media only is affected by this process. Calcium deposits are seen in a hyalinized media, as plate-like or ring-like patches (Figure 3.35). Sometimes the rings and plates coalesce to create a large deposit around the vessel, and bone may even form in the calcified media, as has already been described for dystrophic calcification. The affected arteries appear rigid like 'pipe stems' and often they may be palpated and described as 'gooseneck lamp nodularities'. They are tortuous, hard, calcified vessels but the lumen is not narrowed and the endothelium above in the intima remains intact. There

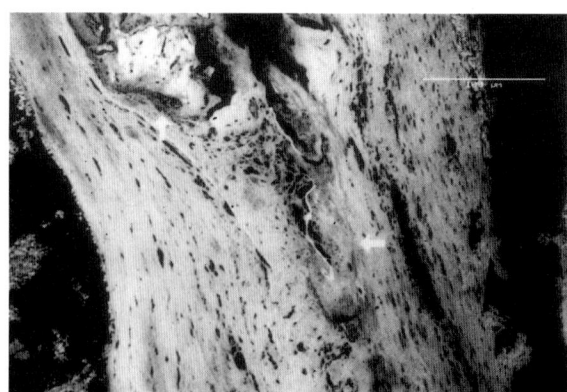

Figure 3.35 *Mönckeberg's medial calcification in a muscular artery. The arrows indicate the regions of calcification deep in the media of the vessel. The lumen is at the left and adventitia at the right (scale bar is 100 µm)*

is minimal inflammatory reaction and the intima and adventitia are largely unaffected by the process.

There are usually no clinical effects in uncomplicated cases of Mönckeberg's as there is no narrowing of the vascular lumen. The condition is often found as an incidental finding at autopsy. However, as the hardened arteries may be palpated during life, and as they are seen on X-ray films, they may give rise to false alarms in some situations. The condition, however, may often be seen together with atherosclerosis, the combination of the two producing ischaemia and other complications already discussed above.

Arteriolosclerosis

Arteriolosclerosis occurs as a result of systemic hypertension or is seen in association with systemic hypertension — either benign or malignant. The vessels affected are small arteries and arterioles. The persistent high blood pressure in the vascular system causes the walls to become thickened with hyaline-degenerating material, fibrinoid necrotic material and the deposition of elastic tissue, having as the result the narrowing of the lumen.

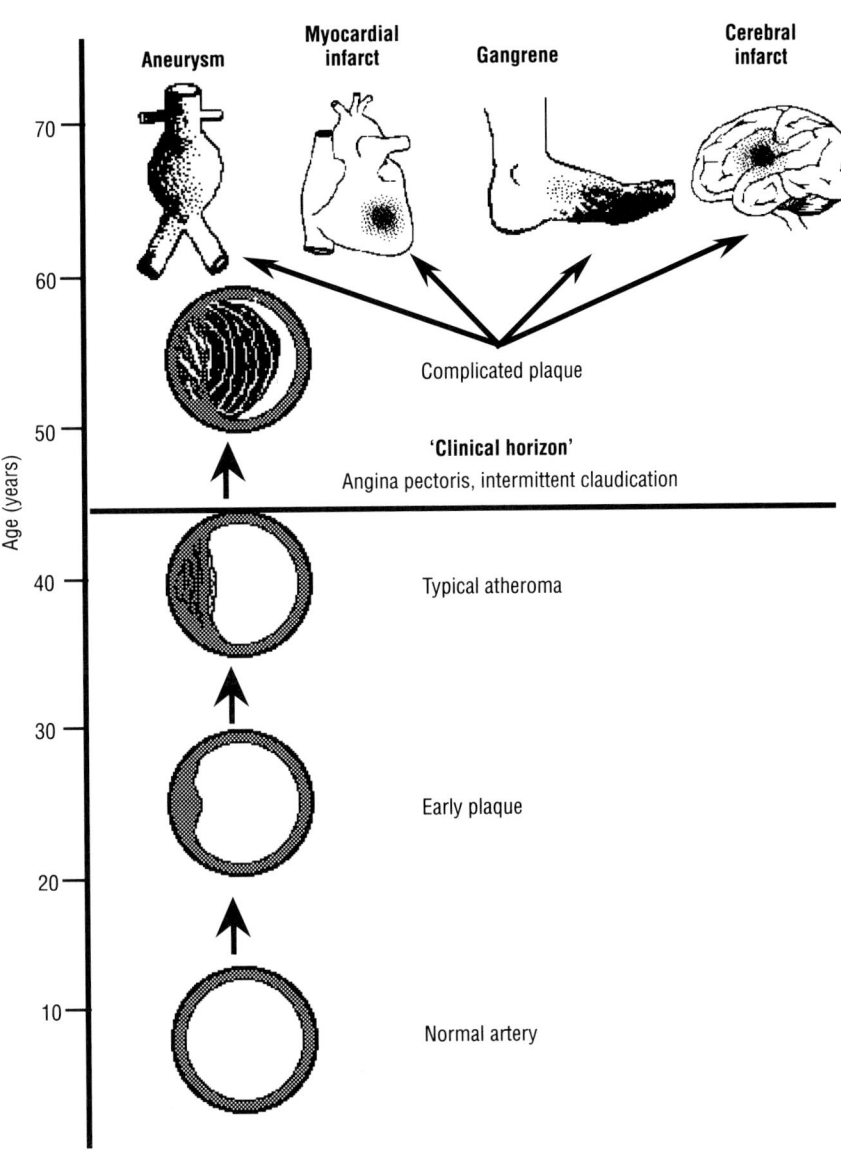

Figure 3.36 *Clinical manifestations of atheroma*

The sites affected are vessels of the kidneys, pancreas, gall bladder, small intestines, spleen, adrenals and retina. When the narrowing of the lumen due to the thickening and degeneration of the wall causes a compromised blood flow to the organ supplied, the cells of the tissue will undergo ischaemia and degenerate. Vascular changes in the retina cause the 'retinopathies' associated with systemic hypertension. The effects on the kidney glomeruli are most important, giving rise to renal disease known as nephrosclerosis, caused by arteriolosclerosis of the afferent arterioles which supply them. The hyaline deposits are composed of proteinaceous material, containing some collagen, immunoglobulins, components of plasma proteins, elastic fibres, basement membrane material, all of which have become denatured.

Arteriolosclerosis is also seen in very elderly patients whether they are normotensive or hypertensive, but its effects are generally more severe and generalized in the latter case. More severe disease is seen the higher the blood pressure and the more prolonged the hypertensive state. Arteriolosclerosis is also seen in diabetics, forming part of the disease process, which reflects the generalised metabolic stress (and consequent deposition of proteinaceous material in vessels) in diabetes mellitus.

Benign nephrosclerosis, hyaline arteriolosclerosis, is seen in benign hypertension. There is a fibrous thickening and hyaline change within the arteriolar walls, causing narrowing of the vascular lumen. Glomeruli are also affected and show hyalinization (glassy appearance) and fibrosis of Bowman's capsule. Small arteries show reduplication of internal elastic laminae. These changes occur over many years and do not initially damage kidneys severely. There may be reduction in glomerular filtration rate (GFR) and mild proteinuria. Benign nephrosclerosis is very common in old age.

Malignant nephrosclerosis, hyperplastic arteriolosclerosis, is seen in malignant hypertension which occurs in approximately 5% of hypertensive patients. This may occur as a result of kidney disease and also may occur as a result of long-standing benign hypertension.

There is oedema of the arteriolar wall with insudation of fibrinogen and plasma proteins into the wall, narrowing the lumen as the wall thickens. Deposition of fibrinogen activates the clotting cascade and microthrombi form in the vessels. The lumen of the vessel becomes narrowed and shaggy due to oedema and microthrombi and there is hyperplasia of the intima (or endothelium). The result is a fall in intrarenal perfusion and there is mechanical damage to red blood cells passing through damaged vessels, causing haemolysis

known as **microangiopathic haemolytic anaemia**. The red blood cell damage leads to further clotting and further fibrin deposition in vessels. The kidneys become ischaemic and renin secretion is stimulated. Angiotensin then further constricts renal vessels, compounding the results. In the end, intimal proliferation and fibrin deposition may obliterate the arteriolar lumen.

Small arteries show concentric, laminated '**onion skin**' thickening due to proliferation of endothelium, intimal fibroblasts and medial smooth muscle cells (smooth muscle hyperplasia). **Fibrinoid necrosis** is seen in arterioles with an intensely pink, smudgy appearance in stained sections.

Haemorrhages may occur into surrounding tissues, for example into glomeruli, and the patient may notice macroscopic haematuria (blood in urine), have headaches, nausea, vomiting and visual derangements. Retinopathy is visible on opthalmoscopy. Consciousness may become impaired and convulsions may follow (hypertensive encephalopathy). Congestive heart failure, renal failure and CVA are the usual causes of death. Untreated, few patients survive for 12 months and with treatment, the 5-year survival rate is only 50%.

Blood Lipids

Blood lipids are a heterogeneous group of substances in the bloodstream that, depending on the method of assay, may be subdivided into a number of subgroups. The major groups of these substances are: cholesterol, triglycerides and phospholipids. All of these circulate within the bloodstream bound to specific proteins that carry them to body tissues where they are needed. The term lipoproteins refers to such blood lipids in their bound form with the carrier proteins. A very common rapid method for separating and assaying the blood lipoproteins is by electrophoresis. From such a separatory technique the following classification of lipoproteins may be given:

• Chylomicrons. These are mainly triglycerides of an exogenous (dietary) derivation. After a lipid-rich meal, chylomicrons will be readily detected in the lacteals (lymphatics) of the small intestine and also within the portal vein.
• Very low density lipoproteins (VLDL). These are primarily endogenous triglycerides, representing body fat which is being mobilized to supply metabolic needs of the tissues.
• Intermediate-density lipoproteins (IDL). A large variety of transitional forms and metabolic intermedi-

ates fall into this group and they are composed of approximately 30% cholesterol and 40% triglycerides.

- Low-density lipoproteins (LDL). These are the more 'sinister' of the blood lipoproteins, being composed of approximately 50% cholesterol. High levels of these substances have been strongly and directly linked with the development of blood vessel diseases and heart attacks (atherosclerosis and myocardial infarction).
- High-density lipoproteins (HDL). These are thought to serve as a means of removal of cholesterol from the tissues, but their exact function remains to be determined. However, it is known that high levels of HDL are inversely associated with risk of vascular disease development. Therefore they appear to have a protective role.

The link between the low-density lipoproteins and vascular diseases is attributed to their high content of cholesterol (see Figure 3.37). While cholesterol is viewed as an offending substance in the development of atherosclerosis and most people regard it as a 'poison' to be avoided at all costs, it must be realized that it is a substance that is useful within the body and is essential for the growth of cells, being a constituent of cell membranes. It is used by the body in the synthesis of various hormones including cortisol, oestrogen and testosterone. Cholesterol is used in the production of bile acids, which by virtue of their emulsifying role in the duodenum aid in the digestion and absorption of fats in the body.

The body is capable of synthesizing the cholesterol it needs in the liver. The raw materials for this process are fats, sugars and alcohol. In addition, this synthesis is supplemented by cholesterol derived from the diet; foods of animal origin are usually high in cholesterol. The fats especially, which are present in animal tissue, are saturated and cholesterol rich. Eggs, milk, butter, cheese and cream are common sources of cholesterol. Ideally, a balance is maintained by the liver between the cholesterol it needs to synthesize and the cholesterol that is derived from the diet. In some people this balance seems to be easily upset or is not maintained by the body's metabolic processes. A genetic predisposition towards the formation of more or less LDL or HDL also operates. These data explain the observations that although some people eat a relatively low-fat diet, they still have a higher level of LDL in their bloodstream than other more fortunate people who, although on a relatively high-fat diet, have near normal levels of LDL.

Plasma cholesterol levels are decreased by a diet which contains a high proportion of polyunsaturated oils and fats such as vegetable oils (olive oil, safflower oil, peanut oil, etc.) and a low proportion of animal fats. Fish oils may not change the plasma cholesterol concentration directly, but they appear to protect against heart disease because they contain polyunsaturated fatty acids that contribute to the reduction of the tendency of blood to undergo thrombosis. An increase in the consumption of unrefined complex carbohydrates and some types of vegetable fibres (e.g. pectin as found in apples) also decreases cholesterol levels. Another fac-

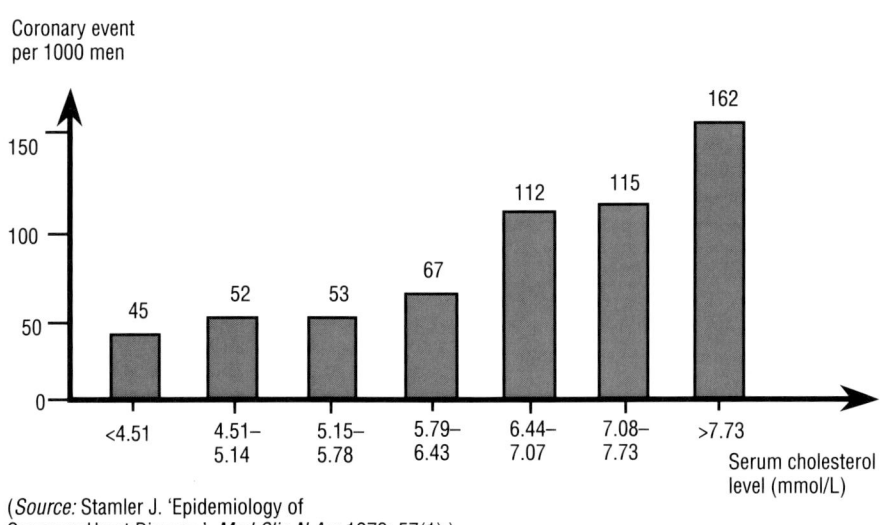

(*Source:* Stamler J. 'Epidemiology of Coronary Heart Disease.' *Med Clin N Am* 1973; 57(1))

Figure 3.37 *The relationship between serum cholesterol levels and the incidence of heart disease*

tor that appears to be important in decreasing blood cholesterol levels is maintaining body weight within the normal range for age and height or reducing body weight to achieve this.

Blood Lipids Tests

With the blood lipids test, the patient's fat metabolism is investigated and the risk of heart disease may be extrapolated from the results of such tests. The blood cholesterol levels are determined as a total cholesterol count, as an LDL cholesterol count and as an HDL cholesterol count. The patient's triglyceride levels are also determined. Increases in the LDL cholesterol count above the normal range are associated with a higher risk of heart disease, while increases in the HDL cholesterol count indicate a reduced risk of heart disease (refer to Table 3.1).

The association between hyperlipidaemia (especially high levels of LDL) and coronary heart disease is very well documented and is more striking the younger the age group of men sampled. It is also well established that lowering abnormally elevated cholesterol levels will also lower the incidence of vascular and heart disease. It is wise to detect such abnormalities early and through the use of dietary measures (or in severe cases both dietary and drug measures) reduce the level of blood lipids. It should be kept in mind that when hyperlipidaemia coexists with obesity, there is commonly an abnormal result for the glucose tolerance test and that fasting blood glucose levels will often confirm the presence of diabetes mellitus. The treatment of the asymptomatic diabetic who presents thus is usually limited to a reduction in weight and management of the elevated blood lipid levels.

In the laboratory, blood lipid levels are now determined using semi-automated and automated techniques of gel electrophoresis in which the patients' blood lipids are rapidly and accurately quantitated. The patients' lipids are identified by comparing against known standards. The fully automated techniques are generally available in only the larger laboratories.

Indications for Patients about to be Tested

The following should be carried out prior to and during the testing of patients for blood lipids:

1. Patients should be advised to eat normally for 3 to 7 days before the test and then eat and drink nothing for 12 to 14 hours before the blood is collected. Explain to the patient that fasting is necessary in order to obtain a useful result. If a blood glucose test is to be performed also, advise the patient to have an average carbohydrate intake.

2. Inform the patient about what is being done and why it is being done. Something like the following should be said: 'A blood sample will be taken from you and will be sent to the laboratory for examination. The laboratory will tell us whether you have a normal cholesterol level, whether your body is able to metabolize fats normally and what your risk of vascular and heart disease is. We may have to take another blood sample in order to make a definite diagnosis.'

3. Collect approximately 10 ml of venous blood and place in a red-topped tube. Fully label the specimen tube and the request form with the patient's name and other details including a list of medications that the patient is currently taking.

4. Have the tube transported to the laboratory immediately. More than one sample may need to be taken because there are often marked fluctuations in the levels of blood lipids in the same patient

Table 3.1 *Normal blood lipoprotein values (all values in mmol/L)*

Age (years)	Total cholesterol	Triglycerides	LDL	HDL
<25	3.5–5.0	0.55–1.6	0.8–1.5	0.3–0.6
25–39	4.0–6.5	0.7–2.75	1.1–2.1	0.3–0.6
40–49	4.2–6.7	0.8–2.75	1.1–2.1	0.3–0.6
50–64	4.5–6.7	0.8–2.25	1.1–2.2	0.3–0.8
>64	4.7–7.2	0.8–2.25	1.1–2.25	0.3–0.8

(*Source:* Levey EI, Feinleib M. 'Risk Factors for Coronary Artery Disease and their Management', in *Heart Disease*, 1980; Philadelphia, WB Saunders and Co.)
NB: Fasting blood glucose levels: 3.9–5.6 mmol/L (70–110 mg/mL).

from day to day any several measurements may be necessary to arrive at a definitive diagnosis of hyperlipidaemia.

Interfering Factors

Various interfering factors may give abnormally high values in the blood lipid determination and these should be kept in mind when interpreting results. The value of repeated tests is also appreciated. Some of these factors are:

1. A high-fat, high-sugar diet.
2. Failure of the patient to comply with the fasting requirements 12–24 hours prior to the sampling of the blood.
3. Drugs that the patient may be taking: aspirin, corticosteroids, oral contraceptives, epinephrine, norepinephrine, bromides, phenothiazines, trifluoperazine (Stelazine), sulphonamides, phenytoin (Dilantin), vitamins A and D.
4. For several days to weeks after a heart attack the patient may show evidence of a raised blood glucose which should not be interpreted as evidence of obesity-associated diabetes mellitus.

Revision Questions and Case Studies

Oedema, Haemostasis, Haemorrhage and Shock

1. Differentiate between local and general oedema. Give two causes for each of the conditions.
2. Define the term 'elephantiasis' and give the commonest aetiology associated with it. What are the underlying mechanisms in the causation of this disorder?
3. What are the common causes of generalized oedema? (Ensure that you explain fully the pathogenesis of the disorder.)
4. Tissue that has undergone hydropic change appears swollen. Is this tissue oedematous? Explain.
5. Write notes on the following:
   (a) Shock
   (b) Haemophilia A
   (c) Haemoperitoneum
   (d) Thrombocytopenic purpura
   (e) Fibrin formation in haemostasis
6. What is meant by the term 'shock'? Discuss the pathological manifestations of the various forms of this condition and cover thoroughly the aetiological and pathogenetic factors associated with each clinically observed type of shock.
7. What are the characteristics of secondary shock? What are the pathological features that you associate with this condition?
8. What do you understand by the term 'haemorrhage'? Discuss the pathological manifestations of the various forms of this condition and cover thoroughly the aetiological and pathogenetic factors associated with each clinically observed type of haemorrhage. In your answer cover the various haemorrhagic diatheses.
10. What is purpura? In your answer include a definition of the word 'petechiae'.
11. In what situations of the body is oedema extremely important clinically? Explain your answer.
12. What is the clinical significance of haemorrhage?
13. Define the following terms:
    (a) Haemarthrosis
    (b) Tachycardia
    (c) Pseudohaemophilia
    (d) Afibrinogenaemia
    (e) Hypersplenism
14. What is thrombasthenia?
15. What are the signs and symptoms associated with shock and what are these due to?
16. Give an indication of the prognosis of the different types of shock.

Case study. A 48-year-old Caucasian man, who has been a heavy drinker for the past 20 years, presents with increasing, painless swelling of both ankles. There is no shortness of breath and physical examination shows: a blood pressure of 135/90 mmHg, pulse rate of 78 beats per minute, temperature of 36.5°C, chest — no abnormal findings, abdomen — a firm, slightly enlarged, palpable liver edge. Urine examination has shown no abnormality present.

(a) What is the cause of the ankle swelling?
(b) Outline the mechanism responsible for the production of the ankle swelling.
(c) How can the swelling of the ankles be alleviated?
(d) What advice should be given to the man?

Thrombosis, Embolism and Infarction

1. Discuss the process of thrombosis, mentioning the predisposing factors, types of thrombi, sites of formation and the sequelae.
2. Discuss the pathology of thromboembolism and infarction. Mention the different types of infarcts,

and sequelae of these processes.

3. What is an infarct? Describe the macroscopic appearances of infarcts in the heart and the brain. Discuss the similarities and differences observed in the two organs.

4. Discuss the pathogenesis of infarction with special reference to the heart, brain and lungs.

5. What is meant by the term 'Virchow's Triad' and to what condition does this predispose?

6. What are the lines of Zahn?

7. What are the clinical factors used in the assessment of a patient's risk of post-operative thrombosis?

8. Define the following terms:
   (a) Thrombocythaemia
   (b) Blood turbulence
   (c) Hyperlipidaemia
   (d) Polycythaemia
   (e) Thrombotic diathesis

9. Outline the sequence of events seen in a venous thrombus that is being recanalized.

10. What occurs in the condition of disseminated intravascular coagulation (DIC)?

11. Explain the pathogenesis of Caisson disease (nitrogen embolism).

12. What occurs in the process of pulmonary embolism and what are the sequelae of this condition?

13. Describe the changes that occur in an infarct that has been caused by arterial occlusion in a tissue such as myocardium.

14. Define the following terms:
   (a) Saddle embolus
   (b) Vegetation
   (c) Dyspnoea
   (d) Propagating thrombus
   (e) Pleurocentesis

15. Differentiate between phlebothrombosis and thrombophlebitis.

Case study 1. Ms Janice V., a 35-year-old Caucasian female office worker, is brought by an ambulance to the local hospital's casualty department immediately after a company lunch. She suffered an acute onset shortness of breath making her feel 'dizzy and confused'. The woman is 165 cm tall, weighs 95 kg and is a smoker (20–25 a day for the past 16 years). She has taken the contraceptive pill for the last 10 years. She has no chest pain and on examination she is cyanotic, has a pulse rate of 110, her blood pressure is 130/90 mmHg and there are no abnormal heart, lung or abdominal sounds.

(a) What is the presumptive diagnosis (with your reasons)?

(b) What tests should be done upon admission to hospital and why?

(c) How is the condition managed?

Case study 2. A 59-year old Caucasian male company manager presents with a dull, constant, crushing chest pain, deep in the centre of his chest. The pain has been present for the past 16 hours. In the hospital the man dies while he is being rushed to the intensive care unit. The cause of the man's death was cardiogenic shock.

(a) What was the chest pain due to?

(b) What changes would you expect to see in the man's myocardium?

(c) What was the cardiogenic shock due to?

Hypertension

1. Write notes on all of the following:
   (a) Phaeochromocytoma
   (b) Auscultatory gap
   (c) Nephrosclerosis
   (d) Oestrogen and hypertension
   (e) Hyaline arteriolosclerosis

2. Discuss the aetiology, pathogenesis and sequelae of the primary hypertensive state with special reference to the major organs of the body that are affected.

3. In order that a patient be diagnosed with systemic hypertension, above what values must the readings for systolic and diastolic blood pressure be?

4. What effect does the secretion of aldosterone by the adrenal gland have on blood pressure and what is the mechanism of this effect?

5. What are the commonest causes of death in hypertension? (Differentiate between benign and malignant forms of the disease.)

6. Define the following terms:
   (a) Papilloedema
   (b) Haematuria
   (c) Mean blood pressure
   (d) Kimmelstiel-Wilson body
   (e) 'Onion skinning'

7. What is the aetiology of secondary hypertension? Explain the pathogenesis of any one cause you have mentioned.

8. Describe the changes that occur in the kidney in a patient with benign hypertension. Briefly mention how the renal changes in the malignant hypertensive state differ from those you have described for benign hypertension.

9. Define the following terms:
   (a) Hyalinization

(b) Elastosis
(c) Protein cast
(d) Nephrosclerosis
10. What are the common clinical findings in hypertension? What are these due to?

Case study 1. A 20-year-old Caucasian female presents for a routine physical examination just prior to her marriage. All results are within the normal range. At this consultation she was prescribed oral contraceptive pills which she started to take immediately. Ten months after her marriage she has another examination on which occasion it is found that she suffers from persistent elevations of the diastolic blood pressure in the region of 105 mmHg. Other results on this occasion were normal.

(a) Explain the abnormal finding and its possible aetiology.
(b) What is the most logical course of action to be taken in this case?

Case study 2. A 60-year-old Caucasian male electrician is referred to his general practitioner because of a blood pressure reading of 210/110 mmHg at his chiropractor's clinic. The doctor after a complete physical examination records the patient's blood pressure as 250/110 mmHg.

(a) Explain the discrepancy in the blood pressure readings.
(b) Which of the two figures is likely to be the more accurate measurement?
(c) If you were told that the patient has a history of slowly and progressively rising blood pressure over a period of several years what is the diagnosis?

Case study 3. Mrs Thelma R., a 29-year-old Caucasian housewife, presents at her doctor's surgery complaining of transient spells of dizziness and headaches. On physical examination the physician records a blood pressure of 142/105 mmHg. After the patient rests in the supine position for 15 minutes an abdominal bruit is heard. Upon questioning, the woman says that in the last 2 months she has felt symptoms on two or three instances and she has had to lie down for a while in order to recover.

(a) What is the presumptive diagnosis?
(b) What tests should be done upon admission to hospital?

Arteriosclerosis

1. Distinguish between the different types of disorders collectively known as 'arteriosclerosis'.
2. Write notes on the following:
   (a) Dystrophic calcification
   (b) Mönckeberg's arteriosclerosis
   (c) Arteriolosclerosis
3. Compare and contrast atherosclerosis and arteriolosclerosis. Discuss macroscopic and microscopic appearances.
4. What are the 'hard' risk factors that are important in the development of atherosclerosis? Discuss how these contribute to the development of the atheromatous plaque.
5. Discuss the 'response to injury hypothesis' of Ross and ensure that you explain how this hypothesis is important in the elucidation of the pathogenesis of atherosclerosis.
6. Some of the major complications of atherosclerosis are responsible for very important diseases in the human body. Discuss these sequelae and use specific examples to lend credence to your arguments.
7. What is a 'musculoelastic lesion'? In what disease process would it be found and what does the lesion progress to?
8. Discuss the various epidemiological factors which predispose to atherosclerosis and describe the mode of formation and the structure of a typical lesion of this disease in a vessel. What are the major theories as to the pathogenesis of this disease process?
9. What is an aneurysm? What is the commonest cause of aneurysms in the abdominal aorta? Give two more causes of aneurysm formation in arteries and indicate the particular artery favoured by each of these.
10. Discuss fully the process of atherosclerosis, giving details about the aetiology, morphology and pathogenesis of the disease.
11. What are the clinical effects of atherosclerosis?
12. Discuss the importance of blood lipid levels in the development of atherosclerosis.
13. Describe the histological appearance of a fully developed atheromatous plaque.
14. Define the following terms:
    (a) Lipophage
    (b) Intimal cushion
    (c) Angina pectoris
    (d) Cerebrovascular accident (CVA)
    (e) Arrhythmia
15. Discuss the pathogenesis of angina pectoris and intermittent claudication.

16. A 59-year-old patient with angina pectoris has been put on a lipid-restricted diet after his blood cholesterol was read at 8.7 mmol/L. After five months of strict adherence to this diet his cholesterol level is tested again and it is found to be 8.1 mmol/L. Explain why there has been minimal change in his blood cholesterol level even after a severely restricted lipid intake.

Case study 1. Mary D., a 67-year-old Caucasian female, 1.65 m tall and 100 kg weight, retired public servant, presents with 'leg pains' that force her 'to sit and rest until they go away'. Upon questioning it is determined that what she experiences (usually after physical exertion, such as walking down to the local milk bar) is a transient, aching pain and numbness in the legs. The pain usually subsides with rest and rarely lasts more than 10 minutes.

(a) What is the presumptive diagnosis?
(b) What laboratory tests would be performed in order to confirm the diagnosis? (List them only.)
(c) What would you predict about the blood lipids profile of the patient?

Case study 2. Mr John H., a 68-year-old Caucasian male, has been diagnosed as having a large aneurysm in his abdominal aorta. He is 1.85 m in height and weighs 119 kg. A blood lipid determination yielded a total cholesterol count of 310 mg/100 ml.

(a) What is the most likely cause of the aneurysm?
(b) What other laboratory determinations should be carried out and why?
(c) What advice should be given to the patient after treatment of his aneurysm?

Case study 3. Thomas D., a 54-year-old Caucasian male sales manager, 1.85 m tall and 115 kg in weight, presents with 'excruciating chest pain'. Upon questioning it is determined that what he experiences (usually after physical exertion) is a transient, sharp pain in the chest which radiates down the left arm. The pain usually subsides with rest and rarely lasts more than 15 minutes.

(a) What is the presumptive diagnosis?
(b) What laboratory tests would be performed in order to confirm the diagnosis? (List them only.)
(c) What would you predict about the blood lipids profile of the patient?

Fluid, Blood and Vascular Disorders Crossword

CLUES

ACROSS

1. Accumulation of excess fluid in extracellular spaces (6).
7. He proposed the 'reaction to injury' hypothesis for the pathogenesis of atherosclerosis (4).
9. A drug enhancing the excretion of fluid from the body by promoting urination (8).
11. One of the risk factors in atherosclerosis (3).
12. Oedema is very serious if in this tissue (4).
14. An infarct of the lung is usually this colour (3).
16. An anticoagulant used clinically (7).
18. Systemic oedema is also so called (8).
21. Oedema in this tissue causes coma and death (5).
22. This organ enlarges if there is excessive breakdown of red blood cells (6).
25. Failure of the circulation to meet the metabolic requirements of the tissue cells (5).
26. A formed element of the blood important in thrombosis and clotting (8).
27. Histamine causes this to form in endothelium (3).
29. An analgesic also having anticoagulant properties (7).
31. Reduced haemoglobin or red blood cells in blood (7).
33. A greenish breakdown product of haemoglobin (10).
34. A thrombus partially blocking the vessel lumen (5).
37. This results after healing of an infarct (4).
38. Lack of factor VIII causes this disease (11).

40. High levels of this lipoprotein is a risk factor in the development of atherosclerosis (1, 1, 1).
41. Lack of this factor causes Christmas disease (2).
42. Carriage of abnormal solid, liquid or gas in the circulation with its subsequent impaction in a vessel (8).
43. A systemic autoimmune disease, involving the connective tissues and associated with a characteristic rash (1, 1, 1).

DOWN

2. An important factor in raising blood lipid levels in atherosclerosis (4).
3. Oedema fluid in the peritoneal cavity is called thus (7).
4. Anaemia is often due to lack of this element (4).
5. The enzyme that breaks down fibrin (7).
6. This insoluble protein is important in consolidating the blood clot in haemostasis (6).
8. This parameter of blood pressure measurements is 1/3 of the systolic plus the diastolic pressure (4).
10. Abnormal immune response causing tissue damage (7).
13. The stoppage of blood flow in acute inflammation (6).
15. A hormone important in causing systemic oedema (5).
16. The process of blood clotting, preventing blood loss from the circulation (11).
17. _ _ _ _ '_ Syndrome is an important cause of secondary hypertension (5).
19. A type of embolus, e.g. as in Caisson disease (3).
20. The commonest type of hypertension (6).
21. A thrombus that is not infected (5).
23. A cerebral infarct or a haemorrhage (1, 1, 1).
24. A mass of clotted blood, as in a bruise (9).
28. Complete absence of urine production (6).
30. A malignant tumour shows this type of growth, destroying and replacing normal cells in the process (8).
32. Widespread coagulation of blood in vessels (1, 1, 1).
35. An infarct of the kidney is of this type (4).
36. High quantities of this substance in the diet are associated with hypertension (4).
37. Factor in causation of post-operative thrombi (3).
38. High levels of this lipoprotein protect against the development of atherosclerosis (1, 1, 1).
39. A thick, yellowish fluid formed in infections (3).

Further Reading

Haemorrhage, Oedema and Shock

Abel FL. 'Myocardial Function in Sepsis and Endotoxin Shock.' *Am J Physiol* 1989; **257**: R1265.

Adamson J, Hillman RS. 'Blood Volume and Plasma Protein Replacement Following Acute Blood Loss in Normal Man.' *JAMA* 1968; **205**: 609.

Dorhout Mees EJ. 'Edema Formation in the Nephrotic Syndrome.' *Contrib Nephrol* 1984; **43**: 64.

Fisher RF, *et al.* 'Toxic Shock Syndrome in Menstruating Women.' *Ann Int Med* 1981; **94**: 156.

Fishman AP, Renkin EM. *Pulmonary Edema*, 1979; Bethesda MD, American Physiological Society.

Hands ME, Rutherford JD, *et al.* 'The In-Hospital Development of Cardiogenic Shock after Myocardial Infarction: Incidence, Predictors of Occurrence, Outcome and Prognostic Factors.' *J Am Col Cardiol* 1989; **14**: 40.

Heikillä J, Slätis P, Valtonen V (eds). 'Shock.' *Ann Clin Res* 1977; **9**: 101.

Lillehei RC, *et al.* 'The Nature of Irreversible Shock: Experimental and Clinical Observations.' *Ann Surg* 1964; **160**: 682.

Mason RG, Saba HI. 'Normal and Abnormal Haemostasis.' *Am J Pathol* 1978; **92**: 773.

McGovern VJ. 'Shock Revisited.' *Pathol Annu* 1984; **19**(1): 15.

Mizock B. 'Septic Shock.' *Arch Intern Med* 1984; **144**: 579.

Mustard JF, Packham MA. 'Normal and Abnormal Haemostasis.' *Br Med Bull* 1977; **33**: 817.

Thrombosis, Embolism and Infarction

Avasthi PS, *et al.* 'Noninvasive Diagnosis of Renal Vein Thrombosis by Ultrasonic Echo-Doppler Flowmetry.' *Kidney Int* 1983; **23**: 882.

Heim CR, Des Prez RM. 'Pulmonary Embolism.' *Adv Intern Med* 1986; **31**: 187.

Kaplan NM. 'Cardiovascular Complications of Oral Contraceptives.' *Annu Rev Med* 1978; **29**: 31.

Mannucci PM, Tripodi A. 'Inherited Factors in Thrombosis.' *Blood Rev* 1988; **2**: 27.

Mustard JF, Kinlough-Rathbone RL, Packham MA. 'Mechanisms in Thrombosis.' *Agents Actions* 1984; **15**: 6.

Nemerson Y, Nossel BG. 'The Biology of Thrombosis.' *Annu Rev Med* 1982; **33**: 479.

Peltier LF. 'Fat Embolism.' *Clin Orthop* 1984; **187**: 3.

Robert A, *et al.* 'Clinical Correlation Between Hypercoagulability and Thromboembolic Phenomena.' *Kidney Int* 1987; **31**: 830.

Strauss RH. 'Diving Medicine.' *Am Rev Resp Dis* 1979; **119**: 1001.

Thomas DP. 'Thrombosis.' *Br Med Bull* 1985; **36**: 39.

Thompson WD, Smith EB. 'Atherosclerosis and the Coagulation System.' *J Path* 1989; **159**: 97.

Vane JR, Ånggard EE, Botting RM. 'Regulatory Functions of the Vascular Endothelium.' *New Engl J Med* 1990; **323**: 27.

Hypertension

Chan JC. 'Renal and Endocrine Hypertension.' *Int J Pediat Nephr* 1983; **4**: 187.

De Swiet M, *et al.* 'Blood Pressure in the First Ten Years of Life: The Brompton Study.' *BMJ* 1992; **304**: 23.

Harris RB. 'Phaeochromocytoma.' *Heart Lung* 1984; **13**: 73.

Haworth SG. 'Primary and Secondary Pulmonary Hypertension in Childhood.' *Curr Topics in Pathol* 1983; **73**: 91.

Heptinstall RH. 'Malignant Hypertension: A Study of 51 Cases.' *J Pathol Bacteriol* 1953; **65**: 423.

Langford HG. 'Salt and Hypertension.' *Ann NY Acad Sci* 1978; **304**: 198.

Laragh JH. 'The Renin System and High Blood Pressure.' *Prog Cardiovasc Dis* 1978; **21**: 159.

Law MR, *et al.* 'By How Much Does Dietary Salt Reduction Lower Blood Pressure? I. Analysis of Observational Data Among Populations.' *BMJ* 1991; **302**: 811.

Lee RM, Smeda JS. 'Primary Versus Secondary Changes in Blood Vessels in Hypertension.' *Can J Physiol Pharmacol* 1985; **63**: 392.

Lindop GBM, Lever AF. 'Anatomy of the Renin–Angiotensin System System in the Normal and Pathological Kidney.' *Histopathol* 1986; **10**: 335.

Morris BJ. 'The Renin Gene in Hypertension.' *Today's Life Sci* 1990: **2**(11): 36.

Porush JC, *et al.* 'Hypertension and the Kidney.' *Am J Kidn Dis* 1985; **5**(4): A1.

Reich IM. 'Renovascular Hypertension.' *Mt Sinai J Med* 1979; **46**: 45.

Swales JD. 'Aetiology of Hypertension.' *Br J Anaesth* 1984; **56**: 677.

Vaughn ED Jr. 'Renovascular Hypertension.' *Kidney Int* 1985; **27**: 811.

Arteriosclerosis

Adams CW. 'Pathological Principles Involved in the Regression of Atherosclerosis.' *Adv Exp Med Biol* 1984; **168**: 1.

Benditt EP, Benditt JM. 'Evidence for a Monoclonal Origin of Human Atherosclerotic Plaques.' *Proc Natl Acad Sci USA* 1973; **70**: 1753.

Chonanian AV. 'The Influence of Hypertension and Other Haemodynamic Factors on Atherosclerosis.' *Prog Cardiovasc Dis* 1983; **26**: 177.

Ginsberg HN. 'Lipoprotein Physiology and its Relationship to Atherogenesis.' *Endocrinol Metab Clin N Am* 1990; **19**: 211.

Libby P, Hanson GK. 'Involvement of the Immune System in Human Atherogenesis: Current Knowledge and Unanswered Questions.' *Lab Invest* 1991; **64**: 5.

Northcote RJ, Todd IC, Canning GP, Ballantyne D. 'Lipoprotein Profiles of Elite Veteran Endurance Athletes.' *Am J Cardiol* 1988; **61**: 934.

Ratliff NB. 'Pathology of Large Vessel Disease.' *Am J Kid Dis* 1985; **5**(4): A93.

Rokitansky C. *A Manual of Pathological Anatomy*, vol. IV, 1852; London, Sydenham Society, 271.

Ross R, Glomset JA. 'The Pathogenesis of Atherosclerosis.' *New Engl J Med* 1976; **295**: 369, 420.

Ross R, 'The Pathogenesis of Atherosclerosis — An Update.' *New Engl J Med* 1986; **314**: 488.

Ross R. 'Mechanisms of Atherosclerosis — A Review.' *Adv Nephrol* 1990; **19**: 79.

Ruderman NB, Haudenschild C. 'Diabetes as an Atherogenic Factor.' *Prog Cardiovasc Dis* 1984; **26**: 373.

Smith EB. 'The Relationship Between Plasma and Tissue Lipids in Human Atherosclerosis.' *Adv Lipid Res* 1974; **12**: 1.

Thomson WD, Smith EB. 'Atherosclerosis and the Coagulation System.' *J Path* 1989; **159**: 97.

Woolf N. 'The Pathogenesis of Atherosclerosis.' *Rec Adv Histopathol* 1978; **10**: 45.

Woolf N. 'Thrombosis and Atherosclerosis.' *Br Med Bull* 1978; **34**: 137.

4

Growth and Differentiation Disorders

Normal growth and differentiation of cells in the body is a process which begins in embryonic life and continues up to the point of death. It is process that we still know remarkably little about and associated with this normal process of growth is the process of cellular and somatic ageing. Important changes occurring in tissues of the body as a function of age are controlled by complex genetic, hormonal, environmental and even social factors. The comprehension of what is known about normal growth and differentiation is essential in the understanding of pathological states involving these processes. Some pathological states, for example the premature ageing seen in **progeria**, may shed light into the normal processes of growth and ageing.

Variations in growth and differentiation may occur in both physiological and pathological situations, thus it is important to be able to differentiate between a normal process and a disease process. Some variations in differentiation have no physiological counterpart and the most important example of such a disorder is that leading to the formation of cancers. Cancer is a major health problem in our community and causes approximately a quarter of all deaths in our society. It is estimated that by the year 2000, cancer will be the major cause of death in Australia.

Although the molecular factors that lead to cancer are understood down to the level of single genes in many cases, it is still far from easy to talk of a 'general cause' for all types of cancer. The aetiology of many types of cancer is still obscure or totally idiopathic and the search for a cause is an ongoing process.

Variations in Cell Growth

Cells adapt to their microenvironment and the demands that are placed on them in the same manner that an individual organism adapts to changes in its macro-environment. For example, shivering is an activity of warm-blooded animals, which has an adaptive role in the face of decreasing environmental temperatures. The increased muscular activity in shivering generates more internal heat to compensate for that lost to the exterior. In the same way, a cell may adapt to stresses placed on it by changes in its immediate environment, or to increased demands placed on it. The increased size of muscles in manual workers is a good example of cellular adaptation to increased work load (stress placed on cells). The total increase in muscle mass that is seen in these people reflects an increase in size of the individual muscle cells, resulting from the synthesis of more intracellular components and organelles. The increased work load is thus shared by a greater mass of cellular elements, so that each individual muscle fibre is spared excessive work, and thus injury to the cell is prevented. In this respect, it is apparent that cellular adaptation to stress is a state intermediate to that of the normal, unstressed cell and the overstressed, injured cell which is undergoing reactive changes and necrosis.

There are many variations in the growth of cells and often these variations will lead to changes in their differentiation which may be totally abnormal morphological variants which will seriously compromise the function of the cell. The variations of cell growth and differentiation show a gradation from an increase or decrease in cell size and/or cell numbers in an organ or tissue, through to a failure of normal organ development in the embryonic or in the adult tissues. Disorders of cell proliferation may be classed as non-neoplastic or controlled proliferations, and neoplastic proliferations, which are uncontrolled. The controlled proliferations and reductions in cell numbers may also be further subdivided into the physiological and pathological changes, reflecting either a normal response by the body to a physiological stimulus or alternatively an abnormal response to a pathological stimulus.

How a cell responds to a stimulus will depend on the growth potential of that cell and the type of cell class that it belongs to as outlined in Table 4.1. Labile cells constantly divide in the normal body and hence will respond very readily to stimuli by undergoing mitosis. Stable cells, although retaining the ability to divide, will only do so under special conditions, while permanent cells are either unable to divide or alternatively will only divide under very special circumstances.

Hyperplasia

Hyperplasia is an increase in organ size due to an increase in the numbers of its specialized constituent cells. Hyperplasia in response to a given stimulus will only persist as long as that stimulus persists. When the stimulus ceases to act, the hyperplasia will cease and the organ will return to its former size. **Physiological hyperplasia** is a reversible increase in the number of cells of an organ as a result of physiological necessity, a good example being the increase in size of the female breast at puberty and during pregnancy and lactation. These changes are in response to changing levels of the sex hormones oestrogen, progesterone and mammotrophic hormone. Another striking example of hyperplasia occurs in the smooth muscle cells of the gravid uterus, resulting in an increase in size of this organ from the size of a small fist to that of a vast voluminous organ which fills most of the abdominal and pelvic cavities.

Compensatory hyperplasia is enlargement of one of a pair of organs or remains of a single organ to compensate for a loss of tissue, either the other organ or from another part of the same organ. Thus if one kidney is removed, hyperplasia and hypertrophy of the remaining kidney may result in an increase in size to approximately 80–90% of the previous total renal mass. The increase is due to hyperplasia and hypertrophy of renal tubular cells. No new nephrons are formed.

Pathological hyperplasia is unwanted or unnecessary increase in the number of cells of an organ. This

Table 4.1 *Cell populations in the body and their regenerative capability*

Cell class	Life span	Turnover mitotic rate	Examples of tissues or organs
Labile	Short	High	Epithelium (skin & hollow organs); lymph nodes; bone marrow
Stable	Long	Low	Epithelium of secretory organs; pancreas; endocrine glands; liver*, kidney*, smooth muscle*
Permanent	Approx. lifelong	None or very low	Neurones; cardiac and skeletal muscle

*These respond to stimuli.

most commonly occurs with excessive and inappropriate hormonal stimulation, for example thyroid goitre. In the presence of LATS (long-acting thyroid stimulating) antibody which mimics TSH (thyroid stimulating hormone), cells of the thyroid increase in number and thyroid hormone levels become pathologically elevated resulting in formation of a goitre and thyrotoxicosis (Graves' disease).

A very important group of pathological hyperplasias occurs in the female breast (refer to Figure 4.1). Fibrous hyperplasia, glandular hyperplasia or fibrocystic disease frequently occur due to hormonal dysfunction and independently of the normal stimuli of lactation. Most 'lumps' seen in the breast are in fact benign lesions corresponding to hyperplasias and benign tumours. In pathological hyperplasia there may be a moderately increased risk of malignant change but less risk than with metaplasia or dysplasia (Figure 4.2).

In the breasts of women between the ages of 35 and 45 years a change known as **adenosis** is seen. This is a pathological hyperplasia or the glandular component of the breast, occurring independently of stimuli causing normal lactation. **Fibrosis** is another such hyperplastic state of the breast, in this case affecting the fibrocollagenous stroma of the breast. It is most commonly seen in women 30 to 35 years of age. Quite often both adenosis and fibrosis occur together in the same breast, giving rise to fibroadenosis. In older women, 45 to 55 years of age, a **cystic hyperplasia** is often seen. In this condition as well as pathological proliferation of breast tissue components many large cysts form in the epithelial component. A true **cyst** is defined as a fluid-filled cavity lined by a layer of epithelial cells. Cysts in breast form by hyperplasia and dilatation of the duct epithelium and as the fibrocollagenous stroma surrounding the ducts also undergoes hyperplasia, the cystic ducts are often com-

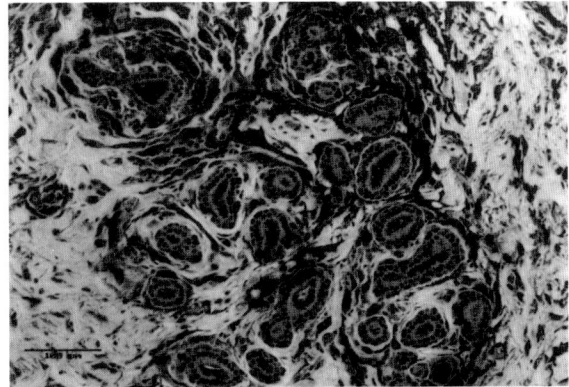

Figure 4.2 *Lobular hyperplasia of the breast showing increased numbers of secretory acini in the lobules (scale bar is 100 μm)*

pressed, appearing as highly contorted, maze-like spaces within the breast tissue. This condition arises because of an imbalance of ovarian hormones. It is not a pre-cancerous condition, although a woman who discovers a lump in her breast caused by a cyst may be greatly alarmed and distressed, often believing that she has breast cancer. All of the breast changes just described may be localized to small areas within the breast, giving rise to a discrete lump or swelling which may be easily palpated, or else they may be more diffuse changes affecting the whole of the breast.

Pathological hyperplasia may also occur in other glandular tissue, a typical, very common example being that of pathological hyperplasia of the prostate gland in elderly men. Between the ages of 40 to 59 years, autopsies shows that pathological hyperplasia is found in 55% of cadavers. In the age group 70 years

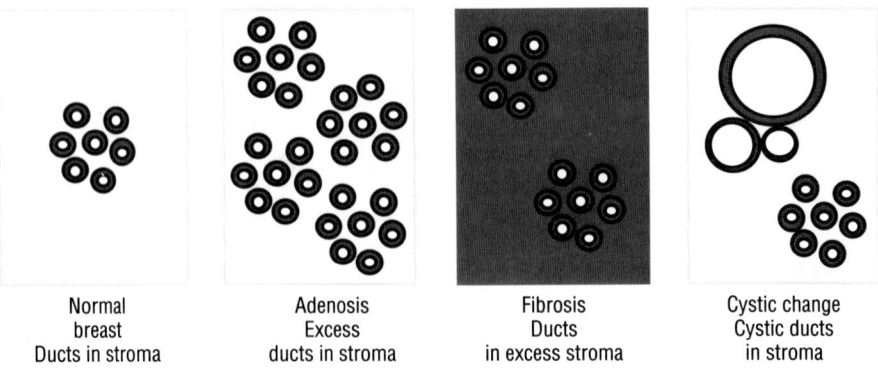

Normal breast Ducts in stroma	Adenosis Excess ducts in stroma	Fibrosis Ducts in excess stroma	Cystic change Cystic ducts in stroma

Figure 4.1 *Some types of pathological hyperplasia in the female breast*

and above, the incidence of the hyperplasia rises to 90% of autopsies. The hyperplasia affects the lateral and median lobes of the prostate and is due to inappropriate oestrogen secretion and reduced testosterone levels. In severe cases the enlarged lobes of the prostate compress the urethra with subsequent retention of urine and a predisposition to infection of the bladder and kidneys (see Figure 4.4). Hyperplasia of the prostate is unrelated to prostate cancer.

Covering epithelia may also undergo hyperplasia, usually as the result of chronic irritation or persisting trauma. Ill-fitting shoes may cause corns or calluses, these being hyperplasias of the skin. Ill-fitting dentures may give rise to gingival hyperplasia. A thorn or splinter lodging deep in the skin may give rise to hyperplasia.

Tissues which are in constant mitosis, such as the bone marrow or lymphoid tissue, may be stimulated to undergo hyperplasia and thus produce a great excess of cells. In an infection for example, there are found numerous neutrophils and metamyelocytes (their immediate precursors) both in the bone marrow and in the peripheral circulation. A peripheral blood smear will show this increased number of neutrophils and their precursors, something which a haematologist describes as a 'shift to the left'. In a chronic infection such as malaria, there is a marked **splenomegaly** (enlargement of the spleen) due to increased proliferation of lymphoid tissue in this organ in response to the presence of *Plasmodium* spp. in the body.

Hypertrophy

Hypertrophy is defined as an increase in the size of pre-existing cells, without an increase in cell number, leading to an increase in the size of the organ. Pure hypertrophy occurs in a tissue which has permanent cells such as skeletal muscle and cardiac muscle, in response to an increased work load. This occurs normally in athletes with increased demand on skeletal and heart muscle. Thus, this type of hypertrophy is said to be physiological. It must be remembered that some tissues are totally unable to respond to stimuli which will cause hypertrophy in other tissues. For example, neurones are never prone to undergo hypertrophy, no matter how hard we think!

Hypertrophy of the heart muscle occurs also in disease states such as heart valve incompetence and hypertension, causing an increased work load on the heart. Such hypertrophy which is caused by pre-existing disease is said to be pathological. Hypertrophy of the left ventricle may be very marked, the hyperplastic heart in some cases of hypertension or valvular insuf-

ficiency weighing up to 1000 grams. This condition is termed **cor bovinum** (literally 'heart of a bullock'). Right ventricular hypertrophy is seen less commonly and is associated with pulmonary problems such as pulmonary valve lesions, chronic lung diseases or pulmonary hypertension. Such hypertrophy of the heart involving the right ventricle is known as **cor pulmonale** (Figure 4.3).

Often, labile and stable tissues respond to a stimulus by undergoing both hyperplasia and hypertrophy together. A very common example of such a tissue is smooth muscle which almost always undergoes both of these changes together. The gravid uterus shows a physiological enlargement caused by hyperplasia and hypertrophy of the smooth muscle cells in its walls. The individual smooth muscle cells may increase in length up to 10 times the normal length. Stimuli causing this change are hormonal and local mechanical ones. Any obstruction in the lumen of a hollow organ the walls of which are lined by smooth muscle layers will lead to hypertrophy and hyperplasia of the smooth muscle lining, causing a thickening of the wall. Cancer of the large intestine is an example of this process. In the case of prostatic hyperplasia and blockage of the urethra mentioned earlier in elderly men, there is attendant thickening of the walls of the urinary bladder caused by the urinary retention and increased pressure inside the lumen of the bladder (see Figure 4.4).

Atrophy

Atrophy is a reduction in the size of a tissue or organ due to a reduction in the size and/or number of the

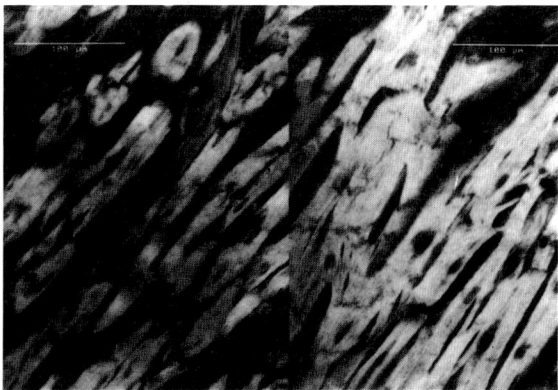

Figure 4.3 *Cardiac hypertrophy in the left ventricle of a patient with systemic hypertension (right), compared to a normal heart (left) (scale bars are 100 μm)*

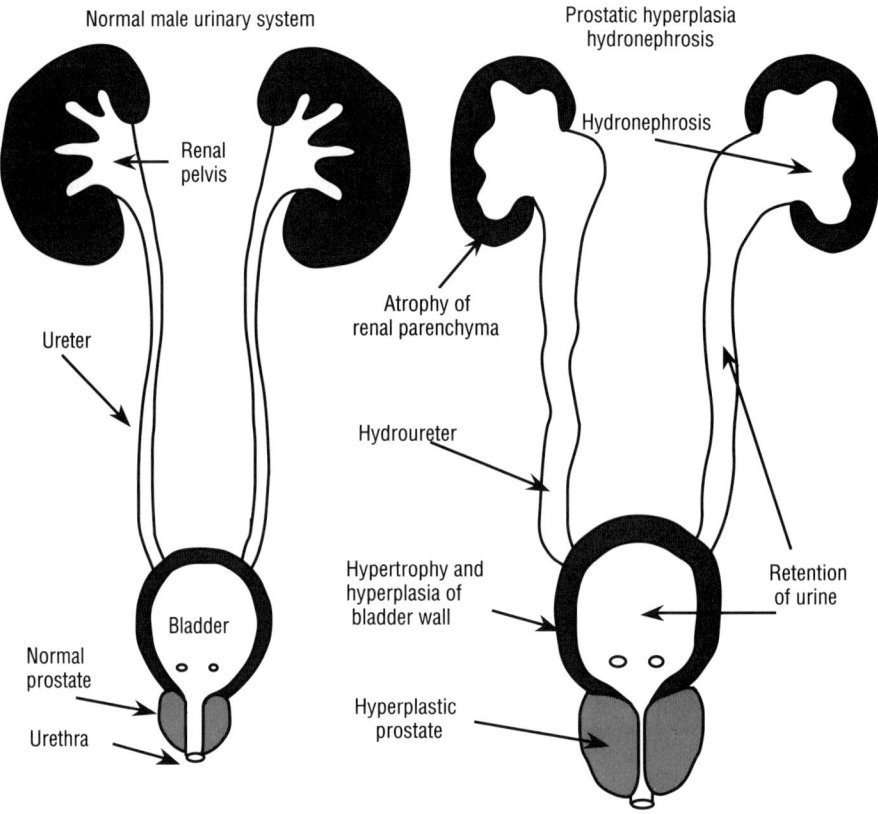

Figure 4.4 *Prostatic hyperplasia, urinary bladder wall hypertrophy and hyperplasia and renal parenchyma pressure atrophy*

cells of a tissue or organ. This occurs, for example, in starvation or ischaemia. Lowered oxygen and essential nutrients cause the cell to shrink as it undergoes autophagy, consuming non-essential cell components in order to maintain its necessary energy level. However, cells may eventually die as they cannot maintain their necessary functions indefinitely without adequate blood supply and nutrients. Thus there is a reduction in cell numbers also.

The mechanism whereby atrophy occurs is **apoptosis** (shrinkage necrosis), a form of cell death which involves individual cells or small groups of cells throughout the affected tissue and which usually occurs over a protracted period. In apoptosis, no inflammatory reaction is seen in the tissue, the apoptotic cells breaking up into fragments and being phagocytosed by surrounding parenchymal cells which use the fragments of the ingested cells as nutrients (Figure 4.5).

Physiological atrophy occurs in many situations in the body when during growth and development some structures shrink or disappear altogether. For example,

the ductus arteriosus, bronchial clefts, notochord and other structures in the foetus, the thymus gland at puberty, the uterus after parturition, the breast after weaning, the gonads and most other organs in old age. Physiological atrophy is known as **involution**.

Pathological atrophy is also seen and may be localized in one tissue or generalized, throughout the whole body. Typical examples of localized atrophy are the following. **Neuropathic atrophy** occurs when there has been damage to motor neurones innervating muscles. Such muscles undergo atrophy because of lack of nervous stimulation and disuse. Muscles undergoing atrophy in poliomyelitis is perhaps the best example. Failure to use a tissue leads to **disuse atrophy**. This may be seen in muscles after a limb has been encased in plaster, but the situation is reversible, the muscles reverting to their original size after the limb is used once again. Exocrine glands may also show this type of disuse atrophy as may occur, for example, after blockage of a duct. Pressure on an organ or tissue will lead to **pressure atrophy**. This is a variant of ischaemic

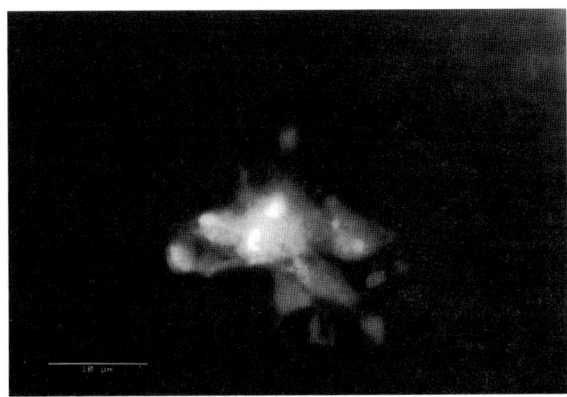

Figure 4.5 *A HeLa cell in cell culture undergoing apoptosis (scale bar is 10 μm)*

atrophy, which occurs when considerable, prolonged pressure is put on a tissue, causing compression of nutritive arteries. Such a situation is illustrated in **hydronephrosis**, a condition in the kidney arising because of inadequate drainage of urine from the renal pelvis. Such a disease process may be seen in severe prostatic hyperplasia, the urine accumulating in the bladder, ureters and renal pelvis. In extreme cases the renal parenchyma atrophies to a thin shell which surrounds the greatly dilated renal pelvis.

The heart in old age may show a localized atrophy known as **brown atrophy**, which is due to the brownish pigmentation in the muscle cells. The heart shrinks in size, often weighing as little as 100 g, and becomes brown due to the accumulation of a brown pigment in the cells. This pigment is **lipofuscin**, which is a lipochrome, very inert and insoluble. It is sometimes called the 'wear and tear' pigment as it accumulates in many of the body's stable and permanent cells with increasing age. It represents indigestible remains of ingested material or fragments of cellular organelles that the cell is unable to break down. The older an individual is, the more lipofuscin will be found in muscle and brain cells.

Generalized atrophy is most commonly seen in **malnutrition** or **starvation** where the body is unable to maintain its mass because of inadequate nutrients. In this case carbohydrate stores are first used up, followed by the fat stores and ultimately muscular proteins. The heart and brain are spared in this process as the body breaks down other non-essential tissues in order to maintain these essential organs. Advanced cancer will lead to generalized atrophy known as **malignant cachexia**. This form of atrophy is a more complex situation due to a combination of factors such

as malnutrition, poor metabolic reserve, competition between cancer and normal cells for nutrients, side effects of treatment (e.g. chemotherapy causes nausea and anorexia). Hormonal disorders on a systemic level will cause atrophy in many situations. In **hypopituitarism** the pituitary fails to produce growth hormone and other important trophic hormones. As a result the adrenal cortex, the thyroid and gonads will undergo atrophy as they depend on pituitary hormone stimulation for normal growth and function. Hypopituitarism at birth and associated genetic factors will cause a generalized atrophy as the child grows, the affected individual showing a stunted and abnormal growth, with premature ageing, such that at 7 to 9 years of age the child will have a biological age of 70 to 90 years with all of the attendant degenerations and diseases of extreme old age. Such a disease process is termed **progeria**.

Aplasia and Hypoplasia

Both aplasia and hypoplasia occur most commonly as developmental cell growth abnormalities, and usually do not occur in previously normal adult tissues. Aplasia is also sometimes used to describe states of extreme hypoplasia.

Aplasia implies a sudden cessation of growth with the affected tissue never reaching its full size or extent, usually as a result of failure of normal differentiation and growth. For example, aplasia of the thymus gland leads to dysfunction of cellular immunity, the individual affected showing a great immunodeficiency, often succumbing to fatal widespread infections. The term aplasia, however, has become almost confined to the condition of **aplastic anaemia** in which the bone marrow fails to produce the blood cells which it does normally. This may be the result of total body irradiation (this condition was seen in the survivors of the atomic bomb blasts in Hiroshima and Nagasaki), or it may be seen after cytotoxic drug therapy for cancer. In advanced malignant disease (widespread cancers in the bone marrow), aplastic anaemia will be seen as tumours replace the normal bone marrow tissue. This is a very severe condition and unless the patients are treated with a bone marrow transplant they will die.

Hypoplasia implies that the organ has failed to attain full size. Such a tissue or organ is much smaller than normal and may be dysfunctional, for example **microcephaly**, in which the foetus has a brain much smaller than normal. Although this condition is not fatal there is usually some mental retardation. An example of hypoplasia occurring after birth is seen in **cryptorchidism** (maldescended or undescended testes). If the testes fail to descend into the scrotum after birth and they remain in the abdomen, at puberty they will undergo hypoplasia, failing to develop into sperm-producing organs, being much smaller than normal. The affected man will be sterile if the condition is bilateral. In other cases hypoplasia may not lead to much harm. For example, it is not uncommon for a person to be born with one kidney much smaller than normal but no disorder is seen as even one kidney is enough for normal renal function. The normal kidney may be somewhat enlarged, having undergone compensatory hyperplasia in order to cope with the increased work load.

Agenesis

In this situation there is complete failure of an organ to develop from its primordia leading to its total absence at birth. For example **anencephaly**, in which the foetus has no brain. In this situation agenesis of the brain is incompatible with life. In other situations agenesis of an organ may be compatible with life, the person not showing any abnormality or dysfunction. For example, agenesis of one of the kidneys is followed by compensatory hyperplasia of the other formed kidney, allowing the individual to carry out a perfectly normal renal function.

Metaplasia

Metaplasia is an adaptive reversible mechanism whereby one fully differentiated adult cell type may replace a less vigorous differentiated adult cell type in the presence of a prolonged noxious stimulus. Usually the stimulus initiating the change is chronic irritation or chronic inflammation. For example, in the case of chronic irritation caused by smoking, the delicate ciliated columnar epithelium and goblet cells lining the bronchi and bronchioles of the lungs are replaced by the more resilient stratified squamous epithelium (Figure 4.6). This causes a physiological disturbance in that the flow of mucus is interfered with in these metaplastic regions, leading to retention of mucus deep in the respiratory tract, causing the person to cough in order to expel the accumulated mucus. The presence of static secretions also increases the risk of respiratory infections.

This type of 're-differentiation' or metaplasia to stratified squamous epithelium is seen in the gall bladder (often associated with gall stones), trachea, bronchi or bronchioles (due to smoking), endocervical glands of the cervix uteri (associated with multiple childbirths or sexual promiscuity) and the excretory

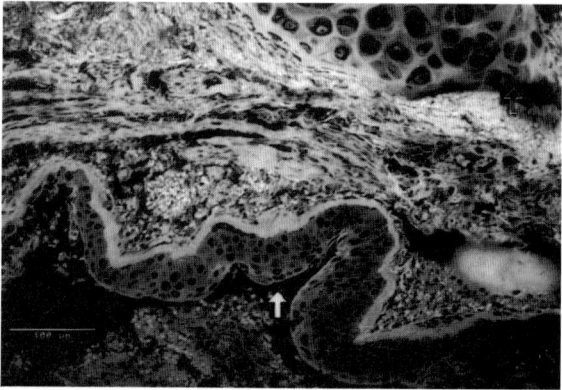

Figure 4.6 *Airway from the lungs of a heavy smoker showing the metaplastic stratified squamous epithelium of the bronchiole (solid arrow). The hollow arrow points to a plate of cartilage in the wall of the airway. Mucus and cellular debris are found in the lumen of the airway in the lower part of the micrograph (scale bar is 100 μm)*

ducts of any exocrine glands of the body, due to chronic inflammation or chronic irritation. It must be remembered that metaplasia is a reversible process and if the noxious stimulus ceases to act the tissue will eventually return to normal.

For reasons that are not clear, vitamin A deficiency is an important contributory factor of epithelial metaplasia in respiratory and transitional epithelia. Although metaplastic epithelium is usually completely differentiated and orderly, in some cases (particularly with chronic irritation, where the noxious stimulation is unrelenting) the metaplastic epithelium is somewhat disorderly. The cells may vary slightly in size, shape or orientation and there may be slight variations in nuclear size and staining properties. This represents atypical metaplasia and is the transitional phase between the normally orderly pattern of metaplasia and the disorderly pattern of dysplasia.

Dysplasia

Of all the non-neoplastic proliferations, dysplasia is the least orderly and it is the frequent forerunner of cancer (malignant neoplasia), although the precise cause of this transition is not clear. It is thus said that dysplasia is a **pre-malignant** (pre-cancerous) condition.

Dysplasia is a disorderly epithelial cell proliferation which is reversible. It comprises a loss in cellular uniformity together with a loss in architectural orientation of individual cells. This leads to a disordered, defective and atypical growth pattern with an associated compromise in function.

Dysplastic cells exhibit **pleomorphism** (variation in size and shape) and possess **hyperchromatic** (deeply staining) nuclei which are abnormally large for the size of the cell (**increased nuclear to cytoplasm ratio**). **Mitotic figures** are more numerous than usual but are normal mitoses although they may occur in abnormal locations within the epithelium. Thus in dysplastic stratified squamous epithelium, mitoses occur in all levels (even in surface cells) and are not just confined to the basal cell layer. There is also an '**architectural anarchy**'. Instead of the usual ordered transition from tall basal cells to flattened surface squames, in dysplastic epithelium dark basal-appearing cells may be seen haphazardly scattered throughout the entire thickness of epithelium.

Dysplasia is seen in the cervix, respiratory tract, oral cavity and gall bladder, in stratified, squamous epithelium (metaplasia), in the presence of chronic cervicitis, chronic bronchitis, bronchiectasis and in smokers; gall stones are the frequent precursor of dysplasia in chronic cholecystitis. Dysplasia is revers-

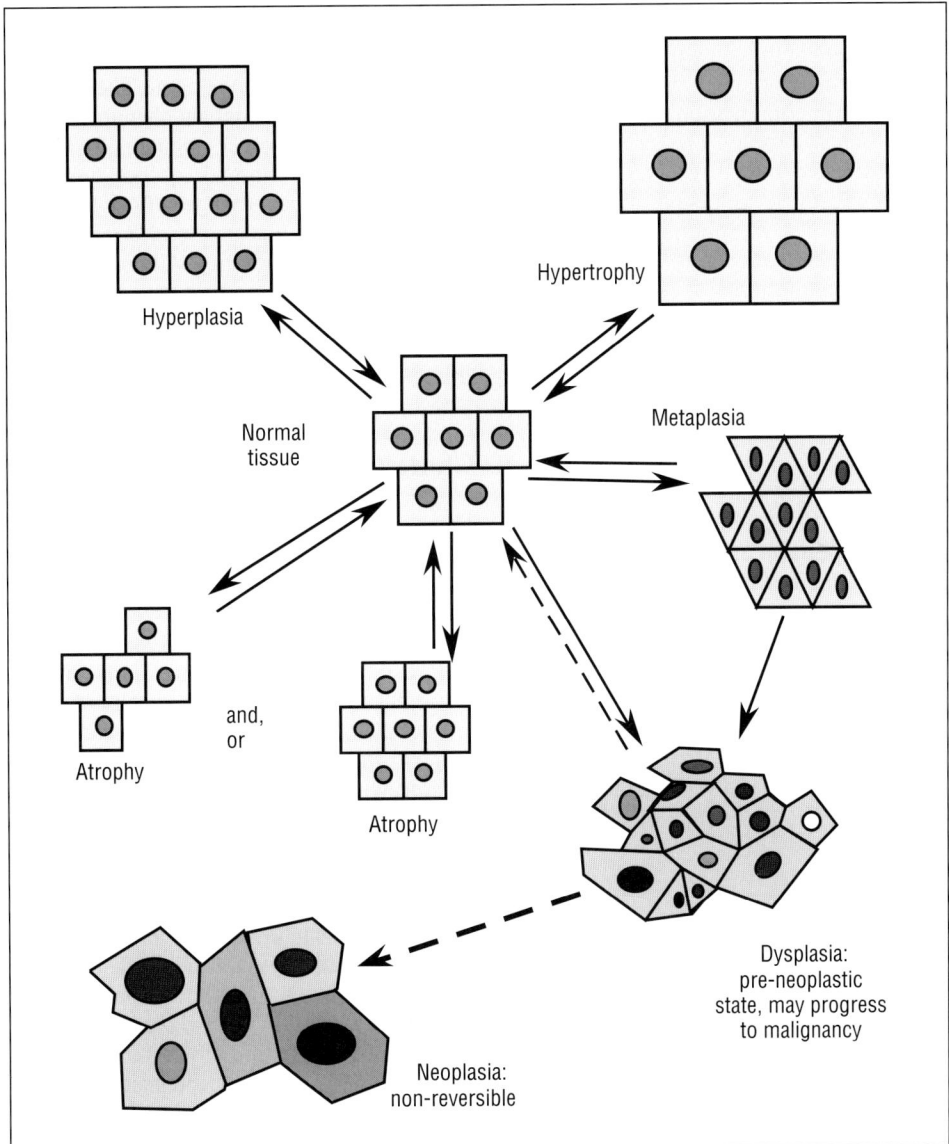

Figure 4.7 *Variations in growth and differentiation*

ible, and therefore presumably a controlled cell proliferation. If the noxious stimulus is removed, dysplastic tissues may revert to normal. If the noxious stimulus persists, however, the cellular abnormalities become more pronounced and frequently malignant transformation (cancer) may supervene (Figure 4.8).

Dystrophy

This term is very loosely used to describe pathological changes in tissues occurring as a result of nutritional or metabolic disturbances which may in a large number of cases be related to genetic disease. Such disturbances in the metabolism of the cell will lead to changes in appearance and architecture of the tissue. The condition may also occur in combination with other variations in growth, such as atrophy. The term dystrophy has now almost exclusively been reserved for conditions in skeletal muscles, and several muscular dystrophies are known. The morphology of such dystrophic cells varies considerably from the normal and each dystrophy has peculiarities of its own. For example, there may be variation in nuclear size, appearance and staining characteristics, the length and width of the muscle fibres and the amount of actin and myosin that they contain.

Hamartoma

This is a focal developmental anomaly which may be seen in any tissue of the body and usually arises be-

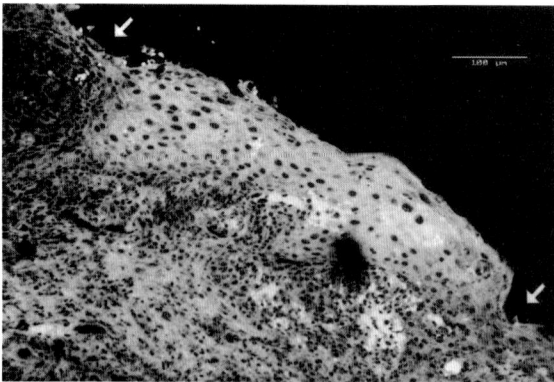

Figure 4.8 *Dysplasia of the uterine cervix. The epithelium shows variation in thickness, ulceration (arrows) and is underlain by a chronic inflammatory infiltrate. The nuclei of the squamous cells show variations in size and staining characteristics (scale bar is 100 μm)*

cause of excessive proliferation of a group of normal cells when the tissue is differentiating or growing. It may be defined as an excessive, focal overgrowth of normal, mature cells or tissues in an organ that is composed of identical cellular elements normally found in that organ. A typical example is a **naevus** ('mole' or 'birthmark') which consists of large nests of normal melanocytes situated in the skin (a tissue in which melanocytes are found normally). This local collection of melanocytes is seen as a dark blemish on the skin and normally gives rise to no disorders. However, because of its situation, this nest of melanocytes may undergo dysplastic changes (when subjected to chronic irritation such as is seen when clothing constantly rubs against a naevus, or if the naevus is exposed to excessive amounts of ultraviolet light). The dysplastic naevus may then undergo malignant change and a cancer may arise at the site. Another example of a hamartoma is a **haemangioma** ('birthmark' or 'port wine stain') which is an excessive focal overgrowth of blood vessels in a tissue, most obvious in the skin. These are normal blood vessels in continuity with the rest of the circulation. They appear as red areas in the skin and may be unsightly but usually cause no other problems. If subjected to trauma they may bleed very easily as they have blood vessels with very thin walls.

Choristoma

This is similar to a hamartoma as it consists of a focal mass of normal cells in a tissue most commonly arising during development but it differs in that these cells are present in a tissue or organ that normally does not contain them. An alternative name for the condition is **ectopia** or **ectopic tissue.** An example of the condition is normal functional glandular cells of the mucosa of the stomach being present in the lower intestinal wall. In most situations such gastric cells are found in association with a developmental anomaly known as **Meckel's diverticulum**, which is a blind-ending tube arising from the small intestine near the ileo-caecal junction and represents a persistence of the omphalomesenteric duct, which in about 1% of the population fails to undergo involution during development and persists in the adult. The mucosa of this diverticulum is lined by the normal intestinal mucosa but most patients also have associated with it choristomata consisting of nests of fully differentiated and functional pancreatic and gastric tissue in the wall of the structure. In some of these patients peptic ulcers may form in the diverticulum as a result of the secretion of acid by the choristoma.

Another example of a choristoma is the condition of

endometriosis in which normal, functioning endometrial tissue (which normally lines the uterine cavity) is found in abnormal sites such as deep inside the myometrium, in the wall of the fallopian tube, in the ovary, the wall of the large intestine, or the wall of the vagina. Since the ectopic endometrium undergoes the normal changes that occur in the normal endometrium during the menstrual cycle, degenerating endometrial cells and blood will be found in cyst-like spaces in the choristomata, causing considerable pain and discomfort. Fibrosis following an inflammatory response at the site may cause strictures and obstruction to form in the affected hollow organs. Table 4.2 summarizes the variations in growth and differentiation that may be seen in the body.

Neoplasia

Neoplasia means 'new growth' and may be more specifically defined as the process which leads to the formation of an abnormal, uncontrolled, new growth of tissue, which will have no co-ordinated, useful function in the body. Rupert Willis, the Australian pathologist, has defined the mass which arises out of the process of neoplasia, the **neoplasm**, as:

> A true tumour or neoplasm is an abnormal mass of tissue, the growth of which exceeds and is uncoordinated with that of the normal tissues, and persists in the same excessive manner after the cessation of the stimuli which evoked the change.

Neoplasms may be benign, which means they are non-invasive, remaining localized to one part of the body, or malignant, which means they are invasive and may metastasize or spread, invading different parts of the body. Malignant neoplasms are often referred to as 'cancer' from the Latin word for 'crab', referring to the macroscopical appearance of the tumour in tissue, as malignant tumours often have a central nodular region like the body of a crab and numerous streamers of cells coming out of the central mass and invading the surrounding tissues, looking much like the limbs of a crab.

Neoplasms attain a degree of autonomy, steadily increasing in size. This increase in size may be ex-

Table 4.2 *Summary of variations of growth (refer also to Figure 4.7)*

Abnormalities of cell growth
(a) Excesses or increases
    (Acquired after full development)
    (i) Hyperplasia — (increase in cell numbers)
    (ii) Hypertrophy — (increase in cell size)

(b) Deficiencies or decreases
    (Acquired after full development)
    (i) Atrophy — (decrease in size due to decrease in cell number or size)
    (ii) Aplasia — (cessation of growth/extreme hypoplasia)

    (Acquired during development)
    (i) Agenesis — (absence of a part due to failure of growth in embryo)
    (ii) Hypoplasia — (relatively deficient growth)

Abnormalities of development
(a) Hamartoma — (nest of overgrown normal components of a tissue)
(b) Choristoma — (nest of overgrown normal components of a tissue present in exotic sites)

Abnormalities of cell differentiation
(a) Metaplasia — (transformation of one mature cell type into another)
(b) Dysplasia — (disordered, defective or atypical growth)
(c) Dystrophy — (a disorder arising from defective nutrition/metabolism)

Neoplasia
(a) Benign — (not life threatening)
(b) Malignant — (virulent, tending to progress from bad to worse)

---

tremely slow, as in the case of many benign neoplasms, or there may be a very rapid and relentless increase in size, as in the case of many malignant neoplasms which grow despite a general wasting of the body known as malignant cachexia. Some neoplasms require endocrine support for their continued proliferation (for example, neoplasms of prostate, breast, uterus) and their growth may cease if this hormonal support is terminated. This is only a temporary effect, however, and most of these hormonally dependent tumours will shortly overcome this hormonal dependence and continue growing indefinitely as other neoplasms.

Thus it is seen that the process of neoplasia differs from that of hyperplasia in the following ways. **Hyperplasia** often results because of the excessive or inappropriate action of a normal stimulus. The degree of growth in this process is directly related to the degree of stimulation, and if the stimulus ceases, the hyperplasia ceases, the tissue going back to its normal size. The component cells of the hyperplastic tissue are normal and show no evidence of dysplasia, the cells having a normal function. **Neoplasia**, on the other hand appears to arise spontaneously, often no stimulus for the change being apparent. If a stimulus is demonstrable, then it is an abnormal stimulus. The neoplasia, once induced, will progress independently of the degree of stimulation. If the stimulus ceases to act, the neoplasm will most often continue to grow in the same excessive manner as before. That is, once a neoplasm is induced, a permanent change has been made in the cells, causing them to proliferate in the excessive, inappropriate manner that they do. The individual cells in neoplasms very frequently have morphological characteristics that are very different from the normal, and display aberrant function.

The study of neoplasms or tumours is termed **oncology**. Neoplasms show a wide diversity of structure but most retain a resemblance to the normal tissue from which they derive. Sometimes neoplasms resemble the precursor cell rather than the differentiated adult type (for example, nephroblastoma, retinoblastoma and blast cells in acute leukaemias). Any cells in the body can give rise to neoplasms, although the transformation occurs more frequently with some cells than with others. Neoplasms arise most often from labile populations of cells which normally have a high cell turnover and are able to proliferate and regenerate rapidly (e.g. skin, epithelium of gastrointestinal tract). Stable cell populations, such as liver cells, which usually do not proliferate but are able to regenerate in some circumstances, may also give rise to neoplasms. The cells which do not undergo replacement or regenerate, i.e. the permanent cells such as neurones and

skeletal muscle cells are the least likely to produce neoplasms, although this may occur rarely, and usually in children (e.g. rhabdomyosarcoma a tumour of striated muscle cells). The adult neurone is probably the only nucleated cell in the body incapable of neoplastic change, but malignant change of embryonic neurones may occur (medulloblastoma, neuroblastoma). Commonly neoplasms may develop in sites of chronic irritation (especially skin, mucous membranes of respiratory and gastrointestinal tracts) though not exclusively so. Generally, more neoplasms occur in those tissues which are in contact with the external environment, that is, the epithelial surfaces of the skin and mucous membranes. The change from a normal to a neoplastic cell appears to take place suddenly and permanently. The neoplastic cell must therefore transmit its new characteristics to its descendants, giving rise to a mass of tissue independent of the cells of origin. This sudden transformation has all the qualities of a **genetic mutation**. Many cancer cells show **polyploidy** (have an increased number of chromosomes) — a fact which supports this view. The cause of this sudden change is still largely unknown even though there is considerable investigation of **carcinogenesis** (cancer causation, see below).

Neoplasia manifests itself as a wide range of diseases in which the common factor is the failure of cells to regulate their proliferation and, in malignant disease, their migration. This change which occurs in the cell is known to be heritable, that is, the progeny of the transformed cell will also possess this characteristic. Many theories have been put forward to explain the property common to all neoplastic cells: the permanent change in growth regulation. There are three probable main mechanisms:

- an abnormal pathway of differentiation;
- mutation in cell genetic material;
- acquisition of viral genes foreign to the cell.

All of these mechanisms may lead to the transformation of a normal cell to a neoplastic one and it is realised now that oncogenes and their interactions with other genetic material in the cell are crucial in the formation of neoplastic cell populations.

Classification and Nomenclature of Neoplasms

Clinical Classification

Neoplasms are broadly classified into two major groups according to their behaviour:

- **benign neoplasms**, which never metastasize; and
- **malignant neoplasms**, which almost always invade and metastasize (spread elsewhere throughout the body, forming secondary tumour masses).

Benign Neoplasms

Benign means 'innocent, non life threatening, not harmful' and the slow, expansile growth and general characteristics of benign neoplasms usually cause little harm to the host unless there are accidental complications such as the tumour swelling compressing a vital structure, such as the brain, or unless the tumour cells secrete substances which in excess may cause harm, for example islet cell tumour of the pancreas producing excessive insulin which causes hypoglycaemia (low blood sugar). When examined microscopically, benign neoplasms tend to reproduce very faithfully the cells of their normal counterparts and combine with normal tissues such as blood vessels, nerves and so on just as in normal tissues. Mitotic figures are uncommon but when seen are normal.

Often a fibrous capsule will separate the tumour mass from surrounding normal cells. Even if there is no capsule, there is usually a clear line of demarcation. Benign tumour cells appear entirely normal, never invade surrounding tissue and never break free and metastasize to other tissue. Surgical removal of benign neoplasms is usually simple because of their encapsulation and obvious demarcation from normal tissue. Benign neoplasms are usually non life threatening and death only occurs if the neoplasm is in a certain position (e.g. in the brain) or because of other accidental complications, such as haemorrhage, infection, strangulation and infarction, ulceration and obstruction of hollow organs. They may also produce excessive quantities of active hormones.

Malignant Neoplasms

Malignant means 'evil, tending to go from bad to worse, life threatening'. Malignant neoplasms will tend to grow more rapidly and extend deeply and widely into surrounding tissue at many points so that no capsule forms around them. As well as displaying this invasive growth, in time, if not excised and treated early, most malignant neoplasms will appear at other sites in the body, forming secondary tumour masses or metastases. Untreated malignant neoplasms which show unrestrained rapid growth, invasion and spread will ultimately interfere seriously with normal body functions and death of the patient will ensue.

On histological examination malignant tumours show a much wider range of cell patterns than benign tumours. Some, which are termed **well differentiated** will resemble closely the tissues from which they arise. Others, which are termed **poorly differentiated** or **anaplastic**, will bear little or no resemblance to the parent cells. There are a range of appearances in between these two extremes and a histological grading of malignant tumours may be carried out (Figure 4.9). Behaviour of the tumour usually closely corresponds to its appearance — so that a well-differentiated malignant neoplasm will often not grow and spread too rapidly and with early treatment there is a better prognosis for the patient. However, a very anaplastic malignant tumour will often grow and spread rapidly, leaving the patient with an extremely poor prognosis. Thus **anaplasia** is that process whereby the malignant tumour cell 'de-differentiates', that is, is converted into a more primitive cell type, showing no resemblance to its tissue of origin and having a rapid growth rate, quickly spreading to other body parts, destroying and replacing the normal tissues.

Even when well differentiated, malignant tumours show many features which distinguish them from normal tissue and benign neoplasms. The malignant cells are not neatly ordered as in normal tissue, often forming disorganized masses of cells. The cells show a wider variation in size both of cytoplasm and nucleus — **pleomorphism**. More than one nucleus may be formed in an individual cell (**syncytium formation**), and there is a tendency for the **nucleus/cytoplasm size ratio** to be greater than normal cells (and benign tumour cells).

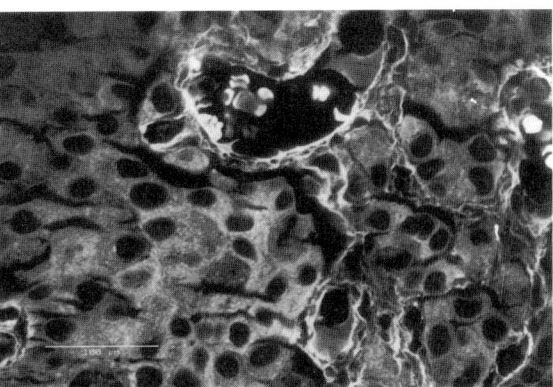

Figure 4.9 *Primary transitional cell carcinoma of the urinary bladder showing the well-differentiated malignant cells which, nevertheless, show considerable pleomorphism, increased nuclear to cytoplasmic ratio and mitotic activity (scale bar is 50 μm)*

The nuclei themselves are usually darker staining than normal (**hyperchromasia**) because they contain a greater number of **abnormal chromosomes**. **Mitotic figures** are more numerous and mostly abnormal, mitosis lasting longer in neoplastic cells than in normal cells.

Because of the rapid, disorderly growth of malignant neoplasms, there is often **poor stromal support** and **fragile blood vessels** which collapse easily under the pressure of the growing malignant cells. Hence **degeneration** and **necrosis** is a frequent finding in malignant tumours. There is usually **no clear demarcation** between the malignant neoplasm and surrounding tissues. Most often clumps of malignant cells are seen **infiltrating** (growing in between) cells of normal surrounding tissue. The malignant cells move along lines of least resistance — lymphatics, thin-walled blood vessels, hollow tubes and through soft tissues. However, malignant cells also show erosion and **invasion** (destruction and replacement) of compact tissues — even bone. Malignant cells may cause pressure atrophy of surrounding tissues and also may produce a hyaluronidase-like enzyme which softens the connective tissue stroma around malignant cells and allows invasion of adjacent tissue. Table 4.3 summarizes the major differences between benign and malignant neoplasms.

Malignant cells adhere less firmly to each other and it is this lack of cohesiveness which allows cells to break free and lodge elsewhere in the body to form secondary tumours or **metastases**. Spread or **metastasis** of malignant neoplasms will be discussed in more detail later.

Histogenetic Classification

As well as being classified as either benign or malignant, neoplasms are classified according to their histogenesis, that is, their tissue of origin. Most neoplasms which are benign are given the general suffix '**-oma**'. Malignant neoplasms of epithelial origin are called **carcinoma**, while those of connective tissue (mesenchymal) origin are called **sarcoma**. The tissue of origin forms the prefix in naming the tumour. For example, osteoma is an benign tumour of bone and

Table 4.3 *Summary of differences between benign and malignant neoplasms*

Benign	Malignant
1. *Structure:* well differentiated, and typical of tissue of origin	1. *Structure:* imperfectly differentiated and atypical of tissue of origin
2. *Histology:* well-formed stroma with little tendency to haemorrhage and no necrosis	2. *Histology:* stroma often poorly formed with haemorrhage and necrosis common. Cells are pleomorphic
3. *Mode of growth:* usually purely expansive and with a capsule formed by the tumour or as a tissue reaction to the tumour	3. *Mode of growth:* infiltrative and invasive as well as expansive, hence not encapsulated
4. *Rate of growth:* usually slow with little mitotic activity	4. *Rate of growth:* may be very rapid and there may be quite a great deal of mitotic activity seen
5. *End of growth:* may stop growing spontaneously	5. *End of growth:* very rarely stops growing spontaneously
6. *Metastasis:* absent	6. *Metastasis:* frequent and often is a diagnostic feature
7. *Clinical significance:* usually not fatal but complications may arise because of: (a) situation (b) accidental complications (c) production of active substances (e.g. hormones)	7. *Clinical significance:* dangerous because it may give rise to all the complications seen with benign tumours, as well as: (a) infiltration and invasion into surrounding tissue (b) metastasis and growth of secondary tumours at distant sites (c) infection, haemorrhage, etc. (d) cachexia due to a combination of factors

osteosarcoma is a malignant tumour of bone. No classification of neoplasms is at present universally accepted, so there is quite often confusion over naming of tumours and there are many inconsistencies in nomenclature and classification of neoplasms. For example a malignant tumour derived from the lymphoid cell line may be called lymphoma, lymphosarcoma or malignant lymphoma. Some neoplasms of infants and children are given the ending **blastoma**, indicating that they are derived from immature or embryonic cells. Typically such tumours are malignant; examples are retinoblastoma, nephroblastoma and neuroblastoma.

The histogenetic classification encounters some difficulties in that sometimes an ambiguity exists as to the classification and nomenclature of a normal body tissue, for example mesothelium — is this an epithelial tissue or should it be defined as a 'connective tissue' element? Are melanocytes a component of the epithelium in which they are found or should their embryonic derivation be considered, in which case they should be classified with the nervous tissue elements of the body? In addition, with anaplastic tumours the tissue of origin may not be determinable as there is total loss of organizational, structural and functional resemblance to the normal tissue. However, given its limitations, the histogenetic classification is a very useful adjunct to the clinical classification of tumours and by combining the two methods much information may be gained about a tumour simply by stating its accepted name, for example 'osteosarcoma' refers to a malignant tumour derived from the osteoblasts of bone. Elements of the histogenetic classification of tumours may be found in Table 4.4.

Table 4.4 *Classification of some neoplasms*

Tissue of origin	Cell involved	Benign neoplasm name	Malignant neoplasm name
Connective tissue and muscle	Fibrocyte	Fibroma	Fibrosarcoma
	Adipocyte	Lipoma	Liposarcoma
	Osteocyte	Osteoma	Osteosarcoma
	Chondrocyte	Chondroma	Chondrosarcoma
	Smooth muscle cells	Leiomyoma	Leiomyosarcoma
	Striated muscle cells	Rhabdomyoma	Rhabdomyosarcoma
	Enamel organ cells	Ameloblastoma	Ameloblastoma
Vascular endothelium	Blood vessels	Haemangioma	Haemangiosarcoma
	Lymphatic vessels	Lymphangioma	Lymphangiosarcoma
Epithelium	Skin	Papilloma	Squamous cell carcinoma / Basal cell carcinoma
	Glandular	Adenoma	Adenocarcinoma
	Transitional — epithelium	Papilloma	Transitional — cell carcinoma
Mesothelium	e.g. Pleura	Benign mesothelioma	Malignant mesothelioma
Nervous system	Glial cell	Glioma	Astrocytoma, etc.
	Nerve	Ganglionic neuroma	Neuroblastoma
	Melanoblast (melanocyte)	Benign naevus	Malignant melanoma ('melanosarcoma')
Meninges	Meningeal fibroblast	Meningioma	Meningosarcoma
Haemopoietic tissue	Lymphocyte	'Lymphoma'	Lymphosarcoma
	Reticulum cell		Reticulosarcoma
	Plasma cell		Myeloma
	Leukocytes		Leukaemia
Embryonal	Pluripotential cell	Teratoma	Malignant teratoma
Placenta	Placental trophoblast	Hydatidiform mole	Choriocarcinoma
Unknown	Unknown	—	Anaplastic tumour

Morphological Classification

Description of appearance of neoplasms is also important in classification. The macroscopical appearance of tumours is often mentioned in the name of the tumour and certain sites in the body may be characteristically associated with giving rise to specific morphological types of tumours (refer to Figure 4.10).

Papillary (or fungating) tumours are tumours which grow outwards from a surface, looking much like a cauliflower. Examples are papillary cystadenoma of the ovary, where neoplastic cell masses project into a cyst-like structure, and papilloma of the skin, where the tumour mass projects from the skin surface in a cauliflower-like growth pattern.

Polypoid tumours are masses found attached to the surface from which they have arisen by a stalk, in this respect resembling a mushroom, for example polyposis coli, in which numerous benign polypoid tumours form on the surface of the large intestinal mucosa.

Most neoplasms show a **nodular** growth pattern in which the tumour presents as 'lump' or nodule in the tissue, for example fibroadenoma or carcinoma of the breast.

Frequently, tumours of glandular tissues in particular will show a **cystic** appearance in that numerous cysts full of fluid will be apparent within the tumour tissue. This type of cystic tumour is very common in the ovaries, for example mucinous cystadenoma.

Many tumours will show prominent **ulceration**, in which the surface of the tumour mass becomes necrotic and sloughs off, leaving a typical ulcer crater. Tumours of the stomach and skin very frequently ulcerate.

Lastly, a tumour may show the **infiltrative** pattern of growth, where the tumour cells become intimately mixed with the normal tissue cell and they rapidly involve the whole of the organ in which they arise. A typical example of this is a cancer of the stomach known as *linitis plastica* in which the malignant cells infiltrate the walls of the stomach, causing them to appear thickened.

In addition a tumour may have varying amounts of stroma (connective tissue elements supporting the tumour cells). Some neoplasms elicit formation of dense stroma, while others have scanty stroma. For example, **scirrhous carcinoma** of the breast has dense stroma and is firm on palpation, while **encephaloid carcinoma** of the breast has less stroma and is mostly composed of gland-like masses of neoplastic cells, hence it is softer on palpation.

Spread of Malignant Neoplasms

Benign neoplasms remain localized at their site of origin, slowly increasing in size by expansive growth, compressing surrounding tissue which regresses due to pressure atrophy. There is often a fibrous capsule around this benign neoplasm. By defintion, a benign neoplasm never moves away from its site of origin.

Malignant neoplasms grow by progressive infiltration (growth between cells and in tissue spaces) and invasion (destruction and penetration of surrounding tissue). They are not encapsulated, although if rapidly growing they may appear to be encapsulated by stroma of surrounding normal tissue. However, microscopy will usually reveal tiny crab-like processes penetrating the margin and infiltrating adjacent structures. The spread of neoplasm cells from their site of origin (referred to as the **primary tumour site**), such that they involve distant organs and tissues, forming deposits and growing there (deposits known as the **secondary tumour sites**) is an important characteristic of malignancy, benign tumours never behaving in this manner. Malignant cells achieve this by growing, invading and destroying normal tissue. Mechanisms of invasion are as follows:

1. **Pressure** generated by the expanding mass.
2. **Less differentiated** tumour cells are more mobile than the differentiated cells that they have arisen from. In the developing tissues of the embryo the dividing and differentiating cells must often move great distances in order to reach the final site where they will settle and organize themselves into an organ. Tumour cells seem to revert back to this highly mobile state and in spreading to distant sites in the body they exhibit this characteristic of primitive cells.
3. **Release of lytic enzymes** (e.g. collagenases and glycosidases) by neoplastic cells which degrade extracellular constituents and make infiltration along tissue planes easier.
4. **Lack of cohesiveness**. Malignant cells have been shown to form pseudopods which insert themselves between and into surrounding normal cells, fragmenting and destroying tissues. There are few tight junctions between malignant cell membranes, allowing a greater mobility. This may also contribute to small masses of cells breaking off and allowing tumour emboli to disperse along lymphatics and via the blood stream, forming distant metastases. Tumour cells have lost the 'contact inhibition' which is seen with normal cells and this is an additional characteristic promoting their spread.

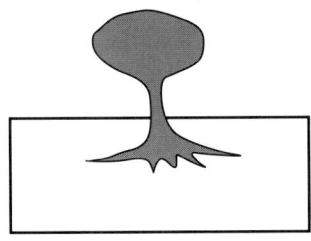

Polypoid neoplasm (polyp): Often forms on free surfaces such as skin or mucosae. It is a 'mushroom-like' growth on a stalk. Examples: polyposis coli, solitary polyp of the large bowel.

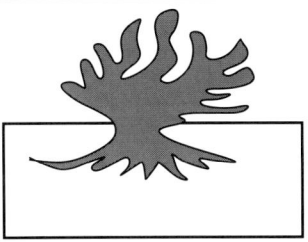

Papillary (fungating) neoplasm: Also forms on free surfaces such as skin or mucosae. Occasionally it may form within cysts, e.g. papillary cystadenoma of the ovary. Other examples: papilloma of the skin, fungating colonic carcinoma.

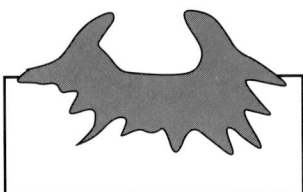

Ulcerating neoplasm: A very common form of neoplasm, the ulcer crater being caused by necrosis and sloughing off in the centre of the tumour mass. Examples are: basal cell carcinoma of the skin, carcinoma of the stomach, carcinoma of the large bowel.

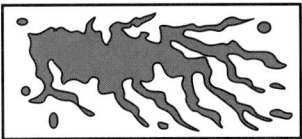

Infiltrating neoplasm: This neoplasm grows within the tissue, intimately mixing with the normal cells as it infiltrates and invades through the tissue. Examples: stomach carcinoma (linitis plastica or 'leather bottle stomach') .

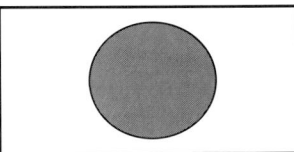

Nodular neoplasm: A very common form of tumour, presenting as a 'lump' in tissue. Examples: fibroleiomyoma of the uterus ('fibroid'), carcinoma of the breast. Many secondary tumours show this nodular pattern when they are found in sites such as lungs, liver or brain, where they are present as multiple deposits.

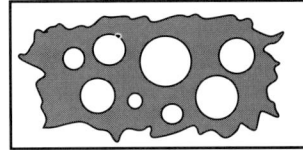

Cystic neoplasm: Often forms in tumours derived from glandular tissue. The cysts may be filled with mucus, serous fluid or secretion. Examples: cystadenoma of the ovary, cystic fibroadenoma of the breast, cystic basal cell carcinoma of the skin.

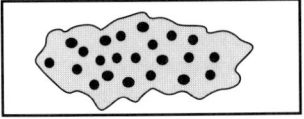

Scirrhous neoplasm: This is a description applying to the texture of the tumour on palpation.It implies a hard mass, which is due to the great amount of fibrous, connective tissue stroma which is present in between the tumour cell masses. For example, most breast carcinoma are scirrhous.

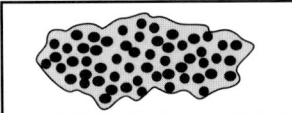

Encephaloid neoplasm: This is a description applying to the texture of the tumour on palpation. It implies a soft ('brain-like' in texture) mass, which is due to minimal amount of fibrous, connective tissue stroma being present in between the tumour cell masses. For example, some breast carcinoma are encephaloid.

Figure 4.10 *Some commonly encountered macroscopic forms of neoplasms*

Mechanisms of Spread

Malignant tumours spread via two routes: **direct invasion routes**, where the tumour cells grow in continuity with one another and the main tumour mass, insinuating their way between normal tissue cells, and **metastatic routes**, where clumps of tumour cells break off and are transported to distant sites mostly in an embolic fashion.

Direct Invasion Routes

Via tissue spaces (intercellular pathways). Tumour cells are seen to infiltrate and occupy intercellular spaces within normal tissues, invading most easily along the line of least resistance, causing pressure atrophy of surrounding cells and eventually replacing them. This is the fundamental way in which malignant tumour cells spread and all malignant neoplasms grow and spread in this fashion. The malignant cells grow in long streamers or tongues and as may be inferred this process is more rapid in loose tissues with many actual or potential spaces, for example in loose connective tissue between muscles, organs of the gastrointestinal tract, the central nervous system and the marrow space. On the other hand, compact, tough tissues such as cartilage, tendons, ligaments, stout visceral capsules, muscular arterial walls all act as barriers to tumour cell spread.

Intracellular pathways (growth within cells, e.g. skeletal muscle fibres). This is an uncommon method of spread and is seen in the spread of malignant tumours in skeletal muscle in particular. The large, thick, long fibres of muscle allow such a process to occur. The invading tumour cells gain entry into the cytoplasm of the muscle fibre, forming long columns of cells that grow inside the cell, eventually replacing all of the sarcoplasm.

Infiltration of lymphatic vessels (lymphatic permeation). The malignant cells in this case invade through the very thin wall of lymphatics and grow by extension within the lumen of the vessel. Lymphatic permeation is a very common way of spread with carcinomata. The tumour cells may permeate lymphatics for considerable distances (Figure 4.11). For example, in carcinoma of the breast, lymphatic permeation may involve the lymph nodes of the axilla or the trunk. It is common to find that the infiltration of lymphatics does not occur in a simple radiating manner from the primary tumour mass. Often some lymphatic vessels allow bet-

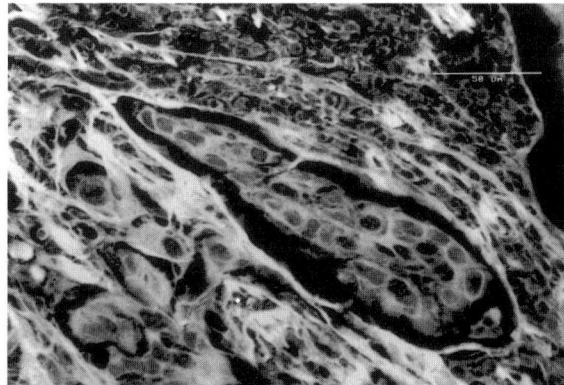

Figure 4.11 *Lymphatic permeation of a malignant tumour. Primary transitional cell carcinoma of the urinary bladder showing invasion into and growth within a lymphatic vessel (scale bar is 50 μm)*

ter spread of tumour cells which then reach regional lymph nodes, grow there as secondaries, occluding lymph flow. After this, tumour cells may then grow backwards, following the diverted lymph flow, showing **retrograde dissemination** into neighbouring lymphatic plexi.

This mode of lymphatic dissemination is not confined to the small lymphatic vessels but may often involve the main lymphatic trunks, including the thoracic duct (which is invaded in approximately 6% of all fatal cases of intra-abdominal carcinoma — e.g. stomach carcinoma).

Via veins, venules and capillaries. Malignant tumours very frequently invade through the wall of blood vessels, mostly venules and capillaries. Large veins, arterioles and arteries are generally resistant to tumour invasion as they have a thick muscular wall not readily invaded by tumour. Both small and large arteries are frequently seen to be totally surrounded by malignant tumours and yet their walls remain intact and resistant to tumour invasion.

Gross invasion of veins is seen in carcinomata of the kidney, lung, thyroid, stomach and liver and this mode of invasion also characterizes many sarcomata (e.g. osteosarcoma). The invading tumour tongues may grow within the vessels for very long distances: it has been recorded for renal carcinoma, for example, that the tumour cells, after invading branches of the renal vein, have grown in continuity up the inferior vena cava, into the right ventricle and then into the pulmonary arteries. Tumour invasion into the vascular system may cause thrombosis with all the sequelae of thrombi that were discussed previously.

Via coelomic spaces. Visceral tumours spread into the serous cavities partly by direct invasion and partly by growth through into the cavity. Some tumours show a special tendency to do this, as, for example, some mucoid tumours of the ovary which may totally fill up the abdominal cavity with tumour cells and mucus (a condition known as **carcinomatosis peritonei**). Mesothelioma of the pleura most frequently grows around the lungs, within the pleural cavity as a sheath, infiltrating within the pleural space.

Via cerebrospinal spaces. The subarachnoid space, the ventricles of the brain and especially the Virchow-Robin perivascular spaces in the central nervous system are particularly prone to become infiltrated by malignancies in these situations (Figure 4.12).

Via epithelial-lined cavities, ducts. Tumours sometimes grow and extend for long distances within the ducts of organs or within other spaces. Carcinoma of the renal pelvis may grow down the ureters, carcinoma of the uterus may grow into the Fallopian tubes and carcinoma of the bronchus may grow and infiltrate along the wall of the airways. Infiltrating tumours of the kidney and testis may grow within the minute epithelial spaces of the tubules found in these organs.

Tumour Metastatic Routes

When tumour cells break away and are conveyed to distant sites forming secondary deposits there, the process operating is that of **metastasis** (literally, 'a change of placing'). The factors which influence the develop-

ment of metastasis are largely unknown though certainly local factors must be important because secondary neoplasms form more commonly in some organs than others. Also the tumour-associated immune response by the host mounted against the primary tumour is important. It has been noted that when there is a good host immune response to the malignant cells the growth of the primary may be limited and secondaries are less likely to develop early. Where there is a deficiency of host immune response, the malignant neoplasm is often seen to be rapidly growing and early to metastasize.

Lymphatic Spread

This is a very characteristic mode of spread of many carcinomata. Malignant tumour cells infiltrate through the thin-walled lymphatic channels in their vicinity, then may either grow along the lymphatics as a solid cord of tumour (as discussed in permeation) or break free and be carried along by lymph to the lymph nodes into which the lymphatics drain (**tumour embolism**). This embolic spread of neoplasms is evidenced by the demonstration of the lack of tumour cells between the primary tumour mass and the secondary which has developed in a lymph node. In early carcinoma of the breast, with axillary lymph node metastasis, no tumour cells may be found between the two sites, a distance of 15 cm or so. Similarly, a malignant melanoma of the great toe may metastasize to the inguinal lymph nodes, a distance of about 80 cm. Microscopically, small clumps of tumour cells may be seen in the cortical sinuses of the lymph nodes. As the neoplasm grows it replaces the lymphoid tissue with malignant neoplastic tissue and extends through the lymph node capsule.

Hence the regional lymph nodes which drain the tissues at the primary site of the malignant neoplasm are often the first site of spread. Malignant cells frequently pass from one lymph node to another, so that it is possible to have a metastasis in a lymph node remote from the primary site, in tertiary or quaternary deposits. Also, retrograde spread of neoplastic cells along lymph channels may often occur because the normal drainage is blocked by lymph node metastases. Malignant cells may eventually find their way into the thoracic duct and thus be disseminated to the lungs by way of the bloodstream. Another way in which tumour cells may find themselves in the bloodstream after having invaded lymph nodes is by direct extension through walls of venules in the node or by invading past the lymph node capsule into the wall of a neighbouring vein. For example, invasion of the jugular vein may occur from deposits of tumour in the cervical lymph nodes.

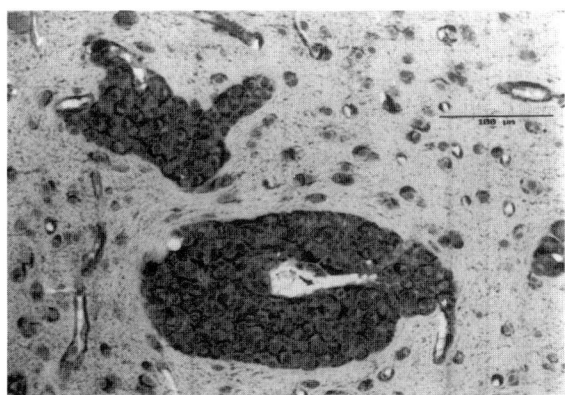

Figure 4.12 *A secondary malignant melanoma of the brain which is showing growth in the Virchow-Robin spaces around the blood vessels in this tissue (scale bar is 100 μm)*

Bloodstream Spread (Haematogenous Spread)

Thick-walled arteries are relatively resistant to infiltration by malignant neoplasms, but thin-walled veins, venules and capillaries are easily infiltrated. When tumour cells penetrate the endothelial lining of these vessels, they also form a nidus for thrombus formation. Fragmentation of these thrombi with malignant cells contained in them is often the starting point of blood-borne metastases, as well as free circulation of individual malignant cells. The commonest size of tumour emboli is between 50 and 200 μm in diameter. The number of tumour emboli found in any case of cancer varies widely and is dependent on the tumour type and various individual factors such as the host response to the presence of the tumour.

The malignant cells are carried along in the venous system either through the right side of the heart to the lung capillaries, or if the tumour arises within the gastrointestinal tract, through the portal vein to the liver sinusoids. Most of these tumour emboli do not survive. However, some proliferate to form metastases. Others permeate along the capillary walls to reach wider distal channels and disseminate further. In the case of the lungs this occurs via the systemic arteries and thus to all parts of the body. In the case of the liver it will be first into the hepatic vein and inferior vena cava, then to the right side of the heart and to the lungs. It must also be kept in mind that tumour which has invaded lymphatics and lymph nodes may then, from that situation, invade blood vessels and hence be carried to distant sites via the bloodstream.

Some blood-borne emboli have unusual destinations: for example, intracardial implantation and growth on the heart valves and cordae may be seen occasionally; in carcinoma of the left kidney there may be invasion of the renal vein, with emboli travelling down to the vaginal, pelvic, spermatic, ovarian or pampiniform plexi, giving rise to secondary deposits in those situations (see Figure 4.13).

Transcoelomic Spread

If a malignant tumour infiltrates through the mesothelial surface of the serous cavities of the body it may appear as secondary nodules elsewhere in that cavity, the tumour cells breaking off and gravitating down to settle on the surface of other organs or on the walls of the cavity. There may be a few nodules or an almost continuous sheet of tumour cells over the surface of the membrane. As the malignant cells penetrate the surface of the cavity, cells may break free and seed elsewhere in the cavity, or perhaps there may be some lymphatic spread via the lymphatic network beneath the membrane surface as well. The development of secondary tumours in the walls of serous cavities is quite a common event, particularly in the peritoneal and pleural cavity. In the peritoneal cavity, the ovaries are prone to become the site of secondary tumours seeded in this way (e.g. **Krukenberg tumours** which are secondary tumours in the ovary, the primary being in the stomach). Seeding of tumours may occur also in cerebrospinal fluid, via the meningeal spaces over the brain and spinal cord.

Some people also believe that malignant cells may break free in the urinary tract, metastasizing further downstream. For example, cells from a carcinoma in the kidney pelvis or ureter break off, seed into the bladder, attach onto the mucosal wall, and then proliferate there as secondary tumour masses. This is not a widely held view, however, and the development of separate primary tumours is the more likely explanation. This is because all the mucosal aspects of the urinary tract are lined by the same epithelium and if this is exposed to carcinogenic agents in the urine, multiple sites are likely to undergo malignant change simultaneously.

Sites of Secondary Blood-borne Metastases

Certain organs of the body are most commonly sites of secondary tumours. This is probably due to many factors: local factors, blood supply to the organ, drainage from other areas and other considerations. There is the so-called '**seed–soil**' concept of metastasis. In other words the malignant cells (the 'seeds') which break free as tumour emboli may lodge in many parts of the body, but many will not survive, and only those that lodge in suitable tissues (the 'fertile soils') will proliferate to become metastases (Figure 4.14).

The main determining factor governing whether or not a tumour cell embolus will 'take' at a certain site is the biochemical environment of that site. Tumour cells have certain metabolic requirements which must be met if they are to grow. Whether a tissue supplies these requirements, whether there is an adequate blood supply, presence or absence of various tissue enzymes and adequate levels of certain metabolites will all influence whether or not a tissue is likely to be favourable to the growth of secondary tumours. Many body parts are virtually never sites of metastases, or very rarely. Such tissues include skin, skeletal muscle, myocardium, spleen and kidneys, despite the fact that these tissues may have large volumes of the blood passing through

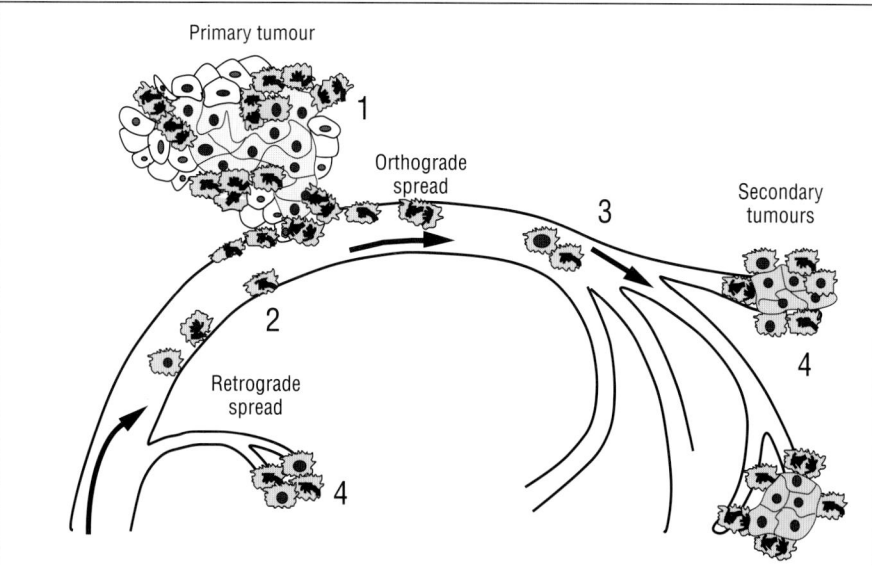

Primary tumour

1

Orthograde
spread

3

Secondary
tumours

2

Retrograde
spread

4

4

Phase 1: Growth, infiltration and permeation of the primary tumour mass, such that normal tissue is pushed aside and undergoes pressure atrophy. As the tumour cells multiply and the tumour grows in size, it replaces the normal tissue and grows around lymphatic and vascular channels.

Phase 2: Invasion of tumour cells into lymphatics and veins but not arteries and arterioles because the latter have a thick wall. Once inside the vessels, the tumour permeates the vessel, growing in a continuous streamer inside the lumen. However, tumour cell clumps break off and are carried as emboli by the fluid inside the vessel.

Phase 3: Embolization transfers the tumour cell clumps to distant sites. This process may be orthograde (going in the direction of fluid flow) or retrograde (going against the flow of fluid). The tumour cell clumps will travel for long distances, being stopped when the lumen diameter becomes smaller than their own diameter.

Phase 4: The arrested tumour cell clumps will develop into new tumour masses, secondary tumours, if the tissue conditions allow the survival of the tumour cells.

Figure 4.13 *The development of metastasis via the tumour metastatic routes*

them. Kidneys, for example, receive 20% of the total cardiac output. Other parts of the body are very common sites of metastases.

The **liver** is the commonest site of secondary tumours. It receives blood from both the portal vein and the hepatic artery, thus tumour emboli may arrive at the liver from the gastrointestinal tract (e.g. carcinomata of the oesophagus, stomach and large intestine) or from the systemic circulation (primary and secondary tumours of the lungs; Figure 4.15). Virtually all the tumour emboli arriving at the liver have been shown to 'take' successfully as the biochemical and metabolic environment of the liver is ideal for tumour cell growth. The liver shows many distinct tumour deposits, each group of cells lodging in the tissue giving rise to a secondary mass (this characteristic is often used to distinguish primary and secondary tumours — primary tumours are usually single masses while secondary tumours are usually multiple masses). The liver often enlarges grossly due to the presence of secondaries; it is not unusual for a liver with secondaries to weigh 10 kg! From the liver malignant cells often enter the hepatic vein, then the inferior vena cava to the right heart and then to the lungs.

The **lungs** are the second most common site of metastatic tumour growth. In this organ, through which blood from every part of the body must pass, bilateral spread is seen and the lungs become studded with multiple tumour masses. Alternatively, there may be only a few large secondary masses with a shower of smaller masses around them. Subpleural sites are commonly affected and intrapleural dissemination often occurs. Any tumour of the body may show secondaries in the lungs but especially common are secondaries from primaries in the breast, bones, kidneys, and squamous cell carcinoma and malignant melanoma of the skin.

The third most common site of metastases are the **bones**, especially vertebrae, sternum, ribs, pelvic bones, diploë of the skull and proximal ends of the humerus and femur (that is, the bones containing red marrow). Metastasis to bone leads to destruction of the bony tissue with rarefaction and resorption (often the patient may show hypercalcaemia and metastatic calcification). Occasionally the bone may become denser as an effect of the tumour. Primary malignant neoplasms of the breast and the prostate commonly metastasize to bone and have this osteoplastic effect. Because of the destruction and replacement of bone marrow by the tumour, anaemia and thrombocytopenia will often result in these patients. Pathological fractures of the weakened bones is also another frequent finding.

The **brain** is the fourth most common site of metastases, especially the cerebrum, with the cerebellum and brain stem occasionally involved. Primary neoplasms of the lungs, breast and malignant melanoma commonly metastasize to the brain.

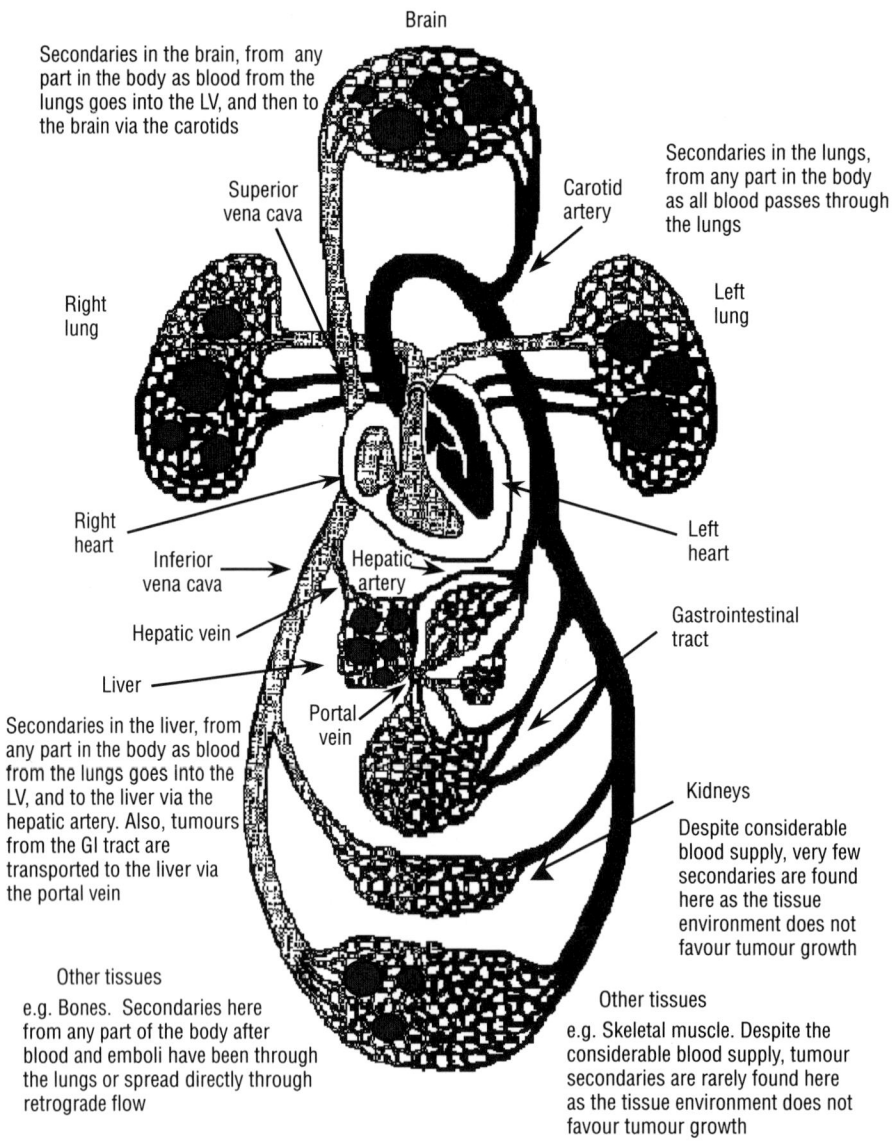

Figure 4.14 *Factors in haematogenous metastasis*

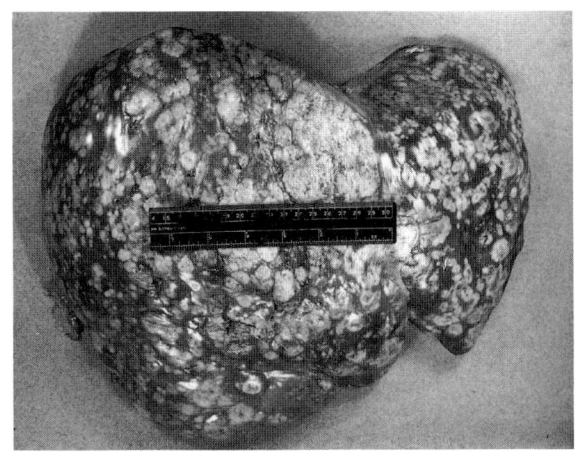

Figure 4.15 *Grossly enlarged liver showing many metastases from an adenocarcinoma of the cardia of the stomach*

The fifth most common site is the **adrenals**. Primary malignant tumours of breast and lungs quite commonly metastasize to the adrenal glands. Studies show that about a third of all fatal cases of lung cancer show adrenal metastases.

Effects of Malignant Tumours

The effects of malignant tumours may be local such as **pressure atrophy** or infiltration of nearby vessels or nerves; may be caused by their secretions such as mucin or hormones; or may be caused secondarily by bacterial infection. **Infection** is not uncommon because there is often **necrosis** in the tumour from ischaemia (pressure on or infiltration of blood vessels). The effects of tumours may also be caused by **failure of the organ** in which they occur. Thus bone metastases tend to form foci for pathological fractures. Infiltration of nerves is often responsible for pain in terminal malignant disease.

General effects of malignant tumours include **pyrexia** due to release of substances from necrotic or infected tissue, and **malignant cachexia** (malignant wasting, generalized atrophy). Reduction of food intake due to nausea may occur in liver failure due to liver metastases or it may be caused by chemotherapy, which may contribute to the body wasting seen in cancer patients. In addition to these factors the host immune response of the body to the malignant cells includes activation of the cell-mediated immune response with secretion of **tumour necrosis factor**. This

is a compound which is very similar in properties to **cachectin**, a compound which adversely affects cell metabolism throughout the body and may be responsible in part for the cachexia seen in advanced malignant disease. Some researchers suggest that cachectin and tumour necrosis factor may be the same substance.

Anaemia is also common in cancer patients, which may be due to haemorrhage from or infection of an ulcerated tumour, replacement of haemopoietic cells of marrow by tumour, or iatrogenic depression of bone marrow by cytotoxic drugs or irradiation therapy. These states also contribute to the cachectic state seen in cancer patients.

Non-metastatic effects of tumours include **depression of immunological defence mechanisms** of the host and occasionally neuropathies or myopathies, multiple venous thromboses (especially in carcinoma of the pancreas) and skin rashes. **Renal disturbances** may result from deposition of tumour antigen–host antibody complexes in glomeruli and may result in the nephrotic syndrome. Hormones may be produced by benign and sometimes malignant tumours, for example inappropriate secretion of ADH and ACTH by bronchogenic carcinoma (oat cell carcinoma), thus giving rise to the so-called **para-neoplastic endocrine syndromes**.

Carcinogenesis

Carcinogenesis is the origin or production of cancer. A **carcinogen** is, therefore, any agent or substance which produces a cancer or acts on a population to change its total frequency of cancer in terms of numbers of tumours or distribution by site and age. Terms that are used synonymously for carcinogen are: cancerogen, tumourigen and oncogen. **Oncogen** is a more generalized term which should be limited to those agents that cause the formation of both benign and/or malignant tumours, carcinogens only causing malignant neoplasms.

As well as carcinogens, which are agents that cause cancer, there are **co-carcinogens**, which are agents that enhance the activity of carcinogens but in the absence of a carcinogen cannot give rise to cancer. Co-carcinogens are also known as **promoters**.

There is no single cause for the formation of all tumours and although some factors in their production are established in humans and animals, the aetiology and pathogenesis of most tumours is still unknown. Where the causes of neoplasia are known, the initiating factors have been proven to produce intracellular, irreversible, heritable changes resulting in the abnormal growth that is recognizable as a neoplasm. The intracellular change which occurs affects the genetic material of the cell, especially the DNA.

Usually when a carcinogenic agent acts it affects many cells. Some of theses cells die, others repair the damage and others change into neoplastic cells. Before the neoplasms develop there may be a variable latent period in which the affected cells do not multiply in the uncontrolled way characteristic of a neoplasm. Some of these abnormal cells may be destroyed by various processes within the body, especially the immune processes that monitor the tissues of the body, searching for 'abnormal' or 'non-self' cells. Therefore in most situations all such abnormal, neoplastic cells will be destroyed. However, it is sufficient for a single neoplastic cell to survive and this will progress through uncontrolled division to the tumour. In fact, the malignancy is derived most usually from a single abnormal parent cell that has undergone the neoplastic change. This initial single cell which has been transformed undergoes multiple divisions, its daughter cells being a **monoclonal population** similar to the initial parent cell and each other.

Various markers of cells have been studied in connection with neoplasia and carcinogenesis, the results of these studies demonstrating that the cells in a given tumour are derived from a single parent cell. One of these markers is the X-chromosome in females. In every normal female there are two X-chromosomes, only one of which is active, the other being inactive and formed into a dense body, set on one side of the nucleus. Which of the two X-chromosomes is to be inactivated is random and occurs very early in embryonic life, usually at about the 20-cell stage of the embryo. This results in approximately half of the cells inactivating the X-chromosome derived from the ovum and the other half inactivating the X-chromosome derived from the sperm. The choice made by each cell is irreversible and therefore when the cell divides the same X-chromosome will be active and the same one inactive in each daughter cell.

Every female is thus said to be a **mosaic**, some cells in her body expressing the paternal X-chromosome, other cells the maternal X-chromosome. When the two X-chromosomes vary in the genetic information that

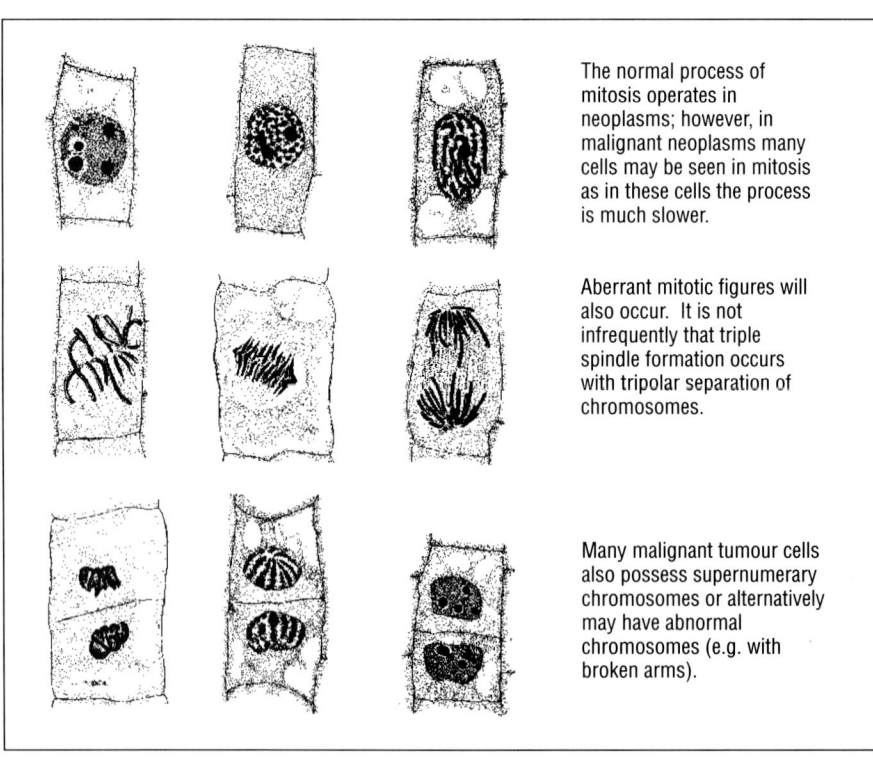

The normal process of mitosis operates in neoplasms; however, in malignant neoplasms many cells may be seen in mitosis as in these cells the process is much slower.

Aberrant mitotic figures will also occur. It is not infrequently that triple spindle formation occurs with tripolar separation of chromosomes.

Many malignant tumour cells also possess supernumerary chromosomes or alternatively may have abnormal chromosomes (e.g. with broken arms).

Figure 4.16 *The process of mitosis*

they carry they may be distinguished by performing various histochemical procedures on them. A common procedure is detecting variants of enzymes coded for by genes on the X-chromosome. If a normal tissue is examined it will be seen that the cells in it express either one or the other X-chromosome in a random manner (refer to Figure 4.17).

If a tumour in a tissue is examined it will be observed that all of the neoplastic cells express only one of the X-chromosomes, evidence that the tumour is derived from a single abnormal parent cell. Other evidence supporting this view is the fact that in certain types of leukaemia there is associated with the neoplastic cells a visible chromosomal abnormality in which a chromosome segment has been translocated onto a different chromosome. All the tumour cells in this case show the same type of abnormality and whenever these cells divide the abnormality is passed on to the daughter cells. It may be said that in a tumour there is a growing family of similar cells all derived from the single abnormal parent cell.

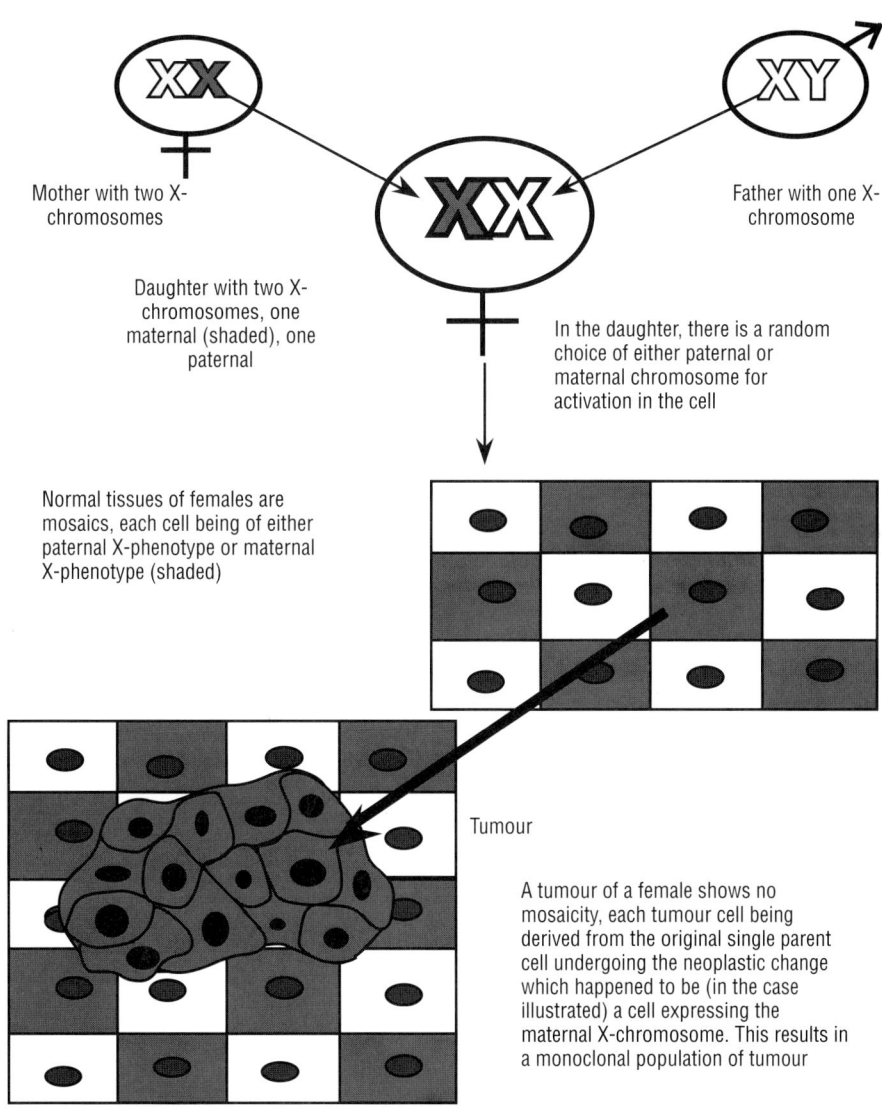

Mother with two X-chromosomes

Father with one X-chromosome

Daughter with two X-chromosomes, one maternal (shaded), one paternal

In the daughter, there is a random choice of either paternal or maternal chromosome for activation in the cell

Normal tissues of females are mosaics, each cell being of either paternal X-phenotype or maternal X-phenotype (shaded)

Tumour

A tumour of a female shows no mosaicity, each tumour cell being derived from the original single parent cell undergoing the neoplastic change which happened to be (in the case illustrated) a cell expressing the maternal X-chromosome. This results in a monoclonal population of tumour

Figure 4.17 *Female mosaicity and monoclonal origin of cancer*

Alterations in the Genetic Material of Cells

The nucleic acids within cells, DNA and RNA, may be altered in a large variety of ways. Changes involving DNA are the most important since this is the nucleic acid that carries information from one cell to another from generation to generation. Every time a cell divides the DNA within it is replicated very accurately with a minimum of errors occurring. Any errors that do in fact occur are not always important because of the degenerate triplet code in the DNA, guarding against such 'chance' mistakes in the replication process. Changes in the DNA that matter and do produce alterations in the expression of the genetic material are termed **mutations**.

Some mutations may once again be unimportant since they may not interfere with the normal functioning of the cell or because they do not involve vital molecules in the cell's biochemistry. On the other hand, some mutations may be lethal, causing the immediate death of the cell. There exist various DNA 'monitoring' and 'correcting' mechanisms in the cell that have evolved specifically to deal with a large variety of such errors in the duplication of DNA or even with damage to the DNA by external factors acting on the cellular level. These correction mechanisms are a complex of enzymes involved with, firstly, detection of the error, secondly, excision of the affected part of the DNA and, finally, replacement with the correct DNA sequence.

The types of mutations that may occur in the cell are multiple and may be very subtle and undetectable unless the DNA is sequenced and compared with the normal sequence, or alternatively they may be gross alterations in the chromosomes easily visible under the microscope. Spontaneous single base changes in the DNA are very rare, with a frequency of less than one mistake for every 100 000 000 bases copied. Chromosomal mutations are more frequent and involve more gross alterations in the genetic material.

Substitutions in the base pairs of the DNA are mutations that involve substitution of one or more pairs of bases with other bases. Such substitutions may not cause any changes in the expression of the genetic material because of the fortuitous coding of several triplets for the same amino acid: for example, UCU, UCC, UCA, UCG, AGU and AGC all code for the amino acid serine. However, substitutions may also cause very serious changes in the cell as the substitution of even a single base pair may lead to dramatic changes in the protein that is coded for by that segment of the DNA: for example UAC codes for the amino acid tyrosine but UAA or UAG both function as stop codons, signalling the end of the protein chain. If we use the example of a simple sentence to illustrate the effects of substitution of base pairs in the DNA it will be seen that this type of mutation can have a variety of effects as is obvious from the analogy illustrated in Table 4.5.

Another class of mutations is that of **deletions**. In this type, one or more base pairs may be deleted from the DNA. The significance of the deletion will vary depending on its position within the DNA and also on the number of bases deleted. Deletions of one or two base pairs, for example, will cause a frame shift in the DNA, altering the way in which triplet codons are read after the deleted bases. Deletion of three (or multiples of three) base pairs will not cause frame shift but may or may not cause serious alteration in the protein coded for by that DNA sequence. Using the example of the simple sentence again, the effects of various types of deletion may be seen in Table 4.6.

Table 4.5 *Mutation through substitutions*

Correct sentence: THE BIG FAT CAT ATE THE RED RAT.
(RAT = Stop sequence)

Substitution 1: THE BIG FAT CAT **EAT** THE RED RAT.
(Ungrammatical but understandable; no change in meaning)

Substitution 2: THE BIG **C**AT CAT ATE THE RED RAT.
(Minimal change in meaning)

Substitution 3: THE BIG FAT **B**AT ATE THE RED RAT.
(Change in meaning)

Substitution 4: THE BIG **R**AT.
(Complete change in meaning as RAT = Stop sequence, which terminates the 'sentence')

Table 4.6 *Mutation through deletion*

Correct sentence: THE BIG FAT CAT ATE THE RED RAT.
(RAT = Stop sequence)

Deletion 1: THE BIG FAT CAT ATE ... RED RAT.
(Ungrammatical but understandable; no change in meaning)

Deletion 2: THE ... FAT CAT ATE THE RED RAT.
(Minimal change in meaning)

Delection 3: THE BIG FAT .... RED RAT.
(Change in meaning)

Deletion 4: THE BIG F.TC ATA TET HER EDR AT
(Nonsense as deletion of 'A' has rearranged the letters of the triplet code and there is now *no stop sequence!*)

Other types of mutations may involve very large pieces of DNA, segments of chromosomes or even whole chromosomes. For example, an arm of a chromosome may break off and may be either lost or joined onto another chromosome (the latter known as a **translocation**). A whole chromosome may be lost or an extra chromosome may be acquired by the cell. Such chromosomal aberrations usually occur during division of cells, especially meiotic division which leads to the formation of gametes.

A large proportion of mutations that occur change genes and the proteins they code for. A protein may be totally abnormal or even totally absent. If that protein is essential for normal cellular function, the cell dies and the mutation is termed a lethal mutation. Other mutations may affect proteins important in the control of various cellular functions. If these proteins are altered or lacking the cell may not be able to modulate some of its functions and may therefore enter an uncontrolled, autonomous growth phase such as is seen in neoplasia.

Changes in the RNA may also lead to heritable changes in the cell if the RNA affected is, for example, the messenger-RNA coding for an important enzyme whose function is DNA replication or DNA repair. Production of an abnormal enzyme of this type may lead to changes in the DNA that will be heritable and once again mutation has occurred.

It is therefore apparent that mutations in the genetic material of cells are extremely important in the causation of cancer. It is demonstrable that in the case of carcinogen–cell interactions the carcinogen effects a heritable change in the genetic material of the cell, that is, a mutation occurs, which has the effect of producing a line of cells that grow excessively and in an uncontrolled manner, showing differences in structure and function from the normal cells.

Aetiology of Cancer

The factors important in the causation of neoplasms are multiple but may be divided into two broad groups. One group is related to the host and consists of various variables inherent in the body of the organism in which the tumour develops. Such host variables are termed **intrinsic** or **endogenous factors**. The other broad group of apparent factors in the causation of tumours is directly related to external, environmental influences on the host and these factors are described as **extrinsic** or **exogenous factors**.

It should be understood that even in the case of a neoplasm the aetiology of which is known, the tumour is the result of the interplay of a multiplicity of factors, often the exogenous factors interacting with one or more of the endogenous variables and therefore leading to a neoplasm in one individual while not leading to a tumour in an apparently identical individual exposed to the same environment. Epidemiological studies on the many neoplasms whose aetiology is not known can indicate the association of these neoplasms with a variety of endogenous and exogenous factors that appear to be linked with those tumours. It is very often difficult to separate these variables and causative agents in individual cases and all of the factors epidemiologically related with a specific tumour are said to be the predisposing factors or risk factors in the development of that tumour.

Intrinsic Factors

Genetic Factors

It is well documented that some human cancers tend to run in families. There are many families in which there is a history showing that there exists a tendency within that family to develop a certain type of tumour. Such evidence favours the hypothesis that heredity plays an important role in the development of these tumours within the affected families. Familial tendencies are known for neoplasms of the breast, stomach, colon, uterus, prostate and lungs and also for certain kinds of leukaemia. The rate of incidence among blood relatives may be as much as 30 times higher than among non-relatives.

Retinoblastoma is a rare, malignant tumour that occurs in infancy, usually before the age of 3 years. Multiple tumours arise in the retina and about 40% of these tumours have been shown to have a hereditary component. These tumours are now cured by surgery or by radiotherapy and chemotherapy and many affected individuals live long enough to reproduce. In the past retinoblastoma was a fatal condition and therefore occurred less frequently than nowadays. Other tumours showing a strong familial predisposition are **Wilm's tumour**, a malignancy of the kidney occurring in infancy, and **neuroblastoma**, another tumour of infancy arising from neural tissue. All of these tumours are rare in occurrence. It is thought that a familial predisposition to these tumours arises because of the inheritance of defective copies of genes coding for regulatory cellular proteins. Mutations that inactivate genes coding for active proteins may also be important.

Cancer of the breast has been shown to have a hereditary component. The chance, on average, of a woman developing breast cancer is about 1 in 17. In women who have had a blood relative (mother, sister, aunt or grandmother) with breast cancer the chance of developing the malignancy is 1 in 5. Women with a family history of breast cancer tend to develop it at a younger age than women who develop the tumour with no previous family history (late thirties or earlier as compared with late forties or later).

Some malignancies showing a genetic predisposition are associated with chromosomal abnormalities. A common disorder of this type is **Down's syndrome** (mongolism) which is due to the presence of an extra chromosome 21 in all cells of the affected individuals. These people show an increased incidence of **leukaemia**. Another chromosomal abnormality seen commonly and predisposing to leukaemia is Klinefelter's syndrome where the afflicted individuals possess three sex chromosomes (XXY).

Another group of diseases where there is an inherited tendency for malignancy is those in which the chromosomes are very fragile and liable to spontaneous fragmentation. Such a disorder is Fanconi's anaemia. Cells of sufferers of this disease are very sensitive

to chromosome fragmentation induced by radiation and they have a high incidence of leukaemia. It is suspected that the breaks and the leukaemia develop because of an underlying defect in DNA repair. The **Philadelphia chromosome** (a portion of chromosome 22 transferred onto chromosome 9) is found in 90% of cases of chronic myeloid leukaemia.

Some other human cancers show an even greater hereditary element in that they are inherited in a Mendelian fashion. That is, the genes for the condition are inherited as a dominant or recessive characteristic. The best example of this is **polyposis coli**, where the inheritance is autosomal dominant. In this disorder multiple benign neoplasms develop all along the length of the colonic mucosa in childhood or young adulthood. All patients will then eventually progress to carcinoma of the colon, about 90% of patients in their fifties having had the malignancy (refer to Figure 4.18). The disease **xeroderma pigmentosum** is inherited as an autosomal recessive trait and causes the patient's skin to be excessively sensitive to sunlight and the affected people have a very high incidence of skin cancer. The basic defect leading to the development of neoplasms in this case is that defective DNA repair mechanisms are involved.

In order to determine the contribution of heredity to the development of a given tumour, the incidence of cancer of the same organ in monozygotic (identical) twins may be compared to the incidence of the tumour in dizygotic (non-identical) twins. One would expect that in monozygotic twins the tumour would affect both twins at the same age and in the same organ more often than it would be seen in the dizygotic twins. Such studies with twins are very difficult to carry out but some epidemiological investigations have occurred. The evidence of most studies points to the general conclusion that identical twins are not much more alike in the cancers they suffer than are non-identical twins. Other studies show that for some tumours at least the incidence in both monozygotic twins is higher than chance would dictate. This reflects the importance of other factors in the causation of tumours. It must be remembered that even if the assortment of genes in an individual may not on its own be sufficient to lead to the development of tumours, it nevertheless may be an important predisposing factor or contributing factor.

Racial factors

These host factors are the most poorly defined and it is suspected that a complex variety of variables may interplay to lead to the differences in the incidence of

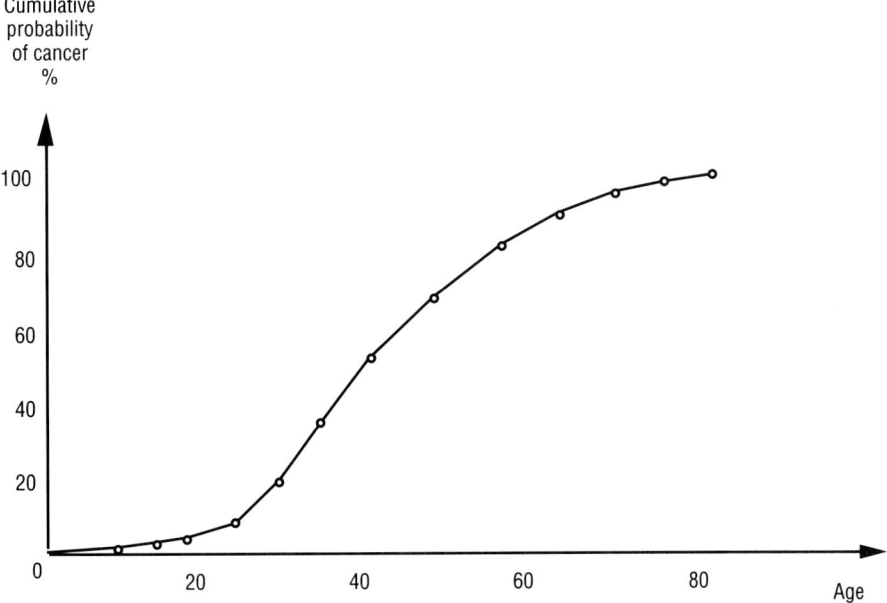

Cumulative
probability
of cancer
%

(*Source:* Fraumeni JF Jr, Mulvihill JJ, in *Cancer Epidemiology and Protection*, edited by Schottenfeld D; Thomas, Springfield Illinois, 1975. p. 405)

Figure 4.18   *Incidence of cancer of the colon in patients with polyposis coli by age*

certain tumours in various racial and geographically defined groups. Some of these variables may indeed be exogenous. Genetic influences, habits and customs, living conditions and socioeconomic factors, diet, soil types, climate, water, etc. may each act alone or in combination. However, whatever factors are operating it is indisputable that considerable differences occur in the incidence of various types of cancer in relation to race and geography. For example, **carcinoma of the breast** is five times more common in Australia than it is in Japan and Taiwan. Conversely, primary liver cancer is very rare in Australia but it is the number one killer in some African and Asian countries. Similarly, the death rate for carcinoma of the stomach in both sexes is approximately seven times higher in Japan than it is in Australia.

It is not known what the proportional importance of exogenous environmental factors and endogenous racial factors may be for these tumours. A strong environmental influence may be important in some cancers as has been shown by studies of people migrating from a country of low incidence of a particular tumour to a country of high incidence. The second generation of the incoming population shows an incidence for the particular tumour that is intermediate to the incidence of the tumour in the parents' country and that in the

children's country. With each successive generation, the incidence more closely approximates that of the general population in the new country.

However, there also exists evidence which does not favour this environmental influence over different racial groups' predisposition or susceptibility to a particular cancer. The rate of cancer of the breast in females is significantly higher in Denmark than in Sweden and yet the environmental differences are negligible. These geographic and racial differences in cancer incidence have attracted great interest and research since they provide clues as to how endogenous and exogenous factors interact in carcinogenesis and they may show significant insight into the causation of cancer.

Immunological Factors

It is thought by some researchers that although cancer cells arise by mutation relatively frequently, they do not develop into tumours in normal, immunocompetent individuals. This has been attributed to the fact that the immune system recognizes the abnormal cells as 'foreign' or non-self through 'immunosurveillance'. That is, immune cells, particularly those of the T lymphocyte group, constantly circulate and come into contact with tissues. They interact with the cancer cells and finding them different from the normal body cells they destroy them. It is known that many cancer cells have unusual surface proteins and these may conceivably be recognized as foreign by the immune system. Further support for this theory is that in individuals with a suppressed immune system the incidence of certain kinds of tumours is much higher than in the general population. For example, in AIDS patients the incidence of **Kaposi's sarcoma** is very high (see Figure 4.19). The same tumour is excessively rare in normal individuals. In some congenital immunodeficiency states the same observations may be made: a much higher proportion of tumours, particularly those of the reticuloendothelial system, occur in these children than in the general population. The same observation may be made on patients who are receiving immuno-suppressive drugs (e.g. kidney transplant recipients). These patients show a high incidence of certain types of tumour, for example reticulum cell sarcomata. The incidence of other types of tumour such as cancer of the breast, however, remains the same as in the general population.

Some experimental studies have attempted to boost the immune response of individuals suffering from widespread malignancy in the hope that the boosted immune system would be better adapted to destroy the malignant cells. Vaccination with the BCG vaccine, vaccination with *Corynebacterium parvum* preparations and adjuvant therapy have all been tried. There have been reports of the slowing of the growth of certain types of tumour, for example malignant melanoma, in the vaccinated individuals, but the results are inconsistent overall and 'miracle' cures have not been achieved.

It is a well-known observation that when tumours are examined under the microscope there are associated with them infiltrates of chronic inflammatory cells, mainly lymphocytes, which are characterized as the **tumour associated immune response**. It is also known that the more pronounced this response is, the more lymphocytes present, the better the prognosis for the patient. This has been quoted as another piece of evidence for the checking of neoplastic cell growth by the immune system. It is argued that the immune system is able to destroy any remaining tumour cells at the site after surgery and therefore prevent the recurrence of the tumour, improving the chances of long-term survival of the patient.

The accumulated evidence seems to support the hypothesis that the immune system is important in responding to tumours, especially certain kinds of tumours. Natural killer cells, activated T lymphocytes, interferons and lymphokines have all been proposed as

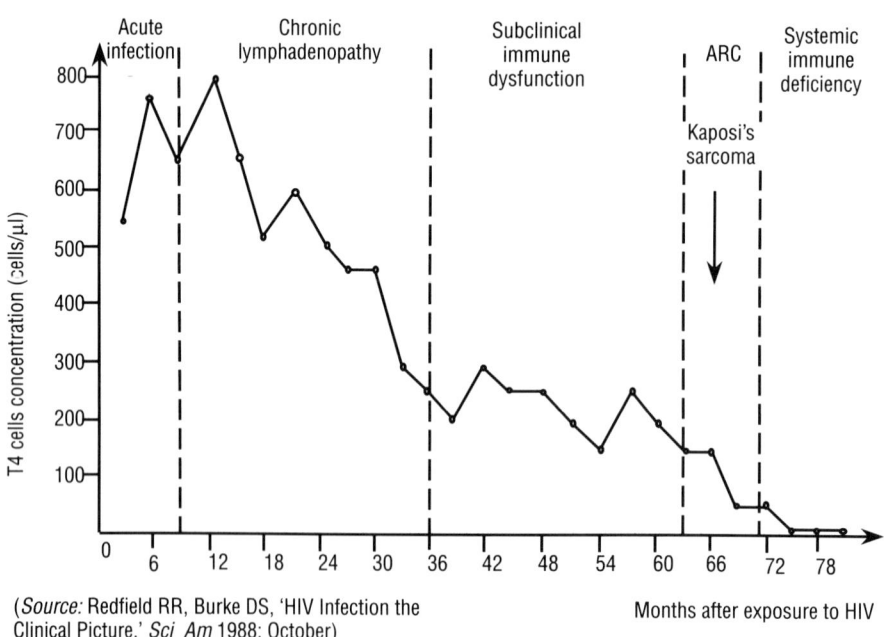

(*Source:* Redfield RR, Burke DS, 'HIV Infection the Clinical Picture.' *Sci Am* 1988; October)

Months after exposure to HIV

Figure 4.19   *The relationship between immunodeficiency and development of cancer*

the effectors of neoplastic cell death. It is not known why some tumours seem to develop in greater numbers in immunosuppressed people and it is also not understood why the boosting of the immune system through adjuvants should decrease the rate of growth of some types of cancer and not others. Current data seem to indicate that most human cancers are not subject to immune surveillance or, if they are, the immune response is unable to limit their growth. Some types of cancer are demonstrably under considerable immune system control and if the immune system is functioning normally such tumours rarely develop, being seen in mainly immunosuppressed individuals.

Sex and Hormonal Influences

Certain types of cancer are more common in males than females, for example carcinoma of the lung, tongue, lip and bladder. Cancer of the breast is more common in women and cancer of the lung in some countries has now become the prime killer of women. This striking sex difference in the incidence of some tumours common to both sexes indicates that sex and hormones are an important factor in the development of some tumours. Although in many tumours the differences between the sexes may be due to other factors

such as heredity and genetics, habits, occupation and environment, the influence of hormones has been indisputably shown to be the main causative factor. Hormonal imbalances, deficiencies and excesses may themselves directly cause the neoplasms or at least contribute greatly in their production. The tumour which has been most extensively studied in this context is **carcinoma of the breast**. This neoplasm has a male to female incidence ratio of 1:125. It is also known that approximately one-third of all human mammary tumours are hormone dependent, that is, their growth is directly related to the amount of hormone controlling their proliferation. Men who develop mammary tumours very commonly show hormonal imbalances, with excesses of oestrogens, and their breasts frequently have undergone gynaecomastia prior to the development of the tumour.

A significant role in the pathogenesis of breast carcinoma is **endogenous hyperoestrinism**. Many of the risk factors of breast carcinoma point to this: long duration of reproductive life, early menarche, late menopause, nulliparity and late age at first child (refer to Figure 4.20). All of these point to increased exposure to oestrogen peaks during the menstrual cycle. Another piece of evidence favouring this hypothesis is that in girls who had their ovaries removed therapeutically before puberty, breast carcinoma is very rare. The same may be observed in males who develop

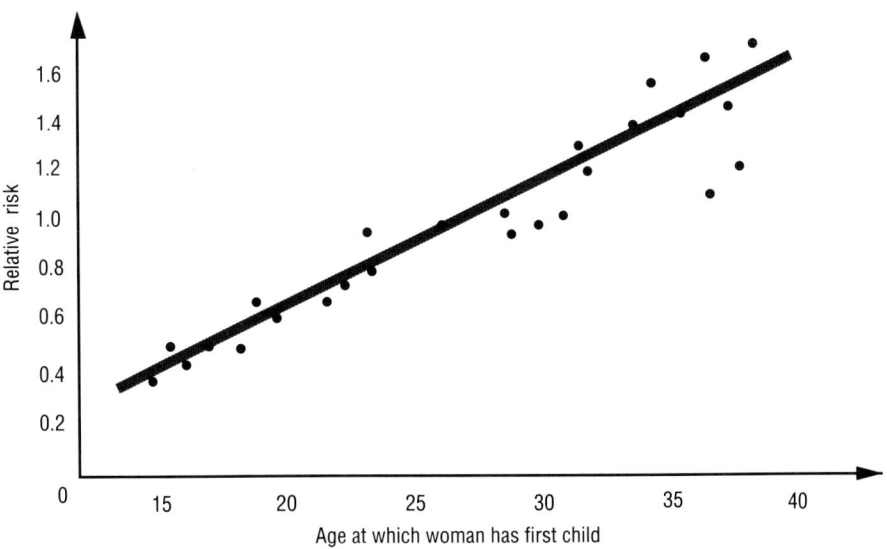

(*Source:* MacMahon B, Cole P, Brown J, *J Nat Cancer Inst* 1973; 50: 21–42)

Figure 4.20 *The probability of a mother developing cancer of the breast, relative to the risk for childless women versus age at which the mother has her first child*

breast carcinoma. Most of these individuals display abnormally high levels of oestrogens, the result of, most commonly, cirrhosis of the liver or Klinefelter's syndrome.

The role of abnormal hormonal levels has been well documented in other neoplastic conditions. Carcinoma of the prostate gland is known to be associated with excessive levels of circulating androgens. The dependence of these tumours on androgenic hormone stimulation is demonstrated by the inhibition of the growth or regression of the tumour that is achieved by orchidectomy or oestrogen therapy. Other tumours that have been associated with abnormalities in hormonal levels in the body are endometrial carcinoma, which shows a higher incidence in women who take various forms of exogenous oestrogens, and vaginal cancer developing in young women whose mothers had taken stilboestrol (a synthetic oestrogen) during pregnancy.

Experiments in animals also support the evidence presented above. Removal of endocrine glands promotes the development of a variety of tumours. In gonadectomized mice, for instance, there is a high incidence of mammary tumours, adrenal tumours and pituitary tumours. Prolonged excessive administration of hormones has also been shown to cause tumours. Thyrotrophic hormone administration over a long period of time has been shown to cause thyroid neoplasms and prolonged oestrogen administration has been observed to cause mammary tumours. The importance of hormones as growth promoters and activators of certain tissues in the normal individual is paramount and it is conceivable that in hormonal dysfunctions and imbalances the tissue may respond abnormally by undergoing a neoplastic change.

Age

Most cancers occur in the older age groups and cancer has been described as a disease of old age. However, a small proportion of generally rare cancers are seen to afflict the younger age groups or to occur primarily in infancy. In the case where the tumours occur very early in life they are almost always seen to be associated with hereditary factors, for example retinoblastoma and Wilm's tumour already discussed above. The reason why other tumours tend to occur in older children or young adults is not clear. Examples of these kinds of malignancy are osteosarcoma, seminoma and leukaemia.

It is not realized, however, just how steeply the incidence of cancer increases with increasing age (see Figure 4.21). For example death due to cancer of the

large intestine increases a thousandfold between the ages of 30 and 80 years. Why the majority of tumours tends to occur in old age is most likely due to a multiplicity of factors. There may be environmental influences. An elderly person has been exposed to a variety of environmental carcinogens for a considerable length of time during life and the cumulative effects of these carcinogens may manifest themselves in old age as a neoplasm. It is thought, however, that a variety of host influences are also very important. As the individual ages, the number of divisions that cells in the body have undergone increases greatly. The daughter cells of these divisions will have a greater chance of expressing heritable errors that have been accumulating in the genetic material of the cell with each division. For example, let us assume for argument's sake that there are ten regulatory genes that prevent a cell from forming an uncontrolled ever-expanding family of progeny. As the cell divides again and again the chance of mutations occurring in all of those ten regulatory genes preventing their anti-neoplastic activity increases with increasing age of the patient.

Several authors have suggested that cancer is seen in old age because it is 'programmed' into our genetic material as part of the general process of 'ageing', having evolved by natural selection and bringing about some general advantage to the species as a whole. The argument is that organisms should live long enough to reach sexual maturity, reproduce, look after their young and when the progeny reaches sexual maturity the parental generation should die off, not competing with their progeny for living space, food, mates, etc. The diseases of old age, therefore, are programmed to cause the death of the parental generation so as not to clutter the ecological niche in which the organism lives, and therefore aiding in the preservation of the species as a whole. There are objections to this theory as it is difficult to account for the fact that there has been selection for a response which brings no benefit to the one who is responding. Also, this theory would suggest that people all over the world should show roughly the same overall cancer incidence for any given age and that changes in habits or environment should have little effect on cancer incidence. This is not true and hence this theory is not supported by much evidence.

Another theory is that the decreased efficiency of the responses of the immune system in old age is largely to account for the increased incidence of neoplasms in old age. Failure or reduction in efficiency of the normal immunosurveillance which occurs constantly and recognizes and destroys abnormal body cells such as malignant cells would certainly mean that the chance of a malignant cell surviving would be

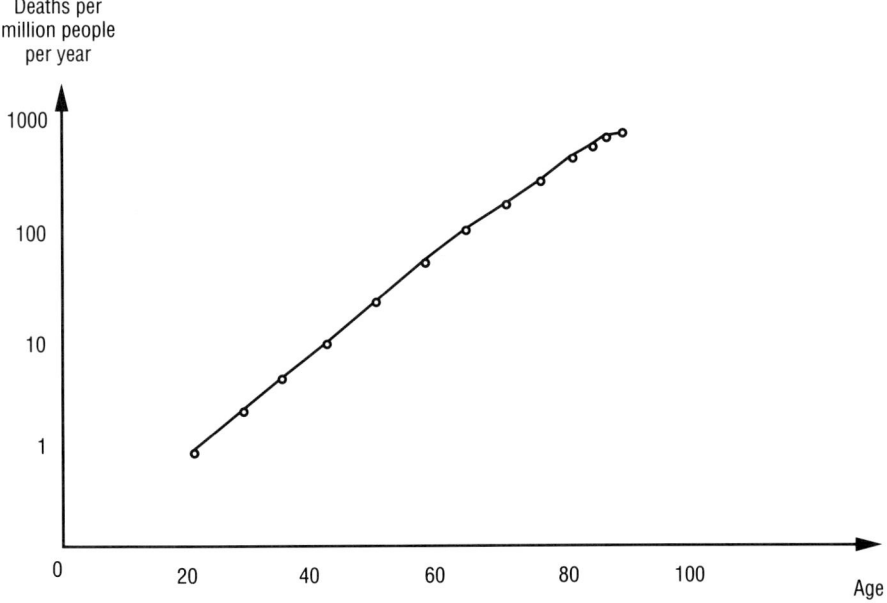

(*Source:* US Department of Health, Education and Welfare, *Vital Statistics of the United States*, Volume II. *Mortality.* US Government Printing Office, 1968)

Figure 4.21 *Annual death rate from cancer of the colon in relation to age, 1968 (NB The y-axis scale is logarithmic)*

greater in those circumstances. It is probable that a combination of many of the above factors contributes to the fact that cancers occur more frequently in the elderly.

Pre-existing Benign Neoplasms

Malignant neoplasms may arise in pre-existing benign neoplasms or other benign, non-neoplastic conditions such as pathological hyperplasias, choristomata and hamartomata. For example, a benign naevus (mole) may give rise to a malignant melanoma. Polyps in the bowel frequently undergo malignant transformation, as may papillomata (polyps) of the nasal sinuses. This may be explained by considering what has occurred in the benign tumour. The genetic material of the neoplastic cells has already undergone a mutation, making it an abnormal cell and thus it may be that such an abnormal cell is more receptive to the effects of other carcinogenic agents or factors. In the case of hyperplasias and other non-neoplastic lesions, the normal cells occur in an abnormal environment, making them more susceptible to carcinogenesis or less amenable to control mechanisms.

Extrinsic Factors

There are many environmental or occupational factors which may result in malignant neoplasms. **Oncogens** are factors which may induce formation of tumours (oncogenesis), **carcinogens** are substances which induce formation of malignant neoplasms (carcinogenesis).

Chemical Carcinogens

The first definitive implication of chemical agents in the causation of human cancer came when **Percival Pott**, a London surgeon, published in 1775 a treatise in which he noted that the incidence of carcinoma of the scrotum was much greater in chimney sweeps than in the general population. He himself notes that the cancer in the trade was called the 'soot wart'. It was correctly suggested that the lodgment of the soot in the rugae of the scrotal skin was the factor that caused the increased incidence of the tumours. Since then, many other workers have found that high incidences of tumours occur in association with exposure to certain compounds which are encountered especially in an occupational context. It was noted, for example, in the 19th century that miners in Austria had a much higher incidence of lung cancers than the rest of the population. Bladder cancer was noted to be of high incidence in workers in the aniline dye industry.

Since then, because of these associations of increased cancer incidence through exposure to various chemical substances, a large variety of specific chemical compounds have been shown to have either directly or indirectly a carcinogenic effect. Many thousands of such compounds, either naturally occurring or synthetic, have been identified and classified according to the tumours that they give rise to, with many more discovered every year (see Figure 4.22). Chemicals that are carcinogenic may be grouped according to their mode of action into three major classes:

- **Direct-acting carcinogens**: these compounds, by virtue of their chemical structure, react irreversibly with various components of the cell, resulting in molecular alterations that can lead to neoplastic transformation. Vinyl chloride would be an example of such an agent, which being highly reactive readily binds to many cellular constituents, including DNA.
- **Procarcinogens**: these are not carcinogenic in themselves but upon metabolism by the host or the bacteria resident in the host, they are converted into active carcinogens. Examples of these are benzopyrene found in soot and tar and also the nitrosamines.

- **Promoters**: these compounds lack carcinogenic or potential carcinogenic activity in themselves but they are important as they enhance or potentiate the carcinogenic activity of either direct-acting carcinogens or procarcinogens. **Croton oil** and phenol are examples of these substances which are frequently used in experimental situations to potentiate the effects of various carcinogenic compounds. The mode of action of promoters is poorly understood.

Another way of classifying the various carcinogenic chemical compounds is to look at their chemical nature, mode of action (where it is known), incidence and use in the community, classify them according to the type of tumours that they cause, whether they are naturally occurring or synthetic and so on. Examples of substances shown to be carcinogenic are:

- **polycyclic hydrocarbons**: benzopyrene, dimethylbenzanthracene;
- **aromatic amines and azo compounds**: aniline and its derivatives, 2-naphthylamine, benzidine;
- **N-nitroso compounds**: N-methylnitrosourea, N-methylnitrosourethane;
- **alkylating agents**: nitrogen mustards and analogues, vinyl chloride;
- **natural products**: safrole (from sassafras), capsaicin (from peppers), aflatoxin (from mould on peanuts);
- **steroids**: oestrogens, anabolic steroids;
- **other organic compounds**: dimethylhydrazine, urethane, carbon tetrachloride, benzene, chloroform;

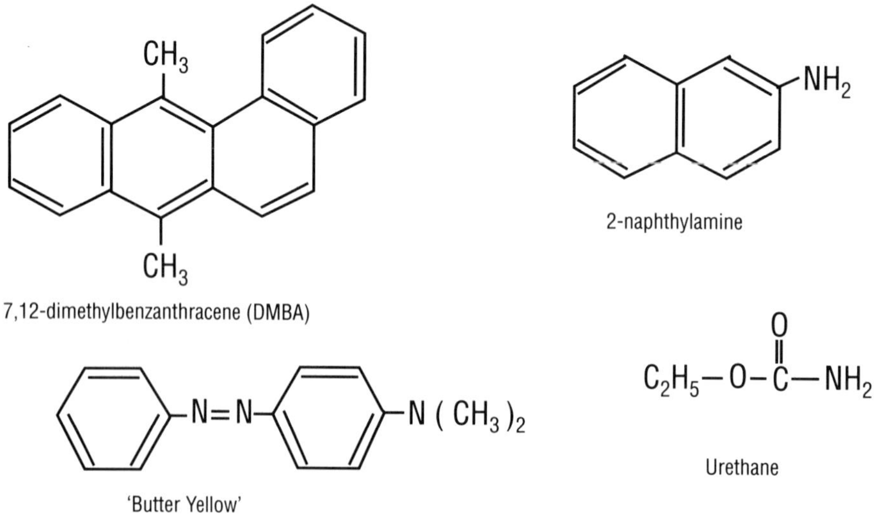

7,12-dimethylbenzanthracene (DMBA)

2-naphthylamine

'Butter Yellow'

Urethane

Figure 4.22 *Some examples of chemical carcinogens*

• **Inorganic compounds**: chromium, nickel, beryllium salts, arsenic, cadmium, cobalt and its salts; asbestos; haematite.

The best-known example of a carcinogen which has been extensively studied is the cigarette (see Figure 4.23). Research has unequivocably shown that cigarette smoke contains many chemical carcinogens. When these are inhaled in cigarette smoke over a long period of time they cause neoplastic change to occur in the respiratory epithelium and also in the mucosal surfaces of the mouth and throat. Components of cigarette smoke with carcinogenic effects include polycyclic aromatic compounds, aromatic amines, nitrosamines, and other components of 'tar'.

Several possible mechanisms exist through which chemical carcinogens exert their effects and ultimately may lead to the formation of the neoplastic cell. Direct-acting carcinogens such as alkylating agents have been shown to bind directly to DNA and other cellular components, causing damage and neoplastic transformation. Procarcinogens are generally chemically inert in their initial form but after enzymatic degradation and metabolism in the body they become highly reactive species that may interact with DNA and cellular components in the same way as direct-acting carcinogens. The binding of active molecules to DNA induces mutations as deletions, substitutions and breaks in the genetic material occur. Chemical carcinogens also bind to cellular RNA and modify it in some way. If the abnormal RNA is transcribed back to DNA via a reverse transcriptase system abnormal DNA will be produced, leading to permanent misinformation stored in the cell's DNA, resulting in a mutation. Also, the altered cellular RNA functions poorly or malfunctions, leading to errors in the translation of genetic material and the formation of abnormal proteins or lack of formation of cellular proteins. This could have profound effects on cellular replication and control mechanisms. If, for example, the aberrant protein produced is a DNA polymerase, it could lead to faulty DNA replication, introduction of errors and mutation.

It is well accepted now that chemical carcinogenesis is a multi-step process. There is a dose-dependent response to chemical carcinogens, implying that higher doses will be more effective in inducing cancers. However, it is also known that a small, 'sub-carcinogenic' dose of a chemical will initiate the cell it enters. This initiation process makes the cell more responsive to subsequent small doses of the carcinogen, each successive dose having, over time, the same effect as a single large carcinogenic dose. Once the cell has been initiated it never reverts back to its normal state; that is, initiation is an irreversible process. Initiated cells are also more receptive to the effects of other chemicals, chemicals that have no effect on normal cells, the so-called promoters or co-carcinogens. If a cell initiated by a very low dose of a carcinogenic compound is not exposed to that chemical again no tumour may develop. If, however, that cell is treated with promoters it will very often undergo neoplastic transformation. It is thought that promoters induce neoplasia in initiated cells by interacting with cell membrane receptors to stimulate cell division. In order for a promoter chemical to be effective it must follow the carcinogenic chemical and not precede it. Also, if repeated

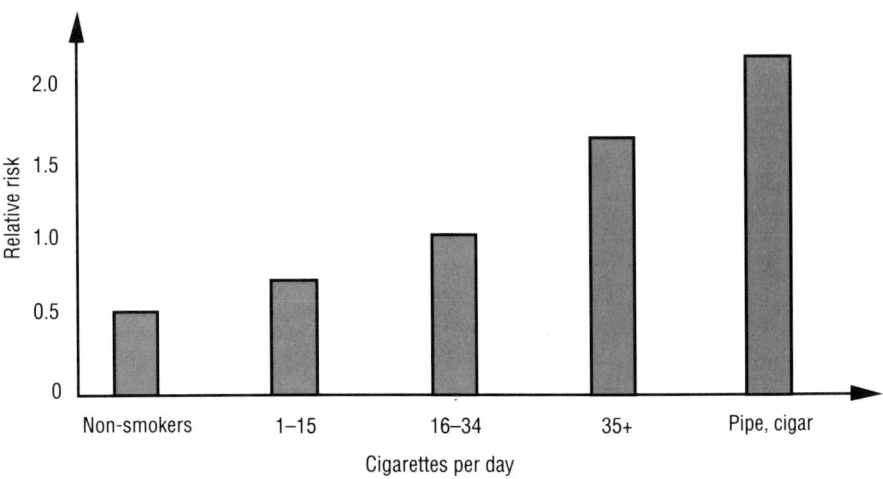

(*Source:* Wynder EL, Bross IJ , Feldman, RM, *Cancer* 1957; 10: 1300)

Figure 4.23 *The relative risk of developing cancer of the mouth, in relation to smoking habits*

doses of promoter are required, the intervals between applications must not be excessively long for tumours to be induced, indicating that the effects of promoters, unlike those of carcinogens, are reversible.

Studies have shown that two or more initiating agents may act on a given cell at the same time, their effects being additive. Different genes may be affected, each mutation helping more and more to 'push the cell over the brink' of malignant transformation. Subsequent interactions with promoters may further increase the probability of malignant transformation occurring. 'Immortalization' of the cells may be the first mutational event induced by the promoters and with each further division of the immortal cell line, the more aberrant, more primitive cells would be selected and would result in the growth of the tumour. It is apparent therefore that small 'sub-carcinogenic' doses of each of the individual compounds involved may in fact interact via a co-carcinogenic effect to produce tumours. It is thus evident that no 'safe' level of exposure to carcinogens exists given their 'co-operative', additive and dose-cumulative effects. Carcinogenesis due to chemicals is a complex process, occurring in many stages, involving many genes and multiple mechanisms (refer to Figure 4.24).

The types of malignant tumours caused by chemical carcinogens are varied and depend on the nature of the agent and how it comes into contact with the tissues. Because chemicals are often used in a variety of occupational settings, occupational cancers are frequently associated with exposure to such chemicals (see Table 4.7). **Skin cancers** may be caused by polycyclic hydrocarbons (coal tars), lubricating oils, shale oils (paraffin hydrocarbons) and arsenic (prolonged dermatitis leads to squamous cell carcinoma). All of these substances tend to produce tumours at the site of contact which is most usually the skin.

Lung, **pleural** and **nasopharyngeal** malignancies may be caused by cigarette smoking (incidence of asbestos carcinoma of the bronchus is 20 times greater in heavy smokers than in non-smokers). Haematite, nickel and chromium workers tend to develop lung cancer, because they inhale the finely divided dusts of these compounds. Asbestos workers tend to develop lung cancer and may also develop mesothelioma of the pleura.

Urinary tract cancer may arise in aniline dye workers, who are prone to β-naphthylamine being present in the urine and causing cancer in the bladder, ureters and renal pelvis.

Physical Agents as Carcinogens

Physical agents are a very well documented cause of

cancer and by far the most important of these is **ionizing radiation**. This includes X-rays, gamma rays, alpha rays, beta rays and ultraviolet radiation. The sources of such radiation are multiple and include nuclear fission, medical diagnostic equipment, sunlight, radioactive substances and industrial equipment. It is known that such radiation can kill cells or cause mutations in them. However, it is also known that the tumours appear after a long latent period during which there have occurred many mitotic divisions in the affected cells. It may be possible that these cell divisions are required in order to 'fix' the radiation-induced damage in the cells or even perhaps to amplify it, resulting in a neoplastic cell somewhere along the line of successive divisions. It has also been observed that the development of tumours is dose dependent, presumably at low doses the radiation-induced damage being amenable to repair. Additive effects are possible and also the affected cells may become more susceptible to other carcinogens after radiation exposure. This makes it virtually impossible to establish 'safe' doses of radiation exposure, this being important in the medical diagnostic and occupational areas where the cumulative effects of exposure may be very important.

There exist many examples of tumours that are indisputably linked with exposure to ionizing radiation and only a few of these will be quoted for illustration. In the early days of scientific research in radioactive substances and Röntgen rays the workers in these areas, unaware of the hazards of exposure, allowed themselves to receive massive doses of ionizing radiation. Skin, lung and bone cancers developed in the majority of them. Madame Curie, the discoverer of radium, and her husband both developed cancers from exposure to this highly radioactive compound. Miners of radioactive elements such as cobalt have a tenfold increased incidence in lung cancer when compared with the general population. In the past when luminous watch and clock dials were painted with a radioactive compound paint to induce the luminescence, most of the workers who applied the paint to the dials died from highly malignant bone tumours. This was due to the fact that as they painted the dials with the radioactive paint they constantly licked the brush to shape it with their lips into a fine point!

Survivors of the atomic bomb blasts in Nagasaki and Hiroshima who were exposed to the radioactive fallout were shown to suffer from a markedly increased incidence of **leukaemia** which developed after a latent period of approximately 7 years. At the present time, many decades later, in these areas of Japan the incidence of leukaemias, mortality rate from cancers of the breast, colon, lung, thyroid and other organs is still significantly higher than in control populations. Therapeutic irradiation has also been shown to be carcinogenic. Thyroid cancers have developed in about 9% of people exposed to head and neck irradiation during infancy and childhood. The treatment of ankylosing spondylitis in the past frequently involved X-ray irradiation, yielding a ten- to twelvefold increase in the incidence of leukaemia in these patients many years later.

But even something that was generally considered innocuous, **sunlight**, has been shown to be linked with cancer. Excessive exposure to the **ultraviolet radiation** in sunlight increases the incidence of skin tumours such as squamous cell carcinoma, basal cell carcinoma and the highly malignant **melanoma**. Fair people, especially redheads, are more susceptible to the effects of ultraviolet light since they have little

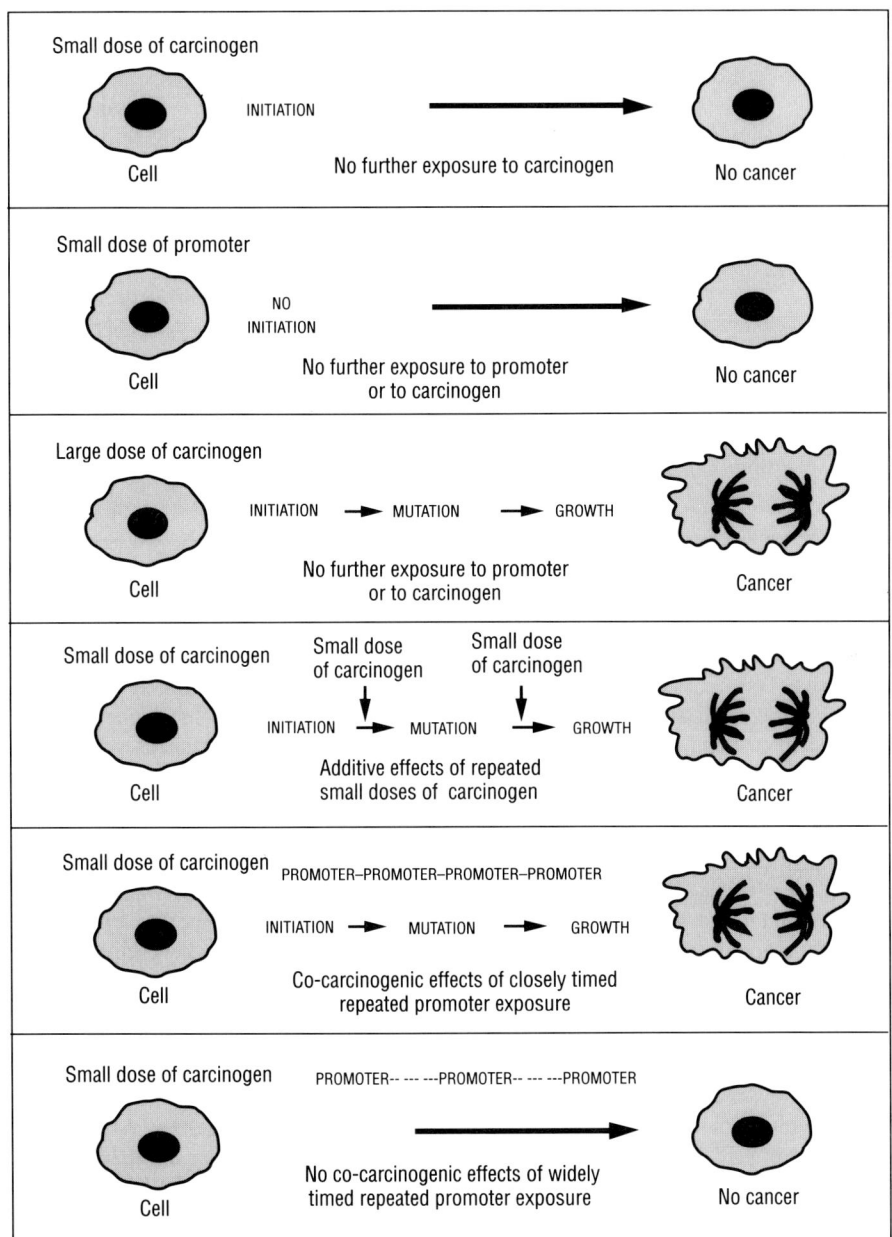

Figure 4.24 *The mechanism of chemical carcinogenesis*

Table 4.7   *Occupational cancers and the agents involved in their causation*

Site	Agent	Occupation
Liver	Arsenic	Tanners, smelters
	Vinyl chloride	Plastics workers
Nasal cavity and sinuses	Chromium	Glass, pottery workers
	Nickel	Battery makers, electrolysis workers
	Wood and leather dust	Wood, leather, shoe workers
Lung	Arsenic, asbestos chromium, coal dust, mustard gas, nickel, ionizing radiations	Miners, asbestos workers, glass and pottery workers, coal tar and pitch workers, iron foundry, radiologists, chemical workers
Bladder	Coal products	Asphalt, coal tar
	Aromatic amines	Dyestuff users, rubber workers, leather and shoe makers, paint manufacturers
Bone	Ionizing radiations	Radium dial painters
Bone marrow	Benzene, ionizing radiations	Benzene workers, dye users, painters, radiologists
Skin	Coal tar, ultraviolet rays, arsenic, ionizing radiations	Stokers, pitch workers, miners, outdoor workers radiologists

Source: Calman KC, Paul J, *An Introduction to Cancer Medicine*, Macmillan, London, 1978.

melanin in their skin, while dark complexioned people and black people have a large quantity of melanin and are therefore protected. The frequency of skin cancer is much higher in the tropical latitudes where the intensity of the sun is strongest and the incidence is also highest in people who expose themselves excessively to the sun. The highest incidence of skin cancer in the world is seen in Queensland, Australia, where the tropical climate, fair complexion and excessive exposure to the sun all interact to give rise to this statistic of dubious honour! Individuals who use tanning lamps extensively also suffer from an increased incidence of skin cancer. Ultraviolet light has been shown to induce breaks and mutations in the DNA of exposed cells. Generally, these damaged and mutated segments of DNA are repaired by the cellular enzymes but cumulative effects and mutations are seen in cells that are constantly exposed to radiation.

Trauma is another physical injury that is often quoted as a cause of cancer. There are many cases heard in courts where people have tried to prove that a single incident of traumatic injury, sustained perhaps in a car accident, has caused a cancer like an osteosarcoma. There is no experimental or epidemio-

logical evidence that indicates that a single case of traumatic injury may predispose to cancer. Some researchers have reported that the incidence of neoplasms in scar tissue is somewhat higher than that in adjacent normal tissues, but in this case the development of the tumour may be attributable to the abnormal environment of a highly collagenous matrix that the cell finds itself enclosed by, initiating or permitting perhaps the changes that lead to malignancy.

A number of **chemically inert substances** such as plastic films, glass spheres, fibres, methylcellulose, metal foils and wires when implanted into the tissues of experimental animals have been shown to cause the formation of tumours, mainly **sarcomata**. It is clear that all of these substances by virtue of their shape, size and other physical properties induce chronic irritation, inflammation and in some cases benign proliferations of tissue before they induce neoplastic change. It is not known whether the malignant changes in the cells are initiated directly by the presence of these materials in the tissue or whether the cells become more susceptible to the effects of other carcinogens because of the irritation they have been subjected to.

There exist some other materials whose carcinogenic effects may be derived from a combination of physical and chemical effects, for example, **asbestos fibres**. Asbestos exposure has been indubitably linked with respiratory system tumours, especially a highly malignant tumour of the pleural cells, **mesothelioma**. The inhaled asbestos fibres are relatively inert and because of their size, shape and very slow chemical degradation may directly cause mutations in the respiratory system cells or alternatively may act in association with other intrinsic and extrinsic factors potentiating the effects of these and leading to the development of the malignancies.

Biological Agents and Neoplasia

There is little evidence that suggests that organisms such as parasites, protozoans and bacteria directly cause human cancer. The implication of these organisms in the process of carcinogenesis is indirect, in cases of protracted, chronic infestations and infections where there is much tissue injury, destruction, inflammation, scarring and repair occurring. **Schistosomiasis** is a parasitic infestation which occurs very frequently in certain tropical developing countries and in these situations the incidence of **urinary bladder carcinoma** is much higher than in countries where the infection is not frequently seen. Causation of cancer by biological agents may be linked with the chemical metabolites that they produce. For example, **aflatoxins** are produced by *Aspergillus flavus* fungi which may infect human food materials, be consumed and hence give rise to tumours through their powerful carcinogenic activity.

The major area of interest in the causation of cancer by biological agents is in the area of virology. **Viruses** are now a well-recognized cause of malignancy in both animals and humans (see Table 4.8). Such agents are called **oncogenic viruses** since they give rise to tumours (*onco-* = tumour). The first indication that tumours could be caused by transmissible agents was in 1907 when it was demonstrated that the common wart could be transmitted to human volunteers by cell-

Table 4.8 *The oncogenic viruses*

	Viruses implicated	Human tumour	Animal tumour
DNA virus family			
Papovaviridae	Papilloma	Warts	Papillomata
	Polyoma	No	Various in rodents
	SV40	No	Sarcomata
Adenoviridae	Adenovirus	No	Sarcomata
Herpesviridae	Epstein-Barr	Burkitt's lymphoma	No
	Epstein-Barr	Nasopharyngeal ca.	No
	Herpes II	Cervical carcinoma	No
	Marekvirus	No	Lymphosarcomatosis
	Lucke	No	Adenocarcinoma
	Herpes saimiri	No	Lymphomata
Poxviridae	Shope fibroma	No	Fibromata
	Yaba monkey	No	Papillomata
Hepadnaviridae	Hepatitis B	Hepatocarcinoma	No
	Woodchuck Hep.	No	Hepatocarcinoma
RNA virus family			
Retroviridae	HTLV I	Leukaemia	No
	Various leukaemia viruses	No	Leukaemia in birds rodents, cats, dogs, rabbits
	Rous sarcoma	No	Chicken sarcomata
	Various sarcoma viruses	No	Sarcomata in cats, dogs, rabbits and cattle
	Bittner, Muehlbock	No	Mammary tumours in mice

free filtrates prepared from cases of the disease. In 1908 Ellerman and Bang demonstrated that an avian leukaemia was transmitted by cell-free extracts. In 1911 Rous showed that an avian sarcoma was caused by a filterable agent. In all of these cases it was correctly assumed that viruses caused the tumours. In the last 20 years intensive research in this field has implicated several viruses as the direct cause of some human cancers, and a very large variety of viruses causing cancers in animals.

Viruses and Oncogenes

The last decade of research has suggested that the genetic information for malignant transformation is mostly encoded within the DNA of normal cells. There is now evidence which shows that certain normal genes in animal cells, including human, may under certain circumstances induce malignancy. These normal genes are termed **proto-oncogenes**. Since they occur in normal cells they are also sometimes referred to as **cellular oncogenes**. The function of these genes in the normal cell is important enough for them to have been conserved during evolution over 600 million years. These proto-oncogenes have also been found in other living organisms such as insects, fish and birds. Their function is essentially concerned with cell differentiation, growth and regulation of cell division.

Viruses have also been shown to possess very similar genes to the cellular oncogenes and these have been termed **viral oncogenes**. It has been shown that it is the viruses that have acquired the cellular oncogenes, incorporating them into their own genome, and not vice versa, since proto-oncogenes in cells are composed of introns and exons like other genes in cells. Viral oncogenes are composed of a single uninterrupted exon sequence and it follows that the viral oncogenes have been acquired by the viruses in the form of processed mRNA transcribed from proto-oncogenes in cells, as is shown in Figure 4.25.

An important group of viruses that contains tumour-causing viruses is that of the retroviruses. These are RNA viruses characterized by their possession of the enzyme reverse transcriptase which is essential in their replication. The enzyme is an RNA-dependent-DNA-polymerase, able to synthesize a strand of DNA from an RNA template. A complementary strand of DNA is synthesized and the double-stranded DNA containing viral genes and viral genetic information may then be inserted ('spliced') into the cellular DNA. When virally coded DNA is inserted into the cell's DNA the viral genes are called progenes. They may be transcribed by normal cellular enzymatic mechanisms into mRNA and translated into viral proteins such as capsomers and reverse transcriptase. The whole of the virally coded DNA segment is termed the provirus and this may be transcribed many times into RNA, each copy of which is the new viral genome (see Figure 4.26).

Cells that have been infected with retroviruses are

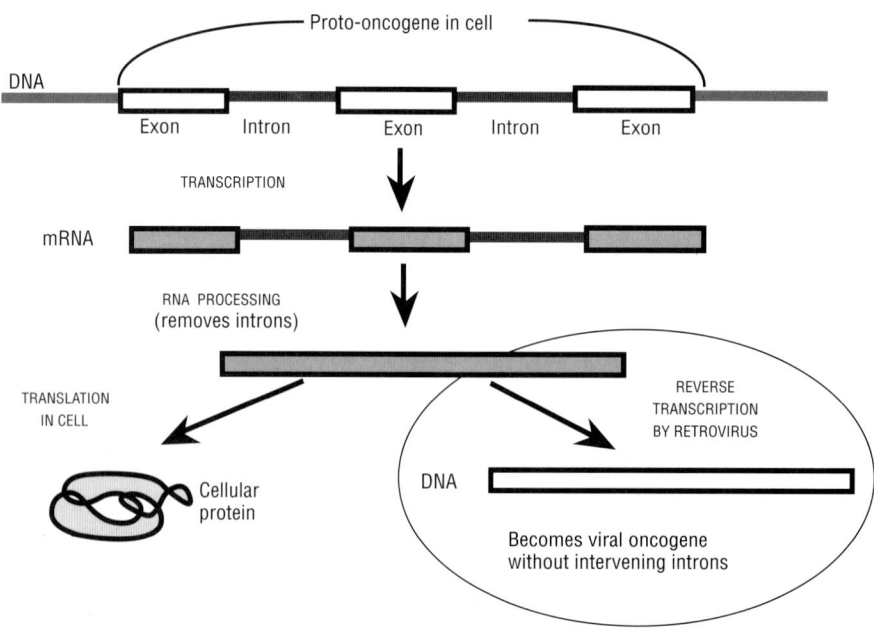

Figure 4.25 *The origin of viral oncogenes*

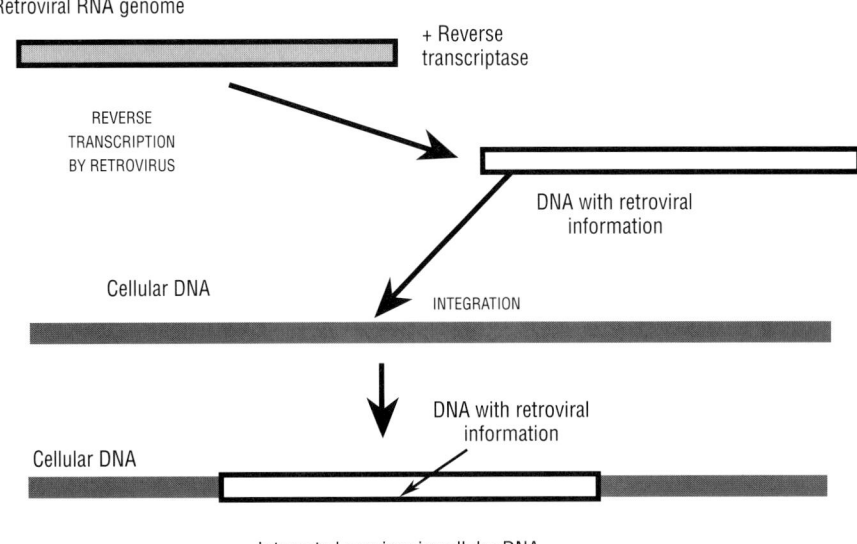

Retroviral RNA genome

+ Reverse transcriptase

REVERSE TRANSCRIPTION BY RETROVIRUS

DNA with retroviral information

Cellular DNA

INTEGRATION

DNA with retroviral information

Cellular DNA

Integrated provirus in cellular DNA

Figure 4.26 *Retroviral genetic material integration into cellular DNA*

termed permissive and non-permissive (see Figure 4.27). Permissive cells allow the replication of a retrovirus which has inserted its genetic material into the cellular DNA (that is, an integrated retrovirus). The result of this process is the formation of retroviral mRNA genome from the provirus DNA and subsequent translation by the cell such that viral proteins are produced. As both retroviral genome RNA is present, together with the complete complement of retroviral proteins, the permissive cell will allow the complete assembly of new retrovirus particles. Non-permissive cells do not allow the replication of integrated retroviruses. However, limited expression of the proviral genes may occur, with fragments of retroviral mRNA produced through cellular transcription processes. Cellular translation of the viral mRNA in the ribosomes will then lead to the production of viral proteins within the cell. These viral proteins cannot aggregate to form complete virus particles as the full complement of retroviral genome and retroviral proteins is not present. Production of foreign, viral proteins in the cellular environment is an abnormal occurrence and these viral proteins may interfere with normal cellular processes and the effects on the cell may be very serious.

When a cell containing an integrated virus divides, as well as replicating its own DNA, it also replicates the provirus. This therefore, is a very effective way for viruses to ensure that they are replicated and that they infect new cells. This is the so-called **horizontal transmission of the virus**. Some proviruses have integrated into the germ cells of the host and are therefore transmitted to the offspring in the same manner as Mendelian genes, this mechanism termed **vertical transmission**. Such viruses transmitted vertically are called **endogenous viruses**. Some animal leukaemia viruses are of this latter type and when passed vertically from parent to offspring they tend to cause long, latent infections in the offspring, in most cases producing no disease at all. This is in contrast to congenital infections with the same viruses (that is, the viruses are not acquired genetically but rather acquired through horizontal transmission at the time of birth), where the offspring develop chronic viraemias and quite commonly leukaemias.

The oncogenic retroviruses may be divided into two groups: the slow oncogenic viruses, which produce tumours after a long incubation period, this oncogenic effect not generally demonstrated in cell culture; and the acute oncogenic viruses, producing tumours within weeks, the oncogenic effect also being demonstrable in cell cultures.

The Slow Oncogenic Viruses
These are viruses that are associated with the leukaemias and the sarcomata, for example the **Feline Leukaemia Virus** (FeLV) and the **Murine Leukaemia Virus**. They show both horizontal and vertical

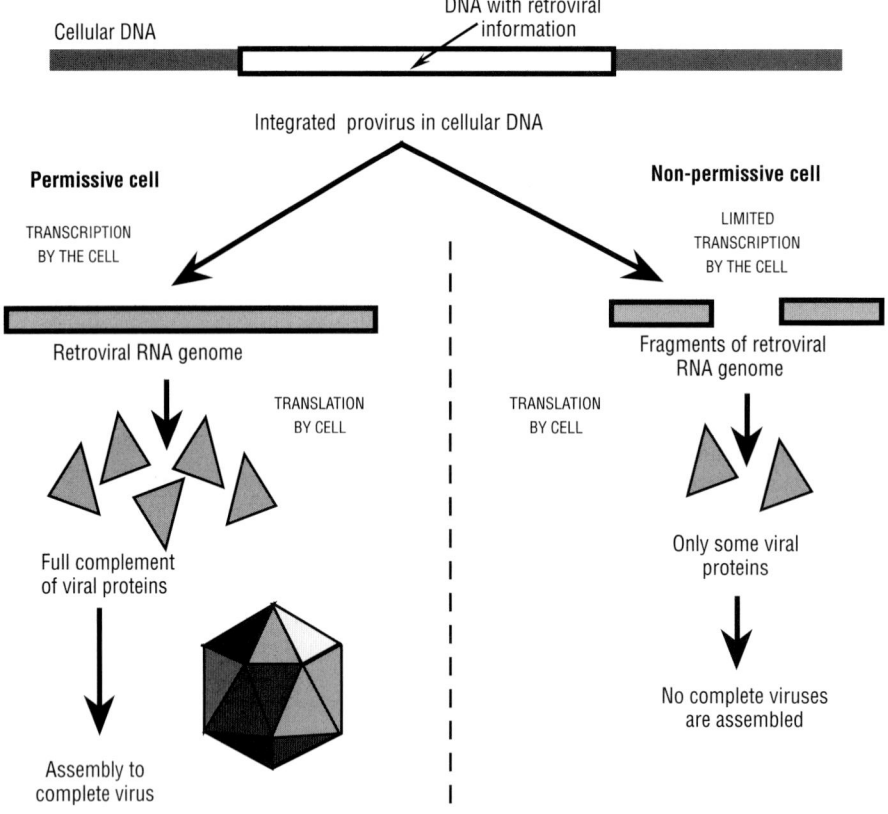

Figure 4.27 *Virus interactions with permissive and non-permissive cells*

transmission. The integrated retroviruses of this type do not need to replicate inside the cell in order to transform it into a malignant cell. The important factor is the integration of one or more copies of the virus genome into the cellular genetic material.

Characteristic of these viruses is not only the long incubation period between infection and development of tumours but also the fact that many infected animals fail entirely to develop tumours. It is known that leukaemias tend to develop in animals receiving large infectious doses of the viruses while still young. The viruses tend to immunosuppress the animal they infect and this is thought to be an important factor in tumour development. In the older animals the viruses infect cells but may remain dormant for many years before they produce tumours or, as was mentioned above, they may not produce tumours at all. It is thought that the immunosuppression by the virus in the older animals is less marked. Immunization of cats against the FeLV is possible and this has a protective effect on the immunized cats even if the immunization is performed after the cat has been infected with the virulent strain of the virus.

A human adult leukaemia/lymphoma syndrome is caused by infection with a human retrovirus, the **human T cell lymphotropic virus type I** (HTLV I). This infection is endemic in the Caribbean islands and certain parts of South-western Japan where at least 12% of the population shows evidence of infection with the virus. The leukaemia due to this virus has a high incidence in these areas but both the virus and the leukaemia are very rare in other parts of the world. Researchers working with the virus are confident that their work will yield a vaccine for this type of leukaemia.

The Acute Oncogenic Viruses
These viruses transform the cells they infect quickly and they differ from the slow oncogenic viruses in possessing a viral oncogene. An example of such an acute oncogenic virus is the **Rous sarcoma virus** which contains the viral-sarcoma gene (**v-src**). The Rous

sarcoma virus was the first to be discovered in this group and the v-src gene it contains is responsible for the tumourigenicity of the virus. There are strains of the Rous sarcoma virus in which, as a result of mutation, the v-src is not expressed. These strains are not acutely oncogenic. Many other acutely oncogenic viruses have now been discovered, each being oncogenic for a particular species. There are viruses infecting monkeys, rodents, poultry and felines and each of these produces a different type of tumour depending on the viral oncogene (v-onc) that is present in the viral genome. There are viruses producing sarcomata, carcinomata or leukaemias. Among all of these acute oncogenic viruses the Rous sarcoma virus is unique in that it is a complete oncogenic virus. Its genome contains the v-src gene in addition to the **Gag** (group-specific antigen gene coding for proteins on the viral capsid), **Pol** (reverse transcriptase polymerase gene) and **Env** (envelope gene coding for viral proteins on the viral envelope) genes. This implies that the Rous sarcoma virus has all the genetic information necessary to invade, multiply in and transform cells into neoplastic cells (see Figure 4.28).

All other viruses of the acute oncogenic group so far discovered are **defective** viruses, meaning that the v-onc gene has replaced other essential genetic material (usually Pol and often parts of Gag and Env). Consequently, such defective viruses cannot replicate inside hosts cells unless the cell is simultaneously infected with a 'helper' virus, this being usually one of the slow leukaemia viruses. Because these viruses are defective they are not infectious under ordinary conditions and do not become endemic in a population. They have been found in individual animals and they have been transmitted experimentally. Under normal conditions, when an animal is infected with such a virus the virus dies out when the tumour it has induced in the animal kills it. It should be noted that no acute oncogenic virus is known that induces a human cancer. However, the study of such viruses and their v-onc genes has elucidated many details in the process of carcinogenesis.

Proto-oncogenes and Cancer

Experiments using DNA isolated from human and animal cells which contain proto-oncogenes have been carried out. When DNA sequences containing proto-oncogenes from normal cells are injected into other cells they will not produce tumours. However, DNA isolated from cancer cells, when injected into normal cells, will effect a transformation of the cells into neoplastic cells. The responsible genes for this neoplastic transformation were isolated and cloned and it was shown that they were genes resembling very closely proto-oncogenes and their corresponding viral oncogenes. Through a series of experiments it was shown that such inactive cellular, proto-oncogenes could be caused to become oncogenic if they were somehow transformed to **activated cellular oncogenes**. That is, the genetic information of the oncogene must be somehow 'tampered with' causing it not to respond to normal cellular control mechanisms. There is a variety of ways in which cellular oncogenes may be activated.

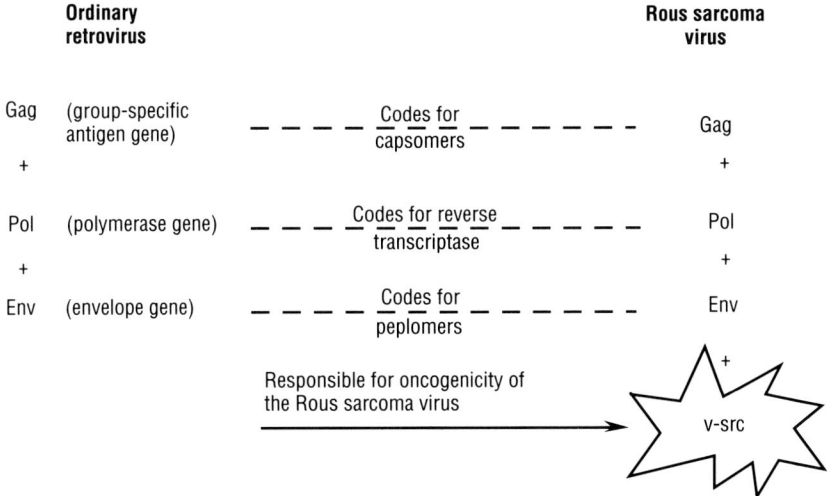

Figure 4.28 *Complete and incomplete oncoviruses*

Point mutations. It has been discovered that even such a subtle change as a single base pair change in a normal cellular oncogene (causing only a single amino acid to be changed in the protein product coded for by that oncogene) may result in inappropriate activity of the oncogene and induction of uncontrolled cellular division and cancer (see Figure 4.29).

Foreign environment. Normally, oncogenes are associated with regions of the DNA that control their expression, allowing the oncogene to be activated under controlled conditions only when the gene products of that region are required by the cells. If the oncogene is removed from that controlling, normal environment of the DNA and is moved to another portion of the DNA it may be expressed without any controlling influences and this inappropriate expression may lead to cancer (see Figure 4.30). This situation arises in some human tumours which result from chromosome translocations, where portions of one chromosome break off and attach to another chromosome, for example the **Philadelphia chromosome** which is found in 90% of cases of myeloid leukaemia. In the case of the Philadelphia chromosome there is a reciprocal translocation between chromosomes 9 and 22. The result is a hybrid gene on chromosome 22 leading to an abnormal protein being produced. The protein has tyrosine kinase activity and is responsible for the neoplastic transformation of the cell.

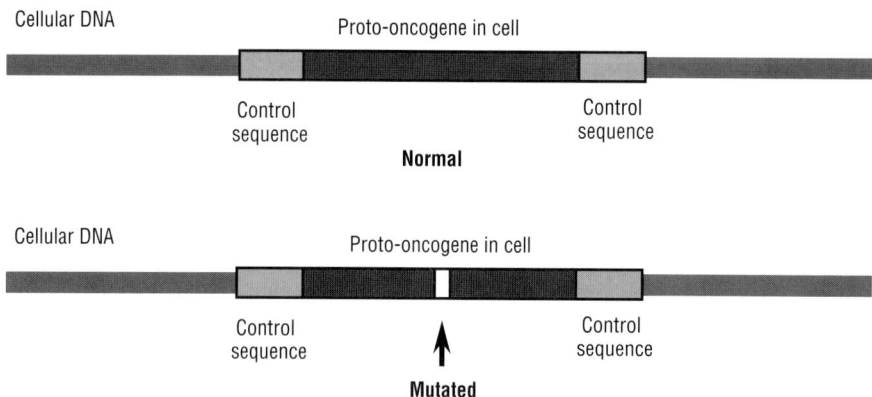

Figure 4.29   *Point mutation of proto-oncogenes may result in neoplasms*

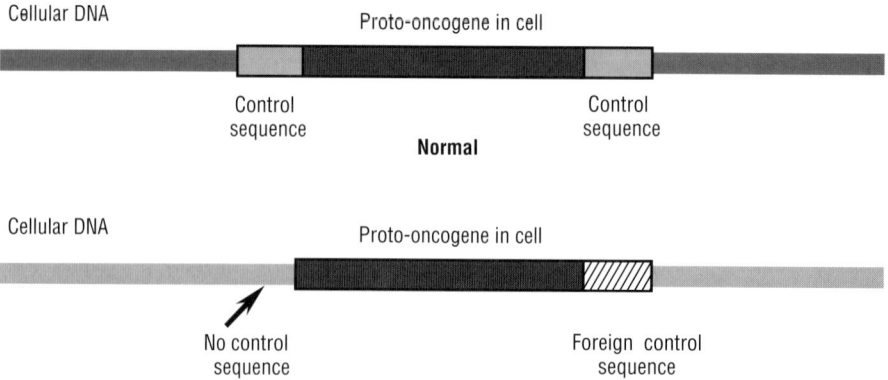

Figure 4.30   *Translocation of proto-oncogenes may lead to cancer*

Gene amplification. In this case many copies of the cellular oncogenes are present next to each other in the DNA. Some tumour cell lines (e.g. human lung cancer) have been shown to have many tens of copies of a cellular oncogene in their DNA. This is presumably what has caused the transformation to a cancer cell (refer to Figure 4.31).

Inappropriate expression. Although oncogenes are present in the DNA of all cells in the body they should only be expressed by some cells at a particular time, always under the control of regulatory DNA sequences. In some tumours the oncogenes have been shown to be continuously activated and expressed in a manner uncharacteristic of the normal cell from which the tumour has arisen. An example is the *c-sis* oncogene which codes for platelet-derived growth factor, a substance produced in platelets through normal activation of the gene. Some human tumours, for example some sarcomata (not derived from platelets or their precursors), show activation of *c-sis.*

Integration of viral genome into the cell. When a virus integrates its genetic material into the DNA of the cell it effects a genetic change in the infected cell. The virus may in fact be a DNA virus such as **Herpes virus** or **Papovavirus** or it may be an **RNA retrovirus**, such as HTLV I. Incorporation of the foreign genetic material into the cell may be in the vicinity of a cellular oncogene and the effect may be one of **promotion** or **enhancement** of the cellular oncogene. That is, insertion of viral genetic material will cause the cellular oncogene to be activated as is illustrated in Figure 4.32.

Oncosuppressor Genes

Oncosuppressor genes are genes whose expression represses the formation of neoplasms. Hence, they appear to function in opposition to the oncogenes. Most of these genes have been identified in connexion with genetically determined neoplasms. An example of such a neoplasm in which oncosuppressor gene failure leads to development of the tumour is retinoblastoma. The gene responsible for tumour production is RB-1 on the thirteenth chromosome and this is a mutated oncosuppressor gene. The tumour does not develop in these individuals as their cells also contain a normal copy of the gene in the sister chromatid. If there is mutation in the RB-1 gene on the sister chromatid, then the person has two altered oncosuppressor genes and this will lead to the tumour. So here is an example of a gene which when **inactivated** (through mutation) will lead to tumour production. Therefore it is the normal functioning of the gene that prevents neoplasia. Other oncosuppressor genes are now being identified in association with other tumours.

Hormonal Factors in Neoplasia

Some tumours are sensitive to sex hormones and their growth can be slowed by hormonal reduction. For example, carcinoma of the prostate can be slowed by removal of the testes. Hyperoestrinism in women (e.g. in oestrogen-secreting granulosa cell tumours of the ovary) appears to lead to increased risk of endometrial carcinoma. There is no evidence of a link between the **oral contraceptive pill** and cancer, although there may be a small increase in incidence of benign hepatic

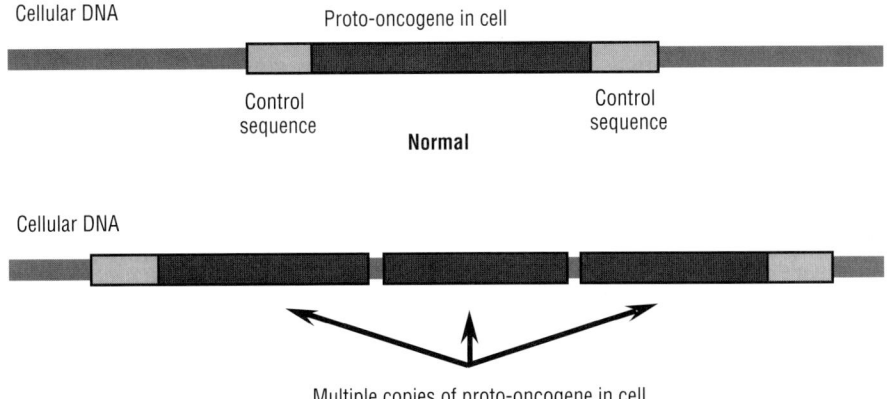

Figure 4.31 *Gene amplification and carcinogenesis*

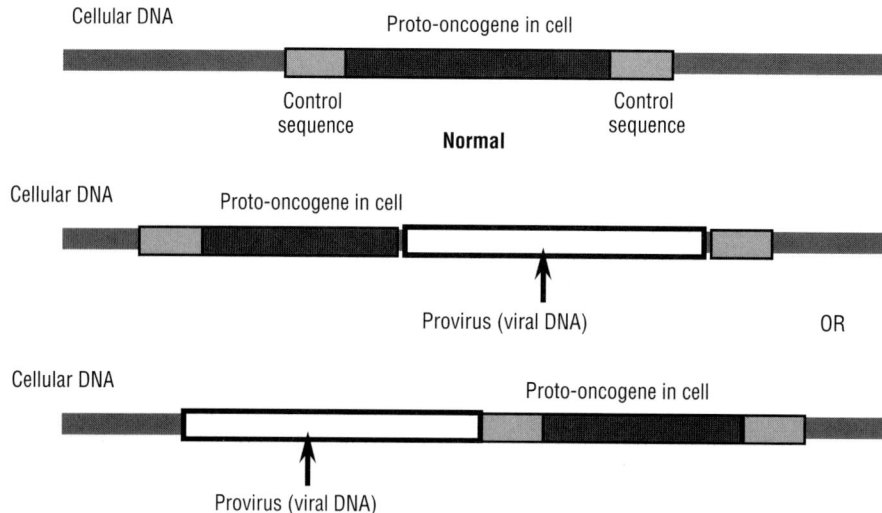

Figure 4.32 *Viral oncogenes and carcinogenesis*

tumours, while the incidence of benign breast lesions is decreased. Numerous studies have failed to find any link between the 'pill' and cancer of the breast or uterus. This is because of the fact that the contraceptive pill contains a balanced amount of oestrogen and progestagen, so no hyperoestrinism is seen.

Dietary Factors and Neoplasia

Certain foods are known or strongly suspected to be carcinogenic. For example aflatoxins, produced by the mould *Aspergillus flavus*, found on mouldy peanuts, may cause liver cancer. It is also known that consuming 'charcoaled' meat such as barbecued meat is carcinogenic. Hot, spicy foods such as chilli peppers are probably carcinogenic if consumed to excess, producing stomach cancer and oesophageal cancer.

It is also known that there is a high incidence of colorectal cancer in countries with **low fibre diets** (see Figure 4.33). Bacterial metabolites of bile acids have been shown to be carcinogens or co-carcinogens in animals. Large amounts of dietary fibre alter the bacterial flora and reduce time of contact of intestinal contents with bowel bacteria, and may be relevant to the lower incidence of bowel cancer in communities in which the diet is high in fibre.

Most probably, the causation of cancer related to specific diets is in part due to ingested carcinogens and in part due to endogenous factors relating to metabolism, normal flora bacteria, intestinal transit times and interactions between luminal contents of the intestine with the lining of the gastrointestinal walls. Other important metabolic/endocrine effects may interact with dietary factors. It is known that obese women have a higher incidence of breast carcinoma, presumably because more dietary fats are being shunted into metabolic pathways that increase hormone levels.

Social Factors in Neoplasia

It has been well established that cigarette smoking is linked to cancer of the bronchi, larynx and oral cavity, and it may also be linked to cancer of the bladder and stomach (see Figure 4.34). Taking up smoking is related to social factors, for example peer group pressure. Remarkable changes in sex incidence of carcinoma of the bronchus in the last few years have largely been the result of more women than men smoking. Aggressive advertising and changes in the status of women are responsible for this. As more women are smoking and they are smoking more and more cigarettes than men, the incidence of 'lung cancer' in this group has risen dramatically. Other 'social' excesses such as alcoholism may also result in cancer. Alcoholics of long-standing with cirrhosis of the liver are predisposed to liver cancer. Carcinoma of the pancreas is also thought to be linked to increased consumption of alcohol.

Many occupations are linked with an increased exposure to carcinogenic substances and influences. Tan-

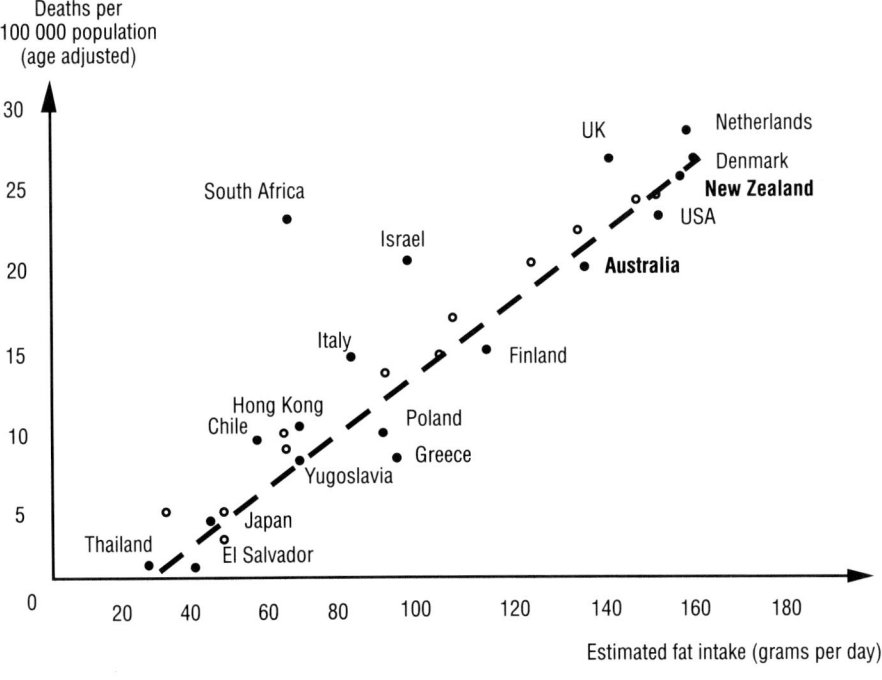

(*Source:* Cohen LA, *Sci Am* 1987; 257; 5: 42–48)

Figure 4.33 *Annual death rate from cancer of the colon in relation to daily fat intake*

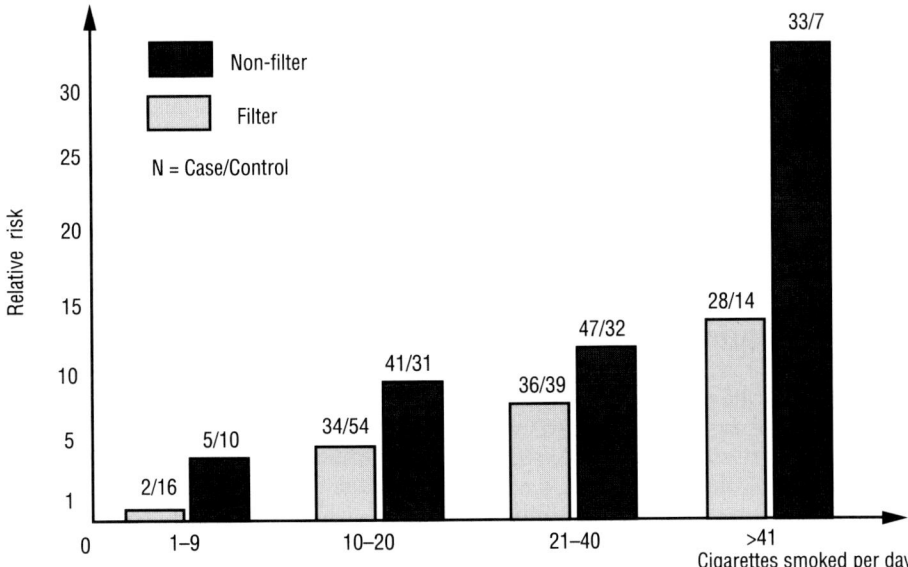

(*Source:* Wynder EI, Mabuchi K, Hoffman D, in *Cancer Epidemiology and Protection*, edited by Schottenfeld D; Thomas, Springfield Illinois, 1975, p. 121)

Figure 4.34 *Relative risk of lung cancer among current smokers, in relation to the number of cigarettes smoked per day (males 1966–1971)*

ners and smelters are exposed to arsenic, plastics workers are exposed to vinyl chloride and both have a higher incidence of liver cancer. Miners and asbestos workers are exposed to a variety of carcinogens such as asbestos, nickel, chromium and coal dust and have a much higher incidence of cancer of the lungs. Radiologists, radiographers and researchers have an increased risk of being exposed to ionizing radiation and have a higher risk of developing bone, thyroid and skin tumours. People who work unprotected in the sun for long periods of time are more likely to develop skin cancers (refer to Table 4.7).

It has become increasingly more important to make workers aware of the risks encountered in their workplace and also employers must provide adequate protection for the employees in the workplace. Most cancers developing in the work environment are preventable, either through the elimination of contact with the offending substance causing the tumour or through adequate protection when exposed to it.

Other Factors which Contribute to Neoplasia

While many other factors have been shown to be epidemiologically linked with cancer, on analysis it is to be seen that most of these factors are related to the intrinsic and extrinsic factors already discussed previously. It must be realized that although we know that cancers result because of a heritable change in the genetic material of cells, many factors may interact to produce that change. Often extrinsic and intrinsic factors react in an additive or multiplicative manner, thus giving rise to the statistically significant increases in the probability of developing a cancer in certain subgroups of populations.

Overview of Malignant Disease

Cancer is a recognized health problem in many countries around the world but especially in the so-called Western-type industrialized nations such as Australia. In the developing countries cancer is not such a major problem as many people there still die young from other causes such as malnutrition and infectious diseases which are relatively rare causes of death in the developed countries. Cancer has been described as a disease of old age and this to a certain extent is true as most cancers have a peak incidence in people over 50 years of age. It is no surprise, therefore, that in the developed nations where people live longer, due to

good nutrition and good health care protecting them from infectious diseases, they succumb to cancers, which in Australia cause approximately 23% of all deaths, as is illustrated in Figure 4.35.

Using statistical studies, it is possible not only to determine the contribution of number of cases of cancer as cause of death but also the type of cancer, as is seen in Table 4.9. When such figures are examined it becomes obvious that the great majority of cancers affecting the body affect the epithelial organs, that is, carcinomata are more common in incidence than sarcomata and the leukaemias.

From these figures it is apparent that the external epithelia are more prone to undergo malignant change. This is understandable since it is these tissues which are more likely to come into contact with environmental carcinogenic agents. It has been determined that the majority of cancers may in fact be preventable through avoidance of such environmental, external carcinogens. For example, diminishing exposure to ultraviolet light (sun tanning) will diminish the incidence of skin cancers, avoiding a high animal fat, low fibre diet will decrease the risk of colonic carcinoma, not smoking cigarettes will diminish the risk of lung cancer.

As far as the cancers of the internal epithelia are concerned, it is here that we are possibly observing more the effect of intrinsic factors such as heredity and hormonal status influencing malignant change. This is not meant to exclude totally the interaction with extrinsic factors, but deep inside the body environmental factors are less important than on the exterior of the body.

The low incidence of malignant change in the connective tissues and blood may be an indication of, once again, the decreased contact that these tissues deep within the body have with extrinsic carcinogenic agents, but it also possibly may reflect the fact that these tissues are somehow better adapted, biologically, to cope with the possibility of malignant transformation.

When the individual organs and tissues are considered with respect to the incidence of cancer at various sites in the body it is possible to construct a table which indicates the most common causes of death among patients with malignant disease (see Table 4.10). By far the most common cancer in this country presently is carcinoma of the bronchus or 'lung cancer'. This is associated with cigarette smoking and before smoking was so popular this was a rare tumour. Carcinoma of the colon is another common tumour which reflects our dietary habits. In women, in this country at present, breast carcinoma is by far the commonest tumour but it seems that it is just about to be supplanted by lung cancer since at present more women

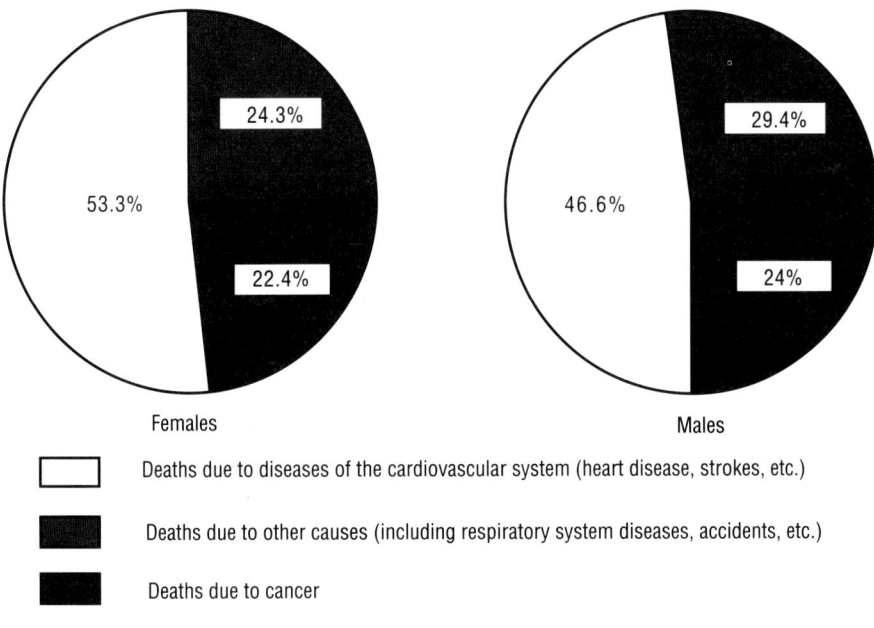

Females   Males

☐ Deaths due to diseases of the cardiovascular system (heart disease, strokes, etc.)

■ Deaths due to other causes (including respiratory system diseases, accidents, etc.)

■ Deaths due to cancer

(*Source:* Based on data from the Australian Bureau of Statistics, 1983)

Figure 4.35 *All deaths, percentage distribution by cause, Australia, 1983*

Table 4.9 *Incidence of cancer in different classes of cells*

Class of cell affected	Percentage of total
Cancers of the external epithelia (e.g. skin, large intestine, lung, stomach, cervix)	56%
Cancers of the internal epithelia (e.g. breast, prostate, ovary, bladder, pancreas, kidney)	36%
Cancers of connective tissues and blood (i.e. sarcomata, leukaemias, lymphomata)	8%

Source: Clemmesen, J, 'Statistical Studies in Malignant Neoplasms.' *Acta Path Microbiol Scand Suppl* 174 (1964), 209 (1969), 247 (1974).

and fewer men are smoking cigarettes. It is very sad to see that most cancer deaths are in fact caused by tumours which are almost totally preventable (i.e. lung cancer and colonic cancer).

When considering individual tumours in the context of pathology, it is necessary to examine each one methodically in a standard manner, a procedure which will consistently give the maximum information about the condition. If we take as an example the commonest tumour in our society presently, carcinoma of the bron-

chus, this standard way of discussing tumours will become apparent.

Incidence of the tumour is first considered. This includes overall incidence in the population (which may be considered as number of people in the population presenting with the tumour or the number of people dying of this condition). In the case of carcinoma of the bronchus the incidence is described as 24% of all cancer deaths, or alternatively, as 5% of deaths from all causes.

Table 4.10   *Mortality from the various cancers (USA, UK and Australia 1976–1981)*

Organ or tissue	Percentage mortality	Percentage incidence
Lungs	25	15
Colon	15	14
Breast	10	14
Lymphoma and leukaemia	7	8
Stomach	6	4
Pancreas	5	3
Prostate	5	9
Cervix	4	10
Bladder and kidney	3	7
Ovary	3	2
Skin	2	2
All else	15	12

Source: Cancer, the Facts, Oxford Univ. Press, Oxford, 1981.

Also, age and sex incidence must be covered. On average most lung cancers are seen around the age of 55 years, but the tumour has been known to occur anywhere between the ages of 15 and 80 years. Currently, the male to female ratio of people presenting with the tumour is 2:1 but epidemiological studies indicate that the ratio tends towards equalizing and in the next few years the tumour will be commoner in females. It may sometimes be relevant in certain tumours to talk of geographical distribution as in certain countries or racial groups the incidence of a given tumour may be markedly higher or lower than in others.

Aetiology and predisposing factors, where known, should then be discussed and also, where known, the pathogenesis of the malignancy. In the case of lung cancer there is one major predisposing factor: the smoking of cigarettes. In addition, irradiation (X-rays, gamma rays, etc.), certain occupational factors (e.g. inhalation of dusts in mining and industry) and possibly atmospheric pollution are also important.

The site in the particular organ that the tumour occurs in should then be discussed as this is important in diagnosis and treatment. Certain tumours show quite a marked predilection for a given area within the tissue they affect. In the lung, carcinoma occurs in most cases (55% of cases) in a central situation, either in the lower trachea or in one of the major bronchi.

Macroscopic and microscopic appearance should then be thoroughly covered, and the two should be correlated. In the case of lung cancer there are many different histological types of tumour which are different in their clinical behaviour. Special imaging techniques which are used to visualize the tumours should

also be kept in mind, for example X-ray, CT scanning and so on.

Spread of the tumour and metastasis should then be examined. In the case of lung cancer, the tumour first spreads locally and very quickly infiltrates the lymphatics, permeating to the draining lymph nodes. Vascular invasion then follows with distant metastases developing in the brain, bones and liver.

Diagnostic techniques for the particular tumour are then covered and in this context, symptoms and signs are important. Carcinoma of the bronchus presents usually with a persistent non-productive cough which quickly changes character to become severe, productive of phlegm and blood. Chest tightness and pain, dyspnoea and cyanosis are usually late features. Symptoms may also arise in association with the distant metastases. Diagnosis is usually by X-ray, CT scanning, biopsy, sputum cytology.

Treatment of the tumour is then described and this can be either curative or palliative. Very often treatment regimes depend on the stage at which the the tumour is diagnosed, and with most tumours various staging systems are in use. One of the commonest is the TNM system, in which T stands for the size of the primary tumour, N stands for the condition of the draining lymph nodes (i.e. whether they contain tumour or not) and M stands for metastasis presence or absence. Another staging system in use classifies tumours from stages 1 to 4, the criteria once again being the extent of tumour growth and spread. The three main ways in which tumours are treated are by surgery (e.g. lobectomy or pneumonectomy in the lung), radiotherapy and chemotherapy.

Finally, the prognosis of the tumour is stated and the

standard way of quoting this is as a 5-year survival figure. That is, what percentage of patients with the tumour are likely to be still alive after 5 years have elapsed from the time the tumour was diagnosed and treated. In the case of lung cancer the prognosis is grave, with an average 5-year survival of 15%. It should also be noted that some cancers are now deemed to be curable with a combination of treatment regimes (refer to Figure 4.36).

Laboratory Investigations of Malignant Disease

Cellular Examinations–Biopsies

The mainstay of diagnostic procedures in malignant disease is clinical symptomatology and the subsequent sampling of the mass by biopsy with examination of the sampled piece of the tumour under the microscope. A typical example of this procedure would be with a suspected cancer of the large bowel. A patient may present with symptoms relating to obstruction of the bowel or alternatively patients may have noticed that lately there has been blood or increased quantities of mucus in their faeces. A **colonoscopy** is performed in which procedure a colonoscope is inserted into the lumen of the large bowel *per rectum* enabling the doctor to inspect the internal mucosal aspect of the large bowel. This instrument is also equipped with a remote control blade which is able to snip off the lesion or a small area of tissue for biopsy purposes. Once the lesion has been located and observed, a biopsy is taken, the tissue fixed, sectioned and stained and then observed under the microscope by the histopathologist, who can tell if the tissue is normal or abnormal, distinguishing between benign and malignant tumours.

An alternative method of diagnosis of tumours by biopsy depends on the skills of the cytologist, and the samples removed from the body are cells that are scraped off body surfaces, or alternatively cells that have desquamated naturally and are present in secretions such as mucus. **Cytology** is that science which examines these cells and relates their morphology and staining characteristics to the functional character of the cells. This procedure can be illustrated by taking the case of suspected carcinoma of the bronchus. The patient is asked to cough up some sputum, in which desquamated epithelial cells, which normally line the respiratory passages, will be found. The sputum sample is smeared on a slide, fixed, stained and examined by the cytologist, who will determine whether malig-

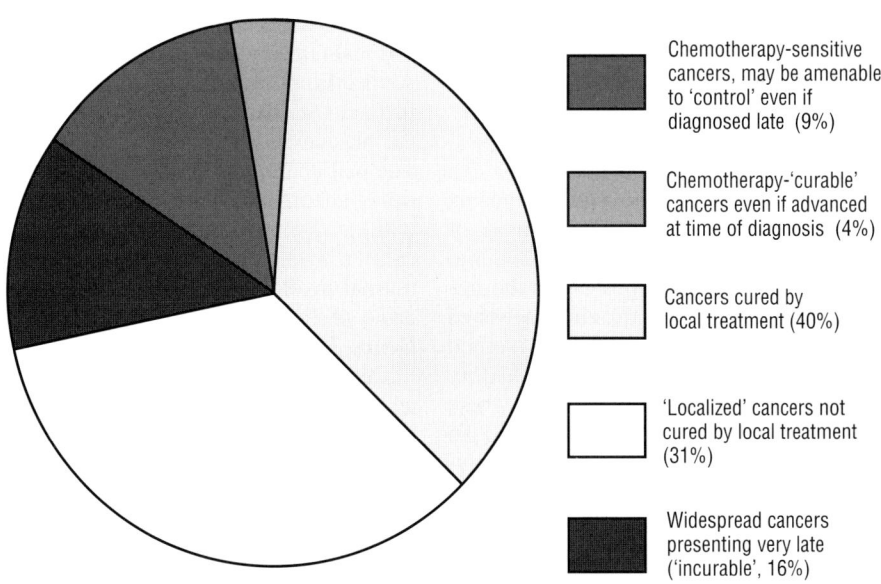

Chemotherapy-sensitive cancers, may be amenable to 'control' even if diagnosed late (9%)

Chemotherapy-'curable' cancers even if advanced at time of diagnosis (4%)

Cancers cured by local treatment (40%)

'Localized' cancers not cured by local treatment (31%)

Widespread cancers presenting very late ('incurable', 16%)

(*Source:* Cancer: Causes and Control Symposium: Cancer Cell Biochemistry and Chemotherapy, MHN Tattersall, May 1980, Australian Academy of Science)

Figure 4.36 *Cancer prognosis*

nant cells are present in the sample. Fluid from the pleural and peritoneal cavities are also frequently examined by this method. Another very frequently performed test utilizing cytology is the **Papanicolaou smear test** ('Pap test'), which is performed on a cell sample removed from the uterine cervix, in an attempt to diagnose at an early stage carcinoma of the cervix. Cells are scraped off the uterine cervix with a special spatula during routine gynaecological examination and the cells are examined under the microscope after smearing on a slide, fixing and staining. This test is very important in detecting dysplastic and early neoplastic changes in the cells lining the cervix and has contributed greatly to the decreased number of deaths due to carcinoma of the cervix, as women are now diagnosed and treated at earlier stages of the tumour than in the past.

Another test in which malignant disease may be diagnosed by biopsy is in the case of the leukaemias and lymphomas. In these neoplasms the abnormality occurs in the blood, bone marrow and the lymphoid tissue. In the case of the leukaemias, a peripheral blood sample may be sufficient to diagnose the disorder. A blood sample is taken, a smear made and the abnormal leukaemic cells may be identified in it. Alternatively, bone marrow specimens may be obtained by operation or via needle biopsies. The needle biopsy may also be of use in removing lymphoid tissue for analysis of primary tumours (lymphomata) or secondary tumours (especially carcinoma of the bronchus, breast and malignant melanoma).

Enzyme Assays

All of the most generally used methods of diagnosing neoplasms depend on direct sampling of the 'lump' of abnormal tissue or some of the tumour cells in order to identify their malignant characteristics under the microscope. These methods have their disadvantages and many researchers have tried to develop a method whereby a tumour is diagnosed early in its history through a simple blood test. However, all of these attempts have met consistently with failure and no reliable alteration of plasma or other enzymatic activity has been found to be diagnostic of early malignant disease. In fact, for the majority of cancers no specific enzymatic changes occur in the body even in advanced cases of the disease. With a small number of tumours, some changes in body enzyme levels are known and are used in the diagnosis of these particular tumours.

Carcinoma of the prostate. In this tumour there are raised levels of *acid phosphatase* in the serum. How-

ever, these increases are predominantly seen in advanced, spreading prostatic carcinoma.

Other tumours (non-specific). In advanced malignant disease of many sites in the body there are increased levels of a *placental-type alkaline phosphatase* (the Regan isoenzyme).

Non-specific increases of other enzymes. In advanced malignancy the levels of specific enzymes may be many times the normal values. In widespread malignant disease and in leukaemia there is often an increase in the levels of *serum lactate dehydrogenase* and in *serum phosphoglucose isomerase*. Increased levels of other enzymes indicating increased cellular proliferation may be associated with certain tumours. For example, increased levels of *β-glucuronidase* in urine may be associated with carcinoma of the bladder and high levels of *6-phosphogluconate-dehydrogenase* in vaginal fluids may indicate carcinoma of the cervix.

Protein Assays

In advanced malignant disease of various primary origins there tends to be a fall in the **albumin** plasma level and a rise in total plasma **globulin** (but especially the α_2 component) and a rise in **fibrinogen**. All of these changes reflect non-specific tissue damage and may be further enhanced by the secondary infections and malnutrition so commonly seen in cancer patients. A specific protein test relating to malignancy is performed with **multiple myeloma**. This is a tumour of the plasma cells which normally produce antibodies. The malignant plasma cells produce excessive quantities of abnormal antibodies (myeloma globulins) which will cause an increased level of total protein and increased levels of **globulins** in the plasma. These abnormal myeloma globulins will also be found in the urine of these patients, giving rise to the so-called **Bence-Jones proteinuria**.

Detection of α_1-**foetoprotein** in patients may give an indication of the presence of malignant disease. This protein is an α globulin which normally disappears after birth. It is found in the serum of 50% of patients with primary hepatocarcinoma and in those with malignant teratoma. Increased levels of this protein may also be found in some cases of carcinomata of the gastrointestinal tract and lungs, and also in neuroblastoma.

Some cancers of the breast are associated with increased serum levels of another foetal protein, known as **carcinoembryonic antigen**. The same protein may also be found in the urine of patients with carcinoma of the bladder. It should be kept in mind that many chronic inflammatory, non-neoplastic diseases may give false positive results.

Hormone Assays

A large number of tumours of the endocrine glandular organs (malignant as well as benign) are associated with production of inappropriately high levels of active hormones. This is because the neoplastic cells remain sufficiently well differentiated so as to secrete hormones, but because they are neoplastic they will secrete the hormones continuously and independently of the normal stimuli which influence secretion of the hormone.

Pancreatic Islet Tissue

Although tumours of this tissue are rare, they are important as they have very important effects because of excessive hormone production. Approximately 60% of all neoplasms of the pancreatic islet tissue secrete active hormones. Of all pancreatic islet tissue neoplasms, 80% are benign while 20% are malignant.

Tumours of the β cells (Insulin Secretors)
These tumours produce large quantities of insulin which results in a low fasting blood glucose level. Not infrequently, these patients show attacks of severe hypoglycaemia with neurological symptoms, sometimes progressing to a hypoglycaemic coma.

Tumours of the G cells (Gastrin Secretors)
The tumours derived from these cells secrete an excessive quantity of the hormone **gastrin** which stimulates the continuous secretion of stomach acid, leading to intractable stomach ulceration (**Zollinger-Ellison syndrome**). The excessive stomach acid may be detected in gastric function tests or the excessive gastrin levels may be detected by radioimmunoassay (RIA).

Tumours of the D₁ cells (Secretors of VIP)
These tumours secrete excessive quantities of vasoactive intestinal peptide (VIP), a substance which inhibits gastric secretion and stimulates water and electrolyte secretion by the small intestine. The patients present with symptoms resembling infectious cholera: watery diarrhoea, hypokalaemia and achlorhydria (**WDHA syndrome**). The excess VIP may be detected by RIA.

Tumours of the α cells (Secretors of Glucagon)
These tumours secrete excessive quantities of glucagon which raises plasma levels of glucose. Characteristically the patients present with **diabetes mellitus**, stomatitis, anaemia and a specific skin lesion known as **necrolytic migratory erythema** (a rash with dermatitis). The diagnosis is confirmed by demonstrating excessive plasma levels of glucagon.

Tumours of the δ cells (Secretors of Somatostatin)
This is a rare tumour, the cells of which produce inappropriately high levels of somatostatin, a substance which normally inhibits the activity of α, β, and G islet cells as well as the secretory activity of pancreatic exocrine cells. The clinical findings of this disorder are non-specific and its diagnosis often comes late. The patients present with gall stones, mild diabetes mellitus, steatorrhoea and hypochlorhydria, all due to the inhibitory effect of somatostatin on other pancreatic cells and their reduced secretion of active hormones.

Adrenal Gland

This gland secretes many important hormones, and increased levels of the hormones will be associated not only with neoplasms but also with hyperplasias of the gland.

Glucocorticoid Excess (Cushing's Syndrome)
In 30% of cases glucocorticoid hormone excess is due to tumours in the adrenal. However, an identical syndrome may be the result of hyperplasia of the gland due to an ACTH-secreting tumour of the pituitary gland. A marked increase in cortisol levels is seen in these patients and the predominant symptoms and signs are the metabolic effects of the cortisol, all other effects seen being secondary. Hyperglycaemia, glycosuria and an insulin-dependent diabetes are due to effects on the metabolism of carbohydrates. Cessation of growth, muscle wasting, osteoporosis and atrophy of the skin are all effects on the metabolism of proteins. The 'moon face' and the 'buffalo hump' that are seen in patients are due to disordered fat metabolism. Owing to the effect of accompanying increases in the levels of mineralocorticoids and androgens there is also hypertension, hirsutism and menstrual disorders (the last two in women only). Typically, in this disorder, the urine corticosteroid levels are more than 25 g per 24 hours, the plasma levels of corticosteroids also being high.

Adrenogenital Syndromes
These may present as androgen excesses or as oestrogen excesses.

Androgen excesses. In the case of these occurring in children, the disorder is almost always due to a neoplasm, whereas in the adult the condition is almost always due to adrenal hyperplasia. The excessive androgens that are produced in both cases are excreted in large quantities in the urine as **17-oxosteroids**. Excess pregnanetriol is also produced and excreted in the urine. The diagnosis of the disorder depends on the collection of 24 hour specimens of urine. In boys the condition results in precocious development of secondary sexual characteristics while the testes remain infantile due to suppression of secretion of pituitary gonadotrophins. In girls there is enlargement of the clitoris, masculine body build and distribution of hair. Puberty is not attained because of depression of pituitary sex hormone secretion. In men the syndrome has no observable clinical effect. In women there is virilization, amenorrhoea, atrophy of the breasts and external genitalia and enlargement of the clitoris.

Oestrogen excesses. This condition is very rare but is always due to neoplasms. Its effects are seen mainly in men and boys where a feminization occurs with gynaecomastia, loss of body hair, etc. In women there may be menstrual cycle abnormalities.

Primary Aldosteronism (Conn's Syndrome)

Adrenal cortical tumours may produce excessive levels of aldosterone thus giving rise to this condition. The syndrome is one of hypertension (usually severe) and hypokalaemia due to urinary and intestinal potassium loss leading to muscle weakness and cramps. Alkalosis, polyuria and increased plasma sodium are also seen. High levels of aldosterone are detected in the urine and in the plasma there will also be seen a decreased level of renin.

Adrenaline/Noradrenaline Excesses

These are produced by a rare tumour of the adrenal medulla, the **phaeochromocytoma**, which secretes excessive quantities of the catecholamines. The syndrome is characterized by paroxysmal hypertension which sometimes is sustained, a raised basal metabolic rate and, often, hyperglycaemia and glycosuria. A major end-product of catecholamine metabolism is **vanilmandelic acid** (VMA) which is excreted in the urine. Normal urinary VMA is less than 7 mg per 24 hours, whereas in phaeochromocytoma, values are raised to 10 mg or more per 24 hours. Note that the urinary concentration of VMA in primary hypertension is normal.

Thyroid Gland

A very small proportion ($\approx 1\%$) of thyroid adenomata produce hormones and give rise to hyperthyroidism. In most cases hyperthyroidism is caused by hyperplasia of the thyroid or alternatively by autoimmune thyroiditis due to LATS antibody (**Graves' disease**). The effects of hyperthyroidism all relate to the metabolic effects of raised thyroxine and triiodothyronine levels. The basal metabolic rate measured as oxygen uptake (assuming a constant respiratory quotient of 0.82) is raised when compared with normal subjects. The test is performed in the morning after the patient has been fasting and at rest for 12 hours. However, it is not a very accurate test and rarely used nowadays. Cardiovascular symptoms include tachycardia and raised cardiac output (predisposing to heart failure). Neurological signs such as exaggeration of mood variations or mania and tremors may be seen. Characteristic eye signs are also useful in diagnosis: exophthalmos and lid retraction are thought to be direct effects of thyroxine excess.

The laboratory findings of diagnostic value are alterations in the iodine metabolism, high plasma levels of protein-bound iodine and thyroxine, high resin uptake, a high 4-hour thyroid uptake of iodine clearance, etc. In severe cases there is demineralization of the skeleton with increased urinary calcium. If secondary renal damage occurs, then hypercalcaemia will be found.

Parathyroid Gland

In this case neoplasms or hyperplasias of the gland will cause a **primary hyperparathyroidism**. The laboratory findings are changes in the levels of many plasma substances directly caused by the increased levels of parathormone produced by the tumour. There is a raised plasma calcium, which may only be obvious if provoked by a low-phosphate diet. Urinary phosphate and calcium levels are increased, with a tendency to form alkaline urine. The calcium is derived from bone breakdown and mobilization of bone calcium. Secondary renal damage leads to increased levels of phosphate and urea in the plasma. If the plasma levels of calcium rise above 13 mg per 100 mL, signs of hypercalcaemia develop: loss of appetite, hypertonicity of muscles, abdominal pain, duodenal ulceration (due to increased acid and gastrin secretion), bone rarefaction and fibrosis, fractures, pain and deformities in bone (**Von Recklinghausen's disease**). Metastatic calcification is also seen.

Polyuria and polydipsia are caused by high levels of calcium and phosphate in the urine. Stones composed of calcium phosphate and calcium oxalate are a very common finding in the urinary tract of such patients.

The laboratory diagnosis of primary hyperparathyroidism is according to the following regime:

1. Measurement of plasma calcium and phosphate levels.
2. Measurement of Ca^{2+} excretion.
3. Phosphate clearance levels.
4. 'Cortisone Test': a patient is placed on a high daily dose of cortisone (150 mg for 10 days). If the patient has primary hyperparathyroidism the serum calcium level (corrected for protein) remains **unaltered**. However, if there is hypercalcaemia due to secondary tumours in bone or due to sarcoidosis, the serum calcium level (corrected for protein) is **reduced**.

The Anterior Pituitary Gland

Six separate hormones have been isolated as products of the anterior pituitary gland: (1) **growth hormone**, GH; (2) **thyroid stimulating hormone**, TSH; (3) **adrenocorticotrophic hormone**, ACTH; (4) **luteotrophic hormone**, LTH; (5) **follicle stimulating hormone**, FSH; (6) **luteinizing hormone**, LH. All of these except GH and LTH act on other endocrine glands, stimulating them to secrete more of their own hormones. There is a feedback control mechanism which limits the secretion of the trophic hormones by the pituitary and secretion of pituitary hormones may also be influenced by injury, anxiety, infection, etc.

Hormone assays for pituitary function may be performed in the laboratory using RIA, enzyme-linked immunosorbent assays (ELISA) or gas chromatography techniques.

Detection of these hormones is particularly important in the case of patients presenting with **gigantism** or **acromegaly** (growth hormone excesses); **thyrotoxicosis** (TSH excesses) and **Cushing's syndrome** (ACTH excesses).

The Posterior Pituitary Gland

The most important hormone secreted here is the **antidiuretic hormone**. When more than 90% of the gland has been destroyed by tumour, the levels of this hormone are almost nil and the patient develops **diabetes insipidus** where very large volumes of dilute urine are produced. Hormone assays in this case will indicate the absence of the hormone.

Predisposing Factors to Diseases of Ageing

The Process of Ageing and Biological Theories of Ageing

Ageing is a very complex process, beginning in adulthood and progressing inexorably into what we know as senescence or 'old age', ending in the death of the individual as a direct result of the many 'degenerative changes' and 'diseases of old age' that are so frequently seen to be afflicting elderly individuals. We know surprisingly little about the normal processes of cellular differentiation and growth and unfortunately even less about the process of cellular and somatic ageing. However, as research progresses we learn more about cellular processes and we begin to understand how the ageing process operates. In the meantime, several theories have been proposed in order to account for the observed data that have been collected in relation to cellular, organic and bodily changes that occur in old age and also in relation to the common diseases that are seen to occur very frequently with advancing years. The main theories of ageing are:

- Free radical theory
- Cross-link theory
- Immunologic theory
- Somatic mutation and errors theory
- Programmed ageing theory
- Popular theory

The theories of ageing attempt to account for the increased or decreased cellular activities and changes that give rise to metabolic errors due to slow repair processes, chromosomal aberrations or accumulation of waste products. As a result of all of these processes, there is an increased risk of degenerative and atrophic changes occurring in tissues and it is this fact that the theories have to take into account.

Free Radical Theory

Free radicals are highly reactive molecules that possess an extra negative electric charge (a free electron). This electric charge causes irreversible reactions which damage or alter structure and function of cell membranes and other cellular components (see Figure 4.37).

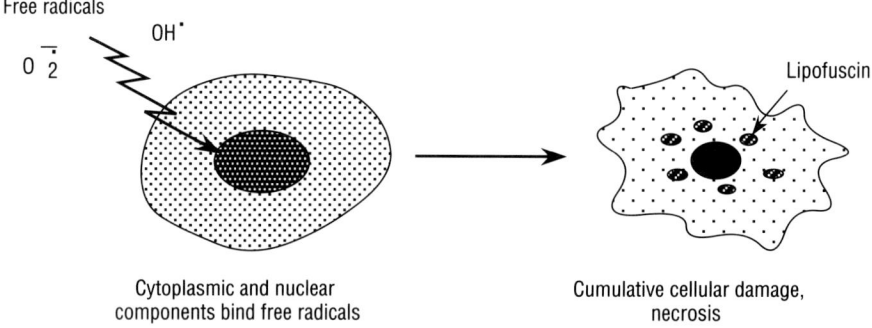

Free radicals

$O_2^{\cdot -}$ OH$^{\cdot}$

Lipofuscin

Cytoplasmic and nuclear
components bind free radicals

Cumulative cellular damage,
necrosis

Figure 4.37 *Free radical theory of ageing*

The **oxidation** of protein, fats and carbohydrates results in free radical formation and formation of unusable compounds, for example oxidation of polyunsaturated fats forms lipid peroxides that **crosslink** proteins, lipids, DNA and other cellular macromolecules. **Lipofuscin** is an ageing pigment which accumulates in body cells (but especially within cardiocytes, hepatocytes and neurones). This substance represents a complex insoluble lipoprotein that is a product of lipid and protein fragmentation from the peroxidation of the cell membrane components. Although the accumulation of lipofuscin in permanent and stable cells in the body is consistent with the free radical theory, it appears that this substance itself is very inert and exerts no toxic effects on cells.

If DNA in cells is **irradiated**, free radicals form and in addition aberrant cell growth and development occurs, both of which processes affect ageing. **Copper**, **iron** and **magnesium** ions increase free radical activity by catalytic activity in oxidation reactions. **Smog** and other environmental factors can increase free radical activity in the body. Some examples of these environmental factors are oxidation of petrol in cars, plastics by-products, drying linseed oil paints and atmospheric ozone.

As the body ages it appears that free radical formation and accumulation becomes too rapid for repair processes in the body cells. Free radicals greatly damage the cell membrane (oxygen diffusion affecting oxidizable lipids). Inside the cell, metallic ions, enzymes and cellular materials combine with O_2 to form free radicals. Oxygenation of water in the cell provides additional radicals and electrons. In arterial walls oxygen reacts with lipoprotein to form radicals.

Certain compounds in the body protect cellular elements from free radical damage and these compounds have generated a great deal of interest as they have the potential to be used in various anti-ageing preparations. **Vitamin E** and **co-enzyme Q** protect mitochondria (major sites of cellular oxidation) from free radical activity. **Vitamin E** acts as an antioxidant and in vitamin E deficiency increased lipid oxidation can be demonstrated in cells. Certain enzymes function to degrade, neutralize or detoxify free radicals that attack the cell membrane. These free radical scavengers are **superoxide dimutase**, **catalase**, and **glutathione peroxidase**. Dimutase activity increased in proportion to metabolic rate results in an increase in the life span of various species of laboratory animals. **Vitamins A, C** and **niacin** also act as free radical scavengers because they possess similar properties to **mercaptans**, which are free radical scavengers. Older people have decreased blood levels of vitamins A and C. Vitamins A and C (both easily oxidized vitamins) form free radical scavengers, binding and neutralizing free radicals in a manner similar to the antioxidant behaviour of vitamin E. Free radical scavengers can be introduced into the body by injection or dietary supplementation. Some of these compounds currently used in this manner are vitamin E, selenium, vitamin C and various food additives (BHT, BHA, etc.).

In summary, it may be said that there are both internal and external sources of free radicals which may contribute to ageing through combination with cellular components leading to cumulative damage in body cells. Such damaged cells are more prone to develop many different types of degenerative diseases and they are also less likely to function effectively in repair processes. All of these factors predispose to cellular and somatic death. Awareness of the importance of free radical damage to cells makes it possible to interfere with this process by attempting to monitor diet and limit the number of environmental factors that predispose to free radical formation.

Cross-link Theory

The cross-link theory ('collagen' theory) proposes that ageing occurs owing to chemical reactions in the cellular environment functioning to create strong bonds between molecular structures that should normally be separate. Cross-linking agents are numerous and diverse and impossible to avoid entirely through the diet and environment. **Aldehydes, minerals** (copper and magnesium), and **oxidizing fats** serve as biological reservoirs of cross-link inducing agents. Body chemicals which become cross-linked are lipids, proteins, nucleic acids and carbohydrates. Cross linkages form especially between saccharides which are important ingredients in collagen, elastin and DNA. Non-enzymatic glycosylation of proteins is another important mechanism of cross-link formation. Linkage can also be attributed to free radicals that function especially as agents that bind DNA molecules together. (see Figure 4.38).

Collagen (25–30% of body protein) is important in the connective tissues of the body. It is a major component of the matrix giving support to the tissues of the body and providing tissue strength. Collagen content is high in skin, tendons, bone, muscle, in blood vessels and the heart. Cross-linkage occurs most actively between the ages of 30–50 years and contributes to ageing of body tissues. During this time, normal collagen and elastin in connective tissue alter by cross-linkage formation. Newly formed collagen in a young individual shows little cross-linkage, but with ageing the collagen shows an increased number of cross-links in its structure. Ageing collagen becomes more insoluble, stable and rigid. Its molecules dehydrate and bond together as glycosylation reactions occur between adjacent strands. As water content of tissues also diminishes as a function of ageing, this produces a higher concentration of calcium, sodium and chloride both extra- and intracellularly. Calcium salt deposits form increasingly commonly with increasing age and are found throughout the body but especially in the cardiovascular system. Deposition of calcium in pericardium and endocardium, in the heart valves and in the major blood vessels is seen with many of the degenerative disorders of old age.

Elastin behaves in a similar way to collagen and is equally prone to cross-linkage. Elastin in youth is a highly elastic and resilient protein while in old age elastin is frayed, fragmented and brittle. Elastin binds calcium due to its molecular charges, and with the changes occurring in it with cross-linkage, more calcium ions are attracted to it, contributing to its brittleness and loss of elasticity. Cross-linkage of elastin and collagen is best illustrated in the skin during ageing. Skin in youth is smooth, soft, silky and firm, becoming drier, saggy and less elastic in old age. The cross-linking in skin is like the tanning of hides by chemicals to form tough leather. Elastin is important in elasticity (distensibility) and tissue mobility and thus cross-linking affects muscle contractions and any tissue pulsations.

Ageing of connective tissues by cross-linkage is important as it affects cell permeability, fibril flexibility of muscles and heart contractility. Tendons become dry and fibrous, teeth may loosen, arterial walls decline in tensile strength, and linings in the lungs and gastrointestinal tract decreased in efficiency. Passage of substances through vessel walls and intercellular spaces is also affected. Gases, nutrients, metabolites, antibodies and toxins are all involved as they must pass through connective tissue to reach blood vessels or to get to cells.

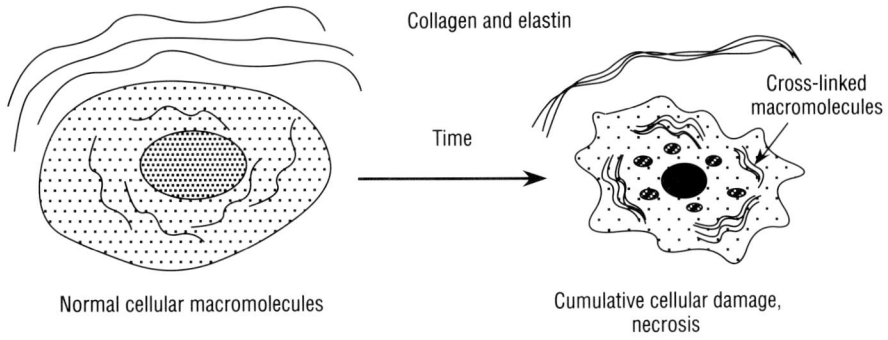

Figure 4.38 *The cross-link theory of ageing*

In experiments with rats it has been shown that restriction of intake of kilojoules (dietary restriction) increases life expectancy and decreases cross-linkage in protein and DNA. **Prednisolone** (a glucocorticoid used therapeutically as an antiallergic and anti-inflammatory agent) has been shown to decrease cross-link formation and prolong animal life. Chemicals known as **lathyrogens** inhibit cross-links forming in collagen, as does β-aminopropionitrile (BAPN) and penicillamine. It should be noted, however, that BAPN inhibits young collagen development. Hence, once again it seems that **diet** becomes important in contributing to the ageing process, and administration of 'anti-link' agents with other dietary modifications may be important in delaying the ageing process.

Immunological Theory

There is a demonstrated link between **autoimmune disease** and the ageing process. In autoimmunity, normal cells of the body are recognized as foreign or 'non-self' by immune system cells and are attacked by the immune system. Alternatively, there is impaired surveillance by immune system cells, allowing adverse immune reactions to occur or causing increased susceptibility to infections and malignant tumours. This results in the so-called **auto-aggression**. In the elderly there is an increased incidence of various forms of autoimmune reactions and autoimmune diseases.

In order to have normal immune function it is important to have balance between the B cells (B lymphocytes, humoral immunity) and T cells (T lymphocytes cell-mediated immunity). Imbalance of B and T cell activity gives rise to increased production of autoantibodies (antibodies which attack self components). Cytotoxic effects occur in host tissue when T lymphocytes are transferred to the peripheral lymphoid circulation. B and T cell imbalance results in compromise of the humoral mechanism resulting in decrease of the body's immune surveillance capability and causing hypersensitivities and the autoimmune phenomenon. Cell-mediated immune reactions mediated by T cells are responsible for hastening age-related changes attributed to autoimmune reactions, where the body is literally fighting against itself.

Sometimes **haptens** (small molecules, normally non-immunogenic, e.g. certain drugs in hypersensitive individuals) may combine with natural body components (for example, cell membranes) and result in an antigen (hapten–protein complex) that can be recognized by antibodies. This results in attack against the body's own proteins and other components.

Another possible mechanism of autoimmunity is release of sequestered antigen previously never exposed to the immune system. This may result from release of protein products normally not exposed to the immune system (e.g. from the lens of the eye following damage there as may occur in later life). Infection may result in release of abnormal proteins as an interaction between microbe and cell occurs. Or, in later life, there may be release of antibodies which have been previously suppressed in the immune system, which may result in autoimmunity (refer to Figure 4.39).

Tissue grafts have been shown to be rejected at a higher rate in older mice than in younger mice. There may be greater cell aberration occurring with age and cell self-regulation may be lacking. This may explain why wound healing and generation of healthy tissue seem to progress more slowly in the aged despite adequate diet, rest and care.

Antibodies or immunoglobulins are part of the humoral system. There is evidence that gammaglobulin, rheumatoid factor, antithyroid and anti-insulin antibody activity increases with age. Hence immune system dysfunction may be a cause of ageing and could explain onset of diabetes and rheumatoid arthritis exacerbations, and other conditions with a strong autoimmune component in older people.

Depletion of immune function may account for some other disorders seen with increasing frequency as an individual ages. Immunodeficiency consequences such as infection, auto-immunity and cancer may be the body's response to several types of events. In mice there are slow viruses which once passed on to newborn animals suppress normal immune function. Leukaemia viruses in mice induce a similar decline in immunity.

In old age there could be an age-related decline in the immune system function (as the function of all systems seems to decline with age) and age-dependent anatomical and physiological changes such as decreased secretions, dry skin and changes in collagen could add to disruption of defence mechanisms. There seems to be a concurrent decline in the immune system and increase in the autoimmune response. A decline in immunity would allow abnormal immune cells to surface or exert themselves. Decreased efficiency of the immune system certainly increases vulnerability to disease and malignancy.

Immune System, Ageing and Disease

Viruses and other antigens and their corresponding antibodies form antigen–antibody complexes. When antigen–antibody complexes lodge in specific body sites such as kidneys and arteries, factors injurious to the tissues are released and initiate deterioration of these tissues. This may contribute to ageing.

Autoimmune disorders and ageing may be correlated. Antigens found in bacteria, fungi, protozoa and many food constituents can induce cross-reactions with components present in the upper respiratory tract, gastrointestinal tract and genitourinary tract. Antigens may be kept from the general immune system by selective local immune mechanisms. There are shared characteristics between autoimmune disease and ageing. Both processes exhibit **lymphoid depletion** and **hypoplasia**, **thymic atrophy**, and increased plasma cells (antibody cells) in lymphoid organs. In the aged, **hypergammaglobulinaemia** is present and tests for auto-antibodies are often positive. Alloantigen response is also decreased (a process that requires B and T cell co-operation). Decline in immunity contributes to infections, autoimmunity and cancer.

Amyloidosis, cancer and adult-onset diabetes mellitus can be considered diseases of ageing emanating from immunodeficiencies or adverse immune reactions. In **amyloidosis** there are fibrillar deposits in various tissues of the body which consist of light chains of immunoglobulins. These are present in various organs of the aged individual. Islets of Langerhans in the pancreas show signs of amyloidosis and complement-fixing anti-insulin antibodies.

Cancer appears to be strongly influenced by immunodeficiencies (especially associated with immunosuppressant drugs). Autoimmune mechanisms contribute also to atherosclerosis, hypertension and thromboembolism. Cardiovascular disease, allergic angiitis and rheumatic heart disease are considered to be the result of immune system dysfunctions. Senile plaque found in ageing, degenerating brain tissue contains amyloid (e.g. Alzheimer's disease).

The immune system is regulated by an aggregate of genes on a single chromosome. This cluster of genes is called the major histocompatibility complex (MHC). Part of the responsibility of the MHC is the self–antiself recognition. The MHC type of a person seems to influence susceptibility to many diseases of ageing such as Alzheimer's disease.

In summary, immune responses are thought to effect age-related changes seen:

- when the immune system begins to decline in adulthood (this decline becoming more marked with increasing years);
- when thymic atrophy occurs, and possibly as soon as there is a decrease in the thymic hormone thymosin in the blood;
- when there is a significant increase in plasma cell activity;
- when circulating lymphocytes with an abnormal number of chromosomes are increased;
- when there is an increase in the immunoglobulins in the blood.

Various diseases may thus be linked to immune dysfunctions seen with ageing. It appears that immune system disorders are of two types, both predisposing to disease. One group is related to the degenerative changes occurring in immune system efficiency and are linked to reduced immunocompetency and decreased immunological surveillance (e.g. development of the various cancers seen in old age would relate to this). The other group of disorders relates to increased destruction of self components due to the development of autoimmune reactions and thus inappropriate immune responses would be responsible for the diseases (e.g. autoimmune thyroiditis). Selective alteration, replenishment or rejuvenation of the immune system are immuno-engineering challenges that will hopefully

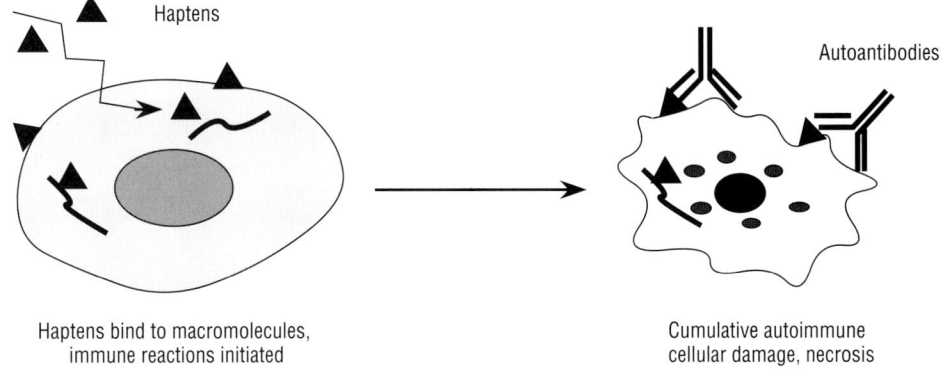

Haptens

Autoantibodies

Haptens bind to macromolecules,
immune reactions initiated

Cumulative autoimmune
cellular damage, necrosis

Figure 4.39 *The immunological theory of ageing*

control, moderate or eliminate effects of autoimmunity, immunodeficiencies and perhaps slow down the ageing process. In the future, genetic engineering and manipulation of the immune system may help maintain normal immune function in old age.

Somatic Mutation and Errors Theories

The somatic mutation theory suggests that cell by cell alteration of DNA by spontaneous hydrolysis, miscoding or irradiation occurs continuously during life. Cumulative effects of DNA mutations may thus occur and also evolve from spontaneous replication of errors. Subsequent replicated cells perpetuate the deleterious effects, which ultimately decrease cellular function and organ efficiency. All of these changes are more marked the older an individual is. Normal somatic cells may become aberrant through error or irradiation, permitting undefined life span and errant cell propagation. Similar behaviour is seen in cancer cell activity.

The errors theory expands the mutation theory to include cumulative mistakes in RNA synthesis, protein and enzyme synthesis. Each cell type has an explicit function in the body providing opportunity for numerous mutations.

In this context, it is interesting to note that some somatic cells are of the non-dividing type (permanent cells) and have a limited life span. These cells are not replaced when they become injured or when they die (heart, muscle, and brain cells). Thus there is a decreased functioning cell population in the tissues containing these permanent cells, leading to a decreased efficiency in the corresponding tissue with increasing age as more and more cells are lost.

The somatic mutation and errors theories are not widely accepted now as the sole cause of ageing processes but as they are thought to contribute to the cellular damage seen with increasing age, they have been incorporated into the other theories of ageing.

Programmed Ageing Theory

This concept of ageing depends on the postulated presence of a biological or genetic clock regulating an intrinsic cellular process, ultimately resulting in the 'winding down' of cellular activities at a certain time after birth. That is, it is an inborn clock within the cellular genetic material that determines ageing. Correlations with time of development, maturation and cessation of activity have been made between the beginning of menopause, thymic atrophy and various other body functions (refer to Figure 4.40).

Human cell culture studies have shown that *in vitro* human cells have a limited number of replications before cell death occurs. Human cells double 40 to 60 times *in vitro* before the ability to replicate is lost. There is gradual and sequential degeneration of cell culture which includes the following:

- An extension of time required for cell doubling.
- A progressive cessation of metabolic activity.
- An accumulation of cellular debris.
- A total degeneration of the cell culture.

Keeping the cells at subzero temperatures for long periods allows preservation of cells and subsequent extension of the duration of their existence. When thawed years later cells continued to double from the point of interruption and the total number of doublings remained constant. Embryonic cells undergo more doublings than adult cells. It is interesting to note that all such findings are difficult to extend from *in vitro* studies to *in vivo* observations and theories.

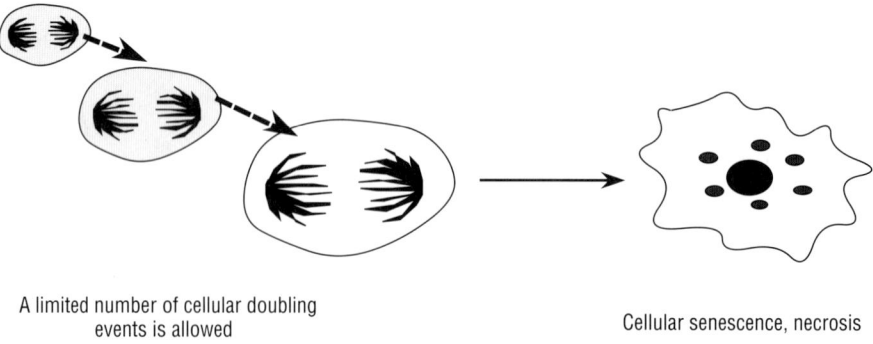

A limited number of cellular doubling events is allowed

Cellular senescence, necrosis

Figure 4.40 *The programmed cellular death theory of ageing*

Popular Theory

The **wear-and-tear theory** and the **stress-adaptation theory** attempt to describe the results of ageing and represent a combination of many of the features outlined in the theories previously considered. In the 'wear-and-tear' theory it is proposed that body structures and functions wear out or are overused or repeatedly injured with increasing years. Therefore, the longer an individual lives the more 'wear and tear' is seen accumulating in the tissues, causing the eventual downfall of the body as a whole. In the stress-adaptation theory it is proposed that effects from residual damage of stresses accumulate until the body no longer resists stress and dies. The stressors are internal and external, and may be physical, chemical, biological, psychological, social and environmental. The damage sustained by tissues as they are repeatedly injured in the various diseases that occur throughout life has a cumulative effect and is sufficient in the long term to produce death through an inability to respond effectively to further stresses that are placed upon the body (see Figure 4.41).

In both of these theories the inducing mechanisms of ageing are based on the gross changes that are observed in the ageing body. Thus, these theories depend on the other theories already considered for the reasons why the body becomes less resistant to wear and tear and stress adaptation in old age.

Revision Questions and Case Studies

Variations in Cell Growth

1. Write short notes on the following:
   (a) Physiological hypertrophy
   (b) Pathological atrophy
   (c) Hypoplasia
   (d) Metaplasia
2. Discuss the process of hyperplasia, distinguishing between physiological and pathological variants. Use examples in different tissues to illustrate your discussion.
3. State what variation of growth the following processes in tissue are examples of:
   (a) The enlarged breast of a woman who has just given birth
   (b) The shrinking thymus gland of a 30-year-old man
   (c) The biceps of a weight lifter who has commenced training
   (d) The heart of a 64-year-old man with systemic hypertension
   (e) The wasting of the body of a child with extreme malnutrition
   (f) A mobile, rubbery breast lump of a non-pregnant woman of 25 years

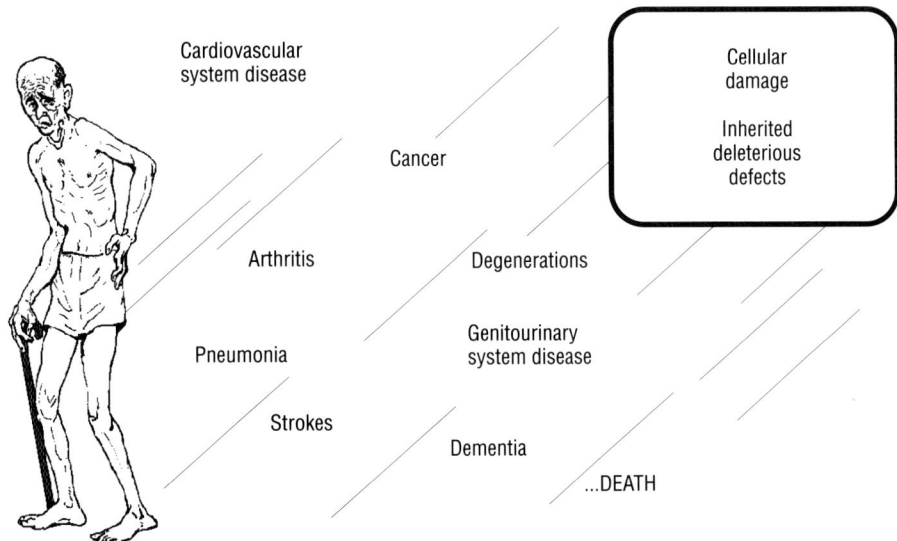

Figure 4.41 *Cellular changes occurring as a result of various insults predispose to the development of degenerative changes and the various diseases commonly observed in old age*

(g) The enlarged heart of an 18-year-old woman who is an Olympic swimmer

(h) The squamous epithelium lining the trachea of a man who has smoked for the last 20 years

(i) The bone marrow of a 12-year-old boy who underwent total body irradiation prior to a bone marrow transplant

(j) The shrinking uterus of a woman who has given birth

4. Atrophy in a tissue occurs by the process of apoptosis. What is the mechanism of this apoptotic process?

5. Define the word 'regeneration' and explain in your answer why tissues with a labile cell population may undergo regeneration while cells with a permanent cell population cannot.

6. What is a 'hamartoma'? Give two examples.

7. What is a 'choristoma'? Give two examples.

8. Distinguish between physiological and compensatory hyperplasia.

9. The uterus in pregnancy undergoes a substantial increase in size. What cells are responding to stimuli in this case and what variation(s) of growth of cells is (are) causing the change?

10. Distinguish between neuropathic atrophy and disuse atrophy.

11. Define the following terms:
    (a) Anencephaly
    (b) Cryptorchidism
    (c) Hydronephrosis
    (d) Meckel's diverticulum
    (e) Hypopituitarism

12. Give an example of a commonly encountered dysplasia and discuss the importance of this condition, indicating possible sequelae.

Case study 1. Mrs Hattie M., a 48-year-old Caucasian, nulliparous woman presents at her doctor's clinic, greatly distressed as she has discovered a breast lump. Upon palpation of the left breast, a mass, approximately 3 cm in diameter, is found in the left lower quadrant. The lump is of a firm and rubbery consistency, freely mobile, not attached to any underlying structures. The breast skin and nipple are normal and there is no pain of the breast, only some tenderness of the breast when the woman is menstruating. All other findings in the physical examination are within the normal range.

(a) What is the presumptive diagnosis?
(b) What advice would be given to the woman?

Case study 2. A 72-year-old South African Black male, resident in the United States for 20 years and in Australia for the past 8 years, presents with urinary frequency, dysuria, nocturia, dribbling of urine and failure to maintain a good stream of urine during micturition. He complains of 'feeling full all the time but even though the urge is there, he cannot pass a large volume of urine, therefore going to the toilet many times'. The man is married with two adult children. Physical examination reveals a blood pressure of 130/100 mmHg and he tells the examining chiropractor that he is on medication for his hypertension. Other values are normal.

(a) What is the presumptive diagnosis?
(b) How would the diagnosis be confirmed?
(c) What advice would you have given to the man?

Neoplasia and Metastasis

1. What is a neoplasm? Distinguish between neoplasia and hyperplasia. Mention in your discussion the histogenetic and clinical classification of tumours, the differences between benign and malignant neoplasms and the nomenclature of tumours.

2. Distinguish between benign and malignant neoplasms.

3. Discuss the various ways in which tumours are classified and named.

4. Write an essay on malignant neoplasms, indicating systems of nomenclature, properties, histological features, clinical behaviour and correlation with patient presentation.

5. Give an account of the spread of malignant tumours. Use examples of the various tumours occurring in the body to substantiate your discussion.

6. Why are secondary tumours more commonly found in some organs than others? Discuss.

7. What are the various tumour metastatic routes? Use specific examples of tumours to support your arguments.

8. Define the term 'anaplasia' and give an example of this process.

9. What occurs in the process of metastasis? Which tumours are likely to metastasize?

10. A benign tumour is usually defined as a 'non life threatening one'. Can a benign tumour ever cause death? If yes by what means?

11. Classify the following tumours into benign or malignant and epithelial or non-epithelial in origin:
    adenoma; carcinoma of the breast; lymphoma; haemangioma; fibroma; fibrosarcoma; keratoacanthoma; osteosarcoma; chondroma;

liposarcoma; malignant melanoma; hepatoma; 'warts'; glioma; meningioma; carcinoma of the stomach; 'lung cancer'; carcinoma of the colon; cystadenoma; leiomyoma; chondrosarcoma; basal cell carcinoma; leukoplakia; lipoma; teratoma of the ovary; papilloma; rhabdomyoma; adeno-carcinoma.

12. What is a 'teratoma'? Is this a benign or a malignant tumour? Explain.
13. Explain the term 'differentiation' in the context of neoplasia. Mention in your answer benign and malignant tumours, anaplasia, cellular mobility and metastasis.
14. Define the following terms:
    (a) Transcoelomic spread of tumours
    (b) Carcinomatosis peritonei
    (c) Retrograde dissemination of tumours
    (d) Malignant cachexia
    (e) Carcinomatosis

Case study 1. A 23-year-old Caucasian male model comes to your clinic complaining of a 'sore leg'. Upon examination of the legs you discover a dark spot on the back of the left lower leg. It is approximately 7 mm in diameter, dark brown in colour, flattened and has an irregular margin. Two smaller, 2 mm and 1 mm, similar lesions are found adjacent to it. On palpation you find that the large lesion is hard, tender and attached to the underlying tissues. There is no bleeding associated with it, but there is a small ulcer present in the centre of the large lesion. The man tells you that he was unaware that he had the lesion there. When the groin is examined you find that the both the left and right inguinal lymph nodes are swollen and firm. Upon questioning the man tells that he has lived nearly all his life in Surfer's Paradise and has been in Melbourne for the past year. He spends a lot of time on the beach and although he is fair he tells you that he 'tans easily and does not get sunburnt'.

(a) Explain the findings above.
(b) What is the presumptive diagnosis?
(c) What advice would you give the man?

Case study 2. A 73-year-old Caucasian male presents because of a severe, lower left limb pain and breathlessness. Although he has had generalized aches and pains in his bones for a year or so, the pain in the left leg has become bad enough to compromise his walking. He complains also of bifrontal headaches, poor hearing and tinnitus. There were no other neurological symptoms, his vision is unimpaired and he is on no medication. On examination, his left leg showed a hard swelling of the anterior half of the left tibia, the skin temperature elevated over the swelling. The swelling was not tender and the range of motion of knee and hip joints was full. His skull appeared enlarged and the response to Rinne's test was normal for both ears. Neither nystagmus nor vertigo was elicited by postural testing. The patient's blood pressure is recorded as 135/70 mmHg and his pulse as 110 beats per minute, irregular, with a pulse deficit of 15–20 beats. A soft ejection systolic murmur was audible in the fourth intercostal space. Blood tests showed urea being 10.4 mmol/L (N = 3.2–7.7 mmol/L), alkaline phosphatase 572 IU/L (N = 30–95 IU/L) and all other values within normal range. An ECG showed atrial fibrillation.

(a) What is the most likely cause of the generalized bone aches and pains that the patient has suffered from for about a year?
(b) What investigations need to be carried out to confirm the diagnosis?
(c) What is the most likely diagnosis of the tibial swelling and pain?
(d) What has predisposed to the development of the tibial 'swelling'?
(e) Explain the symptoms and signs referable to the cardiovascular system in the context of the man's disease.

Case study 3. A 56-year-old Aboriginal male farm worker presents at a community health centre with a sore throat which developed about a month ago. On questioning the man says that he has smoked about two packets of cigarettes a day for about 40 years and that he has been in good health all his life. He was given some antibiotics and was told to come back in 2 weeks. The man did not return until 2 months later, at which time he complained of an increase in tiredness and the onset of some right-sided chest pain, with a feeling of fullness in the right supraclavicular area. He was admitted to hospital and a chest X-ray revealed a right upper lobe lesion, 4.5 cm in diameter, with probable mediastinal adenopathy. A bone and brain scan were ordered.

(a) What is the diagnosis?
(b) Why were the brain and bone scans ordered?

After the brain and bone scans proved negative, the patient did not return to hospital until 2 weeks later, at which time he had developed more severe symptoms. His neck had become engorged, there was severe shortness of breath, marked swelling of the arms and distension of the thoracic and abdominal walls. **Superior vena caval obstruction** was diagnosed. This is a medical emergency and requires immediate attention!

(c) What is the most serious complication of this condition and what would the result be if the patient is not treated immediately?

(d) What is the treatment of this condition?

Case study 4. A 65-year-old Caucasian female and mother of two is admitted to hospital to be investigated for weight loss and generalized unwellness that she has experienced over the past 8 months. Her appetite has been poor, she has lost 10 kg (height is 166 cm, weight 48 kg) and her bowel motions are irregular with hard faeces. There was no abdominal pain, no rectal bleeding, no diarrhoea, no dyspepsia. There was no chest pain, no excessive sweating or heat intolerance and no depression. She has noticed hoarseness for some months, and also she is becoming alarmed as she is losing her hair. When she was examined the hoarseness was apparent but there was no throat abnormality nor lymphadenopathy. Her breasts were atrophic with no masses palpable in them. Her blood pressure was 135/75 mmHg, her pulse 80 beats per minute, no cardiac murmurs auscultated, the respiratory system normal. She had excessive facial and truncal hair and also temporal hair loss. The abdomen was normal with no masses palpated. A pelvic examination showed a firm mobile cervix, atrophic vaginitis and clitoral hypertrophy. Her haemoglobin was 10.2 g/dL (N = 12–16 g/dL); albumin 31 g/L (N = 35–55 g/L); alkaline phosphatase 102 IU/L (N = 30–95 IU/L); serum testosterone 3.1 mg/L (N = 3–19 ng/L); urinary ketosteroids 55 mg/24 h (N = 4–17 mg/24 h); all other findings within normal values.

(a) Explain the clinical findings in relation to the biochemical findings.

(b) What is the most likely diagnosis?

(c) What can cause a similar presentation (differential diagnosis)?

(d) What further test should be performed in this case?

(e) What is the treatment?

(f) What is the prognosis?

Carcinogenesis

1. Discuss the process of carcinogenesis, with special reference to aetiological and pathogenetic factors, both endogenous and exogenous.

2. What are oncogenes? How may oncogenes bring about the formation of a neoplasm in tissue?

3. Identify the type of carcinogen (i.e. physical, chemical or biological) that each of these following examples represents:

(a) Ultraviolet radiation

(b) Beta-naphthylamine

(c) Hepatitis B virus

(d) Blue asbestos fibres

(e) Aflatoxin (*Aspergillus flavus* toxin)

(f) Sodium nitrite

(g) Rous sarcoma virus

(h) X-rays

(i) Radium

(j) Vinyl chloride

4. Write notes on the following topics:

(a) Chemical carcinogens

(b) Oncogenes

(c) Physical carcinogenic agents

(d) Promoters of carcinogenesis and the multi-step theory.

5. What is a co-carcinogen? Give an example of a co-carcinogen important in the causation of human neoplasms.

6. What carcinogen(s) have the following tumours been associated with?

(a) Hepatocarcinoma

(b) Osteosarcoma

(c) Carcinoma of the bronchus

(d) Mesothelioma of the pleura

(e) Leukaemia

(f) Carcinoma of the urinary bladder

(g) Carcinoma of the oral cavity

(h) Malignant melanoma of the skin

(i) Colorectal carcinoma

(j) Carcinoma of the stomach

7. Discuss factors important in the causation of any three human cancers that have been associated with chemical carcinogens. What steps may be taken in the prevention of these cancers?

8. How may viruses bring about malignant transformation in a cell?

9. What is a mutation? What types of mutations do you know of? How do carcinogens bring about mutations in cells?

10. Discuss the endogenous factors important in carcinogenesis. Give examples of human tumours in order to substantiate your discussion.

Case study 1. A 66-year-old Caucasian male has been diagnosed as suffering from advanced carcinomatosis. The history of the patient shows that he was employed for all his working life as a worker in a dye manufacturing plant. He has smoked about 25 cigarettes a day for the past 46 years. The man has been a keen swimmer and says with pride that he rarely missed an opportunity to go the beach and take in the sun and surf (something he does often as he lives in Brisbane). Asked about his general health in the past he mentions some respiratory infections and problems with his bowel but he hastens to add that there have been no serious health problems previously. When he is questioned about his diet he says that he eats 'hearty meals, meat and vegies'. The man drinks about a litre of beer a day and he has not shown any evidence of liver disease in the past. The man has recently moved house as his previous home had to be vacated as asbestos sheeting was used extensively for insulation purposes.

(a) Outline the various carcinogenic agents that the man may have been exposed to during his life and indicate what class they belong to.
(b) List the various tumours that the man may have developed and which have caused the generalized carcinomatosis.
(c) What do you know of the synergistic effects of carcinogens? Give an example of such effects from this case study.

Case study 2. A 45-year-old Caucasian woman, Mrs Anna G., has been diagnosed with breast cancer. The woman's mother died 15 years ago from breast cancer. Mrs G. has an only daughter aged 6 years. A study of the oestrogen receptors on the woman's breast tissue has shown an increased number of receptors on the glandular cells of the breast and the tumour cells. The tumour in the woman's breast, measuring 2.5 cm in diameter, is removed and the axillary lymph nodes (also removed) are clear of cancer cells. The woman also has radiotherapy and chemotherapy treatment.

(a) What, on average, is an Australian woman's chance of developing breast cancer?
(b) What predisposing factors are associated with breast cancer?
(c) What is Mrs G.'s daughter's chance of developing breast cancer?
(d) What is the prognosis for Mrs G.?

Growth Disorders Crossword

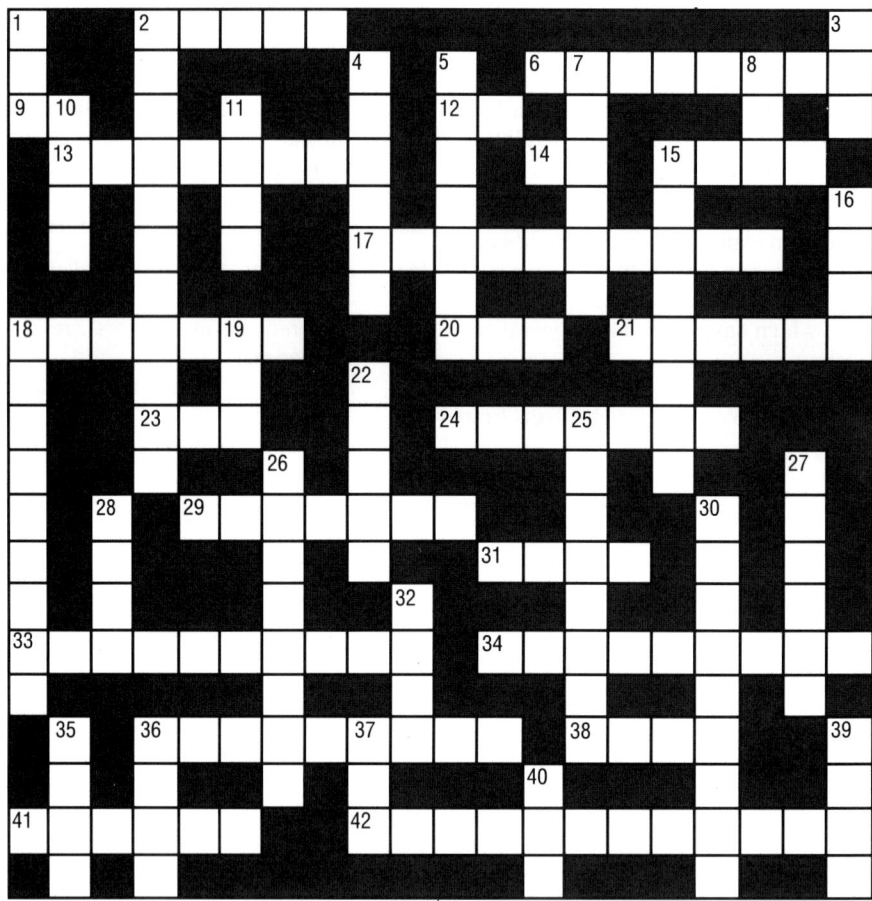

CLUES

ACROSS

2. Organ undergoing hypertrophy in hypertension (5).
6. The study of neoplasms (8).
9. Element hypothesized to be involved in the causation of Alzheimer's disease (2).
12. Element increasing free radical activity by catalyzing oxidation (2).
13. Common type of pathological hyperplasia in the breast of women aged between 35–45 years (8).
14. Element increasing free radical activity by catalyzing oxidation (2).
15. 'Cancer' literally means this (4).
17. The yellow pigment, commonly called the 'wear and tear' pigment that accumulates in cells with old age (10).

18. Reduction in the size of an organ due to a decrease in cell size or cell number (7).
20. An important factor in the development of cancers (3).
21. This type of tumour is usually non life threatening (6).
23. The virus causing warts (1, 1, 1).
24. A sudden cessation of growth, the affected organ never reaching its full size or extent (7).
29. A malignant tumour of connective tissue origin (7).
31. A very common site for secondary tumours to occur (4).
33. The process of physiological atrophy (10).
34. A premalignant disorder of differentiation where

the cells look bizarre, are arranged abnormally and their function is compromised (9).

36. A disorder of growth caused by abnormal or defective metabolism and nutrition (9).
38. A carcinogen associated with scrotal carcinoma as shown by Percival Pott in 1775 (4).
41. Malignant neoplasms tend to _ _ _ _ _ _ to distant parts of the body (6).
42. Focal masses of normal cells in abnormal situations in the body (e.g. masses of endometriosis) (12).

DOWN

1. The genetic material of cells (1, 1, 1).
2. Increase in tissue size due to increase in cell size (11).
3. Retinoblastoma occurs in this site (3).
4. This tissue undergoes pure hypertrophy (6).
5. Condition of normal tissue in an abnormal site (7).
7. A typical hamartoma (= a mole) (6).
8. Suffix denoting a benign tumour (3).
10. This antibody is involved in thyrotoxicosis (1, 1, 1, 1).
11. The third commonest site for metastasis (4).
15. An example of generalized atrophy seen in cancer (8).
16. Tissue prone to carcinogenesis induced by UV light (4).
18. Mechanism of cell number reduction in atrophy (9).
19. Virus associated with carcinoma of the cervix (1, 1, 1).
22. This organ is the site of the second commonest cancer in our community (5).
25. Complete failure of development of an organ leading to its absence at birth (8).
26. The commonest site of hyperplasia in old men (8).
27. Common site of cancer in sexually active women (6).
28. Virus causing a certain type of human leukaemia (1, 1, 1, 1).
30. A focal overgrowth of normal cells in a site that normally contains a fewer number of these cells (9).
32. The standard system of nomenclature of pathology (1, 1, 1, 1).
35. Inhibitor of cross-link formation in collagen; β-aminopropionitrile (4).
36. Important factor in the causation of many cancers (4).
37. The abbreviation for oncogene (3).
39. A physical carcinogenic agent (4).
40. The cause of AIDS (1, 1, 1).

Further Reading

Variations in Cell Growth, Neoplasia and Metastasis

De Wys WD. 'Pathophysiology of Cancer Cachexia.' *Cancer Res* 1982; **42**(Suppl): 721s.

Edelson RL. 'Light Activated Drugs.' *Sci Am* 1988; August: 50.

Feldman M, Eisenbach L. 'What Makes a Tumour Cell Metastatic?' *Sci Am* 1988; November: 40.

Folkman J. 'Tumor Angiogenesis.' *Adv Cancer Res* 1985; **43**: 175.

Folkman J, Klagsbrun M. 'Angiogenic Factors.' *Science* 1987; **325**: 442.

International Union Against Cancer. *TNM Classification of Malignant Tumors*, 1968; Geneva.

Kartner N, Ling V. 'Multidrug Resistance in Cancer.' *Sci Am* 1989; March: 26.

Liotta LA. 'Tumor Invasion and Metastasis.' *Cancer Res* 1986; **46**: 1.

Liotta LA, Steeg PS, Stetler-Stevenson WG. 'Cancer Metastasis and Angiogenesis: An Imbalance of Positive and Negative Regulation.' *Cell* 1991; **64**: 327.

Lugo M, Putong PB. 'Metaplasia.' *Arch Pathol Lab Med* 1984; **108**: 185.

Mackay B, Silva EG. 'Diagnostic Electron Microscopy in Oncology.' *Pathol Annu* 1980; **15**(2): 241.

Nowell PC. 'Mechanisms of Tumour Progression.' *Cancer Res* 1986; **46**: 2203.

Odell WD, Wolfsen AR. 'Humoral Syndromes Associated with Cancer.' *Annu Rev Med* 1978; **29**: 379.

Pennica D, Nedwin GE, Hayflick JS, *et al.* 'Human Tumour Necrosis Factor: Precursor Structure, Expression and Homology to Lymphotoxin.' *Nature* 1984; **312**: 724.

Roos E. 'Cellular Adhesion, Invasion and Metastasis.' *Biochem Biophys Acta* 1984; **738**: 263.

Rosenberg SA. 'Combined Modality Therapy of Cancer: What is it and When Does it Work?' *N Eng J Med* 1985; **312**: 1512.

Rosenberg SA. 'Lymphokine-activated Killer Cells: A New Approach to Immunotherapy of Cancer.' *J Natl Cancer Inst* 1985; **75**: 595.

Rosenberg SA. 'Adoptive Immunotherapy for Cancer.' *Sci Am* 1990; May: 34.

Sobel ME. 'Metastasis Suppressor Genes.' *J Nat Cancer Inst* 1990; **82**: 267.

Tanner JM (ed.). 'Control of Growth.' *Br Med Bull* 1981; **37**: 207.

Theologides A. 'Cancer Cachexia.' *Cancer* 1979; **43**: 2004.

Wallach DFH. 'Membrane Abnormalities of Tumor Cells.' *Prog Exp Tumor Res* 1978; **22**: 1.

Wright NA. 'Cell Proliferation in Health and Disease.' *Rec Adv Histopathol* 1984; **12**: 17.

Carcinogenesis

Anisimov VN. 'Carcinogenesis and Aging.' *Adv Cancer Res* 1983; **40**: 365.

Arends MJ, Wyllie AH, Bird CC. 'Papilloma Virus and Human Cancer.' *Human Pathol* 1990; **21**: 686.

Bishop JM. 'Cellular Oncogenes and Retroviruses.' *Annu Rev Biochem* 1983; **52**: 301

Bishop JM. 'The Molecular Genetics of Cancer.' *Science* 1987; **235**: 305.

Borek C. 'Radiation Oncogenesis in Cell Culture.' *Adv Cancer Res* 1982; **37**: 159.

Brookes P (ed.) 'Chemical Carcinogenesis.' *Br Med Bull* 1980; **36:** 1.

Burch PRJ. 'Pathology, Inference and Carcinogenesis.' *Pathol Annu* 1980; **15**(2): 21.

Comings DE. 'A General Theory of Carcinogenesis.' *Proc Natl Acad Sci USA* 1973; **70**: 2324.

Dausch JG, Nixon DW. 'Garlic: A Review of its Relationship to Malignant Disease.' *Prevent Med* 1990; **19**: 346.

Doherty PC, Knowles BB, Wettstein PJ. 'Immunological Surveillance of Tumors.' *Adv Cancer Res* 1985; **42**: 1.

Fearon ER, Vogelstein B. 'A Genetic Model of Colorectal Tumorigenesis.' *Cell* 1990; **61**: 759.

Hecker E, *et al. Cocarcinogenesis and Biological Effects of Tumor Promoters*, 1982; Raven Press, New York.

Hursting SD, Thornquist M, Henderson M. 'Types of Dietary Fat and the Incidence of Cancer at Five Sites.' *Prevent Med* 1990; **19**: 242.

Jarrett WFH. 'Papillomaviruses and Cancer.' *Rec Adv Histopathol* 1981; **11**: 35.

Jose DG. 'Virus-Associated Malignant Disease in Animals and Man.' *Aust NZ J Med* 1978; **8**: 195.

Karwinski B, Svendsen E, Hartveit F. 'Changes in the Cancer Spectrum at Autopsy: 1975–1984.' *J Path* 1989; **157**: 117.

Klinken SP. 'How Retroviruses Affect Haemopoietic Cells.' *Today's Life Sci* 1990; **2**(7): 28.

Knudson AG. 'Hereditary Cancers in Man.' *Cancer Invest* 1983; **1**: 187.

Kontiris TG. 'The Emerging Genetics of Human Cancer.' *N Eng J Med* 1983; **309**: 404.

Marshall CJ. 'Tumour Suppressor Genes.' *Cell* 1991; **64**: 313.

Rapp F. 'The Challenge of Herpesviruses.' *Cancer Res* 1984; **44**: 1309.

Spandidos DA, Anderson MLM. 'Oncogenes and Oncosuppressor Genes: Their Involvement in Cancer.' *J Path* 1989; **157**: 1.

Varmus HE. 'Viruses, Genes and Cancer.' *Cancer* 1985; **55**: 2324.

Wands JR, Blum HE. 'Primary Hepatocellular Carcinoma.' *New Eng J Med* 1991; **325**: 729.

Weinberg RA. 'The Action of Oncogenes in the Cytoplasm and Nucleus.' *Science* 1985; **230**: 770.

Weinberg RA. 'Finding the Anti-Oncogene.' *Sci Am* 1988; September: 34.

Weinberg RA. 'A Short Guide to Oncogenes and Tumor Suppressor Genes.' *J NIH Res* 1991; **3**: 45.

Ageing

Anisimov VN. 'Carcinogenesis and Aging.' *Adv Cancer Res* 1983; **40**: 365.

Beard K, *et al.* 'Management of Elderly Patients with Sustained Hypertension.' *Br Med J* 1992; **304**: 412.

Chipman JK. 'Mechanisms of Cell Toxicity.' *Curr Opin Cell Biol* 1989; **1**: 231.

Coni N, Davison W, Webster S. *Ageing: The Facts*, 1986; Oxford University Press, Oxford.

Dean R, Simpson J. 'Free Radicals: The Good the Bad...' *Today's Life Sci* 1989; **1**(3): 28.

Fairweather DS, Evans JG. 'Aging.' In Cohen RD, *et al.* (eds) *The Metabolic and Molecular Basis of Acquired Disease*, 1990; Bailliére Tindall, London.

Finch CE, Schneider EL (eds). *Handbook of the Biology of Ageing*, second edition, 1985; Van Nostrand Reinhold Company, New York.

Gleckman RA, Gantz NM (eds). *Infections in the Elderly*, 1983; Little Brown and Company, Boston.

Holliday R. 'Towards a Biological Understanding of the Ageing Process.' *Persp Biol Med* 1988; **32**: 109.

Mack P, Michaelis J, Moss B, *et al.* 'The Use of Peptides as Therapeutics and Vaccines.' *Aust Biotech* 1991; **1**(3): 160.

Mulligan T, Katz PG. 'Why Aged Men Become Impotent.' *Arch Int Med* 1989; **149**: 1365.

Olshansky SJ, *et al.* 'In Search of Methuselah: Estimating the Upper Limits of Human Longevity.' *Science* 1990; **250**: 634.

Overmyer RH. 'Quality of Life in the Elderly may Improve with Human Growth Hormone.' *Mod Med* 1992; January: 48.

Robine JM, Ritchie K. 'Healthy Life Expectancy: Evaluation of Global Indicator of Change in Population Health.' *Br Med J* 1991; **302**: 457.

Schimmel EM. 'The Hazards of Hospitalization.' *Ann Intern Med* 1964; **60**: 100.

Song M. 'Environment and Skin Ageing.' In Krieps R (ed.) *Environment and Health: A Holistic Approach*, 1989; Averbury, Aldershot.

Stykowski PA, *et al.* 'Changes in Risk Factors and the Decline in Mortality from Cardiovascular Disease Framingham Heart Study.' *New Engl J M* 1990; **322**: 1635.

5

Immunopathology

The immune system is the body's means of protecting itself against invasion by pathogenic micro-organisms and foreign cells that may find their way into the tissues. It is a highly specific and complex system capable of mounting specialized responses and retaining in memory a record of previous substances that it has responded to, thus protecting the body during subsequent attacks of organisms that it has encountered before.

It is often described as a 'two-edged sword', which although normally functioning to protect the tissues of the body can also turn against the body causing damage to the tissues it was meant to protect. Manifestations of this undesirable attack of normal tissues by the immune system are considered in immunopathology. Hypersensitivities (allergic reactions) and autoimmune diseases are examples of such diseases. Immunopathology also concerns itself with abnormalities of the immune system that prevent it from functioning normally. Such deficiencies in immunity include the important disease AIDS.

In the last few years the knowledge of normal immune mechanisms and immunopathology states has increased dramatically. Many of the diseases that were considered 40 years ago to be completely idiopathic are now known to have an autoimmune basis. It is not unlikely that many of the diseases that we still know little about may have an important autoimmune component in their pathogenesis.

Immunopathology is a complex subject and knowledge in this field is rapidly expanding. Immunological mechanisms are involved in our defence against infection by micro-organisms and in maintaining a resistance or 'immunity' against re-infection following recovery from infectious disease. Immunopathology is concerned with certain aberrations and adverse reactions occurring in the immune response, examples of which are organ-graft rejection, immunodeficiency states, hypersensitivities and autoimmune diseases.

The Normal Immune System

There are lymphocytes of various types in the body

whose function is dependent on and/or regulated by macrophages. Immunocompetent cells are broadly divided into T lymphocytes and B lymphocytes. The former are concerned with **cell-mediated responses** in which the immune reaction involves specific lymphocytes directly taking part in body defences; the latter differentiate into plasma cells which secrete **antibodies** (immunoglobulins) which are specific proteins. Antibodies react with **antigens**, macromolecules which are foreign, harmful or potentially harmful. The secretion of antibodies by plasma cells is known as the **humoral response.** Most immune responses involve both antibodies and cell-mediated mechanisms, either of which may predominate.

Characteristics of the immune response are:

- ability to recognize 'self' and 'non-self' and react only to foreign materials;
- specificity;
- ability to 'remember' antigens to which there has been previous exposure;
- increasingly active and rapid response on re-exposure to an antigen.

B Lymphocytes

They are so called because in birds their differentiation is dependent on a lymphoid organ, the Bursa of Fabricius. In humans similar differentiation probably occurs in the bone marrow. B lymphocytes have a surface coating on their cell membranes of a large immunoglobulin, IgM, with the smaller immunoglobulin, IgD, also present in small quantities. This membrane-bound immunoglobulin is capable of reacting with a specific antigen. When thus stimulated a **single B cell** becomes activated and divides to form a **clone** of cells all of which are derived from that single precursor cell. These differentiate into a clone of **plasma cells** each of which will secrete specific antibodies which interact only with the antigen that initiated the process. This response of B lymphocytes and the resulting antibody synthesis is modulated and assisted by macrophages and T lymphocytes.

Plasma cells

Plasma cells are the differentiated clonal products of B lymphocyte activation by an antigen. They secrete antibodies. They have a large volume of cytoplasm rich in rough endoplasmic reticulum. The nucleus is placed eccentrically with chromatin in dense clumps about the nuclear membrane, having a 'clock-face' or 'cartwheel' appearance. Malignant change in plasma cells results in the disease **multiple myeloma**. In this condition the malignant cells produce large quantities of abnormal antibodies which are found in the plasma body fluids and urine.

T Lymphocytes

These cells are dependent on the thymus for maturation and acquisition of their specific functional properties. With age, the thymus undergoes involution, and T cell function declines. T cells form the majority of circulating lymphocytes. T cells have surface receptors for, and are activated by, antigens. Several subgroups of T cells exist and these may be recognized serologically through the demonstration of certain specific proteins on their plasma membranes. Important subgroups of T cells are as follows.

Helper T cells, which secrete soluble messenger substances which interact with B cells to enhance antibody production to most antigens, make other T cells better able to react with antigens and also convey messages to other immune cells. These are the cells that 'turn on' the immune response.

Suppressor T cells interact with B cells to inhibit antibody production, particularly to the host's own proteins. Impaired suppressor T cell function is associated with autoimmune disease. Suppressor T cells 'turn off' the immune response.

Cytotoxic T cells can kill target cells to which they are activated through direct contact which inflicts lethal cell membrane damage. These cells destroy tumour cells and virally infected cells.

Delayed-type hypersensitivity T cells are important in some allergic reactions. Their normal function is to perpetuate immune responses against an antigen that persists in the body and is not easily inactivated or destroyed.

Macrophages

The importance of macrophages in acute and chronic inflammation has already been covered. In immunity these cells have numerous roles, which include:

- regulation of T and B lymphocyte proliferation by secretion of monokines (soluble regulatory proteins);
- uptake and processing of antigens, and transfer to lymphocytes;
- direct participation in cell-mediated reactions;
- production of complement components;
- phagocytosis and destruction of pathogens;

- secretion of factors that promote or inhibit replication of many cells;
- secretion of neutrophil chemotactic factor.

Normal macrophage function is essential for normal immune system function as can be seen from the various activities of these cells.

Complement

Complement comprises a series of plasma proteins, most of which are produced by macrophages. It is triggered, amongst other things, by antigen–antibody complexes and plasmin. Complement produces a cascade of reactions which brings about membrane damage resulting in cell death (e.g. of bacteria), chemotaxis of neutrophils, formation of kinins, which help to mediate the vascular responses in acute inflammation, and anaphylatoxin, which produces reactions similar to acute allergic anaphylaxis. Also, some products of the complement cascade are opsonic (they bind to particles such as bacteria, making them more amenable to phagocytosis).

The Nature of the Immune Response

Most **antigens** are large molecules with molecular weights between 10 000 and 100 000 or more and are defined as substances which activate the immune response, either the humoral immunity (dependent on antibody production) or the cellular immunity (dependent on activation of specific antigen-reactive cells, the lymphocytes and macrophages). When these substances enter the tissues they stimulate the immune response. Usually both cellular and humoral immunity occur together, but with a specific type of antigen, one or other of these responses may predominate. For example, in a pneumonia caused by *Streptococcus pneumoniae* it is mainly phagocytosis and humoral immunity that brings the infection under control. In tuberculosis caused by *Mycobacterium tuberculosis* it is mainly the cell-mediated mechanism of immunity that is activated. Micro-organisms may contain many different antigenic components on their surface and infection with a single type of bacterium may give rise to an immune response in which many different kinds of antibody are produced and many different clones of T cells are involved, each specific for a particular antigenic determinant.

Haptens are small molecules (e.g. penicillin) which are not antigenic themselves but in certain individuals can bind to a non-antigenic protein carrier and this combination induces an antibody response specific for the hapten. Haptens can also link to each other and this large combination then stimulates an antibody response. Haptens may link to host proteins and the resultant hapten–body protein complex may stimulate an immune response against the body's own protein, resulting in an autoimmune disease. Penicillin allergy as it occurs in some people is an example of this type of reaction.

Antibody production is complex. The antigen is ingested by macrophages and helper T lymphocytes bind to these macrophages. A specific B lymphocyte then binds to the T cells and under the stimulus of the antigen the B cell is activated to produce a clone of antibody-producing plasma cells. In the initial exposure IgM is produced after a definite lag period, reaches a peak and declines after usually 1–2 months. In subsequent responses IgG is produced after a short latent period, rapidly rises to a very high serum level and persists for years.

Cell-mediated immunity depends on T cells which have been activated by antigen which has been ingested by macrophages. These lymphocytes produce soluble substances (lymphokines) which include **interferon**. Lymphokines attract other lymphocytes, macrophages and neutrophils to the attack. Some T cells are cytotoxic and induce lethal cell membrane damage on target cells through direct contact. Macrophages may also be rendered cytotoxic through the action of certain lymphokines.

Immune Deficiency States

Immune deficiency diseases (immunodeficiencies) are states in which the normal function of the immune system is lacking in some way and thus the body is more susceptible to all kinds of infections. Generally, there exists a great variety of such states and the degree of severity is greatly variable, in some people manifesting as a slightly greater susceptibility to some infections while in others manifesting as widespread, overwhelming, fatal infections. Immunodeficiency may be primary or secondary. Primary immunodeficiency is generally seen congenitally and presents in the newborn or the infant with deficiencies in T cell, B cell or both T cell and B cell function. Secondary immunodeficiency exists in conjunction with and often as a consequence of other disease states and generally appears later in life, being much more common in adults.

Primary Immunodeficiency

Agammaglobulinaemia

This is also known as X-linked infantile agammaglobulinaemia or as Bruton's disease. In the disorder there are no detectable B cells or their differentiated form the plasma cells in the body. Hence, no antibodies at all are produced and none are found in the body fluids. These children still possess T cells, however, and their cell-mediated immune responses are functional and normal. Therefore, these children are susceptible to most bacterial infections while they are protected from viral, fungal and protozoal infections by their T cells.

The affected children (usually male, as the disease is X-linked) are protected by maternal IgG antibody until they are about 5–6 months of age. Following this period, as the maternal antibody levels rapidly fall the infants develop recurrent bacterial infections, especially of the respiratory tract, to which they develop no humoral immunity. In addition to the pulmonary system, infections develop on the skin and in the sinuses, ears, eyes and brain.

Common bacterial causes of these very serious infections in such babies are: *Streptococcus pneumoniae*, *Streptococcus pyogenes*, *Haemophilus influenzae*, *Neisseria meningitidis* and *Pseudomonas aeruginosa*. The infections are treated with antibiotics and the children are protected by injections of gamma globulins purified from pooled, donated human blood. However, the overall incidence of bacterial infections is very high and the recurrent infections cause much distress and tissue damage, generally greatly reducing the life expectancy of these individuals.

Congenital Thymic Aplasia

This disorder is also known as the Di-George syndrome and is a very rare congenital anomaly in which the third and fourth pharyngeal pouches fail to develop embryonically, thus leading to congenital absence of the thymus and parathyroid glands. If the neonate survives the hypocalcaemia mediated by the absence of normal parathyroid function, it is observed that there is total absence of cell-mediated immunity. There is considerable risk of viral, fungal and protozoal infections becoming systemic and overwhelming, and there is a great risk of very serious tuberculous infections. The susceptibility to bacterial infections is slightly increased due to the absence of normal helper T cell function which is important in antibody synthesis.

These children suffer commonly from very serious viral respiratory infections such as measles, and early death is often the outcome of childhood infections such as chicken pox, respiratory syncytial virus infection, mumps, etc. Herpes virus infections, tuberculosis and atypical mycobacterioses are also very common. *Candida albicans* infections may become very serious and systemic (candidaemia) and infections of the brain with *Toxoplasma gondii*, *Cryptococcus neoformans* and Herpes virus are very common causes of death. Treatment of these children is very difficult and antimicrobial drugs with interferon injections and prevention of infections is the only means available.

Combined Immunodeficiency

This disorder was formerly called Swiss-type immunodeficiency. In this extremely rare disorder there is a congenital lack of lymphocyte stem cell precursors in the bone marrow, the affected individuals showing no T cells or B cells. Hence, a combined immunodeficiency results, and no humoral or cell-mediated immunity is observed. The affected babies are susceptible to all infections, due to all types of microbes. The non-specific host defences are insufficient to prevent overwhelming, fatal infections developing in the first few months of life.

In order for these children to survive they must be placed in sterile rooms where micro-organisms are excluded and all the material they come into contact with is sterilized. There is some hope of the treatment of this disorder by bone marrow transplants, but such procedures are limited by the closeness of matching between the donor and recipient marrow tissue type and also by the graft versus host response. In this latter case, when functional immune cells are transplanted from a donor to a recipient and the major histocompatibility complex regions are not matched, the donated cells will start to mount an immune response against the recipient's tissues, which they recognize as 'foreign' and 'non-self', the immune cells having come from another individual. In order to circumvent the mechanisms that lead to this response close matching between donor and recipient is required and to this end bone marrow banks are now in existence in many parts of the world. Normal healthy donors have a minor operation where a small portion of their bone marrow is removed and frozen, the tissue type having been recorded. When there is a need for this sample, it is thawed and transplanted into the awaiting recipient.

Secondary Immunodeficiency

Miscellaneous Secondary Immunodeficiencies

Many disease states in the body are associated with an attendant secondary immunodeficiency which is generally not as severe as that seen in the primary immunodeficiency states.

Ageing. It is known that many elderly people suffer from recurrent infections, which are associated with their increasing years, having previously had a normal immune response. This secondary immunodeficiency is often attributed to atrophy of the thymus gland which begins in young adulthood and progresses as the individual becomes older. There is a measurable decreased T cell function as the thymus involutes to a tiny remnant in old age. The decreased efficiency of the immune system in old age may have a more complex aetiology and may be linked to atrophy of other tissues, decreased cellular mobility and mitotic activity, accumulated effects of environmental toxins and the increasing susceptibility of the body due to the breakdown of the non-specific defences to infection.

Infections. Infection with some microbes greatly decreases the immune response and such infections may be followed by secondary infections. A typical example is infection with the influenza virus which so suppresses immunity that a variety of secondary bacterial infections also develops in the respiratory system. This explains the misnomer of *Haemophilus influenzae*. The early bacteriologists searching for the cause of influenza isolated *Haemophilus influenzae* from nearly every case of influenza that they took specimens from, thus linking this micro-organism with influenza. Of course the *Haemophilus* was only a secondary bacterial infection in the disease which is caused by the influenza virus. The mechanisms via which this secondary immunodeficiency is produced are not clear.

Neoplasms. Some malignant tumours are associated with secondary immunodeficiency. This is especially the case with tumours that affect the thymus, bone marrow or lymph nodes, all of which are very important organs in the immune response. Thymomata are thymus gland tumours which are often associated with a T cell deficiency. Hodgkin's disease is another malignancy in which decreased T cell function may be seen. In multiple myeloma, a tumour of plasma cells, decreased humoral immunity is observed. Leukaemia generally leads to secondary immunodeficiency as do multiple, secondary malignant tumours in the bone marrow.

Immunosuppressive drugs. In certain cases the administration of some drugs leads to a secondary immunodeficiency which is seen as a hypersensitivity reaction to the drug and is reversible on cessation of administration of the drug. Such reactions are not common and are seen in only allergic individuals. In other cases the administration of drugs is meant to produce an immunodepressed state. Immunosuppressive drugs such as steroids and azathioprine are used to depress the immune response in the recipients of transplanted hearts and kidneys and therefore minimize the risk of graft rejection. However, these individuals are more likely to then develop various infections and must be carefully monitored. Generally, the cell-mediated immune response is suppressed, as this is the most important in graft rejection, and the patients are more likely to develop viral and fungal infections rather than bacterial infections.

Effects of Radiation. Patients who have received extensive radiation treatment for malignant tumours or people who have been exposed to radioactivity following atom bomb blasts and nuclear accidents may show a secondary immunodeficiency due to destruction of the stem cells in their bone marrow. Generally, the doses of radiation received to cause such effects will also cause other more acutely serious effects often leading to the death of the patients before they develop extensive, life threatening infections. If the patient survives serious infections do develop.

Acquired Immune Deficiency Syndrome (AIDS)

AIDS is a new disease and was first described in the USA in groups of homosexual males in 1981. It was called acquired since the disease is not in the genes, but appears later on in life due to another cause; it is an immune deficiency, i.e. there is an inability of the immune system to cope with infections, and a syndrome, meaning it presents in all patients with a set of similar symptoms and signs. In 1983, the cause of AIDS was discovered by French and American researchers who found it to be a virus and named it the human immunodeficiency virus (HIV; refer to Figure 5.1). Two types of the virus are known: HIV 1 and HIV 2. The virus originated in Africa and is related to non-pathogenic viruses that are present in African green monkey (*Cercopithecus aethiops*) tissues. The virus crossed into the human population, mutated and infected Africans but also some Haitian workers in Africa who carried the virus back to Haiti. Americans holidaying in Haiti carried the virus back to the east and west coasts of the USA and from there the virus spread worldwide.

The HIV is a retrovirus which means that it carries in its shell a genome consisting of RNA and an enzyme called reverse transcriptase which is not found in human cells. Once the virus has infected a cell, this enzyme transcribes the viral RNA into DNA (a backward step never occurring in human cells) and the viral DNA is then spliced into the cellular DNA where it may remain for many years.

When the HIV enters the body it infects the T4 cells (helper T cells) and also the macrophages and some nervous system cells. A phase of viral replication ensues where the infected cells each produce thousands of new virus particles, each of which then infects more cells. Subsequently, the virus infects more susceptible cells and incorporates its RNA into the cellular DNA, remaining dormant in the body for many years. Upon suitable stimulation (for example, another viral infection or the initiation of an immune response), the dormant HIV is reactivated, goes through another phase of replication, infects most of the cells that it is capable of infecting, destroys the helper T cells and macrophages, thus crippling the immune system, leading to a massive secondary deficiency in the cell-mediated immune response. Multiple life threatening infections and malignancies result, generally causing the rapid death of the affected person.

The symptoms and signs of HIV infection depend on what stage of virus replication most viral particles are in at the time. Generally, the earliest symptoms appear 5 to 10 days after infection and the presentation is very non-specific, most patients complaining of a mild cold-like or glandular fever-like disease, with slight fever, headache, malaise, sweating and dry throat. This symptomatology is due to the first replication of the virus in the body. The immune system responds to this first phase of viral infection by forming antibodies to the virus and detectable levels of antibodies are seen 2 to 3 months after infection. The person is then said to be seroconverted, meaning that an HIV antibody test performed will be positive. However, the antibodies are not able to overcome the infection as the virus is found incorporated into the DNA of the cells it has infected (T cells, macrophages, brain cells) and is out of reach of the circulating antibodies. The infected person is now in the quiescent or latent phase and will remain in this phase for 2 to 10 years. Although such people appear healthy they are infectious and may pass the virus onto others.

Two to 10 years after infection the infected person goes into the persistent generalized lymphadenopathy phase (PGL) in which the lymph nodes around the body swell and become very prominent. This indicates

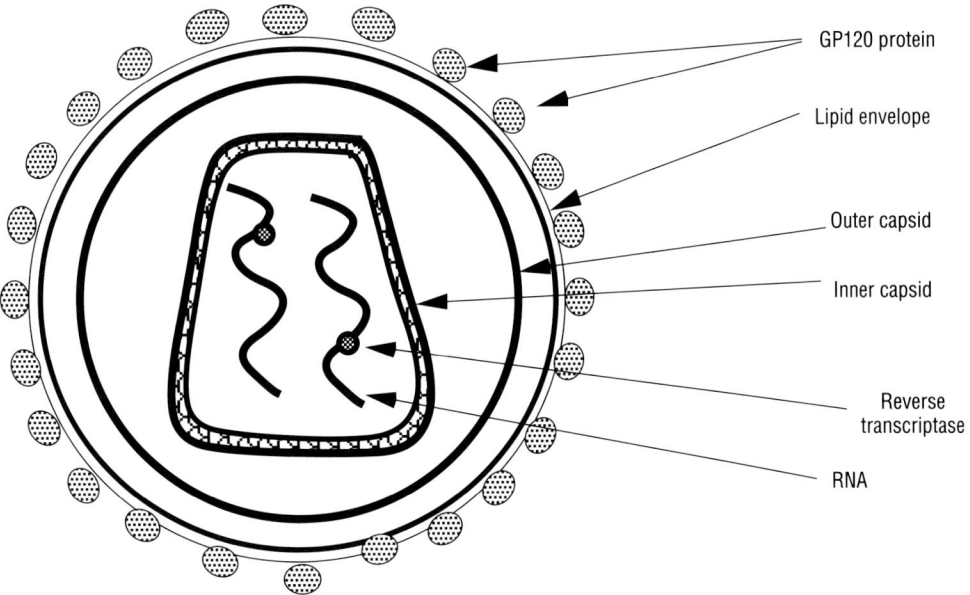

GP120 protein

Lipid envelope

Outer capsid

Inner capsid

Reverse transcriptase

RNA

Figure 5.1 *The human immunodeficiency virus, the cause of AIDS*

the second phase of virus replication and release. Since the virus is destroying the helper T cells, the immune response against it is minimal. The PGL phase is associated with the AIDS-related complex phase (ARC). In the ARC phase the first indications of systemic immunodeficiency become apparent: the patient starts to lose weight, complains of fatigue and weakness, headache, night sweats and continued bouts of diarrhoea, has anaemia and decreased T cell counts in the bloodstream with more suppressor T cells than helper T cells. This phase of the disease is associated with the beginning of many infections. The last phase, full-blown AIDS, is defined as one in which one or more opportunistic infections are present, when there is an increased incidence of malignant disease and lastly where there are positive laboratory tests for HIV. In full-blown AIDS, there are infections with *Candida albicans*, causing thrush (Figures 5.2 and 5.3), *Toxoplasma gondii* and *Pneumocystis carinii*, causing pneumonias, *Cryptococcus neoformans*, causing brain infections, widespread Herpes virus and cytomegalovirus infections. Also common are *Mycobacterium* spp. infections and severe gastrointestinal infections with *Cryptosporidium* and other parasites. Commonly observed cancers are Kaposi's sarcoma, Hodgkin's disease and lymphoma.

The symptoms and signs of full-blown AIDS are associated with multiple infections and cancers and include: debility, emaciation, enlarged lymph nodes, severe continual dry cough, severe diarrhoea, purplish lesions on the skin, white furry tongue, sore throat, fever, night sweat, decreased appetite. The patients may also show the AIDS-associated dementia and other neurological disorders associated with the replication of the virus in the CNS. The progression of the changes seen with HIV infection is often depicted as the 'AIDS pyramid' shown in Figure 5.4, and this shows that as a function of time there are fewer and fewer people in any of the upper phases as progression of the disease means that death will ensue.

AIDS is currently causing a pandemic (that is, a worldwide epidemic) and the recorded number of cases of full-blown AIDS in Australia at the end of July 1993 was 4287 cases. The cumulative number of deaths due to AIDS at that time was 2814. In looking at the epidemiological data concerning the patients who developed AIDS it became obvious that certain factors were very important in spreading the disease. These factors were associated with certain high-risk behaviours which were more common in certain community groups. When the disease was first described it was almost exclusively seen in young, previously healthy, homosexual males. As the disease was further characterized it was also detected in Haitians, bisexual males,

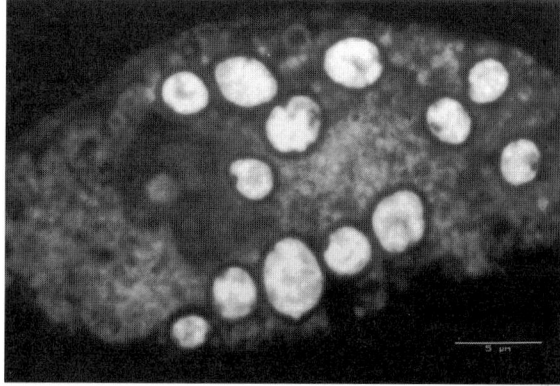

Figure 5.2 *A macrophage from a healthy person in cell culture, which has phagocytosed many* Candida albicans *yeasts (scale bar is 5 μm)*

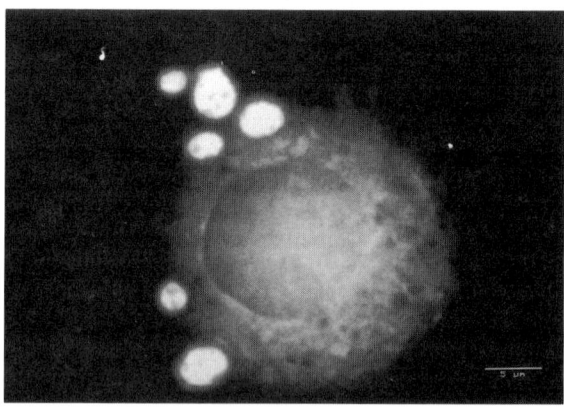

Figure 5.3 *An HIV-infected macrophage in cell culture, which although exposed to many* Candida albicans *yeasts is unable to phagocytose them effectively (scale bar is 5 μm)*

females, haemophiliacs and intravenous drug users. This indicated that the virus was spread by transfer of body fluids and blood between individuals. Specific sexual practices such as unprotected anal intercourse also carry a very high risk as does the sharing of needles and syringes between people. Before the routine testing of donated blood, blood transfusion and the use of blood products also spread the infection (haemophiliacs must inject themselves with purified factor VIII which is derived from donated blood, and in the days before blood testing for HIV, this factor concentrate carried the virus).

All of these routes of transmission spread infected

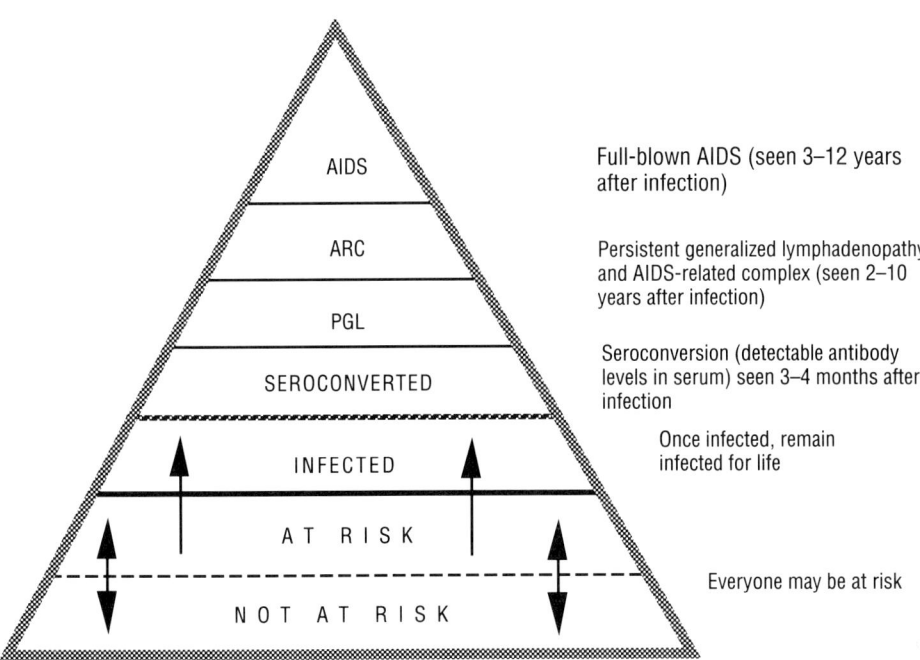

The AIDS pyramid labels, top to bottom: AIDS, ARC, PGL, SEROCONVERTED, INFECTED, AT RISK, NOT AT RISK

Full-blown AIDS (seen 3–12 years after infection)

Persistent generalized lymphadenopathy and AIDS-related complex (seen 2–10 years after infection)

Seroconversion (detectable antibody levels in serum) seen 3–4 months after infection

Once infected, remain infected for life

Everyone may be at risk

Figure 5.4   *The AIDS pyramid*

lymphocytes and free viruses from individual to individual. As the disease established itself, the virus spread to prostitutes (male and female) and generally people with multiple sex partners. Accidental infection of health workers has also been recorded. Pregnant women infected with HIV pass the virus transplacentally to their unborn baby thus when the baby is born it is already infected in many cases (≈ 40%).

Safe sex practices which prevent the exchange of blood and body fluids between individuals reduce the risk of infection. Testing of donated blood is now routinely performed and there is no longer a considerable risk associated with blood transfusions or through the use of blood products. Taking adequate care in the laboratory and health care situations prevents infection there. The virus is definitely not transmitted via: casual social contact, touching, hand shaking, casual kissing, living in the same household as AIDS cases, donating blood, dental procedures, handling money, swimming in public pools and baths, using public toilets, through mosquito bites, rodents, insect stings and so on. Some unconfirmed means of transmission which should be regarded as capable of spreading the virus are: oral sex, anal–oral contact, sexual kissing, toothbrush and razor sharing.

The treatment of AIDS is fraught with difficulties

and currently there is no cure available. It is known that people infected with HIV will remain infected for the rest of their lives and can spread the virus to others. Most treatments are centred around treating the opportunistic infections and cancers when they arise. Antibiotics and antiviral drugs are used for infections while radiotherapy and chemotherapy are in use for tumours. Lately, many anti-HIV drugs have been developed and most of these are directed against the reverse transcriptase of the HIV; a typical such drug is AZT (azidothymidine, Retrovir®). It should be stressed that these drugs certainly prolong the life of patients and improve the quality of their life but they do not cure the infection. Other drugs are currently being developed and tested: soluble CD_4 receptor of helper T cells onto which the virus attaches when it infects the cell, interferon, interleukins, etc. Research into HIV vaccines is also steadily progressing. To date, prevention is the best means of limiting the spread of AIDS in our community.

Autoimmunity

The immune system of the body has very aptly been described as the 'two-edged sword', capable of protecting the body from foreign or abnormal components but also being capable of causing considerable damage to the body's tissues resulting in serious or even fatal disease. Autoimmune disease refers to a group of disorders where the body's immune system is somehow interacting with the tissues, damaging them. This results in destruction and injury that are capable of causing dysfunction at an organic or systemic level, sometimes severe enough to cause the patient's death. Autoimmune diseases include a group of disorders known as the hypersensitivities or allergies, which represent disease caused by an inappropriately mounted or perverted immune response, resulting in damage to the tissues. There is a wide variety of such autoimmune states and they may be classified very diversely.

The Hypersensitivities

The hypersensitivities are a group of autoimmune diseases where the immunological reactions of the body, instead of contributing to recovery from disease, themselves are the cause of tissue damage and form an important or major part of the disease process. The hypersensitivities are commonly called allergies (compare anergy which implies that the immune system is deficient and is incapable of mounting an immune response). There are two major groups of hypersensitivities as shown in Table 5.1. In one group the damage to the tissue is mediated by antibody (humoral response), while in the other group the damage is mediated by cells (cell-mediated response). Generally, in the hypersensitivities mediated by antibody the reactions develop very quickly while in those mediated by cells, the reactions develop over a longer period of time.

The damaging effects of the Group 1 hypersensitivities may be mediated by antibody alone or by a combination of antibody and complement. In many specific forms of such allergic reactions, inflammatory mediators are released and it is the resulting inflamma-

Table 5.1 *The hypersensitivities or allergic responses*

Group 1 hypersensitivities (antibody mediated)	Group 2 hypersensitivities (cell mediated)
Type I: Anaphylactic	Type IV: Cell mediated
Type II: Cytotoxic	
Type III: Complex mediated	
Type V: Receptor mediated	

tion at the site that damages the tissues and causes injury. The antibody produced may bind to specific body cells or proteins and may have a variety of effects: It may, for example, 'block' a cellular receptor, it may cause hyperactivity of a cell or it may destroy a cell by immune lysis in association with complement.

In the cell-mediated hypersensitivities, the interleukins released by activated T cells and macrophages are very important in causing tissue damage through mediating chronic inflammation and tissue destruction. Very often the inflammation that is seen is of a granulomatous nature; also commonly seen are fibrous reactions which represent attempts by the body at healing.

All the hypersensitivities are of common incidence in the population, but fortunately most of them may be effectively controlled. However, sometimes, even nowadays, some individuals may die of very severe hypersensitivity reactions as, for example, in very severe asthmatic attacks or following bee and other insect stings.

Type I — Anaphylactic Hypersensitivity

In 1902, Charles Richet introduced the term anaphylaxis to describe the severe and sometimes fatal reactions of animals to a second injection of foreign protein. He coined the term in order to make it contrast with prophylaxis, which means the normal protective effect observed in animals after injection with foreign material. The severe form of anaphylaxis is called anaphylactic shock and its consequences are so severe that death may result. Anaphylactic shock may be demonstrated in the guinea pig as follows. An injection of foreign protein such as egg albumin is given subcutaneously, a procedure not followed by any ill effects. After a period of 10 to 14 days a second injection of egg albumin is given. It is now observed that even a small dosage will cause the guinea pig to go into anaphylactic shock. It suffers from intense bronchiolar constriction, leading to asphyxia and there is also extreme vasodilatation systemically, which precipitates the shock. In humans anaphylactic shock with fatal results is rare, but it may occur, as, for example, when penicillin is given to individuals who are allergic to it. Anaphylactic reactions may also follow insect stings in certain people. However, localized type I reactions are very common — hay fever, allergic asthma, urticaria (hives), and various food allergies are all examples of anaphylactic reactions. The sensitizing antigen causing the reaction in all of these cases is called the **allergen**.

The mechanism of these type I reactions has been elucidated and is illustrated in Figure 5.5. In certain individuals contact with an allergen (e.g. pollen, house dust, dander, food) stimulates the formation of IgE antibody instead of IgG or IgA. This is an intrinsic reaction associated with the particular person's immune response. The IgE antibody formed is termed homocytotropic antibody or reaginic antibody (= reagin). This reaginic antibody attaches by its Fc end (the non-antigen reacting end) onto the surface of mast cells, which are found in connective tissues throughout the body, and also attaches to the surface of basophils in the blood.

Both of these cell types contain many granules that are full of histamine, serotonin, platelet-activating factor (PAF) and eosinophil chemotactic factor of anaphylaxis (ECF-A). Membrane changes in these cells activate the enzyme phospholipase A2, producing another mediator, slow reacting substance of anaphylaxis (SRS-A). The first time the allergen is encountered by these allergic people, they experience no adverse reactions as the IgE has not formed yet. In the following 7 days their immune system is reacting to the antigen by forming IgE antibody, which attaches to the surface of mast cells and basophils as soon as it is formed. Such cells with the antibody attached to their surface are said to be sensitized, and are found throughout the body. Upon the second encounter with the sensitizing

allergen, when the allergen comes into the body it attaches to the specific IgE antibody which is bound to the surface of sensitized cells. This causes the degranulation of these cells, with the release of all the active compounds that they contain in their granules. These pharmacologically active compounds mediate directly or indirectly the bronchoconstriction, inflammation, oedema, vasodilatation and increased vascular permeability that characterize the anaphylactic responses.

Anaphylactic reactions are controlled naturally mainly through the action of eosinophils that are attracted to the area of mast cell degranulation by ECF-A. The eosinophils release their granule contents, which include substances such as histaminase and other enzymes, which destroy histamine, SRS-A and PAF that have been released by the mast cells. When it becomes necessary to treat patients who are affected by anaphylactic-type reactions, this is achieved mainly through the symptomatic relief of the disorder. The drugs that are used include antihistamines (e.g. asthma inhalers), and also anti-inflammatory drugs such as corticosteroids. Preventative measures may also be used. When the patient feels that an attack is imminent, or is in a situation which consistently precipitates an attack (e.g. asthmatic attacks after exercise), he or

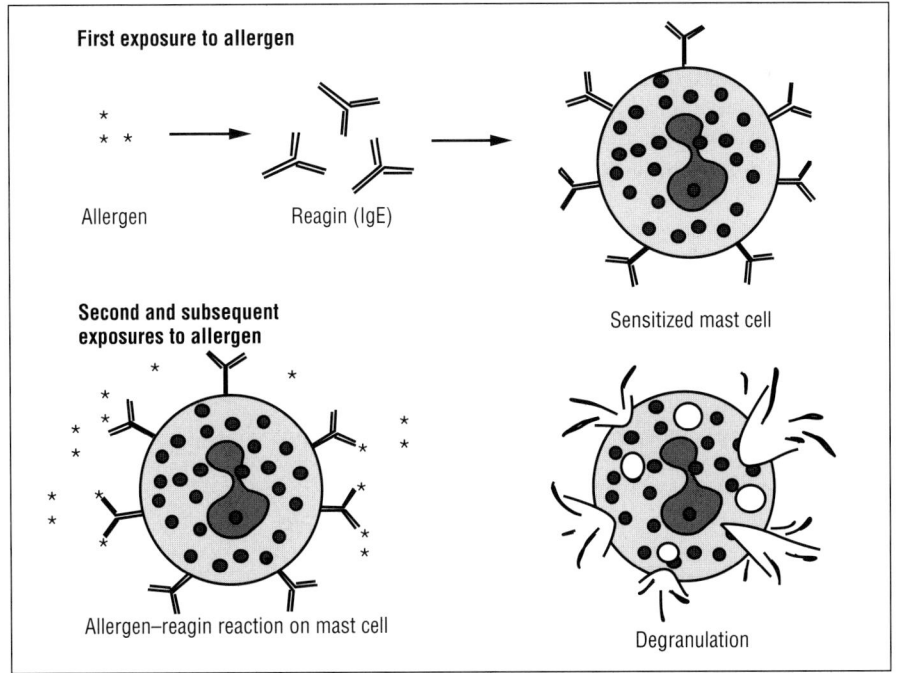

Figure 5.5 *Type I, anaphylactic hypersensitivity*

she may take drugs that prevent the degranulation of mast cells, and hence prevent the attack. One such drug used is sodium cromoglycate, which is used extensively with very good results. The only disadvantage of such treatment is that the patient must be aware of the specific situations that induce the anaphylactic attacks and take the medication before the attacks.

Type II — Cytotoxic Hypersensitivity

Cytotoxic hypersensitivity involves direct damage to cells caused by antibodies, usually of the classes IgG or IgM. The antibody is directed against some cell surface component or against a small molecule that may have attached itself to the cell surface. The cells commonly affected in this hypersensitivity are erythrocytes and platelets. It is therefore common to see type II reactions being the cause of anaemias and thrombocytopenias. The mechanisms responsible for the destruction of the cells involved are many and varied. Usually, they first involve the binding of antibody to the cell surface and consequently there is complement activation and fixation with cell lysis through antibody-dependent cell cytotoxicity. Alternatively, the cell may be phagocytosed by neutrophils or macrophages, which will readily ingest opsonized, antibody-coated cells (refer to Figure 5.6).

Many important human diseases are caused by such hypersensitivity reactions: isoimmune reactions such as **erythroblastosis foetalis** (haemolytic disease of the newborn) and **incompatible transfusion reactions**. Organ and grafted tissue rejections are in many cases due to this type of hypersensitivity as are **autoimmune diseases** such as thyroiditis, some of the **anaemias** and **thrombocytopenias**.

Transfusion reactions rarely occur nowadays because of the close control of transfusion procedures and the careful blood type matching that is carried out before the transfusion. In the past they were commoner, and in some cases the patient who received mismatched blood died as a result of it. An example of a mismatched transfusion, involving the ABO group of antigens, will be given here as an illustration of the principle.

Note that the antibody to the ABO blood group antigens is naturally present in the plasma, just as the ABO antigens are naturally present on red blood cells (see Table 5.2). When mismatched blood is transfused, these naturally occurring antibodies will attach onto the antigens which are expressed by the transfused erythrocytes. If, for example, blood from an individual of type A is transfused into an individual of blood type B, the transfused erythrocytes will express the A antigen. Since the anti-A antibodies are naturally occurring in the blood of the blood group B individual, even without previous contact with erythrocytes of the A type, the anti-A antibodies in the recipient's blood will attach to the transfused type A erythrocytes, complement will be activated and lysis of the red blood cells will occur. Similarly, some of the recipient's own red blood cells, expressing the B antigen, will be lysed by the anti-B antibody present in the transfused plasma; however, this reaction is minimal (see below).

It may now be understood why persons of blood group O are termed universal donors. Their red blood cells possess neither A nor B antigens on their surface, and therefore when these cells are transfused, they will remain unaffected by anti-A and anti-B antibodies. It must also be realized that the number of anti-A and anti-B antibodies that are transfused in the plasma of the donor is not significant enough to cause a problem

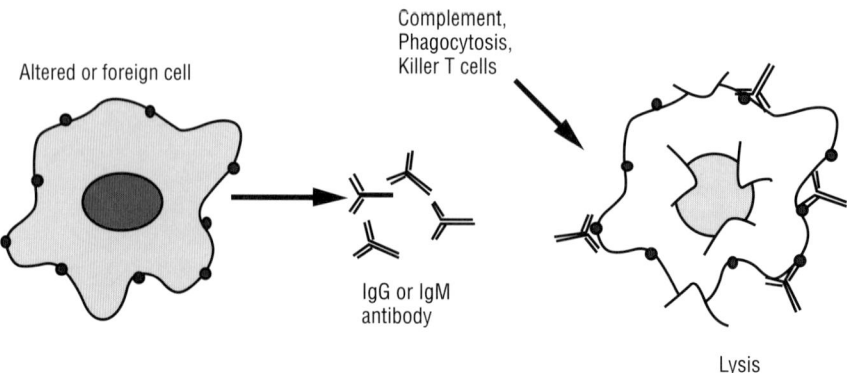

Figure 5.6 *Type II, cytotoxic hypersensitivity*

Table 5.2 *The ABO blood group system*

	Blood group			
	A	B	AB	O
Antigen on red blood cell	A	B	A and B	Nil
Antibody in plasma	Anti-B	Anti-A	Nil	Both anti-A and anti B

with lysis of the recipient's own cells. Similarly, people with blood group AB are known as universal recipients. This is because these people have no anti-A or anti-B antibodies in their plasma and if erythrocytes of any group whatever are transfused into their blood, they will be unable to lyse them. It should be noted that nowadays, blood groups are always matched and transfusions based on these 'universal' donor–recipient rules are not relied upon, except in cases of the utmost emergency.

Erythroblastosis foetalis, also referred to as haemolytic disease of the newborn, depends on the Rhesus blood groups, being independent of the ABO system. The inheritance of the Rhesus antigen on erythrocytes is dependent on Mendelian genetics and the trait is inherited as autosomal dominant as shown in Figure 5.7. The majority of Caucasians (≈ 85% of them) are Rhesus positive, Rh +ve, and their genotype is either DD or Dd (D being the notation for the dominant allele which causes the expression of the Rhesus antigen on the erythrocyte membrane). The remaining 15% of the population are Rhesus negative, Rh –ve, and their genotype is dd. The problem arises when an Rh –ve mother is carrying an Rh +ve baby. The condi-

tion is seen only in the second and subsequent pregnancies when the Rh –ve woman is carrying Rh +ve babies. This is the case because there must first be exposure to the Rh antigen in the mother's bloodstream which stimulates the formation of anti-Rh antibody. This is because contrary to the ABO autoantibodies, anti-Rh antibodies are not naturally occurring in plasma. The first pregnancy therefore initiates a primary immune response against the Rh antigen and the subsequent pregnancies initiate secondary immune responses to the Rh antigen.

In the course of all pregnancies there is normally a small trickle of foetal blood cells into the maternal circulation (refer to Figure 5.8). These erythrocytes are insufficient to cause an immune response to be initiated against them. They are destroyed instead by killer cells and by phagocytosis. During labour and parturition there is a considerable transplacental haemorrhage with leakage of considerable numbers of foetal erythrocytes into the maternal circulation. If the mother is Rh –ve and the baby is Rh +ve, it is these erythrocytes which cause the mother's immune system to form anti-Rh antibodies after the conclusion of the first pregnancy. So at the end of the first pregnancy, both Rh –ve mother and Rh +ve baby are well, but the mother has now been sensitized and has anti-Rh antibodies and anti-Rh lymphocytes in her bloodstream.

Subsequent pregnancies with an Rh +ve baby in the sensitized Rh –ve woman will result in the condition erythroblastosis foetalis. This is because in the second pregnancy, the small trickle of foetal erythrocytes into the maternal circulation, during the course of the pregnancy is sufficient to cause the initiation of a secondary immune response against the Rh antigen on the erythrocytes, with activation of the specific maternal lymphocytes and the formation of many anti-Rh IgG and IgM antibodies by the mother. The maternal IgG antibody crosses the placenta into the foetal circulation where it begins to react with the Rh +ve foetal erythrocytes. These opsonized erythrocytes are then

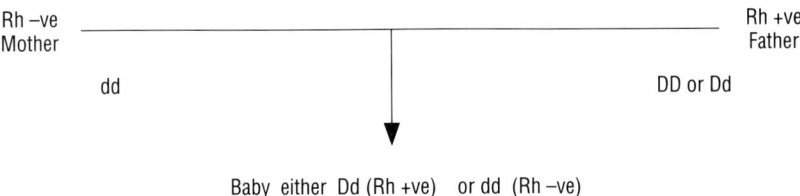

Figure 5.7 *The genetics of the Rhesus (Rh) factor*

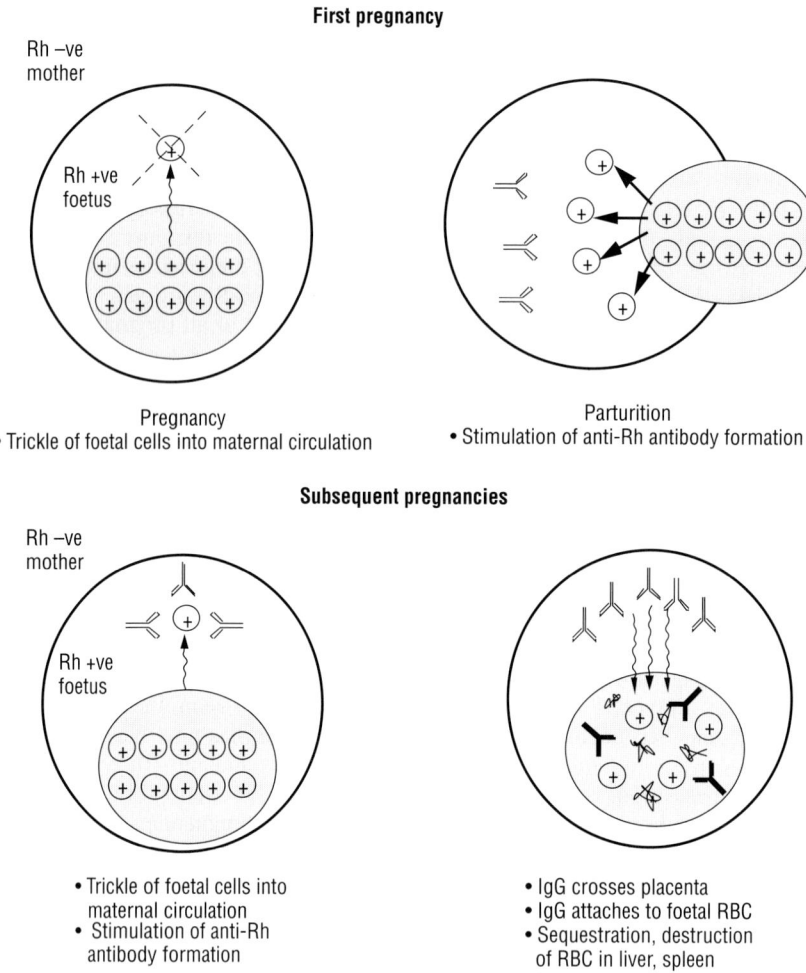

Figure 5.8   *Erythroblastosis foetalis, a type II hypersensitivity*

phagocytosed by macrophages in the foetal liver and spleen (they are not lysed by complement). The foetus is then seen to suffer from a haemolytic anaemia, which may be severe enough to cause its death.

It is important to realize that erythroblastosis foetalis does not occur with ABO blood group incompatibilities between mother and foetus. This is because there are the naturally occurring antibodies against the ABO antigens present in the maternal circulation. Any incompatible foetal erythrocytes which enter the mother's bloodstream during the pregnancy will react with the naturally occurring antibodies and will be destroyed as soon as they enter the mother's bloodstream.

Currently, immunoprophylaxis is carried out routinely on all Rh –ve mothers and this procedure prevents erythroblastosis in all cases. The procedure involves passive immunization of the mother at the time of birth with an intramuscular injection of 200–300 mg of anti-Rh antibody. This is a purified human immunoglobulin which is obtained from Rh immunized donors. It has the effect of attaching to and destroying any foetal erythrocytes that may come into the maternal circulation at the time of birth and therefore preventing the stimulation of an immune response to the foetal Rh +ve erythrocytes that come into the maternal circulation at parturition. In this way, erythroblastosis is prevented at subsequent pregnancies. Immunoprophylaxis must be carried out each of the times the Rh –ve mother has a baby, if erythroblastosis is to be prevented in the following pregnancy.

Type II hypersensitivity reactions are also important in the rejection of grafts and transplants in the following case: long-standing homografts that have survived the onslaught of the cell-mediated reaction (see type IV hypersensitivity reactions below) may stimulate the formation of antibodies in the recipient. These antibodies are directed against the incompatible transplantation antigens (MHC — major histo-compatibility antigens) on the transplanted tissue cells. Once the antibodies to the graft have formed, they attack the transplanted tissue and a type II reaction results in the death of the cells and the rejection of the graft.

Hyperacute graft rejection reactions are also mediated by type II hypersensitivity reactions and they rely on the presence of a preformed specific antibody directed against antigens on the transplanted tissue; i.e. this is an anamnestic response directed against grafted tissue which enters the body for the second time or subsequent times. The first time that the graft enters the tissues it stimulates a primary antibody response against it. This may be sufficient to reject the graft. The following times the same tissue type enters the body it will stimulate a secondary, anamnestic response of antibody leading to a very rapid rejection of the transplant.

Various so-called 'autoimmune reactions' are also based on type II hypersensitivity operating and causing tissue damage. Autoimmune haemolytic anaemia is an example of these. Following a triggered stimulation the patients begin to form antibodies directed against their own erythrocytes. The antibodies attach to the red blood cells, leading to a marked reduction in their life span as they are sequestered and destroyed very quickly after they have been coated by antibody.

The trigger for this disease may be an adverse drug reaction, genetic, hereditary or idiopathic. Hashimoto's thyroiditis is another case in which antibodies are manufactured and directed against body cells, in this case the parenchymal cells of the thyroid gland. The antibodies attach to the thyroid cells and with complement fixation the cells are destroyed, leading to a gross destruction of the gland and hypothyroidism, or in severe cases even myxoedema.

Certain drugs, when administered to some individuals who are hypersensitive to them, will stimulate the destruction of body cells through a type II reaction. In these cases, the drugs act as haptens and they attach to body cells thus being converted into an active antigen, being capable of initiating an immune response. The antibodies formed will react with the drug–body cell complex and the individual is said to be sensitized with respect to that drug. A number of such drugs are known which often lead to hypersensitivity reactions after administration in the people so predisposed. Haemolytic anaemia often is linked with chlorpromazine or phenacetin therapy. Agranulocytosis (reduction in the granulocytic leukocytes in the blood) is seen after administration of amidopyrine or quinidine to some individuals. Sedormid administration may lead to thrombocytopenic purpura.

Type III — Complex-mediated Hypersensitivity

This hypersensitivity results when there are large amounts of soluble antigen in the body. The antigens combine with specific antibodies to form large numbers of immune complexes (see Figure 5.9). The anti-

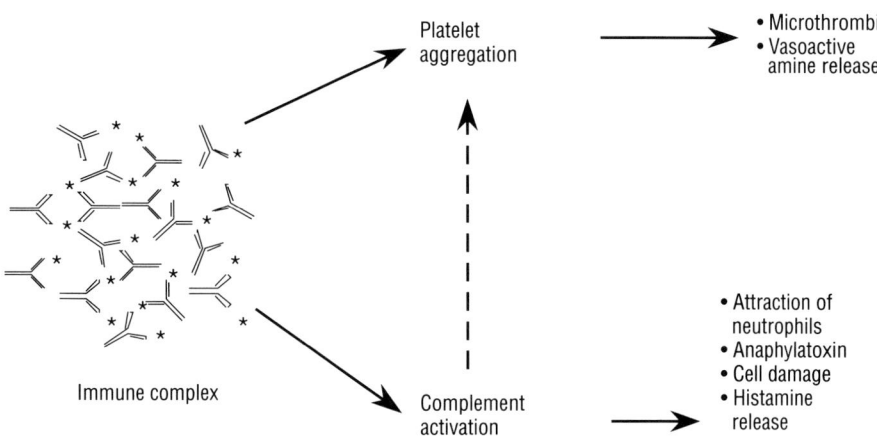

Figure 5.9 *Type III, complex-mediated hypersensitivity*

gen–antibody complexes thus formed circulate around the body and may localize in the walls of blood vessels. The prototype complex-mediated hypersensitivity reaction was described by Maurice Arthus in 1903 and the experiment he performed is still known as the Arthus phenomenon. Arthus injected a rabbit subcutaneously with a foreign protein (e.g. horse serum proteins). The rabbit developed a high circulating level of antibody specific to the horse protein. The next time the horse serum was injected subcutaneously into the sensitized animal, the circulating specific antibodies combined with the horse protein and formed immune complexes locally, around the site of injection. Within 2 to 8 hours a haemorrhagic, oedematous lesion developed on the skin. The inflammation persisted for 12 to 24 hours and in severe cases resulted in extensive tissue necrosis with ulceration and haemorrhage. These necrotic and inflammatory changes are due to destruction of small blood vessels by thrombi and neutrophils, and also through the fixation of complement at the site. Several such localized reactions are known, but these reactions may also occur systemically, initiating a damaging response through complement activation and neutrophil infiltration.

In the past, antitoxin and antibacterial sera were often administered repeatedly to provide passive immunity. These immune sera were prepared in horses and injected into humans after purification to extract the horse antibodies which gave the serum its protective effects. The body reacted to the horse serum since it was a foreign protein. It was common for Arthus-type reactions to develop at the site of injection of the serum. Nowadays such reactions are rare as the risk of sensitizing individuals with foreign protein are known and these injections are avoided. If antiserum need be injected for any purpose it is human antiserum rather than horse antiserum that is used; this way there is less risk of sensitization. Occasionally, frequent administrations of toxoid preparations will cause Arthus-type reactions.

An example of a type III reaction that occurs locally in the lungs is one known as farmer's lung. In this condition sensitizing allergens are contained in dust from mouldy hay. The antigenic determinants dissolve in the lung fluids and initiate a localized type III reaction. Sufferers from this condition are frequently farmers and people in contact with vegetable materials and when they contact the mouldy fibres they experience severe respiratory difficulties, approximately 6 to 8 hours following exposure to the dust.

A typical manifestation of type III reactions on a systemic level is the so-called serum sickness. This once again was commoner in the past when large amounts of horse-derived antitoxin were administered to treat advanced toxaemias in diphtheria and tetanus. Injection of the foreign protein stimulated the production of antibody to it in the body. Whenever there are large numbers of antibodies present in the body, they are in excess in relation to the antigen and they combine with the antigen to give rise to insoluble precipitates which are rapidly phagocytosed and cleared from the body by white cells. However, in the early stages of antibody formation, when there are relatively few antibodies in relation to antigen, the complexes that form are small and soluble, therefore not easily phagocytosed. These soluble complexes circulate in the blood for several days, gradually being deposited around various body sites: the kidneys, heart, joints, skin, etc. The symptoms and signs of such conditions are all associated with the tissue destruction that occurs due to formation of microthrombi in the circulation and the inflammation and complement fixation at the site. Arthritis with painful joint swelling; albuminuria and haematuria indicating renal failure; irregularities in heart beat associated with carditis; oedema, skin lesions, vasculitis and fever are all seen in severe reactions and death may ensue. Serum sickness is not seen at all frequently nowadays since the risks of injections of large amounts of soluble, foreign proteins are realized and avoided.

The mechanisms of type III, complex-mediated hypersensitivity are illustrated in Figure 5.10 in relation to glomerulonephritis, an important type III reaction. The immune complexes form in the circulation and body fluids, and as they circulate in the bloodstream they cause the release of vasoactive mediators from basophils and platelets. Immune complexes in extravascular tissues also cause degranulation of mast cells. These mediators cause gaps to form in the endothelial junctions of the blood vessels and the immune complexes are deposited in the gaps of vascular walls of capillaries and venules. Platelets aggregate at sites of open junctions and complement is activated. Microthrombi are formed in response to the platelet aggregation and the complement-mediated vascular damage. As the complement is fixed, neutrophil chemotactic substances are released and these attract neutrophils to the site. The white cells attempt to phagocytose the immune complexes which are lodged deep inside the vascular wall and out of reach of the neutrophils. As the neutrophils attempt to phagocytose the inaccessible complexes, they release their lysosomal contents in the area and these cause further endothelial cell damage. This last effect is known as 'frustrated phagocytosis' and contributes greatly to the ensuing damage and continued inflammation at the site.

A typical picture of acute vasculitis develops at the site and the reaction may progress for some time as a

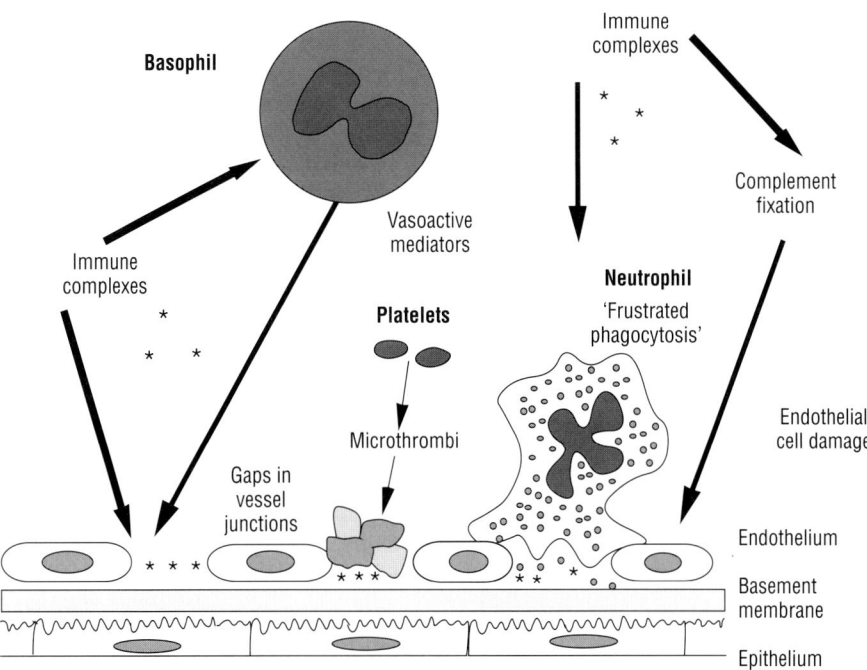

Figure 5.10 *Type III, complex-mediated hypersensitivity — glomerulonephritis*

vicious cycle develops with more endothelial damage causing more inflammation and platelet aggregation. The microthrombi formed may completely block the affected vessels and ischaemic effects may be seen in the tissues irrigated by these vessels.

Numerous examples of important diseases caused by type III reactions may be quoted and some of these are sufficiently severe to cause the death of the patient; post-streptococcal glomerulonephritis is a typical type III hypersensitivity reaction which occurs after infections with *Streptococcus* spp. in the hypersensitive individual. Large amounts of soluble breakdown products of the streptococci combine with specific antibody in the bloodstream and large amounts of immune complexes form. These complexes are filtered out by the kidney glomeruli and they settle in the gaps of the glomerular capillaries where most of the damage occurs. The condition is accompanied by loss of normal renal function which may even be manifested as a renal failure, with massive loss of protein in the urine, oedema, haematuria and uraemia.

Other diseases in which type III reactions are important are systemic lupus erythematosus (SLE), rheumatoid arthritis, rheumatic fever, various reactions to drugs such as penicillin, penicillamine, sulphonamides and streptomycin in hypersensitive individuals and

various manifestations of leprosy, syphilis, malaria, hepatitis B and measles.

Type IV — Delayed hypersensitivity

This type of hypersensitivity is also called the cell-mediated type as no antibodies are involved in the reaction at all. It is called delayed, as the manifestations of the reaction develop in the sensitized individual 24–48 hours after contact with the antigen. This is in contrast to the antibody-mediated reactions (e.g. type I, anaphylactic hypersensitivity) in which the manifestations are evident only minutes after contact of the sensitized individual with the antigen.

The prototype of this hypersensitivity is the tuberculin reaction. This reaction is seen in people who have come into contact with *Mycobacterium tuberculosis*, have become sensitized to it and who are then exposed to tuberculin (extract from *M. tuberculosis* cultures, or a purified protein derivative therefrom) in an intradermal test procedure known as the Mantoux test. In this test, a positive reaction after injection results in an erythematous induration, meaning that there is reddening and firmness in that region of the skin. It is characterized, under the microscope, by an intense infiltration by lymphocytes and macrophages (approximately 85% lymphocytes and 15% macrophages) around blood vessels and throughout the loose connective tissue of the skin.

The process that leads to the formation of this reaction is essentially the same as that of cell-mediated immunity and is illustrated in Figure 5.11. The initial contact with the antigen produces a clone of sensitized T cells. Some of these T cells persist in the blood and tissues as memory cells. When the antigen is re-encountered the memory T cells specific for that antigen migrate to the area, react with it, and produce lymphokines that attract many more mononuclear cells to the area. The principal lymphokines isolated from sites of type IV reactions are migration inhibition factor, monocyte chemotactic factor, skin reactive factor and blastogenic factor. It is interesting to note that delayed type-hypersensitivity may be transferred between experimental animals by transferring T cells from a sensitized animal to a non-sensitized animal. It has also been reported by some researchers that de-

layed-type hypersensitivity may be transferred by a cell-free T cell extract called transfer factor (TF). This TF is a protein of 10 000 Daltons molecular weight and it seems to confer on the recipient the sensitivity to the particular antigen that stimulated its formation in the donor.

Tissue damage in type IV reactions occurs through peculiarities of the antigen that induce these reactions as well as through the nature of the cell-mediated response itself. It is observed that antigens that cause delayed-type hypersensitivity reactions tend to persist in the tissues for long periods. This prolonged presence of antigen in the tissue attracts very large numbers of mononuclear cells. The secretion of interleukins attracts more cells to the area and also prevents cells from leaving the area. Some interleukins stimulate inflammatory changes in the tissues, with increased vascular permeability, exudation and hyperaemia resulting. The presence of large numbers of inflammatory cells in the area is important in causing local ischaemic effects and tissue necrosis. The prolonged

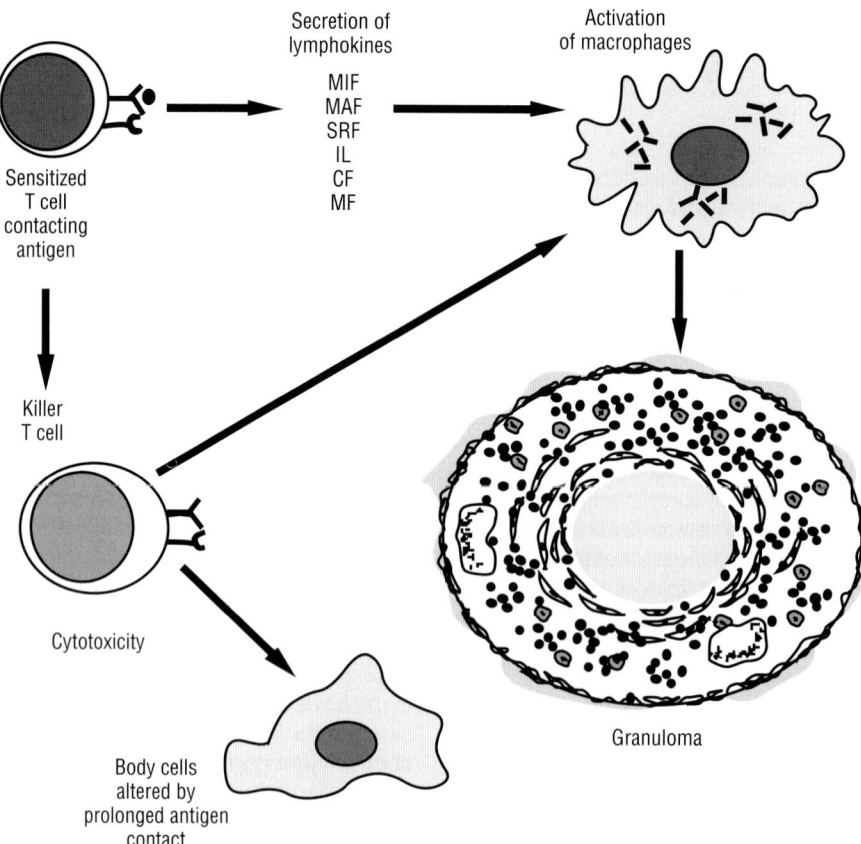

Figure 5.11 *Type IV, delayed-type hypersensitivity*

contact of antigen with body cells may alter their cell surface characteristics, thus making them liable to be attacked by killer T cells and macrophages, causing more tissue damage.

Examples of type IV reactions are seen in many natural infections in people who react to the infecting organisms in this manner instead of in the normal way. For example, in the majority of people who come in contact with *Mycobacterium tuberculosis* the body reacts and there is a rapid neutralization of the bacteria with minimal tissue damage. However, in hypersensitive individuals there is gross tissue destruction with the formation of extensive granulomata, caseous necrosis and even death if the infection remains untreated. Other examples of such infections where there may be severe tissue reactions, depending on the individual's response to the infecting organism's antigenic structure, are viral infections (e.g. with the vaccinia virus), protozoal infections (e.g. leishmaniasis) and some fungal infections (e.g. histoplasmosis).

It is also frequently observed that mosquito and flea bites will initiate delayed-type hypersensitivity reactions at the site of the bite. This finding should be compared with that observed after bee stings which give rise to anaphylactic-type responses. A very common manifestation of type IV reactions is that of contact dermatitis which is essentially a skin reaction to various substances that contact it and which act as allergens. Common allergens include metals such as mercury, nickel and chromium and it is not infrequently that people present with contact dermatitis due to a nickel clasp on some item of jewellery that they have worn. Dyes and other organic chemicals are often the cause of such allergic reactions and cosmetics belong to this class. Inorganic chemicals such as potassium dichromate or plant components and plant products (e.g. poison ivy, primrose leaves) may also be the allergens of type IV reactions.

Type IV hypersensitivity reactions are also very important in another commonly observed situation. Transplantation reactions and graft rejections that are observed after grafting operations are the results of a cell-mediated immune response incited by the persistent presence of the foreign tissue in the recipient's body and generally result in necrosis of the graft, unless immunosuppressive drugs are given.

Graft Rejection

In tissue and organ grafts (transplants) the recipient runs the risk of rejecting the donor tissue if the donor tissue is from another individual. The recipient's immune system recognizes the graft cell antigens as 'foreign', initiating a cell-mediated response leading to the necrosis or **rejection of grafted tissue**.

An exception to this rule is in identical twins who have identical genetic material. Hence their cell surface antigens are also identical and donation of tissue (e.g. a kidney) from one twin to the other does not result in rejection.

In order to prevent rejection of grafts it is preferable to match the tissue as closely as possible between donor and recipient as is routinely performed now for kidney transplants and heart transplants. The matching concerns the **major histocompatibility antigens**. These are inherited and there are six pairs of allelic genes involved (**MHC** — major histocompatibility complex, genes A, B, C, DP, DQ and DR). The antigens which are commonly used in matching are the HLA antigens (human leukocyte antigen system; genes located on chromosome 6). There are two classes of HLA antigens, class I expressed on the surface of all nucleated cells in the body and class II antigens expressed on the membrane of cells reacting with T lymphocytes, for example macrophages. A convenient cell to test for these antigens is the lymphocyte and there are eight MHC antigens present on leukocytes which are not present on red blood cells. A blood sample is taken to match antigens on the leukocytes. As well as these major histocompatibility antigens there are minor histocompatibility antigens on cells so the only complete match is with an identical monozygotic twin. Because of the many different classes and subclasses of major and minor antigens involved in tissue histocompatibility, identical matching is usually not possible and it is essential to use **immunosuppression** (drugs which suppress the immune system) to prevent graft rejection. People who have had organ transplants may now live for many years with daily immunosuppressive drugs (but even though the organ tissue may not be rejected infections may prove fatal).

Certain sites in the body are **immunoprivileged** and thus grafting involving these sites will not need tissue matching. A typical example of this is the cornea of the eye, where lymphocytes of the host do not reach the grafted tissue. Hence, corneal grafts may be effected between strangers without fear of rejection in the uncomplicated case. If the corneal graft becomes vascularized, rejection will occur. In certain other cases of grafts, the tissue transplanted is **non-viable**, that is, the cells are not living cells. This occurs when bone and blood vessels are transplanted between individuals. The tissue is made non-viable before transplant and simply provides a connective tissue network that will allow growth and regeneration of the individual's own tissues.

Type V — Cellular Receptor Hypersensitivity

Many cells receive information or instructions by agents such as hormones through surface receptors on their plasma membranes. The binding of signal substances on the cell surface receptor initiates allosteric changes in the receptor activating it to transmit information to the cell's interior. An example of such a system is seen when thyroid stimulating hormone (TSH), secreted by the pituitary gland, attaches to the surface receptors of thyroid cells. This attachment of TSH to thyroid cells activates the enzyme adenyl cyclase which makes cyclic-AMP from ATP and it is this cyclic-AMP that stimulates the cell's nucleus into a mode which results in secretory activity, with thyroxine secreted. In type V hypersensitivity antibodies are formed to receptor proteins on cell surfaces, but instead of destroying the cell, the attached antibody will stimulate the cell into activity as if it were the signal molecule that normally attaches to the receptor, as is shown in Figure 5.12.

An example of a surface receptor hypersensitivity is seen in the case of some thyroid disorders where there is excessive secretion of thyroid hormone and the patient presents with symptoms and signs of thyrotoxicosis (Graves' disease). In many of these patients it can be demonstrated that there are antibodies to thyroid cells, which persist for long periods of time, constantly stimulating the thyroid to secrete excessive levels of thyroid hormones. These antibodies are known as LATS (long-acting thyroid stimulating) antibodies.

Type V stimulatory hypersensitivity is also thought to be a major mechanism that operates in the causation of some immune system disorders where there is excessive stimulation of immune system cells. For example, there may be antibodies that form against interleukin receptors on immune system cells, and attachment of antibody to such receptors would continuously stimulate the cell into activity, giving rise to an inappropriate immune response.

Another manifestation of type V hypersensitivity is when the antibody formed against the receptor attaches to it but in this case instead of stimulating the cell it causes the destruction of the receptor. This causes a marked reduction in the number of receptors present on the cell surface thus making that cell less responsive to the normal stimuli that interact with it. A typical example of this reaction is myasthenia gravis, where antibodies form against the acetylcholine receptors on the skeletal muscle end plates. The antibodies attach to these receptors and through the mediation of complement destroy the receptors, making the muscle cell less responsive to stimulation when acetylcholine is released from the motor end plate when a nervous signal reaches it. The result is that the muscle does not contract forcefully and the affected person experiences muscle weakness and fatigue.

Autoimmune Disease

The function of the immune system has been described previously as one in which its components distinguish between what is 'self' and what is 'non-self'. Once this distinction has been established in the body, what is recognized as belonging to the body is spared ('tol-

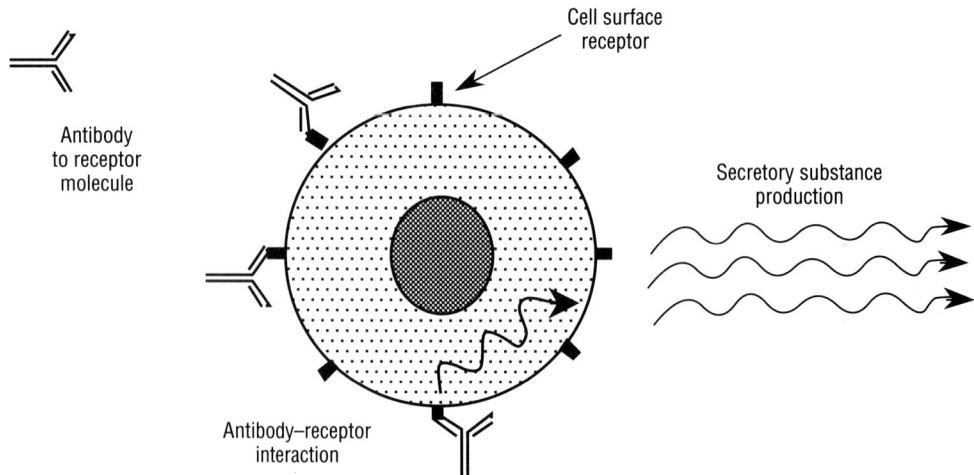

Cell surface receptor

Antibody to receptor molecule

Secretory substance production

Antibody–receptor interaction

Figure 5.12 *Type V, cellular receptor hypersensitivity*

erated') and what is recognized as foreign is destroyed or rejected. However, it is apparent in many disordered states that this system of recognition of self will often break down and the immune system will mount an immune response against components of the body. It is these situations that are referred to as autoimmune disorders. In these diseases the body's normal components, proteins, complex carbohydrates and other macromolecules will function as antigens and are therefore called **autoantigens**. These antigens will stimulate a humoral response against them, thus giving rise to **autoantibodies** (antibodies produced against 'self' components); or they may stimulate a cell-mediated immune response against them with sensitized T cells reacting with and destroying tissues. Not infrequently, both cell-mediated and humoral mechanisms may co-exist in any one autoimmune disorder. The spectrum of autoimmune diseases is very wide and many diseases which in the past were of an unknown cause have now been shown to be essentially due to an autoimmune response. It appears that females are more likely to develop autoimmunity and generally the older an individual is the more chance there is of such autoimmune reactions occurring. Some autoimmune states are very definitely inherited or have some familial association, indicating that a genetic cause may be very important in some of them.

Therefore, human autoimmune diseases have various features in common, including the following:

- They are commoner in females.
- There is frequently a positive family history (relatives and others may show similar genetic trends, e.g. HLA genotype).
- Autoantibodies, sometimes multiple, are present in the blood. Some of these react with the target tissue, but most appear to be without clinical effect. Thus thyroid autoantibodies may be present with or without signs of thyroid disease.
- Circulating harmless autoantibodies are frequently detectable in healthy relatives.
- Lymphocytes and macrophages are abundant in target tissues, especially around blood vessels.
- Vasculitis and arthritis are especially common in autoimmune immune complex disease.
- Immunoglobulin and complement are detectable at sites of tissue damage.
- The disease responds to immunosuppressive treatment.

Autoimmune diseases may be broadly divided into the so-called organ-specific diseases, where the destructive effects of the immune system are confined to one specific organ or tissue type in the body, and the systemic autoimmune diseases, in which the autoimmunity is seen in many tissues and organs throughout the body with, often, quite severe effects. Organ-specific diseases are especially common in the glandular tissues of the body, for example the thyroid gland, pancreas and stomach mucosa. The systemic diseases very frequently affect the connective tissues, with muscles, joints and loose connective tissues predominantly affected. It should be kept in mind that although most of these autoimmune states, be they organ specific or systemic, are associated with the presence of autoantibodies or of sensitized T cells, it is sometimes observed that even in apparently healthy individuals some autoantibodies will be found in the body if they are looked for. This is especially the case in healthy blood relatives of people who suffer from some autoimmune disease. This once again points out the importance of genetic causes for autoimmunity.

Organ-specific Diseases

Many of these disorders are known and although glandular tissues are primarily affected some of these diseases may affect other epithelia such as the skin, or the blood cells. Generally, what occurs is that specific autoantibodies are formed against the tissue components, these components being unique to the specialized parenchymal cells of that tissue. The antibodies react with the tissue cells and through the mediation of sensitized antibody-dependent cytotoxic T cells (and/or complement) the tissue cells are destroyed. The appearance in the tissue is one of chronic inflammation which is followed by a shrinkage of the organ as more and more parenchymal cells are destroyed and are replaced by fibrous tissue (scar). Some examples of these organ specific diseases are discussed below.

Chronic autoimmune thyroidits (Hashimoto's disease). This disorder primarily affects the thyroid gland although in some patients with the disease the salivary glands and lacrimal glands may also be affected. The affected organs are infiltrated by very large numbers of lymphocytes and there is progressive loss of glandular tissue, which in advanced severe cases may altogether disappear. The thyroid in some cases resembles in microscopic appearance a lymph node, the glandular tissue having been replaced by lymphoid follicles. The thyroid gland is enlarged (goitre) but is hypofunctional, insufficient thyroxine being produced, and the person showing symptoms and signs of hypothyroidism (decreased metabolic rate, weight gain, presence of oedema, dullness and slowness, dry skin and puffy face, brittle hair and enlargement of the thyroid). This disease is commoner in females and it has been shown that over 10% of elderly females have some degree of this type of thyroiditis. The incidence also increases with increasing age. It must be mentioned that in many affected women the changes in the gland are not very florid and sufficient thyroid tissue is spared, such that enough thyroxine is produced for the body's needs. These women show only a moderate enlargement of the gland and under the microscope the thyroid shows many normal thyroid glandular follicles and only some areas are affected by chronic inflammation and infiltration by the lymphocytes (Figure 5.13).

Chronic autoimmune atrophic gastritis. This disorder affects the acid-secreting mucosa of the stomach and resembles very much thyroiditis in its epidemiology. It affects women more commonly than men and is seen with increasing frequency with increasing age. The autoantibodies react with the gastric mucosal cells, destroying them, and the stomach mucosa shows atrophy and fibrosis with chronic inflammatory cells in the lamina propria. As the acid-producing cells are destroyed, the patient presents with dyspepsia and when laboratory investigations on gastric function are performed a hypochlorhydria or achlorhydria (less than normal or no HCl produced by the stomach) is found. This may seriously interfere with the digestive process, especially that of proteins.

In a proportion of patients with this disorder autoantibodies are also produced against intrinsic factor which is produced by the stomach mucosa. Intrinsic factor is essential for the absorption of vitamin B_{12} from the intestine and in its absence, pernicious anaemia will result. The patient presents therefore with atrophic gastritis and a severe anaemia.

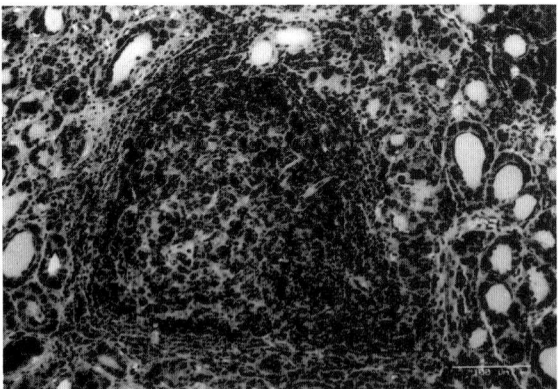

Figure 5.13 *Hashimoto's disease of the thyroid. A large active lymphoid follicle is present in the thyroid parenchyma and the greatly reduced numbers of thyroid acini are infiltrated by lymphocytes (scale bar is 100 μm)*

Autoimmune adrenalitis and autoimmune parathyroiditis. These are much rarer conditions affecting the adrenals or the parathyroid glands and once again autoimmune mechanisms destroy the tissues, with chronic inflammation, fibrosis and hypofunction of the affected glands resulting.

Systemic Diseases

Systemic lupus erythematosus (SLE). This is the typical systemic autoimmune disorder in which many tissues and organs in the body are affected, but in particular the connective tissues seem to suffer the most (SLE was also at one stage called a 'connective tissue' disease). In SLE, a whole series of auto-antibodies are present in the bloodstream and tissue fluids. The autoantigens in this case are: extractable nuclear DNA, nucleoproteins (histones), cytoplasmic soluble antigens, formed elements of the blood, IgG, clotting factors and cardiolipin. The commonest autoantibody present in nearly all cases of SLE is the antinuclear antibody. As is expected from the widespread location of these autoantigens in all tissues of the body, antigen–antibody reactions occur at a systemic level, causing systemic disease.

The patient's skin and connective tissues are affected, with characteristic rashes being apparent on the face and other exposed areas, there is joint and muscle involvement and also, as there are circulating antigen–antibody complexes, there is serious kidney disease (glomerulonephritis) initiated by complex-mediated hypersensitivity reactions at the glomerular level. The commonest cause of death in SLE patients is renal failure, which illustrates the importance of these kidney lesions. As there is widespread antigen–antibody reaction with subsequent complement activation in many parts of the body during the acute phase of the disease, most SLE patients show a marked hypocomplementaemia, which may be associated with an increased risk of infections. There may be platelet destruction with an increased tendency to haemorrhage.

Rheumatoid arthritis. This is another typical systemic autoimmune disorder in which there is marked damage to bones and joints but also other connective tissues throughout the body. The autoantigen in this case is an abnormal form of IgG which is formed throughout the body. That is, an antibody is functioning as an antigen. To this abnormal IgG, the immune system forms an antibody (about 70% of these autoantibodies are IgM antibodies) which is called rheumatoid factor. The IgM (rheumatoid factor) and abnormal IgG react together in a typical antigen–antibody fashion, they are deposited in many body sites, but especially around the synovial membrane of joints. This activates complement fixation and also activation of cell-mediated immune responses, giving rise to tissue destruction and overgrowth of scar tissue, causing fusion of the joint.

The clinical features of the disease are a polyarthritis, with many joints around the body being affected. In addition, subcutaneous and visceral lesions may be seen (rheumatoid nodules), consisting of areas of destroyed collagen and tissue with a marked infiltration by plasma cells, macrophages and T cells. Destruction of connective tissues in the eyes may lead to vision impairment.

Scleroderma. This is another of the 'connective tissue' diseases which has been shown to be due to autoimmune causes. In this disorder there is thickening and damage to the skin and mainly the dermal collagen and epithelial cells of the epidermis are involved. The autoantigens are connective tissue components and also nucleolar components. Many of these patients have antinucleolar antibodies which can be detected by fluorescent staining techniques of the epidermis.

Sjögren's syndrome. In this autoimmune disease there are antibodies against glandular epithelia (especially antithyroid and antisalivary gland antibodies) but also antibodies to nuclear components, mitochondria and IgG molecules. Joint disease and eye changes may also be seen in these patients as well as disorders relating to dysfunctions of the thyroid and salivary gland.

Mixed connective tissue disease. This combines features of scleroderma, rheumatoid arthritis, SLE and dermatomyositis. The autoantigen is nuclear and clinically it resembles the disorders to which it is related.

Aetiology of Autoimmune Disease

There have been many theories proposed as to how the autoimmune disorders arise. However, evidence from various researchers does not seem to support any one particular theory and often a specific disease will show an association with many aetiological factors. It is possible that a multifactorial aetiology is responsible for a great many, if not all, of the autoimmune states.

Cross-reaction of Self Tissues with Foreign Antigens
This is a mechanism which has been studied in relation to some disorders and seems to be a very important feature of many autoimmune states. In this case a micro-organism which enters the body possesses some antigens that are related to the body's own proteins. The immune system reacts to the microbe by producing an immune response against it which destroys the microbe and the infection is overcome. However, the antibodies produced against the microbe also cross-react with some body proteins since these body proteins share some antigenic determinants with the microbe. Hence, the immune response directed against the microbe also destroys body tissues. A typical example of this type of initiating factor in autoimmunity is rheumatic fever, in which an immune reaction to some strains of *Streptococcus* spp. will, in some individuals, also give rise to an autoimmune reaction directed against the connective tissues and heart muscle. This causes damage to the heart muscle and valves every time the person mounts an immune response against streptococci which enter the tissues. It should be noted here that the tissue damage results not from the infectious agent itself (which does not get into the heart and may cause a superficial infection in the throat or skin), but rather to the circulating antibodies to the microbe which also cross-react with and cause damage to body tissues.

Failure of 'Self Tolerance' Mechanisms
The mechanisms whereby we normally tolerate our body constituents and do not mount an immune reaction against them are poorly understood. It is suspected that these mechanisms may have much to do with the suppressor T group of lymphocytes which are the ones that normally suppress immune responses when there is no further need of them. It is thought that these T cells are very important in suppressing immune responses against our own body components, by interacting with the virgin T cells specific to the body proteins, which are present in our body since birth. If the normal regulatory mechanisms exerted by suppressor T cells fail, these virgin T cells specific to body proteins will be activated and lead to autoimmune reactions. Experiments in which suppressor T levels are reduced specifically in experimental animals are associated with an increased incidence of autoimmunity. In some cases of human autoimmune disorders, decreased suppressor T levels have been demonstrated.

Emergence of Normally 'Hidden' Antigens
It is known that sometimes tissue damage or death of cells may release small fragments of cell proteins that were previously sequestered inside the cell and therefore 'out of sight' of the immune system. These protein fragments, once released into the tissue fluid, may

stimulate an immune response, the immunity being directed against all proteins which bear on them antigenic determinants related to the protein fragments that initiated the immune response.

Modification of Self Antigens

This may be an important factor when we consider the increased incidence of autoimmunity with increasing age. The older an individual is the more cumulative tissue damage and alteration of body proteins we may expect to see in their tissues. If body components become sufficiently modified so as to differ from what the immune system regards as 'normal', there may be an autoimmune state. Another causative factor in this respect is that of increased incidence of autoimmune diseases after chronic infections such as tuberculosis. In this case, the persistent presence of poorly degraded antigen in the tissues and its prolonged contact with body cells may initiate changes in the self-determinants on body cells, leading to autoimmunity. Another very frequently encountered mechanism in this respect occurs with various autoimmune states and hypersensitivities resulting after drug administration to susceptible individuals. The drugs in many cases act as haptens, adhering to body proteins, altering them and leading to autoimmunity.

Polyclonal Activation

The presence of some specific types of microbes in the body induces a non-specific activation of humoral and cell-mediated immunity. That is, we see proliferation of many different clones of antigen-reactive cells in the immune system. This is a well-documented effect of *Mycobacterium leprae* infection (leprosy) and also EB virus infection (glandular fever). This non-specific activation has been likened to an adjuvant effect. In this response some of the normally suppressed self-specific clones may be activated and lead to autoimmunity.

Genetic Factors

These must exist as many autoimmune diseases are seen more commonly as running in some families, or are more commonly met in some races. It is a well-known observation that many autoimmune diseases are associated with a particular class of MHC antigen. Also, since females are more frequently affected by autoimmunity, there may be effects of the double X karyotype of females.

It should be remembered that why we do not normally react to our own body proteins is not fully understood and why these mechanisms often break down resulting in autoimmunity is in many cases a complete mystery. As we learn more about the normal immune system, it is hoped that the subject of autoimmunity will become better understood, leading in some cases to prevention of such aberrant immune responses.

Formation of Autoantibodies

Autoantibodies may form due to altered 'self' molecules. Cross-reactive antigens may be introduced from external sources — that is, antigens which resemble 'self' antigens. Antigens may be 'revealed' by tissue damage, allowing formation of autoantibodies. Autoantibodies may be seen in infectious diseases such as syphilis (Wassermann antibody) and other granulomatous diseases (TB, leprosy).

Autoantibodies can occur **normally** in sera. This is found with increasing frequency in ageing. Autoantibodies may be found against several antigens. Examples are rheumatoid factor (anti-IgG) seen in rheumatoid arthritis; antinuclear factors (anti-DNA) seen in SLE; antibodies against thyroid, adrenal or gastric cells or against intracellular organelles. These autoantibodies may be found in 30% of females over 60 years of age. (Most autoimmune disease is seen in early to middle age, however, so there may be genetic predisposing factors.) Often an autoimmune disease may have a superimposed hypersensitivity component. In fact some experts in the field classify all hypersensitivities as autoimmune diseases since in these allergic reactions it is an inappropriate immune response by the host which causes damage to 'self' tissues.

Revision Questions and Case Studies

1. Write an essay on the various forms of hypersensitivity reactions (allergic responses) encountered in the body and explain fully the underlying immune mechanisms responsible for the adverse reactions. Give appropriate examples of human disorders where necessary.

2. Discuss in detail the pathology of autoimmune diseases and give three typical examples of such disorders with their pathogenetic features. What are the theories that have been proposed to explain why such autoimmune reactions arise?

3. What are autoantibodies?

4. What is the mechanism of tissue damage in type IV, delayed-type hypersensitivity (allergy) reactions?

5. What is LATS antibody? What disease does it cause?

6. Rheumatic endocarditis is one of the complications seen in some people after infection with

which group of micro-organisms? What type of autoimmune reaction is this an example of?

7. Outline the secondary immunodeficiencies with special reference to the commonest of these.

8. Define the following terms:
   (a) Persistent generalized lymphadenopathy (PGL)
   (b) Agammaglobulinaemia
   (c) Candidaemia
   (d) Anaphylaxis
   (e) Immunoprophylaxis

9. Discuss one important human disease, the pathogenesis of which is dependent on a type III hypersensitivity.

10. What type of hypersensitivity is Graves' disease an example of? Discuss the pathogenesis of this disorder.

11. Write short notes on the following diseases indicating the factors of autoimmunity that are responsible for their development:
    (a) Rheumatoid arthritis
    (b) Systemic lupus erythematosus (SLE)
    (c) Hashimoto's disease
    (d) Chronic autoimmune gastritis.

12. What is meant by the term 'self tolerance'? Why is it an important consideration in autoimmunity?

13. Discuss the pathogenesis of erythroblastosis foetalis.

14. Define the following terms:
    (a) Mast cell
    (b) Immune complex
    (c) Lymphokine
    (d) Contact dermatitis
    (e) Graft rejection

15. What features do human autoimmune diseases have in common?

16. State what type of hypersensitivity reaction is responsible for the causation of the following diseases:
    (a) Farmer's lung
    (b) Post-streptococcal glomerulonephritis
    (c) Serum sickness
    (d) Allergic asthma
    (e) Erythroblastosis foetalis
    (f) Bee stings
    (g) Mosquito bites
    (h) Thyrotoxicosis
    (i) Transfusion reactions
    (j) Flea bites

Case study 1. A 24-year-old Caucasian woman presents at the physiotherapist with slight neck pain. When she removes her necklet in order to be examined, he notices an erythematous, swollen, indurated patch on the skin on the back of her neck that is in contact with her necklet. The woman says that the lesion feels itchy and she thinks that it is some kind of dermatitis and that she will soon get over it as it often 'comes and goes'.

(a) What is the most likely diagnosis in respect of the skin lesion?
(b) If a biopsy of the skin lesion were taken what would be observed under the microscope?
(c) How is this disorder managed?

Case study 2. A 23-year-old Caucasian man presents at your clinic with a sore throat, generalized malaise, fatigue and joint pains. Upon examination it is found that his cervical and axillary lymph nodes are enlarged and very prominent. There are no lesions on the oral mucosa but the pharynx looks slightly inflamed. There is a red rash over his midriff but this 'has not given him any trouble'. Questioning the man you discover that he has also suffered from 'gastrointestinal upsets' over several weeks but he has 'got over that now'. The man is a homosexual but has been celibate for the past 16 months. Previous to that he had had a single sex partner for 2 years in what was a monogamous relationship. His partner had died of a drug overdose 16 months ago. The patient is not a drug user himself.

(a) What is the most likely diagnosis?
(b) Outline the way in which the disease may be spread, using the case study as an example.
(c) What is the prognosis for this patient?

Case study 3. A 4-year-old Caucasian girl presents with severe proteinuria, haematuria, generalized oedema and low-grade fever. Three weeks earlier the child had developed skin lesions of scarlet fever and was promptly treated with erythromycin as she is allergic to penicillin. The infection regressed and the child was well until the current illness. Kidney function tests show there is evidence of acute renal failure and a renal biopsy shows features typical of acute glomerulonephritis.

(a) What specific tests are available for the diagnosis of the precise aetiology of the child's renal disease?
(b) Outline the pathogenesis of the child's current disorder.
(c) How is this disorder treated?
(d) What is the prognosis?

Immunopathology Crossword

CLUES

ACROSS

1. The disease responsible for the commonest type of secondary immune deficiency (1, 1, 1, 1).
5. Persistent generalized lymphadenopathy (1, 1, 1).
7. A type I hypersensitivity reaction affecting the whole body, may lead to shock and death (11)
9. Disease where type IV responses cause tissue damage (2).
10. The antibody class causing type I allergies (3).
12. Antigen system on erythrocytes important in the causation of erythroblastosis foetalis (6).
13. The liquid part of blood remaining behind after clotting of the blood has been allowed to occur (5).

15. The sex genotype of people affected most commonly by autoimmune diseases (2).
16. Antibody — abbreviation (2).
17. The standard abbreviation for antigen (2).
20. The state whereby the immune system does not mount an immune response against a particular antigen (9).
22. Antigen system on red blood cells important in transfusion reactions (3).
23. The immune system normally recognizes _ _ _ _ components and does not attack them (4).
25. Antibody class found in secretions (3).
26. The _ _ _ _ cavity is involved in thrush in AIDS (4).
28. Type III reaction, also called an _ _ _ _ _ _ reaction (6).

31. A group of cells that are identical in every respect (5).
33. The Epstein-Barr virus (1, 1).
35. An inflammation of the kidney commonly due to type III reactions (18).
38. _ _ _ _ _ _' _ disease is also called agammaglobulinaemia (7).
40. Inflammation of the stomach, sometimes due to autoimmunity (9).
41. A body protein produced in response to an antigen (8).

DOWN

1. A substance which when introduced into the body will cause an immune response (7).
2. Granulation tissue forming over the articular cartilage in rheumatoid arthritis (6).
3. A group of T cells that will destroy abnormal cells (9).
4. An intradermal test for gauging susceptibility to TB (7).
5. Many small haemorrhages present throughout the body, often due to an autoimmune thrombocytopenia (7).
6. The _ _ _ _ antibody causes Graves' disease (4).
7. An antigen causing allergy (8).
8. An autoimmune disease causing thickening of skin and arthritis (11).
11. Haemolytic disease of the newborn, a type II hypersensitivity (16).
14. _ _ _ _ _ _' disease is thyrotoxicosis caused by a type V hypersensitivity (6).
18. _ _ _ _ _ _ are rejected by a type IV delayed type hypersensitivity (6).
19. Inactivated toxin that generates immune responses (6).
21. An antibody produced against self components (12).
22. AIDS-related complex (1, 1, 1).
24. A foreign substance too small to generate an immune response on its own (6).
27. Organ affected by a type of autoimmune cirrhosis (5).
29. A fungal infection of the skin, often seen in AIDS (5).
30. Antibody class that crosses the placenta (3).
32. Viral disease causing secondary immunodeficiency (3).
34. A tumour not usually fatal (6).
36. A pentameric antibody (3).
37. The cause of AIDS (1, 1, 1).
39. Systemic autoimmune disease characterized by a 'butterfly rash' (1, 1, 1).

Further Reading

Bennett JE. 'Searching for the Yeast Connection.' *New Engl J M* 1990; **323**: 1766.
Bodmer WF. 'The HLA System.' *Br Med Bull* 1978; **34**: 213.
Buckley RH. 'Immunodeficiency.' *J Allergy Clin Immunol* 1983; **72**: 627.
Carpenter AB, Rabin BS. 'Autoimmunity in Immunopathology.' *Clin Lab Med* 1982; **3**: 745.
Cohen IR. 'The Self, the World and Autoimmunity.' *Sci Am* 1988; April: 34.
Cohne S, Williamson GM. 'Stress and Infectious Disease.' *Psych Bull* 1991; **109**(1): 5.
Corey L, Fleming TR. 'Treatment of HIV Infection — Progress in Perspective.' *N Engl J Med* 1992; **326**: 437.
David JR, et al. 'Lymphokines and Macrophages.' *Cell Immunol* 1983; **82**: 75.
Fineberg HV. 'The Social Dimensions of AIDS.' *Sci Am* 1988; October: 106.
Geczy CL. 'The Role of Lymphokines in Delayed-Type Hypersensitivity.' *Springer Semin Immunopathol* 1984; **7**: 321.
Haseltine WA, Wong-Staal F. 'The Molecular Biology of the AIDS Virus.' *Sci Am* 1988; October: 34.
Horsburgh CR, et al. 'Duration of Human Immunodeficiency Virus Infection Before Detection of Antibody.' *Lancet* 1989; **ii**: 637.
Husband AJ. 'Psychoimmunology — Frontier or Fantasy?' *Today's Life Sci* 1992; **4**(1): 12.
Ishizaka K, Ishizaka T. 'Mechanisms of Reaginic Hypersensitivity and IgE Antibody Response.' *Immunol Rev* 1978; **41**: 109.
Johnson HM, Russell JK, Pontzer CH. 'Superantigens in Human Disease.' *Sci Am* 1992; April: 42.
Lucke WC. 'Anaphylaxis.' *J Emerg Med* 1983; **1**: 83.
Mobley K, et al. 'Autopsy Findings in the Acquired Immune Deficiency Syndrome.' *Pathol Annu* 1985; **20**(1): 45.
Niedt GW, Schinella RA. 'Acquired Immune Deficiency Syndrome.' *Arch Pathol Lab Med* 1985; **109**: 727.
Redfield RR, Burke DS. 'HIV Infection: The Clinical Picture.' *Sci Am* 1988; October: 70.
Rennie J. 'Overview: Tolerating Self. Experience Teaches the Immune System to Recognize Self.' *Sci Am* 1990; September: 18.
Roitt I. *Essential Immunology*, seventh edition, 1991; Blackwell Scientific Publications, Oxford.
Rosen FS, Cooper MD, Wedgwood RJ. 'The Primary Immunodeficiencies.' *N Eng J Med* 1984; **311**: 300.

Schuurs AHWM, Verheul HAM. 'Sex Hormones and Autoimmune Disease.' *Br J Rheumatol* 1989; **28** (Supp I): 59.

Sprent J. 'The Thymus and T cell Tolerance.' *Today's Life Sci* 1991: **3**(12): 14.

Steinberg AD. 'Autoimmunity.' *Annu Rev Immunol* 1983; **1**: 175.

Suciu-Foca N. 'The HLA Systems in Human Pathology.' *Pathobiol Annu* 1979; **9**: 81.

Sullivan KM, Storb R. 'Allogenic Bone Marrow Transplantation.' *Cancer Invest* 1984; **2**: 27.

Thomas W, *et al.* 'Allergy to the House Dust Mite.' *Today's Life Sci* 1990: **2**(8): 20.

Urmacher C, Nielsen S. 'The Histopathology of the Acquired Immune Deficiency Syndrome.' *Pathol Annu* 1985; **20**(1): 197.

von Boehmer H, Kisielow P. 'How the Immune System Recognizes Self.' *Sci Am* 1991; October: 50.

Wong DJ, Ogra PL. 'Viral Infections in Immunocompromised Patients.' *Med Clin North Am* 1983; **67**: 1075.

Yarchoan R, Mitsuya H, Broder S. 'AIDS Therapies.' *Sci Am* 1988; October: 88.

General Pathology Test

Allow 3 hours for this test.

Part A: Multiple Choice Questions

The following questions or statements have only **one correct response**. Read carefully all choices and indicate the **best** response by marking the letter corresponding to it (allow 60 minutes for this section).

1. Colliquative necrosis is a prominent feature of:
   (a) Tuberculosis
   (b) Central nervous system infarction
   (c) Non-specific granulomata
   (d) Renal infarction
   (e) Secondary syphilis

2. The manifestations of a specific disease that are obvious to the person performing the clinical examination but not necessarily to the patients themselves are called that disease's:
   (a) Pathology
   (b) Symptoms
   (c) Pathogenesis
   (d) Signs
   (e) Aetiology

3. The state whereby intracellular water is increased as a direct result of failure of the ATP-driven cell membrane ion pumps is called:
   (a) Oedema
   (b) Inflammation
   (c) Hydropic change
   (d) Dropsy
   (e) Fatty change

4. When the lungs are no longer air containing, the alveolar spaces having become full of fluid or cells, they are said to be:
   (a) Infiltrated
   (b) Consolidated
   (c) Congested
   (d) Inflected
   (e) Infarcted

5. The commonest cause of delayed fracture healing is:

(a) Infection
(b) Malnutrition
(c) Vitamin C deficiency
(d) Foreign body reaction to suture material
(e) Poor blood supply to the area

6. Thrombocytopenia refers to a decreased number of:
   (a) Red blood cells in the bloodstream
   (b) White blood cells in the bloodstream
   (c) Platelets in the bloodstream
   (d) Helper T lymphocytes in the bloodstream
   (e) None of the above

7. Pale infarcts would be seen most frequently in organs with a good collateral arterial supply.
   (a) True
   (b) False

8. Thromboemboli that have lodged in the lungs are most likely to have arisen in the:
   (a) Liver
   (b) Left ventricle
   (c) Brain
   (d) Arteries of the legs
   (e) Veins of the legs

9. When sectioned, pale thrombi characteristically show:
   (a) Virchow's Triad
   (b) A uniform white-grey cut surface
   (c) Lines of Zahn
   (d) Triple response of Lewis
   (e) A spotty pinkish grey surface with a red centre

10. Hypertensive people rarely die from:
    (a) Cerebral haemorrhage
    (b) Myocardial insufficiency
    (c) Cerebral infarction
    (d) Phlebothrombosis
    (e) Renal failure

11. A localized, abnormal dilatation of any vessel, caused by a weakening of its tunica media, is defined as an:
    (a) Atheromatous plaque
    (b) Atheroma
    (c) Angioma
    (d) Intimal cushion
    (e) None of the above

12. Histamine is a protein found in plasma in trace amounts.
    (a) True
    (b) False

13. The so-called 'soft' risk factors in the development of atherosclerosis are:
    (a) Infections, septicaemia, high-fat diet, pimples
    (b) Hypertension, soft drinking water, myocardial infarction

(c) Thromboembolism, myocardial infarction, cigarette smoking
(d) Hypertension, diabetes, cigarette smoking, hyperlipidaemia
(e) Oral contraception, stress, obesity, lack of exercise

14. The severity of hypertension is enhanced by atherosclerosis.
    (a) True
    (b) False

15. Well-developed cells of one organ found in another unrelated organ constitute a hamartoma.
    (a) True
    (b) False

16 In hypertensive individuals the left ventricle often undergoes hypertrophy as a result of the increased work load.
    (a) True
    (b) False

17. A condition in which a fully differentiated, adult tissue loses its regular appearance and architecture, the individual cells losing their uniformity and regularity, is called:
    (a) Aplasia
    (b) Hypoplasia
    (c) Dysplasia
    (d) Metaplasia
    (e) None of the above

18. The brain of a stillborn baby is found at postmortem examination to be totally absent. This case is an example of:
    (a) Hypertrophy
    (b) Agenesis
    (c) Hypoplasia
    (d) Atrophy
    (e) Aplasia

19. Malignancies of the small intestine are very rare. When they do occur, such tumours would most probably show secondary, haematogenous, metastatic deposits in the:
    (a) Lymph nodes
    (b) Lungs
    (c) Bone
    (d) Liver
    (e) Brain

20. The increase in the size of the female breast that is seen with lactation is an example of:
    (a) Physiological hypertrophy
    (b) Physiological hyperplasia
    (c) Physiological neoplasia
    (d) Pathological hyperplasia
    (e) Pathological hypertrophy

21. A rhabdomyosarcoma is an example of a:

(a) Benign tumour
(b) Malignant tumour
(c) Hypertrophy
(d) Hyperplasia
(e) Reactive inflammatory change

22. A disease caused by a human retrovirus is thalassaemia.
(a) True
(b) False

23. Macrophages have a much longer life span than neutrophils.
(a) True
(b) False

24. Biological carcinogenic agents include:
(a) Plastic films, heat, trauma and X-rays
(b) Procarcinogens, carcinogens and oncogenes
(c) Viruses, and bacteria or fungi causing chronic infections
(d) Croton oil, glass, plastic, asbestos, silicon
(e) Epoxides, nitrosamines, coal tar derivatives, aflatoxins

25. Deposition of calcium in necrotic tissues occurring in an individual with normal blood calcium levels is termed:
(a) Dystrophic calcification
(b) Metastatic calcification
(c) Hypercalcaemic calcification
(d) Metacalcaemic calcification
(e) Osteotic calcification

26. Examples of cytogenetic disorders are the following:
(a) Albinism, six-digit hands, phenylketonuria
(b) Down's syndrome (mongolism), Klinefelter's syndrome
(c) Scurvy, bacterial pneumonia, gout, Klinefelter's syndrome
(d) Scurvy, arsenic poisoning, viral pneumonia
(e) Viral pneumonia, diabetes mellitus, phenylketonuria

27. Atherosclerosis may cause:
(a) Massive peritoneal haemorrhages
(b) Peptic ulceration
(c) Decreased immunity
(d) All of the above
(e) None of the above

28. Increased levels of which lipoprotein are associated with atherosclerosis?
(a) High-density lipoproteins
(b) Low-density lipoproteins
(c) Very low density lipoprotein
(d) Cholesterol esters
(e) Acetate esters of long-chain fatty acids

29. Coronary heart disease incidence is lower in India than in Australia.

(a) True
(b) False

30. Benign tumours are usually not life threatening tumours.
(a) True
(b) False

31. The primary change that is seen in atherosclerosis is:
(a) Adventitial necrosis and intimal fibrosis
(b) Medial calcification and inflammation
(c) Smooth muscle cell proliferation with lipid deposition in the intima
(d) Intimal fibroblast proliferation with adventitial fibrosis
(e) Inflammation of the media with reduction in lumen size

32. Hallmarks of the chronic inflammatory response include:
(a) Redness, heat, swelling and pain
(b) Pleomorphic exudates
(c) An exudative rather than a productive response
(d) A granulomatous form occurring commonly
(e) The presence of large numbers of neutrophils in the tissue

33. The commonest variety of chromosomal disorder is:
(a) Down's syndrome (mongolism)
(b) Turner's syndrome (X/O karyotype)
(c) Klinefelter's syndrome (XXY karyotype)
(d) Trisomy 13/15
(e) Trisomy 16/18

34. Metastatic calcification is *not* usually seen in:
(a) Hypercalcaemia
(b) Hyperparathyroidism
(c) Necrotic tissues
(d) Hypoparathyroidism
(e) Hypervitaminosis D

35. The protein content of inflammatory exudate is:
(a) Equal to that of plasma
(b) About a tenth of that of plasma
(c) About half that of plasma
(d) About twice that plasma
(e) About ten times that of plasma

36. Vinyl chloride is a substance which exerts its carcinogenic effects by acting as a co-carcinogen or promoter of neoplasia when it comes into the body with other carcinogenic substances.
(a) True
(b) False

37. In Mönckeberg's calcification:
(a) There is intimal calcification and degeneration
(b) There are usually marked ischaemic effects
(c) Calcification is the result of fat deposition

(d) Ossification never occurs in the calcium deposits

(e) The arteries of the arms and legs are usually affected

38. The following is *not* a feature observed in the development of the atheromatous plaque.
    (a) Accumulation of lipid in the intima
    (b) Proliferation of smooth muscle cells
    (c) Endothelial injury may be an initiating event
    (d) Muscular arteries are involved
    (e) There is accumulation of connective tissue matrix compounds

39. Benign tumours may cause death by invading a blood vessel and causing a heart or a brain infarct.
    (a) True
    (b) False

40. Fatty change of the liver is characteristically seen in:
    (a) Alcoholics
    (b) Infarction of the liver
    (c) Patients with immune deficiencies (e.g. AIDS)
    (d) All of the above
    (e) None of the above

41. A substance *not* involved in chemical mediation of the acute inflammatory response is:
    (a) Histamine
    (b) Interleukin I
    (c) Bradykinin
    (d) Prostaglandin
    (e) C2-kinin component of complement

42. In chronic inflammation *ab initio*, the inflammation:
    (a) Is a sequela of suppuration
    (b) Can be best described as atypical
    (c) Follows an acute inflammatory response that persists
    (d) Begins as such without an acute phase
    (e) Follows infection with *Staphylococcus epidermidis*

43. The cells that are the most numerous white blood cells in the circulation are the:
    (a) B cells and T cells
    (b) Monocytes
    (c) Neutrophils
    (d) Helper T cells
    (e) Eosinophils

44. In thyrotoxicosis, patients have an enlarged thyroid gland with symptoms and signs indicating a hyperactivity of the thyroid. What is the most likely cause of this type of goitre?
    (a) Hypertrophy
    (b) Hyperplasia
    (c) Atrophy

(d) Neoplasia
(e) Metaplasia

45. A patient presents with evidence of extensive granulation tissue formation on his skin. What is the major pathological process operating at that site?
    (a) Chronic inflammation
    (b) Tuberculosis
    (c) Neoplasia
    (d) Acute inflammation and repair
    (e) Non-specific disease

46. In chronic inflammation the serous form (e.g. bursitis) is very common.
    (a) True
    (b) False

47. Gummatous necrosis is characteristic of leprosy.
    (a) True
    (b) False

48. Damage to blood vessel walls, alteration in the blood constituents and alteration in the flow characteristics of blood in any vessel are all factors predisposing to:
    (a) Thrombosis
    (b) Embolism
    (c) Atherosclerosis
    (d) Hypertension
    (e) None of the above

49. The cause of a disease is also known as its pathogenesis.
    (a) True
    (b) False

50. Genetic factors are important in the development of atherosclerosis.
    (a) True
    (b) False

51. Teratoma of the testis is most commonly a benign tumour.
    (a) True
    (b) False

52. An example of an autoimmune disease is:
    (a) AIDS
    (b) Systemic lupus erythematosus (SLE)
    (c) Di-George syndrome
    (d) Primary agammaglobulinaemia
    (e) None of the above

53. A substance important in type IV hypersensitivity reactions is:
    (a) Histamine
    (b) Macrophage-activating factor
    (c) Bradykinin
    (d) Prostaglandin
    (e) C2-kinin component of complement

54. Type III hypersensitivity is an example of a cell-mediated hypersensitivity.

(a) True

(b) False

55. Histocompatibility testing is not required in grafting involving the following tissue:
    (a) Bone marrow
    (b) Heart
    (c) Blood
    (d) Cornea
    (e) All of the above

56. An example of a type I hypersensitivity reaction is:
    (a) Reaction around a mosquito bite
    (b) Farmer's lung
    (c) Blood transfusion mismatch reactions
    (d) Glomerulonephritis
    (e) Adverse reactions following bee stings

57. Factors *delaying* bone fracture healing include:
    (i) Infection
    (ii) Immobilization
    (iii) Vitamin C deficiency
    (iv) Pre-existing bone disease
    (v) Congenital liver disease

    (a) Choices (i) and (iii) are right
    (b) Choices (ii) and (iv) are right
    (c) Choices (i), (iii) and (iv) are right
    (d) Choices (ii), (iii) and (v) are right
    (e) All choices are right

58. Uterine fibroleiomyomata:
    (i) Are very common in incidence
    (ii) Are benign tumours
    (iii) Very rarely undergo malignant transformation
    (iv) May cause very serious complications
    (v) Regress after the menopause

    (a) Choices (i) and (iii) are right
    (b) Choices (ii) and (iv) are right
    (c) Choices (i), (iii) and (iv) are right
    (d) Choices (ii), (iii) and (v) are right
    (e) All choices are right

59. The features observed in acute inflammation include:
    (i) Chemotaxis
    (ii) Direct vascular injury
    (iii) Increased vascular permeability
    (iv) Neutrophil accumulation in the area
    (v) Diapedesis

    (a) Choices (i) and (iii) are right
    (b) Choices (ii) and (iv) are right
    (c) Choices (i), (iii) and (iv) are right
    (d) Choices (ii), (iii) and (v) are right
    (e) All choices are right

60. Granulation tissue consists of:

(i) Epithelioid cells

(ii) Actively growing capillary loops

(iii) A few acute inflammatory cells

(iv) Dead and dying neutrophils, debris, bacteria

(v) Fibroblasts

(a) Choices (i) and (iii) are right

(b) Choices (ii) and (iv) are right

(c) Choices (i), (iii) and (iv) are right

(d) Choices (ii), (iii) and (v) are right

(e) All choices are right

61. Oedema may result from:
    (i) Primary shock
    (ii) Hypoproteinaemia
    (iii) Hydropic change
    (iv) Increased capillary blood pressure
    (v) Decreases in the microvascular permeability

    (a) Choices (i) and (iii) are right
    (b) Choices (ii) and (iv) are right
    (c) Choices (i), (iii) and (iv) are right
    (d) Choices (ii), (iii) and (v) are right
    (e) All choices are right

62. Hypotension in primary shock is due to:
    (i) Vasodilatation
    (ii) Heart failure
    (iii) Increase in the volume of the peripheral circulation
    (iv) Apnoea
    (v) Decreased blood volume

    (a) Choices (i) and (iii) are right
    (b) Choices (ii) and (iv) are right
    (c) Choices (i), (iii) and (iv) are right
    (d) Choices (ii), (iii) and (v) are right
    (e) All choices are right

63. Benign tumours usually show:
    (i) Many mitotic figures
    (ii) No necrosis
    (iii) No invasion
    (iv) Well-differentiated cell populations
    (v) A pseudocapsule formed by the compression of the surrounding tissues

    (a) Choices (i) and (iii) are right
    (b) Choices (ii) and (iv) are right
    (c) Choices (i), (iii) and (v) are right
    (d) Choices (ii), (iii) and (iv) are right
    (e) All choices are right

64. Oncogenes may be:
    (i) Normal cellular genes
    (ii) Bacterial genes inserted in cells by viruses
    (iii) Important in the process of neoplasia
    (iv) Very important in the process of germ cell production
    (v) Activated by viral infection

(a) Choices (i) and (iii) are right
(b) Choices (ii) and (iv) are right
(c) Choices (i), (iii) and (v) are right
(d) Choices (ii), (iii) and (iv) are right
(e) All choices are right

65. Shock may be due to:
    (i) Purpura
    (ii) Haemorrhage
    (iii) Hypovolaemia
    (iv) Bacteraemia
    (v) Oedema

    (a) Choices (i) and (iii) are right
    (b) Choices (ii) and (iv) are right
    (c) Choices (i), (iii) and (v) are right
    (d) Choices (ii), (iii) and (iv) are right
    (e) All choices are right

66. Chronic inflammation will characteristically be seen in:
    (i) A small pimple
    (ii) A nodule in the skin of a person suffering from leprosy
    (iii) A peptic ulcer that has formed 40 hours prior to examination
    (iv) Sarcoidosis
    (v) The lungs of a patient with pneumonia caused by *Streptococcus pneumoniae*

    (a) Choices (i) and (iii) are right
    (b) Choices (ii) and (iv) are right
    (c) Choices (i), (iii) and (v) are right
    (d) Choices (ii), (iii) and (iv) are right
    (e) All choices are right

67. An infarct of the kidney is characterized by:
    (i) Colliquative necrosis
    (ii) Coagulative necrosis
    (iii) Pale colour (non-haemorrhagic infarct)
    (iv) Common incidence
    (v) Red colour (haemorrhagic infarct)

    (a) Choices (i) and (iii) are right
    (b) Choices(ii) and (iv) are right
    (c) Choices (i), (iii) and (v) are right
    (d) Choices (ii), (iii) and (iv) are right
    (e) All choices are right

68. Factors predisposing to the development of atherosclerosis are:
    (i) Hypercholesterolaemia
    (ii) Undernutrition
    (iii) Stress
    (iv) Diabetes insipidus
    (v) Diabetes mellitus

    (a) Choices (i) and (iii) are right
    (b) Choices (ii) and (iv) are right
    (c) Choices (i), (iii) and (v) are right

(d) Choices (ii), (iii) and (iv) are right
(e) All choices are right

69. A 62-year-old Caucasian male self-employed businessman, 1.9 m tall, weighing 114 kg, presents with a history of sharp pain in the left lower leg which usually manifests itself when he is walking rapidly. He says that he 'just has to sit down and rest until the pain goes away, usually within 5 minutes' but if he exerts himself again the pain returns. The man is a smoker (25 cigarettes a day) and his blood pressure is 170/102 mmHg. Lately, he mentions, he has noticed that he has increased his fluid intake. The man does not drink alcohol. What is the most likely cause of the man's presenting signs and symptoms?
    (a) Malignant tumour
    (b) Metastatic calcification
    (c) Mönckeberg's medial calcification
    (d) Thromboembolism
    (e) Atherosclerosis

70. In the case of the patient mentioned in question 69, additional diseases that need to be considered when treating him are:
    (i) Hypertension
    (ii) Kidney infarction
    (iii) Kidney damage
    (iv) Metastatic tumours in the lung or bones
    (v) Retinal damage

    (a) Choices (i) and (iii) are right
    (b) Choices (ii) and (iv) are right
    (c) Choices (i), (iii) and (v) are right
    (d) Choices (ii), (iii) and (iv) are right
    (e) All choices are right

Part B: Short Answer Questions

Answer all of the following questions lucidly and concisely, covering all of the important main points. You should spend about 70 minutes answering this section. The suggested time you should spend on each question is given after it.

1. What is meant by the term 'fatty change' when it is applied to body cells? Give an example of three tissues which commonly undergo this process and indicate three different aetiologies associated with fatty change. (5 minutes)
2. What is a thrombus? What are the sequelae associated with a thrombus? (7 minutes)
3. What are the features that autoimmune diseases share, and what may be inferred about their aetiology from these features? (10 minutes)

4. Define the term 'anaplasia'. (2 minutes)
5. What occurs in the process of carcinogenesis? What is the result of such a process? Give one example of each of the following major classes of carcinogens: (a) physical agent, (b) chemical agent, (c) biological agent. (6 minutes)
6. What is a 'musculoelastic lesion'? In what disease process would it be found and what does the lesion progress to? (4 minutes)
7. What do you know of the group of conditions known as 'hypersensitivities'? Give an example of a type I hypersensitivity and explain its pathogenesis. How are type I hypersensitivities managed? (10 minutes)
8. Differentiate between localized and generalized oedema. Give two major causes for each of these conditions. (6 minutes)
9. List the various causes of disease (differentiating between intrinsic and extrinsic) and give a disease as an example of each. (10 minutes)
10. What occurs in the process of necrosis? Outline the process of necrosis as it occurs as a result of infarction in the myocardium. Differentiate between the various forms of necrosis as it occurs in various body sites and as a result of various aetiologies. (10 minutes)

Part C: Essay Question

Choose **only one (1)** of the following topics and write an essay, including all relevant information, concisely and thoroughly. (50 minutes)

1. Discuss the process of acute inflammation and indicate its characteristics, various forms, macroscopical and microscopical features. Outline the steps in the formation of exudate and infiltrate and the possible sequelae of the inflammation. Ensure that you cover thoroughly the clinical manifestations of the acute inflammatory response and also that you explain the purpose and advantageous effects of this process.
2. What is meant by the term 'shock'? Discuss the pathological manifestations of the various forms of this condition and cover thoroughly the aetiological and pathogenetic factors associated with each clinically observed type of shock.
3. Discuss the process of neoplasia, fully differentiating it from that of hyperplasia. Mention in your discussion the various systems of tumour classification and nomenclature and indicate the important differences in the behaviour of benign and malignant neoplasms. Give an account of the spread of malignant tumours. Use examples of the various tumours occurring in the body to substantiate your discussion.

Part II

Systemic Pathology

Systemic Pathology

The study of systemic pathology is an application of the basic pathological processes to diseases as they manifest themselves in the various body systems. It is much a case of correlating the basic processes as they have been studied in isolation in typical, specific tissues to the occurrence of such processes in an organ or a body system. Systemic pathology integrates and interconnects all of the basic concepts that have already been covered in general pathology. It is easier for the student who is studying systemic pathology to appreciate the nature of disease on a somatic level, as it is systemic disease that is equated in one's mind with patient presentation at the clinical level.

As a consequence, in this portion of the text, the stress is more on aggregation of the many general pathological processes into a unified whole, relating this to each of the many diseases that may afflict a certain body organ. The patient presentation in terms of signs and symptoms is related to the changes in the tissue brought about by the pathological processes active in a certain disease. In addition, certain disease states that are unique to some body sites are introduced at this level of study, as, for example, is the case with cirrhosis of the liver and the dust inhalation diseases in the lungs. However, it is important to note that even in these cases, it is basic pathological processes that are active in the tissue and this is because the body has only a limited way of responding to an overwhelming diversity of injurious agents. Therefore, even in systemic pathology, basic processes such as necrosis, inflammation, organization and neoplasia, for example, are the basis of the disease states and it is important for the student to be able to associate such general pathological processes with disease as it presents in the various organ systems. The importance of aetiology versus pathogenesis in determining the development of disease in an organ system cannot be stressed enough.

It is therefore essential for the student of systemic pathology to have learnt and to have understood thoroughly the processes that have been covered in Part I. If he or she does not understand how a disease affects an organ system, often this is because he or she does not understand the basic pathological processes active in that disease. The student who is studying systemic pathology may need to revise general pathology.

The significance of various diagnostic tests and laboratory investigations in the diagnosis of disease becomes evident when systemic pathology is studied. Where relevant, various important, common diagnostic procedures are given and their relationship with the various organosystemic diseases is pointed out.

6

Cardiovascular System Disorders

The Normal Cardiovascular System

The function of the cardiovascular system is to circulate blood throughout the body. The normal cardiovascular system comprises: the **heart**, which is the pumping organ, being a specialised, very muscular blood vessel; the **arteries**, which are muscular and elastic vessels conveying blood to the tissues; the **capillaries**, which are very thin, of small diameter and through which diffusion of nutrients and metabolites occurs within the tissues; the **veins**, which are thin walled and have a thin muscular layer in their walls, conveying blood back to the heart; and the **lymphatic vessels**, which convey excess tissue fluid back to the bloodstream, through a system of vessels of increasing diameter, finally emptying the lymph via the thoracic duct into the vena cava.

The heart is divided by a septum into two halves, right and left, each half being separated into two cavities, the upper, termed auricles or atria, and the lower, ventricles (refer to Figure 6.1). The right half of the heart contains venous, unoxygenated blood and the left half contains arterial, oxygenated blood. From the cavity of the left ventricle the blood is pumped into the aorta and thence into smaller and smaller arteries to all parts of the body, until it reaches the capillaries where the gas exchanges occur, where metabolites of tissues diffuse into the blood, and nutrients diffuse out. The unoxygenated, impure blood is collected by venules, and through a system of gradually enlarging veins, this blood is returned to the right atrium of the heart, from where it is emptied into the right ventricle and then pumped via the pulmonary arteries into the lungs. In the pulmonary capillaries, the blood is oxygenated and then passes into the pulmonary veins, the left atrium and left ventricle, where the cycle begins again.

The course of the blood from the left side of the heart, through the body tissues generally, to the right side of the heart is termed the systemic circulation. The course of the blood from the right side of the heart, through the lungs, to the left side of the heart is termed the pulmonary circulation. Because of the intimate interconnection of the circulatory and respiratory systems, disease in one of these systems very frequently will be associated with disease in the other. For example, valvular diseases in the left side of the

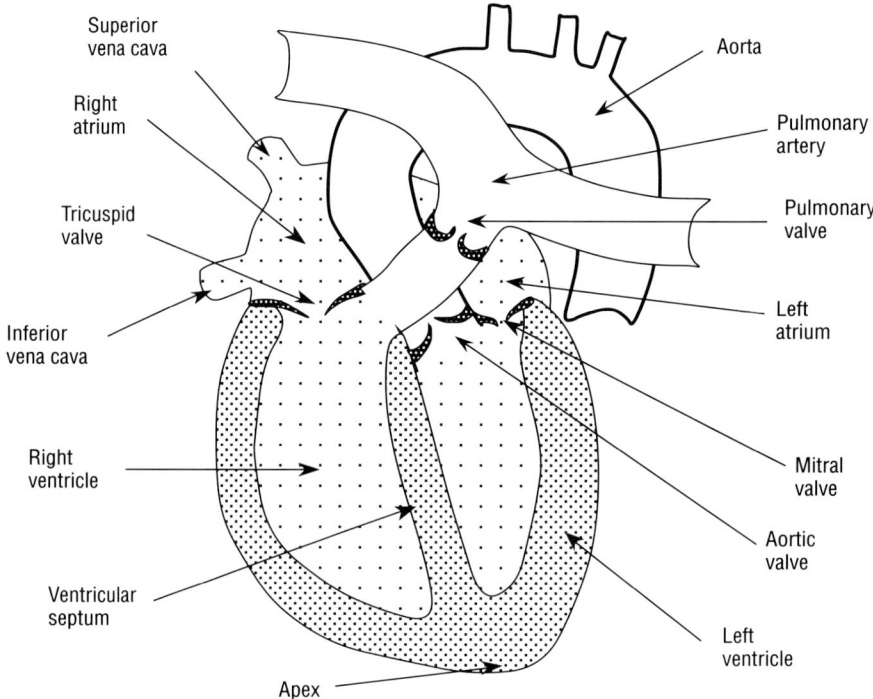

Figure 6.1   *The normal heart*

heart lead to compromise of pulmonary arterial blood drainage from the lungs, which may in turn cause pulmonary hypertension and oedema.

Cardiovascular disease is a major cause of death, especially in the Western world. The major diseases implicated in the cardiovascular system for these deaths are atherosclerosis, thrombosis, embolism and infarction. The left side of the heart, being the side which has the greatest work load and therefore depends much on its extensive blood supply, is the part of the heart most frequently involved in the ischaemic necrosis of infarction. Cardiac muscle is one of the permanent tissues in the body and its necrosis is followed by healing through fibrosis, if the person survives the infarct. Adequate cardiovascular function is essential to life and if the heart stops in its function as a pump for the blood, death will ensue in a few minutes.

Congenital Cardiovascular System Diseases

These are malformations present at birth and often there is more than one present. Some are life threaten-

ing and need urgent investigation and surgical treatment. Most of the other malformations interfere seriously with cardiac function and may lead to early death if not corrected during childhood. Congenital heart disease may be due to complex genetic factors, often arising as a developmental defect due to inappropriate gene action or activation of the wrong gene at the wrong time. Otherwise the defects arise through the interaction of environmental agents with the developing embryo, for example viral infections (rubella virus, cytomegalovirus, etc.), or alternatively through the action of various chemical agents, drugs or radiation. There are many types of congenital heart disease, but only the most common types will be discussed here.

Left to Right Shunts

Atrial Septal Defect

This is a connection between right and left atria due to a hole in the interatrial septum, caused in about 90% of cases by failure of closure of the foramen ovale. The disorder accounts for approximately 15% of congenital heart diseases and is the commonest congenital heart defect found in adults. Surgical correction of such lesions is usually required, although in a small number of cases the greater pressure inside the left atrium keeps the defect functionally closed. A complication associated with untreated cases of this disease is the occurrence of **paradoxical emboli**, implying that venous emboli will find their way into the systemic circulation, bypassing the lungs, and thus causing systemic infarcts in organs. Pulmonary hypertension may also be seen in patients with patent foramen ovale. Treatment of the condition is by surgery at a young age.

Ventricular Septal Defect

This is an abnormal connection between right and left ventricles due to a hole in the interventricular septum. It is the most frequent of the congenital heart defects, accounting for approximately 28% of such diseases. The severity of the disorder depends on the amount of blood shunting from left to right parts of the heart and in severe cases the infant dies at a very young age if the condition is not surgically treated. The prognosis of such operations is now excellent. In smaller lesions the volume of blood shunting is smaller and the condition may be compatible with life, although there are many complications of the disorder, for example vegetations may form on the margins of the defect.

Patent Ductus Arteriosus

This disorder accounts for approximately 18% of congenital heart diseases and may be brought about as a result of maternal rubella infection in early pregnancy. The ductus arteriosus is a structure connecting the distal aortic arch with the left pulmonary artery in the foetus. In the normal infant the ductus arteriosus is converted into a fibrous cord within about two months of birth. In the disorder, the ductus arteriosus fails to close after birth, leading to aortic blood being diverted from the systemic circulation into the pulmonary circulation. The advanced condition is treated by surgery, which is a successful way of effecting a cure. In a small number of cases, therapy with inhibitors of prostaglandin synthesis, such as indomethacin, can facilitate the closure of the ductus arteriosus prior to a fully fledged shunt developing.

Anomalous Pulmonary Venous Drainage

In these defects, one or more pulmonary veins drain into the systemic circulation, as occurs, for example, when they drain into the inferior vena cava and not into the left atrium. There is usually an atrial defect as well, allowing blood to flow into the left side of the heart. Sometimes, an abnormal vein leads from the right lung to the inferior vena cava and shows up in an X-ray as a curved shadow, giving this condition the name of the '**scimitar syndrome**'. All of these conditions involve passage of blood back into the right side of the heart and the pulmonary circulation, without entering the systemic circulation normally. Hence, the pulmonary circulation is overloaded, pulmonary hypertension occurs and the pulmonary vessels enlarge. The heart enlarges also due to increased blood being pumped, with resultant right ventricular hypertrophy.

Pulmonary Stenotic Lesions

This involves narrowing of the pulmonary artery or the pulmonary valve, thus reducing the amount of blood in the lungs. The pulmonary artery enlarges (post-stenotic dilatation) due to turbulent flow. The reduced pulmonary blood flow leads to insufficient oxygenation of blood, so the affected babies appear blue (**cyanotic**), hence the term 'blue babies'.

Pulmonary stenosis may occur as an isolated lesion. However, the condition is often combined with other congenital defects. In **Fallot's tetralogy**, pulmonary stenosis is combined with a high ventricular septal defect, overriding of the septum by the aorta (which is supplied by both ventricles), and right ventricular hypertrophy (because it pumps against the pressure of the left ventricle). This condition accounts for about 10% of all congenital heart defects (see Figure 6.2).

Coarctation of the Aorta

This is the condition where there is narrowing or blockage of the aorta, usually at the distal end of the aortic arch, and accounts for about 5% of congenital heart disease. In about half of cases there is also a bicuspid aortic valve. There are two forms of this disorder. The **preductal (infant) type** has severe narrowing of a segment of the aorta between the origin of the subclavian artery and the ductus arteriosus. A patent ductus allows blood to enter the systemic circulation from the pulmonary circulation. Usually such a condition is fatal in infancy. The **postductal (adult) type** of coarctation is more common and involves a shorter segment of the aorta. Frequently, in this type of the disease a ring of fibrosis occurs in the wall of the aorta just distal to the ductus arteriosus, which is usually

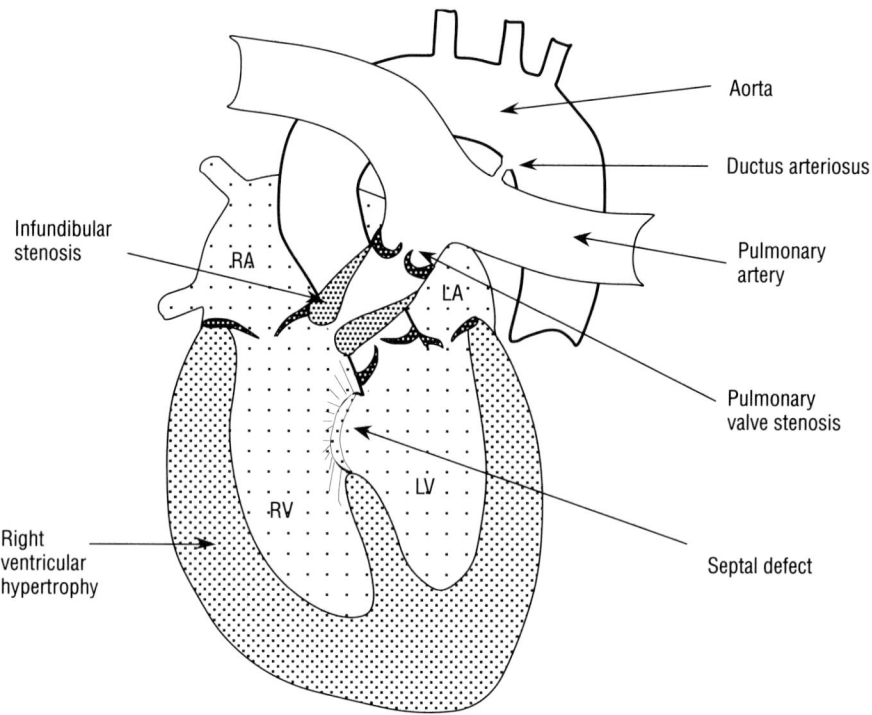

Figure 6.2   *The tetralogy of Fallot*

closed. When the aortic stenosis is severe enough to cause symptoms, these include hypertension proximal to the obstruction (headaches, dizziness) and hypotension distal to the obstruction (weakness, coldness of lower limbs, pallor). Blood pressure measured in the upper limb is much greater than that measured in the lower limb. To supply blood to the lower body many anastomotic vessels develop, including the intercostal arteries, the flow reversing to reach the descending aorta. Complications of the disease include hypertrophy of the heart and cerebral artery aneurysms. Death from untreated coarctation of the aorta occurs before middle age.

Transpositions

These malformations show transposition of the great vessels and account for about 8% of all defects. For example, the pulmonary artery arises from the left ventricle and the aorta from the right ventricle. To preserve life there must also be a septal defect to connect systemic and pulmonary circulations. The affected infants are stunted, cyanotic and dyspnoeic, often suffering from congestive heart failure. Untreated, few children live more than a few months.

Truncus Arteriosus

This is a rare malformation in which a single vessel arises from both ventricles and supplies branches to the lungs and to the systemic circulation. There is usually an interventricular septal defect or the septum is totally absent. Both ventricles are hypertrophied and the orifice of the single vessel has three cusps, but it is not unusual to see four or six cusps in the valve. Few patients survive infancy without treatment. They are cyanotic and suffer from pulmonary hypertension.

Anomalies of Position

The aortic arch may be on the right side, while the descending aorta often remains on the left. The heart may be reversed in position (**dextrocardia**). This may be an isolated anomaly or it may be associated with complete reversal of the position of the liver, intestines and other abdominal viscera (**situs inversus**). The term **dextroversion** of the heart implies that the atria are normally placed but the ventricles are turned to the right.

Acquired Cardiovascular System Diseases

Most heart disease is acquired, congenital heart malformations being comparatively rare. In the following discussion on acquired heart disease, each of the three layers of the heart, the pericardium, myocardium and endocardium (including heart valves), will be considered separately. Some acquired disorders of vessels will also be discussed here.

Diseases of the Pericardium

The pericardium (or epicardium) is a double-walled sac that encases the heart. The visceral layer is an inner, thin, serous layer, adjacent to the myocardium, and the parietal layer is an outer, thicker, fibrous layer. The space between them is occupied by a few millilitres of pericardial fluid, preventing the two layers from rubbing against one another ensuring that there is almost no friction between the layers as the heart beats.

Inflammations — Pericarditis

Acute Pericarditis

Of the inflammatory lesions pericarditis is the most important; however, primary acute pericarditis is rare. Most cases of pericarditis arise from the involvement of the pericardium in some disease process already present in some neighbouring tissue, usually a process of direct extension from myocardial tissue or from the lungs and pleura. Alternatively, the pericarditis may be a manifestation of generalized disease.

The aetiology of acute pericarditis may be divided into the infective and non-infective (or aseptic) types. Of the infective causes, **viral pericarditis** (also called 'idiopathic') is now more commonly seen than bacterial pericarditis in the developed countries. It mostly affects young adults and subsides within two weeks. Some pericardial thickening with adhesions forming is evident but this rarely has any consequence. Viruses isolated from such cases include Group B Coxsackievirus and echovirus, but may include any of the other viruses that cause myocarditis. Viral pericarditis may also occur in association with severe viral infections elsewhere in the body. For example, it may follow acute upper or lower respiratory tract infections with influenza viruses or paramyxoviruses.

Bacterial pericarditis may be seen with pyaemia or septicaemia, pneumonia or penetrating lesions of the oesophagus or bronchi, for example ulcerating carcinoma. Direct spread from adjacent structures is the most common way in which this condition develops. Haematogenous (blood spread) or lymphatic spread may also occur, in these cases the bacteria reaching the pericardium from distant sites of infection. Pyogenic bacteria are often involved, with staphylococci, streptococci and occasionally Gram-negative bacteria isolated. Tuberculous pericarditis frequently complicates chronic pulmonary tuberculosis, the route of spread being through the lymphatics or directly via the infected pleura.

Aseptic pericarditis may be due to rheumatic heart disease and in this case is part of the pancarditis that characterizes this disease. Pericarditis may also occur in **acute myocardial infarction** where the affected muscle is adjacent to the pericardium and where the inflammatory reaction in response to the necrosis in the myocardium also involves the pericardium. In this case the inflammation develops during the first week

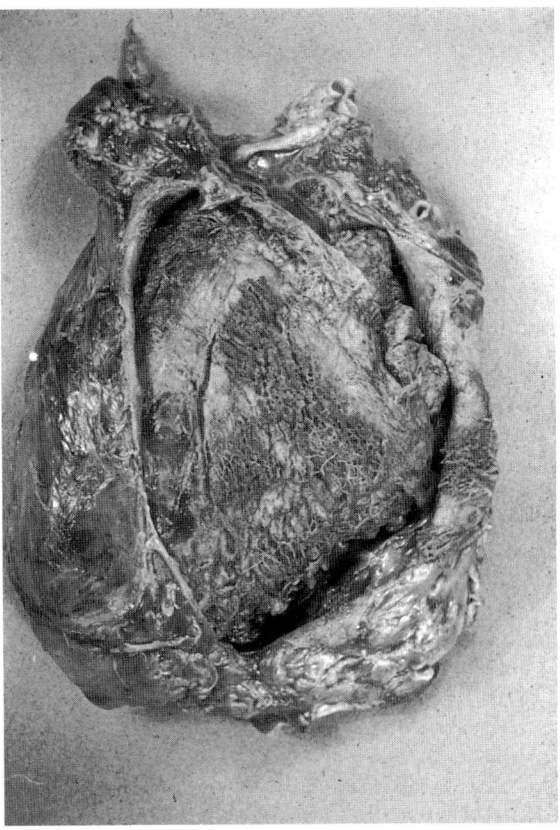

Figure 6.3 *Heart and pericardium from a patient with rheumatic heart disease, showing extensive fibrinous deposits between the two pericardial layers and the typical 'bread-and-butter' appearance*

in patients with transmural myocardial infarcts. Injury or surgery to the heart may also be followed by pericarditis. Other causes of non-infective pericarditis include **uraemia** (as seen in renal failure), or pericarditis due to **neoplasms**, the neoplastic pericarditis resulting mainly from direct or metastatic spread (for example, from mediastinal lymphoma or from bronchogenic or oesophageal carcinomas).

Pericarditis may result from **hypersensitivity reactions** as is seen in rheumatic heart disease (rheumatic fever, Figure 6.3), and from other autoimmune diseases such as systemic lupus erythematosus (SLE), rheumatoid arthritis and polyarteritis nodosa. Allergic pericarditis may also be seen in serum sickness and drug hypersensitivities.

In all cases of acute pericarditis the usual acute inflammatory phenomena occur, with hyperaemia, exudate formation, fibrin deposition, or in some cases, even suppuration. The types of acute pericarditis are often classified on the appearance of the exudate, the forms that are distinguished being:

- **Serous**: This is especially common in viral pericarditis. The exudate that is formed is clear, straw-coloured and has a high protein content. Its volume is usually small (50–200 mL) and this fluid does not interfere with cardiac function. In the cases where a large volume of fluid is formed or where even a small volume is formed very quickly, the pericardial pressure rises sharply, interfering with the filling of the atria, leading to a compromise in the general circulation, the whole syndrome being referred to as a cardiac tamponade.
- **Fibrinous**: This type is the one most frequently seen and is a prominent feature of non-infective aetiologies, for example uraemia. The exudate that is formed contains abundant fibrinogen, which is rapidly converted into insoluble networks of sticky fibrin, gluing the serous and fibrous layers of the pericardium together. On separating these two layers at autopsy, the surfaces present a shaggy, uneven appearance, much like the surface of two buttered slices of bread that have been separated. This justifies the commoner name of the condition, 'bread-and-butter pericarditis'. Fibrinous pericarditis may resolve with total removal of the fibrin and exudate, or alternatively the fibrin may be organized, fibroblasts laying down collagen, resulting in permanent fibrous adhesions of the pericardium. This type of pericarditis is also seen in rheumatic fever, myocardial infarction, some hypersensitivities and some cases of viral pericarditis.
- **Suppurative**: This almost always occurs after septic pericarditis caused by pyogenic organisms. Large volumes of thick, creamy pus may be present from which organisms will be isolated. Death results if the condition is not treated promptly and in survivors, organization and fibrous adhesions of the pericardium are the commonest aftermath.
- **Haemorrhagic**: In this case the inflammatory exudate filling the pericardial cavity is mixed with blood and is usually caused by invasion of the pericardium by tumour or else occurs associated with severe bacterial infections. The condition must be differentiated from haemopericardium. This type of pericarditis is often seen in neoplastic involvement of the heart where there is considerable bleeding within the pericardial sac.

In pericarditis, where large amounts of effusion accumulate, there may be **cardiac tamponade** with impaired diastolic filling of the heart. This arises because the increased pressure around the heart reduces the venous return to the heart. The blood pressure in the atria increases and in the case of the right side, there is increased central venous pressure, the jugular veins becoming distended and the liver congested. On the left side, the raised atrial pressure causes impedance of the circulation through the lungs, with pulmonary hypertension, dyspnoea and sometimes cyanosis occurring. Cardiac output falls dramatically and there is systemic hypotension. Cardiac tamponade is a potentially fatal condition and requires immediate treatment.

Serous and fibrinous pericarditis usually resolve, but sometimes in fibrinous pericarditis there may be a degree of fibrosis, which is usually focal and does not interfere with normal cardiac function. Suppurative pericarditis, however, may lead to more severe fibrosis (scarring) as the exudate organizes. There may be fibrous adhesions between the pericardium and surrounding structures such as the lungs, impairing cardiac function and leading to Pick's disease of the pericardium.

Chronic Pericarditis (Pick's Disease of the Pericardium)

Chronic pericarditis, as such, is quite rare but occasionally may be seen in cases of viral or bacterial pericarditis where these conditions persist for long periods (usually because of individual variation or because of ineffective treatment). The acute pericarditis progresses to a chronic form, scarring in the pericardium being a prominent feature. More frequently the condition results from tuberculous pericarditis, especially the healing lesions in which fibrosis is once again the aftermath of inflammation. Tuberculous pericarditis induces serous exudation, and if the patient survives for a long period of time, a caseous necrotic lesion will develop. Tuberculous pericarditis can cause cardiac tamponade and also tends to scar rather than resolve.

The pericardium in all of these cases is obliterated by dense bands of collagenous fibrous tissue, totally ensheathing the whole heart in severe cases. In addition, there may be areas of calcification and dense fibrous tracts may attach the pericardium to the lungs, chest wall or diaphragm.

Diffuse organization within the pericardial sac can cause **chronic constrictive pericarditis.** This is characterized by encasement of the heart in dense scar tissue. The heart is unable to expand properly during diastole, and thus constrictive pericarditis interferes with normal cardiac function, the abundant tough fibrous tissue encircling the heart impeding venous return during diastole. This results in a direct mechanical obstruction to the cardiac action. The clinical picture is one where there is progressive congestive heart failure, associated with a small heart and a low stroke volume. This may lead to cardiac tamponade. The fibrosis may also constrict the rather soft and pliable walls of the venae cavae as they enter the heart, producing the clinical syndrome known as **Pick's disease.** In this syndrome, venous return from the lower parts of the body is compromised and hepatosplenomegaly with ascites is produced as a result. Treatment of constrictive pericarditis involves resection of the constricting fibrous tissue bands. For most patients this surgical intervention proves adequate and there is good long-term prognosis.

Non-inflammatory Pericardial Disease

Hydropericardium

In hydropericardium there is accumulation of transudate (increased intercellular non-inflammatory fluid) within the pericardial cavity. The fluid has a low protein content and forms in conditions of generalized oedema associated with cardiac failure, chronic renal disease and hypoproteinaemia. The pericardial surfaces remain smooth and glistening. When the primary conditions that cause hydropericardium are treated, the fluid is resorbed, leaving a normal pericardium. However, hydropericardium may cause a cardiac tamponade if the fluid accumulates too quickly or if large volumes of fluid are involved.

Haemopericardium

Haemopericardium is an accumulation of blood within the pericardial sac, usually due to haemorrhage into the pericardium. It occurs as a result of rupture of the heart, either from stab wound or more commonly associated with a myocardial infarct. Alternatively, the intrapericardial portion of the aorta may rupture, usually because an aneurysm is present. Also, in the various haemorrhagic diatheses there may be spontaneous bleeding into the pericardium. In most cases of haemopericardium death occurs because the blood accumulates in the pericardium quite rapidly leading to cardiac tamponade. If the patient survives the haemopericardium, the blood in the pericardial sac will clot and become organized, often with fibrous adhesions forming or obliteration of the pericardial cavity.

Pneumopericardium

Pneumopericardium is air (usually) or other gases (rarely) within the pericardium. This may occur in lung disease when air may pass from damaged lung and pleura through to the pericardium, or as a result of chest trauma (fractured ribs, etc.). Alternatively, bacterial infections with gas-producing bacteria will produce this condition. The bacteria involved are usually anaerobes (e.g. *Clostridium* spp.). Rarely, the pressure of gas within the pericardial sac will be sufficiently high to produce cardiac tamponade.

Tumours

Primary tumours of the pericardium are very rare. When they do occur they are fibromata, lipomata, angiomata, mesotheliomata or, even more rarely, their equivalent malignant counterparts. Mesothelioma of the atrioventricular node is a benign tumour around two centimetres in diameter, consisting of cystic spaces lined by flat epithelial-like cells. Although benign, this tumour can cause complete heart block and death.

Secondary tumours affecting the pericardium are common, resulting when tumours of adjacent organs infiltrate the pericardium (e.g. spread of bronchogenic carcinoma into the pericardium or lymphosarcoma from the mediastinum invading the pericardial sac). Blood-borne metastatic tumour deposits and lymph-borne secondaries also occur, especially when the primary tumours are malignant melanomata and malignant lymphomata. As the tumour invades the tissue it may cause interference with cardiac function, induction of an inflammatory response (pericarditis) or haemorrhage (haemopericardium). Any of the complications of the aforementioned conditions may have a fatal outcome because of interference with the normal functioning of the heart.

Diseases of the Myocardium

The myocardium is the thick muscular layer of the heart which contracts forcefully to circulate blood. This heart muscle has its own blood vessels (coronary arterial supply) supplying the hard-working muscle cells with the large amounts of oxygen and nutrients that they require. The left ventricle is the part of the heart that is affected most commonly by disease as this is the part that has the heaviest work load and that requires the most nutrients and oxygen. Vascular disease of the myocardium will be considered first.

Vascular Disease of the Myocardium

Coronary Insufficiency

The diseases affecting the myocardium are primarily of a vascular origin and by far the commonest disorder is coronary artery insufficiency leading to ischaemic heart disease (IHD). Death rates from IHD have increased dramatically in the first half of the 20th century, especially in the industrialized, developed countries. It has become the prime cause of death in these countries, accounting for about 33% of all deaths. Amongst the countries with the highest incidence of IHD are the USA, Finland, Britain, Australia, New Zealand and Canada. Japan is a notable exception, the rate of IHD there being less than 15% of the rate of IHD in the USA. Males tend to be affected more than females and the rates increase with increasing age, most deaths being recorded above the age of 40 years.

IHD is almost always due to the narrowing of the coronary artery lumen by atheroma, often with complete occlusion of the artery lumen by superadded thrombosis. Two factors are of importance in respect of reduction of blood flow to coronary arteries. First, the **rate** at which blood flow is decreased, that is, a gradual or a sudden occlusion; and, second, the **amount** of decrease in the flow, ranging from low flow to complete stoppage of flow (Figure 6.4).

Coronary insufficiency implies that the coronary arteries are unable to supply the myocardium with its required amounts of nutrients and oxygen.

Gradual Occlusion — Coronary Heart Disease

The most usual occurrence in vascular disease of the heart is a gradual occlusion of coronary vessels due to atherosclerosis which leads to **coronary heart disease** (= ischaemic heart disease). This progressively re-

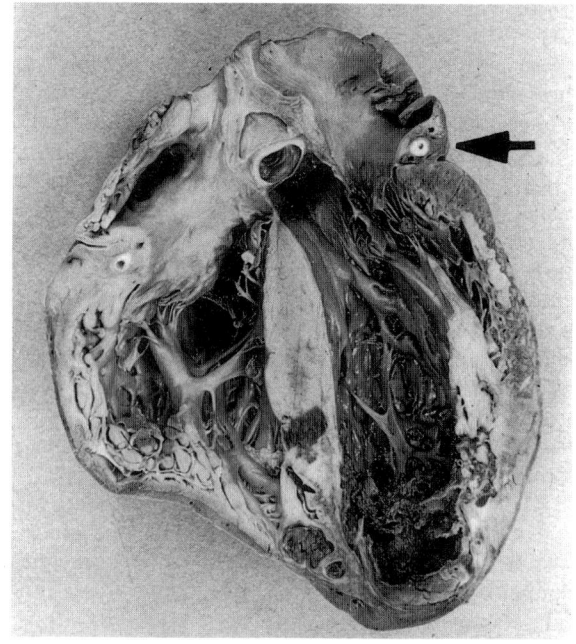

Figure 6.4 *Heart showing marked coronary atheroma (arrow) and large areas of infarction in the left ventricular wall (45-year-old male)*

duced supply of blood to the heart muscle causes a gradual replacement of cardiac muscle fibres by scar tissue. The nature of this disease is a slowly developing ischaemia of the heart muscle, usually due to atherosclerosis of the coronary arteries. The condition is frequently seen in conjunction with hypertension. In the patients suffering from this disorder there is a continuous precarious balance between the perfusion of the myocardium and its metabolic needs. The decreased amount of blood, and hence of oxygen, leads to the progressive necrosis of regions of the myocardium, resulting in replacement fibrosis.

The disease is very common above the age of 50 years, especially in males. Its most important clinical effect is **angina pectoris**. These patients present with a severe, crushing, left-sided chest pain, which often radiates down the left arm. The pain of angina is felt upon exertion, emotional stress, overeating, extremes of temperature or any other cause of increased myocardial activity. As the muscle fibres are consuming increased amounts of oxygen with increased activity and since the coronary arteries cannot supply them with an increased volume of blood (atherosclerosis = hardening, loss of elasticity of arteries and a reduction of luminal diameter), the myocytes utilize anaerobic metabolism, produce metabolites such as lactate to toxic levels, causing the pain. This anginal pain usually lasts about 15 minutes and resolves if the patient rests.

Characteristically the myocardium in coronary heart disease shows diffuse or patchy fibrous tissue replacement of the myocardium which is undergoing a slowly progressive necrosis. The fibrosis may be extensive and the fibrous tracts thick if there is associated hypertension. In patients with coronary heart disease over 90% of cases show atherosclerosis of the coronary arteries with narrowing of the lumen, the change affecting nearly all branches of the coronary vessels, but of variable severity and distribution. The valves are frequently involved and display fibrous thickening which may be complicated by senile calcification, leading to stenosis and incompetence. This may give rise to cardiac failure and death of the patient.

Alternatively, there may be a sudden occlusion of coronary vessels which leads to **myocardial infarction**. The sudden occlusion may be due to a thrombus forming in an already narrowed (partially occluded) coronary vessel, or it may be a thromboembolus lodging in a branch of the coronary artery, both situations resulting in sudden, total occlusion of the vessel, and thus total lack of blood to the area of heart muscle supplied by the blocked vessel. This causes the necrosis of heart muscle and is commonly referred to as a 'heart attack'.

Myocardial Infarction
Myocardial infarction (MI) is a major cause of death and in various industrialized countries it accounts for about 10 to 25% of all deaths. In approximately half the patients who develop MI, the condition is fatal. MI occurs typically in middle-aged males, the sex incidence ratio being about 3 to 1. Predominantly the age group 40 to 60 years is affected but the average age of onset appears to be decreasing so that it is not surprising to hear that 35-year-old people have had an MI. The disease occurs after a major branch of the coronary artery is occluded and the collateral circulation is unable to reach and perfuse the affected part. Some infarcts occur after unaccustomed exercise or physical exertion, after emotional crises, after large meals or extremes of climate but many cases of MI occur during the patient's sleep.

More than 90% of cases of MI are associated with coronary atherosclerosis and superimposed thrombosis, while some are associated with thromboembolism. Contributory factors to the development of MI include vascular insufficiency associated with aortic valve lesions, shock and arrhythmias of the heart. Severe anaemia, anoxia, or hypertrophy of the heart caused by hypertension or rheumatic heart disease are also important factors. Coagulopathies of the blood and the various dyscrasias also lead to an increased risk of MI occurring.

The commonest site of occlusion of the vessels is the second and third centimetres of the left and right coronary arteries. The anterior descending left branch is the most commonly occluded one (50% of MI), followed by the main trunk on the right (30% of MI) and the left circumflex branch (20% of MI). The site in the myocardium most frequently affected is the left ventricle, the right ventricle and atria rarely being involved. The sites within the left ventricle affected depend on the branch of the coronary artery occluded and the level of the occlusion. Generally, occlusion of the anterior descending left branch of the coronary artery causes an anterior infarct with ECG changes in the anterior leads. An infarction resulting from occlusion of the main trunk on the right is an inferior one and causes changes in leads II, III and aVF. Occlusion of the left circumflex branch causes a lateral infarction and ECG changes occur in leads I, aVL and V4–6.

Small infarcts may be confined to a central area of muscle or be principally subendocardial or subpericardial. Quite often the infarct is **transmural**, involving the whole thickness of the left ventricle (see Figure 6.5). The infarcted area presents the typical appearance of tissue that has undergone coagulative necrosis, its fate being the eventual disintegration of necrotic cells by neutrophils and macrophages, with granulation tissue and fibroblastic activity leading to the formation of a fibrous scar. The stages observable at a region of MI as a function of time may be summarized in the following way:

- **0–12 hours**: Slight pallor, flabbiness; coagulative necrosis (after 8 hours).
- **12–24 hours**: Pallor, friable appearance (necrosis).
- **2–4 days**: Yellow-grey colour; red zone of hyperaemia (congested vessels) around it (Figure 6.6); neutrophils infiltrate the region.
- **4–10 days**: (Acute inflammation); soft yellow structureless appearance with surrounding wide, red margin; granulation tissue forms (early scar).
- **2–6 weeks**: Gradual fibrosis replaces necrotic tissue.
- **6 weeks +**: Infarct replaced by fibrous tissue (scar).

In MI, the patient feels a very severe chest pain concentrating in the centre of the chest and radiating outwards. This pain persists for longer than 15 minutes, being unrelieved by rest. The patient may go into shock or lose consciousness, or alternatively suffer from cardiac arrest and die.

The sequelae of myocardial infarction are as follows:

- There may be sudden death.
- Death may occur within 2 days from shock or heart failure.
- There may be congestive heart failure with pulmonary oedema.
- Fibrosis may take place, leading to a healed infarct.

There are several complications of myocardial infarction:

- **Pericarditis** may occur when the infarct occurs adjacent to the pericardium.
- **Rupture of the heart** may occur, particularly at the apical part of the heart where the muscle is thinnest, due to the softening by necrosis. This rupture leads to haemopericardium, cardiac tamponade and death.
- **Mural thrombosis** may occur, that is, thrombus formation on damaged endothelium directly overlying an area of infarcted heart muscle. This mural thrombus may then break free causing thrombo-embolism. This embolus would then circulate and lodge elsewhere in the body, in turn leading to further infarction in other organs and death. Frequently, a cerebral infarction ('stroke') complicates an MI and causes the patient's death.
- An **aneurysm** may form in the ventricle as the weakened myocardium bulges out due to the ventricular pressure. This aneurysm may also rupture at a later stage.

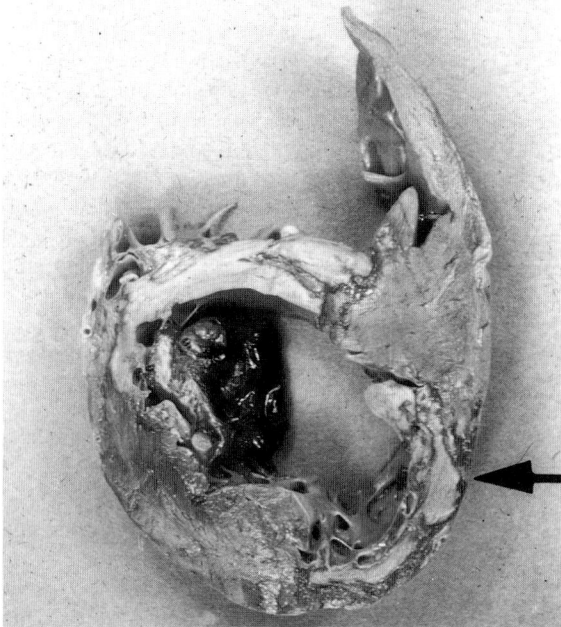

Figure 6.6   *Heart of a 56-year-old male showing large areas of infarction in the left ventricular wall (arrow)*

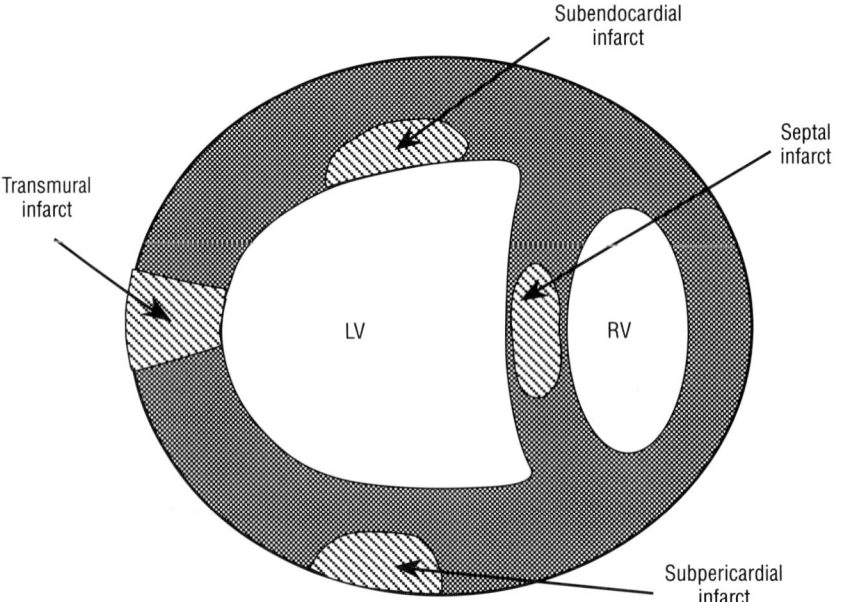

Figure 6.5   *The sites of myocardial infarcts*

- There may be **extension of the infarct** due to further thrombotic occlusion of the coronary vessel, affecting a larger area of adjacent heart muscle. It is not uncommon in a patient with a healing myocardial infarct to die as a result of an extending infarct.
- **Cardiac arrhythmias** may occur, especially with extensive heart muscle involvement where infarction has affected the conducting muscle fibres of the heart which are necessary for normal ventricular contraction. Death may occur when there is ventricular fibrillation.

The results of myocardial infarction are various: 10–24% of patients with myocardial infarcts die within 6 weeks; approximately 20% of patients live for 10 years or more; 50–60% of patients will die from complications of myocardial infarction. The precise sequela of any myocardial infarct will depend on many factors. For instance, age and general health condition of the patient (associated lung problems, for example); extent of the infarct; location of the infarct; promptness and effectiveness of treatment; management of patient and prevention of complications.

Non-inflammatory Diseases of the Myocardium

Amyloidosis

Amyloidosis is a systemic disorder which may be **primary** (unknown aetiology, may be hereditary) or **secondary** (seen after or in association with chronic infections or inflammations such as rheumatoid arthritis, also seen in malignancies, especially multiple myeloma). In this condition, a characteristic proteinaceous substance, **amyloid**, is deposited intercellularly in various tissues throughout the body and may be seen in the heart commonly in the myocardium and the endocardium. Amyloid means 'starch-like' and was initially thus termed because it reacts with iodine to form a reddish brown material. However, amyloid is not chemically related to starch. Amyloid also stains a characteristic red colour with Congo red. The amyloid substance is not a single chemical entity but rather is composed of several major and minor biochemical forms. All of these amyloid proteins are fibrillar in nature, composed of filaments ≈10 nm wide and of an indefinite length, aggregating in tissues in a β-pleated sheet conformation.

There are two major biochemical classes of amyloid:

- **Amyloid light chain (AL) protein**: This is derived from immunoglobulin molecule fragments, i.e. complete light chains (usually λ chains) and/or fragments of these chains. Experiments have shown that proteolysis *in vitro* will yield amyloid substance.
- **Amyloid associated (AA) protein**: This is derived from an apoprotein of a high density lipoprotein (the so-called serum amyloid associated, SAA, protein) and is 8500 Daltons MW. The concentration of SAA rises one thousandfold following an inflammatory stimulus.

There is a multitude of other minor forms of amyloid proteins including AE_t, a calcitonin-like protein, and **P** component, a non-fibrillar part, which is a serum α-glycoprotein.

The classification of amyloidosis is quite complex and generally two major presentations of the disease are recognized, primary and secondary.

Primary amyloidosis. This form of the disease occurs apart from any predisposing factor or cause, appears to arise spontaneously and is focal, not systemic, in nature. The organs are affected in the following order of frequency: skeletal muscles, heart, alimentary tract, tongue, skin, spleen, kidney, liver, lymph nodes and lungs (Figure 6.7). The affected organ becomes enlarged, firm, and displays a waxy cut surface. It will retain its shape and will not easily deform when it is handled. Microscopically, the amyloid is seen to be deposited intercellularly, predominantly around blood vessels, in relation to basement membranes. It interferes with the passage of nutrients and metabolites from and to blood vessels and puts considerable pressure on adjacent tissue cells. There is interference with the normal functioning of the affected tissue and cells undergo reactive changes and atrophy. There may be serious functional disturbance of the organ if the deposition is particularly heavy, for example proteinuria in kidney amyloidosis, and malabsorption with

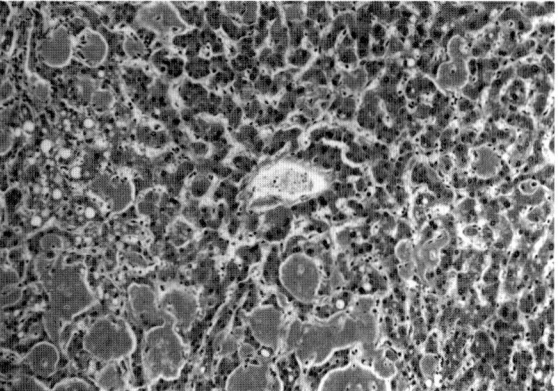

Figure 6.7 *Liver showing extensive deposits of acellular amyloid material (×150)*

amyloidosis in the gut. In the heart, the deposition of amyloid may be quite extensive and is seen especially in elderly people, causing extensive wasting of the myocardial cells and atrophy of the heart.

Secondary amyloidosis. In this type of amyloidosis there is an association with a pre-existing disease. Formerly, chronic inflammatory reactions such as chronic pyogenic osteitis, tuberculosis, syphilis and bronchiectasis accounted for most cases. With the advent of antibiotic therapy and treatment of these diseases, the commonest initiating disease is rheumatoid arthritis. In this type of amyloidosis the spleen (100% of cases show involvement), liver (90% of cases), kidney (90% of cases, Figure 6.8), adrenals (90% of cases), lymph nodes (70% of cases), pancreas (60% of cases) and gut are primarily affected, and usually more than one organ is involved (i.e. systemic in nature). It affects the elderly more than the young and several heredofamilial forms are known, involving certain racial groups, for example the Portuguese type, which is associated with neuropathy, and familial Mediterranean fever, not associated with neuropathy. Another condition which gives rise to amyloidosis is neoplasia of the plasma cell (a cell normally producing antibodies). Multiple myeloma is the prime condition of this last type and amyloidosis is a frequent complication with these patients.

Pathogenesis. The pathogenesis of amyloidosis depends to a certain extent on the initiating stimulus for the disorder and is also reflected by the type of amyloid protein which is deposited in tissues. Deposition of AL

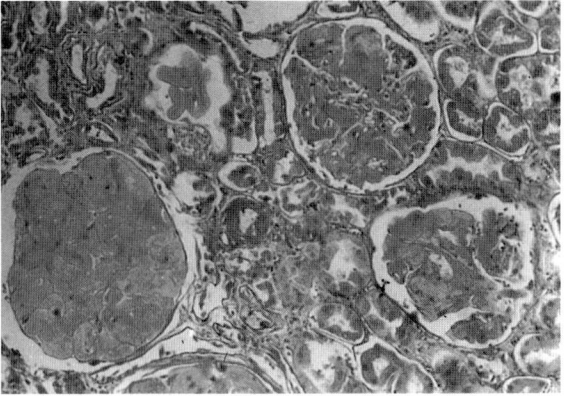

Figure 6.8 *Kidney of a patient exhibiting secondary amyloid deposition (patient was suffering from chronic rheumatoid arthritis) (×350)*

protein is likely to be associated with plasma cell neoplasia whereas SAA protein deposition is associated with chronic inflammatory states.

In all cases, there is an increased elaboration of the amyloid-associated proteins in the body and this is followed by an intercellular deposition in the tissues. It may be observed from Figure 6.9 that in chronic inflammatory states the interleukins mediate both the protraction of the inflammation as well as the stimulation of the liver cells to produce increased quantities of SAA. In multiple myeloma, it is the neoplastic cells themselves that are producing the amyloid protein in excess quantities leading, not surprisingly, to its deposition in the tissues (refer to Figure 6.9).

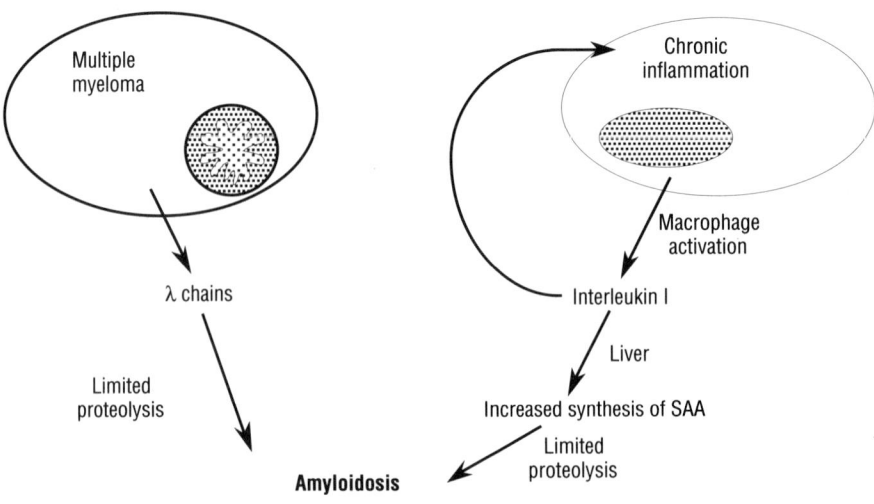

Figure 6.9 *The pathogenesis of amyloidosis*

Clinical findings. Clinically, amyloidosis may have little effect and the patient may live for a long period without being aware of any disorder, the condition being discovered incidentally at autopsy. This is especially the case in senile amyloidosis of the heart. In generalized amyloidosis, the clinical findings vary considerably, depending on the organs involved, the severity and extent of the disease. Early symptoms are weakness and fatigue with loss of weight. Later there may be evidence of renal disease, hepatomegaly and splenomegaly with cardiac abnormalities.

In severe cases of cardiac involvement, the presence of large quantities of amyloid between the cardiocytes interferes with diffusion of nutrients and oxygen and atrophy of the heart may supervene, cardiac failure being evident in the patient. Conduction disturbances are a common presentation and many patients show evidence of cardiac arrhythmias. Heart problems develop in many patients with amyloidosis, and ≈40% of patients die of cardiac disease.

Renal involvement often presents as massive proteinuria with oedema and often the patient will progress to renal failure (≈20% of patients die of renal problems). The hepatosplenomegaly (enlargement of liver and spleen) rarely causes clinical dysfunction but may be important diagnostically.

Diagnosis. The diagnosis of amyloidosis depends on the clinical symptomatology but also on biopsy and biochemical findings. Renal biopsy may be performed and the tissue stained with Congo red, which demonstrates the amyloid material conclusively. In generalized amyloidosis, gingival or rectal biopsies will be positive in 75% of patients. In immunocyte disturbances serum and urinary protein electrophoresis is valuable diagnostically.

Prognosis. In generalized amyloidosis, the prognosis is quite poor with the mean survival time ranging between 1–3 years following diagnosis. In less severe forms, the patients may survive for many years and in mild cases the condition may remain totally subclinical, the patient surviving for his or her normal life span, the amyloidosis often being never diagnosed or discovered as an incidental finding at autopsy.

Fatty Change of the Heart

Fatty change may occur in the heart as one of the reactive changes of cells to injury. This is an **intracellular** accumulation of lipids (the fat accumulating as droplets within the myocardial cells) as a result of some damage or injury sustained by the car-diac muscle fibres. The injury may be the result of any of a number of agents of cell damage including infection, anoxia, nutritional factors, toxins and anaemia. For example, if the blood supply is briefly occluded and then resupplied through clot lysis to an area of heart muscle, the myocardial cells may undergo reactive changes including fatty change. Often, hydropic change is also seen in the same regions of the heart affected by fatty change. In its early stages the fatty change may be reversed by removing the cause of cell damage. In later stages the severely affected cells will degenerate and undergo necrosis, being replaced by fibrous scar tissue.

The heart looks pale and mottled on sectioning, particularly in the region under the endocardium in the left ventricle especially. Microscopically there are fine droplets of fat throughout the cytoplasm of the myocardial cells, sometimes coalescing to form larger droplets. Those fibres closest to the injurious agent and those furthest away from the blood vessels display the most severe fatty change (see Figure 6.10).

Fat Infiltration of the Heart

In obese individuals there is not only a great increase in pericardial fat but also an infiltration of fat into the myocardium. This fat is **intercellularly** placed (found in adipocytes placed between muscle fibres). The fat is stored within normal fat cells and therefore this condition represents an increase in the normal fatty tissue of the heart and is not a reactive change to injury. The cardiac function is not compromised except in very severe cases where there may be interference with the normal cardiac cycle. The myocardial fibres are normal and they show no intracellular deposits of fat (unless there is concurrent ischaemic heart disease).

Brown Atrophy of the Heart

In this condition there is a wasting of the heart so that its size and weight are much lower than normal. Its surface appears wrinkled and there is considerable loss of pericardial fat, tortuous coronary vessels and brown-coloured friable myocardium. The disorder is seen in extreme old age and with wasting diseases such as advanced malignancies. The myocardium atrophies and becomes brown in colour, a change easily discernible with the naked eye at autopsy. As the muscle fibres atrophy they accumulate a brown pigment known as **lipofuscin** (or lipochrome). The pigment is believed to derive from the breakdown of lipid membranes of

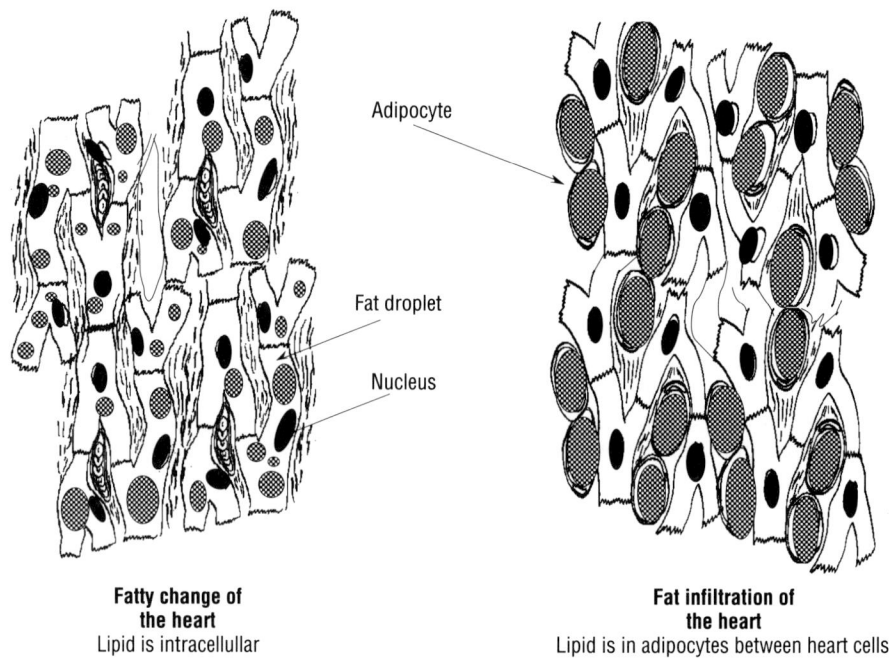

Figure 6.10   *Comparison of fatty change of the heart and fat infiltration of the heart*

cellular components and represents indigestible remains that the cell cannot dispose of. Lipofuscin remains in that cell for the remainder of the life of that cell, and in the case of permanent cells (such as cardiocytes or neurones), increasing amounts of lipofuscin will be seen with increasing age.

Microscopically, the muscle fibres appear shrunken and wasted, containing granules of brownish pigment in the perinuclear region of the cells. In most cases this does not interfere with the function of the heart, the damaged areas being replaced by scar tissue. In some cases, especially with diphtheria, the conducting system of the heart is damaged with heart block, arrhythmias and acute cardiac failure leading to the sudden death of the patient.

Cardiomyopathies

The cardiomyopathies are a broad group of cardiac disorders that are usually not inflammatory but present as myocardial dysfunction not associated with hypertension, coronary heart disease or rheumatic heart disease. There may be both primary and secondary cardiomyopathies. The primary, idiopathic cardiomyopathy (CMP) develops in the absence of ischaemic,

hypertensive, congenital, valvular or other forms of heart diseases that have a known cause and include alcoholism, viral infections, hypersensitivity and connective tissue diseases, neuromuscular diseases (certain muscular dystrophies, Friedreich's ataxia), metabolic disorders (hyperthyroidism, hypothyroidism, beriberi, haemochromatosis), amyloidosis, certain glycogen storage diseases, and drug or chemical toxicities. The patient presents with myocardial dysfunction, chest pain and features of cardiac failure. Sometimes arrhythmias are a prominent feature, or the heart may be enlarged or dilated, or both. Cardiomyopathies may be classed as follows.

Congestive or dilated CMP. In this condition there is dilatation and hypertrophy of both ventricles, with poor systole. The coronary arteries are patent and there is no evidence of aortic stenosis. Often, there are adherent mural thrombi in the ventricles and under the microscope there is evidence of interstitial fibrosis. Although many patients present with an idiopathic disease, there are also groups of patients with alcoholism, viral infections and beriberi that develop this type of CMP. Generally, the prognosis for the condition is rather poor and the best treatment for the patient is a heart transplant.

Hypertrophic CMP. Hypertrophic CMP involves massive increase in ventricular mass, small ventricular cavities, a hypercontracting left ventricle, with or without subaortic stenosis and obstruction. The hypertrophy is especially marked in the interventricular septum. This is an idiopathic CMP that possibly has a genetic basis. It is not associated with hypertension as is the hypertensive hypertrophic disease of the heart. Patients may present with a diastolic murmur as the posterior cusp of the mitral valve is abnormal. Alternatively, sufferers of the conditions may have dyspnoea, chest pain and palpitations. Sudden death brought about by ventricular arrhythmias or atrial fibrillation may be seen. Patients are treated with drugs (e.g. beta-blockers) or surgically where valvular defects are corrected and hypertrophied muscle is removed.

Restrictive and obliterative CMP. Restrictive CMP is a less common cardiomyopathy where the prime feature is restriction of ventricular filling. Examples of restrictive cardiomyopathies are those caused by amyloidosis, other infiltrative disorders such as leukaemia, glycogenoses and also idiopathic forms. Arrhythmias, heart block or heart failure may develop if the heart is extensively involved. Obliterative CMP is caused by a rare fibrosis of the endocardium (endomyocardium). This CMP is seen especially commonly in Africa (Sudan and Uganda) or in other tropical countries. The disease is idiopathic. A feature found in some patients with cardiac failure that has developed in association with this disease is peripheral blood eosinophilia and systemic embolism, usually leading to death.

Inflammatory Diseases of the Myocardium — Myocarditis

The term 'myocarditis' refers to myocardial disorders marked by inflammatory changes. Myocarditis mostly involves microbial infections but also may be caused by hypersensitivities, physical or chemical agents and drugs (e.g. adriamycin and doxorubicin used widely for the treatment of malignant disease) which cause myocardial necrosis and inflammation. There may be primary myocarditis, where the myocardial inflammation is the dominant pathology involved, or secondary myocarditis, where myocardial involvement is only one component of a more generalized disease such as occurs in rheumatic fever. Myocarditis due to any aetiology may proceed to cardiomyopathy and myocardial dysfunction (arrhythmias, etc.). If the myocardial function is severely compromised, it is not unusual for the patient to die.

Bacterial Myocarditis

Myocarditis may result after infection of the myocardium with pyogenic organisms, but this is a rare condition. It is associated with pyaemia or septicaemia and occasionally the organisms spread directly into the myocardium via an infected pericardium or endocardium. The bacteria most usually involved are *Staphylococcus aureus* or *Streptococcus pyogenes*.

Focal areas of inflammation develop around the multiplying bacterial colonies and especially in the case of *S. aureus* localized abscesses may form within the myocardium. Characteristically, as occurs in other tissues, *S. pyogenes* causes a spreading infection with considerable necrosis and haemorrhage. Thus a typical suppurative infection is seen. In syphilis (caused by *Treponema pallidum*) and tuberculosis (caused by *Mycobacterium tuberculosis*) there are characteristic chronic inflammatory lesions (gumma and tubercle formation) in the myocardium. Unless treated early the infections cause extensive destruction of the myocardial muscle, a process which may result in arrhythmias or cardiac failure, both conditions often having fatal outcomes.

Viral Myocarditis

Group B Coxsackieviruses and type 8 Echoviruses give rise to acute myocarditis accompanied by an acute pericarditis. Young adults, especially males, are more prone to this type of infection but outbreaks in nurseries have also been reported. Focal areas of inflammation appear in the myocardium showing infiltration by lymphocytes and macrophages, sometimes plasma cells and eosinophils being also present. The condition is usually mild and complete recovery is the rule. It may occasionally be severe with the extensive involvement of the myocardium leading to death. Many viral diseases such as poliomyelitis, influenza, yellow fever, hepatitis A and intrauterine rubella are accompanied by an acute viral myocarditis with features similar to those already described.

Protozoal Myocarditis

Myocarditis may be seen in *Toxoplasma gondii* infection (toxoplasmosis) and in Chagas' disease (*Trypanosoma cruzi* infection) seen primarily in South America. The multiplying protozoa cause quite considerable destruction of myocardial substance and the inflammation accompanying the infection will further damage the heart. If sufficiently large areas of myocardial tissue are involved by the parasitic infection, cardiac function may be so severely compromised as to cause the death of the patient.

Toxic Myocarditis

Toxic myocarditis often accompanies infections such as diphtheria, typhoid fever, or pneumonia and other streptococcal infections. In this situation no organisms are demonstrable in the myocardium, the injury resulting from bacterial toxic products which damage the myocardial fibres. It is also seen as a result of poisoning with carbon monoxide, arsenic, phosphorus and chloroform.

There are focal areas of degeneration and coagulative necrosis of the myocardium, often fatty change and inflammation accompanying the lesions. Macroscopically, the heart appears firm and waxy, the left ventricle being thickened. The organ retains its shape even after cutting. A thin slice of the tissue looks translucent and the waxy appearance is even more marked. The effects of the disorder are variable depending on its severity and the time course of its development. If the condition is mild or in its early stages it may remain subclinical and both patient and physician may be unaware of its presence. In the severe or rapidly progressive types the heart may enter cardiac failure, the patient often dying.

Idiopathic Myocarditis

Myocarditis may have no known cause as in Fiedler's myocarditis (giant cell myocarditis) which is very severe, causing death within weeks. It is possible that idiopathic myocarditis may be shown to be viral in the future, possibly with hypersensitivity reactions to the viral infection being involved in the pathogenesis.

Syphilis

In the past, cardiac involvement in tertiary syphilis was very commonly seen but nowadays such disease is rarely observed, as syphilis is effectively treated in its primary or secondary stages. The average age of presentation of tertiary syphilis is 50 years, usually 15–20 years after the primary infection. The typical gummata form in the myocardium, either solitary or multiple, of variable size. Very rarely, a diffuse form of interstitial inflammation of the myocardium is seen with involvement of the blood vessels and extensive myocardial and vascular fibrosis.

Rheumatic Heart Disease

Acute Rheumatic Fever

Acute rheumatic fever (RF) is an acute febrile illness in which there are systemic manifestations, with lesions occurring in the connective tissues of the tendons and joints, serosal membranes, skin, in the respiratory system and blood vessels. Joint involvement is the most frequent occurrence but is benign and transient. The heart is very commonly affected with often fatal consequences (the capacity to cause heart damage is the most important factor in rheumatic fever). Most patients (90%) have the first attack between 5 to 15 years of age and the incidence of the disease in the industrialized countries has been reduced due to prompt antibiotic therapy and improved living conditions. RF is still common in India, Africa, the Arab countries and South America. Lesions of the heart due to RF cause up to 25% of all clinical cases of organic heart disease. Thus, it is still an important cause of death in school age children, especially in developing countries. Recently, there has been a resurgence of streptococcal infections in developed countries and this may lead to an increased incidence of RF.

RF occurs as a hypersensitivity response following infection by group A, β haemolytic streptococci, the disease being linked most often with attacks of pharyngitis due to *Streptococcus pyogenes* ('strep. sore throat'). It is also seen after other infections with this organism, for example scarlet fever, but the strongest correlation seems to be with infections of the throat. There is a strong individual predisposition to the disease and it has been shown that more than 75% of the patients with RF share a common HLA antigen on their B cells which has an incidence of 20% in the general population. There is also evidence pointing out that the serotypes of *S. pyogenes* involved are important since some serotypes will not cause RF in the susceptible groups.

The streptococci are not found in the myocardium of the patient with RF and it is unlikely that the disease is caused by circulating streptococcal toxins since RF develops after the infection in the pharynx has subsided and when the antistreptococcal antibody titre is at its highest level. It is the antibody that causes the heart damage and it has been shown that subsequent infections with suitable strains of *S. pyogenes* in sensitized people will lead to episodes of RF with more destruction of the heart and valves.

The pathogenesis of RF is linked with the fact that certain individuals share 'self-antigens' with *S. pyogenes*. That is, when they form antibodies against the bacterium, these antibodies will cross-react with various tissues of their own body, notably myocardium, endocardium, vascular smooth muscle, skeletal muscle and connective tissue components. In this respect RF may be considered to be a type II hypersensitivity in which antibodies and complement cause tissue damage. However, since the antibodies causing the destruction are the patients' own, RF is also classified as an autoimmune disease.

First attacks of RF are rare after 20 years of age, most cases occurring in childhood. The sex incidence of the disease is equal. Clinically, the disease has an insidious onset, the most notable feature being fever 2 to 3 weeks after the streptococcal infection. Most patients develop symptoms of polyarthritis and 65% develop carditis, an inflammation of the heart. With subsequent attacks the risk of developing carditis increases, eventually 75% of all patients having cardiac involvement.

In the heart all three layers are affected, **rheumatic pancarditis** (pericarditis, myocarditis and endocarditis) resulting. Myocardial involvement is responsible for most deaths in the acute phase of RF. The pericardium is thickened and shows a typical fibrinous pericarditis, which may organize so that fibrous adhesions are formed in the pericardium with partial or complete obliteration of the pericardial sac. The myocardium generally shows no evidence to the naked eye of the disease although sometimes there may be pinhead-sized foci of a pale grey colour visible scattered throughout the myocardium. These are the **Aschoff bodies** or **Aschoff nodules**, a feature pathognomonic of rheumatic carditis. Under the microscope the Aschoff nodules are seen to be present in the interstitial connective tissue and the fibrous septa separating the fascicles of the myocardial fibres. Nodules are usually found in close association with blood vessels and are more nu-

merous in the left ventricle and atrium. They are composed of hyaline, eosinophilic material which is exudative in origin and may contain fibrin. There is degenerate collagen appearing very eosinophilic and amorphous. This is surrounded by aggregates of inflammatory cells, a pleomorphic population present although the lymphocytes and macrophages are very prominent. Characteristic of the lesion are the so-called Aschoff giant cells, cells approximately 30 μm in diameter, possessing two to five nuclei. There may be a few fibroblasts present also. In addition, there may be evidence of **Anitschkow myocytes** or 'caterpillar cells'. These are large elongated cells with a central bar-shaped nucleus. The nucleus has fine projections of chromatin all around it mimicking in appearance the legs of a caterpillar, hence the name. It is thought that they are altered myocardial cells but some people believe they may be derived from fibroblasts (the Aschoff nodule is shown in Figures 6.11, 6.12 and 6.13).

The Aschoff nodules progressively heal and are replaced by fibrous tissue, causing a diffuse fibrosis of the myocardium. Death may occur at the acute phase due to the myocarditis, or in the later stages after many attacks of RF, the considerable fibrosis and pancarditis interfering with the heart's function. Generally, the endocardial manifestations of the disease are the ones causing the major problems.

The mural endocardium shows a diffuse inflammation and thickening with Aschoff nodules also forming at this site, especially in the atria. The most serious

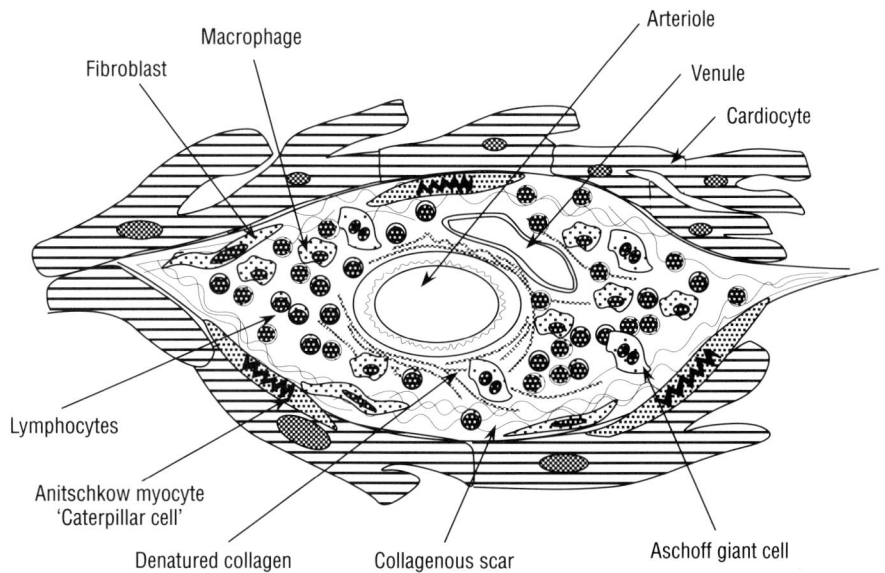

Figure 6.11 *The Aschoff nodule of rheumatic heart disease*

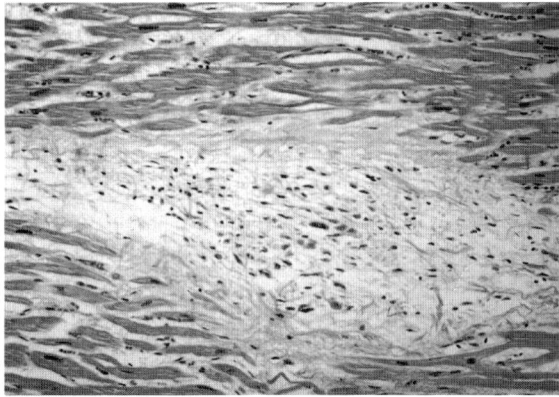

Figure 6.12   *An Aschoff nodule in the myocardium of a patient with rheumatic heart disease (×100)*

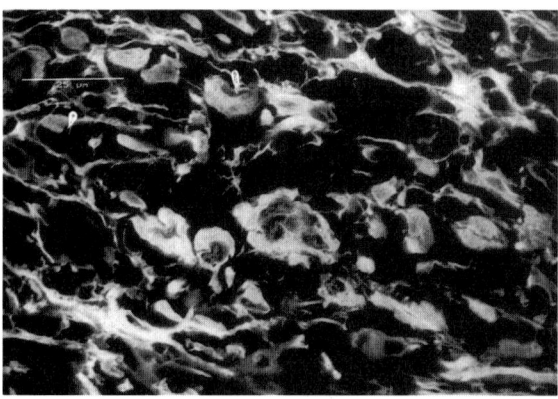

Figure 6.13   *Aschoff giant cells, macrophages and lymphocytes in an Aschoff nodule in the myocardium of a patient with rheumatic heart disease (scale bar is 25 μm)*

lesions are present on the heart valves. The **mitral** and **aortic valves** are mostly affected, occasionally the tricuspid and pulmonary valves also showing damage. The mitral valve alone is affected in 30% of patients, the mitral and aortic valves in 50% and the aortic valve alone in 5% of patients. The appearances are similar for all valves. There is swelling and inflammation with the destructive changes leading to the formation of **vegetations**, excrescences formed of platelets and fibrin. (NB: No bacteria are present in these vegetations.) Organization of the damaged valve cusps and of the vegetations leads to scarring of the valves, with stenosis and incompetence resulting. The mitral valve in particular shows the typical 'button hole' stenosis. The chordae tendinae are also thickened and fused. Calci-fication of the damaged valves is a frequent adjunct. This leads to incompetence of the valves and quite frequently to cardiac failure.

Chronic Rheumatic Heart Disease

Following recovery from the acute phase of RF, the myocardium returns to normal and the heart functions well, although small fibrous scars may be visible at the sites of healed Aschoff nodules. Subsequent attacks of RF will lead to progressively more damage sustained by the myocardium with increasing fibrosis, chronic pericarditis which may progress to constrictive pericarditis, and the very serious valvular lesions causing incompetence of the valves, leading in about 30% of patients to cardiac failure. The risk of developing the chronic, severe manifestations of the disease depends on the age of onset of the disease, the most risk being associated with RF developing in childhood. However, the disease may smoulder undetected for 5 to 30 years before there is clinical evidence of the valvular disease.

Very frequently the cardiac valves (mainly the aortic and mitral valves) are so calcified and fibrotic that these patients must be treated by valvotomy or artificial valves may need to be put into the heart in a valve prosthesis operation. Usually this operation has a good prognosis provided the myocardium and pericardium are relatively healthy.

The sequelae of rheumatic heart disease are as follows:

- 30% of patients die within the first 20 years;
- 30% of patients still show evidence of heart disease after 20 years, leading to reduced life expectancy;
- the remaining 40% show only minor effects, with minimal compromise in life expectancy.

Mechanical/Physical Diseases of the Myocardium

Hypertensive Heart Disease

This term refers to the effects on the heart of long-term **systemic hypertension** (high blood pressure). Hypertensive heart disease is characterized by thickening of the left ventricle (myocardial hypertrophy), enlarging the heart. The chamber of the left ventricle becomes smaller as the wall thickens, leading to **concentric hypertrophy**. Cardiac failure (congestive heart failure) may then occur, causing dilatation of the heart, which stretches the ventricular wall and thins it, leading to **eccentric hypertrophy**.

The majority of people with hypertension suffer from heart failure. The failure may be acute and sudden but is most often of a gradual progression to congestive cardiac failure, eventually affecting both left and right ventricles and culminating in inadequate myocardial contraction, ventricular fibrillation and death.

Myocardial Hypertrophy

Normally, the heart weighs 250–300 g in women and 300–360 g in men. It is roughly the size of a fist, although there is some variation in these normal parameters depending on age, body size, amount of pericardial fat present and dietary factors. Hypertrophy of the myocardium occurs due to an increased work load on the ventricles. This results in increased size of individual myocardial fibres, increased thickness of ventricular wall and increased size and weight of the heart. It is not unusual to see the heart weight reaching 800 g. Systemic hypertension results in left ventricular hypertrophy, sometimes known as **cor bovinum** (heart of a bull). Pulmonary hypertension results in right ventricular hypertrophy, sometimes referred to as **cor pulmonale**. Heart valve disease may also result in myocardial hypertrophy. Concentric hypertrophy occurs when the ventricular wall thickens but the chamber size diminishes, while eccentric hypertrophy occurs when dilatation of the hypertrophied ventricle occurs. Usually, eccentric hypertrophy supervenes on concentric hypertrophy (see Figure 6.14).

Hypertrophy of the myocardium may result in heart failure, with arrhythmias and ventricular fibrillation leading to death. If, however, the cause of myocardial hypertrophy is removed (e.g. heart valve replacement) then the heart may return to normal.

Diseases of the Endocardium

Endocarditis

Endocarditis is an inflammation of the endocardial layer of the heart; however, the term now almost always has been limited to an inflammatory condition of

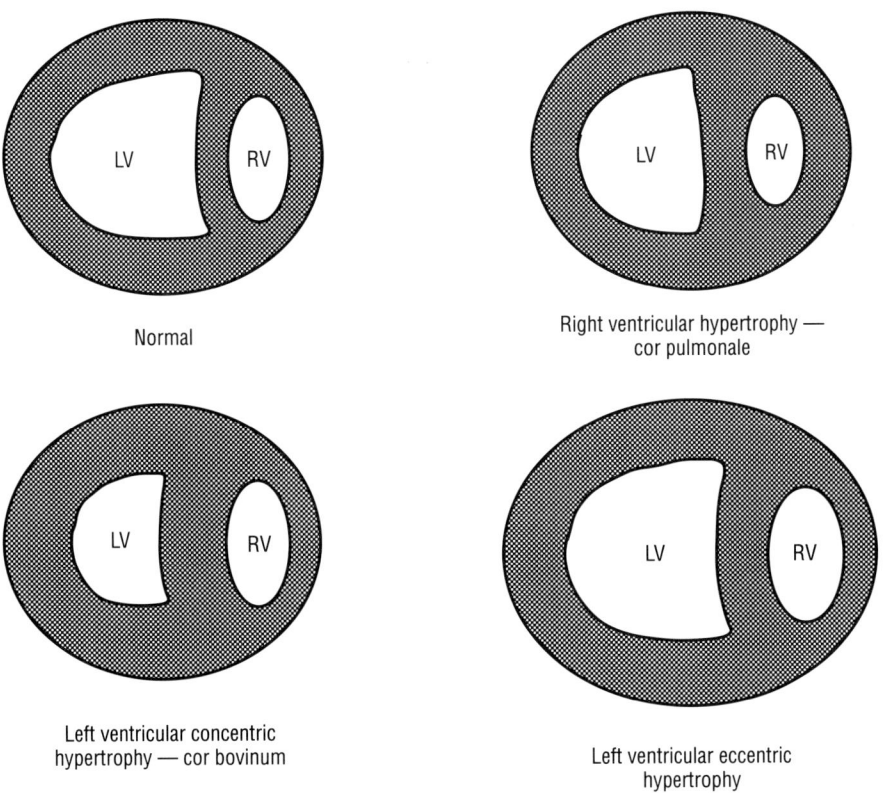

Normal

Right ventricular hypertrophy — cor pulmonale

Left ventricular concentric hypertrophy — cor bovinum

Left ventricular eccentric hypertrophy

Figure 6.14 *Types of myocardial hypertrophy*

the heart valves. The inflammation may be infective or result from a hypersensitivity, as in rheumatic fever. Rheumatic endocarditis may be called aseptic as bacteria are not present on the heart valves (see previous section on rheumatic heart disease). Infective endocarditis (septic) is so called because micro-organisms will lodge on the heart valves, causing an infection. Bacterial infection of the heart valves, may be acute or subacute.

Acute Bacterial Endocarditis

This is a relatively rare terminal event in acute septicaemic infection, the causative bacteria spreading to the heart valves from other sites of infection elsewhere in the body. It is most commonly due to pyogenic bacteria, for example *Staphylococcus aureus* and *Streptococcus pyogenes*, or other bacteria such as *Streptococcus pneumoniae* and *Clostridium perfringens*.

Acute bacterial endocarditis is becoming more common in intravenous drug users due to dirty needles and lack of aseptic techniques. The infection may affect healthy valves or previously damaged valves. The damage on the heart valves leads to thrombosis, the thrombi on the heart valves being called **vegetations**. These thrombi are often large and friable (crumbly), consisting of large numbers of bacteria, platelets, fibrin and inflammatory cells. These vegetations are likely to break free, becoming septic emboli and leading to infected, suppurating infarcts. Untreated, this condition is rapidly fatal, due more to the septicaemia than to the endocarditis.

Subacute Bacterial Endocarditis

This condition is caused predominantly by *Streptococcus viridans,* a less virulent organism than those causing acute bacterial endocarditis. The disease has an insidious onset and affects previously damaged heart valves, being progressive and fatal if untreated (Figure 6.15). *Streptococcus viridans* may seed into the bloodstream, perhaps even through vigorous tooth brushing or chewing an apple. There is greater risk in dental caries so scrupulous dental hygiene is important in people with heart valve damage.

The transient bacteraemia with this relatively avirulent bacterium results in vegetations forming on damaged valves. Embolism from the vegetations tends to dominate the picture, resulting in infarcts, especially in brain, spleen, kidney and skin. Death may occur due to embolism or, less commonly, to heart failure.

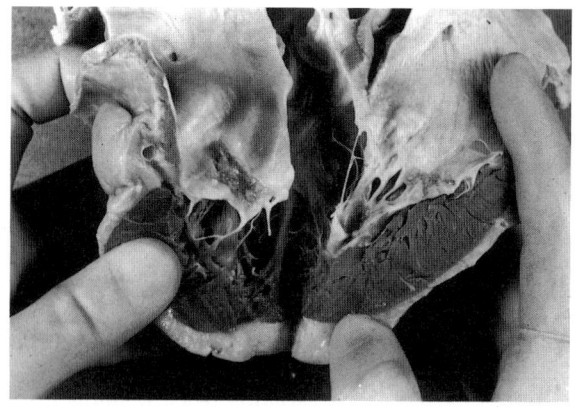

Figure 6.15 *A heart from a 62-year-old female showing mitral endocarditis associated with subacute bacterial endocarditis*

Valvular Lesions

Valve disease may result in **stenosis** (reduction in the size of the valvular opening) and **incompetence** (regurgitation or backflow of blood) of valves. Very frequently, the same valve damaged by inflammation and heavily scarred will show changes characteristic of both stenosis and incompetence (see Figure 6.16):

- 40% of cases of valvular disease show mitral valve involvement only;
- 40% show mitral and aortic valve involvement;
- 10% show aortic valve involvement only (Figure 6.17);
- 10% show tricuspid, pulmonary, aortic and mitral valve involvement in various combinations.

Valve disease may be caused by congenital heart diseases, rheumatic heart disease and infective endocarditis. The effects of valve disease are hypertrophy of the left ventricle, coronary artery insufficiency, pulmonary hypertension and heart failure.

Diseases of the Veins

Veins are thin-walled vessels with a relatively large lumen and are generally involved in fewer pathological processes than the arteries. They have been discussed already in relation to thrombosis, thrombophlebitis and tumour invasion. The other relatively common and important pathological process in which veins are involved is that of varicose veins.

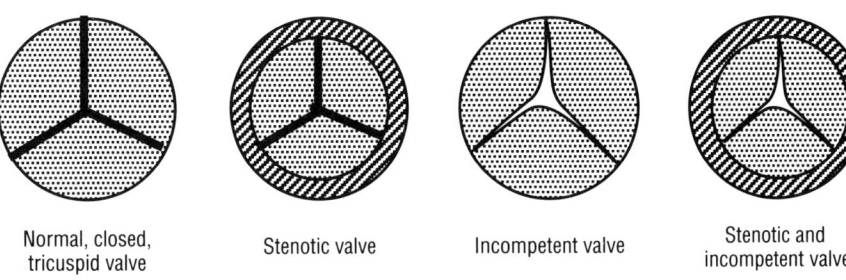

Normal, closed, tricuspid valve   Stenotic valve   Incompetent valve   Stenotic and incompetent valve

Figure 6.16   *Types of lesions commonly encountered in the cardiac valves*

Varicose Veins

This is a condition in which the veins become enlarged and dilated, very tortuous and appear quite prominently below the surface of the skin if they are in a superficial situation. Varicose veins usually occur in the legs. Alternatively, they may be seen in the regions draining the portal circulation with involvement of the lower oesophagus (**oesophageal varices**), of the umbilical veins (**caput medusae**) and of the haemorrhoidal veins (**haemorrhoids**). In these cases, the conditions

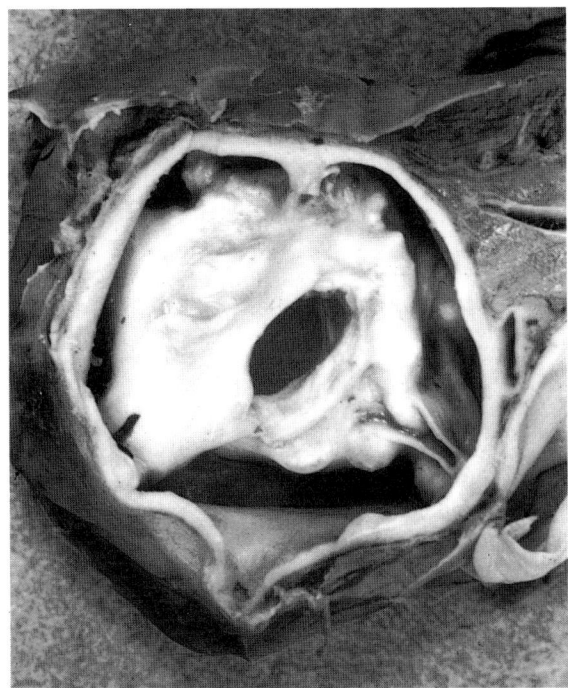

Figure 6.17   *Calcific aortic stenosis from a 65-year-old male. The left ventricular wall was 3 cm thick and the heart weighed 670 g*

are associated with portal hypertension (due to cirrhosis of the liver).

Varicose veins are common in incidence, seen in about 15% of the general population, the incidence increasing with increasing age, most commonly seen above the age of 50 years. Females are affected four times more commonly than males. In the systemic circulation varicose veins develop in those situations where connective tissue support is least and where effects of gravity are considerable, that is, in the superficial veins of the legs. The veins become elongated, dilated, congested and very prominent, and in some cases are very unsightly which is the reason why many patients first present. The walls of the dilated veins are uneven in thickness due to patchy hypertrophy of the muscle layers and the venous valves become incompetent as the vein is misshapen and distorted (see Figure 6.18).

Various factors have been implicated in the aetiology and pathogenesis of the disorder. There appears to be some **familial** predisposition to the disorder in about 40% of cases and this has been linked to a weak venous wall which arises in the later years of the affected individuals. The condition is seen more commonly in the **obese** as the veins of the legs are poorly supported in these individuals, the adipose tissue being less able to support the venous wall than the fibrocollagenous tissue which is seen in lean people. With increasing **age** there is a degeneration of the connective tissues and the wall is less well supported. In the elderly with arthritic conditions that cause pain and a reluctance to move the legs, varicose veins will develop in association with the **decreased muscular activity**. The propulsion of blood in the venous system greatly depends on the action of muscles which compress the venous wall and push the blood along, the venous valves making blood flow one way — towards the heart. If there is less muscular activity the blood is more likely to pool in the veins causing distension and dilatation.

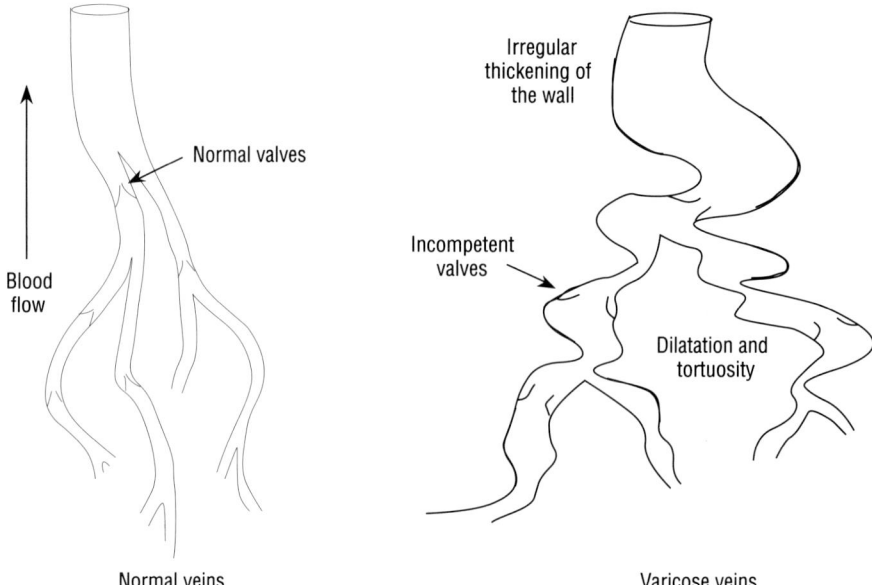

Normal valves

Blood
flow

Normal veins

Irregular
thickening of
the wall

Incompetent
valves

Dilatation and
tortuosity

Varicose veins

Figure 6.18 *Varicose veins*

Increased hydrostatic pressure in the venous lumen also predisposes to the condition and is seen in many cases. Those people who **stand immobile** for long periods of time have a higher hydrostatic pressure in their veins. In **pregnancy**, the gravid uterus compromises venous return from the lower part of the body, thus raising the intravenous hydrostatic pressure. **Thrombotic conditions** in the veins with blockage of channels will cause an increased pressure in the still patent collaterals which will now carry a larger proportion of the blood. **Tumours** around veins (e.g. ovarian tumours) may compress the thin wall and reduce luminal size considerably thus raising the pressure within the lumen.

Various **complications** are seen with varicose veins and these relate to the raised hydrostatic pressure within the veins, the poor flow of blood through them (with ischaemic effects) and the predisposition to thrombosis. **Oedema** and **trophic changes** in the skin of the affected regions are often seen. There may be **varicose ulcers** present on the legs, reflecting the ischaemia. A very common occurrence is **thrombosis** and all of its attendant complications (thrombophlebitis, thromboembolism, infarction). Also, the weakened wall and high pressure within the lumen predispose to **haemorrhages** developing.

Treatment of the condition relies on alleviating if possible any of the predisposing factors (e.g. weight reduction, exercise, thrombolytic therapy, prevention

of further thrombosis). In some cases the varicose veins must be surgically removed, either to prevent or eliminate complications or as is often the case, for cosmetic reasons.

Diseases of Arteries

The most important group of arterial diseases, that of arteriosclerosis, has been discussed already in Chapter 3 and various other less common and less important forms of arterial diseases are treated here.

Raynaud's Disease

Raynaud's disease is a functional disorder of small arteries and arterioles of the extremities in which intense, prolonged vasoconstriction is seen (= vasospasm). The patients affected are mainly young, otherwise healthy, women. The disease affects the peripheral tissues, mainly the fingers and hands, occasionally the toes and feet and sometimes the tip of the nose. Cold and emotional stimuli seem to trigger attacks, although sometimes an attack may be seen without any predisposing causative stimulus. The affected parts become very pale, almost white, then blue and then red.

The aetiology is unknown and it is thought that

there is some form of hyperlability of the autonomic innervation of the affected region. The symptoms described are all due to the extreme vasoconstriction mediated by nervous mechanisms, therefore organic changes in the vessel wall are usually absent. Occasionally, in chronic cases there may be slight intimal thickening and endothelial cell proliferation in the affected vessels. The disease does not usually follow a severe course and there are minimal complications; however, in some severe, chronic cases there may be atrophy of the skin, subcutaneous tissues and muscles, with, in very rare cases, ulceration and gangrene.

Raynaud's Phenomenon

This is a disorder characterized by cold sensitivity in the fingers, pain and colour changes in the skin and the patient may resemble a case of Raynaud's disease. However, in Raynaud's phenomenon, all of the observed changes that develop in the tissue are **secondary** to some underlying, often serious disorder which is causing an organic lesion in the arterial wall. The disorders with which this phenomenon is most commonly associated are: arteriosclerosis, connective tissue diseases (e.g. scleroderma, systemic lupus erythematosus), thromboangiitis obliterans (Bürger's disease), ingestion of drugs or poisons (e.g. ergotamine, lead), prolonged use of vibrating tools (e.g. jack hammers, pneumatic drills), primary pulmonary hypertension, or, rarely, occult carcinoma. Trophic changes develop in the affected parts, with degeneration of the skin, subcutaneous tissues, ulcerations, secondary infections and even frank gangrene.

Arteritis

Arteritis is an inflammation of the arterial walls. Any type of injury to an artery will cause arteritis and this condition is commonly seen associated with infections (e.g. septicaemias), trauma (e.g. following surgery), chemical injury (e.g. at the base of a peptic ulcer) or exposure to ionizing radiation (e.g. following radiotherapy for a tumour). In the acute types of arteritis, a typical inflammatory reaction will be seen in the wall, usually associated with thrombosis. In prolonged cases, the inflammation will be chronic, there will be organization and the lumen of the artery will be progressively occluded, a condition termed **endarteritis obliterans**.

The major complication of arteritis is either partial or complete ischaemia with reactive changes or necrosis occurring in the affected region. Haemorrhages may also occur.

Arteritis may also be seen in many hypersensitivity reactions (e.g. Arthus phenomenon) and autoimmune states (e.g. rheumatoid arthritis). If the disease affects muscular and small arteries in many organs throughout the body it is termed **polyarteritis nodosa**. This disorder occurs mainly in young to middle-aged adults and is more common in males. It is often due to a hypersensitivity reaction to sulphonamides or streptococcal infections. In some cases the initiating factor seems to be rheumatoid arthritis. The kidney, heart, liver, gastrointestinal tract and lung arteries are most commonly involved. Vessels may be extensively inflamed and destroyed with ischaemic effects in the affected organs. Death may be due to renal or cardiac failure or effects of haemorrhage. Many cases undergo spontaneous remissions and in the others there is good clinical remission with anti-inflammatory drug therapy (e.g. steroid preparations).

Aneurysms

An aneurysm is a localized, abnormal dilatation of any vessel or the heart. Although the disorder may develop in any part of the vascular system, it is most commonly seen in the arteries. Most aneurysms occur in the aorta, arteries of the brain and head, iliac arteries and in renal arteries (the last-mentioned are especially involved in the diabetic patient). Aneurysms may be classified according to various criteria:

- **Site**: Whether they occur in veins, arteries or the heart.
- **Aetiology**: The cause that has led to their formation may be atherosclerosis, syphilis, arteritis, medial necrosis, genetic predisposition, etc.
- **Morphology**: The shape and appearance of the aneurysm may be characteristic of a certain site or aetiology. There are saccular, fusiform, cylindroid, dissecting and berry aneurysms (as shown in Figure 6.19).

The force that expands the aneurysm is the blood pressure, but in order for an aneurysm to form there must be a pre-existing arterial lesion which causes a weakening of the media locally. If the patient is also hypertensive, the aneurysm may form more quickly or complications may be seen earlier. As the balloon-like dilatation develops in the vascular wall expansion and stretching cause progressive enlargement of the aneurysm, very often leading to **rupture** of the wall of the dilated vessel with massive **haemorrhage** occurring, usually with fatal results.

Other complications are **thrombosis** within the lu-

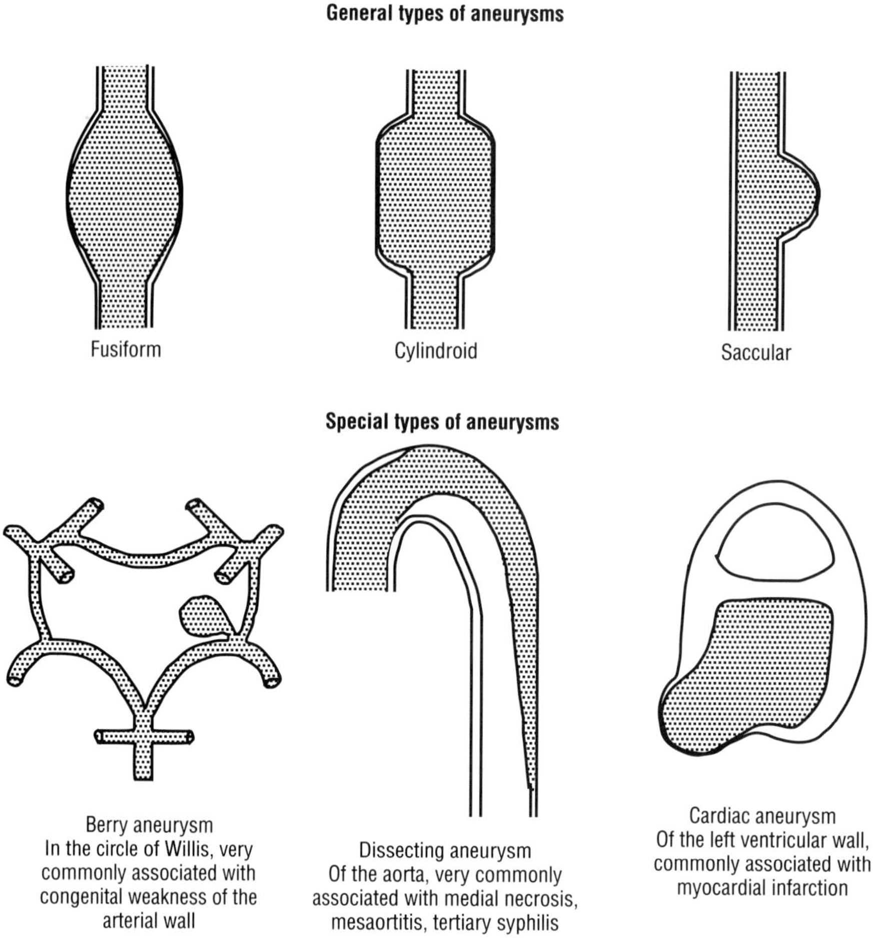

General types of aneurysms

Fusiform   Cylindroid   Saccular

Special types of aneurysms

Berry aneurysm
In the circle of Willis, very
commonly associated with
congenital weakness of the
arterial wall

Dissecting aneurysm
Of the aorta, very commonly
associated with medial necrosis,
mesaortitis, tertiary syphilis

Cardiac aneurysm
Of the left ventricular wall,
commonly associated with
myocardial infarction

Figure 6.19   *Types of aneurysms*

men of the aneurysm with all of the complications of that condition (e.g. embolism, infarction). In dissecting aneurysms, the wall of the vessel (usually the aorta) splits along the damaged media with the blood coursing within the split wall, separating inner and outer layers and forming a false lumen while at the same time obliterating the true lumen. This condition is usually rapidly fatal.

Atheroma is the major cause of aneurysms nowadays and the most commonly affected sites are the abdominal aorta and iliac arteries. These aneurysms are usually fusiform or cylindroid and typically occur in men of 50 years of age and above (Figure 6.20). They form as the result of extensive atrophy and weakening of the media due to pressure put on it by the enlarging intimal atheromatous plaques. Such aneurysms are treated by grafting a dacron tube in the affected region of the artery, which strengthens the

wall thus preventing rupture of the aneurysm and fatal haemorrhages.

Syphilitic aneurysms occur in the tertiary stage of the disease (i.e. 10 to 20 years after infection) and are very rarely seen now. They occur in association with syphilitic aortitis which is seen in the aortic arch and thoracic aorta, rarely extending below the diaphragm. There is ischaemic mesaortitis, destruction of the media and weakening of the wall. A dissecting aneurysm or a saccular aneurysm very frequently results. Dissecting aneurysms also occur with some idiopathic diseases such as **idiopathic cystic medial necrosis of the aorta**, which is an uncommon disorder seen more frequently in males around the age of 40 years (Figure 6.21).

Cerebral aneurysms are usually **berry aneurysms**, being most often within vessels of the circle of Willis. They are the most common cause of subarachnoid

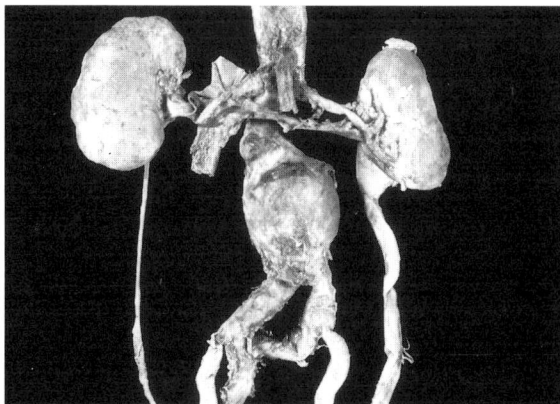

Figure 6.20 *Fusiform aneurysm of the abdominal aorta in a 65-year-old male patient*

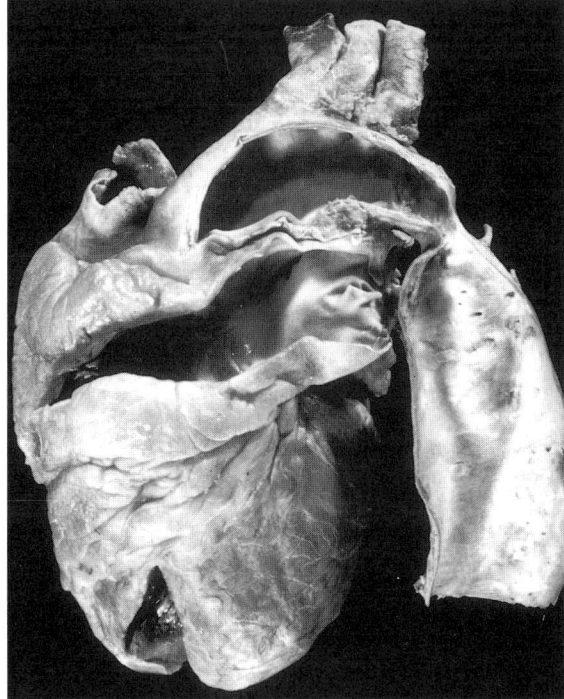

Figure 6.21 *Dissecting aneurysm of the aortic arch in a patient with syphilitic heart disease*

haemorrhage in the brain. They occur usually in the anterior part of the circle and are slightly more common in females. They may occur in children or young adults but mostly are seen in people of 50 years of age and above. The aneurysm most frequently develops because of congenital weaknesses of the wall of these vessels, the defect being in the media of the angles formed by the junctions of the vessels. As the patient ages and becomes more prone to developing hypertension, the risk of aneurysms forming in the weak areas also increases. The prognosis of these patients is poor with more than 60% of them dying when the aneurysm ruptures.

Mycotic aneurysms are formed by the weakening of vascular walls as a result of infection. Almost all cases are associated with subacute bacterial endocarditis with complicating septic thromboembolism. The aorta, coronary, cerebral and mesenteric arteries are most frequently involved and the aneurysms that form are saccular dilatations which are caused by the infection and inflammation that follows impaction of the septic embolus. Associated fibrosis and thrombosis may cause obstruction of the vessel with ischaemic effects seen in the tissue supplied by the vessel.

Revision Questions and Case Studies

1. Write short notes on any three of the commonly occurring, congenital, cardiac diseases.
2. Discuss acute pericarditis, distinguishing infective and non-infective types and classifying them on the basis of their macroscopic appearance.
3. What are the possible sequelae of acute pericarditis?
4. Write notes on Pick's disease of the pericardium.
5. What are the most commonly occurring tumours of the pericardium?
6. Discuss the pathology of myocardial infarction with special reference to age and sex incidence, aetiology, appearance (macroscopic and microscopic), sequelae, complications and results.
7. Compare and contrast the pathology of:
   (a) Fatty infiltration of the heart
   (b) Fatty change of the heart
8. What is meant by the term 'myocarditis'? Give the commonest forms of this disorder, discussing in detail the pathology of any one of these forms.
9. Discuss the pathology of rheumatic heart disease (RHD).
10. Distinguish between cor bovinum and cor pulmonale, giving common aetiologies of each condition.
11. Define the term 'hypertensive heart disease'. What are the typical myocardial changes seen in a patient with this condition?
12. Discuss the pathology of the septic endocarditides.
13. What are the commonest valvular lesions seen in

the heart? Discuss the pathology of any two commonly occurring such diseases of the cardiac valves.

14. How common are primary tumours of the myocardium? What is the commonest primary malignancy associated with this tissue?
15. Discuss the pathology of secondary tumours of the heart.
16. What is Fallot's tetralogy?
17. What is an aneurysm? Discuss aneurysm formation in relation to atherosclerosis of the abdominal aorta and indicate the possible sequelae.
18. Discuss the manifestations of tertiary syphilis in the cardiovascular system and the possible fatal complications of this condition.
19. Write short notes on any four of the following topics:
    (a) Varicose veins
    (b) Phlebothrombosis
    (c) Pulmonary thromboembolism
    (d) Thrombocytopenic purpura
    (e) Cardiogenic shock
20. Discuss the pathology of varicose veins.

Case study 1. A 47-year-old Caucasian male 1.76 m tall and 115 kg in weight presents with a history of a sharp, left-sided chest pain which radiates down the left arm. He states that the pain is brought on by effort and stress, mainly, but he has also noticed that it occurs during very hot weather, which the man does not like at all. The pain usually lasts until the exertion stops and disappears within 5 minutes. When questioned further the man admits to smoking approximately 25 cigarettes a day. He is a public servant and says that he leads a sedentary life, not exercising much at all. His blood pressure is 175/105 mmHg. Lately, he mentions, he has noticed that he is drinking more fluids.

(a) What is the diagnosis?
(b) What tests or investigations are advisable in this case? (List only).
(c) How should this man's condition be managed?

Case study 2. A 60-year-old Caucasian male is admitted to hospital after a suspected 'heart attack' which happened the previous night. The patient's wife gives the following history: 'He has had chest pain for the past two weeks and he has been complaining of feeling tired. Yesterday evening he was out in the garden and I heard him call out. I went out and found him sitting holding his chest. He had quite considerable difficulty breathing and he kept clutching his chest, being in pain. He was very pale and in a cold sweat. The pain lasted for about forty minutes and we managed to get him to bed. This morning we convinced him that he should come to the hospital.' Physical examination shows that the patient is hypotensive with a weak rapid pulse. A pericardial friction rub is heard and there is evidence of mitral regurgitation. Crepitations of the lung at the lung bases are present. On questioning, the man says that he has had 'twinges of chest pain' in the past but not as bad as this attack. The examining clinician notices the patient's fingers are tobacco stained and she elicits the information that the man smokes about 40 cigarettes a day. He is a plumber but his apprentices 'do most of the heavy work'. An ECG shows the pattern below:

(a) What is the diagnosis?
(b) What further laboratory tests would confirm this diagnosis?
(c) Discuss the management of this disorder.

Case study 3. Mr Stephen P., a 32-year-old Caucasian shop assistant, was rejected after a life insurance physical examination and was referred to his family physician. She noted on three separate examinations that Mr P.'s blood pressure was: 160/100, 140/90 and 185/98 mmHg. His resting pulse rate was 92 per minute and he had a strong cardiac apex impulse. The other values of the physical examination were normal. The patient was aware that his father suffered from 'high blood pressure'. Further questioning elicited the information that when Mr P. was at business school he was excluded from sporting activity as a diagnosis of 'vascular instability' was made.

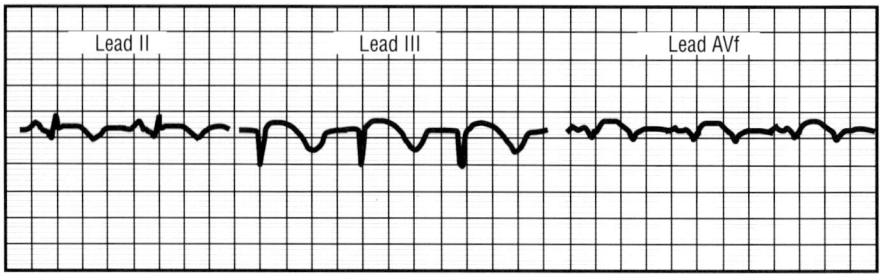

For *Case Study 2*

(a) What is the diagnosis?
(b) What other tests or examinations should be done?
(c) How is the condition managed in cases such as this?

Case study 4. A 74-year-old retired Caucasian male electrician presents at his doctor's surgery and complains of respiratory difficulty and increasing shortness of breath at rest. Up to three months previously, the man had enjoyed a daily walk in the park with his dog but he found that he had to give this up as it became impossible to exert himself due to his breathlessness. He has no history of past respiratory disease and he has been a non-smoker and a teetotaller all of his life. His abdomen is swollen and on palpation the doctor determines that ascites is present. She also notes that the liver is not enlarged. The man's blood pressure is 110/60 mmHg, heart sounds were soft and it was noted that there was an early diastolic sound. Blood tests showed: haemoglobin content 8.2 mmol/L (N = 8.1–11.2 mmol/L), white cell count 8.2 × 10^9/L (N = 4.3–10.8 × 10^9/L), sodium 138 mmol/L (N = 135–144 mmol/L), potassium 3.8 mmol/L (N = 3.1–4.8 mmol/L), urea 5.2 mmol/L (N = 3.2–7.7 mmol/L), serum albumin 38 g/L (N = 36–48 g/L), serum globulin 34 g/L (N = 24–37 g/L), lactate dehydrogenase 120 IU/L (N = 100–300 IU/L) and bilirubin 12 μmol/L (N = up to 17 μmol/L).

(a) What is the differential diagnosis?
(b) What is the most likely diagnosis?
(c) How is this disorder treated and how effective is the treatment?

Further Reading

Ackman RG. 'Variability of Fatty Acids and Lipids in Seafoods.' *Omega 3 News* 1990; **5**(4) 1.
Bloor K, Humphreys WV. 'Aneurysms of the Abdominal Aorta.' *Br J Hosp Med* 1979; **21**: 568.
Chen Z, *et al.* 'Serum Cholesterol Concentration and Coronary Heart Disease in Populations with Low Cholesterol Concentrations.' *BMJ* 1991; **303**: 276.
Coffman JD. 'Raynaud's Phenomenon: An Update.' *Hypertension* 1991; **17**: 593.
Crawford ES. 'The Diagnosis and Management of Aortic Dissection.' *JAMA* 1990; **264**: 2537.
Davies MJ. 'The Cardiomyopathies: A Review of Terminology, Pathology and Pathogenesis.' *Histopathol* 1984; **8**: 363.
Gotto AM. 'Cholesterol Intake and Cholesterol Level.' *New Engl J M* 1991; **324**: 912.
Ikonomidis JS, *et al.* 'Thoracic Aortic Surgery.' *Circulation* 1991; **84** (suppl): III, 1.
Jackson R, *et al.* 'Alcohol Consumption and Risk of Coronary Heart Disease.' *BMJ* 1991; **303**: 211.
Kleijnen J, Knipschild P. '*Gingko biloba*.' *Lancet* 1992; **340**: 1136.
Markowitz M. 'Reappearance of Rheumatic Fever.' *Adv Pediatr* 1989; **36**: 39.
Northcote RJ. 'Editorial: Cardiac Disease and Exercise — A Modern Paradox.' *J Path* 1989; **157**: 93.
Olsen EGJ. 'Myocarditis — A Case of Mistaken Identity?' *Br Heart J* 1983; **50**: 303.
Olson LT, *et al.* 'Surgical Pathology of Pure Aortic Insufficiency — A Study of 225 Cases.' *Mayo Clin Proc* 1984; **59**: 835.
Pepine CJ. 'New Concepts in the Pathophysiology of Acute MI.' *Am J Cardiol* 1989; **64**: 2B.
Radack K, Wyderski RJ. 'Conservative Management of Intermittent Claudication.' *Ann Intern Med* 1990; **113**: 135.
Rastam L, *et al.* 'Seasonal Variation in Plasma Cholesterol Distributions: Implications for Screening and Referral.' *Am J Prev Med* 1992; **8**: 360.
Sinclair AJ. 'The Good Oil: Omega 3 Polyunsaturated Fatty Acids.' *Today's Life Sci* 1991: **3**(8): 18.
Stehbens WE. 'Relationship of Coronary Artery Thrombosis to Myocardial Infarction.' *Lancet* 1985; **ii**: 639.
'The Management of Hyperlipidaemia: A Consensus Statement.' *Supplement, Med J Aust* 1992; 3 February.
Thomas AC, *et al.* 'Community Studies of Causes of "Natural" Sudden Death.' *BMJ* 1988; **297**: 1453.
Waller BF. 'The Pathology of Acute Myocardial Infarction: Definition, Location, Pathogenesis, Effects of Reperfusion, Complications and Sequlae.' *Cardiol Clin* 1988; **6**: 1.
Watkins H, *et al.* 'Characteristics and Prognostic Implications of Myosin Missense Mutations in Familial Hypertrophic Cardiomyopathy.' *N Engl J Med* 1992; **326**: 1108.

7

Respiratory System Disorders

The Normal Respiratory System

The normal respiratory system comprises the upper respiratory system (consisting of the nose, nares, sinuses, larynx, upper trachea) and the lower respiratory system (consisting of the lower trachea, bronchi, bronchioles and alveoli). The function of the respiratory system is gas exchanges between the bloodstream and the air. The blood is oxygenated in the lungs and carbon dioxide is removed from the blood. The lungs are paired organs, one in each side of the chest, separated from each other by the heart and other contents of the mediastinum. Each lung is conical in shape and is composed of lobes. The right lung comprises three lobes and the left lung comprises two lobes. The apex of each lung extends into the base of the neck at about the level of the first rib, while the base of each lung rests upon the diaphragm. Each lung is invested on its external surface by a thin, delicate serous membrane, the visceral pleura, which encloses the organ as far as its root, and this membrane is then reflected upon the inner surface of the thorax to line it becoming the parietal pleura. The space between the two layers of pleura is the pleural cavity and is normally filled with a few millilitres of serous fluid that allow the lung lobes to slip effortlessly past one another during breathing.

The surface of the lung is smooth, shining and on close examination seen to be marked out into numerous polyhedral compartments that are an indication of the lobular structure of the organ. The substance of the organ is of a light, spongy texture which is air containing and the organ floats if placed in water. The pulmonary tissue is highly elastic in texture and rapidly collapses once it is removed from the thoracic cavity. The bronchi, once they enter the lungs, ramify considerably such that they may convey air into all parts of the organ. Each of the smaller subdivisions of the bronchioles ends in a lung lobule which is composed of a group of cup-shaped air spaces, the alveoli, in which the gas exchanges occur. The surface area of the alveoli when normally distended is estimated at 63 000 square metres. The alveoli are lined by type I pneumocytes, flattened cells about 0.05 μm thick that abut onto the endothelium of the alveolar capillaries. A thin basal lamina exists between the two cells, bringing the total thickness through which gas exchanges occur to 0.3 μm. Type II pneumocytes are also found interspersed between the type I cells, and these are cuboidal and contain inclusions of surfactant. The surfactant is secreted and coats the outer aspect of the alveolar cells, reducing surface tension and aiding in alveolar recoil during expiration.

In order that the respiratory system functions normally the following factors must be maintained:

- Normal muscle function
- Nervous supply
- Patent airways
- Intact thoracic wall (negative pressure)
- High blood flow
- Adequate drainage of fluid
- Secretion of surfactant
- High surface area at the alveolar level
- Maintenance of thin alveolar walls
- Expulsion mechanisms for inspired particles (sneezing, coughing, 'mucociliary escalator')

When any of the above factors is not maintained at a normal level, a respiratory disorder develops with subsequent compromise of gas exchanges occurring in the lungs. Respiratory distress will then be observed and pathological changes will develop.

Circulatory Disorders

Chronic Venous Congestion

As the term implies this is a disorder of the circulation arising in the lungs as a result of a passive pooling of blood within the pulmonary circulation. The vessels become congested since the blood is not adequately removed from the lungs by the left ventricle. The aetiology of the condition, then, is associated with chronic failure of the left side of the heart. Mitral stenosis and incompetence, chronic hypertensive heart failure and rheumatic heart disease are all conditions frequently giving rise to chronic venous congestion of the lungs.

To the naked eye the lungs look brown and fibrous, are quite firm and are described as having undergone **brown induration**. Under the microscope, in the first stages there is a prominent congestion of the vessels, with stagnant anoxia and parenchymal cell destruction. The walls of the pulmonary veins thicken as a result of the increased pressure and they resemble pulmonary arteries. Haemorrhagic areas develop as a result of the necrosis and raised venous pressure and many red blood cells are found within the alveoli. This may give rise to the coughing up of blood-stained

sputum, but more frequent is the ingestion and breakdown of the erythrocytes by the alveolar macrophages which thus contain large amounts of haemosiderin. These are the so-called '**heart failure cells**' (Figure 7.1). In later stages there is widespread fibrosis of the alveolar walls and their gas exchange capacity is greatly hampered.

Chronic venous congestion occurs in chronic left-sided heart failure, for example due to mitral valve stenosis or chronic hypertensive heart failure. Chronic left-sided heart failure results in chronic venous congestion of the pulmonary circulation. There is associated congestion of alveolar vessels, vascular thickening, fibrous thickening of alveolar walls and development of atheroma in larger pulmonary arteries.

Pulmonary Embolism

Pulmonary embolism is a common cause of sudden death or pulmonary infarction, usually complicating deep venous thrombosis of pelvic or leg veins. Rarely, a thrombus in the lung circulation may arise *in situ*. Such indigenous thrombi most commonly form in relation to atherosclerosis and hypertension. Other types of emboli which may impact in pulmonary vessels are fat emboli following bone fractures or amniotic fluid emboli during childbirth (especially with protracted, difficult labour).

Pulmonary thromboembolism is thought to cause about 5–10% of post-operative deaths and most of the thromboemboli arise from the deep leg veins. The thromboembolus has the dimensions of the vein it

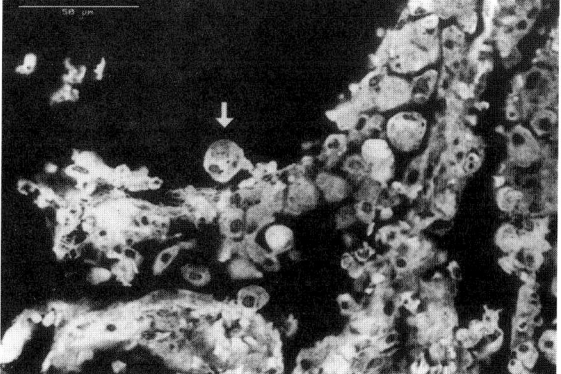

Figure 7.1 *Heart failure cells (arrow) in a patient with chronic venous congestion of the lungs. Many such cells are found scattered in the alveoli and lining the alveolar walls. Granules of haemosiderin are seen in the cytoplasm of these alveolar macrophages (scale bar is 50 μm)*

formed in and, travelling through the venous system and the right heart, it finally lodges in the pulmonary arteries or one of their branches. It may form a **saddle embolus** in which case it sits astride one of the major bifurcations of the pulmonary artery. Large emboli which obstruct blood flow considerably may cause sudden death. Smaller emboli may cause regions of infarction. Even smaller emboli may cause no appreciable degree of damage, especially if the person is young and otherwise healthy; alternatively in the older patients who already have some respiratory disease, even small emboli may cause infarcts.

Pulmonary Infarction

Pulmonary infarction occurs usually due to embolism or, rarely, due to pulmonary vascular thrombosis associated with abnormal circulation, for example pulmonary hypertension and atheroma of pulmonary arteries. Approximately 75% of pulmonary infarcts occur in the lower lobes of the lungs. The infarct is haemorrhagic (red infarct) because of the dual blood supply in the lungs (refer to Figure 7.2). It is usually pyramidal in shape with its base at the pleural surface. Microscopically there is coagulative necrosis of the lung tissue, red blood cells filling the alveolar spaces and an inflammatory response occurring at the margins. The infarct later heals by fibrosis, such that necrotic lung tissue is replaced by scar tissue. Scarring resulting from larger infarcts or from multiple infarcts may seriously interfere with normal lung function. Large infarcts may cause right ventricular strain, leading to right heart failure, or pulmonary hypertension.

Following pulmonary infarction a patient may experience dyspnoea and may appear cyanotic due to reduced oxygenation. There is often pleuritic pain. If the infarct subsequently becomes infected (septic infarct) or results from a septic embolus, there may be abscess formation.

Pulmonary Hypertension

Pulmonary hypertension can occur as a primary disease with no known pre-exiting condition. This primary, idiopathic condition is rare. Most commonly, pulmonary hypertension occurs secondarily to a known disease. Pulmonary hypertension occurs owing to:

- **Excessive pulmonary blood flow**, for example congenital heart defects which shunt excessive blood into the pulmonary circulation (left to right shunts).
- **Chronic passive venous congestion** in which blood stagnates within the pulmonary circulation thus considerably increasing the blood pressure.
- **Obstructive lung disease** with obstruction of pulmonary vessels, for example pulmonary fibrosis due to pneumoconioses and other lung disorders, emphysema, etc.
- **Idiopathic** disease.

Pulmonary hypertension results in thickening of the walls of pulmonary arteries and also contributes to the development of atheroma of pulmonary arteries.

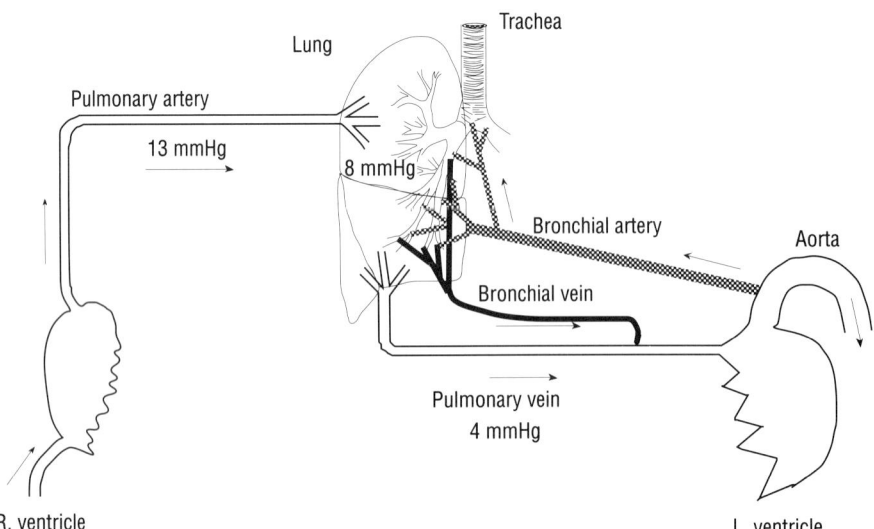

Figure 7.2 *The pulmonary circulation. Arrows indicate direction of blood flow; values in mmHg refer to the mean pressure inside the blood vessel they are closest to. Note the slight mixing of unoxygenated blood from the bronchial vein and the oxygenated blood of the pulmonary vein*

Pulmonary Oedema

Pulmonary oedema is the passage of large amounts of fluid transudate from pulmonary vessels into the alveoli. The lungs become firm like a 'wet sponge' and the alveolar fluid accumulation interferes seriously with normal lung function (lowered gas exchange, increased risk of infection, pH changes, etc.).

Common causes of pulmonary oedema are:

- acute left ventricular failure;
- early acute infection (pneumonia);
- conditions causing generalized oedema, for example renal failure;
- inhalation of chemical irritants;
- hypersensitivity reactions, for example Farmer's lung;
- aspiration of gastric contents, vomitus, food material, etc.;
- raised intracranial pressure.

In acute heart failure, pulmonary oedema results in breathing difficulties and the passage of air through the oedema fluid is heard as a gurgling sound known as **rales**. The oedematous fluid in the alveoli often results in infection known as **hypostatic pneumonia**. This is an infection of the stagnating pools of fluid and is contributed to by the poor mucociliary function associated with the oedema in the affected lung areas.

Mechanical Disorders

Atelectasia (Atelectasis)

Atelectasia, strictly speaking, refers to the failure of the lungs to aerate at birth. This failure of the lung to aerate may result from brain damage causing respiratory failure or may occur owing to bronchial obstruction by mucus or aspirated amniotic fluid. If the whole lungs are involved in this process the baby may die of asphyxia. However, only a lobe of the lungs may be affected, the remaining lung tissue being normal.

At autopsy atelectatic lungs look small, grey and airless and if placed in a bucket of water they will sink to the bottom, unlike normal lungs which will float to the top. The cut surface looks bluish-grey and may show evidence of haemorrhage, the airways often showing the cause of the obstruction. Microscopically, the alveolar walls look thicker than normal and they are crowded together with very inconspicuous alveolar spaces. There are congested vessels and airways may show debris from the amniotic fluid in the lumen.

Pulmonary Collapse

Collapse of lung occurs when air normally contained in the alveoli becomes absorbed and is not replaced through respiration. The volume of lung which has collapsed is less than normal, such that the overlying pleural surface becomes wrinkled. The collapsed area of lung appears more solid and is firmer than normal. If this collapsed area fails to re-aerate it will organize, the process being known as **carnification**. This causes the cut surface of the lung to assume a firm, meaty appearance.

Collapse arises as a result of obstruction of the bronchial tree supplying the area. Causes of this obstruction are:

- undrained bronchial secretion in the form of viscous mucus plugs;
- pus or exudate in airways;
- aspirated vomitus;
- foreign bodies (e.g. peanuts in child's lung);
- depressed cough reflex (post-operative);
- compression of bronchi by tumours, aneurysms, cysts, enlarged lymph nodes, etc.

Compression of the lung due to pneumothorax, pleural effusions, tumours, etc. will also result in pulmonary collapse. An area of pulmonary collapse which fails to re-aerate may result in bronchiectasis at a later stage. If the area of lung collapse is great, the condition may be fatal, otherwise there may be compromise of respiratory function and unless the cause of the collapse is not dealt with, carnification of the lung will cause permanent loss of that region of lung tissue.

Emphysema

Emphysema is defined as the permanent increase, beyond the normal, in the size of air spaces distal to the terminal bronchiole, either from dilatation or destruction of their walls (Figure 7.3). Often, both destruction and dilatation of the alveolar walls may be seen. Nomenclature of different forms of emphysema depends on the distribution of dilated air spaces within the lung lobule or whether destruction of alveolar walls may be demonstrated, but the severity of the disease and the effects on the respiratory function of the patient are more important, therefore a clinical classification is a more useful way of approaching the disease.

Classification of emphysema depends on whether there is dilatation of air passages and spaces alone or whether there is destruction of the cross-walls of air passages and spaces. The anatomical region of the lung lobule affected is also used in classifying the

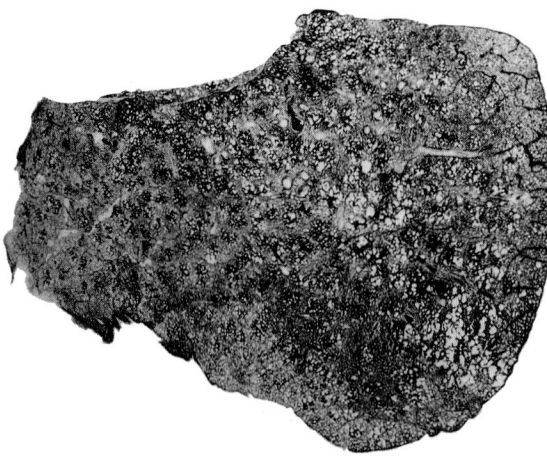

Figure 7.3 *Large lung section (showing a whole lobe) of a coal miner with focal emphysema*

disease and the different types of emphysema which may occur in the lobules are:

- **Centrilobular emphysema**: This shows dilatation or destruction of air spaces around the terminal and respiratory bronchioles.

- **Panacinar (panlobular) emphysema**: This shows these change throughout the lobule.
- **Irregular (mixed) emphysema**: This shows a mixed, irregular distribution of emphysema, often seen with great regions of fibrosis.
- **Paraseptal emphysema**: This is a rarer variety which is confined to the paraseptal region of the lobule (see Figure 7.4).

Although the aetiological factors associated with emphysema are well documented it should be noted that there is great individual variation in the observed emphysematous changes in persons exposed to the same aetiological agent as genetic/familial factors are also important in the development of the disease. It should also be noted that often there is poor correlation between the various anatomical types of emphysema and the various aetiologies associated with the disease. Often the length of time exposed to an agent or the amount of injury the lungs suffer is more important in the development of a particular type of emphysema than the nature of the aetiology itself. However, centrilobular emphysema, which is the commonest form of emphysema, most often occurs in association with cigarette smoking, dust inhalation diseases (pneumoconioses) and urban pollution. It is more

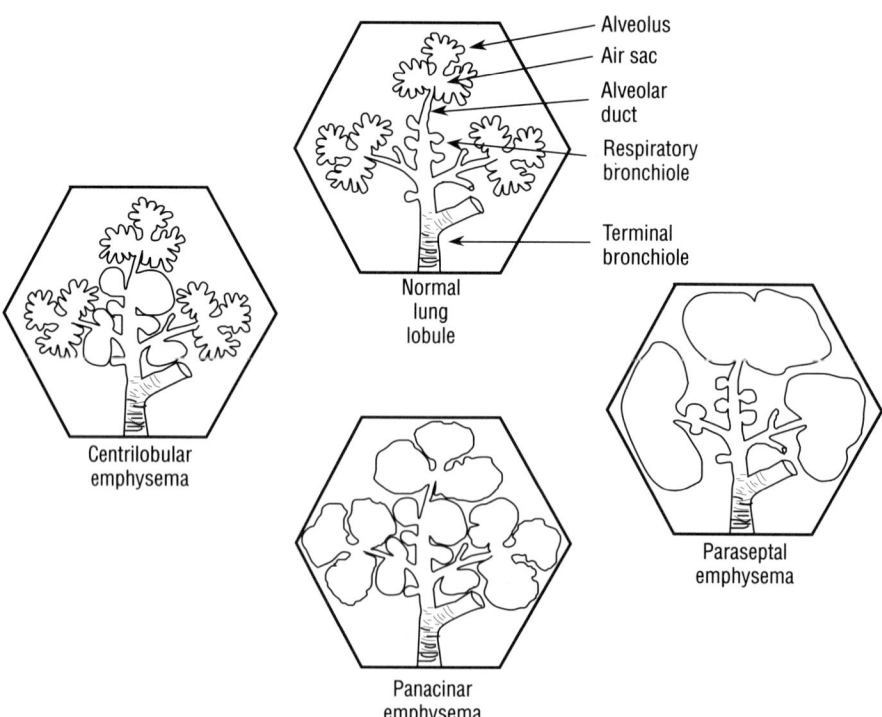

Figure 7.4 *Classification of emphysema*

common in males, often seen together with chronic bronchitis, and most commonly involves the upper zones of the lungs.

Panacinar emphysema occurs with chronic obstructive diseases such as asthma or in association with inhaled foreign bodies and lung collapse. It may also develop with smoking, chronic bronchitis and dust inhalations, especially after heavy exposures or prolonged contact time with aetiological agents. It is most commonly seen and most severe in the lower lobes of the lungs.

Familial factors are important in the development of emphysema and the great severity of the disease seen in some patients is due to an inherited defect in circulating α-1-antiproteinase (= α-1-antitrypsin deficiency). Over 30 different alleles are now recognized as being important in the control of levels of antiproteinase in the body and the most severe deficiency occurs in about 5% of the population, commoner in those of Scandinavian origin and rarer in Jews, black people and the Japanese. Normally, there should be adequate levels of α-1-antiproteinase in the alveolar spaces to protect against damage. The function of the antiproteinase is to destroy any free serine elastases in the alveoli which are derived from the lysosomes of phagocytic cells (mainly neutrophils) in the lungs.

Large amounts of elastases are released in the lungs when smoke or other particulate material is inhaled and the phagocytic cells attempt to phagocytose and inactivate the particles. The elastases are inactivated by the α-1-antiproteinases, thus preventing the destruction of elastic tissue in the alveolar walls (refer to Figure 7.5). It should be noted that cigarette smoke, pollutants, free radicals and other damaging agents inhibit the functioning of the α-1-antiproteinases. If inhalation of these irritants is coupled with a hereditary decrease in α-1-antiproteinase levels in the alveoli, then large amounts of free elastases are released and they will cause destruction of the elastic tissue of the alveolar sacs, contributing to the development of emphysema. The disease will be much more severe the lower the level of circulating α-1-antiproteinases and the more aetiological factors the patient is exposed to.

In all forms of emphysema, as the disease progresses, more and more lung is affected resulting in the same appearance, and the effects of emphysema depend on the severity of the disease and the amount of lung tissue involved rather than the specific anatomical subtype. As the distal air spaces enlarge and the cross-walls are broken down, the surface of the alveoli available for gas exchanges decreases and there is inadequate ventilation and lowered oxygenation of the blood. There

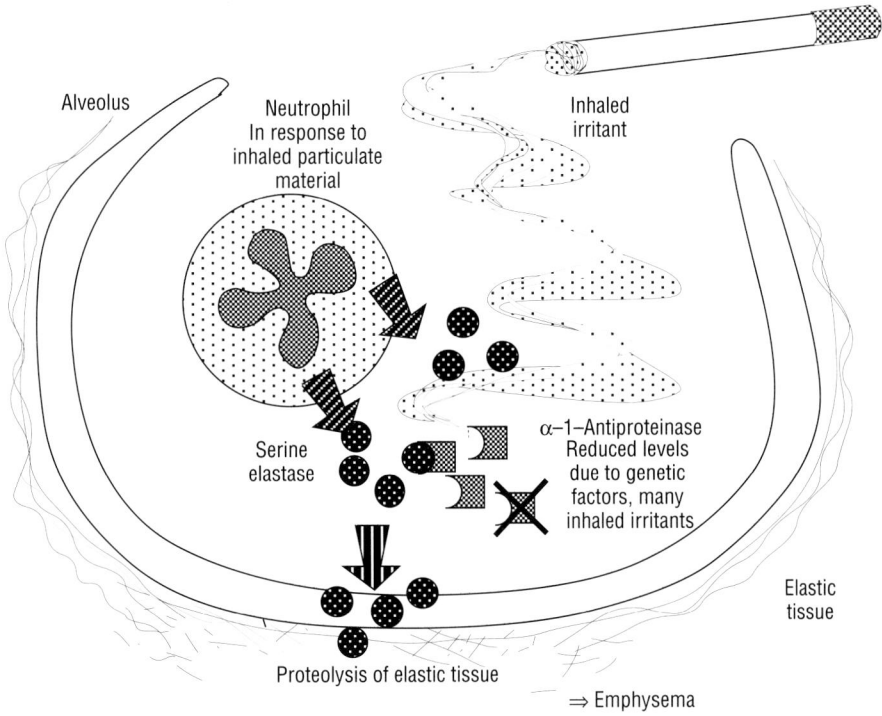

Figure 7.5 *Pathogenesis of emphysema*

is an increase of physiological 'dead space' and chronic bronchitis is almost always associated with emphysema, both of which factors contribute to the chronic airflow obstruction seen in the disease. The increased alveolar pressure compresses the capillaries in the alveolar walls, which results in pulmonary hypertension. Pulmonary hypertension leads to right ventricular hypertrophy, cor pulmonale and right heart failure. When emphysema is severe, **bullae**, large cyst-like areas, may form. Bullae may rupture and cause pneumothorax.

The typical patients with emphysema present with the disease in their fifties with a history of dyspnoea of insidious onset, evidence of chronic bronchitis and often with weight loss. They are usually smokers, or have an occupation in which they are chronically exposed to irritant chemicals, air pollutants or various finely divided dusts (e.g. SO_2, NO_2, coal dust and smog). Radiological findings include overinflation of the lungs, depressed diaphragm levels and an inversion of the convexity of the diaphragm. These patients are frequently described as having a 'barrel chest'.

As far as clinical presentation relating to respiratory function of individual patients goes, they may be placed anywhere between the two extremes of a spectrum of presentations, these two extremes being known as the 'pink puffers' and the 'blue bloaters'. The blue bloater is so described as he or she is hypoxic and hypercapneic, has peripheral oedema associated with heart failure and a rate of ventilation that is lower than would be expected. At the other extreme, the pink puffer is usually thin and has normal levels of blood gases maintained by hyperventilation.

Bronchiectasis

Bronchiectasis is defined as a permanent, abnormal dilatation of the bronchi and bronchioles, this enlargement of airways occurring above the level of the terminal bronchioles. It is a common disease found in all age groups including childhood. The basal segments of the lower lobes, middle lobe and lingula are the regions of the lung most commonly affected (Figures 7.6 and 7.7).

The main aetiological factors in the disorder are infection associated with bronchial obstruction. Obstruction may be due to the presence of intraluminal foreign bodies such as mucus, inflammatory exudates, pus or tumours, and strictures of the wall. Pressure from outside the wall may cause the obstruction. The disease is very often seen in association with chronic infectious/inflammatory states, for example as a sequela of whooping cough (*Bordetella pertussis* infection),

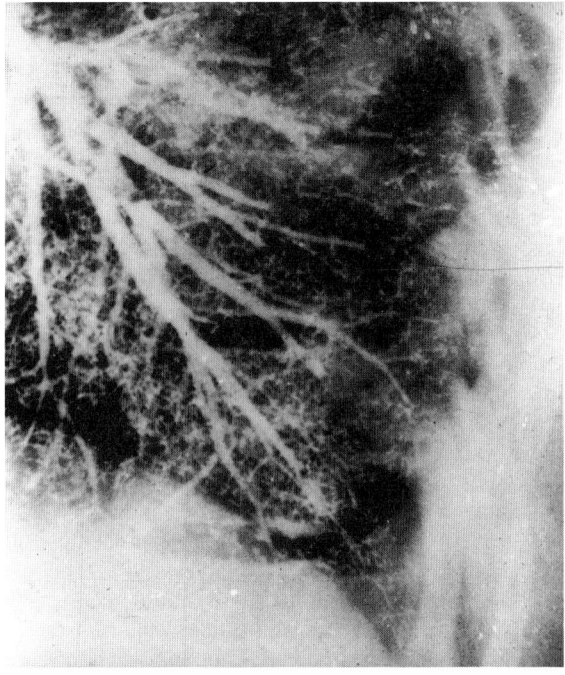

Figure 7.6   *X-ray of lungs demonstrating normal airways*

adenovirus infection and measles. It may also be caused by obstructive lesions (chronic obstructive airways disease, COAD), scarring (TB, dust inhalations), tumours, strictures, emphysema, pressure anomalies, cystic fibrosis, etc.

The pathogenesis of the disorder involves the partial or complete obstruction of airways by any one of the aetiological factors listed above. In the portion of lung distal to the obstruction there is resorption of air with an area of pulmonary collapse developing. Accumulation and stasis of secretions within the obstructed bronchi then ensues leading to a great probability of infection occurring with extension into the bronchial walls. There follows dilatation of the damaged wall by the effect of negative intrapleural pressure transmitted through the collapsed lung tissue and by the distension effect of retained excessive secretions in the blocked bronchi.

Bronchiectasis may be classified according to the aetiological factor that has caused it, anatomically, depending on which regions of the lungs are affected, or quite commonly on the morphological type encountered. The airways may show **saccular**, **cylindroid** or **fusiform** distension. Inflamed walls are characteristic of the condition with the adjacent lung tissue and

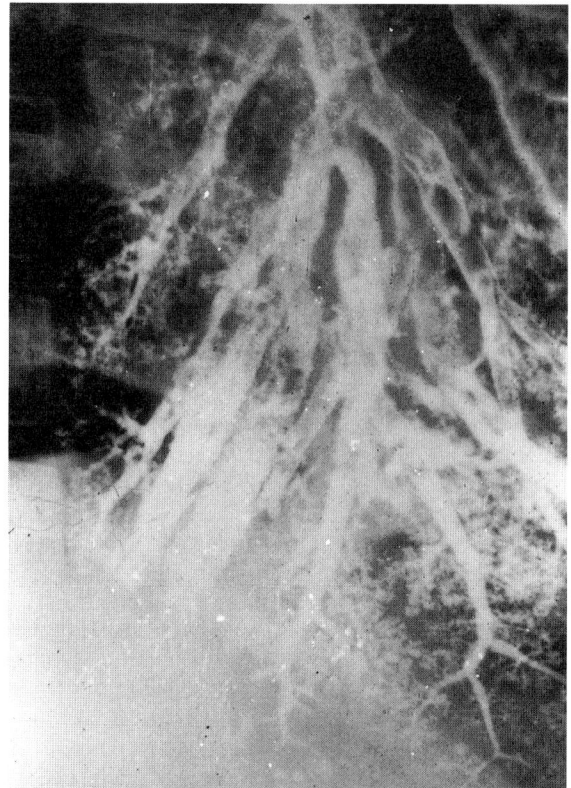

Figure 7.7 *X-ray of lungs demonstrating bronchiectasis of the airways of the lower left lobe (lateral view)*

pleura being frequently fibrous due to organized collapsed regions and chronic inflammation.

Microscopically, there is variable infiltration of part or all of the bronchial wall by chronic inflammatory tissue with fibrous replacement (Figure 7.8). The mucosa is usually replaced by inflammatory tissue with foci of respiratory mucosa and areas of squamous metaplasia. The lumen is filled with a mucopurulent exudate and debris in which bacteria may be demonstrated.

Characteristic of the disorder is the production of copious purulent sputum with respiratory dysfunction due to pulmonary fibrosis. The patient may present with dyspnoea and a chronic cough productive of mucopurulent, foul-smelling sputum. The condition greatly predisposes to repetitive inflammatory episodes due to aspiration of infected material into other areas of the lungs, so that chronic bronchitis may be perpetual or bronchopneumonia may develop. Abscesses, fibrosis and respiratory dysfunction with development of COAD are commonly seen sequelae.

Bronchial Asthma

Bronchial asthma is a condition characterized by widespread bronchial obstruction due to muscular spasm, producing expiratory wheezing with prolongation of expiration. Typically, a thick, white mucus is produced by the respiratory epithelium of the bronchi and this leads to plugging and distension of the airways, the patient experiencing considerable difficulty in breathing. There are two forms of asthma when the age of presentation is considered: childhood asthma, which affects 9% of children, and adulthood asthma, which affects 5% of adults. Furthermore, the disease is classified on aetiological grounds into the **extrinsic** and **intrinsic** types according to whether the aetiology is environmental in origin or whether the patient's own idiosyncrasy is more important in the causation of the disorder.

Extrinsic type (environmental/allergic). This accounts for 10% (or less) of all cases and is usually seen in childhood. It is more frequent in individuals with atopic allergies with a well-defined family history of allergies. It begins in childhood or early adult life and is usually of an allergic type. It frequently occurs in people who suffer from other allergies also (e.g. dermatitis, hay fever). It is due to an atopic (type I) hypersensitivity. This is an immediate-type hypersensitivity in which the primary encounter with the allergen is followed by the formation of IgE antibody. This antibody attaches to the surface of **mast cells** throughout the body, including the lungs. When the antigen is next encountered, it binds to the IgE anti-

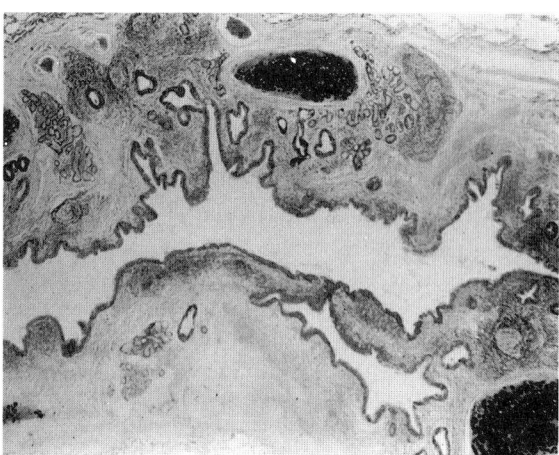

Figure 7.8 *Bronchiectasis displaying dilatation of the airways, mucous gland hyperplasia and focal accumulations of chronic inflammatory cells (×100)*

bodies that are attached to the mast cell surface. The allergen-antibody binding induces degranulation of the mast cell with release of histamine, serotonin and other biological amines. In the lungs these compounds cause an increased vascular permeability with exudation, vasodilatation, congestion and hyperaemia. Eosinophils accumulate at the site and the bronchial smooth muscle contracts, causing the bronchospasm characteristic of the attacks.

Allergens associated commonly with extrinsic asthma include various pollens, animal dandruff (dander), house dust containing house mites (*Dermatophagoides* spp.) and various types of fungi and their spores. Pulmonary attacks may also be precipitated by ingestion or injection of various substances that will act as allergens in the asthmatic patient; for example various drugs and foods.

Intrinsic type (idiosyncratic/psychological). Intrinsic asthma can occur at any age and tends to be more frequently recurrent and severe. This form of asthma may result from some abnormality of parasympathetic control of airway function but the mechanism through which an attack begins is unknown. Once the stimulus acts on the lungs, the attack is mediated by the degranulation of mast cells in a similar way to the extrinsic type of asthma. Stimuli responsible for initiating intrinsic asthma are: infection, exercise, aspirin ingestion, air pollution, cold temperatures and psychogenic (emotional) factors. Intrinsic asthma is often associated with chronic bronchitis. The chronic infection in the bronchial tree has been thought to be a factor in the development of atopic hypersensitivities but this has seldom been established in cases of the disease. Adulthood asthma is described frequently as a typical intrinsic asthma but there are almost certainly interactions between intrinsic and extrinsic asthma as many asthmatics react to both allergic and non-allergic stimuli. This type of asthma usually develops later in adult life and the affected individuals have no previous family history of atopic allergies. No allergen responsible for the attacks may be demonstrated. Polyps in the nose are frequent findings and these growths are densely infiltrated with eosinophils. The prognosis is worse than in extrinsic asthma and treatment is usually more difficult. Drug hypersensitivities may develop in people with intrinsic asthma, in particular allergies to aspirin and penicillin. Administration of these substances to affected people will be followed by anaphylaxis or anaphylactic shock and death.

In both extrinsic and intrinsic asthma it is well documented that psychological factors are important in precipitating the attacks. For example, it is known that asthmatic attacks occur more commonly during periods of anxiety, stress or emotional disturbance.

Asthmatic attacks are acute and involve a tightness in the chest, dyspnoea and difficulty during exhalation, which is accompanied by wheezing and coughing. As the attack subsides, copious, viscous, white sputum is coughed up. Attacks may last for a few minutes to days, and may vary in severity from very mild to the so-called **status asthmaticus**, which is a severe, prolonged, unremitting attack leading to grave mental and physical exhaustion or even death.

The asthmatic lungs may appear normal or may show one or several of the following features: viscous mucus in the bronchi and bronchioles, thickening of the bronchiolar walls, focal areas of lung collapse, emphysema and bronchiectasis. Secondary infection may also be present. Histologically there is marked thickening of the bronchiolar walls due to smooth muscle hypertrophy and hyperplasia of the mucous glands. There is marked eosinophil infiltration. In the lumen of the airways there are eosinophils, desquamated epithelial cells, abundant mucus and **Charcot-Leyden** crystals derived from eosinophils. There may also be seen the so-called **Curschmann's spirals**, which are twisted strips of desquamated epithelium (Figure 7.9).

Treatment of the disease may be preventative or symptomatic. In preventative treatment drugs are administered immediately prior to an impending attack and mostly are drugs that interfere with the degranulation of mast cells and therefore prevent the release of histamine and other substances into the lung tissue. Such a drug is disodium cromoglycate, which through its action on mast cells prevents degranulation and hence the attack. Alternatively, the drug may be

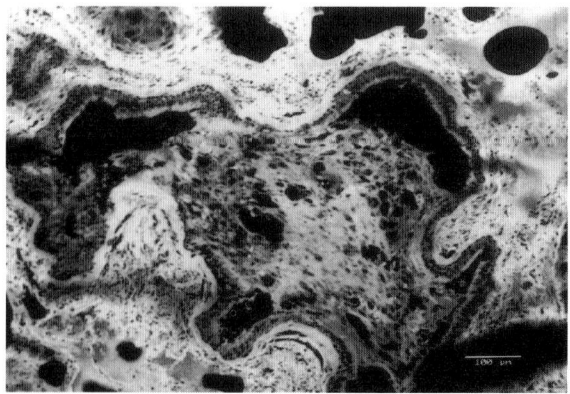

Figure 7.9 *Section from the lungs of an asthmatic patient showing a dilated airway filled with mucus and a few inflammatory cells. There are increased numbers of goblet cells in the lining epithelium (scale bar is 100 μm)*

given during an attack in an attempt to try to relieve the symptoms. Most drugs of this sort are antihistamines that counteract the effects of histamine which is the compound that causes the bronchospasm and hence the obstruction of the airways.

Death from asthma is seen rarely with adequate treatment, but it may occur during a prolonged severe attack (a status asthmaticus) or may be caused by massive pulmonary collapse due to bronchial obstruction by mucus. The pulmonary lesions predispose to infection, and this, together with the bronchiectasis and emphysema, may lead to a reduction in the life span of the sufferers.

Infections and Inflammations

Non-specific Laryngitis

Infection of the larynx is relatively uncommon and more often there is secondary infection and inflammation at this site as a result of spread of infection from the upper respiratory tract. The condition commonly follows the common cold, rhinitis, mouth and throat infections. The laryngeal mucosa shows typical acute inflammatory changes with redness, swelling and often this causes laryngeal stridor which may progress to obstruction. Typically the condition resolves spontaneously.

Acute Tracheobronchitis

This is a typical acute inflammatory response of the airways, common in occurrence and due to a variety of aetiologies. Infective agents may cause it and such organisms as *Streptococcus* spp., *Haemophilus influenzae* and *Bordetella pertussis* have been commonly isolated. Viruses, especially the influenza, parainfluenza and measles viruses, have also been implicated. Non-infective agents may also precipitate the disorder and the most important of these are mechanical, chemical (e.g. dust, pollution, cigarette smoking) and allergic causes (e.g. pollen, or pulmonary manifestations of a systemic allergy). In the non-infective inflammations there is a tendency for secondary infection to occur.

Macroscopically the mucous membranes of the airways show the typical appearance of acute inflammation: a swollen, red surface with production of much mucus or pus. Sometimes fibrinous or membranous tracheobronchitis occurs, but also in some cases haemorrhage may be a feature. Under the microscope a typical acute inflammatory response is seen with vasodilatation and congestion, oedema, infiltration by neutrophils and also ulceration of the respiratory epithelium and suppuration or haemorrhage.

The disease may regress with prompt, appropriate antibiotic treatment and also patient co-operation in limiting exposure to irritants and allergens. The mucosa may recover and resolution is usually seen; however, in some cases, although the epithelium is restored the cilia on the regenerated cells are lacking, therefore predisposing to recurrences of the infection. If the condition is left untreated it very often progresses to **chronic bronchitis** or, with spread of the infection to deeper tissues, **bronchopneumonia** may result.

Chronic Bronchitis

Strictly speaking, chronic bronchitis is a term that should be reserved for a prolonged inflammation of the bronchial tree, but the term is frequently used to include all disorders where the clinical presentation is one of a long-standing cough, resulting from a chronic irritation of the bronchial epithelium. Cigarette smoke, heavy atmospheric pollution and certain occupational factors are common irritants whose effects on the airways are aggravated by dampness and fog.

Chronic bronchitis is a very common disorder in temperate and cool climates and is seen especially frequently in heavy smokers and in industrialized areas. Males are rather more prone to develop the condition, which begins in early adulthood. The disease is slowly progressive with exacerbations in the winter months. Each of the attacks in successive years becomes more severe.

The disorder has a complex aetiology and several factors are thought to be important in its development. Repeated attacks of acute bronchitis produce damage to the protective mechanisms of the lungs and make them more prone to infection. Infection may remain at a low level over a long period of time and may lead eventually to bronchiectasis and failure of normal mucus expulsion. To these factors are added the irritating effects of inhaled particulate matter and chemicals, cigarette smoking and a cold damp climate. Due to the inefficiency of respiratory function and the failure of the 'mucociliary escalator' the airways become infected. The infection is most commonly caused by *Haemophilus influenzae* and *Streptococcus pneumoniae* both being bacteria that tend to produce chronic, low-grade infections in this situation. These bacterial infections often extend deep into the respiratory bronchioles and alveolar sacs, which are clogged by mucus. This leads to acute exacerbations of the disease.

The bronchi are dilated and the mucous membrane is roughened, thickened, red and granular, being bathed by copious mucous secretions. The trachea and bronchioles show a similar appearance. In advanced cases emphysema and bronchiectasis are almost always present. Microscopically the major change discernible is an increase in the mucous glands of the submucosa with a variable chronic inflammatory cell infiltrate. Some fibrosis is also a feature of the disorder. The epithelium lining the airways shows loss of cilia and thickening and a squamous metaplasia may have occurred. Frequently, especially during exacerbations, there will be seen foci of acute inflammation and suppuration.

Unless the multiple aetiological factors are controlled, the disease progresses over many years with episodes of bronchopneumonia, development of emphysema and bronchiectasis all due to bronchial obstruction. As a result, there may be a strain placed on the right ventricle with development of cor pulmonale and heart failure. Air flow in the lungs is impaired as is normal ventilation and all of these factors combined lead to a shortened life span and considerable distress to the sufferers from this condition.

Pneumonia

The term 'pneumonia' implies an acute inflammatory disorder of the lung, characterized by **consolidation** due to the presence of acute inflammatory exudate and infiltrate within the alveolar spaces. A large number of infective agents may cause pneumonia and these include protozoa, fungi, bacteria, mycoplasmata and viruses. Pneumonia may also be caused by aspiration of material into the lungs, for example food or drink. The bacterial pneumonias are the most characteristic and common of these lesions and they have been divided into lobar pneumonia and bronchopneumonia, depending on their distribution in the affected lungs. Viral pneumonia is also commonly seen especially in the elderly and debilitated, and increasing in incidence nowadays are the protozoal pneumonias in association with AIDS. Therefore, pneumonia is not a single entity but takes many forms, the appearance of the inflamed lung tissue and the clinical symptomatology depending on the infecting organism. There are many different types of pneumonia; for example:

- Lobar pneumonia — most often caused by *Streptococcus pneumoniae*.
- Bronchopneumonia — caused by a large variety of micro-organisms.
- Atypical pneumonia — caused by such organism as *Mycoplasma pneumoniae*.
- Viral pneumonia — caused by many viruses, for example, influenza virus.
- Tuberculous bronchopneumonia — caused by *Mycobacterium tuberculosis*.
- *Pneumocystis carinii* pneumonia — seen in AIDS patients.

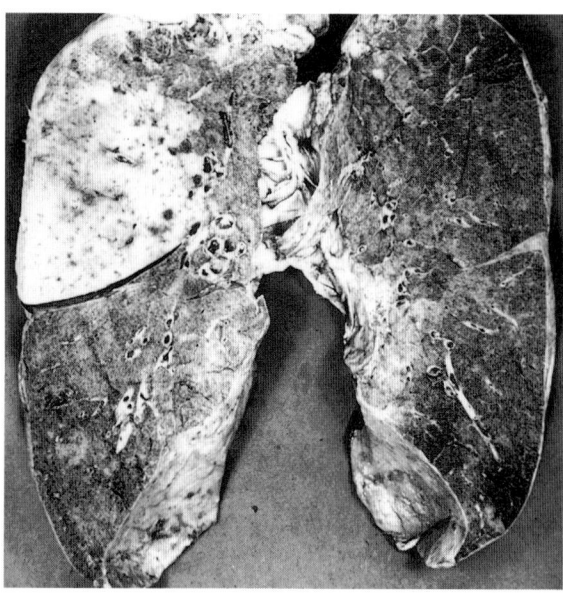

Figure 7.10 *Lobar pneumonia showing the grey hepatization stage involving almost all of the upper lobe.*

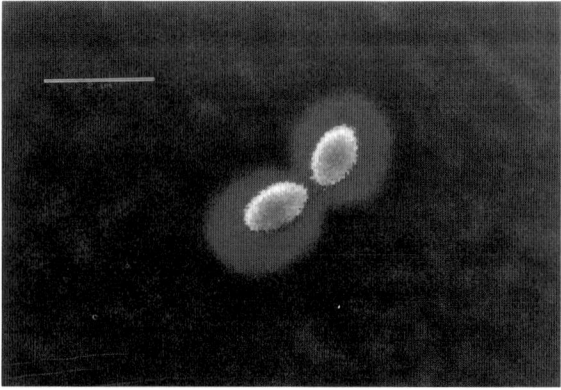

Figure 7.11 Streptococcus pneumoniae, *the causative agent of lobar pneumonia, showing the capsule surrounding the organisms (scale bar is 2 μm)*

Lobar Pneumonia

In lobar pneumonia the inflammation is sharply confined to one or two lobes, which are diffusely affected (Figure 7.10). Rarely, larger areas of the lungs may be involved. More than 90% of cases of lobar pneumonia are caused by *Streptococcus pneumoniae* ('pneumococci') with different specific antigenic types affecting different age groups (Figure 7.11). However, the disease is primarily one of previously healthy young adults.

The infection is acquired by inhalation of the bacteria into the lung via the bronchial tree. If the dose of pneumococci inhaled is the infectious dose or over, if the pneumococci are virulent and if the patient is susceptible, the disease process commences and runs a very well defined course. It has been suggested that a local hypersensitivity reaction to the organism in the lung as well as a quick spread of the bacteria into the alveoli via the pores of Kohn are important factors in the rapid consolidation of the whole lobe (illustrated in Figure 7.12). The stages of the disease in an untreated case are very well characterized and a classical pneumococcal pneumonia progresses as follows.

Days 1–2, acute congestion. This is the first stage of the disease commencing as soon as the organisms have lodged in the lungs and lasts for approximately 1–2 days. It is characterized by vasodilatation, hyperaemia and congestion of the vessels at the site. Oedema fluid is formed in great volumes. The affected lobe is red in colour, firm and heavy (see Figure 7.13). The alveolar capillaries are engorged with blood and although many alveoli contain fluid which can be squeezed out of the lung at autopsy, the majority of alveolar spaces are still air containing. Erythrocytes will be found in the alveolar spaces at this stage, having been passively squeezed out of the alveolar capillaries, through the interendothelial gaps, by the high blood pressure in the congested, hyperaemic vessels.

Days 2–4, red hepatization. This is the stage beginning at about the second day and lasting two days. The vessels are still congested at this stage and exudate is still forming. The pleural surface of the affected lobe shows signs of pleurisy (inflammation of the pleura), and is covered by exudate and greyish white networks of fibrin which cause the visceral and parietal layers of the pleura to adhere to one another. The cut surface of the lobe now looks deep red, dry, firm and consolidated (airless). It is heavy and if placed in water it will sink, unlike normal lung which will float. This appearance justifies the term 'hepatization', which means 'looking solid like liver' (refer to Figure 7.14).

Microscopically, the alveolar congestion persists but the alveolar spaces are now all filled with inflammatory exudate, containing much fibrin, visible as thin branching networks. Many extravasated erythrocytes are still present in the alveoli and are being phagocytosed by alveolar macrophages. As the disease progresses there are increasing numbers of neutrophils migrating from the vessels into the alveolar spaces.

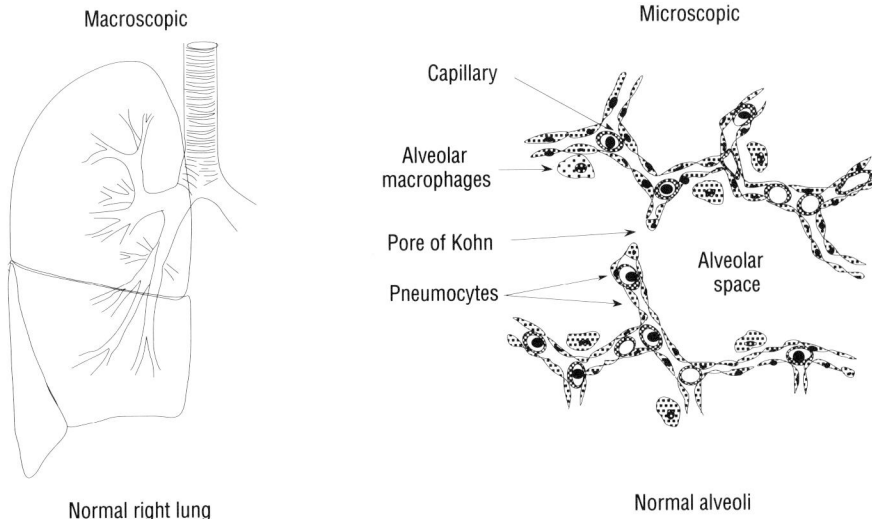

Figure 7.12 *Normal lung morphology*

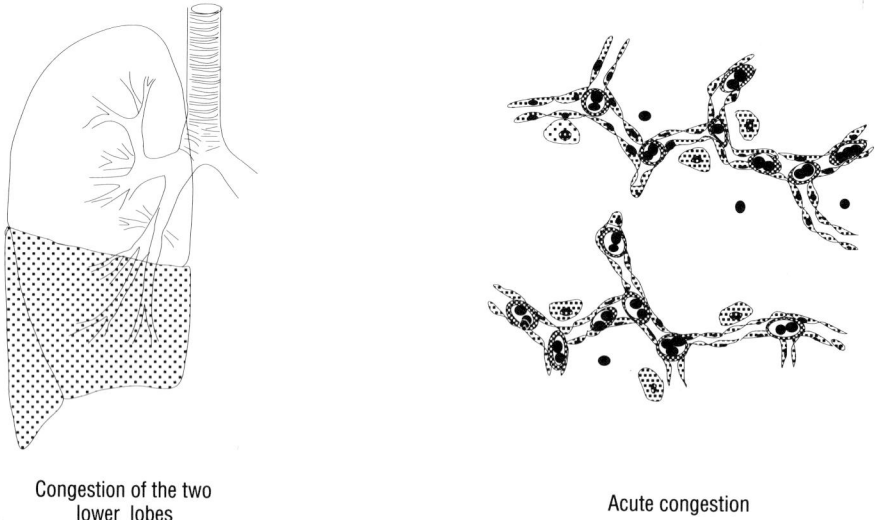

Congestion of the two
lower lobes

Acute congestion

Figure 7.13   *Acute congestion stage of lobar pneumonia*

Days 4–8, grey hepatization. This stage lasts from the fourth day to the eighth day and is the stage of late consolidation, the lung having increased in weight considerably. Fibrinous pleurisy is now marked over the inflamed lobe. The cut surface of the lung is firm, grey, dry, granular and consolidated. The alveoli are distended and full of large numbers of neutrophils amidst dense networks of fibrin. Many of the inflammatory cells are dead and disintegrating, yet no pus forms as the alveolar walls remain intact, the neutrophil enzymes not destroying the walls. The erythrocytes in the alveoli have all been lysed and the alveolar macrophages are already ingesting the dead red blood cells. It is at this stage that antibodies to the pneumococci start to appear in the plasma and the infection begins to subside. Few streptococci will now be found in the alveolar spaces, the majority of bacteria having been ingested and destroyed by the neutrophils. Increasing numbers of monocytes begin to migrate into the alveoli as fewer neutrophils are needed (see Figure 7.15).

Day 8, resolution. This is the usual outcome of lobar pneumonia and commences on the eighth day, lasting approximately one to three weeks. It is characterized by the influx of macrophages into the alveoli from the alveolar septa. They begin to disrupt the fibrin network and remove the exudate and debris. Fibrinolytic enzymes and macrophage phagocytosis have an important role in clearing the alveolar spaces rapidly.

The debris is removed, the fluid is returned to the circulation and sputum is coughed up. At first, the cut surface of the affected lobe looks mottled red and grey and is friable. The lung then progressively becomes air containing and returns to normal. The alveolar walls are not involved in the inflammation, and not damaged in any way, therefore the inflammation resolves without fibrosis or scarring. In approximately 3% of cases, the exudate of lobar pneumonia is organized within the affected lobe and is converted into scar tissue. The lobe becomes fibrous, tough, grey, airless and contracted. The exudate covering the pleura over the affected lobe in lobar pneumonia will also frequently undergo organization and as collagen is laid down **fibrous pleural adhesions** will form, causing the two layers of the pleura to adhere permanently to one another.

Clinically, lobar pneumonia presents with chills, a high fever, headache, cough and chest pain. As the disease progresses, breathing becomes more difficult, painful, shallow and rapid. Sputum is coughed up, becoming thick and purulent as the disease progresses. Other signs and symptoms may be profuse sweating, cyanosis and gastrointestinal disorders. On the eighth day, by the end of the stage of grey hepatization, the affected regions of lung are non-functional and the patients have considerable trouble breathing if much tissue is involved. They reach a point called a **crisis**. In the past, this was the crucial stage where patients either

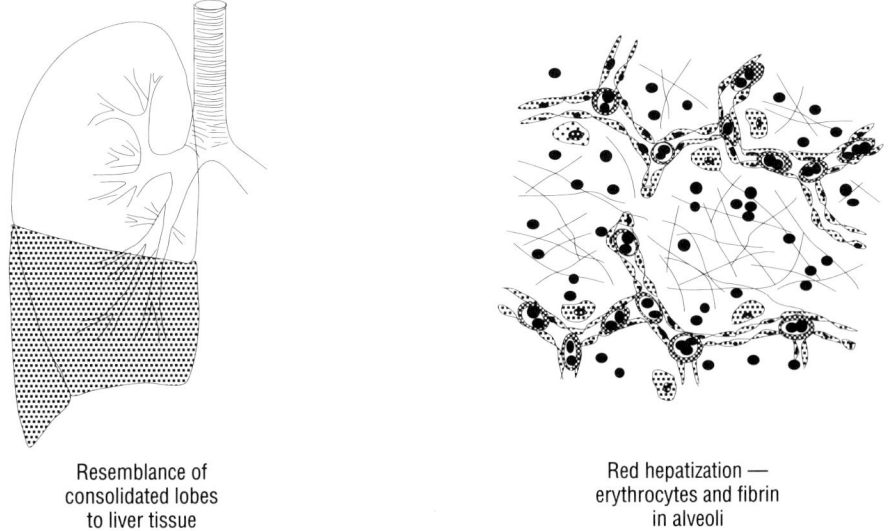

Resemblance of
consolidated lobes
to liver tissue

Red hepatization —
erythrocytes and fibrin
in alveoli

Figure 7.14 *Red hepatization stage of lobar pneumonia*

survived and progressed to resolution or died of respiratory failure. At this stage, if the patient survives, there is a rapid improvement in his or her condition, with alleviation of the discomfort and fever, the patient feeling much better within a few hours.

The above account refers to an untreated case. Before the advent of antimicrobial drugs the disease often had fatal results. Today with prompt treatment the disease hardly shows the same course as that described above and is limited to its first stages, resolution occurring rapidly after antibiotic therapy. Penicillin is the drug of choice as pneumococci are still very susceptible to it. Other antibiotics may be prescribed to individuals hypersensitive to penicillin.

Occasionally, there may be various complications in the case of lobar pneumonia. Cardiac complications of a mechanical nature may occur because of the strain placed on the heart, or pericarditis may develop by direct extension of the infection into the pericardium. Septicaemia may occur with complications such as meningitis, multiple pyaemic abscesses or a suppurative arthritis. Empyema of the pleura or lung abscess with suppuration occur in less than 1% of untreated cases.

Bronchopneumonia (Lobular Pneumonia)
Bronchopneumonia is an acute inflammatory condition of the lungs occurring when organisms primarily colonize the airways, gradually extending into the adjacent alveolar sacs, resulting in numerous discrete foci of consolidation occurring throughout the lungs

(Figure 7.16). It is a patchy lesion, which is multifocal and frequently bilateral. Bronchopneumonia is caused by a large variety of bacteria, for example *Streptococcus pneumoniae, Staphylococcus aureus, Haemophilus influenzae, Klebsiella pneumoniae*. Viruses and organisms of low pathogenicity may also cause chronic bronchopneumonia and *Mycobacterium tuberculosis* causes the so-called 'tuberculous bronchopneumonia'.

The disease is characteristically one which affects age extremes: the very young or the very old and debilitated. The general resistance of the host in these groups is very low and therefore the individuals are more susceptible to the organisms of generally low virulence that cause bronchopneumonia. Other states which lower the general or local resistance of the host to infection will predispose to bronchopneumonia, hence it is often seen in patients suffering from diabetes mellitus, malignant disease, anaesthesia, malnutrition and exposure and also in alcoholics and drug addicts.

The lobular consolidation in the lungs may be patchily distributed in one lobe, but is most often multilobar and frequently bilateral and basal because of the tendency of secretions to gravitate to the lower lobes. Confluence of the individual lesions in the later stages of the disease may give rise to an appearance resembling lobar pneumonia. The infection is a pyogenic one and the exudate consisting of plasma and fibrin fills the affected alveoli around the airways. There is infiltration by large numbers of neutrophils and there

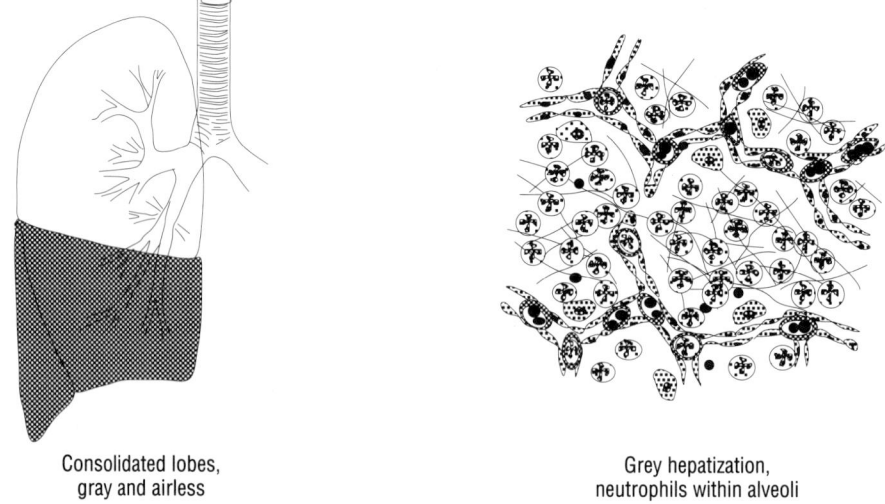

Consolidated lobes,
gray and airless

Grey hepatization,
neutrophils within alveoli

Figure 7.15 *Grey hepatization stage of lobar pneumonia*

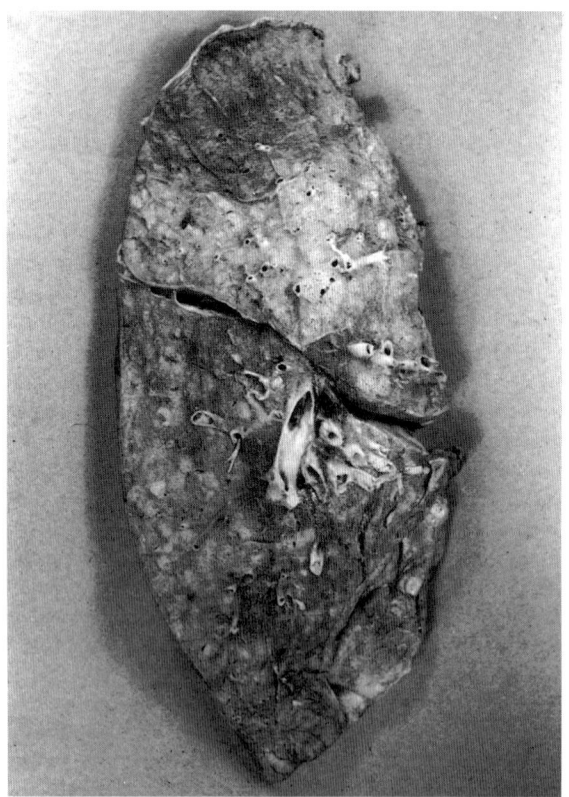

Figure 7.16 *Bronchopneumonia in a female of 76 years who had suffered from rheumatoid arthritis for many years. Many islands of consolidation are found scattered throughout the lungs with a region of confluent lesions in the left upper lobe*

is destruction of the alveolar walls in the inflamed areas, with frank suppuration. This last feature differentiates this type of pneumonia from lobar pneumonia where the alveoli remain intact and there is no suppuration. The pleura may show a fibrinous pleurisy or areas of suppuration which may progress to empyema of the pleural cavity.

Multiple areas of consolidation are seen around the bronchi, which are inflamed and filled with mucopurulent exudate. Pus may exude from the cut surface of the lung on pressure. The lung tissue between the lesions may appear normal but as the disease advances these areas may be involved in the infection also, with coalescence of the lesions. Microscopically the disease resembles lobar pneumonia in that there is fibrin, exudate and acute inflammatory infiltrate in the alveoli. However, in bronchopneumonia there is destruction of alveolar walls, suppuration and a suppurative bronchitis and bronchiolitis.

Complete resolution is very rare in bronchopneumonia and is almost always seen when there has been prompt treatment of the disease with the appropriate antibiotics, early in the infection before any structural damage to the lungs has been done. In most cases of the disease there is a variable amount of damage to alveolar walls and airways and this together with the organization of the exudate lead to considerable fibrosis, with scarring being the commonest sequela to bronchopneumonia (Table 7.1 outlines the major differences between lobar and bronchopneumonia). In children especially, scarring of the bronchi and imperfect mucosal regeneration predispose to further infection and bronchiectasis. Other

Table 7.1 *Comparison of lobar pneumonia and bronchopneumonia*

Lobar pneumonia	Bronchopneumonia

Caused by:
  Streptococcus pneumoniae
	Caused by:
	  S. pneumoniae, Haemophilus influenzae,
	  S. aureus, etc.

Distribution:
  Whole lobe(s) affected usually more in lower lobes
	Distribution:
	  Patchy lesion, near airways

Ages affected predominantly:
  Previously healthy young adults,
  the immunosuppressed or debilitated
	Ages affected predominantly:
	  Infants, the elderly, the debilitated

Course:
  Clear-cut course.
  Acute congestion (1–2 days)
  Red hepatization (2–4 days)
  Grey hepatization (4–8 days)
  Resolution (8–16 days)
	Course:
	  Course not as clear cut.
	  Microscopical changes are at different
	  stages in various parts of the lungs at
	  the same time

Characteristics:
  Alveolar walls remain intact, no pus is formed,
  resolution is the rule
	Characteristics:
	  Alveolar wall destruction, pus is formed,
	  foci of fibrosis is the rule

Results, sequelae, complications:
  Right heart strain, pericarditis, suppuration,
  empyema, septicaemia, rarely fibrosis,
  rarely death
	Results, sequelae, complications:
	  Pericarditis, suppuration, abscess formation,
	  empyema, lung fibrosis, bronchial damage,
	  bronchiectasis, commonly death

complications of the disease are the formation of multiple pulmonary abscesses, involvement of the pleura and empyema of the pleural cavity. Rarely, direct extension of the infection may produce a suppurative pericarditis.

Bronchopneumonia is a very common cause of death, especially in the elderly and also in patients suffering from chronic, debilitating diseases. It is also quite common to see death resulting even in the absence of other disease if the bronchopneumonia is quite extensive and is caused by an organism which is virulent or to which the host is highly susceptible.

Tuberculosis

Tuberculosis is an infection caused by *Mycobacterium tuberculosis*, which is a typical chronic granulomatous inflammation *ab initio* (Figure 7.17). The granuloma is called a tubercle. Although any site of the body may be affected pulmonary tuberculosis is by far the commonest encountered. The disease is still seen in con-

siderable numbers (six new cases per 100 000 population per year in Australia), so the idea that it is a 'disease of the past' is not justified. Aggressive treatment of tuberculosis with chemotherapeutic agents at an early stage has minimized the number of deaths due to the disease and immunization with the BCG vaccine in endemic areas has decreased the incidence of the disorder. This infection has been described in detail earlier (see under 'Chronic Inflammation' in Chapter 3).

Sarcoidosis (= Boeck's Sarcoid)

This is an idiopathic granulomatous inflammation which, although systemic, most commonly affects the lungs. Other sites in the body very frequently affected include lymph nodes, skin, eyes, salivary glands, spleen, liver and the bones. Microscopically, the lesions are typical granulomata, each one appearing almost identical to the tubercle of tuberculosis. However, in sarcoid granulomata there is no caseation as seen with tuberculosis (Figure 7.18).

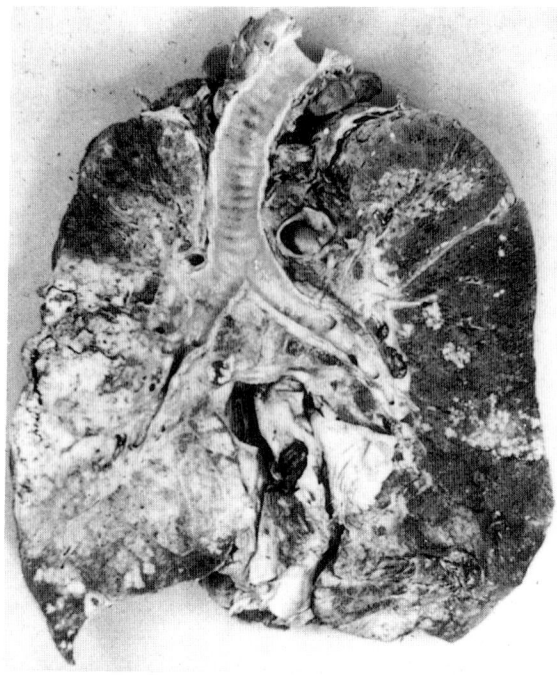

Figure 7.17   *Tuberculosis in the lungs of a 54-year-old man with extensive regions of caseation (pale areas)*

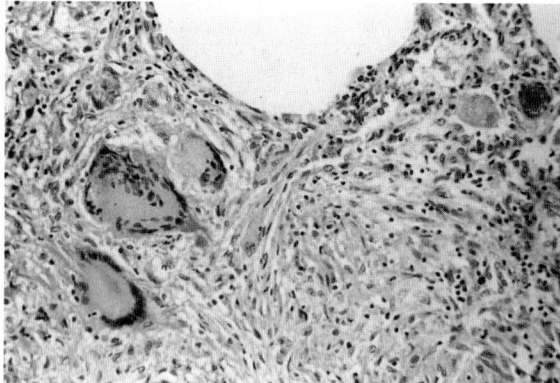

Figure 7.18   *Pulmonary sarcoidosis showing the typical granuloma and giant cells (×180)*

There is some evidence for genetic and racial factors being important in the development of sarcoidosis but there is still no clear-cut proof. The disease is more frequent in Caucasians than Asians, common in the Scandinavian countries, Caribbean and USA, in the last two locations black people being more commonly affected than white people.

As granulomata form systemically in sarcoidosis it is suspected that the disease is due to an immune system abnormality. This is supported by the numerous abnormal immunological findings that characterize the disease. The patients with active sarcoidosis have depressed cell mediated immunity, a finding which can be demonstrated by the **anergy** (lack of reaction) to common challenge allergens in cutaneous tests. The number of helper T4 cells is decreased in the circulation when compared with suppressor T8 cells, but the opposite is true in sites of active disease (in the granulomata, for example), where the helper T4 cells are greatly in excess. There are increased numbers and increased activity of B cells and plasma cells, which give rise to hypergammaglobulinaemia and also to circulating immune complexes. These effects are thought to be mediated by some stimulus, possibly an antigen, as yet unidentified. Various workers have sug-

gested a virus but there is no evidence of an infectious agent causing sarcoidosis; others have suggested an allergen with possibilities being clay dust, pine pollen, resin or metal dusts. However, no such antigenic stimulus has been demonstrated without doubt to be associated with the disorder. Once the immune system is stimulated there is macrophage activation with production of interleukin 1. This causes activation of T cells with production of interleukin 2, further enhancing the proliferation of helper T4 cells. There is production of lymphokines which stimulate the immune response with formation of granulomata, stimulation of B cells polyclonally with elaboration of antibodies of different specificities causing the hypergammaglobulinaemia and formation of immune complexes (Figure 7.19 outlines the pathogenesis of the disease).

During the active phase of the disease there is frequently **hypercalciuria** and **hypercalcaemia, elevated immunoglobulin levels** and **raised serum levels of angiotensin converting enzyme**. A skin test, the **Kveim-Siltzback test**, is positive in about 80% of patients with sarcoidosis. In this test, a suspension of human sarcoid tissue (from a positive case of the disease), is prepared in saline and injected subcutaneously. A positive test is seen to occur within two days and is characterized by reddening, inflammation and induration. It should be noted that false positives may be seen in this test with some other autoimmune diseases such as Crohn's disease.

The non-specific granuloma of sarcoidosis may be confused with that of tuberculosis as the two lesions are very similar. In tuberculosis there is caseous necrosis in the central region whereas in sarcoidosis there may

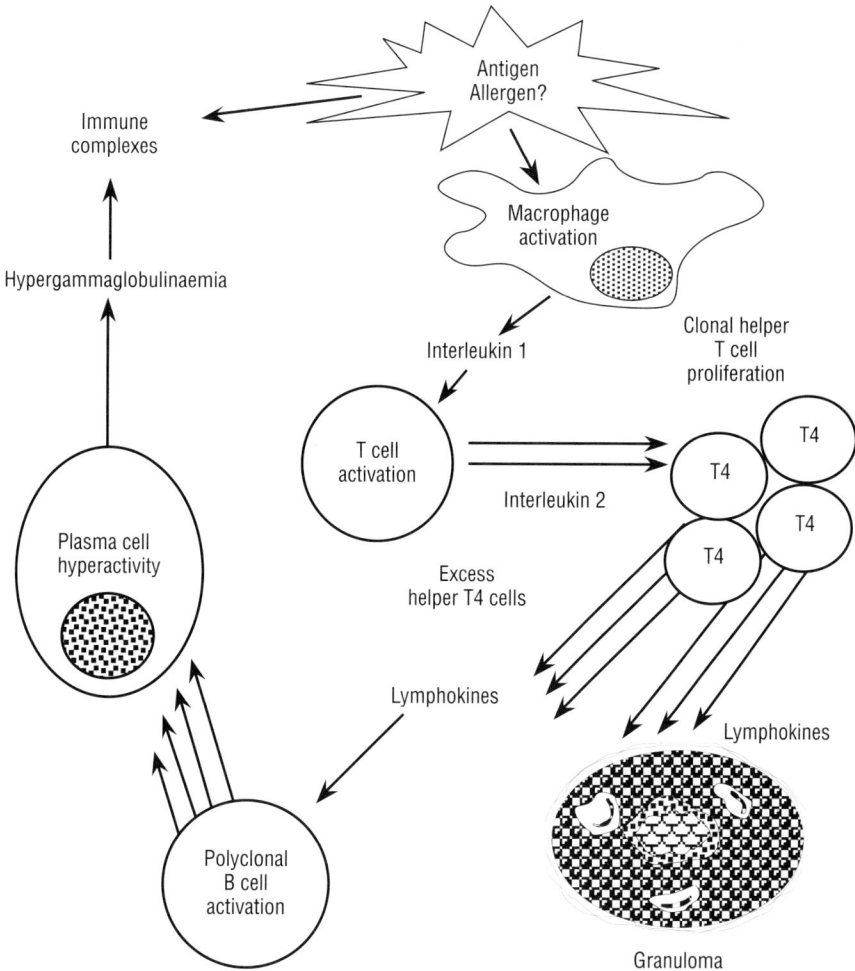

Figure 7.19 *The pathogenesis of sarcoidosis*

be coagulative necrosis in the larger granulomata. In both lesions there are macrophages, epithelioid cells, giant cells and lymphocytes. The giant cells of sarcoidosis may contain inclusions which are termed **Schaumann bodies** (≤ 10 μm in diameter, basophilic laminated bodies consisting of iron and calcium deposits) and **asteroid bodies** (which are star-shaped eosinophilic structures composed of lipoproteins). Fibrosis becomes marked around the granulomata as the disease progresses and in the lungs it may be very severe. The lungs may become diffusely involved with quite severe compromise of respiratory function. Approximately 25% of all patients with sarcoidosis show marked, permanent respiratory dysfunction that may contribute to their death (Table 7.2 compares TB to sarcoidosis).

In the skin, sarcoidosis gives rise to subcutaneous nodules, slightly elevated reddened plaques and scaling lesions. There may be similar lesions in the mucous membranes. Eye involvement occurs in many cases with **iritis** and **iridocyclitis, choroiditis** and **retinitis**. These inflammatory changes are associated with granuloma formation and, later in the disease, scarring. There may be loss of vision or blindness if the changes are widespread. If the eye disease (particularly uveitis) is associated with inflammation of the salivary glands the disorder is called **Mikulicz's syndrome**.

Approximately 5–10% of patients will show bone involvement, especially in the short bones of the hands and feet. The granulomata that form in the bone marrow create regions of bone resorption with reactive

Table 7.2   *Comparison of tuberculosis and sarcoidosis*

Tuberculosis	Sarcoidosis
Caused by: *Mycobacterium tuberculosis*	Caused by: Cause unknown, idiopathic disease
Nature: Chronic granulomatous infection, specific granulomata, tubercles form	Nature: Chronic granulomatous disease, non-specific granulomata form
Ages affected predominantly: Young adults, children more susceptible	Ages affected predominantly: Adults under 40 years, females in their reproductive years mostly affected
Predisposing factors: The pneumoconioses, especially silicosis; hypersensitivity	Predisposing factors: Genetic factors relating to race and geography, immune factors
Course: Primary pulmonary infection developing in the upper lobes = Ghon focus, usually heals, may be reactivated at a later stage. Hypersensitivity induces great damage and caseation. Miliary TB and tuberculous bronchopneumonia may develop. Almost any other organ of the body may be affected.	Course: 90% of cases involve lungs. Non-specific granulomata form, 25% of cases show respiratory dysfunction. Skin lesions. Eye involvement. Spleen, kidney, bone, liver, heart, CNS and endocrine glands may show disease. Many cases respond well to corticosteroid therapy
Characteristics: Development of caseous necrosis in lesions older than 12 days. Ziehl-Neelsen stain positive, growth of bacterium in culture	Characteristics: Hypergammaglobulinaemia, hypercalcaemia, hypercalciuria, non-caseating granulomata, positive Kveim-Siltzback skin test
Results, sequelae, complications: Lung fibrosis, spread to involve other body sites, cavitating lesions. Pott's disease of spine. Congenital infections. Renal TB	Results, sequelae, complications: 'Honeycomb lung', fibrosis, Mikulicz's syndrome, cor pulmonale, cardiac failure, renal calculi, visual problems

new bone formation on the outer regions of the bone shafts with widening of the cortical bone. Granulomata may also form in the liver, spleen, kidneys, heart, CNS and pituitary.

The results of the disease are extremely variable and it should be noted that in about 75% of cases sarcoidosis may exist in the patient without any major symptoms and signs associated with it, only being discovered as an incidental finding. Because of the significant involvement of the lungs in other patients, however, the disease may manifest itself as a severe pulmonary dysfunction and overall about 10% of patients will die of respiratory system disease, pulmonary fibrosis and severe COAD ('honeycomb lung') or cardiac problems such as cor pulmonale and cardiac failure.

Treatment and prognosis of the disease depends on the degree of involvement and sites affected in the body. Generally in patients under 30 years where the onset is acute with fever, malaise, lymphadenopathy and little lung involvement, response to corticosteroid therapy is good and the disease may often go into permanent remission. In patients over 40 years where the disease has an insidious onset, with significant lung involvement and with also other tissues showing signs of the disease, corticosteroids are less effective and the disease usually relapses and progresses slowly with more and more damage occurring in all affected parts of the body. Overall, about 5% of patients die as a direct result of their sarcoidosis.

Pulmonary Abscess

Pulmonary abscesses caused by pyogenic bacteria may occur as a complication of pneumonia (especially bronchopneumonia), in bronchiectasis, as a result of septic emboli, pyaemia, etc. Pulmonary abscesses are typical acute abscesses which may persist causing chronic suppurative inflammation. This results in loss of lung tissue and as healing occurs large scars will form which interfere with normal lung function. In addition, bacteria may spread from the lung abscesses to other body sites such as the brain, causing the development of metastatic abscesses in these locations. Aggressive treatment with the appropriate antibiotics at an early stage is required for lung abscess, but in certain cases this treatment may need to be combined with surgical drainage of the pus.

Clinically, patients with lung abscess present with fever, malaise and loss of weight. As the lesion enlarges, it may rupture into an airway, in which case the patient will develop a cough and this may produce copious, purulent, foul-smelling sputum. There may also be haemoptysis if there is erosion of small blood vessels, something that is seen in about half of the cases. Pleurisy with pain will also be seen in a considerable number of patients. In some patients, chronic lung abscess will produce clubbing of the fingers.

Other Infections

Mycoplasma pneumoniae causes primary atypical pneumonia or **pneumonitis**, which is an inflammation of the alveolar walls. The alveolar spaces show little exudate or infiltrate while the alveolar walls are grossly thickened and infiltrated by large numbers of inflammatory cells. This condition presents as an insidious disease with fever, malaise, cough, headache, fatigue and respiratory distress. Radiographic examination of the lungs usually shows evidence of pneumonia well before clinical symptoms and signs suggest it. Involvement is mostly confined to one of the lower lobes and occasionally the pneumonia may show involvement of alveolar spaces, giving a picture similar to a bronchopneumonia.

Treatment of this infection is with broad-spectrum antibiotics. A treatment of patients with tetracycline combined with erythromycin has been shown to be very effective in limiting the course of the disease. Patients, however, consistently show a long convalescence, often extending to 6 weeks after the infection. In a small number of cases there may be complications such as central nervous system disease (the Guillain-Barré syndrome, encephalitis and aseptic meningitis), pericarditis, pancreatitis and anaemia.

Legionella pneumophila causes 'Legionnaire's disease', which is an alveolar pneumonia with predominance of macrophages and fewer neutrophils in the affected region of the lung. It is a bronchopneumonia which often becomes confluent, resembling a lobar pneumonia. It is more common in middle-aged or elderly men with a history of cigarette smoking and moderate to excessive alcohol consumption. The early symptoms and signs of the disease are headache, malaise, myalgia, cough which may be non-productive, or, uncommonly, a frankly purulent or mucopurulent sputum may be produced. Within 24 hours of infection there is dramatic fever followed by chills or rigor. Diarrhoea or abdominal pains may also be present. On X-ray the lungs show patchy consolidation which may involve both lungs as the disease progresses. Approximately 25% of patients may show neurological symptoms and signs such as confusion and delirium or ataxia.

After serological diagnosis of the infection, it is treated with antibiotics, the most effective being erythromycin, either alone or in combination with a variety of others. Occasionally rifampin is used in cases where erythromycin is not effective.

Pneumocystis carinii is a parasite which causes an interstitial pneumonia with a foamy exudate. This is an infection seen in infants, very debilitated patients and immunodeficient patients, being the commonest cause of death in AIDS patients. In many cases of the disease, associated viral and bacterial infections are also present. The patient presents with a rapidly worsening illness over a period of days to weeks, although in the AIDS patient the disease may be more lingering, developing over weeks to months. There is dyspnoea, cyanosis, fever and on X-ray examination there is considerable opacity of both lung fields. Histologically, the alveoli are full of a foamy exudate that on silver staining is seen to be teeming with cysts of the organism (Figure 7.20).

Diagnosis may rarely be made on sputum examination, but rather depends on alveolar lavage or on open lung biopsy. The infection is treated with pentamidine or trimethoprim-sulfamethoxazole, however, it is still a disease carrying a high mortality as the immune deficiency in the host allows very rapid proliferation of the organism and its rapid dissemination in the tissue.

Klebsiella pneumoniae causes a slowly progressive lobar pneumonia which accounts for about 3% of pneumonia cases. The organism causes extensive damage in the lungs and over 90% of untreated cases are fatal. Lungs infected with *Klebsiella pneumoniae* may show

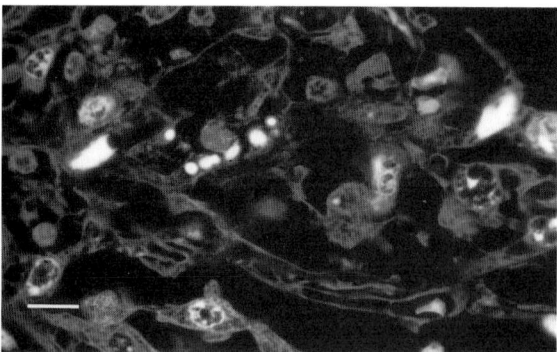

Figure 7.20   *Section from the lungs of a patient with AIDS and pneumocystosis. The* Pneumocystis carinii *organisms are the bright spots in the centre of the micrograph (scale bar is 10 μm)*

extensive involvement with abscess formation and large amounts of frankly purulent secretions in the airways. The disease is more common in alcoholics and the elderly and debilitated, sometimes being acquired as a nosocomial infection. The infection is treated aggressively with antibiotics, combined treatments usually given, for example clavulanic acid and amoxycillin.

Viral pneumonias are a rather uncommon manifestation of the most common of respiratory infections, the upper respiratory viral infection group. If viruses involve the lower respiratory tract they cause a pneumonitis, which most often is transient and not associated with much disease or complications, but on occasion it may be a very severe or fatal disease. The latter is especially true with infants, the elderly and the debilitated. Typical viruses involved are: influenza viruses, Coxsackieviruses, adenoviruses, echoviruses cytomegaloviruses, respiratory syncytial viruses.

In severely affected lungs there is much inflammation and oedema of the alveolar walls and there may be evidence of haemorrhage and regions of lung collapse. An infiltrate of lymphocytes and macrophages is present, and the number of cells present may range from very few to many. Viral inclusions and cytopathic effects on lung cells may be seen with cytomegalovirus, herpes virus and adenovirus pneumonias, but usually they are not prominent features in the affected tissue. Necrosis of infected cells will usually occur and the most important complication is secondary bacterial infection. Superinfection with *Haemophilus influenzae, Streptococcus pneumoniae* or *Staphylococcus aureus* is very common with influenzal pneumonia.

The patient with viral pneumonia presents with fever, muscular aches and pains and headache caused by the viraemia. There is also a sore throat, rhinitis and upper respiratory tract involvement. A dry, unproductive cough with a burning discomfort in the region of the sternum is associated with the tracheitis. There is usually no cyanosis or severe dyspnoea as the pneumonia is patchy and allows sufficient aeration of the lungs. Usually, the disease is self-limited and most patients recover spontaneously within two weeks. Antibiotic therapy is usually administered prophylactically to prevent bacterial superinfection. The prognosis for viral pneumonia is good, unless the patient is at the extremes of age, debilitated or immunosuppressed. The immunization of the elderly in the face of influenzal epidemics has saved the life of many millions worldwide in the last few decades.

Pneumoconioses

The pneumoconioses are a group of disorders caused by inhalation of organic or inorganic finely divided dusts. They are usually diseases of occupational or industrial association. The dust particles inhaled must be less than 5 μm in diameter to reach the alveolar level. The pneumoconioses often appear as granulomatous lesions within the lung, forming hard, rounded fibrotic nodules and replacing normal lung tissue. They are associated with emphysema, COAD, cor pulmonale and heart failure. Certain pneumoconioses, such as asbestosis, are associated with a much higher incidence of lung malignancies.

Anthracosis

This is a pneumoconiosis caused by the inhalation of carbon particles (cigarette smoke, polluted air, smog, industrial fumes). It is a fairly harmless disease and is seen in almost every city dweller, but is especially severe in smokers. The carbon particles at alveolar level are phagocytosed by alveolar macrophages, which subsequently migrate to the local lymph nodes. There is blackening of the lungs due to carbon contained in macrophages, in the subpleural lymphatics and hilar lymph nodes.

There is no significant fibrosis associated with this type of carbon deposition and the pathological effects are minimal. In heavy smokers, anthracosis coupled with the continual irritant effect of having particulate matter in the bronchial tree predisposes greatly to the development of chronic bronchitis and emphysema.

Silicosis

Silicosis is a pneumoconiosis due to the inhalation of silica (SiO_2) or silicate (SiO_3^{2-}) particles. In the past it used to be known as 'knife-grinders' disease' as these individuals used to breathe in the silica dust as they ground the blades on the whet stone. Nowadays, this pneumoconiosis may be seen in sand blasters, quarry workers, stone masons and miners.

Particles of silica 3–5 μm find their way to the alveolar level where they are ingested by alveolar macrophages. These cells then proceed to the lymphatics, which become blocked. The presence of silica in the lungs causes a pronounced fibrotic reaction as the particles are not broken down by the body. It is thought that several mechanisms probably contribute to this fibrosis. Silicic acid, being formed very slowly in the tissue, is the irritant substance acting as a tissue poison evoking necrosis and a strong fibrotic, chronic inflammatory reaction in the lungs. Silica or silicic acid may combine with tissue protein and initiate an autoimmune response. Individuals with silicosis show a marked tendency to contract tuberculosis as the two agents causing these diseases have a synergistic effect.

The pleura in a case of silicosis are greatly thickened by tracts of fibrous tissue. In the lung parenchyma there are several large nodules of fibrosis of varying size (Figure 7.21). Within the nodule are degenerating collagen centres, surrounded by fibroblasts and collagen with a few chronic inflammatory cells. The particles of silica within the nodules are not readily seen. However, when the lungs are incinerated an analytical determination will yield values of silica content as high as 1.6%, whereas normal lung silica content is 0.2%. The silicotic nodules are mainly in the upper lobes of the lungs and associated with them are regions of bronchiectasis and emphysema, with the pulmonary arteries showing hypertensive changes, all indications of COAD. Many individuals (as many as 60%) also have the characteristic changes of tuberculosis in the lungs.

Silicosis is a slowly progressive lung disease which eventually produces a patient who is a 'respiratory cripple'. Such patients experience severe respiratory distress upon the slightest exertion and often have to breathe in oxygen in order to cope with the reduced surface area and increased dead space in their lungs caused by the bronchiectasis and emphysema. Commonly they suffer from cor pulmonale and many die of cardiac failure.

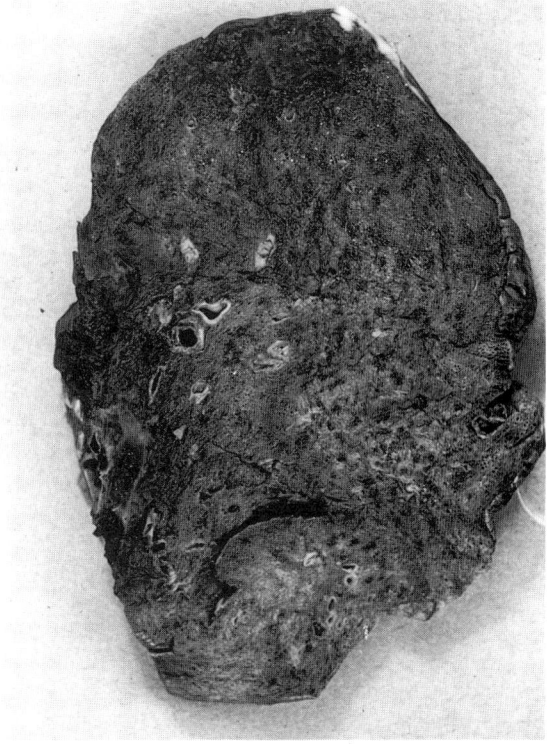

Figure 7.21 *Silicosis of the lungs in a 75-year-old male. Numerous regions of consolidation and darker regions of anthracosis are seen throughout the lung. A pale region of extensive pleural fibrosis is seen in the upper right of the pleura*

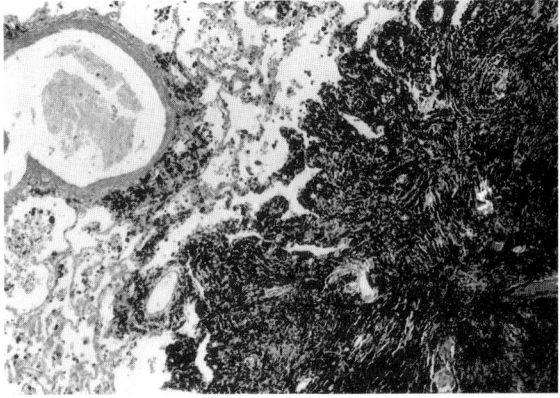

Figure 7.22 *Anthracosilicotic nodule in the lungs of a coal miner (×80)*

Coalworkers' Pneumoconiosis (= Silicoanthracosis)

This type of pneumoconiosis is almost exclusively found in coalworkers who suffer from extremely heavy anthracosis due to carbon dust inhalation from the coal they mine. In addition, these miners may have associated silicosis in their lungs due to the presence of silica in the inhaled mineral dusts. The carbon particles are mainly found in the respiratory bronchioles and surrounding centrilobular areas of lung parenchyma, where there is also emphysema and bronchiectasis (Figure 7.22).

The disease may not cause extensive fibrosis unless the quantity of silica inhaled with the carbon is considerable or unless there is associated infection present (especially tuberculosis, present in about 30% of patients). This has led to the naming of the disease as a 'simple coalworker's pneumoconiosis' or alternatively as an 'infected' or 'complicated coalworker's pneumoconiosis'.

In the simple type of pneumoconiosis the patient may not experience severely debilitating disease but rather the symptoms and signs commonly called 'miner's asthma', due to the focal emphysema and bronchiectasis. As the disease progresses to the complicated form, with increasing fibrosis and lung damage there is the development of severe emphysema, pulmonary hypertension and bronchiectasis, with the patients often progressing to respiratory and cardiac failure.

Berylliosis

This is a pneumoconiosis caused by the inhalation of beryllium-containing dusts. It is seen in miners and refiners of beryllium ores, metal welders in the electronics industry and in the workers involved in the manufacture of fluorescent light tubes. The beryllium causes a fibrotic reaction in the lungs without much pleural involvement, eventually leading to the production of emphysema and COAD. Microscopically, typical 'beryllium granulomata' will be seen which resemble those of sarcoidosis. Thus, often, a definite diagnosis cannot be made unless the lung is analysed chemically. Other organs such as lymph nodes, spleen and liver may show granulomata but the disease is usually most serious in the lungs and the patient may die of respiratory or cardiac failure.

Silicosiderosis (Haematite Lung)

This type of pneumoconiosis results from inhalation of iron oxide dust (Fe_2O_3, haematite). It is seen in quarry workers and miners where the inhaled dusts are rich in iron oxides. The lung becomes a rusty red colour and shows a severe fibrotic change. Iron is also present in the lymph nodes and liver where it may be demonstrated by Perls' staining. The condition is associated with cor pulmonale and heart failure but may also lead to a higher incidence of tuberculosis and lung cancer.

Asbestosis

Asbestosis is caused by inhalation of asbestos fibres, a complex magnesium silicate [$CaMg_3(SiO_3)_4$]. There are two major varieties of asbestos, white asbestos and blue asbestos. Of the two, blue asbestos (crocidolite) is the most harmful fibre and is associated with the most severe tissue reaction and complications. Asbestosis is now a well-documented hazard wherever asbestos has been used in manufacturing, construction of buildings, fire-proof insulating, brake-lining, etc. The disease has been mainly encountered in people contacting the fibres in an occupational setting but some cases have occurred where people have inhaled the asbestos simply by living in houses where the fibres were used in insulating materials.

With extensive exposure to asbestos a typical severe, diffuse, fibrous reaction occurs in the pleura and lung parenchyma, especially in the lower lobes. The asbestos fibres are long, needle-like and cannot be broken down by the body. They become surrounded by a protein sheath to give rise to the characteristic dumb-bell-shaped 'asbestos bodies' in the respiratory bronchioles, which are diagnostic of the disease (Figure 7.23). Surrounding the asbestos bodies are macrophages and giant cells.

Severe asbestosis in the lungs causes widespread fibrosis and COAD with many patients suffering from cor pulmonale and heart failure. Patients are also more likely to contract tuberculosis. However, even more sinister is the fact that asbestosis has been very strongly linked with the development of lung cancer or pleural mesothelioma, especially if the patient is also a smoker, the two carcinogens having a multiplicative effect. There are documented cases of tumours developing even after one exposure to asbestos. However, the latent period between exposure and development of the tumours is very long, up to 40 years elapsing before the cancers arise.

Organic Pneumoconioses

These occur after inhalation of dusts composed of organic particles. As a group, the organic pneumoconioses are all rather less severe in effects and com-

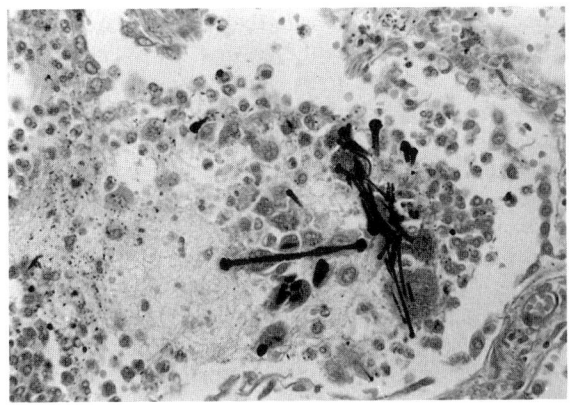

Figure 7.23 *Asbestos bodies in the lungs of a patient with asbestosis (×400)*

plications than the inorganic pneumoconioses already discussed. Most of them tend to give rise to allergic-type responses in the lungs with an immediate effect mediated by acute inflammatory changes, pulmonary oedema and bronchoconstriction. These effects are reversible upon removal of the irritant and fibrosis does not result. Several such pneumoconioses have been described.

Byssinosis occurs in cotton mill workers who breathe fine dusts laden with cotton proteins. Prolonged exposure leads to chronic bronchitis, an asthmatic type of disease, emphysema and manifestations of COAD.

Bagassosis results in people exposed to dried sugar cane refuse ('bagasse') which is used in manufacturing insulating material. The causative agent is most likely a mould growing on the sugar cane. A similar type of allergic, bronchitic, asthmatic presentation develops as that already described for byssinosis.

'Farmer's lung' is a pneumoconiosis occurring after inhalation of mouldy hay dust, the causative agents being the mould spores. It is a typical type III hypersensitivity caused by the dissolution of antigenic material from the mould spores into lung fluids and the subsequent elaboration of antibodies to those antigens with the production of immune complexes. An inflammatory reaction develops which is self-limiting with no fibrosis seen.

Primary Tumours

Benign primary tumours of the lung are rather uncommon, although there exists a wide variety of such lesions, and often included in the classification are tumour-like lesions such as hamartomata. The most frequently encountered benign lesions are the so-called 'tumourlets' that are found near the walls of the bronchi or bronchioles. The term describing these tumours indicates that they are of microscopic dimensions and not visible to the naked eye. The lesions form in association with chronic damage, inflammation and scarring of lung tissue and consist of small groups of elongated epithelial cells in a collagenous stroma.

Another rather commonly occurring benign tumour of the lungs is the so-called 'adenoma' of the lung, but this is a misnomer, as the tumour often follows a malignant course after it has been present in the body for a length of time and also it may be of several subtypes. Adenoma of the lungs arises around the age of forty years and affects the sexes equally. It may be found in the trachea or major bronchi and rarely may arise in peripheral situations. The tumour may be of a mucous gland type (often described as a salivary gland tumour of the lungs) or it may be of a carcinoid type (and thus resembling the intestinal carcinoid tumours). Of the two tumours, the former is more sinister, as it may undergo malignant transformation after it has been growing for several years. Carcinoid tumours of the lungs follow a typically benign course, although some of them may secrete large quantities of serotonin and thus give rise to the carcinoid syndrome (see Chapter 8, under 'Small Intestine').

Benign tumours of the lungs may cause obstruction and infection of the airways and are thus treated by bronchoscopic surgical excision, although there is a high recurrence rate after such treatment. More aggressive surgery such as lobectomy and pneumonectomy is usually curative. If left untreated benign tumours (especially those of the mucous gland type) may cause the death of the patient after many years.

The remaining important primary tumours of the respiratory system are malignant and of quite high incidence. These tumours are: carcinoma of the larynx, carcinoma of the bronchus ('lung cancer', bronchogenic carcinoma) and mesothelioma of the pleura.

Carcinoma of the Larynx

Incidence. This tumour causes ≈1% of malignant deaths and is seen more commonly in males (M:F ratio is 8:1) around the age of 60 years.

Aetiology. Carcinoma of the larynx often arises in pre-existing benign lesions such as leukoplakia but there are also certain factors which have been shown to be important epidemiologically and may lead to the cancer without a pre-existing premalignant lesion. These are:

- smoking of cigarettes;
- drinking of excessive quantities of alcohol (especially if the person is a smoker also);
- presence of benign tumours, papilloma;
- geographical, racial factors — the tumour has a higher incidence in Puerto Rico, India and Sweden. France has the highest incidence of cancer of the vocal cords.

Sites affected. Approximately 70% of the tumours arise on the vocal cords, the reminder arising from the adjacent tissues such as the epiglottis or aryepiglottitic region (Figure 7.24).

Morphology. This tumour frequently forms diffuse, nodular, papillary or ulcerated growths arising from the mucosa, growing along the mucosa and invading into the wall. Microscopically, most of the tumours are keratinizing, squamous cell carcinomata, although occasionally, anaplastic forms will be seen.

Spread. Spread of carcinoma occurs directly to involve the vocal cord in which it arises and across the commissure to involve the other cord. The laryngeal cartilages tend to confine the tumour for a period of time and hence the tumour spreads more in the vertical direction to the epiglottis or the subglottic area. Lymphatic spread involves the cervical lymph nodes and blood spread tends to occur late, especially to the lungs, forming secondaries there.

Signs and symptoms. Cancers arising on the vocal cord frequently present early as they cause a persistent hoarseness or alteration in the voice characteristics rather soon in the course of the disease. There may also be obstruction and difficulty in breathing, patients often complaining of 'a lump in the throat'. Occasionally there are unexplained earaches or a soreness in the throat. Frequently, secondary infection of the ulcerated tumour occurs and bronchopneumonia is a relatively common finding.

Diagnosis. The vocal cords are first examined by using a mirror, and a biopsy may be obtained under local anaesthesia if the tumour is easily accessible. If the tumour is not easily reached, then a biopsy will have to be taken with a laryngoscope under general anaesthesia. Histology will determine whether the tumour is malignant and how well differentiated it is.

Treatment and prognosis. The tumour is treated solely by radiotherapy if it is small but needs to be surgically excised if larger, a laryngectomy being carried out, with radiotherapy used as an adjunct. There is minimal response to chemotherapy, and this is a treatment used in terminal cases to relieve symptoms. Generally, the tumour has a very good prognosis, carcinoma of the vocal cords diagnosed and treated early having a 5-year survival of 85–90%, while in those patients where treatment is initiated after lymph node involvement the 5-year survival is 33%. On average the 5-year survival is 45%.

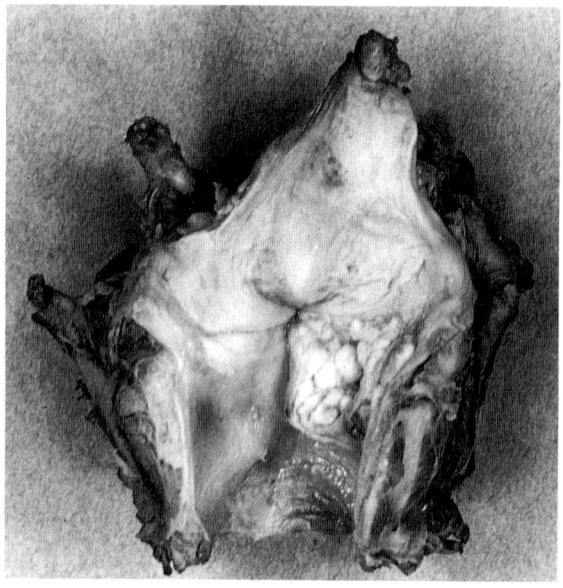

Figure 7.24 *Carcinoma of the right vocal cord in a male 74-year-old smoker*

Carcinoma of the Bronchus

Incidence. There has been a great increase in incidence of bronchogenic carcinoma over the last 30–40 years. Bronchogenic carcinoma is responsible for approximately 25% of all cancer deaths, and approximately 5% of deaths from all causes. In many countries carcinoma of the lungs is the major cause of death due to cancer.

The average age of incidence is 55 years, but carcinoma of the bronchus may occur in an age range of 15–80 years. The male to female ratio is 2:1. However, the tumour is becoming more common in females, (since more women than men now smoke cigarettes). In the United States, carcinoma of the bronchus is now commoner in women than in men.

Aetiology. Many aetiological and predisposing factors have been implicated in this carcinoma. These are:

- **Cigarette smoking**: This is the major causative factor, due to carcinogenic hydrocarbons ('tar') in the combustion products of tobacco. A very large epidemiological study in Britain clearly demonstrated the association between smoking and lung cancer in the early 1950s. Since that time more and more data and evidence have accumulated clearly implicating cigarette smoking as the major causative agent in this tumour.
- **Irradiation**: The incidence of carcinoma of the bronchus is much higher in mine workers where radioactive ores are mined, for example in cobalt and radium mines, where it is mainly through the inhalation of the radioactive gas radon that the bronchial epithelium is thought to be affected and the neoplastic process begun. X-ray therapy in the chest region for prolonged times is avoided for fear of inducing lung cancers.
- **Occupational**: Prolonged exposure to various elements and ores mainly in an industrial or mining environment may cause carcinoma of the bronchus to develop. The incriminated substances are nickel, arsenic (used in weed killers), haematite, asbestos, chromates. Very often the tumour develops in lungs that are damaged by pneumoconiosis.
- **Atmospheric pollution**: There appears to be a higher incidence of lung cancer in city dwellers. This is related to heavy pollution and the inhalation of diesel, petrol and other fumes, as well as inhalation of carbon in the form of finely divided particles (smoke and soot). Other compounds released in combustion processes may also be involved.

It should be kept in mind that when more than one aetiological factor is acting in the same lung simultaneously, the risk of developing the tumour increases much more steeply than if a simple additive effect were operating. For example, in patients who have been exposed to asbestos and who are smokers the risk of developing lung cancer is many times greater than in people who are smokers only or who have been exposed to asbestos only.

Sites. **Central**: 55% of lung cancers arise in the main, lobar or segmental bronchi and about 75% of the tumours are visible at bronchoscopy. Most tumours tend to be in the right bronchus and its subdividing branches (Figure 7.25). **Peripheral**: 40% of the tumours arise in the small bronchi or bronchioles. **Diffuse**: 5% of lung cancers are multifocal, or of indeterminate origin.

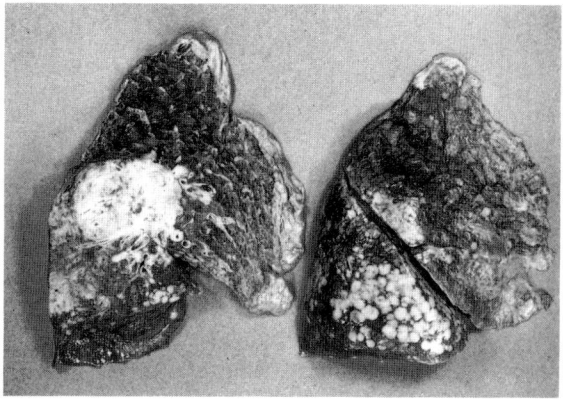

Figure 7.25 *Carcinoma of the bronchus with extensive perivascular and peribronchial lymphatic spread in a 55-year-old male smoker. The cut surface shows the large mass of the primary tumour and the pleural aspect shows the many deposits of subpleural neoplasms that have subsequently spread there via the lymphatics*

Macroscopic appearance. The tumour begins as a localized small, pale, rough patch on the mucosa of the bronchus, very quickly ulcerating and spreading by infiltration to the local lymphatics. As the tumour grows into the lumen of the airway, it narrows the lumen and may in certain cases cause considerable difficulty in the passage of air through the affected airway. The surrounding lung tissue is invaded by a pale mass of tumour which may undergo necrosis, haemorrhage or become infected, with subsequent abscess formation. The lung tissue distal to the tumour may show collapse, bronchiectasis or abscess formation, effects mainly mediated through obstruction of airways. Characteristically the tumour cells invade the lymphatics very early in the course of the disease, and the hilar lymph nodes are almost always affected at the time of diagnosis. In addition the tumour invades blood vessels, and very frequently infarcted areas are found both in the tumour and adjacent lung tissue.

Histopathology. Approximately 40% of the tumours are **squamous cell carcinomata** arising in metaplastic respiratory epithelium. Chronic irritation of the delicate respiratory epithelium by substances such as smoke, dusts and chronic infections leads to metaplasia which is reversible upon removal of the offending irritating stimulus. If the irritation persists, the metaplasia becomes atypical, progresses to dysplasia and ultimately to neoplasia. The squamous cell carcinoma occurring in the bronchus is usually a poorly differentiated one with little or no keratin formation.

About 15% of the tumours are **adenocarcinomata** which are papillary and secrete mucus. Tubular and gland-like structures are found within the tumour masses. These types of tumour are slightly commoner in female patients.

Approximately 0.5% of tumours are the so-called '**alveolar cell carcinoma**' which originates in the bronchioles but rapidly spreads into the alveolar spaces, using the alveolar walls as a scaffold onto which it grows in sheets which have papillary projections (Figure 7.26). The tumour is often an adenocarcinoma, secreting mucus. It is often bilateral and appears to arise multifocally.

By far, the majority of cases of lung carcinomata (> 45%) are **undifferentiated carcinomata** which may be subdivided into two groups depending on the cellular morphology of the tumour cells. About 30% of these are '**large cell' tumours** with the cells being large and polygonal, arranged in solid sheets, or sometimes attempting to form irregular groups. These tumours are thought to represent very undifferentiated squamous cell carcinomata and adenocarcinomata. Approximately 15% are '**small cell' carcinomata** ('**oat cell' carcinomata**) composed of small hyperchromatic cells with scanty cytoplasm. They have been likened to oat seeds in appearance, hence the alternative name. The cells may be arranged in sheets or irregular rosettes. These are very rapidly growing and invading tumours which usually have a small primary lesion but at the same time quite extensive and massive involvement of the draining lymph nodes, as well as invasion of the pleura, lung tissue and pericardium. Involve-

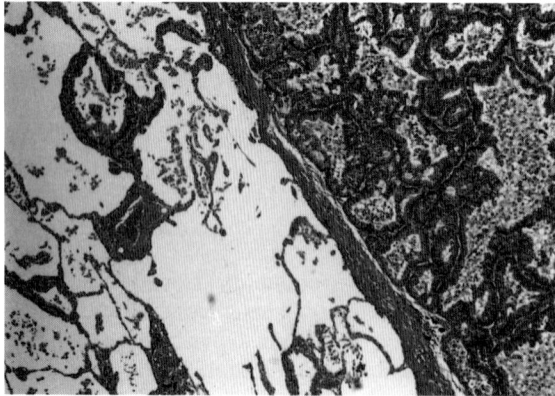

Figure 7.26 *Alveolar cell carcinoma demonstrating the ability of the tumour to utilize the alveolar walls as a scaffold for its growth (×300)*

ment of the oesophagus may give rise to a broncho-oesophageal fistula.

Spread. The tumours spread **directly**, to involve the surrounding lung tissues and grow in the bronchial tree. Invasion and permeation of the **lymphatics** usually occurs early in the disease and the lymph nodes affected are the hilar, mediastinal and cervical nodes. The tumour then spreads into the bloodstream, the **haematogenous** spread resulting in secondary tumour masses in the **bones**, **liver** and **brain**. As the tumour spreads outwards and involves the pleura, **transcoelomic** spread occurs in the pleura with seeding of tumour within the pleural cavity. The tumour may involve the pericardium and heart, as well as the oesophagus. When the tumour spreads locally, it invades the pleura, recurrent laryngeal nerve, pericardium, oesophagus and brachial plexus (in the last-mentioned case called **Pancoast's tumour**). Involvement of the mediastinal lymph nodes may be considerable which will cause compression of the vena cava with gross oedema and cyanosis of the face and upper limbs (superior vena cava syndrome).

Symptoms and signs. Patients with carcinoma of the bronchus may present with signs and symptoms relating to the primary growth of the tumour, and hence due to local factors: cough, which tends to be persistent and associated with haemoptysis, dyspnoea or lung infections. Secondaries, which mainly occur in the brain, adrenal gland, liver and bones, may produce the following signs and symptoms due to disease in these parts: neurological disorders, pathological fractures, jaundice and hepatomegaly, or adrenal cortical failure. Finally, the patient may present with generalized signs and symptoms, common to all malignant diseases: loss of weight, cachexia, anaemia, peripheral neuropathy, endocrine disturbances and myopathies. In some types of lung cancers there is secretion of ACTH by the tumour cells which may lead to considerable endocrine abnormalities. There may be involvement of the laryngeal nerve, with hoarseness arising, invasion of the pericardium and heart, with fibrillation or cardiac failure resulting.

Diagnosis. Various investigations in the clinic, hospital and laboratory confirm the presumed diagnosis which may have already been made on clinical grounds. A **chest X-ray** usually shows opacity in the lung involved with associated lymphadenomegaly. **Bronchoscopy** is the procedure where a special instrument is inserted into the airways and the surface of the trachea and bronchi examined visually. During this procedure the tumour may be seen directly (visible in about 75% of cases) and small pieces of the tumour are **biopsied for histological examination**. The affected lymph nodes (especially cervical nodes) may also be biopsied for evidence of tumour. **Cytological examination of sputum** will often show the presence of malignant cells in the smear. In the same way, pleural fluid aspirate may also be examined by cytology.

Treatment and prognosis. The treatment of lung cancer is fraught with difficulties, as even in the case of surgical removal of the tumour (pneumonectomy/lobectomy) there is only a 30% 5-year survival rate. In addition, by the time the tumour is diagnosed, it is usually quite incurable, about half the cases proving to be inoperable at the time of diagnosis, and suffering from no symptoms at all. Radiotherapy prolongs survival by about 14 months and can also considerably alleviate some of the most distressing symptoms for the patient, such as superior vena caval obstruction, relief from cough, dyspnoea and haemoptysis, and relieve the pain of secondary bone growths. Chemotherapy is not very effective for these tumours and is seldom of use. The average, overall 5-year survival is ≈ 7–10%, hence the prognosis for lung cancer is very poor.

Mesothelioma of Pleura

Incidence. This is a malignant tumour of the pleura which until the 1960s was a rare tumour. However, the general incidence of this tumour is increasing and we must expect to see a lot of these tumours as we go into the 21st century. It is a tumour more commonly seen in males because of occupational factors and they generally present between 55 and 80 years.

Aetiology. Mesothelioma of the pleura has been shown to be associated with asbestos exposure. During the 1950s asbestos use increased greatly and until the 1960s not many cases of mesothelioma were seen at all. In the late 1970s, the incidence of mesothelioma of the pleura increased greatly with over 90% of cases of mesothelioma showing an occupational exposure to asbestos. Asbestos miners, workers in the building industry, workers in fire-proof insulation, automotive workers associated with brake-lining and also plumbers and 'laggers' who insulated hot water pipes with asbestos are likely to present with the tumour. The incidence of the tumour increases greatly if the person is also a cigarette smoker. Exposures of as little as 3 months duration have been shown to be sufficient to

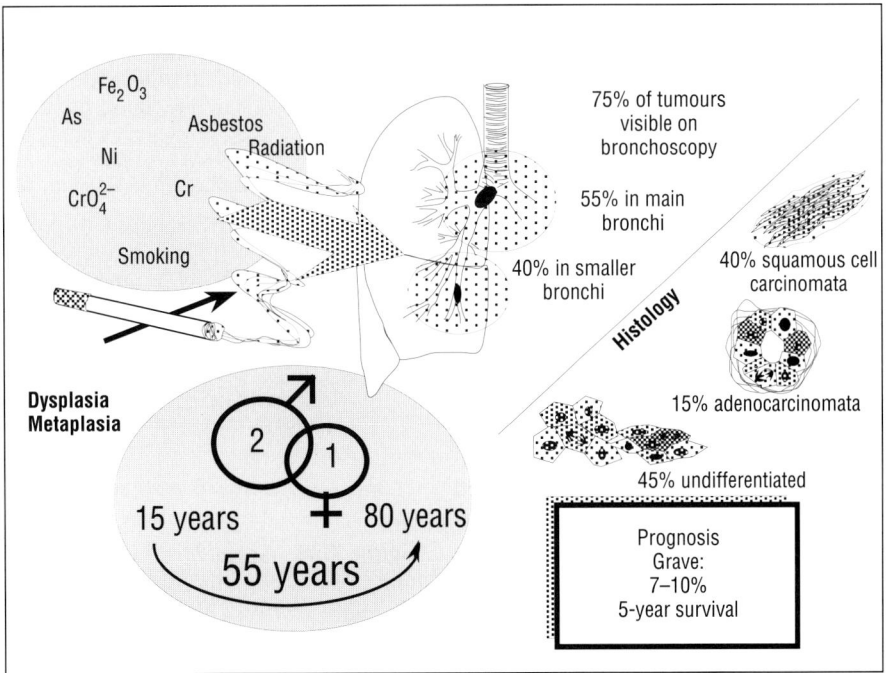

Figure 7.27 *Pathology of carcinoma of the bronchus*

cause the tumour; however, the tumour may take 20–40 years after exposure to develop. Most cases of mesothelioma of the pleura develop in patients who are already suffering from asbestosis and have a long history of exposure to asbestos.

Sites affected. Most of the cancers affect both visceral and parietal layers of the pleura arising from the mesothelial cells lining the pleura. Occasionally other sites in the body possessing mesothelial lining may show this tumour, that is, the peritoneum, pericardium and synovium.

Morphology. The tumour grows within the pleura, forming a dense layer with abundant fibrous stroma, encasing and compressing one or both lungs, extending into the interlobar spaces. It is a grey-white tumour and usually does not invade deeply into the lungs until late. It may form a thick layer 0.5 to 1 cm thick around the lungs and often there is associated haemorrhage and exudate within the pleural space. A variable histological picture is seen with tumour cells that are very pleomorphic. Areas of necrosis are observed and cystic spaces full of mucinous fluid are a common feature. The tumour may contain papillary or tubular structures within a sarcomatous, spindle cell populated stroma. Asbestos bodies and changes characteristic of asbestosis may be seen in the lungs, although asbestos bodies are not seen in the tumour itself.

Spread. Mesothelioma spreads early directly to involve the pleural spaces and subsequently lymphatic spread occurs with the hilar and abdominal lymph nodes involved. Later in the course of the tumour there is involvement of the lung parenchyma and haematogenous spread to the other lung, liver, thyroid, adrenals, bones and brain.

Signs and symptoms. The patient usually presents with signs and symptoms relating to the asbestosis which predates the carcinoma. There may be respiratory distress and signs of heart failure. When the tumour involves more and more tissue there may be weight loss, anaemia, fatigue and other generalized effects of malignancy. Patients with asbestosis may be monitored for the development of mesothelioma but even tumours that are diagnosed early are difficult to treat.

Diagnosis. X-ray films of the lungs will show the asbestotic changes and the presence of the tumour. Biopsy of the tumour mass through thoracocentesis will confirm its presence.

Treatment and prognosis. Treatment of the tumour is centred around palliation of the symptoms, for example with chemotherapy, as surgical treatment is not feasible. Prognosis is very poor, death of most patients usually occurring within a year of appearance of symptoms.

Secondary Tumours

The lungs are a favoured site for the development of secondary tumours from other parts of the body, being only second to the liver in this respect. The primary sites for these metastases are usually the breast, kidney, bone and skin (e.g. malignant melanoma, Figure 7.28). Spread to the lungs results from direct vascular haematogenous spread, or alternatively from retrograde lymphatic permeation from involved mediastinal lymph nodes (lymphangitis carcinomatosa).

Secondary tumours in the lungs usually present in the form of multiple deposits of various sizes, scattered throughout the lung parenchyma, the appearance of the masses having given them the name of 'cannonball lesions'. Frequently encountered, such lesions in

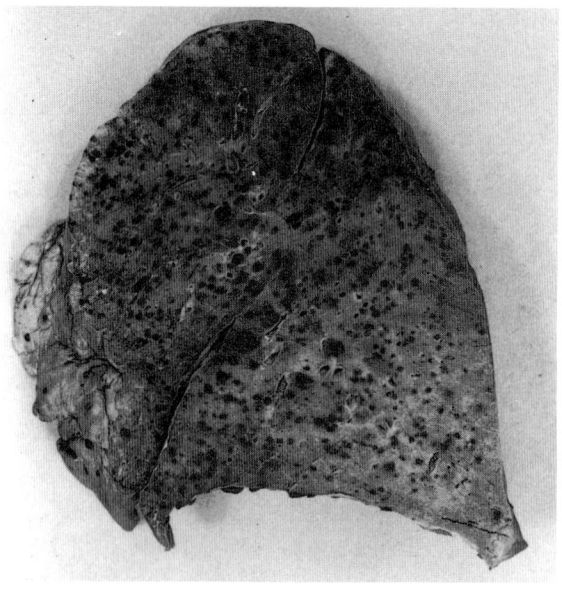

Figure 7.28 *Secondary malignant melanoma of the lungs. Numerous, round dark deposits of the tumour are found scattered throughout the lung tissue. A 43-year-old male who showed extensive involvement of almost all organs by the tumour, the primary site of origin of the melanoma being undetermined*

the lungs are secondaries from primaries of the breast and bone. Alternatively, a single mass within the lung parenchyma may be a secondary tumour.

Since secondary tumour deposits are so common in the lungs, a chest X-ray is standard practice with most forms of malignant neoplasms. The patient may present with similar signs and symptoms as a patient with primary carcinoma of the bronchus.

Revision Questions and Case Studies

1. Discuss the pathology of atelectasia and distinguish this condition from lung collapse.
2. Compare and contrast the macroscopic and microscopic appearance of:
   (a) Emphysema
   (b) Bronchiectasis
3. What disease states are encompassed by the term 'chronic obstructive airways disease' (COAD)?
4. How could a lung abscess develop? What organisms would most commonly be isolated from it? What are its complications?
5. Compare and contrast the related conditions of:
   (a) Bronchopneumonia (lobular pneumonia)
   (b) Lobar pneumonia (a table may be used)
6. Discuss the pathology of atypical pneumonia (pneumonitis).
7. Differentiate chronic bronchitis from asthma.
8. Describe the microscopic structure of a typical, fully developed, mature tubercle. What gives rise to such a lesion?
9. Differentiate miliary tuberculosis from tuberculous bronchopneumonia. How does the pathogenesis of the two conditions differ?
10. What are the similarities and differences in the microscopic structure of a sarcoid granuloma and a typical tubercle? What is the aetiology of these two granulomata? Name two other types of specific granulomata.
11. What are the pneumoconioses? Name four important pneumoconioses caused by inorganic particles and two pneumoconioses caused by organic particles. Give the complications of any one of the more serious pneumoconioses that you have mentioned.
12. To what sites do bronchogenic carcinomata metastasize and by what routes?
13. How are bronchogenic carcinomata diagnosed? What symptoms and signs do they give rise to? Explain these symptoms and signs in relation to the pathological changes occurring in the body of a patient with bronchogenic carcinoma.
14. What are the predisposing factors in the development of bronchogenic carcinoma? Discuss the pathogenesis of the tumour in relation to the most commonly encountered aetiological agent in the causation of this tumour in our community.
15. Describe the microscopic types of bronchogenic carcinoma and relate these different types to prognosis for the patient.
16. What is meant by the term 'honeycomb lung'?
17. The lungs are a very frequent site in which secondary tumours occur. What primary tumours commonly metastasize to the lungs and by what route? Explain why the lungs are such a common site in which metastatic neoplasms are found.
18. What are 'cannon-ball lesions' in the lung?
19. Define the term 'pleuritic fibrous adhesions'.
20. Define the term 'consolidation'.

Case study 1. A 62-year-old Caucasian male presents at the doctor's surgery complaining of attacks of respiratory distress which occur two to three times weekly and which last for a few hours. Each attack is characterized by tightness in the chest with inspiratory and expiratory difficulty. Sometimes there is a cough which is usually dry but in the last two attacks was productive of phlegm. The man tells the doctor that the attacks are most frequent during the winter months and are often associated with colds. An audible wheeze on expiration is a feature of the attacks. The man's granddaughter suffers from hives.

(a) What is the presumptive diagnosis?
(b) What are the complications of this condition? (List them only).
(c) How is the condition managed?

Case study 2. Mr Kevin H. is a 64-year-old tradesman who has always been very fit. He presents at your clinic complaining of severe low back pain which he has had for approximately one month. He has vomited over the past two days and has become progressively more weak and anorexic over the past two months, sometimes experiencing vague abdominal pain, and has noticed changes in his bowel habits. He has not had a bowel motion for the past 10 days. He mentions that he has had attacks of breathlessness on exertion for two months and he can no longer walk for more than a few metres without becoming dyspnoeic. This has been of some trouble to him and often he has had to stop during work in order to catch his breath. He has been a smoker in his youth but gave up smoking 15 years ago. On examination you notice that he is breathing rapidly. Over the trachea and left bronchus loud inspiratory and expiratory rhonchi are heard. There is no adenopathy in the cervical or axillary regions. The heart is normal, his blood pressure 125/85 mmHg and his pulse rate 80. Blood investigations were carried out as he appeared anaemic. His haematocrit was 0.40 (0.45–0.52) and haemoglobin was 7.1 mmol/L (8.1–11.2 mmol/L). On palpating the abdomen there is a marked hepatomegaly. The patient is 186 cm tall and weighs 67 kg.

(a) What are the differential diagnoses?
(b) What further investigations would need to be carried out in order to diagnose the condition conclusively?
(c) If the patient's faeces contain red blood what would be the most likely diagnosis for the lung condition?

Case study 3. A 24-year-old Caucasian male presents because he is feeling very debilitated and has respiratory difficulty. He also suffers from malaise, fatigue, anorexia and he has lost considerable weight lately. His weight is 66 kg and his height is 1.75 m. During the past three months he has been coughing, the sputum being mucoid and sometimes flecked with blood. The blood pressure is 110/83 mmHg and the pulse rate is 80 beats per minute. His temperature is 37.9°C and examination of the lungs shows that there are apical crepitations on both sides with some cavitation and pleural effusion on the right side. The abdomen is normal. The man is a non-smoker but drinks one to two bottles of beer a day. He is unemployed and lives in a disused factory with several other unemployed people. A Mantoux test is positive.

(a) What is the diagnosis?
(b) How would the diagnosis be confirmed?
(c) How is this disorder treated?

Case study 4. Mrs Francine P., a 59-year-old Caucasian female and mother of three daughters, visits her doctor complaining of a cough which has been troubling her more and more over the past month. Initially it was a nagging, dry, morning cough and has now changed to become more severe and productive of phlegm. Occasionally, after coughing violently for some time she has noticed that the phlegm contains flecks of blood. Mrs P. has always been active and all her working life she has been working as a factory worker in an industrial estate. She retired when she became 55 years of age and now says that she is often short of breath and tires easily, not being able to cope with looking after her eldest daughter's two young sons. Upon ques-

tioning the doctor elicits the information that Mrs P. started smoking as a teenager, smoking about 30 cigarettes daily for about 40 years. Blood pressure and pulse rate are normal but the patient is tachypneic.

(a) What is the diagnosis?
(b) What laboratory determinations should be carried out and why?
(c) What is the prognosis for this patient if you were given the additional information that she has a palpable hepatomegaly with moderate ascites? What are these findings due to?

Case study 5. Mr Jack N., a 45 year-old Torres Strait Islander and quarry worker, presents at the occupational health centre because lately he has had a cough and has felt a tightness in the chest. On physical examination at the clinic it is found that the man is 1.85 m tall and weighs 88 kg. The abdomen is normal and the blood pressure is 130/78 mmHg, a pulse rate of 82 beats per minute being recorded. His body temperature is 37.3°C. On examination of the chest it is found that there is bilateral focal consolidation of the lungs and rhonchi may be heard on both sides. The man has smoked about 35 cigarettes a day for the past 30 years. It is found that the man is slightly tachypneic. When asked about his job, Mr N. says that he has worked in a coal mine from when he was 16 years old until his late thirties and then 5 years ago he started to work in the quarry where he is employed currently. He has a history of respiratory infections which were treated successfully with antibiotics. On chest X-ray the pleura are greatly thickened and in the lung parenchyma there are several large nodular shadows of varying size. A Mantoux test is weakly positive.

(a) What are the differential diagnoses?
(b) What further tests should be done upon admission to hospital?
(c) What are the predisposing factors that led to the development of this disorder in this man?
(d) What are the complications of conditions of this nature?

Case study 6. A doctor was called urgently to make a house call at night in order to see a Caucasian boy aged 9 years. On arriving at the house he is told that yesterday the boy had come back from school early, complaining of chills and a sore throat. That afternoon he was put to bed and his temperature was noted as being 38.1°C. The boy was given hot herbal teas. Later on in the afternoon he developed a cough which became progressively worse and more persistent as the evening progressed. A naturopath friend of the family gave the boy some antitussive herbal remedy which improved the boy's condition during the night. That morning, the boy began to cough once again and his voice became hoarse. His fever became more severe, at lunchtime 38.7°C being recorded. All offers of hot soup were refused and it was with difficulty that hot lemon drinks with honey and herbs were consumed by the boy. As the evening progressed, the boy's breathing became more laboured and the attending naturopath suggested that a doctor be called in immediately. On examination, the boy was markedly dyspnoeic and cyanosis was evident. The tonsillar area and the pharynx were covered by a whitish grey exudate which resembled a membrane in parts. On questioning, the parents stated that their child had not received any of the common childhood vaccines as they were opposed to their use. The boy was given antitoxin immediately and an intramuscular penicillin injection. An ambulance was called and the boy transferred to hospital for emergency surgery. A throat swab was taken immediately prior to this and was sent to the microbiology laboratory.

(a) What is the diagnosis?
(b) What surgical procedure was performed upon admission to hospital and why?
(c) How is this condition prevented normally?
(d) What are the complications of this condition?

Further Reading

Abrahamson M, Voigt T. 'Ambient Air Pollution and Respiratory Disease.' *Med J Aust* 1991; **154**: 543.

Adams VI, *et al.* 'Diffuse Malignant Mesothelioma of the Pleura: Diagnosis and Survival in 92 Cases.' *Am J Clin Pathol* 1984; **82**: 15.

Bellomo R, *et al.* 'Two Consecutive Thunderstorm Associated Epidemics of Asthma in the City of Melbourne.' *Med J Aust* 1992; **156**: 834.

Craighead JE. 'Current Pathogenetic Concepts of Diffuse Malignant Mesothelioma.' *Hum Pathol* 1987; **18**: 544.

Heppleston AG. 'The Pathology of Honeycomb Lung.' *Thorax* 1956; **11**: 77.

Hoge CW, Breiman RF. 'Advances in the Epidemiology and Control of *Legionella* Infections.' *Epidem Rev* 1991; **13**: 329.

Howard JK. 'Man-Made Mineral Fibres. A Perspective.' *Patient Management* 1986; **10**(12): 15.

Kerstjens, HAM *et al.* 'A Comparison of Bronchodilator Therapy with or without Inhaled Corticosteroid Therapy for Obstructive Airways Disease.' *N Engl J Med* 1992; **327**: 1413.

McKinnon L. 'Upper Respiratory Tract Illness during Training and Competition.' *Sports Coach* Vol 15; **4**: 22.

Murray JF. 'The White Plague: Down and Out, or Up and Coming?' *Am Rev Respir Dis* 1989; **140**: 1788.

Rennick GJ, Jarman FC. 'Are Children with Asthma Affected by Smog?' *Med J Aust* 1992; **156**: 837.

Rhodes GC, Tapsall JW, Lykke AWJ. 'Alveolar Epithelial Responses in Experimental Streptococcal Pneumonia.' *J Path* 1989; **157**: 347.

Robertson CF, *et al.* 'Prevalence of Asthma in Melbourne Schoolchildren: Changes Over 26 Years.' *BMJ* 1991: **302**: 1116.

Shields SD, *et al.* 'The Relationship of Pertussis Immunization to the Onset of Neurological Disorders: A Retrospective Study.' *J Ped* 1988; **113**: 801.

Spitzer WO, *et al.* 'The Use of β-agonists and the Risk of Death or Near-death from Asthma.' *New Engl J Med* 1992; **326**: 501.

Swartz MN. 'Stress and the Common Cold.' *New Engl J Med* 1991; **325**: 654.

Tannock G. 'Living Attenuated Vaccines Against Influenza.' *Today's Life Sci* 1991: **3**(12): 34.

Thurlbeck WM. 'Pathophysiology of Chronic Obstructive Pulmonary Disease.' *Clin Chest Med* 1990; **11**: 389.

Warner JO, *et al.* 'Management of Asthma: An International View.' *Arch Dis Child* 1989; **64**: 1065.

WHO. *Histological Typing of Lung Tumors*, 2nd edition, *Am J Clin Pathol* 1982; **77**: 123.

Wiley JC, Harris CC. 'Cellular and Molecular Biological Aspects of Human Bronchogenic Carcinogenesis.' *Crit Rev Oncol Hematol* 1990; **10**: 181.

Williams GT, Jones-Williams W. 'Granulomatous Inflammation — A Review.' *J Clin Pathol* 1983; **36**: 723.

8

Gastrointestinal System Disorders

The Normal Gastrointestinal System

The normal gastrointestinal system is essentially a long open-ended tube with associated glands, the function of which is the ingestion and digestion of food, absorption of nutrients and egestion of the wastes. It comprises the:

- Mouth, teeth, tongue, salivary glands
- Oesophagus, stomach, duodenum
- Pancreas, liver, gall bladder
- Jejunum, ileum, appendix
- Colon, anus

The mouth is at the beginning of the alimentary canal and is an oval-shaped cavity in which the mastication of food takes place. Lubrication of the food is by the secretion of saliva by the parotid, submaxillary and sublingual salivary glands. The pharynx is the part of the digestive tract that is placed behind the nose, mouth and larynx and leads into the long muscular tube of the oesophagus. The oesophagus begins at the upper border of the cricoid cartilage, descends along the front of the spine, through the posterior mediastinum, passes through the diaphragm and ends at the cardiac orifice of the stomach.

The stomach is the major organ of digestion. It is a pear-shaped organ, with the large end (fundus) directed upwards and the small end bent to the right, terminating in the pylorus, where the stomach communicates with the duodenum. The stomach wall is thick and muscular and, unlike the other parts of the alimentary tract where there are two muscular coats (external longitudinal and inner circular), it has three muscle coats (superficial longitudinal, middle circular and a deeper oblique layer). The mucous membrane of the stomach secretes mucus, hydrochloric acid and pepsin, the last two being important in the digestive process.

The small intestine is a tube, approximately 7 m long, and is subdivided into the following regions, beginning at the junction with the stomach and ending at the junction with the large intestine. The **duodenum** (25 cm in length) is a U-shaped portion that is rather wide and fixed, receiving the secretions from the liver and pancreas via the common bile duct. It is here that the acid secretions of the stomach are neutralized and the bile begins to emulsify the fats such that they are broken down by the lipases of the pancreatic juice. The **jejunum** is the middle part of the small intestine (two-fifths of the length) and the **ileum** is the last part (three-fifths of the length). The small intestine functions largely in the absorption of nutrients, in this function being greatly helped by the numerous finger-like processes, the villi, that line the mucous membrane and greatly increase its surface area.

The large intestine extends from the ileocaecal valve to the anus and is about 1.5 m long. It is largest in diameter at its beginning in the caecum and it is here that the blind-ending vermiform appendix is found, varying in length from about 2.5 to 22.5 cm. The large intestine describes an arch, which surrounds the convoluted small intestine. It is divided into the caecum, ascending colon, hepatic flexure, transverse colon, splenic flexure, descending colon, sigmoid colon, rectum and ends at the anus. The function of the large intestine is to absorb water from the wastes that pass through it and temporarily to store these until they are egested at the anus at defaecation.

Diseases of the Oral Cavity

Stomatitis

This is an inflammatory condition of the oral cavity which may be associated with **glossitis** (inflammation of the tongue), **gingivitis** (inflammation of the gums) and **cheilitis** (inflammation of the lips). Although it may arise non-specifically it is often seen in association with infections. A common agent causing stomatitis is *Candida albicans* which causes oral 'thrush'. This infection is seen especially after antibiotic therapy when the normal flora is reduced and the resistant *Candida* grow unchecked causing the infection. A whitish membranous growth appears on the oral mucosa and may extend downward to involve the pharynx. Oral candidiasis is also seen in immunosuppressed patients, such as people with AIDS. In this case the infection may be very severe, extensively involving mouth, throat and oesophagus, and is difficult to treat.

Viral infections may also cause stomatitis, the prime example being herpes simplex virus infection. Although this virus most commonly causes a skin infection around the mouth ('cold sores' or 'fever blisters'), the infection may spread to involve the oral cavity. This is especially seen in the very young, perinatal infections of this type being common in babies. The infection may spread to the eyes and brain. Other viruses may cause manifestations of infection in the oral cavity, for example with measles virus infection there appear on the buccal mucosa raised, erythematous, small, round lesions known as **Koplik's spots**. In chickenpox, there may be small vesicles and papular eruptions in the oral mucosa.

Bacterial infections are also commonly seen in the oral mucosa, most frequently being associated with dental caries, dental extractions and gum diseases. The infecting organisms are normal flora streptococci and anaerobic bacteria. Such infections are easily treated with penicillin and adequate dental hygiene. A rather less commonly seen infection is 'trench mouth;' or **Vincent's angina** which is caused by commensal spirochaetes (*Borrelia vincentii*) and anaerobic fusiform bacilli, resulting in a mixed infection. There is widespread and irregular, quite painful ulceration of the gum margins with necrosis and an acute inflammatory response with many neutrophils. There is also associated halitosis and difficulty in chewing and eating. If the infection remains untreated it may spread and cause extensive destruction of gum tissue. It is easily treated with antibiotics but may recur.

Other less commonly seen infections of the oral cavity include **actinomycosis**, caused by *Actinomyces israeli*, where there is infection of the gums and tooth sockets, with spread to involve the skin, leading to abscess formation. The 'sulphur granules' visible in the pus are a characteristic feature of this infection. Cervicofacial actinomycosis accounts for about 50% of cases of this disease and from this location the infection may spread to involve the lungs, liver and other organs. **Diphtheria** caused by *Corynebacterium diphtheriae* is associated with a grey pseudomembrane which forms on the mucosa of the oropharynx. This may cause severe difficulty in breathing or asphyxia and there are also very serious systemic effects due to the potent exotoxin which the organism elaborates. Vaccination has greatly reduced the number of diphtheria cases seen nowadays. **Cancrum oris** is a rare gangrenous condition of the mouth, a mixed infection with commensal anaerobes especially seen in children who are malnourished or debilitated. There is massive infection of the mouth, facial muscles and overlying skin, giving rise to a rapidly progressive, highly disfiguring, destructive lesion, which may prove fatal in untreated cases. In **scarlet fever** caused by *Streptococcus pyogenes* the tongue may be involved in the inflammation, becoming very red, with prominent papillae, giving rise to the characteristic 'strawberry tongue'.

Carcinoma of the Mouth

Incidence. Tumours of the mouth including tongue, lip

and pharynx account for ≈2% of all malignancies. Therefore, this is a rather uncommon tumour which is seen more commonly in males (M:F ratio is 8:1) around the age of 60 years.

Aetiology. The tumour is linked with chronic inflammatory conditions of the oral cavity and also chronic irritation and exposure to carcinogenic substances. It has a high incidence in smokers as compared with non-smokers and is also more common in pipe and cigar smokers as opposed to cigarette smokers. Some cases have been associated with ill-fitting dentures which have not been rectified for many years, while in some countries where betel nut chewing is practised there is a higher incidence of the tumour. In females, there is an association of carcinoma of the mouth with the Plummer-Vinson syndrome.

Morphology. The first indication that a malignancy is about to occur is in many cases **leukoplakia** of the membranes lining the oral cavity, commonly seen in the internal aspect of the cheek. This presents as a raised, whitish plaque which on microscopy shows typical dysplastic changes. The lesion then progresses to a typical, keratinizing, squamous cell carcinoma. Rarely, the tumour may be undifferentiated.

Treatment and Prognosis. The tumour is surgically excised but also radiotherapy is recommended for many cases. Generally, the tumour has a poor prognosis with a 5-year survival of about 15%.

Carcinoma of the Tongue

Incidence. This is a relatively uncommon tumour seen more commonly in males (M:F ratio is 8:1) around the age of 55 years.

Aetiology. The aetiology of carcinoma of the tongue is very similar to that of carcinoma of the mouth described above.

Morphology. **Leukoplakia** is commonly seen on the tongue before the malignancy develops and in the tumour, leukoplakia will be seen around the tumour margins. Macroscopically, the cancer shows a papillary, nodular or diffuse habit and the mass is frequently ulcerated. The tumours are typically keratinizing, squamous cell carcinomata, although occasionally they may be undifferentiated (e.g. 'lymphoepithelioma' of the tongue).

Spread. The tumour spreads directly to involve the submucosal tissues of the tongue, there is invasion of the muscle and then quite quickly lymphatic invasion and spread to the cervical and other regional lymph nodes. Blood-borne metastasis to lungs and liver is also commonly seen, especially in the more advanced cases.

Treatment and Prognosis. The tumour is surgically excised but also radiotherapy may be recommended. The tumour tends to have a poor prognosis with a 5-year survival of approximately 15%.

Adamantinoma

This is a tumour derived from remnants of the enamel organ around teeth (the rests of Malassez). The tumour is sometimes also called an **ameloblastoma**. It is rather rare in occurrence and is seen primarily in adolescents and young adults up to the age of about 35 years. Most of such tumours are seen in the lower jaw. They present as swellings in the jaw which cause local destruction of the bone and replacement with whitish, cystic areas of tumour. Microscopically, the tumour resembles the enamel organ, with epithelial-covered processes around a core of stellate reticular cells. Cysts form due to the breakdown of the core. These are locally invasive tumours of low-grade malignancy, which if left untreated will cause extensive destruction of the jaw. They grow slowly and only rarely metastasize, being curable by local excision.

Diseases of the Oesophagus

Hiatus Hernia

A **hernia** may be defined as a protrusion of a body viscus outside its natural cavity and may be internal (within the body) or external (into the exterior environment). A hiatus hernia is an internal hernia where part of the stomach herniates into the thoracic cavity through the oesophageal hiatus. A hiatus hernia may be a 'rolling hernia' (25% of cases) or a 'sliding hernia' (75% of cases) as illustrated in Figure 8.1. A hiatus hernia may develop because of congenital weakness in the diaphragmatic muscle, because of neuromuscular incoordination, or abnormalities of the crura. Very frequently the condition is brought about by obesity and overloading of the stomach. It may also be seen in late pregnancy.

The disorder is commonly asymptomatic but usually presents with upper abdominal pain in obese people or pregnant women. Patients will often present

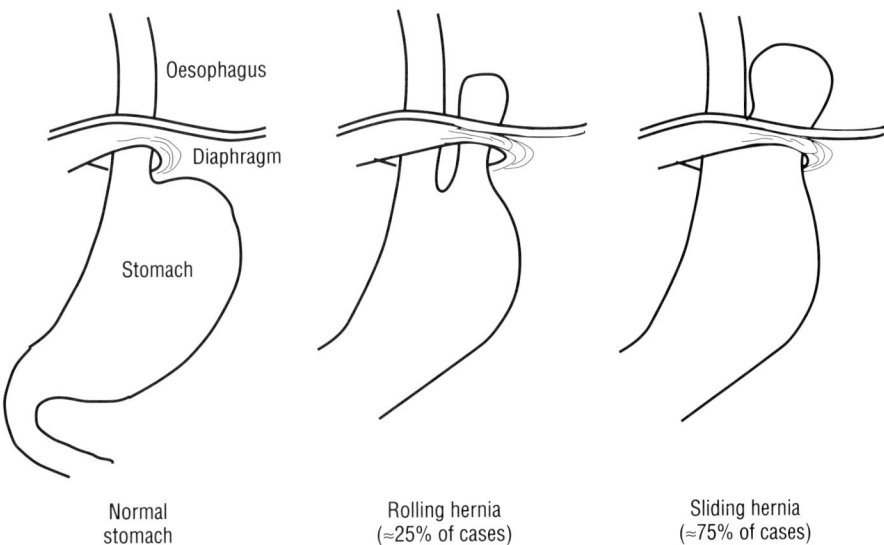

Figure 8.1 *Hiatus hernia*

with oesophagitis and oesophageal reflux with ulceration of the lower oesophagus, all of which present clinically as **dysphagia** (difficulty in swallowing/eating). Neglected cases will progress to fibrosis and narrowing of the lower oesophagus, with an oesophageal **stricture** developing. This further aggravates the dysphagia. Continuous bleeding from the oesophagus leads to a chronic iron deficiency anaemia.

Hiatus hernia is treated by weight reduction, avoidance of alcohol and overloading of the stomach with large meals. Often beneficial is raising the bed head of the patient 20–25 cm (by placing bricks under the bed legs!), a procedure which may be effective in preventing oesophageal reflux when the patient is lying down. Drugs may also be used, especially antacids but also those with action on the cardiac sphincter. As a last resort, surgery may be the only recourse for complicated or intractable cases. A balloon dilatation may be required in the lower oesophagus or a surgical resection of fibrous tissue bands which cause the stricture.

Oesophagitis

Inflammation of the oesophagus may result from infection (e.g. *Candida albicans* infection which causes oral 'thrush' often extends downwards to involve the oesophagus). Also, hot, caustic and corrosive substances will cause inflammation, ulceration and fibrous stricture.

A common cause of oesophagitis is reflux of gastric contents into the oesophagus, **oesophageal reflux**. This occurs commonly with hiatus hernia. The hallmarks of acute inflammation are seen in this condition with oedema, hyperaemia and leukocyte infiltration, all caused by the chemical injury which is mediated by the stomach acid that damages the oesophageal mucosa. Chronic oesophagitis may become complicated by ulceration and stricture of the lower end of the oesophagus, a typical example of the chronic fibrous form of the inflammatory response.

Achalasia of the Cardia

This is a disorder of motility affecting the entire oesophagus. Peristalsis is ineffectual in the lower two-thirds of the oesophagus and the cardiac sphincter remains tonically contracted. Thus the oesophagus empties incompletely and tends to enlarge due to accumulation of food. The patient experiences dysphagia, pain and discomfort at meals. This often leads to anorexia (loss of appetite) and wasting of the patient. There is some abnormality of autonomic nerves and ganglia in the muscle coat of the oesophagus in these cases.

Oesophageal Varices

Oesophageal varices; (varicose vessels) arise in cases of **portal hypertension** (increased pressure in portal circulation), most frequently as a result of **cirrhosis of the liver**. The varicosities occur in the submucosal veins near the cardiac orifice of the stomach (Figure 8.2). This is a region where the portal venous circulation anastomoses with the systemic venous circulation and portal hypertension forces blood from the portal system into the systemic venous system, thus causing the varicosities. These structures may subsequently become ulcerated and cause severe haemorrhage and even death.

Plummer-Vinson Syndrome (Sideropenic Dysphagia)

This is a rather rare, congenital condition of the oesophagus which is seen primarily in females (M:F = 1:9). The patients present with dysphagia, glossitis (inflammation of the tongue), koilonychia (spoon-shaped nails), achlorhydria (failure of HCl secretion by stomach mucosa) and iron deficiency anaemia. There is abnormal oesophageal peristalsis coupled with oesophageal strictures due to fibrosis in the post-cricoid region. This causes the dysphagia which is made more severe by the abnormal projection of mucosal folds or webs into the oesophageal lumen (see Figure 8.3).

There is a constant relationship in these patients with a severe iron deficiency which causes an anaemia (an indication of which is the koilonychia). Complications of the condition are oesophagitis and dysphagia, weakness and lassitude, a high incidence of carcinoma of the tongue and carcinoma of the oesophagus.

Carcinoma of the Oesophagus

Incidence. This tumour causes ≈2% of malignant deaths and is seen more commonly in males (M:F ratio is 8:1) around the age of 60 65 years.

Aetiology. The aetiology of carcinoma of the oesophagus is not very clearly elucidated but there are certain factors which have been shown to be important epidemiologically.

- The Plummer-Vinson syndrome greatly predisposes the female patient to this cancer.
- The consumption of very hot drinks (coffee, tea, soups, etc.).
- Smoking, especially of pipes, cigars, and also tobacco chewing.
- Carcinogenic foods? (Rather debatable as food spends very little time in the oesophagus.)
- Chronic oesophagitis of long duration which shows

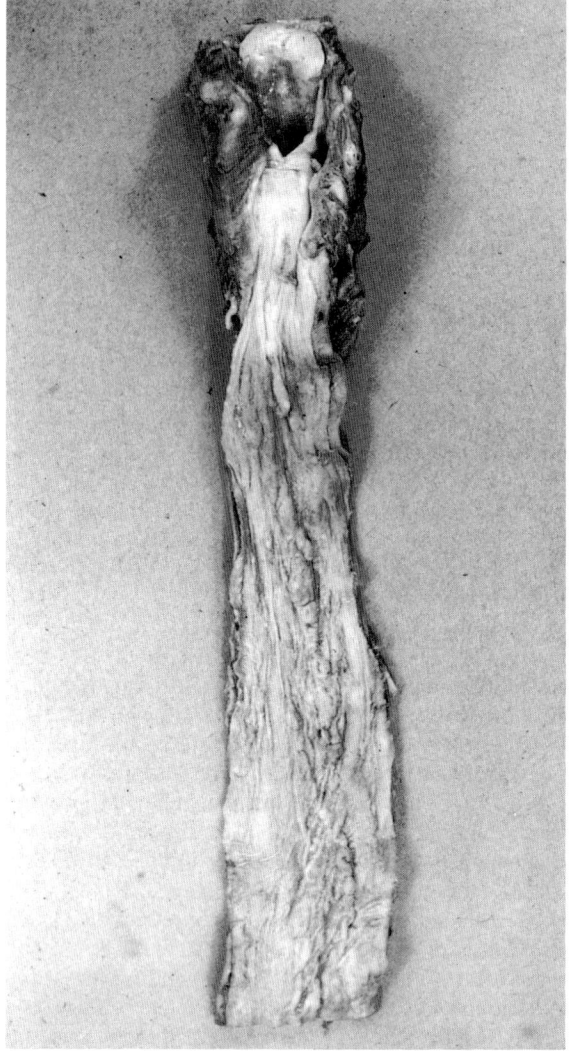

Figure 8.2 *Oesophageal varices in the lower two-thirds of the oesophagus in a 72-year-old male*

evidence of dysplasia and leukoplakia may progress to the carcinoma, hence association with chronic reflux oesophagitis, dysphagia hiatus hernia, achalasia, ulcerated diverticula, etc.
- Geographical, racial factors may be important as the tumour has a higher incidence in Puerto Rico, Bantus in South Africa, France, Switzerland, Honan province in China, and Japan.

Sites affected. Primarily the middle third of the oesophagus, followed by the lower third and finally less commonly seen to be affected is the upper third (middle:lower:upper = 3:2:1).

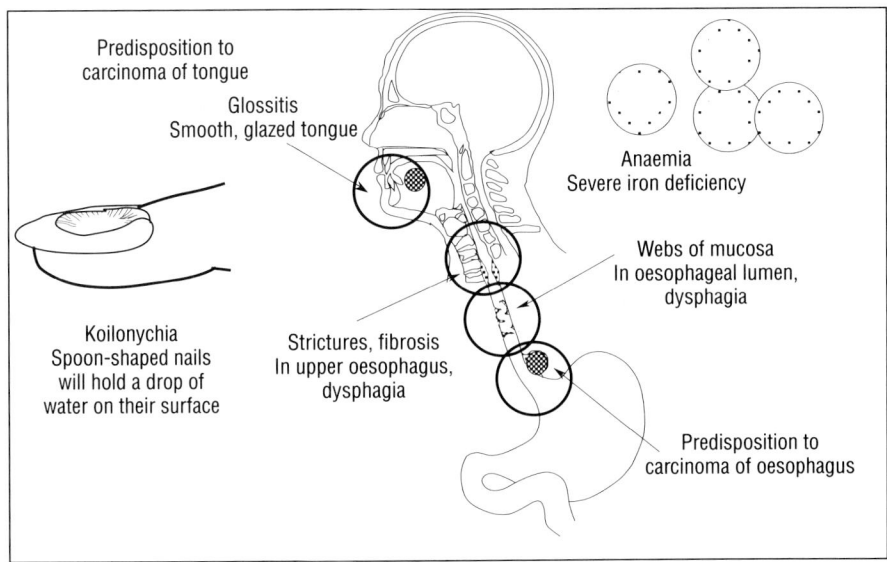

Figure 8.3 *Pathology of the Plummer-Vinson syndrome*

Morphology. The tumours most frequently form nodular growths arising from the mucosa and usually growing along the mucosa with invasion into the wall and beyond the serosa. Less frequently they may grow as an intraluminal nodule, the latter tumour associated with a slightly better prognosis as the patient presents earlier due to the obstruction and dysphagia caused by the growing cancer. The mass may occasionally show a diffuse habit and is frequently ulcerated.

Microscopically, the tumours are typically keratinizing, squamous cell carcinomata, although a minority component may be adenocarcinomata (in which case they may arise out of ectopic gastric mucosa in the oesophagus). Such adenocarcinomata are usually in the lower third of the oesophagus near the stomach.

Spread. Spread of carcinoma occurs directly to involve the oesophageal wall, rapidly invading past the serosa and into adjacent structures such as the trachea. Cervical, mediastinal and abdominal lymph nodes are affected rather early in the course of the condition by lymphatic spread. Blood spread also tends to occur early, especially to the brain and liver, forming secondaries in these organs.

Signs and Symptoms. There are no reliable early warning symptoms and signs for this cancer. Obstruction and difficulty in swallowing are frequent later symptoms. There may be haematemesis (vomiting of blood-

stained material) and the patient may become anorexic with resulting malnutrition. There is pain, choking sensations during attempts to drink fluids and gradual but extreme loss of weight in the late stages of the disease. Frequently, pneumonia results from aspiration of food.

Diagnosis. Diagnostic X-rays are taken while the patient swallows a barium meal. This is usually sufficient to distinguish benign from malignant conditions; however, if a cancer is suspected, a biopsy is taken via an oesophagoscope while the patient is lightly anaesthetized. Histology will determine not only whether the tumour is truly malignant but what histological type it is and how well differentiated it is.

Treatment and prognosis. The tumour is surgically excised but also radiotherapy may be recommended. There is no response to chemotherapy. Generally, the tumour has a very poor prognosis, even in operable cases, with a 5-year survival of ≈5%. There is a slightly better prognosis for the tumours which grow intraluminally and present earlier.

Oesophageal Obstruction

This may result through the impaction of swallowed foreign objects within the lumen, which may also cause damage and perforation of the oesophagus, for example swallowed fish bones and dental prostheses. Alternatively it may result from lesions which occur within the wall or which compress the wall of the organ from the surrounding tissues. Examples of the last two mentioned cases are:

- Fibrosis, either congenital or the result of injury, damage and inflammation.
- Achalasia of the cardia (= Cardiospasm).
- Hiatus hernia.
- Carcinoma of the oesophagus.
- Pressure from diseases of surrounding organs, for example goitres, tumours, aneurysms.

Depending on the cause, oesophageal obstruction may be a temporary event, resolving away, but most frequently will progress to an almost complete obstruction with progressive dysphagia, such that in untreated cases not even liquids may be swallowed.

Diseases of the Stomach and Duodenum

Gastritis

Gastritis is an inflammation of the stomach mucosa which may be acute or chronic. Often the term is used vaguely and is applied to any clinical syndrome which presents with pain or discomfort in the left, upper abdominal quadrant, whether or not there is any indication of pathological changes in the gastric mucosa.

Acute Gastritis

This is common in a mild self-limiting form and may be produced by ingestion of irritants such as alcohol, aspirin, bacterial toxins (e.g. *Staphylococcus, Salmonella*; Figures 8.4 and 8.5). There may be ulceration of the surface epithelium along with evidence of acute inflammation. Frequently, gastric erosions form where the superficial layers of the gastric mucosa slough off. However, these are very superficial lesions and do not progress beyond the *muscularis mucosae.*

Recently, there has been an association of gastritis and peptic ulceration with a bacterium which may in fact infect the gastric mucosa and cause gastritis *de novo.* This bacterium, *Helicobacter pylori*, is unlike most other bacteria in that it can survive the very acidic condition prevalent within the stomach, whereas most other ingested bacteria are killed or their colonization of the stomach is effectively prevented. *Helicobacter pylori* gastritis may start off as an acute attack, then progress to a chronic gastritis and produce

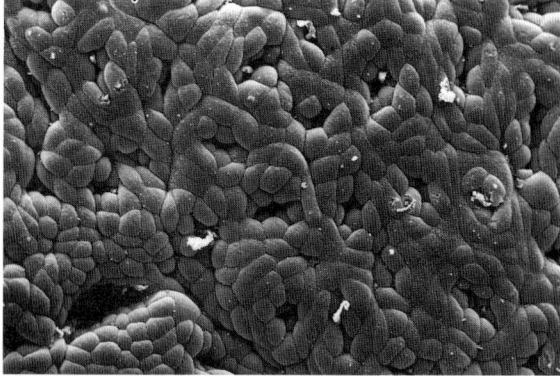

Figure 8.4 *Scanning electron micrograph of the normal stomach surface showing the gastric mucosal cells and gastric pits (×1500)*

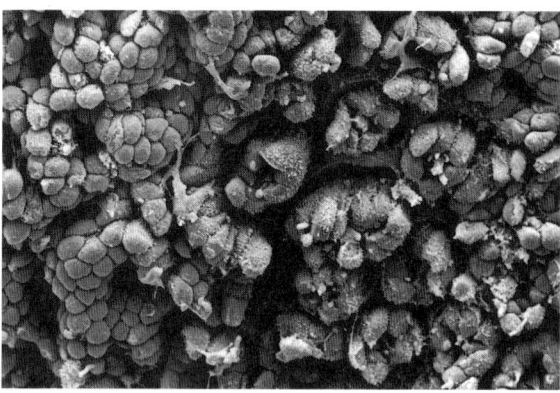

Figure 8.5 *Scanning electron micrograph of the stomach surface after application of 30% alcohol showing the gastric mucosal cell damage, necrosis and denudation of the epithelium with exposure of the underlying connective tissue (×1200)*

peptic ulceration. Antibiotic treatment of these cases of gastritis and peptic ulcer is essential.

The inflamed stomach shows a thickened, swollen appearance with very prominent congested vessels. The mucosa in particular is very hyperaemic with erosions and small haemorrhages seen on the tips of the rugae. Under the microscope, there is swelling and hyperaemia of the mucosa with areas of necrosis and haemorrhage associated with the erosions, and the submucosa is oedematous, congested and infiltrated by neutrophils.

The effects of acute gastritis are those of 'indigestion' with mild to severe abdominal pain. There may be haematemesis and usually the patient will refuse food. The stomach most frequently returns to normal with resolution of the inflammation and regeneration of the damaged mucosa. Occasionally, very severe acute gastritis ('phlegmonous gastritis' where the inflammation is very severe and extends down into the muscle coats) may lead to death and in certain cases of acute gastritis there may be a progression to chronic gastritis with peptic ulceration.

Chronic Gastritis

In chronic gastritis the inflammatory infiltrate consists of lymphocytes and macrophages and there may be several characteristic changes of the gastric mucosa, thus leading to the division of chronic gastritis into two main types.

Atrophic gastritis. This is an autoimmune disease and antibodies are found against the parietal cells. It is more common in females, its incidence increasing with increasing age. Familial/genetic factors also appear to be involved in its development. It should be noted that many patients who have evidence of this disease in a biopsy specimen will not experience any symptoms or signs, their disease being subclinical.

In advanced or severe cases of the disorder, the mucosa of the body of the stomach shows marked atrophy and thinning of the stomach wall, especially in the fundus, the mucosa becoming thin and losing its rugae. There is loss of the parietal cells and chief cells, resulting in **hypochlorhydria** or **achlorhydria** (little or no HCl secreted). The remaining mucus-secreting cells undergo hyperplasia and this change is termed **intestinal metaplasia**.

Atrophic gastritis and intestinal metaplasia may predispose to gastric cancer. People with chronic atrophic gastritis have 5 to 10 times the risk of developing gastric carcinoma when compared with the normal individual. Iron deficiency anaemia or pernicious anaemia may occur due to loss of intrinsic factor, normally secreted by the gastric mucosa. The disease may respond to corticosteroid therapy, and often dietary supplements of vitamin B_{12} and iron may be needed. Alcohol and erosive analgesics should be forbidden as they aggravate the condition.

Hypertrophic gastritis. This condition may be seen in alcoholics, or after repeated attacks of acute gastritis, or in *Helicobacter pylori* gastritis. In this case, the wall of the stomach is thickened with associated thickening of the gastric mucosa. There may be excessive mucus secretion and lymphoid follicles often develop in the deeper layers of the stomach wall. The disorder may have variable effects on the function of the stomach: no change may be seen with normal acid levels secreted, or alternatively hyperchlorhydria (excessive acid secretion) or achlorhydria (no acid secretion) may be observed.

Peptic Ulceration

A **peptic ulcer** is a benign, localized defect consisting of a deep excavation of any part of the gastrointestinal tract mucosa that is in contact with acid and pepsin. The defect extends beyond the muscularis mucosae, which is contrary to the shallower and more superficial **erosions**, the latter not extending beyond the muscularis mucosae (see Figure 8.6). Sites of occurrence of peptic ulcers are the duodenum mainly, stomach frequently, and sometimes the lower oesophagus. Rarely, other sites may be involved, for example the jejunum in the case of patients who have had a gastrojejunustomy operation (attachment of the stomach to the jejunum after removal of part of the small intestine), these ulcers being referred to as stomal ulcers. There is also the occurrence of peptic ulcers in association with Meckel's diverticulum which very frequently possesses fully functional gastric mucosa in its wall as a choristoma. In this case, a peptic ulcer may occur in the ileum.

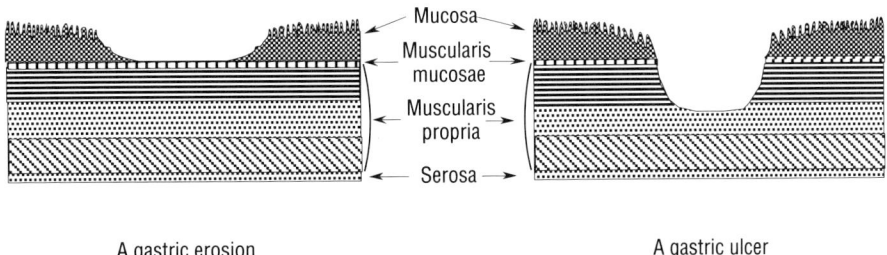

A gastric erosion   A gastric ulcer

Figure 8.6 *Comparison of gastric erosions and ulcers*

Acute Peptic Ulcers

This type of peptic ulceration does not frequently present clinically, most cases remaining subclinical or most patients attributing the symptoms they experience to 'indigestion', putting up with the often transient and self-limiting 'stomach ache'. However, acute peptic ulcers may produce very severe symptoms and the person is then forced to seek medical advice. Most acute peptic ulcers occur in young adults. The site most frequently affected is the stomach, sometimes the duodenum.

The causes of acute peptic ulceration are varied and by far the commonest aetiology is due to ingested substances which irritate and injure the stomach mucosa directly. Aspirin and alcohol are the most frequent offenders in this group. Some acute ulcers are associated with severe burns (Curling's ulcer), others with cerebral haemorrhages, steroid therapy, pituitary tumours (Cushing's ulcer) or uraemia. Mostly, the causes are unknown. The patients usually present with considerable pain in the epigastric region and they may bring up blood-stained vomitus or blood depending on the severity of the ulceration.

Single or multiple gastric ulcers may be present, beginning as only surface erosions, which then become deeper to form typical ulcers. Any region of the stomach or duodenum may be affected. Surrounding the ulcers are zones of acute inflammation. Most of these ulcers heal without much scarring (unless the ulcer is very deep), with the mucosa regenerating quite rapidly to cover the defect. Occasionally with large, deep or multiple ulcers the patient may present with haematemesis, perforation of the ulcer through the stomach wall or through an artery, peritoneal involvement (a sterile peritonitis is seen due to the injurious effects of stomach acid) and occasionally a severe gastric or peritoneal haemorrhage may cause shock or death.

Chronic Peptic Ulcers

Incidence. Approximately 10% of the adult population have or have had a peptic ulcer at some stage. It is uncommon below the age of 25 years, most commonly seen between the ages of 30 to 45 years. It affects males three times as commonly as females (M:F = 3:1). In Australia, gastric ulcers are more prevalent in women than men. (See Figure 8.7.)

Aetiology. Peptic ulcers form due to imbalances between the pepsin and acid on the one hand and mucosal protective factors on the other. The aetiology of the condition is associated with a variety of factors which have been shown to be important statistically.

- Greatly at risk are those with **hypersecretion of acid**. This may be due to a variety of causes and appears to be a very important factor in the development of the ulcer. Increased secretion of acid is seen in the **Zollinger-Ellison syndrome** where a pancreatic tumour is secreting great quantities of gastrin which stimulate acid secretion by the stomach mucosa. Intractable peptic ulcers form in this condition. Another important factor in the development of peptic ulcers is **neurogenic stimulation** of hypersecretion of acid. This may be important in situations of **stress**, and in the laboratory, stress ulcers may be induced in animals. However, there is no convincing evidence that there is any higher incidence in people of different personality types or that the disease is confined to the 'stressed, fast-living, business executive', patients often being in the lower socioeconomic groups.
- The mucosal **protective factors** greatly depend on a good blood supply to the mucosa with production of adequate quantities of mucus. If there is direct injury to the mucosa or if there is vascular disease present, reduced mucus production results, with an appearance of an increased incidence in peptic ulceration.
- Studies have shown that **diet** is not an important factor in the development of the disease and the only association between ulcers and diet seems to be the discomfort the patient with the condition may feel after consuming a certain food. This is an individual matter and patients know which foods to avoid.
- **Cigarette smoking** greatly predisposes to the condition.
- **Genetic factors** are very important and it appears that many cases of peptic ulceration **run in families** with concordance in twin studies. There is a slightly higher incidence of chronic peptic ulcers in subjects with **blood group O**.

Sites affected. Peptic ulceration is now more prevalent in the region of the duodenum (73% of cases), followed by the stomach (25% of cases), the remaining number of cases being seen in other parts of the gastrointestinal tract (e.g. lower oesophageal and stomal ulcers). In the duodenum they may be found on the anterior or posterior wall, very frequently in both situations, forming the so-called 'kissing ulcers'. In the stomach, the ulcers are most frequently found astride the lesser curvature.

Morphology. The ulcers are large, round or oval, 'punched out' deficiencies in the wall of the stomach, extending beyond the muscularis mucosae for a considerable depth. They have a straight wall and the mucosa around the ulcer is not greatly raised as around a malignant 'ulcer cancer'. They are usually less than 3 cm in diameter, although occasionally they may be larger. The floor of the ulcer is smooth, showing perhaps some evidence of necrosis or haemorrhage. The lesion is indurated due to the deposition of fibro-collagenous scar tissue (Figure 8.8).

The microscopic appearance of the ulcer is quite characteristic and shows a base with a superficial necrotic layer often with haemorrhagic areas and damaged blood vessels which may be thrombotic. Beneath this there is an active, non-specific acute inflammatory response with granulation tissue formation. Underlying this is a region of dense collagenous scar tissue. The scar tissue often extends up the walls of the ulcer and deep down into the muscular layer, or even to the serosa.

Signs and symptoms. Chronic peptic ulcer patients often present with **dyspepsia** (uncomfortable fullness after meals, with nausea, heartburn, belching and often abdominal distention). The patients with gastric ulcer complain of a **gnawing pain** in the left upper quadrant of the abdomen or epigastric area, 1 to 3 hours after meals and they will often describe it as a burning feeling which is relieved by food or antacids. Abdominal pain due to duodenal ulcer is a steady, aching pain (often compared to hunger pangs) which occurs high in the mid-epigastrium or slightly off centre to the right. It usually does not radiate backwards unless penetration and pancreatic involvement occur. The pain begins 2–4 hours after meals and may wake the patient

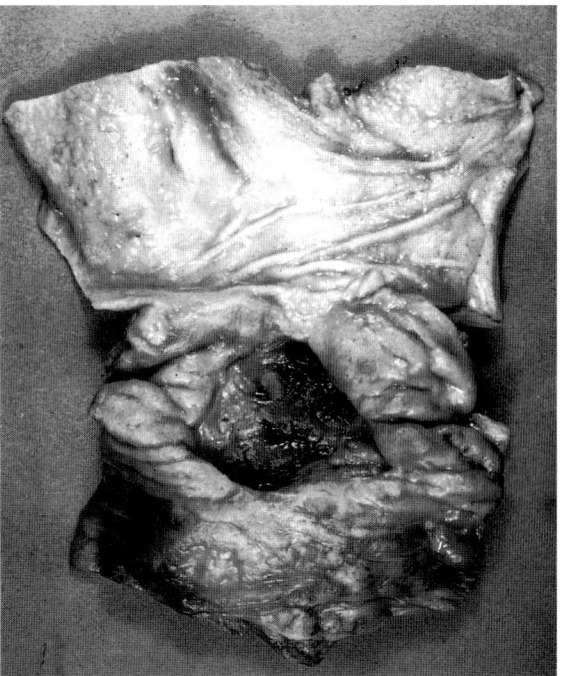

Figure 8.8 *Chronic duodenal ulcer in a 75-year-old male*

at night. It is relieved by food or antacids and the patient may present with weight gain. A **succussion splash** (a splashing sound over a hollow organ) may be auscultated over the epigastrium and this finding often indicates obstruction. **Vomiting** may be seen,

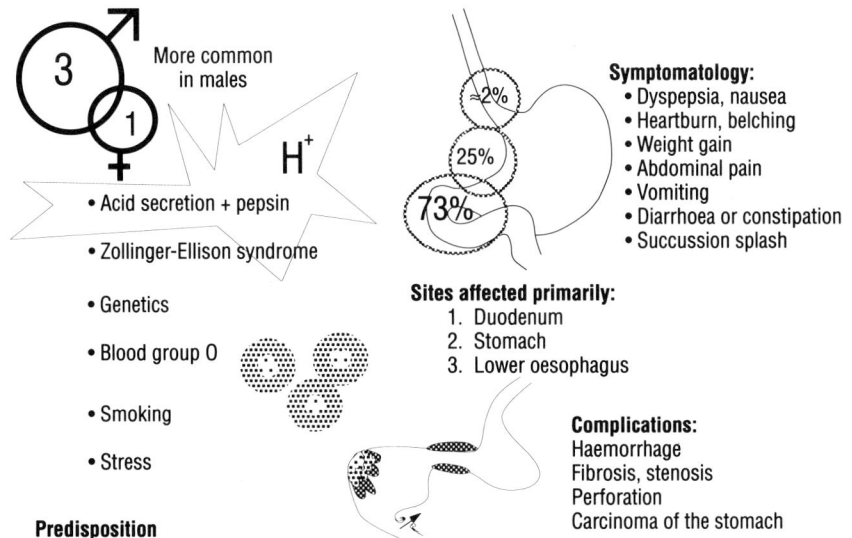

Figure 8.7 *Pathology of chronic peptic ulcer*

associated with severe pain or obstruction. **Diarrhoea** or **constipation** may occur in association with excessive antacid consumption. About 25% of patients will show very severe symptoms, 50% show moderate symptoms and 25% show minimal symptoms.

Diagnosis. Presumptive diagnosis depends largely on clinical findings. Diagnostic X-rays are taken for confirmation while the patient swallows a barium meal. This procedure will outline the ulcer niche in the stomach. A radiologist can generally distinguish with 95% efficiency whether a benign ulcer or an ulcerating carcinoma is present in the stomach. A biopsy may be taken via an endoscope while the patient is lightly anaesthetized. Histology of the biopsy will determine whether the ulcer is malignant. Occasionally, gastric secretion studies may be required, especially if the Zollinger-Ellison syndrome is suspected. For duodenal ulcers, the X-ray plates will show deformity of the duodenum due to stenosis by fibrosis, with duodenoscopy indicated.

Results and complications. The majority of peptic ulcers **heal** with only bed rest and approximately only 15% of them fail to do so. However, a large number of them recur, with 50% of cases showing recurrence within 3 years. Healing of the ulcer is by scarring and re-epithelialization, the mucosa above the healed area often puckered up into a star-shaped region. Stenosis of the stomach or duodenum may result as a consequence of the extensive scarring and contraction around the healed ulcer. Often, a large ulcer may extend quite deeply into the muscularis propria and erode through large arteries or perforate through the entire thickness of the wall of the stomach. In summary:

- **haemorrhage** may occur if a vessel is eroded, patients presenting with **haematemesis** or **melaena**, in the case of a major haemorrhage, they may go into **shock**;
- **penetration** of the stomach wall with **perforation** may occur, the sudden exit of the acid stomach contents into the peritoneal cavity causing acute, severe abdominal pain, vomiting and shock;
- **sterile peritonitis**, associated with perforation and chemical injury due to acid may occur;
- **scarring**, **stenosis** may occur in the parapyloric region of the stomach ('hour glass stomach', fibrous tissue constricting the stomach into two halves), or in the duodenum;
- **malignancy** may supervene ('ulcer cancer', only in stomach or oesophageal ulcers).

Treatment and prognosis. The majority of peptic ulcers heal when the patient is admitted to hospital or rests. Some drug therapy may also be instituted, which not only provides relief of symptoms but also promotes healing of the ulcer. The drugs prescribed include **cimetidine**, which is a histamine antagonist, preventing histamine stimulation of acid secretion, and **colloidal bismuth**, which promotes healing by undetermined mechanisms. Carbenoxolone sodium and aluminium antacids may also be used in some cases. Generally, the prognosis of peptic ulcer disease is very good with such treatments alone.

As there may be recurrence in 50% of cases within 3 years and 75% of cases within 5 years, sometimes the recommended treatment is surgical, especially in the 'high risk patient' (such as seamen, for example, who are often away on long voyages and the complications of the peptic ulcer may cause death on board). Surgery is also recommended for ulcers complicated by stenosis, strictures, gross haemorrhage, suspected malignancy, etc. Several surgical procedures are carried out, from the simple dilatation of strictures, to partial or complete resections of the stomach or upper duodenum. Denervation of the stomach may be performed with partial vagotomy, a procedure which reduces the amount of acid secreted by the mucosa.

Carcinoma of the Stomach

Incidence. Gastric carcinoma is a common cancer, causing approximately 10% of all cancer deaths. However, the general incidence of this cancer has been decreasing, an effect thought to be due to changes in diet. It is rare below the age of 30 years, most commonly seen between the ages of 55 to 65 years. It affects males twice as commonly as females (M:F = 2:1).

Aetiology. The aetiology of the tumour is associated with a variety of factors and conditions which have been shown to be important statistically.

- Greatly at risk are those with **pernicious anaemia**, hence the patient suffering from atrophic gastritis is at risk. The Plummer-Vinson syndrome predisposes females to this cancer.
- Carcinogenic foods. Numerous studies have shown that **diet** is an important factor in this disease and those who consume smoked foods, preserved meats and pickled foods are at risk.
- **Chronic gastritis** of long duration may progress to the carcinoma, hence association with chronic gastritis (atrophic or hypertrophic), **benign chronic ulcers** (5–10% of gastric cancer is associated with this), metaplastic and dysplastic changes.

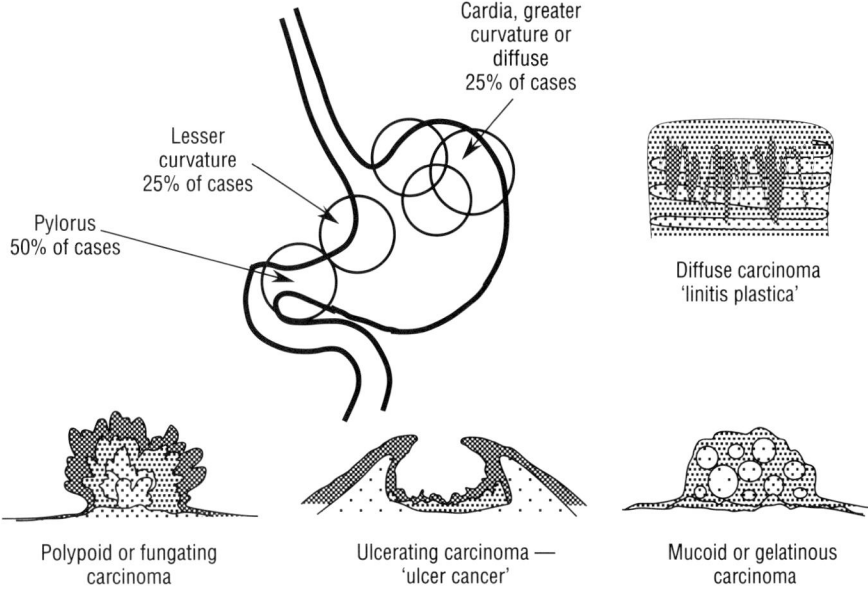

Figure 8.9 *Carcinoma of the stomach*

- **Genetic factors** are important as studies show that the tumour is slightly more prevalent in people with **blood group A**.
- **Benign tumours** (papillomata, adenomata) predispose to the malignancy.
- **Geographical**, **racial factors** are important as the tumour has a higher incidence in **Japan**, Finland, Iceland, Austria and Chile. The tumour has a relatively low incidence in Australia, the USA, UK and Canada. These effects are thought to relate to dietary factors.

Sites affected. The tumour occurs primarily in the region of the pylorus (50% of cases), followed by the mucosa of the lesser curvature (25% of cases), the remaining number of cases being seen in other parts of the stomach but also diffusely throughout the whole organ (see Figure 8.9).

Morphology. The macroscopic appearance of carcinoma of the stomach is very variable and commonly seen are nodular growths arising from the mucosa and which frequently ulcerate to give rise to the 'ulcer cancer'. Polypoid or fungating masses may also ulcerate and occasionally some adenocarcinomata produce large quantities of mucus, giving rise to the 'gelatinous' or 'mucoid' forms. Some types of the tumour grow very rapidly into and along the mucosa, invading into the wall and beyond the serosa, involving the wall of the whole organ very quickly. This last-mentioned type is the **linitis plastica** variant of the neoplasm which thickens and contracts the wall of the stomach, giving rise to the sobriquet 'leather bottle stomach'.

Microscopically, the tumours are typically adenocarcinomata of varying degrees of differentiation. Spheroidal cell carcinomata and papillary carcinomata may be seen, while a small number are squamous cell carcinomata, in which case they arise out of regions of squamous metaplasia of the gastric mucosa. Highly malignant tumours may be anaplastic carcinomata and these are usually very aggressive, spreading extensively quite early.

Spread. Spread of this carcinoma occurs directly to involve the mucosa and stomach wall, rapidly invading into the serosa. The coeliac and other abdominal lymph nodes are affected rather early in the course of the condition by lymphatic spread and the cervical and mediastinal nodes also contain the tumour in many cases. As the tumour invades past the serosa, transcoelomic spread occurs with seeds of tumour lodging and growing in the omentum, the peritoneal wall and abdominal organs. In females, the ovaries are commonly involved and the stomach cancer secondaries in the ovary are termed **Krukenberg tumours**. Blood spread also tends to occur early, especially to the liver, but also to the lungs and bones, forming secondaries in these organs.

Signs and symptoms. Cancer of the stomach gives no reliable early warning symptoms and in Japan where the cancer has a high incidence people often choose to have routine gastroscopies in order to diagnose the tumour, if it is present, at an early stage. The patients with stomach cancer may complain of a gradual onset of deterioration of appetite with a slow weight loss. They may experience irregular and mild upper abdominal discomfort or pain (usually they call this 'indigestion'). Later on there may be haematemesis (vomiting of blood-stained material) and also there may be blood detected in the faeces (melaena), with resulting anaemia. The patient may experience nausea and may vomit. Abdominal swelling and ascites suggest liver secondaries while epigastric pain which often radiates to the back frequently implies that there is pancreatic involvement.

Diagnosis. Diagnostic X-rays are taken while the patient swallows a barium meal. This is usually sufficient to distinguish between stomach carcinoma and benign peptic ulceration in the duodenum, which often produces similar symptoms. If an ulcer is seen in the stomach or if cancer is suspected, a biopsy is taken via a gastroscope while the patient is lightly anaesthetized. Histology will determine not only whether the tumour is truly malignant but what histological type it is and how well differentiated it is.

Treatment and prognosis. The only effective treatment for carcinoma of the stomach is surgical excision; however, more than 50% of stomach cancers are inoperable at diagnosis. Depending on the extent of spread of the tumour and involvement of surrounding tissues, the whole stomach, the spleen and a portion of the duodenum may need to be removed (= complete gastrectomy). With smaller tumours which have not spread far, only a partial gastrectomy is carried out. Radiotherapy and chemotherapy are ineffective and not frequently used in treatment, although they may be the only recourse in advanced cases.

When patients have been treated by complete gastrectomy, they will not be able to eat large meals, but rather many small meals; there may be difficulties with vitamin absorption, and in particular vitamin B_{12}, with pernicious anaemia resulting from that deficiency. Carbohydrates may also be more difficult to digest. The tumour has a very poor prognosis, even in operable cases, with a 5-year survival of around 10%. The patients usually die of widespread metastatic disease and malignant cachexia.

Other Malignancies of the Stomach

There are many other types of malignancies which may arise in the stomach but these are very rare. A few typical examples are **fibrosarcoma**, **leiomyosarcoma** and **neurofibrosarcoma**, all of which produce fungating masses and are associated with a very poor prognosis. Slightly better in prognosis is **lymphosarcoma** (which is a diffuse, locally invasive malignancy), as this tumour responds rather well to chemotherapy and radiotherapy.

Diseases of the Small Intestine

Diverticula

Diverticula are outpouchings in the walls of tubular organs, commonly occurring in the intestines. They may be **true diverticula**, which are most commonly congenital anomalies and the wall of which contains all layers of the gut wall, or **false diverticula** in which case they are usually acquired and the pouch wall contains only the mucosal layer which herniates through a weakness in the muscularis propria (refer to Figure 8.10).

Meckel's diverticulum is the most common congenital anomaly of the gastrointestinal tract, found in 2–3% of the population and arising from persistence of the proximal end of the omphalomesenteric (vitellointestinal) duct. It is a solitary, true diverticulum usually within 60 cm of the ileocaecal valve. It varies in appearance from a fibrotic cord to a pouch with a lumen larger than the ileum and up to 6 cm in length. The wall of the diverticulum is like that of the small bowel. However, it is usual for the wall of the diverticulum to contain nests of fully functional gastric or colonic mucosa or even pancreatic tissue with exocrine and endocrine portions. These rests of foreign tissues are examples of typical choristomata.

In the majority of people with Meckel's diverticulum, the condition produces no symptoms, often presenting as an incidental finding in a laparoscopy or at an autopsy. Complications include severe haemorrhage *per rectum,* associated with **peptic ulceration** in the diverticulum due to the presence of acid-secreting gastric mucosa. There may be progression to perforation with adhesions, internal haemorrhage or peritonitis commonly complicating such diverticular ulcers. The symptoms resemble those of appendicitis but the pain is often in the left, lower abdominal quadrant. The diverticulum may be the site where **intussusception** begins and **diverticulitis** may also be present.

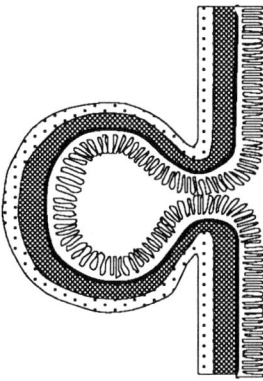

True diverticulum
Contains all layers of the
gut wall, usually congenital

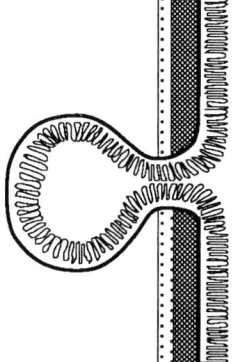

False diverticulum
Contains only mucosal layer
herniating through muscle,
usually acquired

Figure 8.10   *True and false intestinal diverticula*

Duodenal diverticula are also congenital, occurring rather rarely. These pouches also contain all layers of the small bowel wall and are thus another example of true diverticula. Usually, they are asymptomatic as the intestinal contents are fluid, but occasionally an **enterolith** (bowel stone) may form due to inspissation of bowel contents. This may cause obstruction if extruded into the bowel.

In **diverticulosis/diverticulitis**, a condition which is often referred to as 'diverticular disease', multiple false diverticula form in the bowel. In the small bowel, the commonest are jejunal diverticula which are solitary or few in number and mostly symptomless. Occasionally they are numerous and cause malabsorption, with B_{12} deficiency anaemia rarely. Diverticulosis refers to the presence of diverticula without clinical symptoms and signs, whereas, diverticulitis refers to the presence of inflamed diverticula, the patient presenting with clinical disease.

The symptomatic cases are often associated with diverticula that are confined to one small loop of bowel and these patients present with the so-called '**stagnant loop syndrome**', symptoms and signs of which include abdominal pain, diarrhoea, steatorrhoea, haemorrhage *per rectum,* megaloblastic anaemia and nutritional deficiencies. In this case, surgical treatment may be undertaken, which is highly successful as the affected loop of bowel is resected. In most cases of diverticulitis, however, the diverticula are scattered throughout the bowel and treatment is mainly supportive and centres on antibiosis.

Volvulus

Volvulus is the twisting or rotation of a loop of bowel and mesentery through at least 180°, resulting in vascular obstruction which may then progress to gangrene of the bowel (see Figure 8.11). Rarely, two loops of bowel may twist about one another bringing about the same effect. The condition may develop if there is a congenital, incomplete attachment of the mesentery, and in this case, the whole of the small bowel undergoes torsion, a condition known as **volvulus neonatorum**. The neonate will then rapidly die unless immediate surgery corrects the condition and secures the intestines.

Alternatively, and more commonly, the disorder develops in the sigmoid colon and small intestine when there is heavy loading of the intestines with faeces or food. It is also more likely to occur if there are fibrous adhesions (as occur after bowel surgery) or calcified lymph nodes in the mesentery. It is slightly more common in children and presents as a typical 'acute abdomen', with abdominal pain which may be severe, abdominal tenderness and distension.

The effects of volvulus are mainly vascular, with intestinal obstruction and bowel lumen obliteration of secondary importance. As the loops of bowel twist about themselves, the blood vessels in the mesentery will also be strangulated. The veins are primarily affected and phlebothrombosis may supervene within the twisted veins. If the condition is not treated promptly, the arteries will also be obliterated and the

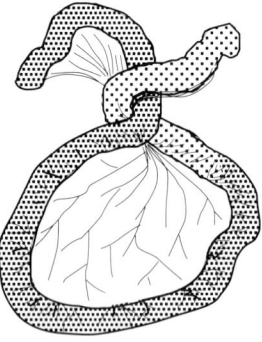

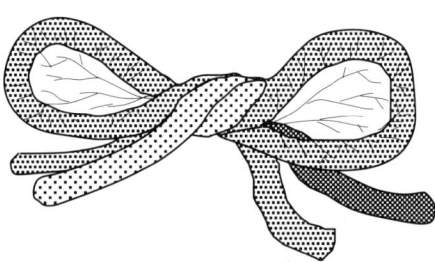

Single loop of bowel   Two loops of bowel

Figure 8.11   *Volvulus with associated ileus*

bowel undergoes septic infarction. The affected parts of the bowel are plum coloured and show extensive haemorrhages, these changes sharply confined to the segment involved in the torsion. Gangrene, perforation of the bowel, peritonitis and peritoneal haemorrhage will then occur, and unless emergency surgery is carried out the death of the patient is inevitable.

Intussusception

This is the invagination of one portion of the intestine into the lumen of the bowel immediately distal to it (a 'telescoping' effect, illustrated in Figures 8.12 and 8.13). The apex of the entering layer, called the intussusceptum, passes down the intestinal lumen, dragging mesentery and its vessels with it, being ensheathed by another layer of bowel, called the intussuscipiens. A sausage-shaped mass of intestine forms and causes obstruction and important vascular effects as blood vessels in the trapped mesentery are occluded.

Causes of the condition depend on the age of the patient. For example, a form of intussusception occurs in babies and infants and seems to be idiopathic, although in a number of cases a change of diet seems to have triggered off the disorder. In children, the condition is frequently associated with intestinal infections which cause a lymphadenitis of the mesenteric lymph nodes. The swollen lymph nodes act as points around which the intestine pivots and peristaltic waves propel the nodes into the portion of bowel distal to them, initiating the process of intussusception. Sometimes a Meckel's diverticulum may invert into the intestinal lumen and act as the apex of the intussusceptum. Tumours of the bowel wall are the most frequent cause of intussusception in adults and in this case it is the

tumour mass which initiates the vigorous peristalsis which carries the mass and intestine wall into the lumen.

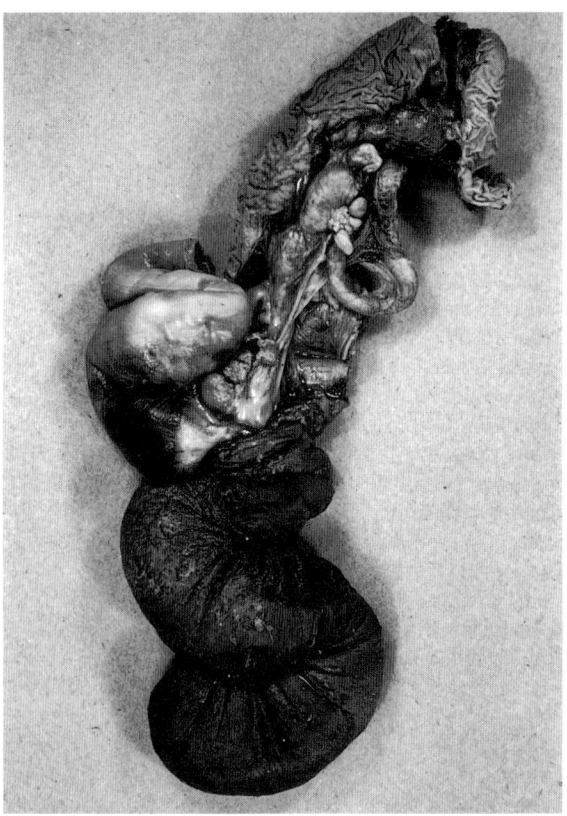

Figure 8.12   *Intussusception of the small bowel in a 14-year-old male*

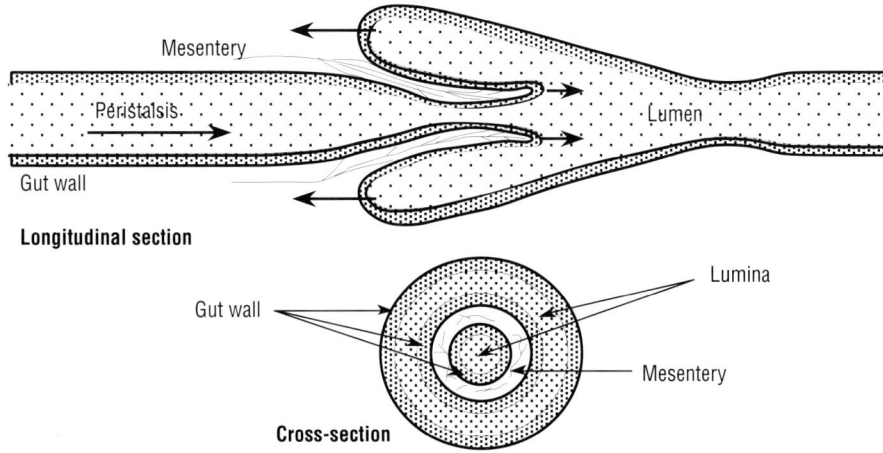

Mesentery

Peristalsis

Lumen

Gut wall

Longitudinal section

Lumina

Gut wall

Mesentery

Cross-section

Figure 8.13 *Intussusception*

The condition is most often seen at the region of the ileocaecal valve and it is occurs more in children. The major complications and effects of intussusception are obstruction and vascular occlusion, with clinical effects and sequelae very similar to those discussed already with volvulus.

Ileus

Ileus is intestinal obstruction due to any cause, including those discussed already above under volvulus and intussusception. Intestinal obstruction may occur because of intraluminal masses such as gall stones, **enteroliths** ('intestinal stones' formed by inspissation of intestinal contents), swallowed foreign objects and also as a result of **cystic fibrosis**. In this last-mentioned case the intestinal obstruction is known as **meconium ileus** and develops in the first or second day after birth, the affected neonate failing to produce faeces in this time. The intestines are obstructed by meconium (thick viscous mucus, amniotic fluid, epithelial cells, bile pigment and debris), usually close to the ileocaecal valve.

Alternatively, the obstruction is caused by lesions in the wall of the intestine, such as inflammatory disease, diverticulosis, tumours and intussusception. Lastly, external factors may cause compression of the intestine from the outside as, for example, occurs with volvulus, bands and adhesions of fibrous tissue, herniations, external tumours compressing the gut and neuromuscular disorders. In the last-mentioned case **paralytic ileus** is said to occur, in which the obstruction is seen without any mechanical defect demonstr-

able. This is caused by peritonitis, severe abdominal trauma, vascular disease (obstruction of the superior mesenteric artery or vein) or neuromuscular dysfunction.

Regional Ileitis (Crohn's Disease)

This is a relapsing–remitting, chronic granulomatous inflammatory disorder of the alimentary tract of worldwide incidence. It may occur anywhere in the alimentary tract and therefore it is termed regional enteritis, regional gastritis, regional colitis, or simply Crohn's disease, the last term describing its occurrence in any site.

Incidence. This is a common disease which appears to be increasing in incidence. The male to female incidence ratio is 1:1.6, and the disease is primarily seen in young adults. Approximately one to five people per 100 000 population are affected.

Aetiology. Crohn's disease is an idiopathic disease but various theories about its cause have been proposed and statistical data have been provided in their support. It is possible that the disease is due to a multifactorial aetiology. In approximately 5–10% of cases the disorder has a genetic/familial association and it is possible that certain HLA antigenic types (e.g. some studies implicate HLA A2, others HLA B27) predispose towards the development of the disease by contributing to allergic/autoimmune-type reactions. If ulcerative colitis is also included in the statistical data, it is apparent that patients with Crohn's disease have a familial association in as many as 40% of cases. Other studies have shown that psychological factors may be important and aggravation of the disease may be psychosomatic. Other researchers have prepared homogenates from intestine with Crohn's disease and have shown in many cases that an infective agent may be involved. Autoimmunity may be a very strong candidate as the prime damaging agent in the disease as dysfunction in the natural killer cell activity can be demonstrated in patients with the disorder.

Sites affected. Although any part of the gastrointestinal tract may be affected the disease is most commonly observed in the terminal ileum (regional ileitis), followed by the colon (regional colitis), with involvement of the jejunum sometimes seen (regional jejunitis) or rarely the stomach (regional gastritis). In some patients the intestinal involvement is associated with inflammation of joints, eyes, skin and liver, further incriminating autoimmunity as a possible pathogenetic mechanism. In the colon, the disease is similar in presentation to idiopathic ulcerative colitis and it is sometimes difficult to differentiate the two disorders clinically.

Morphology. Crohn's disease is characterized by segmental areas of involvement which are abruptly demarcated from contiguous normal gut, the affected regions often referred to as 'skip lesions' (see Figure 8.14). In 80% of cases the terminal ileum is involved, often with more lesions in the upper intestine. In all sites of involvement the wall is thickened and inflexible and likened to a 'rubber hose'. The inflammation is transmural and granulomata form in approximately 60–75% of cases, these lesions developing in the gut wall, lymph nodes, mesentery and anal region. The

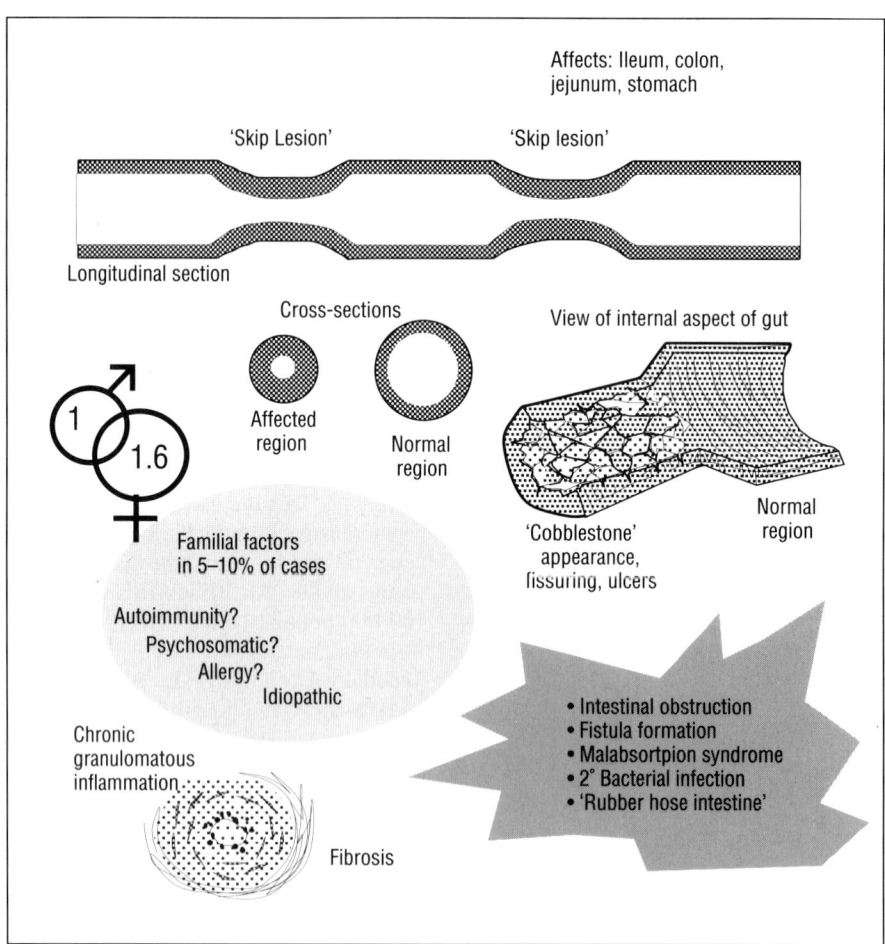

Figure 8.14 *Pathology of Crohn's disease*

chronic inflammatory cell infiltrate is most concentrated in the submucosal regions of the affected portion of the intestine. There may be oedema due to lymphatic obstruction. Fibrosis of the wall becomes more prominent as the disease progresses. The lumen is narrowed and there may be ileus. There are varying degrees of mucosal ulceration and fissure formation with which are associated foci of secondary infection and suppuration (Figure 8.15).

Course and complications. The first attack usually occurs between the ages of 20–30 years. The disease then progresses and may present acutely or insidiously but the characteristic features of transmural, chronic inflammatory, 'skip lesions' inexorably develop. In a small number of cases the lesions may regress and the disease goes into permanent remission. More frequently, however, although some of the lesions may regress, others develop at other sites, at irregular time intervals. Lesions progress, coalesce and give rise to the 'rubber hose' intestine. Adhesions form in association with the affected regions of intestine and these, together with the thickened wall, lead to obstruction of the intestine. Linked with the transmural inflammation and tissue damage, fissures develop in the mucosa and are complicated by secondary infection, the whole luminal aspect of the affected region resembling a 'cobblestone' pavement. Fistula formation is a common complication in advanced, severe cases and the abnormal communications develop between ileum and colon, ileum and exterior or between different loops of the ileum. Abscesses may form and involve the fistulae. Rarely haemorrhage and perforation of the gut occur. In the late stages of the disease where considerable regions of small intestine are involved, the malabsorption syndrome develops and thus in this case, malnutrition may cause death.

Extraintestinal complications include eye disease such as episcleritis, iritis or uveitis, arthritis in medium sized joints and erythema nodosum in the skin, secondary amyloidosis, ankylosing spondylitis, various renal disorders including urolithiasis and urinary tract infections, pericholangitis, cholangitis and cirrhosis of the liver.

Signs and symptoms. Most patients ($\approx$75%) present with abdominal pain and slight fever. Intermittent diarrhoea and weight loss are also commonly encountered. In most cases the disease onset is insidious, but less commonly an acute onset may mimic appendicitis, especially if the caecum is involved. A tender abdominal mass, usually in the right, lower quadrant of the abdomen is found in 33% of patients. Recurrent

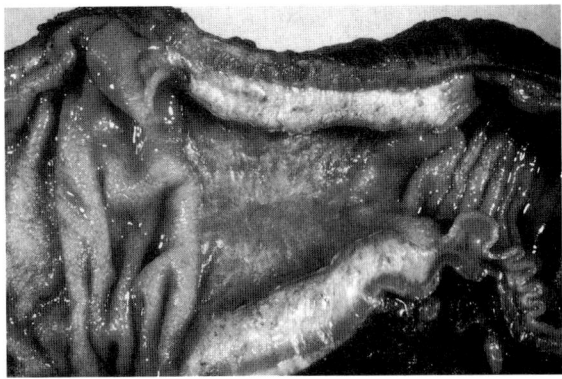

Figure 8.15 *Crohn's disease of the sigmoid colon. The affected parts of the intestine are thickened and rigid*

anorectal fistulae may also be a sign of the disease as is sometimes steatorrhoea.

Diagnosis. Clinical symptomatology may be indicative of the disease and further laboratory tests that aid in diagnosing it are: a raised ESR and leukocytosis due to infection, anaemia due to blood loss and vitamin B_{12} deficiency. Endoscopic biopsy may confirm the diagnosis but it may also prove to be negative in a patient with Crohn's disease as the lesions are patchy and may be missed. Barium enema and a barium small bowel series will not only prove to be diagnostically useful but also indicate the extent of involvement of intestine, the sites affected and the degree of obstruction present.

Treatment and prognosis. The disease is treated rather conservatively at first, with bed rest to settle acute episodes and antibiotics to control the secondary infections. Corticosteroids may also prove useful in managing the acute phase but prove useless in the long term. The disease may then regress but when it relapses the same treatment may prove inadequate to control its progression. Vitamin B_{12} supplementation is required in extensive ileal involvement, parenteral feeding may be given and in the complex, extensive cases the only option may be surgery, which sometimes requires a colostomy to be performed. Surgery is usually required by over half the patients at some stage of their disease but it does not protect the patient from recurrence of the disease, even if all of the diseased segment was removed at the initial operation. It should be noted that Crohn's disease of the large bowel is a premalignant lesion and patients with the chronic disease have a risk of developing carcinoma that is three times the risk of the normal subject.

Malabsorption Syndrome (and Steatorrhoea)

This syndrome is associated with poor absorption, from the intestine, of foodstuffs and products of their digestion. Particularly important are minerals, vitamins, salts, protein and fat. The disorder is observed as a complication of other diseases of the intestine and the patient presents with many signs and symptoms reflective of multiple dietary deficiencies (Table 8.1).

Causes of the syndrome include mucosal disease as is seen in Crohn's disease, TB, amyloidosis and diffuse villous atrophy of the intestine, autoimmune diseases, for example Whipple's disease and hypersensitivities, a typical example of the last being gluten enteropathy. Alternatively, pancreatic and biliary disease may cause malabsorption as occurs with biliary obstruction or pancreatitis. Occasionally infections and infestations may cause the syndrome as is seen with the parasitoses or tropical sprue. Drug-induced causes

for the syndrome may also be quoted, as is the case with laxative abuse, neomycin treatment or colchicine administration.

The clinical features of the syndrome depend very much on which substances are not absorbed but the commonest presenting symptom is chronic diarrhoea. The patient may suffer from malnutrition and appear very thin and wasted, while small children or infants may fail to thrive. There may be atrophy of muscles, oedema and ascites, hypotension, dehydration and manifestation of vitamin deficiencies such as anaemia, haemorrhagic diatheses, skin and eye changes, etc. Failure of fat absorption results in pale, bulky, greasy, offensive stools, known as **steatorrhoea**.

Treatment of the condition depends very much on the underlying cause and if this cause can be treated, the secondary malabsorption will regress (as occurs after drug treatments for a parasitosis, or surgery for biliary anomalies). Often, however, the cause may be impossible to treat adequately (e.g. Crohn's disease,

Table 8.1   *The malabsorption syndrome*

Substance malabsorbed	Effect/disorder noted
Fats	• Steatorrhoea
Proteins	• Loss of weight • Muscle wasting, atrophy • Hypoproteinaemia, oedema, ascites • Osteoporosis
Calcium and vitamin D	• Rickets (in infants and children) • Osteomalacia (in adults) • Hypocalcaemia, tetany

Vitamins
  Vitamin A
  Vitamin B$_1$ (thiamine)
  Niacin (nicotinic acid)
  Vitamin B$_2$ (riboflavin)
  Vitamin B$_{12}$ (cobalamin)
  Vitamin C (ascorbic acid)
  Vitamin K
	
	• Skin changes, infections, eye opacities
	• Beriberi (CNS, GIT, CVS disorders)
	• Pellagra (CNS, muscular, skin disorders)
	• Skin changes, cheilosis, mental changes
	• Anaemia, peripheral nerve damage, paralysis
	• Scurvy (poor wound healing, haemorrhages)
	• Haemorrhages

Minerals
  Potassium
  Iron
  Magnesium
  Manganese
  Iodine
  Copper
	
	• Hypokalaemia
	• Anaemia
	• Tetany, increased irritability of nerves
	• Testicular atrophy
	• Hypothyroidism, myxoedema
	• Anaemia

villous atrophy) and the effects of the malabsorption may need to be alleviated through dietary supplementation or parenteral feeding.

Intestinal Infections

Infections of the intestine are commonly seen and present as a typical attack of gastroenteritis, which may vary in severity from almost subclinical to fatal disease. Protozoa, fungi, bacteria and viruses may cause these conditions. A typical example of intestinal infection caused by protozoa is **amoebic dysentery** (or sometimes referred to as specific ulcerative colitis) where numerous ulcers form in association with the colonization of mucosa and submucosa of the colon by *Entamoeba histolytica* which is ingested in contaminated food or drink (Figure 8.16). Bloody, mucous, diarrhoea is seen in this condition. **Giardiasis** caused by *Giardia lamblia* is an infestation of the duodenum and proximal small intestine, acquired after ingestion of contaminated food or water. It may be associated with diarrhoea and malabsorption.

Bacterial infections seen commonly include the following. **Typhoid fever** caused by *Salmonella typhi* is a very severe, or fatal, intestinal infection in which the bacteria invade the bloodstream and are found in numerous other body sites also. Diarrhoea, fever, severe abdominal pain, bowel haemorrhage and perforation may occur associated with other severe effects in other organs. 'Food poisoning' is in most cases a mild gastroenteritis associated with diarrhoea and abdominal pain, caused by many bacteria but very commonly by species of *Salmonella*, for example *S. typhimurium, S. enteritidis* and *S. newport*. Also, various so-called **enterotoxigenic** and **enteropathogenic** *Escherichia coli* (**ETEC, EPEC**) serotypes may cause such presentations. **Bacillary dysentery** is characterized by diarrhoea, blood and mucus in the stools and is caused by *Shigella dysenteriae, Shigella flexneri* and *Shigella sonnei*. The terminal ileum and colon are infected with mucosal necrosis and ulceration, without invasion of the bloodstream by the organisms. **Cholera** is a very severe gastroenteritis which is associated with necrosis and ulceration of bowel mucosa. The aetiological organism is *Vibrio cholerae*. Violent, watery diarrhoea ('rice water stools') is characteristic of the infection and toxaemia with electrolyte disturbances and dehydration often cause death.

Viral infections of the gastrointestinal tract are much more common than protozoal or bacterial infections in Western-type countries, and are often epidemic in nature. They affect infants and children especially, and usually are mild, characterized by diarrhoea, abdomi-

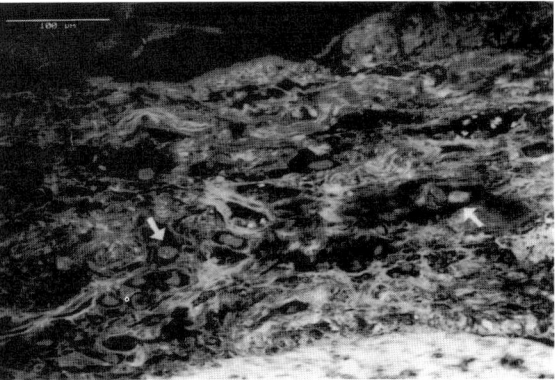

Figure 8.16 *Amoebic ulcerative colitis. The large cells of* Entamoeba histolytica *(arrow) are prominent in the exposed submucosa of the ulcerated regions (scale bar is 100 µm)*

nal tenderness or pain, perhaps fever and malaise. Typical aetiologies of these viral infections are **rotavirus** (especially in children < 5 years of age), the **Norwalk agent** (more so in older children and adults) and **rheovirus** of which numerous serotypes exist.

Small Intestine Tumours

Small intestinal tumours are very rare, constituting less than 2% of all intestinal tumours. Malignant tumours such as the primary lymphosarcoma are the least frequently seen and the tumours which are the most frequent, the carcinoid tumours, are either benign in behaviour, locally invasive or sometimes behave like malignant tumours and metastasize to the liver.

Carcinoid tumour (argentaffinoma). This is an uncommon tumour derived from the amine precursor uptake and decarboxylation (APUD) cells which have a local endocrine function in the intestine. These tumours are commonest in occurrence in the appendix where they are slowly growing and locally invasive, not metastasizing from that site usually. They may also occur in the ileum and rarely in the colon. In the ileum they are frequently multiple and although slow growing they are likely to metastasize. The tumour forms small button-like swellings in the mucosa which later may ulcerate and encircle the intestinal wall, having spread out to the serosa by the time of diagnosis. The tumours are yellow in colour as the cells contain large amounts of lipid in their cytoplasm.

As the tumours grow and increase in size they may

produce intestinal obstruction with symptoms such as a colicky abdominal pain, vomiting and diarrhoea. The neoplasms are treated by surgery and the prognosis is good if the tumour has not spread to the liver at the time of diagnosis. It should be noted, however, that even with metastasis many patients survive for 10 years or more as the tumours are very slowly growing.

The carcinoid syndrome. This develops if sufficient mass of carcinoid tumour is present in the body and usually occurs when there are liver metastases of ileal tumours present in a patient. The patient presents with flushing of the face (which may be associated with alcohol consumption), cyanosis, diarrhoea, ascites and oedema, bronchospasm (resembling an attack of asthma) and signs of pulmonary valve stenosis. These symptoms and signs are related to an excess of serotonin (5-hydroxytryptamine, 5-HT) secreted by the tumour cells. The 5-HT is a potent vasodilator and smooth muscle constrictor and mediates the effects seen in the patients. The pulmonary valve stenosis is due to fibrous thickening.

Patients with the carcinoid syndrome possess large quantities of 5-hydroxyindole acetic acid (5-HIAA) in their urine which is of diagnostic significance as the amount of this substance that they excrete is proportional to the amount of tumour they have in their body. Normal levels of 5-HIAA in the urine are 5–10 mg/24 hours, whereas in a patient with advanced disease the levels may be as high as 400 mg/24 hours. If testing for this substance in urine, the patient is put on a low serotonin diet (no tomatoes, walnuts, bananas, etc.) prior to the test.

It should be noted that the carcinoid syndrome will sometimes be seen in patients who have the rather rare tumours of the lungs known as bronchial adenomata, which are of the same cell origin as the intestinal tumours.

Diseases of the Vermiform Appendix

Acute Appendicitis

Acute appendicitis is a typical, acute inflammatory disorder of the appendix, a common disease that often presents as a surgical emergency. It is by far the commonest disorder of the vermiform appendix.

Incidence. It is a common disease that occurs at any age but is less frequent in infancy and advanced age. It tends to be more prevalent in young adults, with peak incidence at approximately 25 years of age. The sex

incidence is equal, and due to unknown reasons the disease seems to be declining in incidence.

Aetiology. The aetiology of the disease is essentially infectious, normal flora bacteria such as *Escherichia coli*, *Enterococcus faecalis* and β-haemolytic streptococci being very commonly isolated from cases. It is also known that obstruction of the appendix is a very important pathogenetic factor. Intraluminal obstructing bodies such as foreign bodies (swallowed indigestible objects), parasites (*Oxyuris* spp. etc.), faecoliths (inspissated and hardened faecal material) or alternatively swelling of the lymphoid tissue in the wall of the organ are often associated with the disease. The exact pathogenesis remains unclear but it is thought that in most cases, the obstruction occurs first and the bacterial infection is a secondary phenomenon.

Morphology. The whole thickness of the organ is affected by the inflammatory process and the gross swelling associated with the inflammation may decrease the luminal size considerably, or even totally obliterate it. The cause of the initiating obstruction may be seen in the lumen, but in just under half of the cases of appendicitis no obstruction may be demonstrated. The mucosa of the organ is hyperaemic, oedematous, ulcerated and haemorrhagic, changes which may also be seen in the muscular layers and serosa. The inflammation often extends to the peritoneum and the mesoappendix, with fibrinous exudate and congestion of vessels being prominent features.

Three gross variants of acute appendicitis are distinguished and which one develops depends on the severity of the injury. **Simple acute appendicitis** is by far the commonest presentation and in this type the injury to the appendix has been moderate and the organ shows mainly mucosal necrosis and ulceration. **Acute suppurative appendicitis** develops after more extensive injury and as well as most of the mucosa the submucosa is involved in the inflammation, which is characterized by an extensive purulent infiltrate, forming frank pus within the lumen of the organ. Perforation of the wall is commonly seen in this type. **Gangrenous appendicitis** develops with severe injury and extensive infection of the whole of the organ, associated with septic thrombosis. Gangrene develops and the whole of the appendix may disintegrate leading to peritonitis.

Microscopically, there is acute, non-specific inflammation of all three layers of the organ. There is mucosal necrosis and ulceration, oedema in the submucosa, and often haemorrhage. Neutrophils are scattered throughout all layers and characteristically the muscularis is oedematous and infiltrated by large numbers of neutrophils. The serosa is oedematous and contains a fibrinous exudate.

Signs and symptoms. Early in the disease there may be abdominal or periumbilical pain which may be diffuse or around the region of the right lower abdominal quadrant. This pain is often described as cramping. As the inflammation involves more of the organ, there is vomiting and nausea, fever and leukocytosis. The pain now becomes confined to the lower right abdominal quadrant and there is point tenderness over the inflamed organ. Retrocaecal appendices may give atypical symptoms and it should also be noted that in the elderly, symptoms and signs may only develop much later in the course of the disease, often not apparent until after the organ has perforated.

Diagnosis. The disease is largely diagnosed on the clinical presentation which tends to be indicative for the disorder. However, even in the hands of the best clinicians, it should be expected that 10% of cases of resected appendices may be totally normal. Other conditions which may give rise to similar symptomatology are ovulatory rupture of an ovarian follicle ('mittelschmerz'), Meckel's diverticulitis, mesenteric adenitis in children, intussusception or volvulus.

Treatment and prognosis. The standard treatment is surgical resection of the inflamed and infected organ at laparotomy. Sometimes a ruptured or perforated organ may require emergency surgery which may save the life of the patient. Occasionally, where the facilities for laparotomy are not available antibiotic treatment has been attempted but this not very effective. Generally, surgery will be carried out even if the clinical diagnosis of acute appendicitis is not one of 100% accuracy because the complications of the condition are much more serious than laparotomy and appendectomy. Untreated, appendicitis may be fatal but with surgical treatment there is almost 100% survival and recovery.

Sequelae and complications. The condition may uncommonly resolve without any treatment, or alternatively, there may be healing with fibrosis. In the latter case chronic appendicitis may rarely be seen. Localized abscess formation often occurs and the resultant portal pyaemia will lead to pylephlebitis and liver abscesses. Perforation or rupture of the organ will lead to peritonitis or occasionally, because of the inflammation and fibrinous exudate, the infection may be localized to adherent areas of omentum around the ruptured appendix with subsequent healing and intestinal adhesions forming. Septicaemia may occasionally be seen and with gangrenous appendicitis a massive peritonitis may have fatal consequences.

Mucocoele of the Appendix

Occasionally, when the appendix becomes obstructed, instead of infection the condition of mucocoele will develop. Mucus secreted by the mucosal glands will fill the lumen and distend the organ such that it may be palpable. If the obstruction resolves the appendix will go back to normal; if it persists, the mucocoele may become secondarily infected and lead to rupture of the organ. At surgery, a ruptured mucocoele has to be differentiated from pseudomyxoma peritonei and ruptured cysts of ovarian cystadenoma or cystadenocarcinoma.

Diseases of the Large Intestine

Ulcerative Colitis

This is a chronic inflammatory condition affecting the mucosa and submucosa of the large intestine and clinically it may be difficult to differentiate from other inflammatory bowel disease such as Crohn's disease or infections.

Incidence. The disease has an annual incidence of one in 10 000 in Western-type countries, its prevalence being one in 1000 individuals. It affects males and females equally and is a disorder of young adults, most patients being between the ages of 20 and 40 years. All races seem to be affected equally, although data from the USA have shown that the disease is more common in Jews than in non-Jews (the incidence in Israel is comparable with that elsewhere) and more common in white than in black people. These data have been cited as support for the theory that genetic influences are important in the aetiology of the disease.

Aetiology. The aetiology is unknown, but in approximately 15% of patients there is a familial association, with a history of ulcerative colitis or Crohn's disease in the family. Most of the experimental data suggest that the disease is autoimmune in nature. Natural killer cells from patients with ulcerative colitis have been shown to be cytotoxic for colonic cells from those patients, *in vitro*. There have also been studies showing that a cross-reacting antibody exists in some patients, and that this acts as an autoantibody. The antibody forms in response to *Escherichia coli* serotype 0119B14 and subsequently cross-reacts with intestinal

318 Pathology for the Health Sciences

epithelial cells. This may give rise to hypersensitivity reactions and damage to the mucosa. Some researchers have suggested that these immunological reactions may be secondary phenomena and not necessarily part of the disease pathogenesis.

Other theories suggest that a transmissible agent may be involved (possibly a virus) and animal experiments have shown that the disease may be transmitted in some cases. Epidemiologists have pointed out data that suggest the disease is primarily one seen in affluent, Western-type countries and hence it may be related to dietary factors, lifestyle, etc.

It should be noted that histologically and clinically non-specific (idiopathic) ulcerative colitis resembles amoebic dysentery, which also affects the colon, and this latter type of colitis is termed **specific ulcerative colitis**. Specific ulcerative colitis is not as common in Western countries as non-specific ulcerative colitis and *Entamoeba histolytica* can be readily demonstrated in the tissue under the microscope, whereas in the non-specific form these micro-organisms are lacking.

Sites affected. The rectum is always affected by the disease and then in descending order, other sites involved are the sigmoid, the descending colon, or alternatively the whole of the colon. Essentially, it may be regarded as a diffuse condition which begins at the rectum and which may involve more and more of the large intestine proximally. If only the rectum is involved the condition is termed a proctitis. If the sigmoid and descending colon are also affected, it is termed a left-sided ulcerative colitis of substantial involvement. It should be noted that the small intestine is not affected.

Morphology. In the early stages of the disease there is congestion of the mucosa with petechial haemorrhages developing. The haemorrhages are associated with pin-point ulcers which develop on the ridges of the mucosal folds. The ulcers enlarge and many more form. In the later stages of the disease there are multiple regions of ulceration, the ulcers usually linearly arranged and of variable size and distribution (Figures 8.17 and 8.18). Haemorrhage and secondary infection are frequently seen in these areas. Varied degrees of healing by granulation tissue and re-epithelialization are seen. New crops of ulcers may then develop in these healed sites.

In long-standing disease the ulcers are separated by regions of surviving, hyperplastic and inflamed mucosa which may give the appearance of polyps, hence the term **pseudopolyps** to describe them (see Figure 8.17). Scarring develops in areas of long-standing ulceration, damage and secondary infection, and the fibrosis may

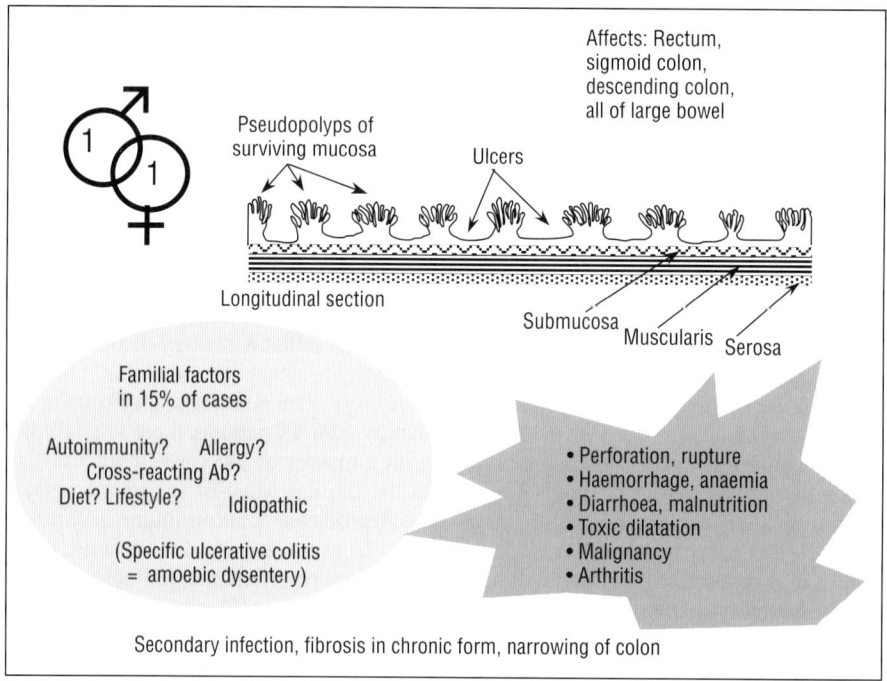

Figure 8.17 *Pathology of ulcerative colitis*

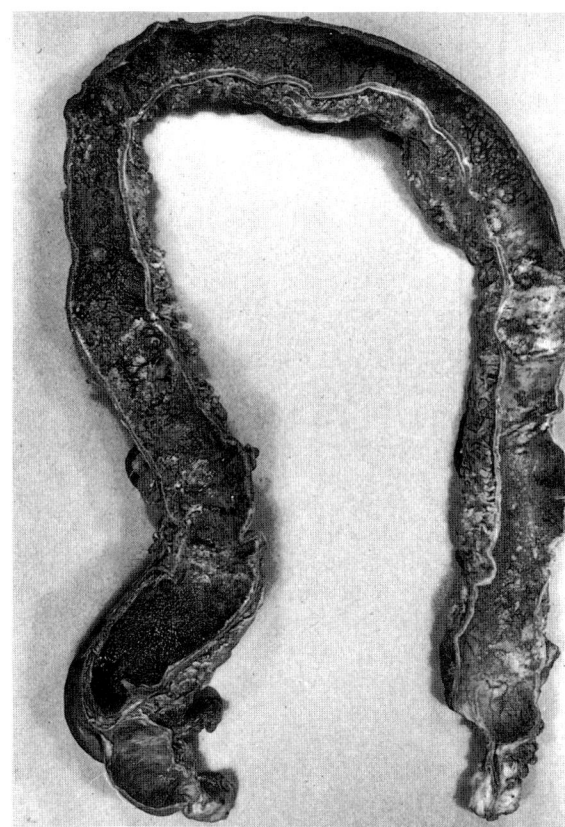

Figure 8.18 *Chronic, non-specific ulcerative colitis in a 70-year-old female who had suffered from the disease for many decades*

eventually involve the whole wall, causing hardening and thickening of the wall, with a narrowed lumen.

Signs and symptoms. About half of the patients with ulcerative colitis present with mild disease characterized by diarrhoea, rectal bleeding and tenesmus. Many patients ($\approx$40%) present with moderate disease complaining of modest or severe (cramping) lower abdominal pain associated with mucous, bloody diarrhoea. The more distal the lesions, the more urgent and frequent is the diarrhoea. However, if only limited involvement of the rectum is seen then the patient may present with constipation, presumably because the inflamed regions of rectum resist the passage of faeces. Low-grade fever, leukocytosis and moderate anaemia may also be observed in all of these patients.

In more chronic cases of the disease and with more extensive involvement of the colon, the patient may present with a history of intermittent diarrhoea, chronic ill health, anaemia, dehydration because of sodium and potassium loss, malnutrition, hypoalbuminaemia and oedema associated with extensive inflammation and loss of protein in the exudate, and there may be palpable mucosal thickening or narrowing of the rectal lumen upon digital rectal examination.

Course and complications. The disease may be seen as an acute incident which causes few symptoms and signs and then goes into remission (<10% of cases). Although there are cases of permanent remission, in most patients the disease relapses after a few years. The patients most often complain of months or years of ill health with symptoms and signs referable to the disease lasting days to weeks, interspersed with short remissions ($\approx$70% of cases). Other patients complain of continuous disease which is unremitting and may progress to involve more and more of the colon ($\approx$20% of cases).

A few cases will develop the so-called **fulminant ulcerative colitis** which is a rapidly progressive form of the disease, the patient having 5 to 15 bowel motions daily, the diarrhoea being bloody and mucous. Dehydration and electrolyte depletion may cause prostration. Patients are feverish and show systemic manifestations such as anaemia and leukocytosis. A massive haemorrhage may be fatal. **Toxic megacolon** may develop in such cases and this refers to extreme dilatation of the colon and toxaemia, abdominal distension and pain. This is a surgical emergency and 15% of patients may die of complications such as colonic rupture or haemorrhage.

Systemic involvement of other tissues may be seen in patients with ulcerative colitis and this includes arthritis and ankylosing spondylitis (25% of cases), skin lesions and rashes (10% of cases), eye changes such as uveitis (10% of cases), and liver disease (3% of cases). A very important complication is that of bowel malignancy. Approximately 30% of patients who have the disease for over 10 years will develop carcinoma of the large bowel and hence ulcerative colitis must be considered as an important premalignant lesion of the large bowel.

Diagnosis. Clinical symptomatology is important in the diagnosis of the disease but several other diagnostic procedures may be required to differentiate this condition from other inflammatory disease of the bowel (refer to Table 8.2). Sigmoidoscopy or colonoscopy will identify the lesions and indicate the extent of involvement. Straight X-rays and barium enema may be of use. The exclusion of Crohn's disease by biopsy and demonstration of normal small intestine may also be of diagnostic significance. Stool examination and culture should be performed to exclude amoebic and bacterial colitis.

Treatment and prognosis. Medical treatment of the disease includes the following: a high-calorie, high-protein diet. Limiting or abolishing milk intake may control the diarrhoea and the secondary alactasia (lack of lactase leading to lactose intolerance) which may have developed. Corticosteroids administered orally, or in enemas, or in suppository form, decrease the inflammation and are continued until the patient is

Table 8.2 *Comparison of ulcerative colitis and Crohn's disease*

Ulcerative colitis	Crohn's disease

Caused by:
  Entamoeba histolytica (specific form).
  Most cases cause unknown, idiopathic disease
  Autoimmune? Abnormal cell-mediated
  immunity (non-specific form)
	Caused by:
	  Cause unknown, idiopathic disease.
	  Autoimmune/hypersensitivity reaction?
	  Abnormal cell-mediated immunity

Nature:
  Disease in continuity.
  Ulcerated, mucosa, acute episodes of
  mucosal, submucosal inflammation.
  No granulomata form.
  Pseudopolyp formation.
  Rectum almost always affected
	Nature:
	  Disease discontinuous.
	  Chronic granulomatous disease,
	  non-specific granulomata form.
	  Ileum most commonly involved (50%),
	  also in jejunum (15%), colon (20%);
	  stomach and rectum uncommonly affected

Ages affected predominantly:
  Young adults, mainly between
  20–40 years; male:female = 1:1
	Ages affected predominantly:
	  Young adults most commonly affected;
	  male:female = 1:1.6

Predisposing factors:
  Familial in ≈ 15% of cases.
  Presence of *E. coli* type 0119B14
  in faeces. Diet? Lifestyle?
	Predisposing factors:
	  Familial in 5–10% of cases.
	  Other autoimmune diseases;
	  e.g. ankylosing spondylitis

Course and characteristics:
  Acute inflammation of mucosa,
  ulceration of the tops of the mucosal
  folds, progressing to long, linear
  ulcers. Haemorrhage, suppuration.
  Pseudopolyp formation.
  Relatively little fibrosis.
  Continuous or intermittent diarrhoea,
  20% of patients present with fever,
  bloody diarrhoea, toxaemia.
  Non-specific inflammatory lesions
  in anal region in 25% of patients
	Course and characteristics:
	  'Skip lesions' in gut wall. Transmural
	  chronic inflammation, with 60% of cases
	  showing typical granulomata in gut,
	  lymph nodes and mesentery.
	  Ulceration and fissure formation.
	  Narrowing, obstruction of gut lumen.
	  Episodic lower abdominal tenderness or
	  pain, intermittent diarrhoea, weight loss.
	  Abdominal mass in 33% of patients.
	  Sarcoid-like granulomata in anal region
	  in 75% of patients

Results, sequelae, complications:
  'Toxic dilatation', megacolon.
  Perforation of colon, haemorrhage,
  anaemia, protein and electrolyte loss.
  Malignancy in long-standing cases.
  Arthritis, ankylosing spondylitis in
  15% of cases. Fistulae, strictures rare
	Results, sequelae, complications:
	  Intestinal obstruction, thickening of bowel,
	  'rubber hose' gut. Malabsorption
	  syndrome, 2° infection, suppuration.
	  Fistulae (ileocaecal, ileocolic, external),
	  ankylosing spondylitis, 2° amyloidosis.
	  Haemorrhage, perforation very rare

well. Blood transfusion, electrolyte replenishment, parenteral nutrition and corticosteroids may be required in a severe case of the disease.

Surgical treatment of the disease may become necessary in severe or prolonged cases of the disorder which are either life threatening or make life intolerable for the patient. The colon and rectum are excised and an ileostomy is performed. Surgical treatment is indicated if the patient presents with carcinoma, perforation, toxic megacolon or intractable diarrhoea, continued ill health, anaemia or other complications of the disease. The prognosis of the disease is influenced by the extent of involvement of the colon, the severity of the disease and age of the patient. Ulcerative colitis is a life threatening disorder as it may give rise to numerous complications and the disease is most likely to cause death in an elderly patient if toxic megacolon, perforation, haemorrhage or carcinoma develop.

Diverticular Disease of the Colon

This condition is very common in the colon, affecting as much as 30% of the population over 60 years of age. Males and females are affected equally. Numerous false diverticula form in the disorder which almost always involves the left side of the colon, especially the descending and sigmoid portions. The basic defect is most likely an abnormality of the muscular layer of the bowel, incoordination of contractions leading to irregularities of pressure, forcing the mucosa through the weakest areas, which are the points where blood vessels enter through the intestinal wall. The abnormal movements of the muscular layer lead to segmental hypertrophy of the circular muscle, this further increasing the likelihood of diverticulum formation. Hernial protrusion of the mucosa occurs between the taenia, forming the diverticula, while the intervening bowel is normal.

It is thought that a major aetiological factor in the disease is diet. The Western-type diet which is often very deficient in fibre, high in simple carbohydrates, fats and processed foods predisposes to a prolonged transit time of faeces in the intestine, constipation and abnormal segmenting movements of the bowel wall. Abnormal movements of the bowel wall have also been shown to occur in response to anxiety, emotional states and other causes of neuroendocrine stimulation.

The uncomplicated condition is termed **diverticulosis** and is most commonly symptom free. A small number of patients with diverticulosis may present with vague abdominal pains and alterations in bowel habit. Frequently, the pouches may fill with faecal matter and a considerable proportion of patients

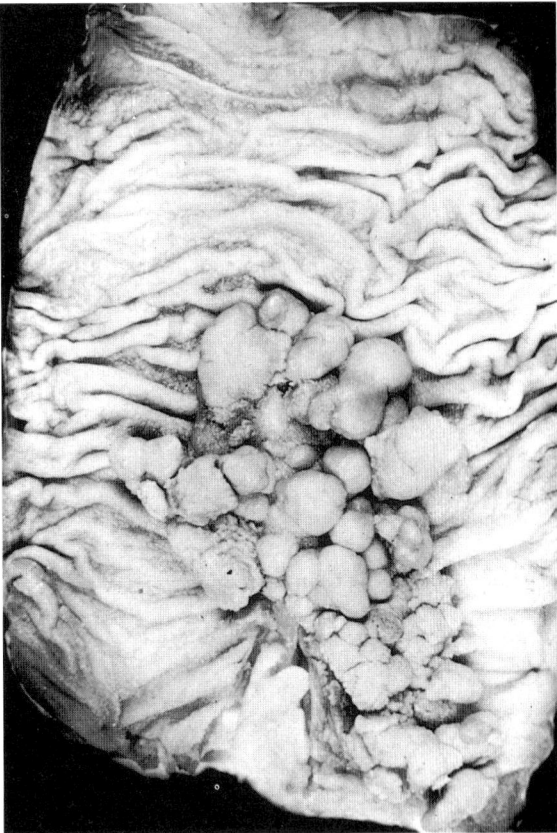

Figure 8.19 *Polyposis of the sigmoid colon*

develop infection and inflammation around the diverticula, giving rise to the condition of **diverticulitis**. The patients then present with intermittent abdominal discomfort or pain and tenderness which seems to be relieved by defaecation. There may be diarrhoea alternating with constipation and the patients may note blood or pus in their faeces. This chronic condition may be present for many years and the patient frequently does not present until there are complications such as perforation and peritonitis or an acute attack of diverticulitis. Acute diverticulitis presents with a constant lower abdominal pain, fever, anorexia, occasional vomiting and usually constipation (occasionally diarrhoea will be seen). There is tenderness over the left iliac fossa and a mass of thickened colon may be palpable abdominally or on rectal digital examination. Peritonitis and abscess formation may lead to the patient becoming very ill with symptoms of an acute abdomen.

Complications of diverticulitis include perforation

of the colon, peritonitis, abscess formation, fistula formation (most usually into the bladder with pneumaturia being a common symptom), intestinal obstruction (due to adhesions forming and compressing the small intestinal wall), rectal haemorrhage. The disease is diagnosed on clinical symptomatology but two procedures may give confirmation: sigmoidoscopy (which also excludes rectal carcinoma and ulcerative colitis) and barium enema with associated radiological examination.

Treatment of the condition involves changes in diet, increasing dietary fibre which generally alleviates the constipation (if it remains a problem laxative preparations containing hydrophilic granules of methylcellulose may be prescribed). Such dietary reform may also relieve much of the pain involved with the condition. Surgical treatments are reserved for the complicated cases but the best prognosis for surgery occurs if the patient has the surgery done electively rather than at the time of one of the complications. The segment of bowel involved in the disease is resected and an end to end anastomosis re-establishes continuity. A temporary colostomy may be needed to protect the anastomosis from the passage of faecal material.

Benign Colonic Polyps

Neoplastic conditions of the large intestine are extremely common when compared with those occurring in the small intestine. Such neoplastic lesions are derived mostly from the epithelium and may be benign or malignant. Most benign lesions are the polyps which are essentially adenomata, well differentiated and functional, secreting much mucus. The size of the lesions varies from 0.2 cm to 3 cm or more in diameter (Figure 8.19). Approximately 5% of the adult population develop colonic or rectal polyps. The lesions are most commonly found in the sigmoid colon and rectum and they are often multiple. The male to female sex ratio is 2:1 and the typical age of presentation is around 55 years.

Colonic polyps may be subdivided into two major groups. The first is the **adenomatous polyps**, which are the most commonly encountered, 90% of all benign neoplasms being of this type in the bowel. These are small lesions, usually 1 cm or less in diameter, having a smooth lobulated surface, resembling the normal mucosa of the bowel. The second group is the **villous adenomata** (or papillomata), which constitute

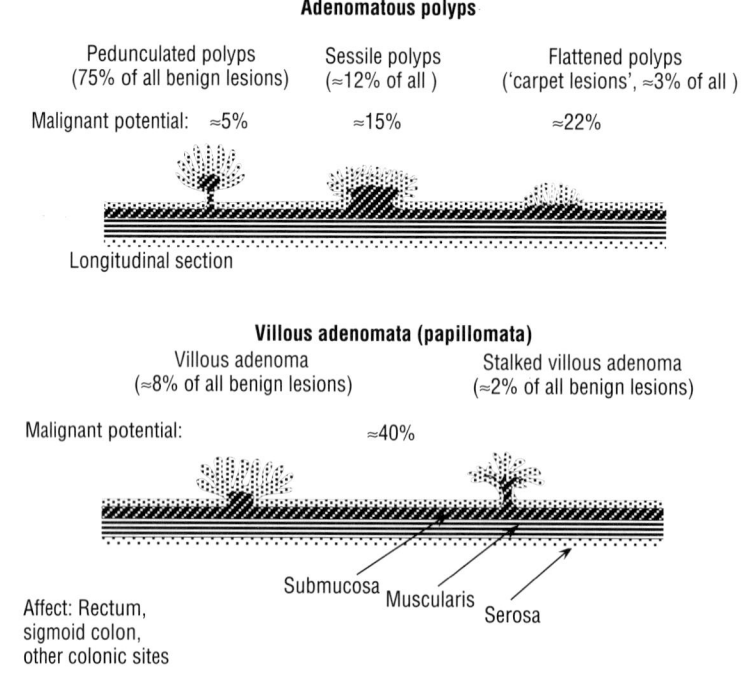

Figure 8.20 *Benign colonic polyps*

close to 10% of the benign neoplasms. These tend to be larger lesions, 1–3 cm in diameter, having a cauliflower-like growth pattern with many finger-like papillae of mucosa projecting into the lumen of the bowel (as shown in Figure 8.20).

The adenomatous polyps may be subdivided into three major forms depending on morphological criteria and malignant potential. **Pedunculated adenomatous polyps** comprise 75% of all benign lesions and they have the least malignant potential, a person's risk of developing cancer on one of these lesions being 5%. These pedunculated lesions appear as toadstools, with a slender stalk on which the mass of tumour is situated, projecting into the lumen of the bowel. **Sessile adenomatous polyps** constitute approximately 12% of benign lesions and they appear as solid nodules with a warty surface and no stalk. Their malignant potential is about 15%. **Flattened adenomatous polyps** or 'carpet lesions' grow very close to the surface of the bowel and are only slightly raised. They are the least common of the adenomata but they have a malignant potential of 22%.

Villous adenomata are subdivided into two major types: the **sessile villous adenoma**, which is the most commonly seen, constituting approximately 8% of all benign lesions, and the **stalked villous adenoma**, constituting 2% of all benign lesions. The malignant potential of these two lesions is 40%.

Microscopically all polyps are typical adenomatous growths with the epithelial components resembling the normal colonic mucosa. However, there may be irregularity in the size and shape of tubules, thickening of the polypoid mucosa with cell populations that are rather atypical in appearance. In villous adenomata especially, the surface epithelium may appear poorly differentiated with evidence of mitotic activity which indicates malignant transformation. As there is a considerable risk of cancer developing in all of these benign neoplasms they are removed as soon as they are diagnosed.

Patients with benign neoplasms of the colonic mucosa often show no associated signs and symptoms and the lesions are discovered incidentally during a routine colonoscopy. Often, the patient presents with a history of haemorrhage *per rectum* as the pedunculated polyps may be mechanically damaged, with ulceration and haemorrhage occurring from the damaged surface. There may be alteration of bowel habit as there is often excessive loss of electrolytes and fluid from multiple polyps. The faeces may contain much mucus as the polyps are functional (especially the villous adenomata). Occasionally, the patient may complain of colicky pain and abdominal distension and tenderness, symptoms which indicate that obstruction is occurring.

Rarely, a large rectal polyp may prolapse through the anus.

Several complications are associated with benign colonic lesions, the most important of which is malignant transformation. The risk of malignancy supervening is directly related to the nature of the lesion as discussed previously but also another important factor is the size of the lesion. If the adenoma is greater than 2 cm in diameter the malignant potential is ≈50%, if the lesion is between 1 and 2 cm in diameter the malignant potential is ≈10%, and if the lesion is less than 1 cm in diameter the malignant potential is ≈1%. Other complications include strangulation of pedunculated lesions around the stalk, with subsequent infarction, secondary infection and haemorrhage. Obstruction of the bowel, and electrolyte–water disturbances may be observed because of the excessive secretory activity of these neoplasms.

Diagnosis of the lesions is performed through the sigmoidoscope or colonoscope, or alternatively barium enema and X-rays may demonstrate the lesions. Treatment is excision of the lesion, which is very easily performed on pedunculated lesions through a diathermy snare on a colonoscope. This is an electrically heated coil of wire which is looped tight around the stalk of the lesion. The electric current cuts through and cauterizes the stalk and the lesion may then be removed intact for histological examination. If the polyp is anaplastic or malignant, bowel resection is then advisable. With large or sessile lesions colectomy is the mode of treatment.

Polyposis Coli (Familial Adenomatous Polyposis)

This is a hereditary disorder which is usually transmitted as a Mendelian dominant trait by either sex, but in some families the condition is of very poor penetrance or appears to be transmitted as a recessive character. In this disease hundreds of adenomatous polyps form in the large intestine. The condition does not appear until adolescence or early adult life. If the polyps have not developed by the age of 40 years, they most probably will not develop after that.

The polyps usually involve the whole of the large bowel but they also may extend into the small intestine and rarely even the stomach may be involved. Many hundreds of polyps develop and each of them is similar in appearance to the single pedunculated adenomatous polyp already discussed. Sometimes when the polyps are particularly dense the surface of the mucosa looks 'furry' or resembles shag pile carpet! A small number of patients with the condition may also present with extracolonic lesions, especially common being osteomata of the mandible.

This condition predisposes to cancer of the colon, the carcinoma being almost inevitable, usually presenting after 15 years of the polyps first developing (see Figure 8.21). Very often the carcinoma will develop well before the patients are in their forties. The entire colon must be excised as soon as the condition is diagnosed. Generally, if polyposis is known to occur in a family, regular colonoscopies at 6 monthly intervals are performed on the offspring from late childhood in order to diagnose and treat the condition early.

Other Inherited Benign Neoplasms

Several other inherited conditions are known which involve the development of benign neoplasms in the gastrointestinal tract. The **Peutz-Jeghers syndrome** is an autosomal dominant disease that is characterized by the presence of small numbers of intestinal polyps and increased melanin pigmentation in the mucocutaneous junctions. The polyps are found most frequently in the small intestine, but may also be present in the stomach and colon. The pigmentation is macular and is seen in the face, lips, buccal mucosa, anogenital areas, hands and feet; it tends to fade at puberty except in the buccal region, where it persists. The polyps that occur in this syndrome are considered to be hamartomatous and not true neoplasms. Patients with the disorder may present with intussusception, intestinal obstruction, upper gastrointestinal tract haemorrhage, occult faecal blood and anaemia. In many cases, the patient is asymptomatic and the only indication that the condition is present is the pigmentation. Although the polyps are considered benign and remain benign for the individual's life, the patient has an increased risk of developing carcinoma of the large bowel (not necessarily at the site where the polyps are).

Gardner's syndrome is an autosomal dominant disorder which greatly resembles familial polyposis in that multiple benign polyps develop mostly in the colorectal area, the small intestine and stomach being less frequently affected. Associated lesions in this condition are osteomata of the mandible, skull and long bones, exostoses and dental abnormalities. This condition is associated with a high risk of malignant transformation to carcinoma of the large bowel. **Turcot's syndrome** is reputedly an autosomal recessive disorder, although the evidence for this mode of transmission is scanty. It is a rare disorder of familial colonic polyposis in which the gastrointestinal lesions are as-

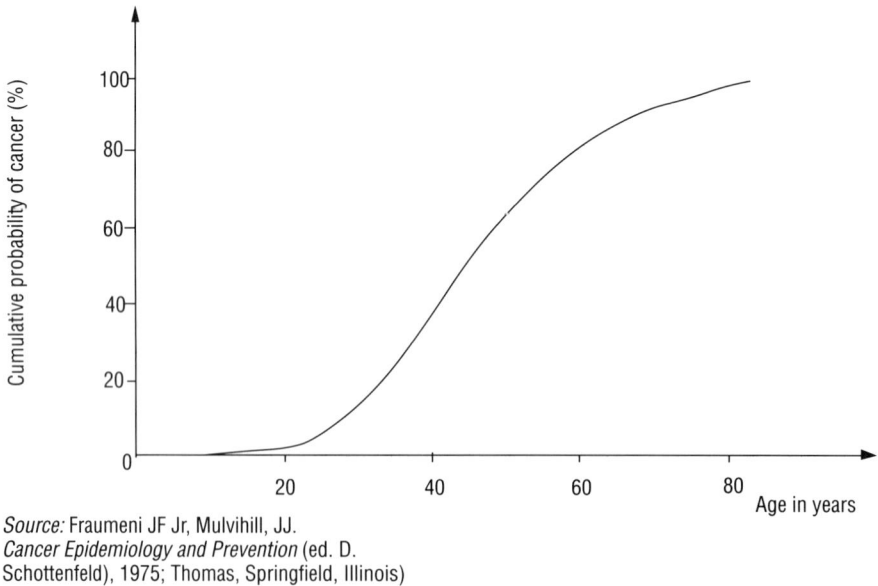

Incidence of cancer of the colon in patients with polyposis coli by age

Source: Fraumeni JF Jr, Mulvihill, JJ.
Cancer Epidemiology and Prevention (ed. D. Schottenfeld), 1975; Thomas, Springfield, Illinois)

Figure 8.21 *Polyposis coli and carcinoma of the colon*

sociated with malignancies of the central nervous system, especially gliomata.

Carcinoma of the Large Bowel ('Colorectal Cancer')

Incidence. Colorectal carcinoma is the second most important cause of death from cancer (16% of malignant deaths). The usual age of presentation is 55–60 years (except in patients with familial polyposis or ulcerative colitis where it may develop at the age of 20–40 years). The incidence in the sexes varies but may be up to twice as common in men (M:F = 2:1).

Aetiology. This tumour has a greater incidence in Western countries. In the majority of cases there is no known predisposing cause; however, epidemiological studies show that diet is very important. People with a high animal fat, low-fibre diet have a much higher risk of developing this cancer. It appears that such diets slow down the passage of faeces through the intestine and thus allow much more time for interaction between any carcinogens in the faeces and the mucosal cells. It has been shown that people with the tumour have a high content of faecal bile acids with *Clostridium paraputrificum* also found in their faeces. This is a bacterium which can metabolize bile acids into cocarcinogens. Chronic constipation is also thought to be a factor.

There are several precancerous lesions which occur in the bowel and people with these diseases have a high risk of developing bowel cancer:

- Familial polyposis coli (100% of sufferers will develop cancer if the condition is untreated).
- Gardner's syndrome (inherited multiple polyps carrying an increased risk of 10–50%).
- Peutz-Jegher's syndrome (inherited hamartomata carrying an increased risk of up to 10%).
- Benign, solitary tumours (e.g. polyps carrying an increased risk of 10–50%).
- Ulcerative colitis (30 times the risk of a normal person).
- Crohn's disease of the colon (3–5 times the risk of a normal person).
- Previous colonic cancer.

Sites affected. These are, in order of decreasing frequency of involvement: the rectum, sigmoid colon, descending colon, caecum, transverse colon and flexures. In approximately 5% of cases of colonic carcinoma, the cancers are multiple, occurring in many sites.

Morphology. The tumour may be **fungating**, cauliflower-like, growing into the lumen; **polypoid**, resembling the mushroom-like polyp growths, on a stalk; **ulcerating**, where tumour necrosis produces an ulcer with overhanging margins; **infiltrating**, invading diffusely into the wall; **mucoid**, producing much mucous secretion; or **annular** ('purse-string' tumours), growing in a ring around the bowel wall (Figure 8.22). Microscopically, most of the tumours are adenocarcinomata, many being very well differentiated and functional (Figure 8.23). Some tumours are anaplastic and thus highly malignant. Rarely, squamous metaplasia may precede the neoplasia and a squamous cell carcinoma will result.

Spread. The tumour first grows into the surrounding mucosa and underlying submucosa through direct invasion of the surrounding tissue. Invasion and infiltration then progresses from the mucosa and submucosa through to the muscle and serosa. Lymphatic invasion and spread to the regional, draining lymph nodes then occurs. The veins are subsequently invaded and haematogenous spread to the liver is characteristic.

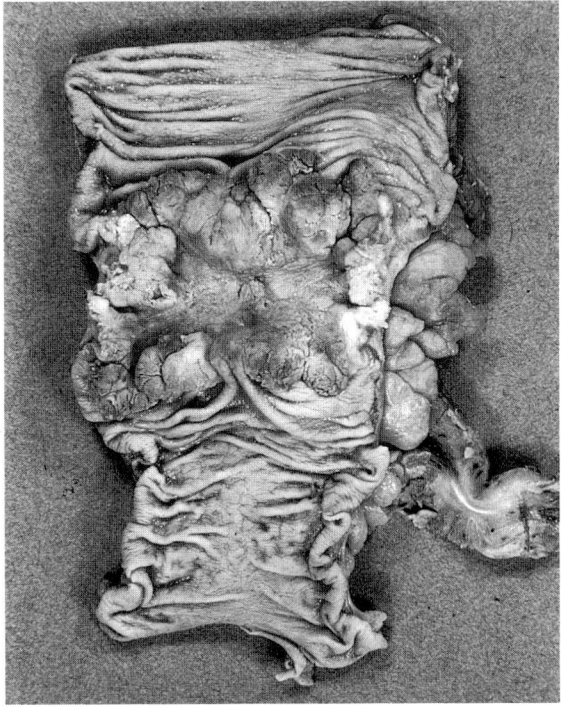

Figure 8.22 *Adenocarcinoma of the rectum showing an extensive fungating lesion with central ulceration. Paler necrotic areas are also evident within the tumour*

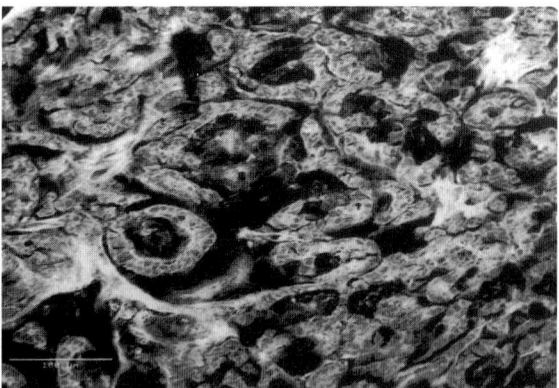

Figure 8.23   *Adenocarcinoma of the colon showing the well-differentiated cells of the neoplasm forming nests of cells and acinar structures (scale bar is 100 μm)*

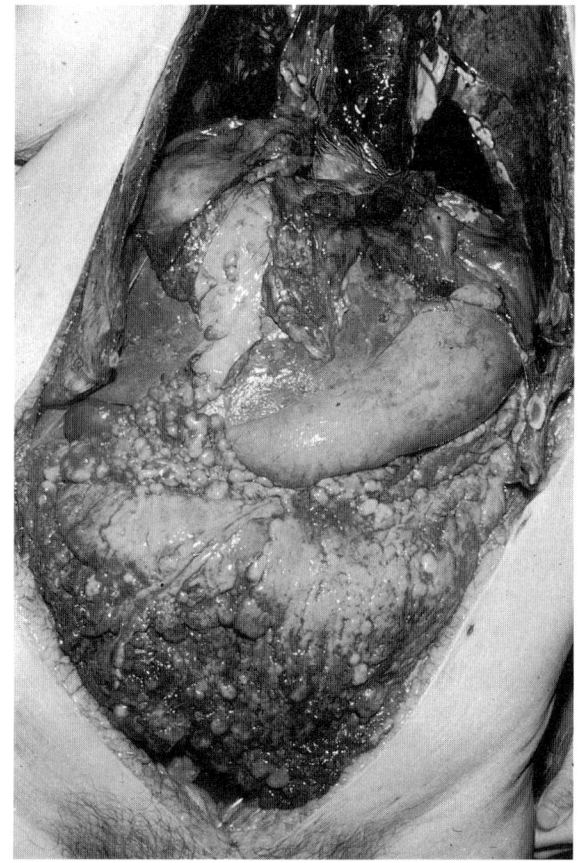

Figure 8.24   *Carcinomatosis peritonei. Numerous tumour nodules are seen studding the surfaces of all of the abdominal organs and omentum*

The tumour may spread to the other organs in the peritoneum by transcoelomic spread. Tumours of the colon that have invaded through to the serosa may cause the condition of **carcinomatosis peritonei** where numerous tumour deposits occur throughout the peritoneal cavity (Figure 8.24).

Signs and symptoms. The earliest symptoms the patients may notice are changes in their bowel habit, dyspepsia and vague abdominal pain. The patients may note large quantities of mucus in their faeces as the majority of tumours are functional adenocarcinomata. Intestinal obstruction may occur, especially with some types of tumour (e.g. annular carcinomata). The patients may see obvious, red blood in their faeces or blood may be demonstrated in the faeces in the laboratory after special treatment of the faeces (**occult blood**). This haemorrhage indicates damage to the tumour and ulceration. Anaemia with fatigue, lassitude and weakness are associated with chronic blood loss from the tumours. Perforation of the wall of the gut, peritonitis, fistula formation and secondary bacterial infection of the tumour may also occur. Later in the disease the patient's general health will deteriorate rapidly and dramatic loss of weight will be seen.

Diagnosis. Most of the tumours are situated in the rectosigmoid area and therefore very accessible to direct observation through sigmoidoscopy. The tumour may then be biopsied with the instrument and the histological type may be determined. A barium enema and abdominal X-rays are of use, especially with the

tumours situated further up the colon. Clinical signs and symptoms are also of importance. Family and patient history of polyposis coli, ulcerative colitis, Crohn's disease should be investigated.

Treatment and prognosis. Treatment of the cancer is by surgical excision with or without a colostomy being performed, depending on where the tumour has arisen and how much of the bowel is removed. For very low situated tumours in the rectum a colostomy may be the only available option. Stapling anastomosis of the bowel after tumour excision has been of importance in maintaining normal defaecation in patients with rectosigmoid tumours. Previous to this technique being developed, such patients had to have colostomies performed. Prognosis of the tumour depends very much on the stage at which the tumour is diagnosed and treated. **Duke's staging** is one staging system widely used:

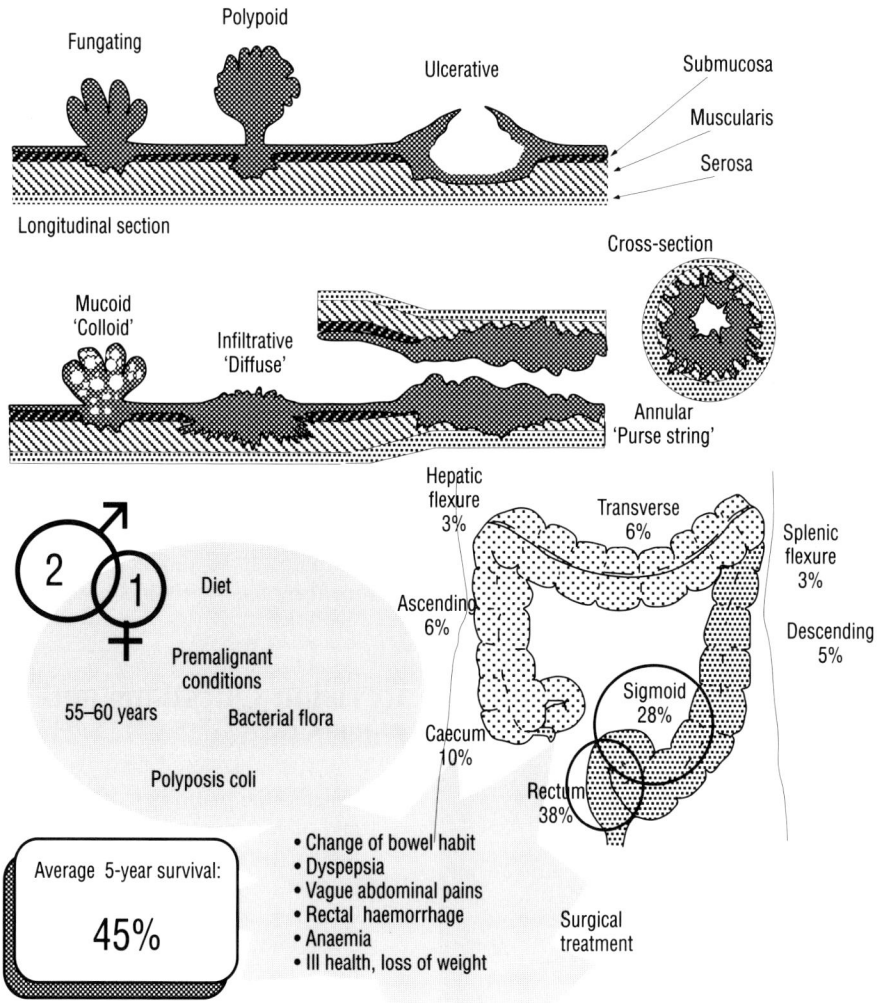

Figure 8.25 *Pathology of carcinoma of the colon*

- Stage A: The tumour is confined to the wall of the bowel. The 5-year survival of patients treated at this stage is more than 80%.
- Stage B: The cancer has spread through the wall and into the serosa, bringing the 5-year survival of patients treated at this stage to approximately 60%.
- Stage C: The tumour can be found in the regional lymph nodes of the bowel. The 5-year survival of patients is about 30%.
- Stage D: When there are distant metastases (e.g. in the liver), the treatment is mainly palliative and the 5-year survival is 5% or less.

The overall, average 5-year survival for the tumour is approximately 45%.

It should be noted that bowel cancer is one of the tumours that is in many cases preventable through early treatment of benign tumours of the bowel, alterations in diet such as decreasing meat and fat consumption and increasing fruit, vegetable and complex carbohydrate (fibre) intake.

Carcinoma of the Anal Canal

This is a relatively rare tumour when compared with

colorectal carcinoma. It occurs mainly in patients between 55 and 65 years of age and affects males and females equally. It is a typical squamous cell carcinoma which arises from the squamous epithelium of the anal margin.

Lymphatic metastases occur early in the history of the tumour and thus it is associated with a poor prognosis.

Haemorrhoids

Haemorrhoids are varicose veins occurring in the venous channels of the internal haemorrhoidal plexi (Figure 8.26). Two types of haemorrhoids are distinguished, internal and external, depending on whether they arise from the superior haemorrhoidal plexus, above the pectinate line or whether they arise out of the inferior haemorrhoidal plexus, below that line. The condition is very common in Western countries, as many as 40 to 50% of people above the age of 50 years being affected to some degree. The rarity of the condition in developing countries seems to suggest that dietary factors are an important factor in the aetiology. Low-fibre diets and constipation are certainly associated with the disorder, as the straining at stool causes great pressures in the anal area with compression of the venous plexi and development of great hydrostatic pressures within their lumina that predispose to dilatation and tortuosity. Pregnancy predisposes to the condition, presumably because of the increased abdominal pressure that is present. Portal hypertension may also predispose to the development of haemorrhoids.

The patient with haemorrhoids presents clinically with bleeding and often chronic bleeding may be associated with iron deficiency anaemia. Rectal prolapse is another common presentation. The dilated, engorged venous plexi that constitute the haemorrhoids may protrude through the anus and thus become strangulated and thrombotic, a condition associated with exquisite pain. It is such cases that require surgical treatment by haemorrhoidectomy.

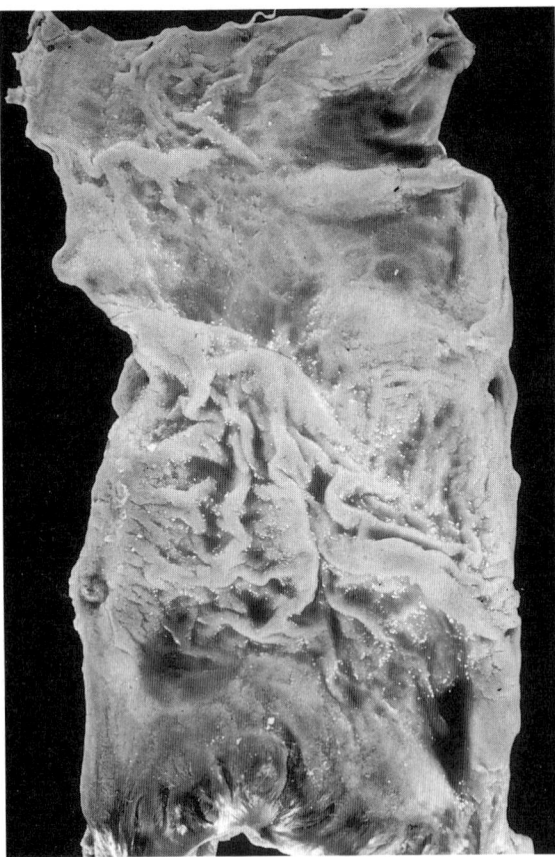

Figure 8.26 *Haemorrhoids. The dilated, congested venous channels of the internal haemorrhoidal plexi are very prominent*

Revision Questions and Case Studies

1. Discuss the pathology of carcinoma of the mouth and of carcinoma of the oesophagus. What aetiological factors are common to both of these tumours?
2. Compare and contrast the macroscopic and microscopic appearance of:
   (a) Chronic peptic ulcer of the stomach (benign)
   (b) Ulcerating carcinoma of the stomach ('ulcer cancer')
3. What are the predisposing factors of chronic peptic ulceration? What are the complications and prognosis of chronic peptic ulcers?
4. What is a hiatus hernia?
5. Write short notes on the following:
   (a) Volvulus
   (b) Intussusception
   (c) Meckel's diverticulum
   (d) Primary tumours of the small intestine
6. What are the complications of ulcerative colitis? (Discuss both specific and non-specific forms.)
7. What is the commonest aetiology of specific ulcerative colitis? Discuss the macroscopic and microscopic appearance of the intestine in this condition.
8. Distinguish between diverticulosis and diverticulitis.

9. Compare and contrast the pathological features of:
   (a) Non-specific ulcerative colitis
   (b) Crohn's disease of the colon (regional colitis)
10. What is familial polyposis coli? Discuss the major features of this disorder.
11. What is a sessile polyp and what is a colonic papilloma? Discuss these two conditions with respect to their premalignant potential.
12. What are the predisposing factors to the development of carcinoma of the colon?
13. What are the commonest sites in which carcinoma of the large bowel is found?
14. What are the symptoms and signs associated with tumours of the large bowel?
15. What are the sequelae and complications of large bowel malignancies?
16. What is the prognosis of cancer of the large intestine? Refer to Duke's staging system of the tumour in your answer.
17. What are haemorrhoids and what predisposes to their formation?
18. Discuss the pathology of diverticular disease.
19. Write short notes on any three of the following:
   (a) Spread of large bowel carcinoma
   (b) Argentaffinoma
   (c) Predisposing factors to the development of stomach carcinoma
   (d) Occult faecal blood
20. Discuss the pathology of acute appendicitis.

Case study 1. A 39-year-old Caucasian male of Spanish origin complains of an epigastric, steady, aching pain which is periodic in nature, often waking him 'in the middle of the night'. He has thought it to be indigestion as the pain is relieved by antacids, which he self-administers liberally. He says that diarrhoea has been an intermittent problem. Lately he has been vomiting about 6 hours after meals. This relieves the discomfort and pain he has been feeling and he mentions that lately he even thought of inducing vomiting to ease his discomfort. Physical examination of the patient show him to be 1.72 m tall, weighing 75 kg, blood pressure 135/80 mmHg, pulse rate 80 beats per minute, temperature 37.0°C. When asked to point out the region of the pain he points to his epigastrium. A succussion splash is heard over the epigastrium. The man admits to eating a lot of 'junk food' but he justifies himself by saying that he is a self employed tradesman, often forced to keep odd hours and to miss meals. He smokes 30 cigarettes a day.

(a) What is the presumptive diagnosis?
(b) What confirmatory investigations are required?

(c) How is this condition managed?

Case study 2. A 66-year-old Caucasian female presents at your clinic requesting dietary advice as she believes her diet may be affecting her bowel habits. She is a lean, pale individual, 168 cm tall, weighing in at 52 kg. Physical examination reveals a blood pressure of 150/92 mmHg and a pulse rate of 82 per minute. Her temperature is 37.8°C. Chest and abdominal examinations are normal. She is a widow and has been living alone ever since the younger of her two daughters was married seven years ago. She has been a housewife all her life. Questioning the patient more closely about the symptoms the following information is elicited: although she has suffered from constipation for many years, in the past three months she has been suffering from bouts of constipation and diarrhoea and on at least two occasions she has noticed some blood in the stool. She often feels bloated, especially several hours after meals. She says this is indigestion and has taken antacids to relieve it, but usually the symptoms persist. When you tell her her weight she is surprised and says that maybe she should not be asking you about a 'diet' as she has 'lost a bit of weight'. The woman is a non-smoker and teetotaller. She has been trying to stay on a vegetarian diet (that her daughter suggested) for the past few months without much success, finding that she just gives up and 'sends out for the take-aways'.

(a) What is the presumptive diagnosis?
(b) Outline the features of the case study which influenced your decision in making the above diagnosis.
(c) What tests should be performed in order to confirm the diagnosis?
(d) What is the prognosis of this condition if it is still limited to the organ in which it has arisen?

Case study 3. A 23-year-old Caucasian woman of Polish origin presents at your clinic because for the past 5–6 months she has been feeling poorly, having had attacks of abdominal discomfort or pain. Lately she has noticed that she is having problems with her vision, with clouding of vision and problems with focusing, but she has attributed this to eye strain and over-work as she is a book keeper. She has also suffered from intermittent diarrhoea which on occasion has had much mucus and sometimes flecks of blood in it. Her appetite has been affected and she has lost some weight because she 'does not feel like eating very often'. Upon physical examination she is seen to be 1.70 m tall, with a weight of 50 kg, her blood pressure is 170/78 mmHg, pulse rate 78 per minute and her temperature is 37.9°C. Her lungs are normal, but in the right, lower quadrant of the abdomen there is a palpable, tender mass. Her last attack was about a week ago and she had some cramping abdominal pain on this occasion, in association with the diarrhoea. The woman eats a balanced diet with a lot of roughage and fibre and meat is eaten only once a week. Enquiring about disease in the woman's family, you learn that the woman's maternal grandmother died at 68 years from severe rheumatoid arthritis and that her mother suffers from skin allergies and hay fever. The patient has looked up her symptoms in a 'home doctor' type of book and is extremely tense and anxious, fearing malignant disease.

(a) What is the differential diagnosis?
(b) Colonoscopy and other tests performed have excluded malignant disease and inflammatory lesions of the colon. What is the presumptive diagnosis if you were given the additional information that there is no evidence of infectious disease causing her symptoms?
(c) What is the treatment for this disease?

Case study 4. A 72-year-old Caucasian male presents with abdominal discomfort, pain and tenderness which has been troubling him periodically over the past two or three years. He has interpreted this as 'indigestion' and has been taking antacids. He often is constipated also, and the symptoms are relieved by defaecation. What has forced him to seek advice is an episode of pain and abdominal discomfort over the last few days and the observation of pus in his faeces. When questioned, the man tells the examining physician that he has experienced a loss of appetite in the past 6 months but this has been related to his episodes of pain and 'indigestion' which have given him increased trouble. Questioned about his diet he says that he eats 'balanced meals with meat and three vegies every day'. Physical examination shows him to be 1.85 m tall, weighing 79 kg. His blood pressure is 140/88 mmHg and pulse rate is 82 per minute. Temperature is 37.9°C. The lungs are normal and abdominal examination shows tenderness over the left iliac fossa and a rather tender mass is palpable abdominally over the left lower quadrant of the abdomen. An appendectomy scar is clearly visible. The man is slightly anaemic and there is occult blood in his faeces.

(a) What is the diagnosis?
(b) What features of the case indicate this diagnosis?
(c) What advice would be given to the man if the condition you diagnosed is confirmed?
(d) What is the prognosis of the condition?

Case study 5. A 60-year-old Japanese male who has been visiting his daughter in Australia for the past three months presents with epigastric discomfort and mild pain especially after meals. He has interpreted this as 'indigestion' and has been taking antacids. What has forced him to seek medical advice is an episode of haematemesis which occurred the previous evening. When questioned, the man tells the examining physician that he has experienced a loss of appetite in the past 6 months. Physical examination shows him to be 1.75 m tall, weighing 65 kg. His blood pressure is 135/85 mmHg and pulse rate is 75 per minute. Temperature is 37.2°C. The lungs are normal and abdominal examination shows tenderness in the epigastrium with slight abdominal distension and a slight hepatomegaly. The man is anaemic and there is occult blood in the faeces. His blood group is A.

(a) What is the diagnosis?
(b) What features of the case indicate this diagnosis?
(c) What is the prognosis of the condition?

Further Reading

Antonioli DA. 'Gastric Carcinoma and its Precursors.' *Monograph Pathol* 1990; **31**: 144.
Ashwell N. 'Is Colon Cancer Really Linked to a Daily Diet of Red Meat?' *BNF Nutr Bull* 1991; **16**: 60.
Black RE. 'Epidemiology of Traveler's Diarrhea and Relative Importance of Various Pathogens.' *Rev Infect Dis* 1990; **12**(Suppl 1): S73.
Blaser MJ. 'Epidemiology and Pathophysiology of *Campylobacter pylori* Infections.' *Rev Infect Dis* 1990; **12**(Suppl 1): S99.
Brocklehurst JC. 'Colonic Disease in the Elderly.' *Clin Gastroenterol* 1985; **14**: 725.
Bruce WR. 'What Chemicals are Responsible for Colon Cancer?' *J Cell Physiol* 1986; **4**(Suppl): 47.
Butkus SN, *et al.* 'Food Allergies.' *J Am Diet Assoc* 1986; **86**: 601.
Cant AJ. 'Food Allergy in Childhood.' *Hum Nutr Appl Nutr* 1985; **39**: 277.
Cummings M. 'Laxatives Rarely Needed.' *FDA Consumer* 1991; April: 33.
Flock MH. 'Fiber, Foods and Gastrointestinal Microecology.' *J Environ Pathol Toxicol Oncol* 1985; **5**: 233.
Friedman G. 'Peptic Ulcer Disease.' *Clin Symp* 1988; **40**: 2.
Fung WP, Papadimitriou JM, Matz LR. 'Endoscopic,

Histological, and Ultrastructural Correlations in Chronic Gastritis.' *Am J. Gastroenterol* 1979; **71**: 269.

Goodwin CS, Armstrong JA, Marshall BJ. '*Campylobacter pyloridis* Gastritis and Peptic Ulceration.' *J Clin Microbiol* 1986; **39**: 353.

Hodgson HJ. 'Inflammatory Bowel Disease and Food Intolerance.' *J Roy Coll Physic Lond* 1986; **20**: 45.

Hogewind WF, *et al.* 'Oral Leukoplakia with Emphasis on Malignant Transformation: A Follow-up Study of 46 Patients.' *J Facial Maxillofac Surg* 1989; **17**: 128.

Hughes NR, Newland RC. 'Colorectal Polyps in an Australian Population. A Histological and Immunohistochemical Study.' *J Path* 1990; **160**: 41.

Ivy AC. 'The Problem of Peptic Ulcer.' *JAMA* 1946; **132**: 1053.

Lee A. '*Helicobacter pylori* and Gastroduodenal Disease.' *Today's Life Sci* 1990; **2**(11): 12.

Lennard-Jones JE. 'Cancer Risk in Ulcerative Colitis.' *Br J Surg* 1985; **72**: S64.

Manousos ON. 'Diverticular Disease of the Colon.' *Digest Dis* 1989; **7**: 86.

Mucha P Jr. 'Small Intestinal Obstruction.' *Surg Clin N Am* 1987; **67**: 597.

Podolsky DK. 'Inflammatory Disease of the Bowel.' *N Eng J Med* 1991; **325**: 929, 1008.

Ravdin JI. '*Entamoeba histolytica*: From Adherence to Enteropathy.' *J Infect Dis* 1989; **159**: 420.

Riboli E, *et al.* 'Cancer and Polyps of the Colorectum and Lifetime Consumption of Beer and Other Alcoholic Beverages.' *Am J Epidem* 1991; **133**: 157.

Rich AM, Radden BG. 'Squamous Cell Carcinoma of the Oral Mucosa: A Review of 244 Cases in Australia.' *J Oral Pathol* 1984; **13**: 459.

Watne AL. 'Sydromes of Polyposis Coli and Cancer.' *Curr Probl Cancer* 1982; **7**: 1.

Weisburger JH. 'Role of Fat, Fiber, Nitrate and Food Additives in Carcinogenesis.' *Nutr Cancer* 1986; **8**: 47.

Willet WC, *et al.* 'Relation of Meat, Fat and Fiber Intake to the Risk of Colon Cancer in a Prospective Study Among Women.' *N Eng J Med* 1990; **323**: 1664.

Willson JKV. 'Biology of Large Bowel Cancer.' *Hemato Oncol Clin N Am* 1989; **3**: 19.

9

Hepatobiliary System and Pancreatic Disorders

The Normal Liver

The liver is the largest gland in the body, weighing normally between 1400 and 1700 g. It is situated in the right, upper, abdominal quadrant and has a double blood supply. The **portal vein** supplies 75% of the liver's blood and this is the vein that drains the intestinal system. This blood therefore is unoxygenated but is rich in nutrients that have been absorbed in the intestine. The **hepatic artery** branches from the aorta and supplies 25% of the liver's blood, this blood being oxygenated. Both of these blood vessels empty their blood into the liver **sinusoids** and all of the hepatic blood is then drained by the **hepatic vein** which empties into the inferior vena cava. Thus, the liver is interposed between the intestinal and systemic circulation and can extract substances from the intestinal blood, metabolize them, store them, or somehow modify them and then secrete them back into the bloodstream. The liver is also important in detoxifying many substances (e.g. alcohol) that are absorbed by the gut and it also filters the blood, such that any bacteria that have entered the blood in the gut will be retained by the hepatic phagocytic cells resident in the walls of the sinusoids (**Kuppfer cells**, which are resident, fixed macrophages).

The main function of the liver is a secretory one and it is able to synthesize and secrete many substances both into its ducts and into the circulation. Therefore, it functions both as an exocrine and as an endocrine gland. The main exocrine function of the liver is the secretion of **bile** into the bile ducts. Bile is an important substance acting as an emulsifying agent, subdividing the dietary fat into tiny droplets, making it more accessible to the action of lipases. Bile is also the way in which the liver rids the body of excessive waste substances such as urea, cholesterol, calcium and bile pigments. The normal brown colour of faeces is due to the presence of biliary pigments. If no bile enters the intestine the faeces are very pale (**china clay stools**; **steatorrhoea**), as occurs in disorders causing obstructions of the biliary tree. Bile is stored in the gall bladder and when it is required it is released from there into the intestine via the common bile duct.

The liver also functions as an endocrine gland as it secretes many substance directly into the bloodstream. For example, most of the **plasma proteins** (e.g. albumin) are synthesized in the liver. The **clotting factors** (e.g. fibrinogen), essential in haemostasis, are also made in the liver. In addition to these functions, the liver has a multitude of **metabolic functions**, storing and processing many substances including glycogen, fats, vitamins (especially vitamins A, D and B$_{12}$), iron and heparin.

The liver is an organ essential to life and in its absence death ensues in about two to three days due to **hepatic coma**. As can be expected with its multitude of metabolic functions, the liver may show many abnormalities as a result of disease and many such derangements may be detected in the laboratory through investigations involving the so-called liver function tests.

The Normal Gall Bladder

The gall bladder is a small saccular organ located posteriorly to the liver and communicating with the common bile duct via the cystic duct. Its functions are to serve as a reservoir for bile secreted by the liver. The liver secretes 600–900 mL of bile daily, and the gall bladder holds 60 to 90 mL. This bile is concentrated ten times within the organ and its discharge into the duodenum is regulated by the muscular wall of the gall bladder, the pressure within the biliary tract also dependent on the activity of the organ. Bile is a complex mixture of substances and includes bile pigments (especially bilirubin), bile acids and salts, cholesterol and mucin. The functions of bile are:

- to emulsify fats in the intestine and thus help in their absorption;
- to aid in the absorption of calcium and fat-soluble vitamins;
- to excrete bile pigments, cholesterol, some drugs and poisons (e.g. heavy metals, strychnine, quinine).

The Normal Pancreas

The pancreas is a loose glandular tissue, approximately 20 cm long, situated in the mesentery of the loop of the duodenum. It is a gland with both exocrine and endocrine functions. The majority of pancreatic tissue comprises the **exocrine part** which is a typical serous gland arranged in secretory lobules and acini. It is in this region that various digestive enzymes and bicarbonate ions are elaborated and released into the intestine in the form of the alkaline pancreatic juice which neutralizes stomach acid as it enters the duodenum, but which also enzymatically degrades the chyme. The chief enzymes of the pancreatic juice are **trypsin**, **amylase** and **lipase**. It also contains the enzyme-like **rennin** and is made alkaline by **HCO$_3^-$** ions. These secretions are conveyed to the intestine via the pancreatic duct which merges with the common bile duct, opening into the duodenum through the ampulla of Vater. The endocrine portion of the pancreas is situated in small aggregates of cells, the **islets of Langerhans**. The cells here secrete important metabolic hormones: **insulin**, which lowers blood sugar, **glucagon**, which raises blood sugar, and **gastrin**, which increases the secretion of HCl by the stomach mucosa.

Diseases of the Liver

Congenital and Metabolic Disorders

Polycystic Disease of the Liver

This is a congenital disease in which multiple cysts form in many organs throughout the body, the kidney, liver and pancreas being the most commonly affected. The disease is not very common in incidence. It occurs in two major forms, the neonatal form inherited as an autosomal recessive trait and in which the kidneys are always affected (the liver only affected in a third of cases), and the adult form, caused by an autosomal dominant gene. In the neonatal form the cysts begin to form *in utero*, the newborn baby already having signs and symptoms attributable to the disease, while in the adult form the cysts develop later in life, symptoms beginning to appear at around the age of 40 years. The sex incidence ratio of the disease is equal.

Multiple true cysts form throughout the organ affected, greatly enlarging it. The kidneys may attain a length of 30 cm while the liver may also be involved in a gross hepatomegaly palpable through the abdomen. The cysts may be so numerous that no normal tissue is seen between them, the organ assuming a spongy appearance. A single layer of epithelium lines the cysts and the lumen is filled with a clear serous fluid.

In the neonatal form of the disease, the effects may be very severe while the foetus is still in the uterus. The abnormality in the affected tissues causes great dysfunction and very often, stillbirth results. The kidneys of the baby may be so large that a caesarean section may be required as the baby has an abdomen that is too large to pass through the birth canal. These infants may live for a few months and then usually die owing to renal failure.

The adult form most commonly presents with haematuria due to kidney cysts. Acute pyelonephritis with secondary infection of the cysts often occurs and repeated bouts of infection and scarring of the kidney lead to renal failure. Hypertension is seen in 75% of the cases and is due to the kidney damage. A combination of the kidney disorders most often causes death in renal failure. Patients usually present with few liver symptoms, the normal liver parenchyma between the cysts being able to cope with the functions of the liver.

Amyloidosis of the Liver

Amyloidosis commonly affects the liver in its secondary form (liver affected in 90% of cases) and less commonly in its primary form. The amyloid is deposited intercellularly, close to the hepatic vessels and sinusoids, and causes pressure atrophy of the hepatocytes. The liver is converted into a firm, pale, enlarged organ with a rather waxy cut surface, the tissue at autopsy being firm enough to retain its shape and resemble fixed tissue. The patient presents with a hepatosplenomegaly without any significant functional abnormality. Clinically evident disease is most likely to develop when the heart, kidneys or adrenals are involved and any of these organs may fail.

Vascular Disorders

Chronic Passive Venous Congestion of the Liver

Chronic passive venous congestion of the liver (CVC) is a condition in which there is pooling of blood in the liver due to inadequate venous drainage of the organ. The condition is also commonly called 'nutmeg liver' due to the resemblance of the cut surface of the liver to a bisected nutmeg which has a creamy brown mottled surface. The disorder occurs primarily in right ventricular failure which is most often brought about by mitral stenosis, pulmonary hypertension ('cor pulmonale') or tricuspid incompetence. In these cases there is prolonged embarrassment of the venous return to the heart and a systemic venous congestion results in the venous system. In the liver this is manifested as CVC with pooling of blood predominantly around the central veins.

In the early stages of CVC there is hyperaemia and congestion of central veins and adjacent sinusoids. The stasis of blood progressively worsens and reactive changes to anoxia begin to develop in the hepatocytes of the centrilobular regions. With prolonged CVC, the anoxia becomes more marked and there is progressive centrilobular necrosis of hepatocytes. Midlobular fatty change will also be seen as the anoxia progressively damages more areas of the lobules. The periportal area remains normal as it is still oxygenated from blood which irrigates the region from branches of the hepatic artery. The liver at this stage shows a variegated, mottled appearance with deeply congested, red-brown centrilobular areas and paler centrilobular regions with fatty change, a classical 'nutmeg liver'. In unrelieved, chronic cases of CVC, **cardiac cirrhosis** will supervene. If the condition which causes the CVC is treated promptly, the liver tissue will return to normal, the reactive changes to injury being reversible.

Infarction of the Liver

Infarction of the liver is an extremely rare condition due to the double blood supply of the organ. There is a mixing of hepatic arterial and portal venous blood down at the lobular level and it is exceedingly rare to see a condition in which both blood vessels are obstructed. When the condition does occur, it is associated with primary or secondary neoplasms growing within the liver. These rapidly growing tumours will cause pressure effects on blood vessels, with invasion of vascular spaces, leading to ischaemia and infarction of regions of tumour and also regions of liver tissue. Typical regions of coagulative necrosis will develop in the infarcted liver parenchyma (Figure 9.1).

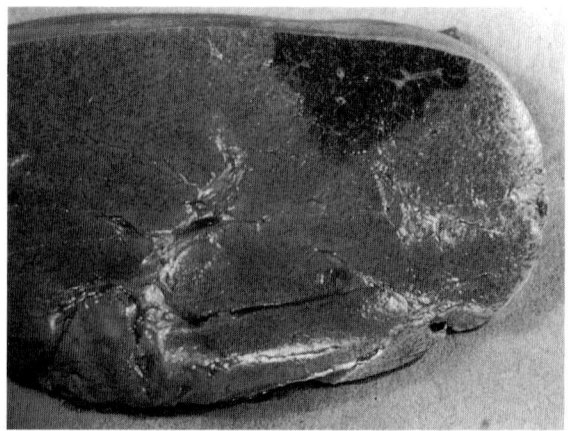

Figure 9.1 *A haemorrhagic liver infarct showing the typical wedge-shaped, subcapsular lesion*

Liver Cell Injury and Necrosis

The liver is one of the major sites in which the metabolism of a wide variety of ingested substances occurs. Many drugs and toxins are converted by the hepatocytes to polar, water-soluble derivatives, which unlike the parent compounds cannot be reabsorbed by the renal tubules and bile ducts, and are therefore excreted. Metabolism occurs in the endoplasmic reticulum, and is mainly carried out by the microsomal enzyme oxidation system (MEOS), where the modification of the parent compound occurs in two phases, firstly a modification of the compound by oxidation or demethylation and secondly a conjugation with polar groups such as glucuronide, sulphate or glutathione. Often the metabolites formed after this phase are very unstable or highly reactive and therefore quite damaging to the liver cells. This may occur with highly toxic compounds, overdoses of drugs or even with therapeutic doses of drugs in some individuals due to '**metabolic idiosyncrasies**'. That is, there are important differences between individuals that are mediated by genetic and environmental influences. Some people possess a more effective MEOS and are therefore better equipped for metabolism of various substances, a typical example being the idiosyncratic response to some therapeutic agents, for example methyldopa leads to abnormal liver function in 5% of patients and to clinical hepatitis in 0.5% of cases. Exposure to the substance in question habitually in other individuals may induce a 'tolerance' to it, that is, an increase in the ability of the MEOS to cope with that substance, the best example in this instance being alcohol.

Fatty Change of the Liver

Fatty change implies the presence of demonstrable fat within the hepatocyte cytoplasm. This change is also commonly seen in cardiocytes and renal tubular cells. The presence of fat indicates injury to the cell and fatty change reflects a reactive change of the hepatocyte to that injury. The fat is derived from fat depots and it comes to the liver via the bloodstream. The lipid may be in the form of multiple small globules or a single droplet, distending the cytoplasm and pushing the nucleus to the side of the cell. The hepatocytes resemble adipocytes (Figure 9.2). The hepatocyte nuclei may show degeneration, and often regions of necrotic cells will also be seen. The central and middle zones of the liver lobule are most commonly affected. Grossly, the liver is enlarged and may be palpated through the abdomen. At autopsy, the organ is very pale with a

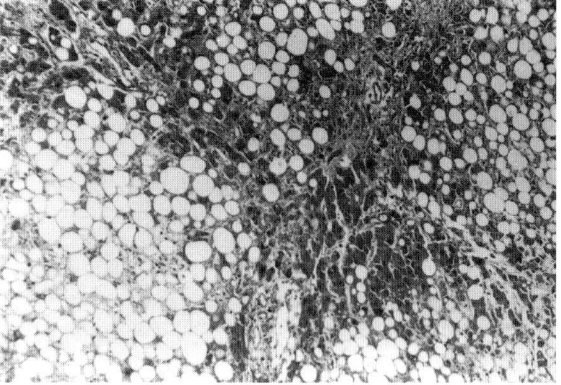

Figure 9.2 *Alcoholic hepatitis and fatty change of the liver (×150)*

smooth, greasy, cut surface, the parenchyma bulging out from the incised capsule.

Fatty change may be produced by many types of injury to the hepatocytes, common forms of injury including infections and various physicochemical factors such as anoxia, nutritional factors and drugs. Hepatocytes perform a central role in lipid metabolism and therefore injury to the cell will be particularly conducive to the development of fatty change. Fatty change is a prominent feature of many disease states:

- **'toxic' conditions and infections** (e.g. toxaemia of pregnancy, hepatitis);
- **poisoning** — organic chemicals (e.g. $CHCl_3$ (chloroform), CCl_4 (carbon tetrachloride), CH_3CH_2OH (alcohol)); inorganic chemicals (e.g. phosphorus);
- **anaemia**, iron deficiency;
- **nutritional factors** — excess fat intake, obesity; pancreatic insufficiency (e.g. pancreatitis); metabolic disorders (e.g. diabetes); inadequate diet (e.g. low-protein diet, vitamin deficiencies).

By far, the commonest cause of fatty change is **alcohol abuse**. The degree and severity of fatty change are related to the amount and duration of alcohol abuse. Hepatic fatty change may be detected after only two days of alcohol excess. When a single large dose of alcohol is taken, fatty acids are mobilized from the fat depots and taken to the liver, whereas when multiple doses are taken (as seen in alcoholism) fatty acids are predominantly of dietary origin. Alcohol is broken down in the liver cell by alcohol dehydrogenase (ADH), involving a change in redox potential due to H^+ generation. Some ethanol is also broken down by the MEOS. Normally, when small amounts of alcohol are consumed, the ADH to MEOS ratio of alcohol breakdown is 3:1. When excessive quantities of alcohol are consumed over a period of time, there is a massive increase in the smooth endoplasmic reticulum of the hepatocyte with a corresponding greatly increased MEOS metabolism of alcohol. This is thought to interfere with fat metabolism by the smooth endoplasmic reticulum.

Mitochondria are also damaged directly by alcohol and this contributes to the mechanism of the fatty change as inadequate ATP is being formed by the damaged organelles. All of these injuries have cumulative effects and relate to alcohol being present in large quantities in the liver almost constantly. The amount of fatty acids that enter the citric acid cycle is subsequently decreased leading to an increased quantity of intracytoplasmic triglycerides and also a hyperlipidaemia. There is an accumulation of cholesterol in the smooth endoplasmic reticulum and also a reduced breakdown of cholesterol which contributes to the hyperlipidaemia (refer to Figure 9.3).

The overall effects of fatty change may be summarized as:

- increased lipogenesis;
- accumulation of fatty acids — NADH/NAD redox changes inhibiting citric acid cycle breakdown of lipids, mitochondrial damage inhibiting citric acid cycle breakdown of lipids, trapping of triglycerides in liver;

- increased lipoprotein synthesis;
- hyperlipidaemia;
- accumulation of cholesterol esters.

If the cause of fatty change is corrected at an early stage, the changes observed in the liver are completely reversible. However, if the injury is of a chronic nature, necrosis of hepatocytes results. Alcoholic hepatitis is seen in association with the necrotic changes and numerous inflammatory cells will infiltrate degenerating regions of parenchyma. Neutrophils will surround regions of hepatocytes which show degenerative changes such as pyknosis of nuclei and hydropic change. Regions of necrotic hepatocytes will also be present, becoming more common the longer the liver is exposed to alcohol.

Other characteristics of alcoholic hepatitis are seen ultramicroscopically and histologically. Giant mitochondria and proliferated smooth endoplasmic reticulum are seen, and **Mallory bodies** (eosinophilic intracytoplasmic aggregates) representing damaged cytoplasmic components of hepatocytes are characteristic of this type of hepatitis. Cholestasis is indicated by bile pigment within the bile canaliculi and macroscopically by a tawny discolouration of the liver. Cirrhosis eventually develops and the patient may then go into liver failure and death.

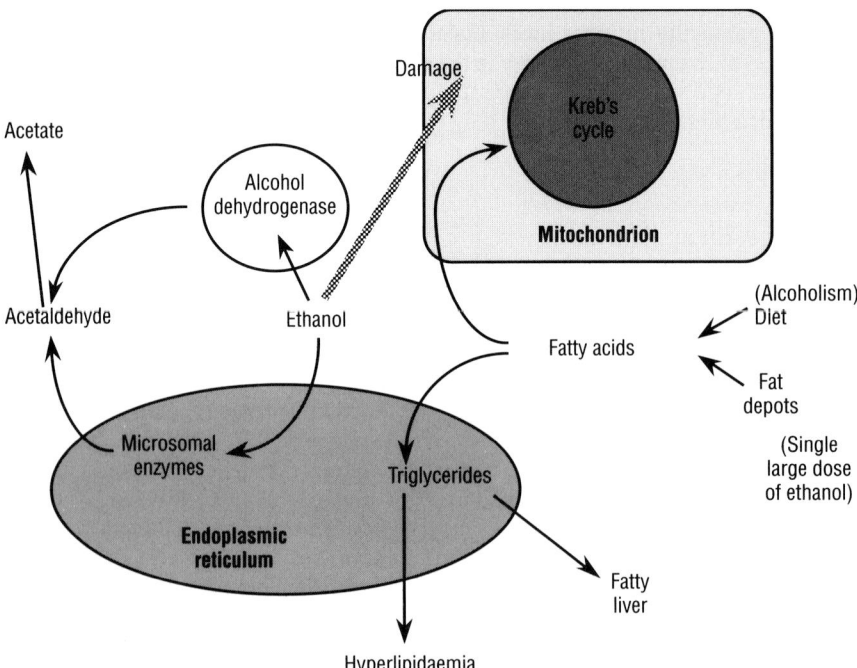

Figure 9.3 *The pathogenesis of fatty change*

Necrosis of the Liver

The death of hepatocytes occurs with many disease processes. Necrotic processes may be divided into **diffuse** (with a further subdivision into zonal diffuse necrosis or massive necrosis) or **focal** (which may affect small groups of cells, or single cells, in the latter case representing a non-pathological mechanism for the control of the hepatocyte population, apoptosis accounting for this loss of cells). Figure 9.4 illustrates the various types of zonal necrosis in the liver.

Focal Changes
Apoptosis. This is a process affecting single hepatocytes and occurs throughout the liver normally. It is a control mechanism whereby senescent hepatocytes are disposed of, with new, regenerating cells taking their place. '**Councilman bodies**' are eosinophilic bodies found in the liver and correspond to the greatly shrunken and dehydrating cytoplasm of cells undergoing apoptosis. Under the electron microscope characteristic changes of apoptosis may be recognized in hepatocytes of normal livers.

Focal necrosis. Focal areas of necrotic hepatocytes with no relationship to lobular architecture will be found in the liver in a variety of conditions. Infections, especially bacteraemias and toxaemias such as typhoid fever, diphtheria and peritonitis, will often lead to this change in the liver. Viral hepatitis and drug-induced liver damage may also present in this manner. Foci of necrotic liver cells are seen with a mild inflammatory reaction surrounding them. A haphazard arrangement of groups of necrotic cells is observed microscopically while macroscopically the liver may appear normal. Generally this is not a severe disorder and there is minimal disturbance to hepatic function. If the necrotic areas are numerous there may be a compromise of liver function, but this seldom occurs. Regeneration of hepatocytes follows the removal of the cause and generally little or no scarring is seen.

Diffuse Changes — Zonal Necrosis
Centrilobular. In this type of change, the necrosis develops in the hepatocytes immediately around the central vein and may then spread around the centre of the lobule as more and more cells are affected. Severe, chronic passive venous congestion of the liver will lead to this type of necrosis, as will viral hepatitis, poisoning (e.g. $CHCl_3$, CCl_4) and miscellaneous other causes.

Midzonal necrosis. Yellow fever characteristically produces midzonal necrosis. Regions of haemorrhage and fatty change may be seen in association with the necrosis. The necrotic cells contain eosinophilic inclusions in their cytoplasm. Cirrhosis does not follow this type of liver necrosis.

Peripheral (periportal) necrosis. Necrotic hepatocytes around the region of the portal tracts typically develop in some toxic conditions such as phosphorus poisoning. Eclampsia (toxaemia of pregnancy) will lead to periportal necrosis of the liver.

In all types of zonal necrosis the organ is diffusely affected and a variable appearance will be seen macroscopically. There may be a blotchy, haemorrhagic or fatty appearance with pallor. Bile-stained necrotic areas may also be apparent. Microscopically, the characteristic zonal areas of necrosis will be seen, with the dead cells surrounded by regions of inflammation, haemorrhage and exudation. The results of zonal necrosis are varied and range from complete recovery and regeneration of hepatocytes, focal post-necrotic scarring or post-necrotic cirrhosis, to massive necrosis of the liver.

Diffuse Changes — Massive Necrosis of the Liver
This is a confluent necrosis affecting nearly all of the hepatocytes of all lobules, thus involving the liver massively. It is also called **acute yellow atrophy of the liver**. It is a relatively uncommon condition, seen as a rare sequela to hepatitis and after some poisonings, for example phosphorus, CCl_4 or muscarine. It may occur in severe eclampsia or severe drug injury, for example paracetamol overdose or hypersensitivity.

The liver is small, wrinkled, flabby and soft, of a yellow colour, frequently haemorrhagic and bile stained. There is a loss of the normal cut-surface pattern. Necrosis of liver cells is seen throughout the parenchyma and some surviving hepatocytes may show evidence of fatty change. If the patients survive for any length of time following the necrosis, inflammation and some bile duct proliferation will be seen. However, in most cases, the condition is rapidly fatal with the patient dying in hepatic coma, the mortality being greater than 80%. In the survivors, cirrhosis will develop.

Infections and Inflammations

Hepatitis

Hepatitis is a term used generally for any inflammatory lesion of the liver. In practice it is used for any diffuse involvement of the liver parenchyma by an inflammatory process. It may occur in acute and chronic

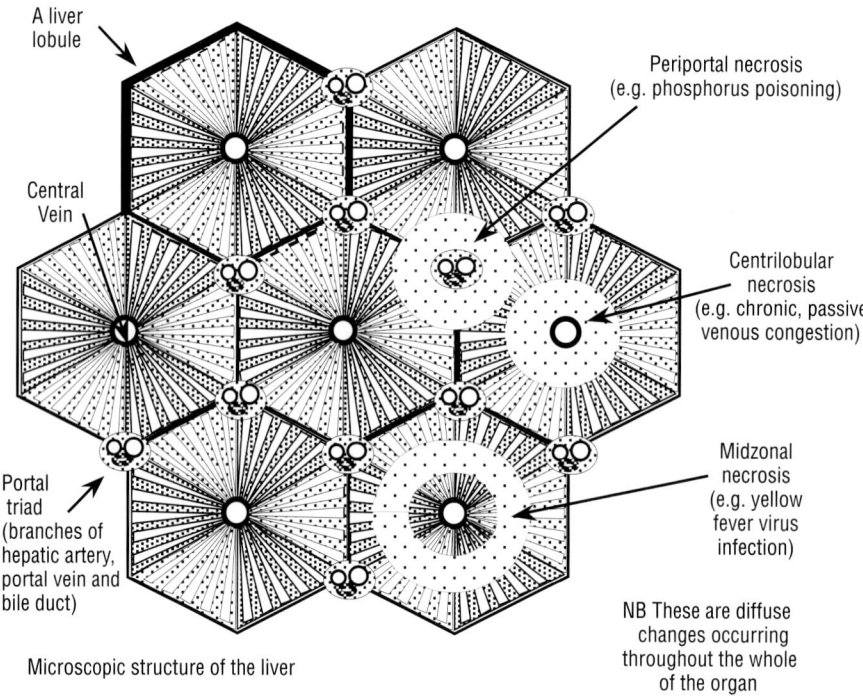

Figure 9.4 *Patterns of hepatic zonal necrosis*

forms and it may be classified also on aetiological grounds. The term hepatitis is often used loosely and it is then understood to mean viral hepatitis, usually serum hepatitis (Hepatitis B). The most common forms of hepatitis are:

- Alcoholic hepatitis
- Drug-induced hepatitis
- Viral hepatitis
- Autoimmune hepatitis
- Idiopathic (or cryptogenic) hepatitis

Viral Hepatitis
Viral agents causing infections of the liver are numerous but the most commonly involved are the hepatitis viruses. These are a variable group of viruses belonging to different families and having different characteristics, the only common factor between them being that they cause liver infections and may give rise to very similar histological changes in the infected tissue. The most important of the hepatitis viruses and their most significant properties are shown in Table 9.1.

The hepatitis viruses have a worldwide distribution and it is observed that hepatitis A virus (HAV) and hepatitis E virus (HEV) infections are commoner in developing countries, often seen in children and young adults, in whom the infection is very mild. The older people are when they first contract these viruses, the more likely it is for the disease to be of a more serious type. HEV infection is particularly serious in pregnancy. In developed countries the infections are prevalent in the institutional setting (mental homes, prisons, barracks) and also in people who engage in specific sexual practices. From 1 January 1991 to 16 July 1991, there were 118 notified cases of hepatitis A in Victoria, 84 of these in males. Of these males 35 were homosexuals, suggesting that sexual practices rather than food sources were more important in spreading the virus.

Hepatitis B virus (HBV) infection is seen to occur endemically in many parts of the world (China and other Far Eastern countries, the Middle East, Eastern and Southern European countries). In these situations the virus is often spread congenitally with a high incidence of chronic infection and carrier states. In the developed countries it occurs sporadically and is seen particularly in intravenous drug abusers, male homosexuals, health and emergency personnel and in the institutional setting. The total number of new, reported cases of HBV infection in Australia for the year ending 17 November 1992 was 2159; for the same period there were 2253 cases of hepatitis C and 332 cases of HAV infection.

Table 9.1 *The viral hepatitides*

Disease	Hepatitis A	Hepatitis B	Hepatitis C	Hepatitis D	Hepatitis E
Synonym	Infectious hepatitis	Serum hepatitis	Transfusion hepatitis	'Delta' hepatitis	New type of infectious hepatitis
Agent	27 nm RNA Picornavirus	42 nm DNA Hepadnavirus	30–60 nm RNA Flavivirus-like	36 nm RNA defective virus (requires HBV to infect)	34 nm RNA virus
Transmission	Faecal–oral	Parenteral	Parenteral	Parenteral	Faecal–oral
Incubation period	15–45 days	40–180 days	15–30 days	30–50 days	30–50 days
Chronicity	None	5% adult carriers 90% neonates carriers	6–60% of cases chronic carriers	79–90% of cases chronic carriers	None
Mortality	0.1%	1–3%	1–2%	up to 20%	20% in pregnancy
Prevention	No vaccine, hygiene, passive immunization	Effective vaccine, safe sex, hygiene, screening blood	No vaccine, safe sex, hygiene, screening blood	No vaccine, safe sex, hygiene, screening blood	No vaccine, hygiene

Hepatitis C (HCV) was named 'Transfusion Hepatitis' as before the routine testing of donated blood for antibody to the virus began it caused over 90% of cases of hepatitis following blood transfusion. In Australia, 0.5% to 1.0% of the adult population is infected with HCV. The infection is very prevalent among intravenous drug addicts (62% of addicts in Victoria are infected and 100% of long-term addicts are infected in NSW), haemophiliacs (76% are infected in Victoria), homosexual men (9–34% infected in Victoria), prostitutes (10% are infected in Victoria) and prisoners (31% in the Victorian study).

Hepatitis D virus (HDV, the δ agent) is a defective virus that cannot cause an infection alone, but needs to infect an individual already infected with HBV. The HBV acts as a 'helper virus', supplying HDV with some genetic information. It is interesting to note that HDV is encapsulated by the coat protein of HBV (HBsAg = HDV surface antigen) but also possesses unique antigens of its own (HDAg). Areas of high incidence include the Amazon basin, equatorial Africa, Middle East, Eastern USSR and Mediterranean basin. In industrialized nations, HDV infection closely follows that of HBV in its selection of victims.

Macroscopically, all of these different types of hepatitis due to the hepatitis viruses show a similar appearance and are described as **acute viral hepatitis** when they first involve the liver. There is diffuse involvement of the organ, although the liver morphology may appear normal. There may be large regions of necrosis and bile staining, or occasionally haemorrhagic regions. In general, HAV and HEV infection cause less damage than the other types of hepatitis viruses.

Microscopically, a great variation in the degree of necrosis is apparent, from almost no necrosis of hepatocytes observed in some cases, to massive, 'panacinar' necrosis involving the whole organ. The type of virus involved and various individual factors are important determinants of how much liver damage will be seen. Zonal necrosis in the centrilobular areas is a commonly observed feature in HBV infection and in some cases this will progress to 'bridging' necrosis between different lobules. More extensive necrosis is commoner with HCV and HBV infection than with HAV infection. Inflammation, with lymphocytes, plasma cells, macrophages and few polymorphs is seen in response to the necrosis. Also apparent is blockage of bile ducts, bile staining and cholestasis. The disease may then regress and the liver will regenerate, the hepatitis resolving (this is most often seen in HAV infection), or the hepatitis may progress to more damage.

In the more damaging, later stages of the disease, if the patient survives, there will be fibrosis, regenerative nodule formation, bile duct hyperplasia, recurrence of necrosis and a typical post-hepatitic cirrhosis will develop. With HBV and HCV infection many of the patients will remain life-long carriers of the virus and in some of these patients a chronic hepatitis will develop causing increasingly more damage to the liver, eventually progressing to liver failure and death (refer to Table 9.2).

The signs and symptoms associated with acute viral hepatitis include, firstly, malaise, fatigue, weakness, nausea, vomiting (may be induced by fatty food), distaste of cigarettes, right upper quadrant abdominal pain, bowel disturbances, diffuse aches and pains, myalgia, headache and fever. These symptoms may be

followed by an icteric phase in which jaundice is seen, with some relief of the initial symptoms. The jaundice deepens for 5–10 days and the anorexia and fatigue may worsen, with some weight loss. Jaundice is more likely to occur with HAV infection. The patients may present with a hepatosplenomegaly, tenderness of the liver or a skin rash. As the patient recovers, the appetite returns to normal with malaise persisting for some time. Exercise tolerance is decreased and depression may be a prominent feature (see Figure 9.5).

Diagnosis of the various types of hepatitis depends considerably on the clinical symptomatology the patient presents with and any relevant medical, family or social history which may be indicative of hepatitis. Laboratory tests for liver function may provide strong evidence for the infection but the full confirmation is dependent on serological profiles in most cases of viral hepatitis, with either antibody seroconversion being noted or alternatively the antigen being detected in the body.

Table 9.2   *Clinical features of the viral hepatitides*

Disease	Hepatitis A	Hepatitis B	Hepatitis C	Hepatitis D	Hepatitis E
Onset	Acute	Insidious	Acute/insidious	Insidious	Acute/ insidious
Severity of disease	Mild	Severe	Moderately severe	Severe	Moderately severe
Jaundice	In ≈50% of cases	In ≈30% of cases	In ≈20% of cases	In ≈30% of cases	In ≈40% of cases
Antigens (+antibodies)	HAAg (Anti-HAV)	HBsAg (Anti-HBs) HBeAg (Anti-HBe) HBcAg (Anti-HBc) HBxAg (Anti-HBx)	No Ag identified (Anti-HCV)	δAg (Anti-HDV)	No Ag identified (Anti-HEV)
Treatment	IgG in severe cases(?), rest, no alcohol	IgG in severe cases, rest, no alcohol	α-interferon, rest, no alcohol	IgG in severe cases, rest, no alcohol	IgG in severe cases(?), rest, no alcohol
Recovery	99% of cases	85% of cases	≈40–50% of cases	≈70% of cases	≈85% of cases
Prognosis	Good, few complications, no carriers	Less favourable chronic hepatitis, cirrhosis, carrier state, carcinoma	Poor, chronic hepatitis, 20% cirrhosis, carrier state, carcinoma	Poor, chronic hepatitis, carrier state, carcinoma	Moderate, no carriers, no chronic hepatitis

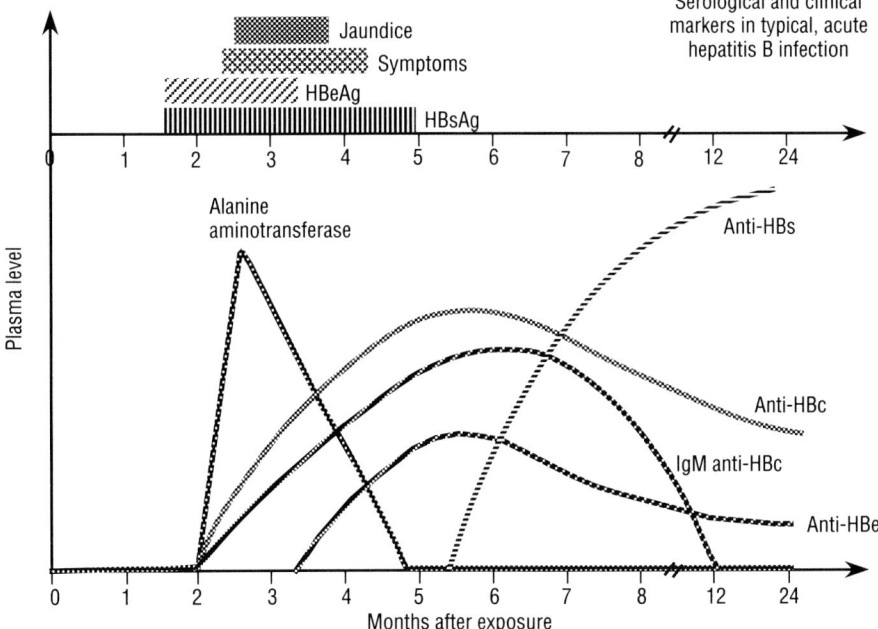

Figure 9.5 *Characteristics of hepatitis B*

Hepatitis Due to Other Viruses

Yellow fever. Yellow fever is caused by a group B Arbovirus of the family Flaviviridae. The virus is transmitted by mosquitoes of the genus *Aedes*. The disease is prevalent in the tropics, often seen in Africa, the Caribbean, Central and South America. The disease varies from an acute febrile illness to a massive liver necrosis with a fatal outcome. Characteristic midzonal necrosis of liver lobules develops and jaundice is what has given the disease its name. The kidneys are also affected with proximal tubular necrosis. The mortality of the disease varies from 20–70% in different epidemics. The surviving patients recover completely with no post-necrotic cirrhosis.

Other types. Herpes virus, rubella virus, Epstein-Barr virus and cytomegalovirus may cause a hepatitis rather similar in appearance to that caused by the hepatitis viruses but liver involvement is an unusual complication of these infections. The infection of the liver occurs especially in immunosuppressed patients and if the disease is very severe may cause the death of the patient.

Weil's Disease

This is a bacterial infection of the liver caused by the bacterium *Leptospira icterohaemorrhagica*, a spirochaete whose natural reservoir is rats and other rodents. Transmission occurs when humans contact rat excreta or urine, more rarely if humans are bitten by rats. The bacteria can penetrate intact skin and mucous membranes and therefore may be acquired by drinking contaminated water. The disease has an incubation period of 2–21 days and the patient presents with hepatosplenomegaly, haemorrhages into mucous membranes and jaundice, which develops in ≈60% of cases. Oliguria may also be observed.

The liver in Weil's disease shows haemorrhages with centrilobular necrosis, ranging from mild to severe. Cholestasis, inflammation and oedema are also seen. The organisms may be demonstrated when sections of liver are stained with silver. The kidneys are also involved with tubular necrosis and haemorrhages. Culture of the organism on special media may be attempted from the blood of the patient in the first week of infection or from the urine in the second week. The disease has a mortality of approximately 10%, patients dying from renal or hepatic failure.

A related disease is **canicola fever** caused by *Leptospira canicola*, whose natural reservoir is dogs. Humans are infected by the bite of the dog, contact with water and food contaminated with dog faeces or urine. The disease resembles Weil's disease, but is rather milder, rarely fatal.

Hydatid Disease

Hydatid disease is an infestation by the cysticercus stage of the tapeworm *Echinococcus granulosus* which is prevalent in sheep-raising countries, therefore very common in Australasia, Africa, the Middle East, South America and the Mediterranean basin. In South America, the disease may also be caused by *Echinococcus multilocularis.* The dog is the definitive host and other related animals such as foxes, jackals and wolves may also act as the definitive hosts. In South Australia half of the dogs are infected with *Echinococcus granulosus.*

Humans are only accidentally involved in the life cycle of the parasite when they come into contact with the ova, which are found on grass, wool or fur contaminated with dog faeces. Children are particularly at risk because of lack of hygiene. The disease is also very common in sheep graziers who contact the parasite daily. Once the ova are ingested they will pass into the intestine where the embryo will form. This will then invade the portal vein and arrive at the liver where most organisms will lodge and form hydatid cysts. The liver is involved in hydatid disease in 70% of cases. Some embryos will negotiate the liver sinusoids and arrive at the lungs where most of them will be trapped by the alveolar capillaries (the lungs being involved in 20% of cases of hydatid disease). Rarely, some embryos will pass through the lungs, into the left ventricle and thence into the systemic circulation with cysts developing in any organ of the body. In the remaining 10% of cases hydatid disease is in evidence in the kidney, bones, heart, spleen, brain, etc. (see Figure 9.6).

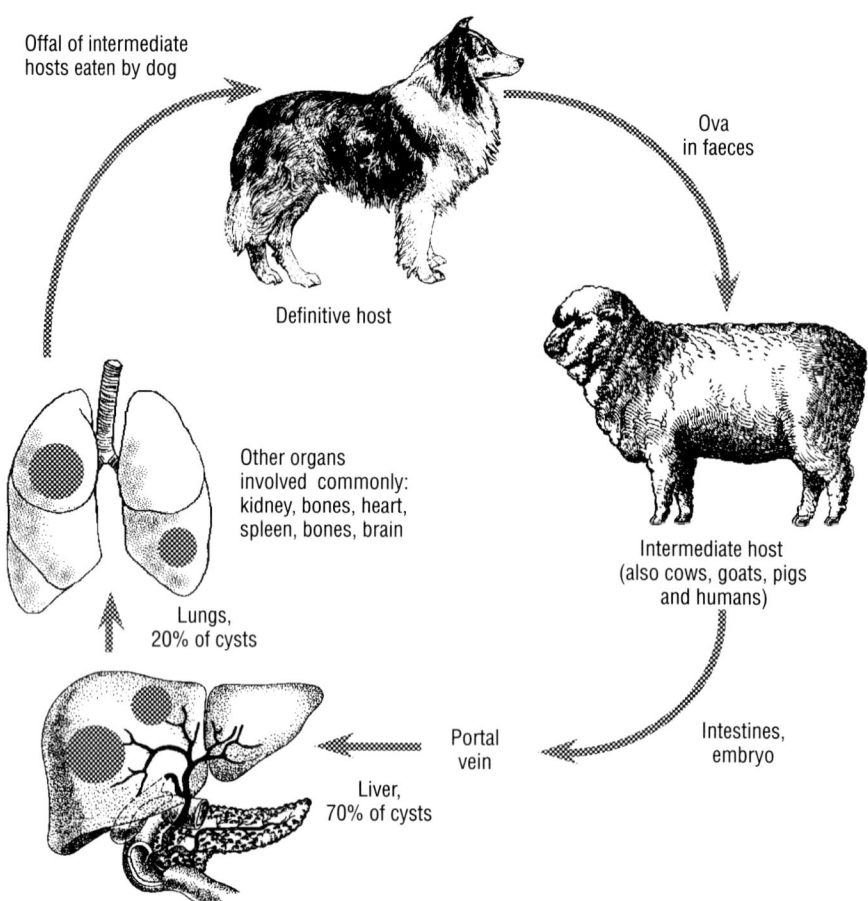

Figure 9.6   *The life cycle of* Echinococcus granulosus

The parasite develops into the typical cystic form the structure of which is the same whatever the site they form in. Hydatid cysts attain a size of 1–5 cm in diameter by 6 months, their final size being 5–20 cm in diameter, or rarely larger. In the liver, the cysts are usually single and in the right lobe and they may cause considerable, palpable hepatomegaly. The host response to the cysts is a chronic non-specific inflammatory response with granulation tissue formation around the cyst and the laying down of a scanty fibrous capsule. Some eosinophils may be seen around the zone of inflammation and an eosinophilia is usually seen in peripheral blood smears. The parasite lays down a thick cystic wall around itself, the inner layer of which is lined by a germinal membrane from which numerous daughter cysts bud off and float free within the cyst fluid, constantly enlarging and becoming filled with scolices (refer to Figures 9.7 and 9.8).

The results of the disease are usually a slowly progressive increase in the size of the cysts which may cause dysfunction in the organ where the lesion is found. The patient may present with dyspnoea and cyanosis due to lung involvement, jaundice due to cholestasis or fever due to secondary infections. Sequelae of hydatid disease include:

- aseptic degeneration followed by calcification;
- secondary infection and abscess formation;
- rupture into the: peritoneum with multiple peritoneal cysts; biliary tree with biliary obstruction; intestine with the parasite excreted in the faeces; chest with multiple pulmonary cysts developing; bloodstream

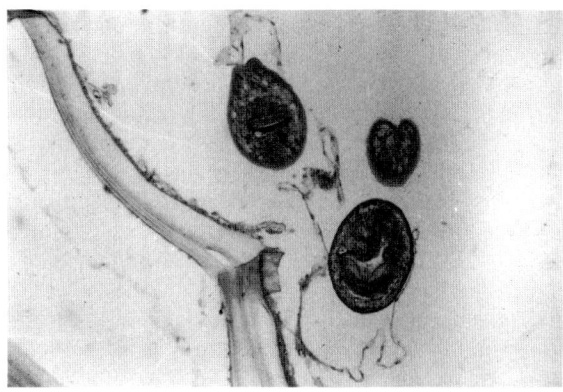

Figure 9.8 *Hydatid cyst within the liver showing the scolices within the cyst cavity (×200)*

with multiple metastatic cysts developing in many organs; external environment through a fistula in the subcutis and skin;
- organ compression and pressure atrophy with dysfunction.

A very important complication of hydatid cyst disease is the development of an allergy (type I anaphylactic response) on a systemic level which may be severe enough to be an anaphylactic shock. The patient experiences dyspnoea, shows cyanosis and circulatory collapse, and may die. The overall mortality of hydatid disease is 10%.

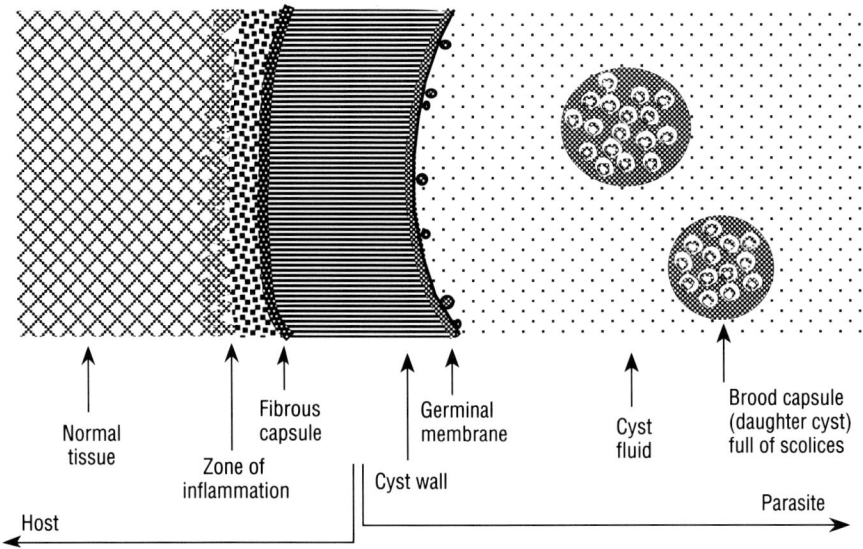

Figure 9.7 *Structure of a typical hydatid cyst*

Diagnosis of the disease is via serology and radiology, but under no circumstances should a biopsy of the mass be tried as the cyst may rupture and thus precipitate an anaphylactic reaction or death. An intradermal sensitivity test may occasionally be used in diagnosis and this is the **Casoni test**. A suspension of purified hydatid antigenic material is injected intradermally and if the patients have contacted the parasite in their tissues, they will develop a localized erythematous area at the site of injection. Treatment of the disease is mainly surgical, with cyst excision and tissue reconstruction. In patients on whom surgery is inadvisable, long-term treatments with scolicidal drugs (e.g. high-dose mebendazole or albendazole) are tried. Prevention of the disease is an extremely important factor in its control and in some countries (e.g. New Zealand), the dog population is treated routinely and regularly for hydatid disease.

Hepatic Amoebiasis

Hepatic amoebiasis is an infection of the liver caused by *Entamoeba histolytica* that occurs mainly in tropical climates, the countries of high incidence being Mexico, Africa and Southeast Asia. The disease typically occurs in 20–50-year-old males. Hepatic amoebiasis develops when the amoebae causing an amoebic dysentery in the large bowel spread via the portal vein into the liver. Diffuse hepatomegaly is usually the first sign associated with the infection and is due to the death of hepatocytes and inflammation, or alternatively due to the liberation of toxic metabolites from the colonic sites of involvement.

Abscess formation in the liver is seen subsequently in many cases and in 75% of cases the abscess formed is single and in the right lobe of the organ. Within the abscess there are many organisms, necrotic hepatocytes, acute inflammatory cells and erythrocytes. This material is a rusty or brownish colour, and the lesion is often known as an 'anchovy paste' abscess. Most patients present with pain in the upper, right, abdominal quadrant and 80% of them also have fever. The pain is worse on moving, breathing or coughing and may be referred to the right shoulder, back or neck. Jaundice is only present in about 5% of cases and is due to abscesses located near the hilum of the organ. Fever and leukocytosis are also evident.

The disease is diagnosed by serology, radiology and microbiological methods. Ultrasonography is increasingly used in the diagnosis; however, differentiating amoebic abscesses from infected hydatid cysts or pyogenic cysts may be difficult with this last-mentioned method. Treatment consists of drainage of the pus (usually percutaneously) in very large lesions, metronidazole administration with rest and other support measures.

Pylephlebitis

This is a suppurative infection of the portal vein and its branches, often spreading into the liver substance with the formation of multiple abscesses. The infection occurs when septic emboli derived from the gastrointestinal tract lodge in branches of the portal vein. Common sites of origin for the septic foci are acute appendicitis, diverticulitis of colon, small intestinal infections, infected haemorrhoids or any other suppurative intestinal infections. Enteric commensal bacteria are usually involved. Multiple liver abscesses will then form if the intrahepatic branches of the portal vein are involved. These abscesses show structures and sequelae typical of abscesses elsewhere in the body (Figure 9.9). The patient presents with symptoms and signs similar to those already described for amoebic abscess above.

Cholangitis

Cholangitis is an inflammation of the liver characterized by an ascending pyogenic bacterial infection of the intrahepatic bile ducts. Common causes are *Escherichia coli*, *Streptococcus faecalis* and other commensal, enteric bacteria. The pathogenesis of the disorder has not been elucidated but several theories exist:

• Ascending infection from an infected gall bladder
• Lymphatic spread
• Direct intraductal spread
• Blood-borne spread

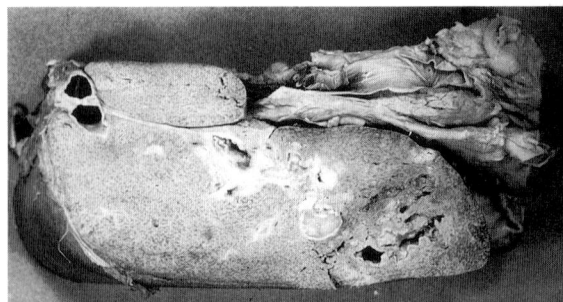

Figure 9.9 *Liver abscess displaying suppuration and involvement of a large amount of the parenchyma of the tissue*

However, the mechanism of infection is not clear, especially in the case where lymphatic and blood spread is involved. Obstruction of bile ducts is thought to be an important factor in pathogenesis The condition causes the patient to present with hepatomegaly, tenderness in the liver, the disease following a septic febrile course. Grossly, pus can be expressed from the cut surface of the liver and is seen to ooze out of the larger bile ducts. Characteristics of the condition microscopically are numerous polymorphs within the intrahepatic bile ducts and cholestasis. Multiple abscesses may form within the liver in this condition. Clinically, cholangitis resembles other septic conditions of the liver.

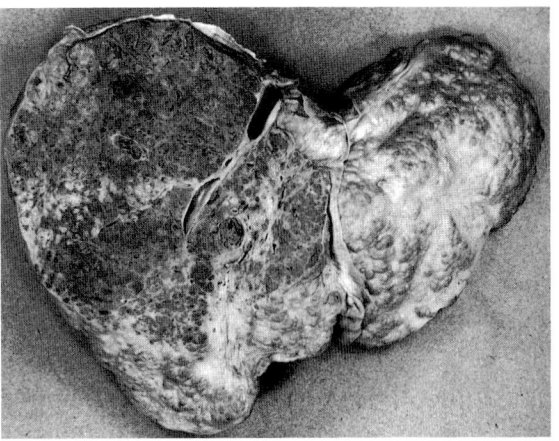

Figure 9.10 *Cirrhosis of the liver and multiple foci of primary hepatocarcinoma in a 56-year-old male heavy drinker*

Cirrhosis of the Liver

Cirrhosis is a condition unique to the liver. It is a disorder affecting the whole of the liver diffusely in which there is gross disruption to the liver architecture, the functioning parenchyma changing into a large number of lobules separated by branching sheets of fibrous tissue (Figure 9.10). The word cirrhosis is derived from the Greek *kirrhos* (tawny) and this colour is due to bile staining of the fibrotic liver tissue that does not allow normal draining of the bile formed by the hepatocytes. The disease may be caused by a variety of different factors and presents with similar end appearance and results, despite the underlying aetiologies. The condition may be classified in two ways, aetiologically or morphologically. It should be noted, however, that there is a poor correlation between aetiological and morphological classifications, different aetiologies being capable of giving rise to similar morphological types of cirrhosis. The aetiological classification of cirrhosis is summarized in Table 9.3. It

should be noted that acquired cirrhosis is more common in incidence than congenital cirrhosis.

The morphological classification of cirrhosis depends mainly upon the gross appearance of the liver tissue. **Micronodular cirrhosis** implies that small nodules, ≈3 mm in diameter, are present in the liver. The nodules are all roughly the same size, giving the liver a regular, granular appearance. This type of cirrhosis was also termed the 'Laennec' or 'portal' type. **Macronodular cirrhosis** implies that larger nodules, up to 3 cm in diameter, are present in the liver, showing some variation in size, giving the liver a nodular, irregular appearance. **Mixed cirrhosis** shows areas of micronodular and macronodular cirrhosis within the affected liver, giving it a great irregularity of appearance (see Figure 9.11).

Table 9.3 *The aetiological classification of cirrhosis of the liver*

Congenital cirrhosis	Acquired cirrhosis
Due to errors of metabolism	Toxic effects
Haemochromatosis	Alcoholic
Wilson's disease	Drug related
Thalassaemia	Post-infectious
Galactosaemia	Post-viral (post-hepatitic)
Glycogen storage disease	Cardiac cirrhosis
α_1 antitrypsin deficiency	Biliary cirrhosis
Others	Autoimmune ('Lupoid hepatitis')
Idiopathic (= cryptogenic)	Idiopathic (= cryptogenic)

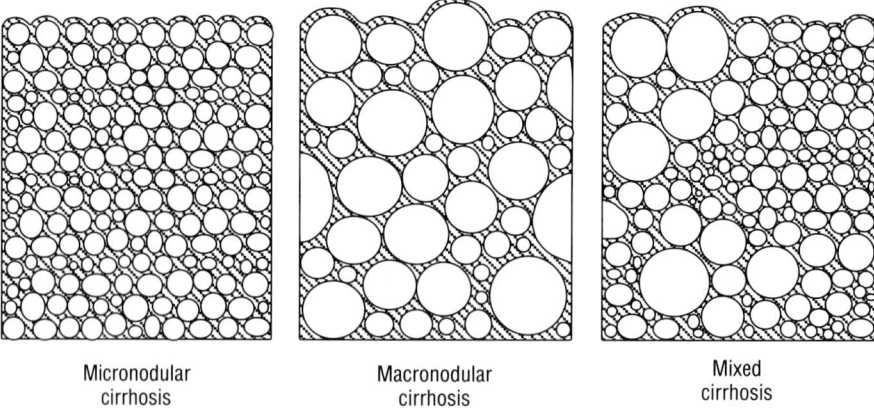

Micronodular   Macronodular   Mixed
cirrhosis   cirrhosis   cirrhosis

Figure 9.11   *The morphological classification of cirrhosis of the liver*

Morbid Anatomical Criteria for Diagnosis of Cirrhosis

In order to diagnose cirrhosis in a liver the following criteria are used. When the features described are present in a liver specimen, it is possible to diagnose cirrhosis with confidence.

- Diffuse involvement of the whole liver must be present.
- Disorganization of the lobular architecture must be demonstrated.
- Necrosis of liver cells must have occurred at some stage.
- Regenerative nodules of hepatocytes must be present.
- Diffuse fibrosis must be in evidence.
- Bile duct hyperplasia and dysplasia (aberrant bile ducts) may be present.

In addition, certain clinical features which may be present will further consolidate the diagnosis. These include:

- evidence of hepatocellular failure;
- hepatic encephalopathy or coma;
- evidence of portal hypertension;
- ascites.

Alcoholic Cirrhosis

Cirrhosis due to the excessive consumption of alcohol over a long period of time is one of the commonest (if not the commonest) forms of cirrhosis in our community. Chronic alcohol abuse is defined as more than 100 g of alcohol (2 litres of beer or one bottle of wine

or five large whiskies/spirits) daily over a period of years. It is important to note that some individuals, but especially females, are more at risk in developing cirrhosis with even smaller quantities of alcohol. Various undefined host factors influence susceptibility in different individuals. Fatty change is the first indication of liver damage by alcohol and as more hepatocytes undergo necrosis, an alcoholic hepatitis will develop. Alcoholic hepatitis is seen 3 to 5 years after sustained alcohol abuse in 35% of alcoholics. On average, it is known that approximately 15% of alcoholics will progress to cirrhosis.

Alcoholic liver disease is associated with fatty change of the liver, the organ being large, pale and fatty. In its early stages, alcoholic cirrhosis presents a fine regular appearance characteristic of a micronodular cirrhosis. This occurs as the hepatocytes are damaged, undergo necrosis and become replaced by fibrous scar tissue. The small nodularities present represent surviving hepatocytes undergoing mitotic divisions and regenerating the lost mass of tissue. Scattered throughout the liver will be seen evidence of continuing damage to hepatocytes, with fatty change and hydropic change observed. In later stages the liver becomes shrunken, tough and markedly nodular. More fibrous tissue is laid down and the regenerative nodules enlarge, with a mixed type of cirrhosis seen (Figure 9.12).

Clinical Effects. The effects of cirrhosis are manifold (refer also to Figure 9.13) and include **hepatocellular failure**. This is a change which develops as progressively more hepatocytes undergo necrosis, the regenerating cells being insufficient in mass and function to replace the cells lost. The patient is aware of fatigue, loss of weight and a general deterioration in health

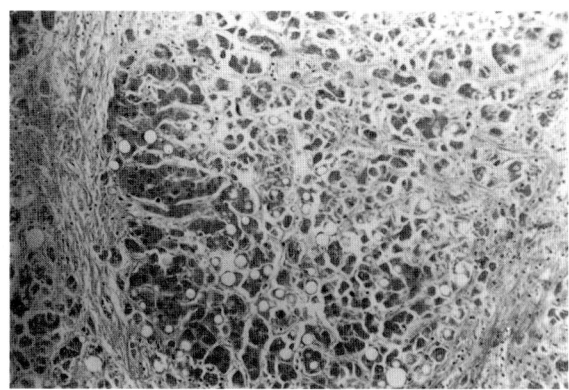

Figure 9.12 *Cirrhosis of the liver showing extensive scarring replacing the necrotic foci of hepatocytes, fatty change of surviving cells and darker cells in a regenerative nodule (×100)*

state. **Low-grade fever** may be present due to the inflammatory changes and necrosis within the liver. Physical symptoms and signs of liver cell failure are as follows.

- **Jaundice**: This occurs as the damaged liver cells fail to excrete normal amounts of bilirubin. The bilirubin enters the bloodstream and is deposited within many tissues including skin. It may be visible only in daylight and indicates a serum bilirubin of over 34 µmol/L.
- **Foetor hepaticus** (= 'liver breath'): This develops as the liver cells fail to detoxify certain compounds and fail in their normal metabolic functions. Substances which would normally have been catabolized in the liver are now present in the blood and diffuse out into the alveoli. The musty odour is related to altered methionine metabolism by intestinal bacteria, leading to expiration of mercaptans in the breath.
- **Endocrine disturbances**: The liver normally catabolizes oestrogens. In cirrhosis, excess oestrogens will be present. In both sexes this will cause **spider naevi**, which are dilated superficial small arterioles, especially in the upper trunk and face, and 'liver palms' which are reddened palms due to dilated vessels, both manifestations of the effects of high levels of oestrogens on the vasculature in these sites. There are also changes in distribution of body hair and infertility. In women there may be changes in the breasts and disturbances in the menstrual cycle. In men high levels of female sex hormones cause **gynaecomastia** (enlargement of breasts), testicular atrophy and decreased libido.
- **Neurological disturbances**: These are related to

the increased ammonia being present in the circulation due to non-inactivation by the damaged hepatocytes. Ammonia is neurotoxic and brain damage may cause drowsiness, 'flapping' tremor, mental changes; hyper-reflexia, rigidity and seizures, or even coma and death. All of these changes are believed to be due to high levels of ammonia or other nitrogenous metabolites in the plasma, circulating as they are unable to be detoxified by the liver.
- **Metabolic effects**: The liver is the site of major metabolic activity and hepatocellular failure will result in many important aspects of metabolism becoming compromised. As the level of albumin synthesized by the cirrhotic liver decreases, generalized **oedema** will be seen. Muscle wasting develops as the circulating albumin is the building block protein of all body proteins. **Haemorrhages** will develop as the clotting factors synthesized by the liver (fibrinogen, prothrombin, etc.) diminish in the circulation. An increased susceptibility to toxic effects of drugs and toxins may be seen as fewer hepatocytes are present to cope with toxin metabolism and as there is also liver dysfunction.

Another important cluster of complications and effects of cirrhosis relate to the development of **portal hypertension** in the cirrhotic patient. This occurs as the fibrous tissue tracts within the liver interfere with the flow of portal blood through the liver.

- **Splenomegaly**: This occurs because there is passive congestion of the spleen with excess blood which is not passing fast enough through the liver.
- **Circulatory disturbances on a systemic level**: A hyperdynamic circulation develops with a high cardiac output. This change is related to portal hypertension and interference with normal venous return to the heart.
- **Oesophageal varices**: Varicosities develop in the lower oesophageal veins as more blood from the portal circulation is attempting to bypass the liver by flowing into communicating systemic venous channels which anastomose with portal venous channels at this location.
- **Haemorrhoids**: Varicosities develop in the haemorrhoidal veins as more blood from the portal circulation is attempting to bypass the liver by flowing into communicating systemic venous channels which anastomose with portal venous channels at this location.
- **Caput medusae**: This is prominence of periumbilical veins seen in those patients in whom the foetal umbilical vein has remained unobliterated and allows communication between systemic venous channels and portal venous channels.

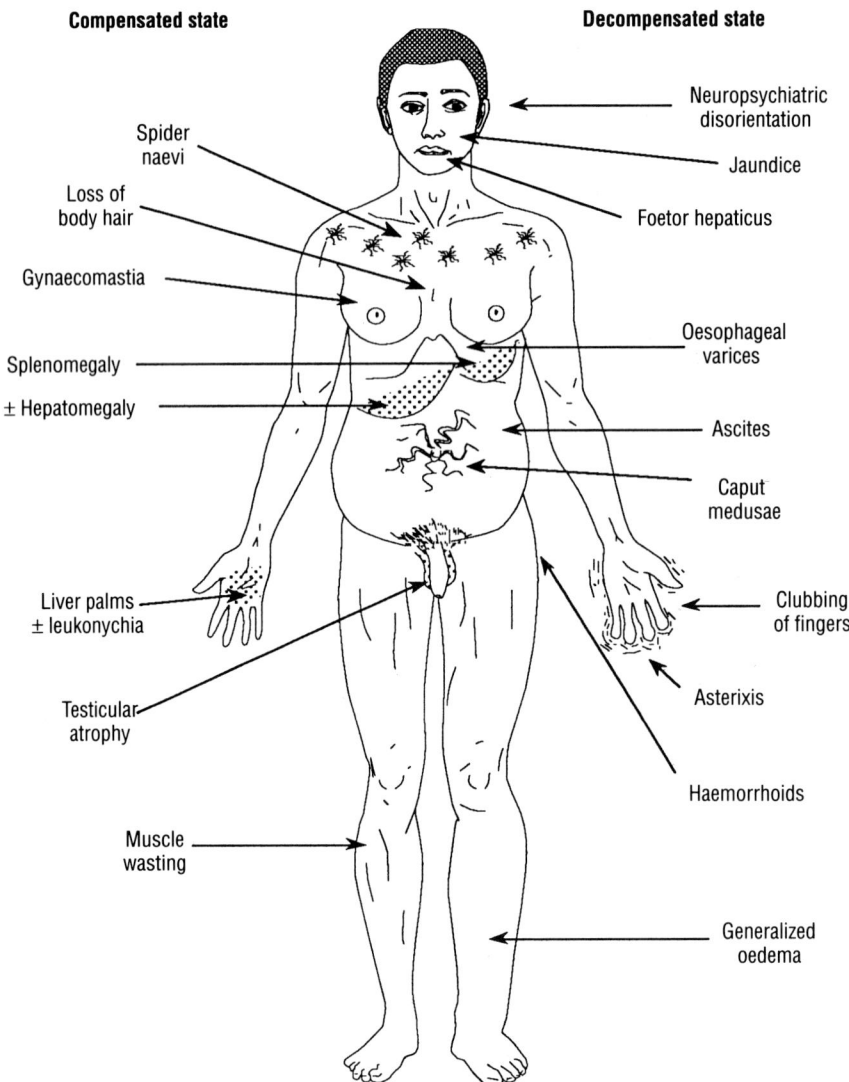

Figure 9.13 *Clinical features of cirrhosis of the liver*

- **Ascites**: This is due to a combination of factors, including portal hypertension, hypoalbuminaemia and compromised lymphatic drainage of the liver, sodium and water retention with secondary hyperaldosteronism. It is clinically evaluated by the sign of 'shifting dullness' in the abdomen.

  Secondary effects of cirrhosis may also give rise to important indications clinically.

- **Anaemia**: This is often seen because of chronic blood loss from small mucosal haemorrhages and also because of the malnutrition. Clubbing of fingertips and **leukonychia** (white fingernails) may be seen in association with the anaemia and malnutrition, but other poorly understood factors may also be responsible for these changes.

- **Xanthelasmata**: These are due to chronic cholestasis and are deposits of cholesterol within macrophages of the skin, especially around the eyelids (if present on the elbows and palms a primary biliary cirrhosis is indicated).

- **Hepatocarcinoma**: Cirrhosis is a premalignant state and 5% of patients with cirrhosis will develop the primary malignancy in their liver. A rapid deterioration of hepatic function is seen in the cirrhotic patient who also develops the carcinoma.

Result. Cirrhosis may be present in patients for many years in a '**compensated state**', a term which implies that there is a precarious balance struck between the number of hepatocytes being destroyed and the number regenerating. The liver still manages to function well enough such that major ill effects are not seen. It should be remembered that in the compensated cirrhotic state, the liver function tests may be normal; however, this does not imply that the liver is normal or that it is functioning very efficiently. The disease then usually progresses to the '**decompensated state**' where the number of functioning hepatocytes is insufficient to cope with the liver's functions. More serious clinical symptoms and signs will then develop and the patient becomes very ill. Death due to hepatocellular failure complications or due to portal hypertension complications may then result.

Diagnosis. Clinical symptomatology is an important factor in the diagnosis of cirrhosis and a presumptive clinical diagnosis is usually made after physical examination of the patient with many of the signs of the disease of cirrhosis. A high index of suspicion is necessary for diagnosing the disease in many cases and the history of the patient should be examined thoroughly. Liver function tests are then performed, but they may be normal. In some patients or in later stages of the disease there may be raised levels of serum alkaline phosphatase and γ-glutamyltransferase. CT scanning will show the fibrotic and nodular liver very clearly and biopsy of the organ will show the severity of the disease and degree of damage.

Treatment. Various behaviour modification therapies and drug treatments are attempted in order to relieve symptoms and to prevent further damage to the body. Alcohol intake is forbidden and various other drugs which are hepatotoxic are avoided. Diuretics may be prescribed for the ascites and oedema. Reduction of the absorption of ammonia in the gut through dietary modification is undertaken. Vasopressin is prescribed or portacaval anastomosis is undertaken for portal hypertension and its effects. Increasingly, liver transplantation is being indicated for patients with very severely damaged livers.

Prognosis. This varies considerably according to whether the patient abstains or not. The outcome is much improved if patients abstain, and the likelihood of complications is decreased. The 5-year survival of abstainers is 60% while the 5-year survival of non-abstainers is 40%. It should be noted that these figures are worse than those for some types of cancer. Patients with cirrhosis and liver cell carcinoma have a grave prognosis with less than 5% surviving for 5 years.

Other Conditions Precipitating Cirrhosis

A variety of other aetiologies will precipitate a cirrhotic state and the appearance of the liver is very similar to that already described in association with alcoholic cirrhosis. As the final results on liver morphology and function are similar, the patient will present with clinical signs and symptoms identical to those of the alcoholic cirrhotic patient. However, as these aetiologies of cirrhosis are associated with some other agents or predisposing causes, there may also be other indications in the patients' presentation which will point towards the precise aetiology of the cirrhosis. Thus, differential diagnosis in a cirrhotic patient is of prime importance. For example, questioning the patient about family history, country of birth, medical history (e.g. has the patient received a blood transfusion?) or sexual orientation may lead to a diagnosis of cirrhosis associated with viral hepatitis infection. Examining the patient for evidence of skin pigmentation or performing tests for diabetes may be important in cases of cirrhosis due to haemochromatosis. Serological tests may identify autoantibodies to hepatocytes and thus a diagnosis of autoimmune cirrhosis may be arrived at.

Post-hepatitic Cirrhosis
This accounts for approximately 20% of cases of cirrhosis and is mainly associated with infections caused by HCV and HBV. The cirrhosis develops as a consequence of necrosis caused by the viruses acutely or, alternatively, instead of a true cirrhosis the liver may show post-necrotic scarring which involves regions of focal scarring in an otherwise normal liver. In most cases, the cirrhosis is associated with cases of chronic hepatitis caused by these viruses.

Haemochromatosis ('Bronze Diabetes')
Haemochromatosis is an inborn error of metabolism involving iron absorption. The defect has been linked to the HLA A3 locus on chromosome 6. Normally, iron is absorbed from the intestine according to the needs of the body; however, if iron is not needed a blocking mechanism operates and no more iron is absorbed. In the patients with haemochromatosis this blocking mechanism does not operate and iron is absorbed continuously from the intestine. The disease is ten times more common in males than females (women presumably protected from the iron overload by their menstrual blood loss). Although the defect is present

at birth, patients do not present with symptoms of the disease until their fourth decade, the iron accumulating in the body over those years until, instead of the normal 2 to 3 g, the body may contain up to 30 g of iron.

Iron is stored in the tissues within parenchymal cells and macrophages in the form of haemosiderin. The tissues affected are the liver, pancreas, spleen, heart, skin, testes and endocrine glands. The liver shows massive deposition of iron and is a rusty red colour, enlarged, wrinkled and nodular. Microscopically it shows the characteristics of a pigment **cirrhosis** (with haemosiderin pigment in hepatocytes and Kupffer cells but also intercellularly), fibrous tracts, large regenerative nodules and bile duct hyperplasia (Figure 9.14). The incidence of hepatocarcinoma is much higher in these patients than in patients with other types of cirrhosis (Figure 9.15). The pancreas is brown and firm and also contains large quantities of haemosiderin. There is considerable pancreatic damage and degeneration with fibrosis. The islets of Langerhans are affected, thereby leading to diabetes mellitus in many cases. In the spleen, there is marked enlargement with firmness and pigmentation. The heart shows pigmentation, atrophy of cardiocytes and severe atherosclerosis of the coronary arteries. In the skin, the iron is deposited in the dermis around the skin appendages and its presence stimulates the melanocytes to produce more melanin, leading to a 'bronzing' of the skin caused by the increased melanin production and iron deposition. As these patients are often also diabetics, the alternative name of haemochromatosis reflects these changes. Iron deposition in the testes leads to testicular atrophy, infertility, decrease in libido or impotence. Endocrine problems may also be seen if the deposition in the glands is very severe and the patient may present with

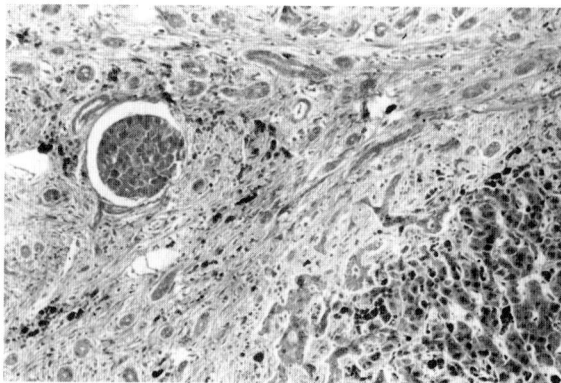

Figure 9.15 *Haemochromatosis of the liver with embolus of hepatocarcinoma in a vessel*

symptoms relating to hypoadrenalism, hypothyroidism or hypopituitarism.

Diagnosis of the disease is confirmed by laboratory investigations which demonstrate a high serum iron level, complete or almost complete saturation of the serum iron-binding capacity and an elevated serum ferritin level. Liver biopsy will show hepatic fibrosis or cirrhosis with deposition of iron. Tests for diabetes often prove positive and a glucose tolerance test is the most useful diagnostically.

Treatment of the disease is by regular venesection with removal of 0.5 to 1 litre of blood weekly. This mobilizes iron stores with considerable improvement in the manifestations of the disease. Iron in the diet may be lowered and many treatments also consist of administration of iron chelating agents which will bind to and remove iron from the body. Prognosis of the disorder improves with these forms of treatment, although the risk of development of primary hepatocarcinoma appears to remain high.

Kinnier-Wilson's Disease (Hepatolenticular Degeneration)
This is another form of congenital pigment cirrhosis, inherited as an autosomal recessive trait. There is a deficiency of the copper-binding protein in the plasma, **ceruloplasmin**. There is an excess of copper in the body and the exact mechanism of the copper metabolism defects is not known. Excess copper is deposited in many tissues including the liver (the copper deposition causing a portal cirrhosis); the brain, especially in the basal ganglia (with degeneration causing tremor, rigidity, dysarthria and other neurological manifestations); the cornea (the copper deposited in the margin of the cornea giving rise to the **Kayser-Fleischer ring**,

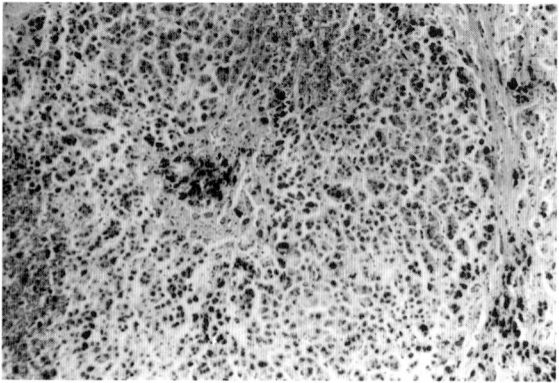

Figure 9.14 *Haemochromatosis of the liver prepared with Perl's stain to demonstrate the iron (dark particles) (×100)*

which is a brownish green line in Descemet's membrane in the eye); and the kidney, in the glomeruli and tubules (causing renal damage and aminoaciduria).

The disease is diagnosed from its familial nature, the clinical presentation and laboratory investigations which show increased urinary copper excretion, low plasma ceruloplasmin (normal = 250–500 mg/L), low plasma copper (normal 11–24 μM/L) and high copper content in the liver. Treatment consists of chelating excess copper by administering penicillamine and this results in marked clinical improvement. However, there is progressive damage and generally the life span of these patients is greatly reduced. Death usually results from intercurrent infections in association with the neurological disturbances and in some patients the liver damage is severe enough to cause liver failure.

Biliary Cirrhosis

Another type of pigment cirrhosis is associated with biliary obstruction, which may be extra- or intrahepatic. The obstruction has as a result the accumulation of bile pigment in the liver. The patient presents with characteristics of obstructive jaundice and if the condition is unrelieved cirrhosis will develop. Most cases of biliary cirrhosis are of a secondary nature, the cause of the obstruction being readily demonstrable and may be due to calculi, strictures, tumours or fibrocystic disease. The liver is enlarged and green in colour with regions of fibrosis and nodular regeneration. Distension of bile ducts is seen and the cause of the obstruction may be demonstrated. Hepatocellular failure and portal hypertension develop later in this type of cirrhosis and treatment of the cause of the obstruction will cause improvement of liver function, even if much necrosis of hepatocytes has already occurred.

In a small number of cases, **primary biliary cirrhosis (Hanot's cirrhosis)** is seen and in this a progressive non-suppurative cholangitis of unknown cause develops, mainly in females between 35 and 70 years. Pruritus and jaundice are brought on in many cases by the oral contraceptive pill. There is hepatosplenomegaly, increased levels of serum alkaline phosphatase, skin pigmentation and xanthomata. The disease has an autoimmune component and anti-mitochondrial antibodies can be demonstrated in these patients. The prognosis is generally poor, most patients dying within 5 to 10 years of development of the condition.

Cardiac 'Cirrhosis'

This condition develops in association with severe chronic passive venous congestion of the liver seen in chronic cardiac failure, unrelieved by treatment for a long period of time. The pooling of blood in the liver leads to firstly fatty and hydropic change and then to a predominantly centrilobular necrosis and fibrosis. Regenerative nodule formation is never prominent in this type of cirrhosis. This lack of liver regeneration is what has led some hepatologists to regard this disease as not being a typical cirrhosis. It is very rare to see hepatocellular failure and portal hypertension in this condition, and in most cases it does not cause clinical effects. The progress of liver damage may be checked by adequate and prompt treatment for the heart failure.

Nutritional Cirrhosis

Nutritional factors may be important in causing liver damage and dietary disturbances are often coupled with alcoholism. Many alcoholics exhibit a dietary deficiency of protein with the lack of choline and methionine causing fatty change and contributing to the liver damage. In very fatty diets of extremely obese people, fatty change may be seen in the liver.

Autoimmune Cirrhosis

Chronic active hepatitis due to autoimmune disease may lead to significant prolonged destruction of the liver, culminating in cirrhosis. This classically presents in women at the time of puberty or the menopause, males only affected in a quarter of cases (M:F = 1:3). Antinuclear antibodies are present in the serum of such patients in high titres and there are also antibodies to mitochondria and smooth muscle cells. Lupus erythematosus cells are present in ≈15% of patients but this disease shows no other relationship to SLE. Corticosteroid therapy, with or without azathioprine, has been shown to be very effective in limiting the extent of the disease, inducing remission and generally prolonging the life expectancy of the patient. The treatment usually has to be given over years (at least two years), but following this period, cessation of drug treatment often leads to complete remission with no relapse.

Cryptogenic Cirrhosis

Approximately 20 to 30% of cases of cirrhosis are of unknown causes and no aetiological factors may be demonstrated in these patients. Control of the disease in these cases is difficult and liver damage may be extreme.

Neoplasms of the Liver

Hepatocarcinoma

This is the primary malignant tumour derived from liver cells and is also called 'malignant hepatoma', 'hepatocellular carcinoma' and 'primary liver carcinoma'. Such liver tumours are rare in Western countries, accounting for approximately 1% of deaths from malignant disease. However, in Asia and Africa they may account for about 30% of all malignancies and in some Southeast Asian countries they are the prime cause of cancer deaths.

The aetiological and predisposing factors associated with these tumours have been identified in most cases and include:

• hepatitis B infection (and cirrhosis);
• haemochromatosis (and cirrhosis);
• alcoholic cirrhosis (5% of cirrhotic patients develop the tumour);
• chronic parasitic liver disease, for example *Clonorchis* spp. infestation;
• ingestion of mycotoxins, metabolites of fungi (**aflatoxin**, produced by *Aspergillus flavus*, is commonly ingested in foodstuffs in Asia and Africa and hepatocarcinoma causes 50% of cancer deaths in African Bantus and 40% of cancer deaths in Javanese Malays);
• ingestion of carcinogens, for example azo-compounds ('butter yellow' was used in the past as a colourant of margarine);
• exposure to ionizing radiation;
• genetic and congenital factors (e.g. in a small proportion of tumours, the **malignant hepatoblastomata**, that arise in neonates).

The appearance of the tumour varies somewhat when examined with the naked eye. Hepatocarcinoma may occur as a single brown mass of irregular outline in the right lobe of the liver, often haemorrhagic, necrotic or bile stained. Alternatively, there may be several such tumour masses, thought to represent multicentric primary tumours arising at approximately the same time in the liver, or, alternatively, a single primary tumour with numerous intrahepatic metastases. The tumour cells microscopically resemble normal hepatocytes although pleomorphism and giant forms are seen. There is an irregular arrangement but there is some attempt by the malignant cells to line blood spaces and they may also secrete bile.

Symptoms and signs associated with the tumour are not very characteristic and may be confused with other liver diseases. Patients complain of vague gastrointestinal complaints, usually referred to as 'indigestion'. There may be weakness, lassitude and loss of weight. A hepatomegaly and ascites are noted during the physical examination and there may be right upper quadrant tenderness or pain. A friction rub or bruit may be auscultated over the liver. Conclusive diagnosis of the tumour is made by ultrasonography, hepatic scintigraphy, selective coeliac angiography and demonstration of raised levels of α-foetoprotein in the plasma of many of these patients (in 75% of cases, levels of 500 ng/mL occur).

Hepatocarcinomata are rapidly growing tumours which invade the liver tissue and replace it, however, extrahepatic metastases are rare. These are rapidly fatal tumours and the majority of patients survive only a few months from time of diagnosis. Treatment of the tumours may be a problem as hepatocarcinomata are not responsive to chemotherapy and the only effective treatment is surgery, with removal of the mass and affected lobe, or hepatectomy and liver transplantation. There is a slightly better prognosis in patients with a single tumour mass, but on average, 5-year survival is less than 5%.

Cholangiocarcinoma

This is the primary malignant tumour of the intrahepatic bile ducts and is also called a 'malignant cholangioma'. It accounts for 20% of all malignant primary liver tumours, but is very rarely seen, causing only 0.2% of all deaths from malignant disease. There is a slight male preponderance of the tumour. Cholangiocarcinoma is less frequently associated with cirrhosis but otherwise there is a similar aetiology to hepatocarcinoma.

Cholangiocarcinoma is a dense white tumour that infiltrates along biliary channels or more rarely as a single nodular mass or many masses. Microscopically, it is a typical columnar cell adenocarcinoma often forming tubules. There is no bile secretion but mucus production may be prominent as is also the abundant stroma which is formed to support the tumour cells.

These are rapidly growing tumours which invade into the surrounding tissues but also rapidly metastasize to the abdominal lymph nodes, bones and lungs. Jaundice is clinically very prominent as the growth of the tumour within the bile ducts causes obstruction. A biliary cirrhosis does not develop in most cases as the patient dies rapidly. The 5 year survival for the tumour is less than 10%.

Secondary Liver Neoplasms

Secondary neoplasms of the liver are extremely common, much more frequently encountered than primary tumours. In about a third of all cases of malignant deaths, secondary tumours are found in the liver. The tumours that are found in the liver as secondaries may arise in any part of the body and they migrate to the liver via three routes:

- via the portal vein (primaries of the colon, stomach and pancreas often using this mode of spread);
- via the hepatic artery (primaries of the lung, breast and malignant melanoma arriving at the liver through this vessel);
- via direct spread (primaries of stomach, pancreas and gall bladder spreading to the liver directly).

Once the tumour cells reach the liver they form multiple deposits of tumour that are paler than the liver tissue, often having necrotic and haemorrhagic centres. The liver attains an enormous size, sometimes up to 10 kg, occupying two-thirds of the abdominal cavity.

Clinically the patient presents with abdominal distension due to hepatomegaly and ascites caused by portal hypertension. There may be jaundice due to biliary obstruction. Liver failure and liver infarcts may result as the tumour compresses and invades into blood vessels. There may develop obstruction and thrombosis of the portal vein, which causes splenomegaly, portal hypertension and haemorrhages. Symptoms and signs of the primary tumour may also be present (e.g. respiratory distress, cyanosis, coughing and haemoptysis associated with a primary carcinoma of the bronchus or, alternatively, bowel disturbances, faecal blood and bowel obstruction associated with colorectal carcinoma). The patient with secondary liver tumours has an extremely poor prognosis, only surviving for a few weeks or months after diagnosis.

Diseases of the Gall Bladder

Infections and Inflammations

Cholecystitis is an inflammation of the gall bladder usually associated with gall stones and the production of abnormal bile. It may be acute or chronic in form. As with most disorders of the gall bladder, cholecystitis is much more frequently seen to occur in middle-aged females. This association of gall bladder disease with a common presentation of patient has given rise to the mnemonic that '**fat, fair, fertile, females over forty**' are likely to present with gall bladder problems.

Acute Cholecystitis

This is a typical acute inflammatory condition of the gall bladder, in which during the early stages 90% of cases are sterile. By 24 hours 35% of cases are infected

and by the third day 90% of cases are infected. The secondary infection which develops is caused by streptococci, coliforms, clostridia and other intestinal anaerobes. *Salmonella typhi* may occasionally cause a primary infection of the gall bladder and *Salmonella* carriers have the organism inhabiting the gall bladder. In most cases, the inflammation is associated with the obstruction of the cystic duct by a calculus (96% of cases). Other important factors leading to a predisposition to the development of the disorder are production of abnormal bile, pancreatic reflux or infarction of the gall bladder wall with subsequent bacterial infection. The routes of infection are via the blood, from infections of the liver and intestine, or direct spread through the biliary tree.

The inflamed organ shows congestion, oedema and distension. Small haemorrhages are often observed and the bile is turbid or frankly purulent. In severe infections the interior of the gall bladder becomes filled with pus, leading to **empyema**. Ulceration of the mucosa with exudation and a fibrinous serosal exudate are seen and, uncommonly, in very severe cases gangrene is found. Microscopically a typical acute inflammatory response will be observed.

Patients with acute cholecystitis present characteristically with pain which is centred around the right upper abdominal quadrant and which often radiates to the right scapula or shoulder. The pain is worse with moving or coughing. Sweating is common but vomiting is unusual. Associated with the infection there will be fever, chills and shivering. On palpation, tenderness over the gall bladder area is elicited.

Complete resolution of the condition is very rare and in most cases the suppuration or empyema will lead to healing by organization and fibrosis, even when treatment with appropriate antibiotics is given. Rarely, especially with neglected, severe cases, gangrene, perforation and peritonitis will result. Chronic cholecystitis is likely to occur as a sequela in large numbers of cases and in these patients, subsequent attacks of acute cholecystitis are a common occurrence.

Chronic Cholecystitis

This is a chronic inflammatory condition of the gall bladder, which although may occur as a sequela of acute cholecystitis, is most often a separate clinical entity of insidious onset. It is associated with gall stones in over 90% of cases and usually no organisms are isolated from the affected gall bladders.

Chronic cholecystitis is a typical example of the chronic fibrotic form of inflammation and the affected organ is markedly contracted, with considerable thickening and fibrosis of its wall. Normally, the gall bladder wall is quite thin and translucent such that the bile in the organ may be discerned through the wall. In chronic cholecystitis the wall is ten times its normal thickness and quite opaque. The mucosa is scarred and atrophic and often is found to grow deeply into the wall, with cystic spaces formed by these invaginating islands of mucosa. When this change is very marked the mucosal invaginations may reach the serosal layer and are termed **Rokitansky-Aschoff sinuses**, the gall bladder being referred to as one exhibiting **cholecystitis glandularis proliferans**. It is very important in this case to differentiate this condition from a carcinoma, which the dysplastic invaginated mucosal cystic spaces may superficially resemble. Other features of the condition are a chronic inflammatory infiltrate throughout the thickened wall and the presence of biliary calculi or a very thick and viscous 'biliary mud' filling the lumen of the organ.

Symptoms of the condition are very ill defined and many cases may be asymptomatic. Some patients complain of vague discomfort in the right upper abdominal quadrant, especially after very large or fatty meals. Definite signs and symptoms are mostly related to acute exacerbations of inflammation which may occur frequently to occasionally. If a gall stone lodges in the cystic duct a biliary colic will result and the patient complains of an excruciating pain lasting for several hours.

Complications associated with the condition almost always relate to the inconvenience, discomfort and pain associated with the recurrent attacks of acute cholecystitis or the blockage of the biliary tract by calculi. Rarely, carcinoma of the gall bladder may be seen to complicate the condition, especially in patients who have suffered from cholecystitis for many decades. The most effective treatment for the disease is **cholecystectomy**, which relieves all of the symptoms and prevents all complications of the condition.

Cholelithiasis

Cholelithiasis is the condition associated with the formation of biliary calculi (gall stones) within the gall bladder, caused by the bile solids coming out of solution and precipitating around foci of crystallization (Figure 9.16). The condition is a very common one and is found in 10% of the adult population and in 25% of routine autopsies. It is more frequently seen in females (M:F= 1:4).

The aetiology of the condition is not precisely known but in all of the cases an abnormal bile composition may be demonstrated, with alteration of biliary choles-

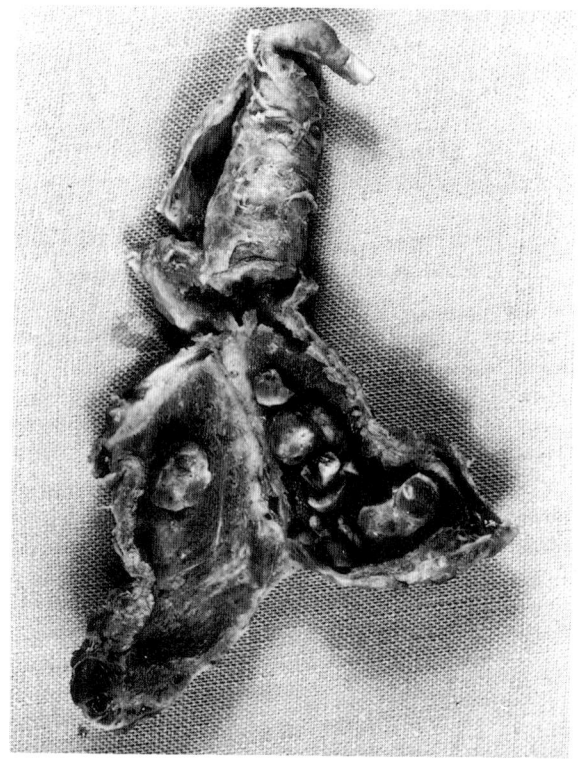

Figure 9.16 *Cholelithiasis in a 45-year-old female patient who suffered from attacks of cholecystitis*

terol levels (normally 60 mg of cholesterol per 100 mL of bile). Calcium salts, biliary pigments or bile acids may also be present in abnormal amounts. In some cases, infection may cause the condition. Stasis of bile is another important factor which causes supersaturation of the bile. Deposition of stones occurs by precipitation from this supersaturated solution.

Two types of gall stones are formed in cholelithiasis. **Pure stones** (found in 10% of all cases) are composed of a single substance and can be cholesterol calculi, calcium bilirubinate (pigment) calculi or calcium carbonate calculi. **Mixed stones** (90% of all cases) are composed of mixtures of cholesterol, bile pigment and calcium salts in a protein matrix. They most often show a laminated structure when they are bisected. These calculi are associated with cholecystitis and are often multiple (up to about 50–60 within the gall bladder); they vary in size from a few millimetres to 5 cm. They are usually dark on the exterior due to bile staining and are faceted as they rub against each other.

The condition of cholelithiasis is frequently associated with attacks of cholecystitis. However, if there is no coexistent acute inflammation in the gall bladder and if the stones remain in the gall bladder there are usually no symptoms. If a stone is passed through the neck of the gall bladder or duct an excruciating pain (biliary colic) occurs acutely and lasts for 12 to 15 hours. The pain may radiate to the right scapula and the patient often suffers from episodes of vomiting and sweating.

The effects of cholelithiasis depend on whether the stones remain in the gall bladder or whether they pass into the biliary tract. If the gall stones remain *in situ*, no clinical symptoms or complications may result, the condition often discovered as an incidental finding during an unrelated examination. Alternatively, in some patients, biliary calculi may cause acute cholecystitis or potentiate chronic cholecystitis. If the stones pass into the cystic or common bile ducts, they will cause obstruction and obstructive jaundice may develop. Calculi may pass into the duodenum where they may block the pancreatic duct and precipitate acute pancreatitis. A gall stone ileus may develop if multiple stones are passed into the intestine.

Diagnosis of the condition may be made on clinical presentation of the patient or occasionally a plain abdominal X-ray will demonstrate gall stones; however, only 10% of gall stones contain sufficient calcium to be radio-opaque. Ultrasonography is the most reliable and most commonly used method for confirming diagnosis. A cholecystogram or intravenous cholangiography and endoscopic retrograde cholangiopancreatography are also used sometimes, especially if obstructions are suspected.

Treatment of the condition is by cholecystectomy, especially if complications have occurred. Fragmentation of the stones by ultrasound (**lithotripsis**) may also be used and, depending on the type of stone formed, drug treatment may prevent the formation of some biliary calculi. Generally, the prognosis of the condition is excellent with treatment.

Miscellaneous Conditions

Cholesterosis

Cholesterosis is a condition resulting from the deposition of cholesterol esters in the mucosal macrophages of the gall bladder in a patchy fashion leading to distinct yellowish flecking of the reddened, inflamed mucosa, producing the so-called 'strawberry gall bladder' (Figure 9.17) The condition is found in 10% of autopsies performed.

The aetiology is not definitely known, but it is not associated with generalized disorders of cholesterol metabolism, so local factors are thought to be impor-

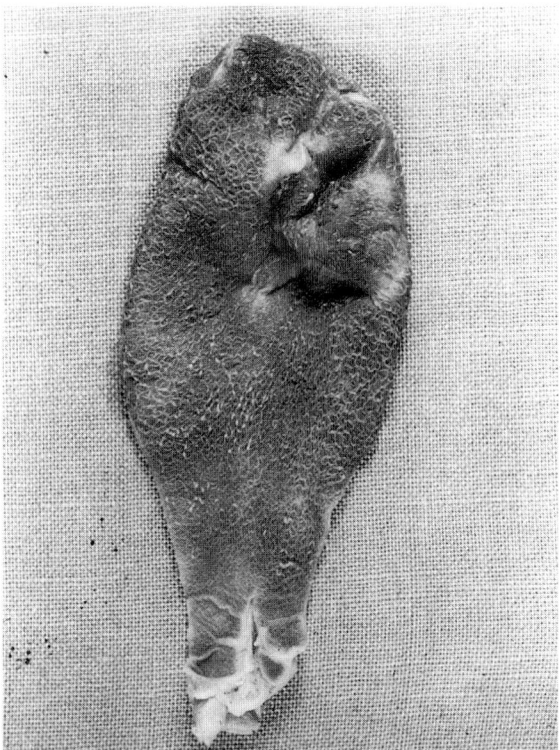

Figure 9.17 *'Strawberry gall bladder' found incidentally at the autopsy of a 31-year-old woman*

tant. It is suspected that excessive absorption of cholesterol from bile occurs and deposition of this then occurs in the mucosa. Alternatively, failure of mucosal secretion of cholesterol into the bile may be the major factor, leading to localized deposition in the mucosa.

The internal aspect of the organ shows enlargement and distension of the mucosal folds with the characteristic appearance of the yellowish flecks of cholesterol on red background. Many foam cells (macrophages laden with lipid) are found in the submucosal layer with a chronic inflammatory infiltrate. The condition is normally symptomless, although it has been shown to precipitate cholelithiasis. It often coexists with cholecystitis, although it does not predispose to it.

Mucocoele of the Gall Bladder

Mucocoele of the gall bladder implies a gross distension of a mucus-filled organ. It is usually caused by a stone impacting in the cystic duct, in the absence of infection. The mucosa secretes copious mucus which fills the lumen, greatly increasing the intracystic pressure. The wall is thin with a smooth, luminal aspect and atrophied mucosa. Evidence of previous cholecystitis may or may not be present and within the mucus more stones may be found. If infection supervenes, empyema may develop in the organ.

Neoplastic Conditions

Carcinoma of the Gall Bladder

The condition is rare, accounting for approximately 1% of all cancers. It occurs more commonly between 60 and 70 years of age and it affects females four times more commonly than males. The aetiology of the condition is not definitely known, although biliary calculi are found in more than 80% of cases of carcinoma (however, less than 2% of patients with stones will develop carcinomata). Some researchers maintain that long-standing chronic cholecystitis may be a predisposing factor. It should also be noted that cholic acid derivatives are amongst the most potent experimental carcinogens known.

Carcinomata in this site are infiltrating tumours causing a diffuse thickening of the wall with invasion to involve the whole of the organ and adjacent tissues. Ulceration and necrosis are common findings. Papillary tumours with areas of necrosis and haemorrhage may also occur. Microscopically, 90% are well-differentiated adenocarcinomata that may secrete mucus, while the remaining 10% are squamous cell carcinomata. The tumours spread locally, involving the liver and bile ducts and causing obstructive jaundice. Lymphatic invasion and blood spread give secondaries in the regional lymph nodes, liver and lungs. The tumours have a very poor prognosis, as they tend to present late and are also quite malignant in behaviour, tending to spread quickly. The average duration of life from diagnosis is one year, with the 5-year survival being less than 8%.

Jaundice (Icterus)

Jaundice is a yellow colouration, first noted in the skin and sclerae, due to deposition of bilirubin in many tissues in the body. This deposition begins to occur if the serum level of the pigment exceeds 34 μmol/L (= 2 mg/100 mL; normally it should be less than 12 μmol/L). The superficial tissues may be stained a yellow to deep orange colour. Olive-green tints are seen in severe chronic conditions due to the formation of biliverdin.

Most bilirubin in the body (85% of it) comes from the splenic breakdown of red blood cells, the remainder coming from bone marrow and metabolism of cytochromes and myoglobin in various body sites. The amount of bilirubin produced in the body daily is 300 mg. Upon release from macrophages in the spleen, bilirubin is in the unconjugated form (or pre-hepatic bilirubin) which is lipid soluble and hydrophobic. In this form it circulates in the blood, bound to serum albumin, and passes into the liver where it is taken up by hepatocytes and conjugated to form the diglucuronide. This conjugated form (or post-hepatic bilirubin) is secreted into bile, passes into the intestine, is converted to stercobilinogen and excreted in the faeces, finally forming stercobilin. In the gastrointestinal tract some of the stercobilinogen is deconjugated by bacteria, the free bilirubin being in part reabsorbed and made available to the liver (enterohepatic portal circulation) and in part broken down by bacterial enzymes to urobilinogen, some of which appears in the urine (refer to Figure 9.18).

Types of Jaundice

In liver disease, jaundice indicates a failure of 80% or more of hepatic function. Several different types of jaundice are known, and if normal bile metabolism is taken into consideration when interpreting laboratory results valuable information may be derived about the possible disease processes which have caused the jaundice (Table 9.4).

Haemolytic (pre-hepatic) jaundice is due to the rate of bilirubin formation being greater than the rate of conjugation and excretion by the liver cells. It is usually caused by conditions where there is an increased breakdown of haemoglobin (such as may occur in a haemolytic anaemia). There is retention of unconjugated bilirubin in the body.

In **parenchymatous (hepatocellular) jaundice** bilirubin production is normal but the hepatocytes are functionally incapable of excreting all of the pigment which arrives in the liver. It is generally caused by damage to hepatocytes (e.g. hepatitis, cirrhosis), and the excess of bilirubin will be a mixture of unconjugated and conjugated forms.

In **obstructive (post-hepatic) jaundice** bilirubin production is normal but the pigment excreted by the liver is prevented from reaching the intestine. Any obstruction of intrahepatic bile ducts or the common bile duct will cause the condition (e.g. gall stones, tumours). There is an excess of mainly conjugated bilirubin which may pass into the kidney and urine.

The pathological effects of jaundice are usually

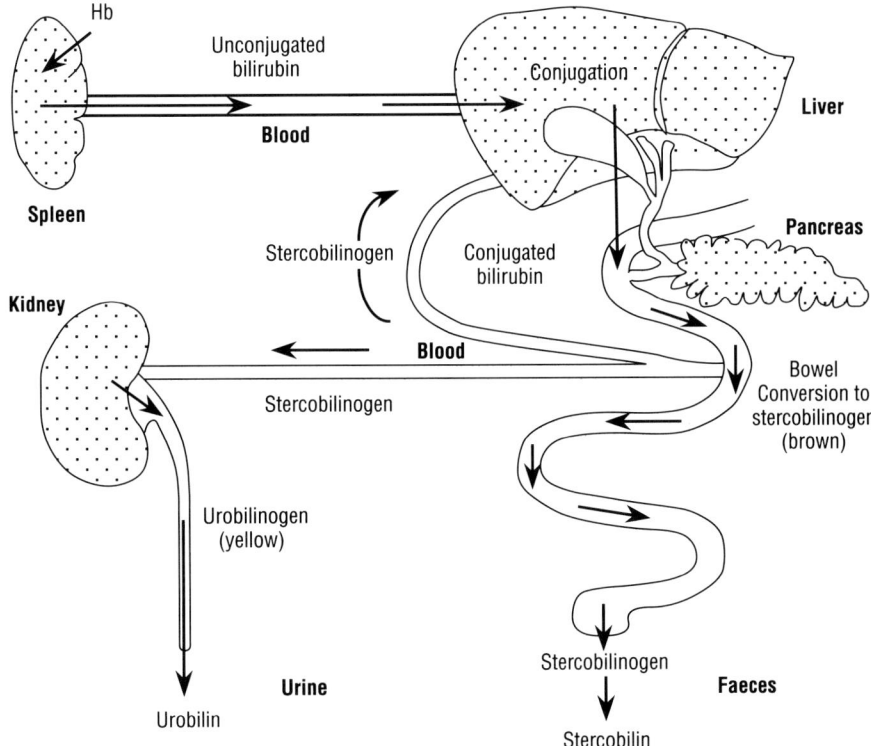

Figure 9.18 *Normal bile metabolism*

minimal if the condition which precipitates is of short duration. Jaundice is a useful sign which may provide clues as to the disease process which is associated with it. With haemolytic jaundice, the patients may have excessive biliary pigments in their bile, causing pigment calculi to form, and all of the complications of cholelithiasis may then occur. Increased iron deposition will also be seen in the liver due to the increased breakdown of haemoglobin. This is termed **haemosiderosis** and will not cause liver damage as does haemochromatosis.

Unconjugated bilirubin, being lipid soluble, may produce central nervous system toxicity, especially in the newborn where it is concentrated in the basal ganglia to produce a severe brain disorder called **kernicterus**. This may be seen in premature infants especially, where the liver is still not fully capable of carrying out its functions and much unconjugated bilirubin is found in the circulation. Unconjugated bilirubin is bound to albumin and is not filtered in the glomeruli. Thus it does not appear in the urine even if the serum level is high (**acholuric jaundice**). Under these conditions more diglucuronide is also produced

by the liver, leading to a high urinary urobilinogen. Conjugated bilirubin, being water soluble, is relatively non-toxic and readily excreted by the urine.

In **cholestatic jaundice** the retained bile eventually causes some hepatocellular damage, or metabolic shift, so that ultimately 20 to 40% of unconjugated bilirubin accompanies the predominantly conjugated hyperbilirubinaemia. A secondary biliary cirrhosis may develop in the liver and the stools become pale and putty-like ('**China clay stools**') due to fat malabsorption. Reduced fat absorption will also include malabsorption of fat-soluble vitamins, the most common and serious of which is vitamin K deficiency, leading to decreased clotting factor formation and haemorrhage. Bile salt overflow from the hepatocytes leads to deposition in skin where irritation causes intense itching. Plasma cholesterol levels rise in cholestasis, leading to xanthomatosis and atherosclerosis.

Hepatocellular jaundice will result with pre-existing damage to the hepatocytes, this being associated with hepatitis or cirrhosis mainly, and in these two conditions the jaundice may serve as an important diagnostic tool.

Table 9.4 *Laboratory findings in jaundice*

Effect on:	Haemolytic jaundice	Hepatocellular jaundice	Obstructive jaundice
Urine bilirubin	Absent	Often absent (may be present, esp. with HBV infection)	Present, increased
Urine urobilinogen	Increased	Increased or decreased	**Not** increased
Colour of faeces	Dark	Pale or normal	Pale (steatorrhoea)
Faecal occult blood	Absent	May be present (esp. with cirrhosis)	Often present (esp. with tumours)
Alkaline phosphatase	Normal	Usually <200 IU	Often >200 IU
Blood bilirubin	2–5 mg/100 mL (unconjugated mainly)	0–8 mg/100 mL (conjugated mainly)	3–30 mg/100 mL (conjugated mainly)
Prothrombin time	Normal	Prolonged, not corrected by IV vitamin K	Prolonged corrected by IV vitamin K
Serum proteins	Normal	Raised γ globulin (hepatitis); reduced albumin (cirrhosis)	Usually normal (may see slight increase in α_2 and β globulins)
γ-Glutamyl-transferase	Normal	Raised usually	Normal

Diseases of the Pancreas

Congenital Disorders

Fibrocystic disease (mucoviscidosis) is a congenital, generalized disease due to the accumulation of thick, viscid mucus in the mucous glands of many organs including the pancreas, lungs, biliary tract and bowel. It is an autosomal recessive trait, with a gene frequency of 1 in 30, 4% of the adult population being carriers and 1 in 2500 children affected. Affected families have a 1 in 4 chance of producing an affected child. The disease causes 3 to 4% of all deaths in children's hospitals. The sex ratio is equal.

The condition is brought about by the excessive formation of abnormal mucus and is assisted by the failure to produce normal mucolytic enzymes. The affected babies often die young because of involve-ment of many organs. The disease should be suspected in the newborn with meconium ileus and intestinal obstruction, indicated by a failure to defaecate in the first 48 hours of life. Infants may present with marked emaciation, wasting of muscles, skin lesions and steatorrhoea. The pancreas is shrunken, fibrous and its ducts are blocked by thick mucus. There is lymphocytic infiltration but the islet tissue is spared. The lungs are affected in 80 to 95% of cases and these children suffer from recurrent respiratory infections, presenting with lung collapse, bronchiectasis, emphysema, bronchopneumonia, abscesses, mucous plugs in airways and often severe respiratory distress. The bile is viscous and often causes obstruction leading to biliary cirrhosis.

The diagnosis is confirmed by finding a high so-dium chloride level in the sweat (levels greater than 60 mEq/L are diagnostic of the condition) and also by pancreatic function tests, which will be abnormally low. Treatment consists of antibiotic therapy for the lung conditions, pancreatic replacement therapy, high-protein, low-fat diet, fat-soluble vitamin supplements and a high salt intake. Bowel obstruction may need treatment with an enema. Increasing numbers of affected people are now surviving into adulthood, but the general prognosis is poor with infant mortality very high.

Infections and Inflammations

Acute Pancreatitis

The term 'pancreatitis' covers a wide range of non-bacterial, inflammatory conditions of the pancreas, ranging from acute fulminating, to mild, or even to symptomless, disease. The pathological features are very diverse. Acute and acute relapsing pancreatitis imply that the pancreas may go back to normal once the initiating stimulus has been removed. If damage is not severe, sequelae do not usually occur. Acute haemorrhagic pancreatitis involves severe damage to the pancreas and its vessels, with necrosis, haemorrhage and fat necrosis being very prominent. Fibrosis, relapsing or chronic pancreatitis are common sequelae of this latter type.

Although acute pancreatitis is not very common in incidence, it is important as it may be fatal. Its incidence is also apparently increasing. It is usually seen in people over the age of 40 years and females are slightly more frequently affected than males. It is commoner in obese individuals in Western countries but acute pancreatitis is also seen in Africa and Asia associated with malnutrition.

The pathogenesis of the disease is the same whatever the aetiology, the tissue damage and inflammation that cause the attack of acute pancreatitis being caused by the release of the pancreatic digestive enzymes into its own substance, with subsequent autodigestion. The release of enzymes into the tissue may be triggered by a variety of aetiological agents or factors:

- gall stones with obstruction of pancreatic or common bile ducts (common);
- alcohol consumption (not very common);
- idiopathic (very common);
- vascular/ischaemic effects (atherosclerosis of abdominal arteries);
- traumatic, post-infectious, post-surgical.

A combination of these may be responsible for the attack.

As the enzymes are released into the pancreatic substance they digest the walls of the arteries and arterioles, this necrosis of vascular walls leading to haemorrhage. The peritoneum may become full of blood-stained fluid or a massive haemoperitoneum and shock may result. The vascular damage causes thrombosis and ischaemia with coagulative necrosis of the parenchyma. Release of lipases causes areas of omental and mesenteric fat necrosis. Soap formation and calcification in the necrotic areas is a prominent feature. At autopsy, the pancreas is swollen and firm, haemorrhagic and necrotic (Figure 9.19). Inflammation and neutrophil infiltration is usually not marked. As enzymes are released, there will be raised serum and urinary amylase levels in the acute phase of the attack.

Depending on the severity of the attack and the amount of tissue involved in the necrosis and inflammation, the patient with acute pancreatitis will present with widely different symptomatology. A mild attack may cause little pain or mild tenderness and discomfort in the epigastrium. With moderate and severe involvement there is sudden onset of severe abdominal pain located in the epigastrium, the left or right upper abdominal quadrants. The pain may be so severe as to cause the patients not to tolerate the weight of a sheet on their abdomen. The pain persists for days and may radiate to the back. Vomiting is common and it aggravates the pain. Tachycardia, pyrexia, jaundice, and glycosuria are also often observed.

Resolution may occur in very mild cases but usually, even with minimal tissue damage, the inflammation fails to resolve completely, organization and fibrosis being the end effect. Chronic pancreatitis may follow an organized acute pancreatitis. Suppuration and gangrene of the organ may occur if secondary bacterial infection follows the necrosis. Death occurs

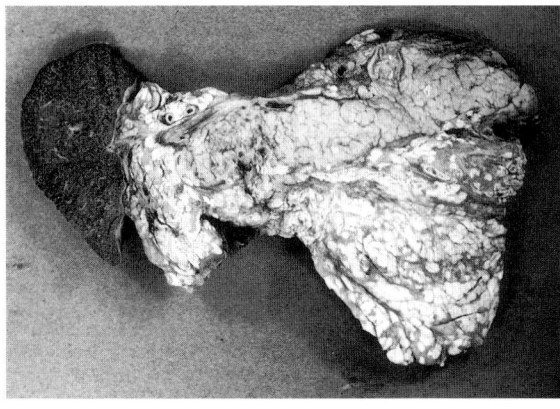

Figure 9.19 *Acute pancreatitis showing extensive areas of fat necrosis in a 51-year-old female*

in 15 to 20% of severe cases, associated with haemoperitoneum and shock.

Chronic Pancreatitis

Young and middle-aged males are more affected by this disorder and it is more prevalent in affluent societies. The aetiology is very frequently alcohol consumption, generally described as 'dedicated drinking' (small to moderate quantities of alcohol over 5–15 years are sufficient in some patients to cause this pancreatitis). The term '**executives' pancreatitis**' is often applied to this condition as this is a social group commonly presenting with the condition, the quantities of alcohol consumed being well within the socially acceptable levels. The condition may also develop as a sequela of acute pancreatitis and in some cases arteriosclerosis of abdominal arteries is demonstrable. Idiopathic disease is also common in occurrence.

The pancreas in this condition is firm, shrunken and often extremely calcified (especially so with the alcohol-induced disease). Areas of fibrosis, duct dilatation or cystic change are very common and the ducts are often blocked by inspissated secretion. Calculi may be present and the fibrous replacement of necrotic tissue is marked. There is focal and interstitial lymphocytic infiltration. The islet tissue is usually spared until the last stages and advanced chronic pancreatitis may only show scattered islet tissue embedded in a sea of fibrous scar. A comparison between the findings in acute and chronic pancreatitis is shown in Table 9.5.

Symptoms and signs of the condition vary between individuals and depend to a certain extent on the severity of disease and degree of pancreatic involvement. Patients often present with recurrent attacks of pain, at intervals of months to years. The pain is mild to moderately severe and the attacks may be precipitated by alcohol or heavy meals, in particular, fatty meats such as pork. The length and severity of the attack is variable. It usually starts suddenly as a discomfort which progresses in several hours to maximal pain, lasting for 3 to 7 days. If the attack is brought on by an alcoholic binge, the pain usually starts 18 to 48 hours later. The pain is epigastric or in the right upper abdominal quadrant and commonly radiates to the back. Nausea and vomiting are common, mild jaundice is sometimes observed and the attack may precipitate steatorrhoea and diabetes mellitus.

Calcific pancreatitis is a common aftermath of recurrent episodes of pancreatitis and is usually associated with alcoholic disease, developing approximately 8 to 10 years after the first attack. The calcium deposits are easily observed in a plain abdominal X-ray. Steatorrhoea is seen in 25 to 50% of cases and most patients will continue to suffer from recurrent attacks of pancreatitis of variable severity with gradual loss of pancreatic function. Obstructive jaundice may develop

Table 9.5 *Comparison of acute and chronic pancreatitis*

	Acute pancreatitis	Chronic pancreatitis
Age	Usually middle aged to elderly	Usually young to middle aged
Sex	Commoner in females	Commoner in males
Alcohol intake	Usually none or low	Usually moderate to high
Attack brought on by	Cholecystitis, cholelithiasis, heavy meals	Alcoholic excesses, heavy, fatty meals
Jaundice	May be marked	Mild, if present
Pancreatic cysts	Rare	Common
Calcification	Occasionally	Commonly
Steatorrhoea	Rare	Common
Diabetes mellitus	Not due to pancreatitis, may be due to obesity	Often due to pancreatitis, patient shows loss of weight
Serum amylase	Markedly elevated	Slightly to markedly elevated
Ultrasound	Cholelithiasis often present	Abnormal pancreas, pancreatic calculi

as fibrosis involves the ducts and diabetes mellitus may occur in the final stages. Death may result from weight loss, frail metabolic reserve, diabetes and various medical and surgical complications.

Neoplastic Conditions

Carcinoma of the Pancreas

This is the commonest tumour of the pancreas, an adenocarcinoma of the exocrine tissue. It is a moderately common tumour causing 3 to 4% of deaths from malignancies and it appears to be increasing in incidence. Patients are 45 to 65 years of age on presentation and the tumour is twice as common in males as it is in females. The aetiology of the tumour is largely idiopathic although some epidemiologists suggest that alcohol consumption and chronic pancreatitis may be important predisposing factors. Ingested carcinogens may also play a role in the causation of the tumour.

The sites involved by the tumour are the head of the pancreas and ampulla in 75% of cases, the body of the organ in 15% of cases and the tail of the pancreas in 10% of cases. The tumour forms infiltrating, hard, white, irregular masses that show early involvement of surrounding tissues. The primary tumour may be surprisingly small at autopsy, but already showing extensive metastases. Occasionally, the tumours are cystadenocarcinomata and large cystic spaces will be seen in the substance of the tumour. Histologically most are adenocarcinomata and they may show mucus secretion or may exhibit an acinar pattern without mucus secretion. Rarely, spheroidal (anaplastic) cell tumours may be observed.

The symptoms and signs attributable to the tumour vary somewhat depending on whether the head or the body and tail of the organ are involved. Carcinoma of the head of the pancreas presents with painless obstructive jaundice in about 25% of patients. Pruritus due to the jaundice may also be present. Gall bladder enlargement and hepatomegaly may be due to the biliary obstruction but the liver will also show enlargement if secondaries are present. Abdominal pain, anorexia, weight loss, malabsorption may be noted and on rare occasions the tumour may be palpated. Carcinoma in the region of the ampulla of Vater shows in almost all cases an early obstructive jaundice and is thus the most amenable to early treatment, having the best prognosis. Carcinoma of body and tail on the other hand may remain undiagnosed for months due to lack of symptoms. If jaundice does develop, it is a late feature indicating that secondaries are present in the liver. The chief symptom is pain referred to the back

and eased somewhat by learning forward. Unexplained lassitude, fever or bleeding in the gastrointestinal tract, mild diabetes mellitus, and a palpable left upper abdominal quadrant mass may be present. A symptom common to both types of tumour is mild to moderate, persistent abdominal pain similar to that of chronic pancreatitis. Approximately 70% of patients present with this pain (refer to Figure 9.20).

The tumour spreads directly into the surrounding tissues with invasion of the duodenum, common bile duct, spine and omentum. Lymphatic spread occurs early and is found in 75% of fatal cases. Early haematogenous spread occurs commonly, with secondaries in the liver and lungs usually. Transcoelomic spread causes carcinomatosis peritonei, occurring especially with tumours of the tail. Effects of the tumour include biliary obstruction, jaundice, biliary cirrhosis (if the patient survives for that long). Pancreatic obstruction may occur with fat malabsorption and steatorrhoea. Portal vein obstruction and thrombosis are common, with diabetes occurring in 5% of cases.

The prognosis of the tumour is, on average, extremely poor, with a 5-year survival of 3%. Most patients are dead within six months of diagnosis. A few long-term survivors following surgery have been reported, especially with early diagnosed and treated cases of carcinoma of the ampulla of Vater region (5-year survival is approximately 30% in this case).

Islet Cell Tumours of the Pancreas

These are tumours of the cells of the endocrine glandular tissue of the islets of Langerhans and may be either adenomata or carcinomata. They are rather rare tumours but important because of their secretory effects. Most of the tumours occur in people between 30 and 50 years of age and they are slightly commoner in males. They are idiopathic in origin.

The tumours usually appear as solitary masses, but in 20% of cases they may be multiple. They form small, firm, circumscribed yellowish brown or reddish nodules. Although they may occur anywhere in the pancreas, they are found most commonly in the tail of the organ and may be so small that they are difficult to see macroscopically in some cases. Microscopically, the tumours bear a striking resemblance to their parent, islet tissue cells, the tumour being composed predominantly of α or β cells. Histologically, it may be difficult to distinguish between benign and malignant tumours, the clinical effects important in the distinction (i.e. if invasion can be demonstrated or if metastasis is present with obvious clinical effects). Rare anaplastic tumours are obviously malignant.

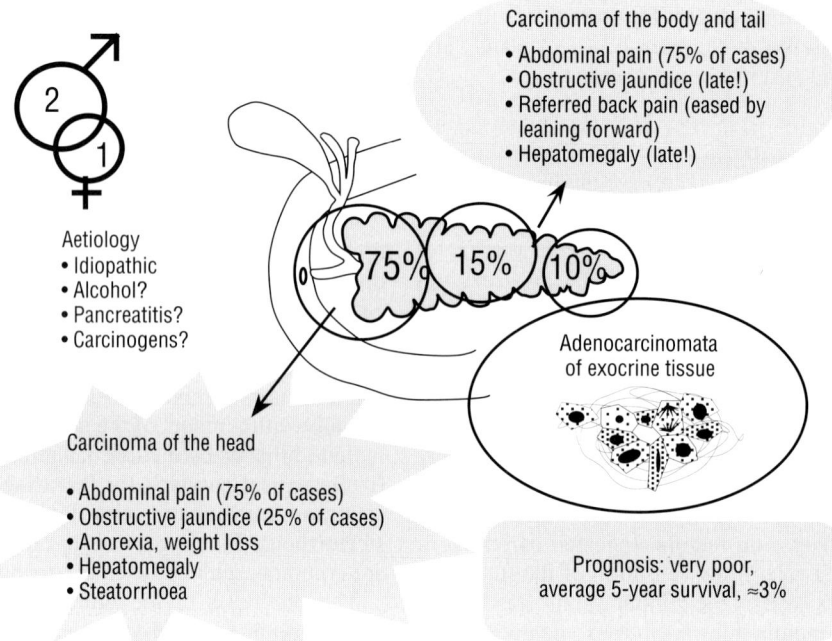

Figure 9.20 *Carcinoma of the pancreas*

Endocrine effects of the tumours are extremely important clinically as 60% of the neoplasms (malignant as well as benign) produce excessive, active hormones. Four different types of tumours and clinical syndromes are distinguished, although other extremely rare tumours may also arise in this tissue.

Insulin-secreting tumour (insulinoma). This is a tumour composed of β cells and it manifests itself by attacks of hypoglycaemia. The patient presents with confusion, disorientation, irritability, sweating, headache or hunger after fasting, typically occurring in the morning before breakfast. The patient has a fasting blood sugar of less than 50 mg/100 mL and symptoms are immediately relieved by glucose consumption.

Gastrinoma. The tumour is one composed of G cells which produce an excess of gastrin. Zollinger and Ellison described the syndrome which bears their name in 1955. The Zollinger–Ellison syndrome develops as excessive quantities of gastric acid are produced, with intractable, progressive, peptic ulceration. The patient presents with signs and symptoms of the peptic ulcers or their complications. Diagnosis is confirmed by a very high acid production in gastric secretion tests and a high serum gastrin content. Almost 60% of these

tumours are malignant but metastases are very slowly growing and patients may survive for many years even with secondaries present.

VIPoma. Tumours of cells secreting vasoactive intestinal peptide (VIP) produce this tumour, which was first described in 1958 by Verner and Morrison. VIP inhibits gastric secretion and stimulates water and electrolyte secretion by the small intestine. The Verner–Morrison syndrome is also termed the WDHA (watery diarrhoea, hypokalaemia, achlorhydria) syndrome named after the major manifestations of the disorder. The patient presents with episodic diarrhoea (even when fasting), high electrolyte loss in the stools, hypokalaemia and metabolic acidosis.

Glucagonoma. These tumours develop from the α cells which secrete glucagon. The patients present with diabetes mellitus, stomatitis, anaemia and a characteristic skin lesion, necrolytic migratory erythema. Diagnosis is confirmed by identifying high circulating levels of glucagon.

In 20 to 30% of cases islet cell tumours of the pancreas are accompanied by adenomata of one or more of the other endocrine glands. The parathyroid, pituitary, adrenal and other glands may be involved and this presentation is known as the **multiple endocrine adenoma syndrome**. The behaviour of these tumours is extremely variable with:

- 80% of tumours being morphologically and clinically benign;
- 10% of tumours being morphologically malignant but clinically benign;
- 10% of tumours being morphologically and clinically malignant.

The malignant tumours invade locally but also spread via the lymph and bloodstream with metastases in the lymph nodes, liver, lung and bones. Treatment of the tumours is surgical extirpation, if possible, and in the case of malignant tumours streptozotocin treatment may be of use. Corticosteroids, indomethacin and nutmeg extracts have also been of some benefit in the treatment. If excision is not possible, inhibitors of gastric secretion for the gastrinomata, replacement of fluid and electrolytes for the WDHA syndrome and insulin administration for the diabetes are given.

Secondary Tumours of the Pancreas

These are infrequent and most arise by direct spread from carcinoma of the stomach. They may produce the obstructive effects of a primary pancreatic tumour. Haematogenous secondaries are rare in this tissue.

Diabetes Mellitus

General Characteristics

Diabetes mellitus is a disease of disordered metabolism due to a relative or absolute lack of insulin in the body. Diabetes literally means 'siphon' in Greek and is in reference to the polyuria of the disease. Mellitus means 'honeyed' and refers to the glycosuria of the disease. Polyuria and wasting away of the body tissues were noted as features of diabetes even in ancient times and Aretaeus in the second century AD described the disorder as '...a melting down of the flesh and limbs into urine...'. Thomas Willis observed in the 17th century that the urine of diabetics was sweet. It should be noted that **diabetes insipidus** is a different disorder in which the urine is not sweet but insipid. It is a rare disease in which there is loss of hypothalamo-hypophyseal tracts in the neurohypophysis leading to many litres of dilute urine being produced. The effects of insulin in the body are many and include **lowering blood sugar** by inducing more sugar

to be taken up by cells by enhancing membrane permeability, inducing more sugar to be more effectively used by cells and inducing more sugar to be stored as glycogen in muscle and the liver. Insulin **inhibits gluconeogenesis** by inhibiting protein and fat conversion into glucose. These effects of insulin are opposed by **glucagon**, and **adrenal corticosteroids** and **pituitary growth hormone**, which increase gluconeogenesis, raising the blood sugar. Normally, a homeostatic balance is struck between insulin and its antagonists, the end result being an almost constant, stable blood glucose level even if the individual is fasting.

Incidence of Diabetes Mellitus

The disease is commoner in females, the sex ratio being 1:3. The disease is of much higher in Australian Aborigines (8–16% incidence) than in Caucasians (3–4% incidence). There is also a higher incidence in the Maltese (Malta = *Mellita*, meaning sweet!), in the Welsh, Polynesians, Micronesians, Flemish and Dutch, and in Jews. The disease has a higher incidence during pregnancy, approximately 1 in 200 pregnant women developing it. When the age incidences are examined it is seen that there are two peaks: the larger group comprising middle-aged to elderly patients and a smaller group of neonates, infants and children.

Aetiology

Diabetes is caused by either less than the normal amount of insulin (or perhaps none at all) being produced by the islets of Langerhans, or less insulin being present in or acting on the body compared to levels of antagonists. The first may be brought about by pancreatic destruction, the other by a variety of disorders of other organs such as adrenal disorders, pituitary disease, heritable or other factors.

Pancreatic destruction is caused by the following disorders and patients with these diseases may present with diabetes mellitus:

- chronic pancreatitis;
- haemochromatosis (Figure 9.21);
- malignant tumours (e.g. carcinoma of the pancreas);
- severe infections;
- autoimmune disease (autoantibody to the islet tissue may be demonstrable);
- pancreatectomy.

Adrenal causes of diabetes are mediated by excessive secretion of glucocorticoid hormones which may

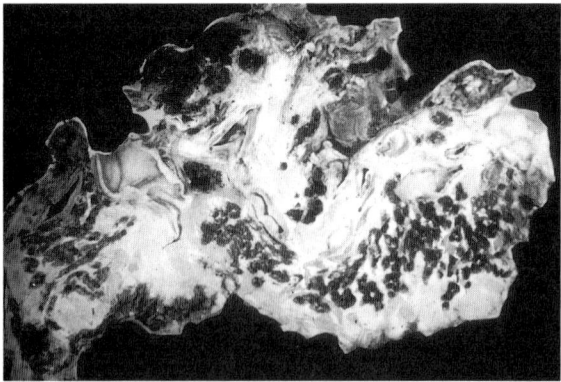

Figure 9.21 *Haemochromatosis of the pancreas stained with the Perl's reaction, demonstrating the large quantities of iron in the organ*

precipitate a hyperglycaemia even if normal levels of insulin are being secreted by the islets. This type of diabetes is seen in association with the adrenal hyperfunction of Cushing's syndrome, or with phaeo-chromocytoma. Alternatively, excessive therapeutic administration of cortisone may have a similar effect. **Pituitary causes** of diabetes may be demonstrated in diseases such as gigantism and acromegaly where an excess of growth hormone is found to be responsible for diabetes. Tumours of glucagon-secreting cells (**glucagonomata**) may produce excess glucagon and hence diabetes.

   Heredity is an important factor in the causation of diabetes and it is known that a familial history is found in approximately 35% of diabetic children. In adults who present with the disease, the epidemiological data suggest that a single recessive trait with poor penetrance may be responsible for this disease; however, other factors may ultimately determine whether or not an individual will develop the disorder. For example, it is known that **obesity** predisposes to the development of the disease as do frequent and large meals. An interesting factor which is becoming recognized in the pathogenesis of the disease is the number of receptors that are available for binding insulin on various body cells. It is suspected that genetic factors may be important determinants of whether adequate receptors are available on a cell's surface.

   It is important to realize that genetic factors and environmental factors interact in complex ways. For example, in an individual who is genetically predisposed, obesity will cause diabetes, whereas obesity will not result in diabetes in non-genetically predisposed individuals. It should be noted that 80% of cases

of NIDDM (see below) are obese, and 60% of obese people have an abnormal glucose tolerance test. Weight loss often corrects or ameliorates the carbohydrate intolerance. All forms of metabolic stress, including pregnancy, will precipitate or worsen carbohydrate intolerance in the genetically predisposed. In IDDM (see below), it is possible that autoimmunity plays a part in destruction of islet cells. An autoimmune aetiology is supported by lymphocytic infiltration of the islets, circulating islet cell antibodies, and the frequent coexistence of multiple endocrine disturbance believed to be autoimmune (Addison's disease, myxoedema, Graves' disease).

Clinical Types of Diabetes Mellitus

Diabetics present in two broad clinical groups:

* Type 1 or **insulin-dependent diabetes mellitus** (IDDM, 'juvenile onset'), 10 to 20% of cases of the disease, and
* Type 2 or **non-insulin-dependent diabetes mellitus** (NIDDM, 'mature onset') 80 to 90% of cases of the disease.

The type of diabetes a patient presents with depends very much on the various aetiological factors that are associated with the disease. In IDDM there is almost always a demonstrable lack of pancreatic islet β cells, and therefore an absolute lack of insulin. Insulin dependence implies that the patients must inject themselves with supplementary insulin daily due to its absolute lack in the body. This type of diabetes is characteristically seen in the younger age group who without treatment lose weight and develop ketosis. In NIDDM, some insulin is still being produced by the islets and therefore the lack of insulin is only relative. Non-insulin dependence implies that the hyperglycaemia of the patient may be controlled by other factors (e.g. carbohydrate-restricted diet or weight reduction) and such patients may avoid the daily injections of insulin. This latter type of diabetes develops more commonly in the adult patient, who is frequently obese or has a family history of diabetes.

Pathological Changes in the Tissues

The **pancreas** will usually show minimal changes, unless primary pancreatic disease has led to diabetes. There may be evidence of chronic pancreatitis and scarring, presence of malignant tumour, or the characteristic changes of haemochromatosis. In a small number of cases the lack of pancreatic islet β cells may be demonstrated microscopically, in an otherwise normal pancreas.

Changes developing in the **kidneys** are important and many diabetics die of renal failure. As diabetics suffer from recurrent infections, evidence of pyelonephritis and papillary necrosis of the kidney will often be found. A diabetic nephropathy develops with evidence of arteriosclerosis, benign nephrosclerosis and approximately 40% of diabetic kidneys show a focal glomerulosclerosis which is pathognomonic for diabetes. The glomeruli affected by glomerulosclerosis show focal regions of hyalinization known as **Kimmelstiel-Wilson lesions** (Figure 9.22). The renal tubules may show increased glycogen content and fatty change.

In the **cardiovascular system** very important changes occur and they secondarily involve many other tissues and organs. Atherosclerosis develops earlier and in a more severe form in the diabetic patient. This has been linked to abnormalities in carbohydrate, fat and protein metabolism, due to metabolic imbalances mediated by the abnormal gluconeogenesis and glucose levels. The diabetic shows hypercholesterolaemia, altered platelet function and increased plasma levels of low-density lipoproteins. Hypertension is also common in diabetics, affecting adversely both heart and kidneys. The **heart** shows evidence of coronary atherosclerosis, left ventricular hypertrophy, myocardial fibrosis and infarcts. In the brain, there may be haemorrhages, thromboembolism and cerebral infarcts. In the **limbs** there is arterial narrowing due to atheroma, trophic changes in the skin, ulceration, infection and gangrene. In the **liver** there is fatty change and an increased amount of glycogen in hepatocytes. The **eyes** show cataracts, glaucoma and in the retina there is microangiopathy with microaneurysms, haemorrhages and degeneration, changes termed **diabetic retinopathy**. Retinal detachment and degenerative changes may lead to blindness. Basement membrane thickening in the small vessels of many body organs is characteristic of diabetes. When such a change occurs in capillaries, it is called **microangiopathy**. It reduces capillary exchange in skin, skeletal muscle, the retina, renal glomeruli and renal medulla. The single basement membrane layer is widened and duplicated forming concentric layers of hyaline collagen. The capillary lumen is narrowed.

In the **skin** there are trophic changes, infections and ulcers. Boils and carbuncles are commonly seen, reflecting the increased susceptibility to infection. Due to the hypercholesterolaemia xanthelasmata form especially on the eyelids. The **lungs** show evidence of infections, especially tuberculosis and bronchopneumonia. The **nervous system** is affected by peripheral symmetrical sensory and motor neuropathy. Autonomic neuropathy also occurs. These changes are probably due to microangiopathies of capillaries that supply these nerves. A peripheral neuritis develops with pain, muscular weakness and paraesthesiae.

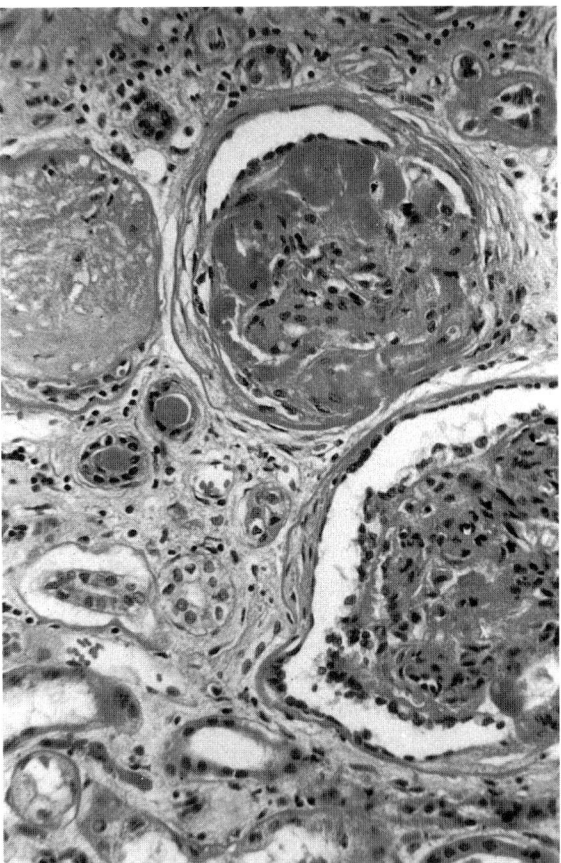

Figure 9.22 *Kimmelstiel-Wilson lesions in a diabetic kidney. The focal regions of acellular fibrinoid material may be easily discerned in the central glomerulus (×250)*

Diagnosis

The condition is diagnosed almost exclusively through the demonstration of raised glucose blood levels. A fasting blood glucose level of >5.5 mmol/L is indicative of the condition. Also, a 2 hours post-prandial blood glucose of >9 mmol/L is suggestive of the condition. However, by far the most reliable method is the glucose tolerance test in which 50 g of glucose is given orally to the patient and blood glucose levels are subsequently determined. A diabetic subject reaches peak values of ≥8.8 mmol/L, with this high level persisting and falling slowly. The diabetic and normal subject's responses are compared in Figure 9.24.

Urine examination of the diabetic subject may also be useful as a screening test and in most diabetics there is glycosuria, ketonuria and acetone in urine.

Symptoms and Signs

Most of the symptoms and signs associated with the disease are related to the hyperglycaemia and diabetic acidosis that the patient invariably suffers from in the untreated case. These symptoms and signs are of slow onset and some variability may be seen between different cases. Generally, these include the following:

- Polydipsia, polyuria, nocturia
- Weakness, abdominal pain, generalized aches

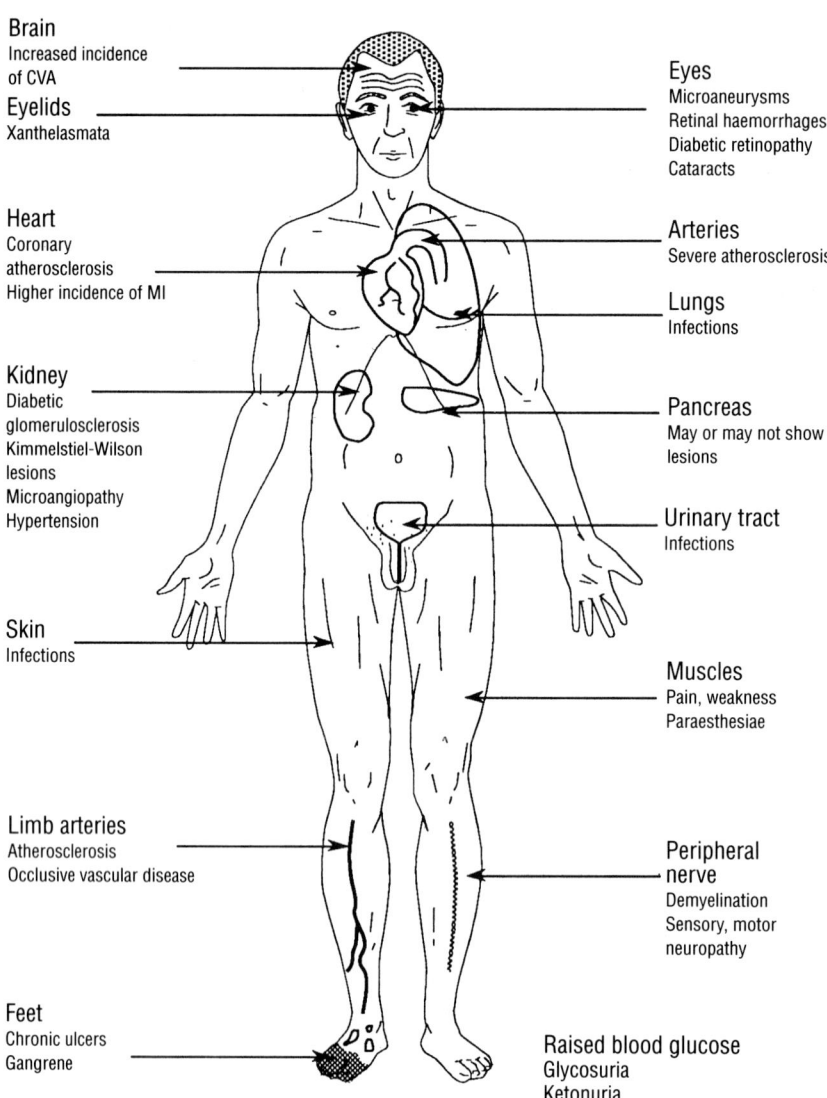

Brain
Increased incidence
of CVA

Eyelids
Xanthelasmata

Heart
Coronary
atherosclerosis
Higher incidence of MI

Kidney
Diabetic
glomerulosclerosis
Kimmelstiel-Wilson
lesions
Microangiopathy
Hypertension

Skin
Infections

Limb arteries
Atherosclerosis
Occlusive vascular disease

Feet
Chronic ulcers
Gangrene

Eyes
Microaneurysms
Retinal haemorrhages
Diabetic retinopathy
Cataracts

Arteries
Severe atherosclerosis

Lungs
Infections

Pancreas
May or may not show
lesions

Urinary tract
Infections

Muscles
Pain, weakness
Paraesthesiae

**Peripheral
nerve**
Demyelination
Sensory, motor
neuropathy

Raised blood glucose
Glycosuria
Ketonuria

Figure 9.23   *The complications of diabetes mellitus*

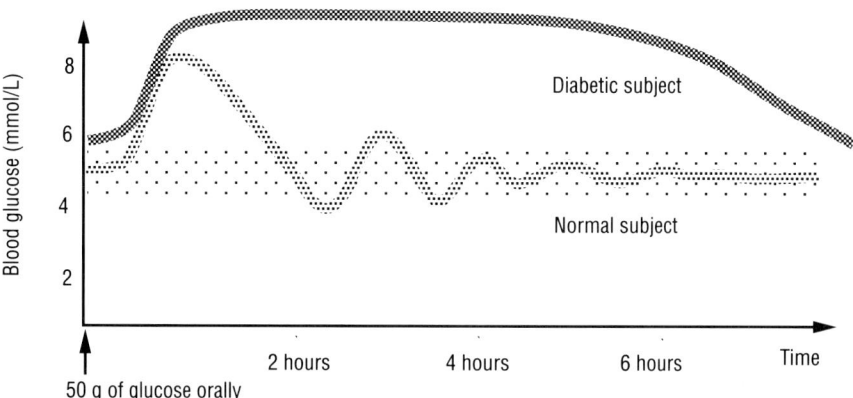

Figure 9.24 *The glucose tolerance test*

- Loss of appetite, nausea, vomiting
- Heavy laboured breathing
- Blurred vision
- Glycosuria, ketonuria
- Persistent skin infections
- Hypertension
- Vascular disease

In the case where the patient is receiving insulin it is also important to recognize the effects of hypoglycaemia, brought about by overdosing with insulin ('insulin reaction'). These symptoms and signs are of a rapid onset and include:

- Excessive sweating
- Weakness, faintness, syncope
- 'Pounding of heart', trembling
- Headache, impaired vision
- Hunger
- Not able to be awakened easily
- Irritability
- Personality changes

Treatment of Diabetes

For type 1, IDDM, insulin injections are required daily and the patient also benefits greatly by exercising regularly and eating balanced meals. Two forms of therapy are available to the patients.

Therapy A:
- A long-acting insulin injection at bedtime which accounts for approximately 40–50% of the body's needs of insulin. This maintains normal glucose levels during the night and between meals.

- Additional 'bolus' injection of short-acting insulin 30 minutes before meals to lower the post-prandial rises in blood glucose.
- Blood glucose testing forms an integral part of the treatment

Therapy B:
- A once or twice daily injection of insulin.
- Regular meals with balanced carbohydrate.

For type 2, NIDDM, insulin injections may not be required until late in the disease when the patient has suffered from it for a number of years. Exercise is beneficial and balanced meals are essential.

Therapy A:
- Weight reduction if obese.
- Regular, moderate, balanced meals.
- Carbohydrate control.

Therapy B:
- As above, plus
- Medication (in tablet form, e.g. promide, tolbutamide, to lower blood glucose levels).

Prognosis

In babies and infants with congenital diabetes mellitus the prognosis is very poor. In young adults death usually occurs ≈15–25 years after onset. Mature onset diabetes mellitus has the best prognosis with only slight depreciation of life expectancy. Causes of death in diabetics are:

- Myocardial infarction (50% of cases)
- Cerebrovascular accident (12% of cases)
- Renal failure (12% of cases)

- Various cancers (10% of cases)
- Bronchopneumonia, pyelonephritis (6% of cases)
- Congestive heart failure (common)
- Gangrene (common)
- Diabetic coma (rare)
- Hypoglycaemic coma (rare)

Hepatic and Pancreatic Function Tests

Hepatocarcinoma

This is a primary malignant tumour of the liver derived from the hepatocytes. It is diagnosed by a variety of methods, including biochemical techniques, visualization and imaging techniques. However, the definitive diagnosis of the tumour depends on **liver biopsy** followed by histopathological evaluation of the tissue by a pathologist. The commonest methods of diagnosing hepatocarcinoma biochemically are the evaluation of **α-foetoprotein** and **carcinoembryonic antigen (CEA)** levels, both of which are usually much elevated in these patients. Alternatively or additionally, the tumour may be directly visualized by **isotopic liver scanning angiography** or by **computerized tomography (CT) scanning** methods. The size of the tumour and extent of the spread may be seen with these last two methods. Biopsy of the tumour will be needed to determine whether it is a primary or a secondary tumour.

Cholelithiasis (Gall Stones)

Cholelithiasis very often produces a well-characterized syndrome of right upper quadrant abdominal pain, nausea and vomiting. However, after history taking and physical examination, several laboratory tests may be performed in order to conclusively diagnose the condition. The commonest and most effective test performed is **ultrasonography**, where ultrasound is used to obtain a view of the gall bladder and stones. Ultrasonography not only indicates the presence of calculi, but also the presence of obstruction in the biliary system caused by stones. **Radiological examination** of the abdomen for other diseases may sometimes give an additional diagnosis of cholelithiasis as a small proportion of calculi contain calcium and are therefore radio-opaque and easily detected on the X-ray film. **Percutaneous transhepatic cholangiography** may also be performed and in this case a fine needle is inserted into the biliary tree through the skin and liver under the guidance of a fluoroscope and

subsequently contrast medium is injected into the biliary tree. X-rays are then taken and obstructions, dilatations and stones in the biliary channels will be seen, as this method permits direct visualization of the biliary tree. In addition to these tests for cholelithiasis, biochemical liver function tests may be carried out and these may show evidence of bile anomalies and gall bladder disease.

Obstructive Jaundice

Obstructive jaundice results whenever there is obstruction of the biliary tree, the most common precipitating disease being cholelithiasis. Other causes include tumours of the liver, gall bladder, pancreas and of other surrounding organs. Cirrhosis may also give rise to this condition and therefore jaundice may be seen in alcoholics, hepatitis patients and in some cases of congenital disease. **Endoscopic retrograde cholangiopancreatography (ERCP)** or **transhepatic cholangiography** are two methods most commonly in use for the diagnosis of obstructive jaundice. **Ultrasound examination** may also be of value. ERCP is examination of the extrahepatic biliary tract by the insertion of a fiberoptic endoscope via the mouth. This has the advantage of also being able to take biopsy samples if they are required, as well as examining the morphology of the area directly. In addition, certain specific therapies may be accomplished via this procedure: **sphincterotomy**, where the ampulla of Vater and sphincter of Oddi are resected, such that there is spontaneous passage of gall stones into the intestine, and **balloon dilatation**, where the biliary canals or ducts are dilated by means of an inflatable catheter, once again allowing the spontaneous passage of gall stones into the intestine.

Liver Function Tests

Serum bilirubin. Normal values are: conjugated, up to 5 µM/L, and unconjugated, up to 17 µM/L. The serum bilirubin levels rise when the liver is unable to conjugate bilirubin or when it is unable to excrete bilirubin. When the bilirubin level rises above 40 µM/L, jaundice is noted. The three most common causes of jaundice are:

- *Excessive haemolysis (haemolytic jaundice)* — The breakdown of red blood cells is releasing more unconjugated bilirubin than the liver is able to excrete. Hence, unconjugated serum bilirubin is increased, whereas conjugated bilirubin levels are normal.

- *Liver cell damage (hepatic jaundice)* — In this case the liver cells are damaged and both conjugated and unconjugated bilirubin levels rise as the liver cells are unable to excrete the bilirubin.
- *Biliary tract obstruction (obstructive jaundice)* — The liver conjugates the bilirubin normally but is unable to excrete it because of intrahepatic or extrahepatic obstruction; therefore, the conjugated bilirubin levels in the serum rise.

Urinary bilirubin. Normally bilirubin is not detectable in urine when using the routine diagnostic tests. Urinary bilirubin levels rise when the liver is not functioning normally and the bilirubin causes the urine to become a deep yellow, smoky or brownish colour ('tea-coloured' urine). The tests that are used to detect urinary bilirubin are:

1. A colour reaction using a test reagent strip (e.g. Multistix®).
2. The foam test.
3. The Harrison spot test.
4. The Ictotest® tablet.

When bilirubin is found in the urine it is usually of the conjugated type since unconjugated bilirubin is tightly bound to serum albumin and is therefore not found in the urine (presuming normal renal function). Bilirubin testing of the urine should be performed while the urine is freshly voided as bilirubin decomposes on exposure to light or at room temperature in approximately 30 minutes.

Plasma ammonia. Normally present in plasma at the concentration of 12–55 µM/L. Ammonia levels in the plasma rise when the liver is unable to form urea from ammonia which comes mainly from the gastrointestinal tract. Excessive ammonia in the bloodstream will cause acid–base imbalances and may also bring about the so-called **hepatic encephalopathy** or **coma**, where there is brain damage caused by ammonia. The plasma ammonia levels rise only when there has been extensive liver damage and liver failure has set in.

Serum alkaline phosphatase. Normal values for the enzyme are 217–650 nM/s/L. This is an enzyme found in the hepatobiliary tract, bone, placenta and intestine. It has important functions in calcification of bone, transport of metabolites across cell membranes and in lipid transport. This test is very useful as it is an index of hepatobiliary disorders and bone disorders:

1. Elevation of enzyme 3–5 times normal levels:
   Secondary liver tumours (in about 80% of cases)
   Other space-occupying lesions in the liver (e.g. abscesses, granulomata, hepatocarcinoma, etc.)

2. Elevation of enzyme less than 3 times upper limit of normal levels:
   Cholangiolithic hepatitis
   Cirrhosis of liver with active hepatitis
   Active liver cell damage
3. Extreme elevation of enzyme levels with other liver tests normal:
   Bone disease

Serum 5'-nucleotidase. Normal levels of the enzyme are 17–183 nM/s/L. 5'-nucleotidase is an enzyme formed mainly in the hepatobiliary tract. The enzyme levels are determined in order to differentiate between liver disease and bone disease as the alkaline phosphatase levels may be raised in both disorders. Abnormalities in 5'-nucleotidase levels indicate liver disease. About 10 mL of venous blood is withdrawn and handled with care so as to prevent haemolysis (the enzyme is also found within blood cells).

Serum aspartate aminotransferase. Normal values of the enzyme are 117–450 nM/s/L. This is an enzyme found in myocardium, liver, skeletal muscle, kidney and pancreas. Elevated levels of the enzyme will be found in the serum 8–12 hours after injury involving any of these organs. The peak of the enzyme will occur approximately 30 hours after injury and the levels return to normal 4–6 days later. About 10 mL of venous blood is withdrawn and handled with care so as to prevent haemolysis. Many antibiotics and other drugs (e.g. salicylates) will influence the test results, as also will intramuscular injections prior to the test. Extreme elevations of this enzyme occur with severe liver necrosis or in the acute phase of hepatitis. The test is also used to diagnose myocardial infarction and skeletal muscle damage. Minor elevations of the enzyme may indicate cirrhosis, metastatic tumours in the liver and a variety of other diseases in many other organs.

Serum alanine aminotransferase. Normal values of the enzyme are 17–350 nM/s/L. Although this enzyme is found mainly in the liver, it is also present in lower levels in the kidney, myocardium and skeletal muscle. Raised levels of this enzyme with concomitant raised aspartate aminotransferase levels are an indication of liver disease. About 10 mL of venous blood is withdrawn and handled with care so as to prevent haemolysis. Many antibiotics and other drugs (e.g. salicylates) will influence the test results.

1. Elevated levels together with elevated aspartate aminotranferase:
   Viral hepatitis
   Infectious mononucleosis
   Drug-induced acute liver injury

2. Elevated levels independent of aspartate aminotransferase:
    Acute alcoholic liver disease
    Active cirrhosis
    Chronic passive venous congestion of the liver
    Metastatic tumours in the liver
    Long-standing extrahepatic biliary obstruction

Serum albumin and globulin. Normal levels of albumin, 35–50 g/L, and of globulin, 23–35 g/L. Total levels of protein in the plasma may vary to a considerable extent with a variety of physiological and pathological states and the commonest and most accurate method of determination of levels of serum proteins is **electrophoresis**. This test provides a 'fingerprint' of the proteins and specific diseases will cause specific alterations in this fingerprint pattern. About 10 mL of venous blood are withdrawn and handled with care to prevent haemolysis. The serum is removed from this and is put onto a gel across which a potential difference is applied. The serum proteins will travel across the gel at different rates depending on their charge. Comparisons with standards identify levels and types of proteins present.

In cirrhosis, the entire gamma globulin zone increases while the beta globulin zone almost disappears. In advanced cirrhosis, there is decreased albumin, increased gamma globulin and the beta globulin peak is incorporated into the gamma peak.

Clotting factors. The liver synthesizes many of the clotting factors — fibrinogen, prothrombin, accelerator globulin, factor VII and several other less important blood coagulation factors. Extensive liver disease with loss of liver parenchyma (e.g. hepatitis or cirrhosis) will lead to depletion of these factors and therefore disorders of blood coagulation. Many tests that are performed to assess the bleeding disorders will also be relevant to liver function, for example **fibrinogen levels**, **prothrombin time** and **bleeding time**.

Blood lipids. The liver has an important role in lipid metabolism and disease in the liver will interfere with lipid levels in the blood. Blood lipids are assessed when liver disease is suspected.

Pancreatic Carcinoma

Carcinoma of the pancreas is an insidious tumour with vague and easily overlooked early symptomatology. It is therefore usually diagnosed late in its course and usually by that time no effective treatment may be given. The prognosis for the condition is therefore very poor. Carcinoma of the head of the pancreas has a marginally better prognosis than carcinoma of the body or the tail of the organ, this being due to earlier symptoms being caused by carcinoma of the head of the pancreas. Incidental examinations such as **computerized tomography** (**CT scans**) of the abdomen or **endoscopic retrograde cholangiopancreatography** (**ERCP**) can be of value in diagnosing this tumour.

Pancreatitis

Acute pancreatitis. The commonest known causes of acute pancreatitis are alcoholism and cholelithiasis. In order to diagnose this condition, in addition to history and clinical and physical examination, tests will have to be carried out evaluating hepatobiliary and pancreatic function. A **complete blood examination** will usually show a leukocytosis associated with infection. **Amylase** and **lipase levels** should also be evaluated. ERCP is not performed routinely as it may precipitate a severe attack of this condition.

Chronic pancreatitis. This condition is more frequently diagnosed from clinical history and physical diagnostic methods. An **X-ray** of the abdomen will often show pancreatic calcification associated with the regions of necrosis in the organ, while an ERCP will often show the pathological changes associated with the pancreatic duct in this condition.

Pancreatic Function Tests

Serum amylase and lipase. Normal values for amylase, 4–25 Units, and for lipase, 2 Units. Amylase is an enzyme secreted by the pancreas, salivary gland, female genital tract and the intestine. Lipase is secreted specifically by the pancreas and abnormalities in its secretion parallel those of amylase in pancreatic disease.

In **acute pancreatitis** the levels of both enzymes are raised. It should be kept in mind, however, that mumps, ischaemic bowel disease and pelvic inflammatory disease (PID) will raise the levels of amylase only.

In **chronic pancreatitis** the enzymes are not elevated. In the case of long-standing chronic pancreatitis resulting in a 'burnt-out' pancreas, the levels of both enzymes are decreased as the organ has been sufficiently damaged such that its ability to secrete these enzymes has been seriously compromised. Drugs that the patient is taking may cause increased levels of the enzymes, for example narcotic analgesics, oral contraceptives and some diuretics.

Faecal fats. Normal value of faecal lipids is less than 7 g per 24 hours. In the normal individual the dietary fats are emulsified by the bile, acted upon by the pancreatic lipases and almost completely absorbed by the small intestine. Faecal fats consist of unabsorbed dietary lipids, intestinal secretions and bacterial and cellular debris. For the test, the patient should consume more than 50 g of lipid daily and should abstain from alcohol. All stools are collected for a period of 3 days and no urine or toilet tissue must contaminate them. Between collections the faeces are refrigerated.

Excessive fat in the faeces is known as **steatorrhoea** and if the quantity of faecal fats is great, the faeces are bulky, pale, light and have a very offensive smell. The malabsorption syndrome due to coeliac disease or cystic fibrosis is the commonest cause of steatorrhoea in children. In adults, steatorrhoea is most commonly caused by pancreatic disease and sprue.

A Guide for Treatment of Problem Drinkers and Alcoholics

There are many difficulties in the treatment of problem drinkers but following treatment, counselling and rehabilitation there are two important goals that may be recommended for each individual patient. These are: complete abstinence from alcohol; and drinking of alcohol as part of a closely controlled programme. The two goals are designed for two different types of problem drinkers. To be successful with treatment, one must attempt to classify the patient into one of two groups which best suits these goals and thus rehabilitation.

Patients who meet the following criteria are best suited to a controlled drinking programme:

- are relatively young;
- are socially stable (married or in a stable relationship; employed; living with relatives or friends who can provide support);
- have a relatively brief history of alcohol abuse;
- have not suffered severe withdrawal symptoms while becoming abstinent;
- prefer trying to drink in moderation and have not made a commitment to do so as a goal;
- have no or little family history of alcoholism;
- show few signs of addiction or medical dependence;
- have no liver, pancreatic, gastric or brain damage.

Patients who require complete abstinence as a goal are:

- older;
- socially unstable (single; unemployed; living alone);
- have a long history of abuse;
- suffer severe withdrawal symptoms;
- have a long family history of alcoholism;
- show liver, pancreatic, gastric or brain damage.

People in the latter category should be directed to **Alcoholics Anonymous** for treatment as this is an organization whose specialised area is the treatment of the severely dependent patient. As a practitioner you may help a patient achieve controlled drinking by getting them to see a qualified counsellor dealing with these problems. Also be aware of the following:

- Fully inform them of the medical effects of continued excessive drinking, explaining the risks they run in developing liver, pancreatic, gastric or brain disorders.
- Fully inform them of the social effects of continued excessive drinking, explaining the risks they run in the areas of family life, social stigmatization, legal issues, etc.
- Ask them to consider the benefits and costs in the short and long term of continued excessive drinking.
- Ask them to keep a diary of drinking to provide a record of progress in treatment.
- Decide upon limits of drinking, formulated into a written contract which may include circumstances where drinking is not to take place.
- Formulate methods to achieve agreed limits, such as:
  drinking only low-alcohol beverages;
  interspacing alcoholic with non-alcoholic beverages;
  avoiding high-risk situations and handling peer pressure.

For further information, contact the places below:

- AA — The Melbourne Clinic
  658 Bridge Road
  Richmond 3121
  Phone (03) 429–1833

- AA — Moreland Hall
  26 Jessie Street
  Coburg 3058
  Phone (03) 386–2876

- Alcohol and Drug Foundation
  153 Park Street
  South Melbourne 3205
  Phone (03) 690–6000

- Alcoholism Rehabilitation Programme
  Marshall Hall,
  Cranbourne Road
  Frankston, 3199
  Phone (03) 776–6155

- Alcohol and Drug 'DIRECTLINE'
  Phone (03) 482–2711

Revision Questions and Case Studies

1. Discuss the pathology of fatty change of the liver in relation to excessive alcohol consumption.
2. Compare and contrast neonatal and adult forms of polycystic disease of the liver.
3. What is chronic passive venous congestion of the liver, what is its aetiology and what are its sequelae?
4. Differentiate between the various forms of liver cell necrosis, describing in detail the aetiology and morphology of each type, with a brief mention of the sequelae of each.
5. What is hepatitis? Discuss the development of alcoholic hepatitis and its sequelae.
6. Discuss the pathology of hydatid disease of the liver.
7. Differentiate between pylephlebitis and cholangitis.
8. Cirrhosis of the liver is seen to be increasing in incidence in our country. Discuss the pathology of this important disease with special reference to its major aetiologies in Australia and relate these to the increasing incidence of the disorder.
9. Discuss the pathology of portal hypertension.
10. Compare and contrast:
    (a) Hepatocarcinoma
    (b) Cholangiocarcinoma
    (c) Secondary liver tumours
11. What is jaundice and how does it arise?
12. Discuss the pathology of acute and chronic cholecystitis.
13. Cholelithiasis is a common condition. Discuss its general incidence in the community, its age and sex incidence, aetiology, morphology, signs and symptoms, diagnosis, sequelae and treatment.
14. Compare and contrast acute and chronic pancreatitis.
15. Discuss the pathology of carcinoma of the pancreas.
16. What are the various tumours associated with the islet tissue of the pancreas? What is their clinical behaviour? To what clinical syndromes do they give rise?
17. Write short notes on the following conditions:
    (a) 'Strawberry' gall bladder
    (b) 'Nutmeg' liver
    (c) 'Anchovy paste' lesions in the liver
    (d) Soap formation in the pancreas
18. Discuss the lesions of haemochromatosis in relation to hepatic and pancreatic disease.
19. Discuss the pathology of carcinoma of the gall bladder.
20. Discuss the pathology of hepatocarcinoma.

Case study 1. A 20-year-old Caucasian male presents at your clinic complaining of malaise and fatigue. He has suffered from vague abdominal pains and slight discomfort lately. Physical examination shows that he is slightly jaundiced. When the abdomen is palpated the liver is firm but not tender or enlarged. The blood pressure is 120/75 mmHg and the pulse rate is 80 beats per minute, his temperature is 37.8°C. When you question the man he tells you that he has been using heroin in the past but has been participating in a rehabilitation programme for the past 4 months together with his girlfriend and neither has taken any drugs intravenously for that period of time. Previously, when they were using drugs, they had shared syringes between themselves and with others.

(a) What diseases could the man be possibly suffering from, consistent with the history and presentation (differential diagnosis)?

Liver function tests are performed and the following results are obtained: raised serum bilirubin (conjugated and unconjugated), raised urine bilirubin, raised serum 5'-nucleotidase, serum alanine aminotransferase is 470 nmol/s/L, serum aspartate aminotransferase is 525 nmol/s/L, serum alkaline phosphatase is 1200 nmol/s/L. All other values are within the normal range.

(b) What is the diagnosis? Would any other specific tests be done?
(c) How is this disorder treated and what is the prognosis?
(d) What other steps should be taken in this case?

Case study 2. A 48-year-old Caucasian male publican, Mr Roy D., is admitted to hospital with extremely severe abdominal pain, shock and vomiting. Minimal tenderness and rigidity are present on examination of his abdomen. His wife says that he is a heavy drinker and she has been worried for the past few months that he may have become an alcoholic. Liver tests show normal values. Pancreatic function tests show amylase to be 38 Units (N = 4–25 Units) and lipase 3 Units (N ≈2 units).

(a) What is the diagnosis?
(b) What other investigations should be carried out and why?
(c) What are the sequelae of this condition?

Case study 3. Mr Trevor W. is a 45-year-old Caucasian builders' labourer with 5 children who presents at your clinic because of weakness, loss of weight, general debility and repeated minor skin infections over the last month or two. On questioning he recalls that he has been drinking much more than usual lately. He now supplements his nightly bottle or two of beer with a daily two bottles of lemonade and has to stop for a glass or two of water at least hourly. When asked if he passes much urine he replies: 'Well, you would do too if you drank as much as I do!'. He smokes up to two packets of cigarettes a day. On physical examination you notice that there is no evidence of jaundice or anaemia, but Mr W. is deeply tanned although it is mid-winter. He has not been out of Melbourne for years and puts his skin colour down to his occupation. He is 175 cm tall and weighs 85 kg (92 kg at previous visit 4 months ago). His blood pressure is 140/85 mmHg and his pulse rate 70 per minute and regular. His temperature is 36.5°C. Examination of the chest shows no crepitations but there are a few scattered rhonchi. The apex beat is heard in the fourth left inter-costal space in the midclavicular line but no cardiac bruits are heard. There is no ankle swelling. The abdomen reveals a 7 cm smooth, firm, non-tender hepatomegaly but no splenomegaly. There are no spider naevi, no gynaecomastia and no testicular atrophy. The CNS is grossly intact. When questioned further Mr W. admits that there has been a reduction of his libido.

(a) What is the presumptive diagnosis?
(b) What further investigations are mandatory?
(c) What treatment is appropriate?
(d) Should other members of his family be investigated?

Case study 4. A 46-year-old Caucasian female, Mrs Joyce B., presents at your clinic requesting treatment for her back pain. When you ask her to point out the area which troubles her the most, she points to the right scapular area and says that frequently 'the pain comes right down the right side'. She is 167 cm tall and her weight is 87 kg. The chest is normal and she tells you proudly that she gave up smoking 15 years ago when she took up cake decorating (it helped her quit). Examining her abdomen you elicit tenderness in the right upper quadrant of the abdomen and this seems to be the source of the pain radiating to the back. Questioning the woman further you learn that the pain gives her a great deal of trouble periodically but espe-cially, she says, 'when she gets indigestion or food poisoning'. Asked to qualify the last remark she says: 'I often seem to get pains and vomiting, especially if we eat take aways. But it's odd the rest of the family don't seem to be affected as much. Of course, I've

always had a sensibility in the bowel...'. You deter-mine that fever and chills often accompany these at-tacks of 'indigestion and food poisoning'. Asked about her family the woman becomes quite loquacious talk-ing at length about her 'happy home life' (she is a housewife), 'absolutely wonderful husband' and her 'four lovely children' (Jenny, Brett, Jason and Kylie).

(a) What is the presumptive diagnosis?
(b) What further investigations are required for con-firmation of the diagnosis?
(c) What treatment is appropriate?
(d) What are the complications of the untreated con-dition?
(e) Should other members of her family be investi-gated (for ...indigestion perhaps)?

Case study 5. A 45-year-old Chinese man, recently returned from Hong Kong where he visited relatives presents with a rather tender liver over the past 2 weeks. During his stay in Hong Kong he had suffered from dyspepsia and had taken a Chinese herbal rem-edy for it, which sometimes relieved the symptoms. In the past 2 weeks in Australia he has noticed that his abdomen is rather painful and he feels very poorly, tiring easily. On examination, a rather enlarged liver is palpated and the right upper quadrant of the abdomen is painful on palpation. Evidence of ascites is seen. The man on questioning says that he is a non-smoker and does not drink alcohol. He is married with two young daughters, 10 and 12 years of age. He has lived in Australia for the past 15 years. In his youth he had been treated for 'jaundice'.

(a) What is the presumptive diagnosis?
(b) What tests are required for definitive diagnosis? (List them only.)
(c) What is the treatment and prognosis in this case?

Case study 6. A 50-year-old Caucasian man presents with abdominal discomfort and swelling and a feeling of weakness and 'no pep'. He is the owner of a grazing property close to Mount Gambier and he tells the doctor that he raises sheep and he has recently also gone into goat farming. He and his wife are visiting his daughter in Melbourne who is getting married next week. He has taken the opportunity to have a general check up and he says that he has been feeling rather unwell for the past few months. On examination he is seen to be a tall, thin man 192 cm tall and weighing 68 kg. He has rather marked jaundice most visible in his conjunctivae and mucosae as he is rather sun-tanned. The chest is normal and the man is a non-smoker. On examining the abdomen there is marked hepato-splenomegaly. When questioned about his drinking he says that he occasionally has 'a few beers with the boys in the pub', but that he does not drink a lot. His wife corroborates this. Liver ultrasonography is performed and three space occupying lesions are found, each approximately 10 cm in diameter. A medical student viewing the ultrasonogram suggests that if a biopsy is performed it will identify the lesions as tumours but the clinician in charge reprimands the student, saying that in this case an attempted biopsy may cause the death of the patient, suggesting that serology will be of more use.

(a) What is the presumptive diagnosis?
(b) What is the aetiology of this disease?
(c) Explain the significance of the conversation between the student and the clinician.
(d) What is the recommended treatment and prognosis in this case?
(e) What are the sequelae of untreated cases?

Further Reading

Cameron AS, Weinstein P. 'Alternative Hepatitis for Alternative Sex.' *CDI* 1991; **15**(15): July, 244.
Castano L, Eisenbarth GS. 'Type I Diabetes: A Chronic Autoimmune Disease of Human, Mouse and Rat.' *Ann Rev Immunol* 1990; **8**: 647.
Chalmers TC (ed.). 'Gallstones.' *Semin Liver Dis* 1983; **3**: 87.
Condon R. 'A Cluster of Cases of Hepatitis A in Western Australia.' *CDI* 1991; **15**(15): July, 247.
Craig JR, Govindarajan S, DeCock KM. 'Delta Virus Hepatitis.' *Pathol Ann* 1986; **21**(2): 1.
Crosby WH. 'Haemochromatosis: Current Concepts and Management.' *Hosp Pract* 1987; **22**(2): 173.
Cuthbert JA. 'Hepatic Transplantation.' *Am J Med Sci* 1986; **291**: 286.
Døssing MJ. 'Occupational Toxic Liver Damage.' *J Hepatol* 1986; **3**: 131.
Driver HE, Swann PF. 'Alcohol and Human Cancer.' *Anticancer Res* 1987; **7**: 309.
Eisenbarth GS. 'Type I Diabetes Mellitus: A Chronic Autoimmune Disease.' *N Eng J Med* 1986; **314**: 1360.
Foulis AK. 'Acute Pancreatitis.' *Rec Adv Histopathol* 1984; **12**: 188.
Galambos JT. 'Portal Hypertension.' *Semin Liver Dis* 1985; **5**: 277.
Galambos JT. 'Transmission of Hepatitis B from Providers to Patients: How Big is the Risk?' *Hepatology* 1986; **6**: 320.
Gardner I, Wan X, Mathews J. 'Hepatitis B in Australian Aboriginals.' *Today's Life Sci* 1990: **2**(9): 16.
Greenberger NJ. 'Etiology and Pathogenesis of Chronic Pancreatitis.' *Hosp Pract* 1985; **20**(9): 83.
Gust ID. 'Control of Hepatitis B.' *Today's Life Sci* 1990: **2**(9): 4.
Hall P de la M. 'The Pathological Spectrum of Alcoholic Liver Disease.' *Pathol* 1985; **17**: 207.
Hambridge M. 'Intellectual Impairment in Male Alcoholics.' *Alcohol and Alcoholism* 1990; **25**(5): 555.
Helmrich SP, Ragland DR, Leung RW, Paffenbarger RS. 'Physical Activity and Reduced Occurrence of Non-Insulin-Dependent Diabetes Mellitus.' *New Engl J Med* 1991; **325**(3): 147.
Howard CR. 'Hepatitis B Vaccines.' *Today's Life Sci* 1990: **2**(9): 8.
Kraegen E, Storlien L. 'Diabetes: Lifestyle Factors and Insulin.' *Today's Life Sci* 1989: **1**(4): 16.
Lafferty KJ. 'Diabetes: The Disease Process.' *Today's Life Sci* 1991; **3**(6): 16.
Lieber CS. 'Biochemical and Molecular Basis of Alcohol-Induced Injury to the Liver and Other Tissues.' *N Eng J Med* 1988; **319**: 1639.
Liguory C, Canard JM. 'Tumours of the Biliary System.' *Clin Gastroenterol* 1983; **12**: 269.
MacSween RNM, Burt AD. 'Histologic Spectrum of Alcoholic Liver Disease.' *Semin Liver Dis* 1986; **6**: 221.
Matolo NM, LaMorte WW, Wolfe BM. 'Acute and Chronic Cholecystitis.' *Surg Clin N Am* 1981; **61**: 875.
McGlashan ND. 'Primary Liver Cancer and Food-Based Toxins.' *Ecol Dis* 1984; **1**: 37.
Merimee TJ. 'Diabetic Retinopathy: A Synthesis of Perspectives.' *N Eng J Med* 1990; **322**: 978.
Okuda K. 'Primary Liver Cancer.' *Dig Dis Sci* 1986; **31**(Suppl): 133S.
Phillips MJ, Poucell S. 'Modern Aspects of the Morphology of Viral Hepatitis.' *Hum Pathol* 1981; **12**: 1060.
Ruebner BH. 'Collagen Formation and Cirrhosis.' *Semin Liver Dis* 1986; **6**: 212.
Sarles H. 'Alcohol and the Pancreas.' *Acta Med Scand* 1985; **703**(Suppl): 235.
Sherlock S (ed.). 'Alcohol and Disease.' *Br Med Bull* 1982; **38**: 1.
Sing SM, Reber HA. 'The Pathology of Chronic Pancreatitis.' *World J Surg* 1990; **14**: 2.
Steer ML. 'Classification and Pathogenesis of Pancreatitis.' *Surg Clin N Am* 1989; **69**: 467.
Steffes MW, Mauer SM. 'Toward a Basic Understanding of Diabetic Complications.' *N Eng J Med* 1991; **325**: 883.
Stewart T. 'A Cluster of Cases of Hepatitis A in Victoria.' *CDI* 1991; **15**(15): July, 246.

Tucker RA. 'Drugs and Liver Disease: A Tabular Compilation of Drugs and the Histopathological Changes that can Occur in the Liver.' *Drug Intell Clin Pharmacol* 1982; **16**: 569.

Ueo CJ, Pitt HA, Cameron JL. 'Cholangiocarcinoma.' *Surg Clin N Am* 1990; **70**: 1429.

Wands JR, Blum HE. 'Primary Hepatocellular Carcinoma.' *N Eng J Med* 1991; **325**: 729.

Watson K. 'Hepatitis C in Australia.' *Mod Med Aust* 1991; July, 18.

10

Urinary System Disorders

The Normal Urinary System

The kidneys are paired, bean-shaped organs situated in the posterior part of the peritoneal cavity in a position close to the aorta (Figure 10.1). One kidney is capable of carrying out all functions of the urinary system, therefore congenital absence of a kidney remains undiagnosed during life. Functions of the kidney include:

- control of fluid and electrolyte balance;
- control of acid–base balance;
- excretion of waste products;
- elimination of drugs and toxins;
- control of blood pressure (and volume), secretion of renin;
- control of red blood cell production (haemopoiesis), secretion of haemopoietin (erythropoietin).

The kidney is surrounded by a thin, fibrous capsule that may be easily stripped off its surface. A concave indentation in the middle of the organ, the hilum, contains the renal artery and vein and the renal pelvis. The interior of the kidney is almost all parenchyma.

There is an external granular part, the cortex, and an internal part, the medulla, which is made up of a number of dark-coloured masses, the medullary pyramids. The apices of the pyramids are called the renal papillae and converge towards the hilar aspect to meet the calyces of the renal pelvis, which then lead into the ureter.

The functional unit of the kidney is the nephron, an unbranched tubule, approximately 35 mm in length, extending from the cortex to the medulla (see Figure 10.2). There are about 1.3 million nephrons in each kidney, their combined length in each kidney being 61 km. The nephron begins at the glomerulus, which is a ball of capillaries that originate from the afferent arteriole and are drained by the efferent arteriole. Surrounding the glomerulus is the Bowman's capsule, comprising the visceral and parietal layers of epithelial cells, the Bowman's space being between the two layers. It is at the glomerulus that the passive process of filtration of the blood occurs. The Bowman's space, which contains the glomerular filtrate, leads through the urinary pole to the proximal tubule. In the proximal convoluted tubule, active resorption of glucose and amino acids occurs from the glomerular filtrate,

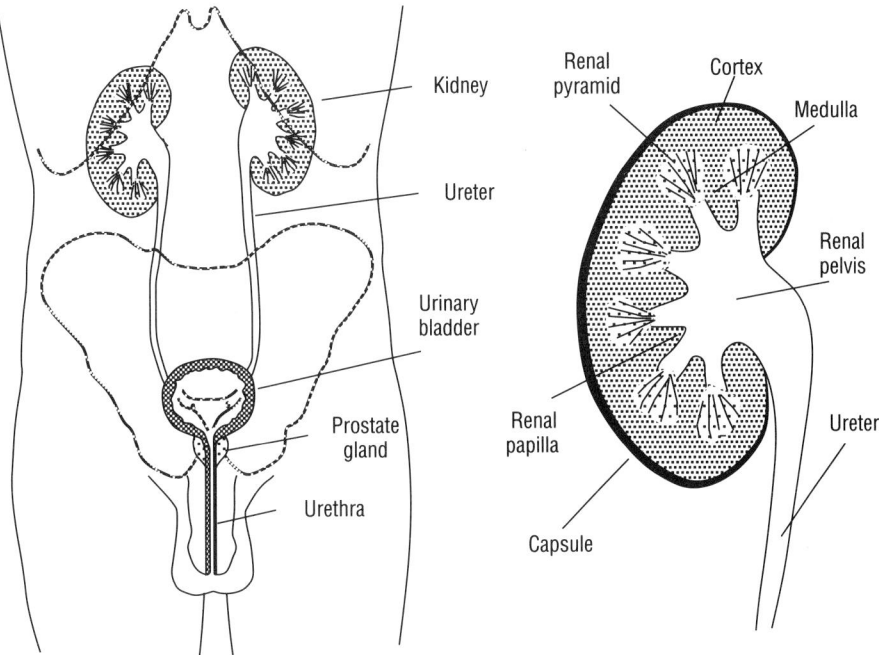

Figure 10.1 *The urinary system*

urea and other wastes not being absorbed from it. At the same time, some secretion of organic acids and bases occurs at this site, the urine being isosmotic to blood. The urine then passes into the loop of Henle where, in the thin, descending limb, water is removed and sodium is added and the urine becomes hypertonic. In the thick, ascending limb, sodium is lost, the urine becoming hypotonic. The urine then passes into the distal convoluted tubule where more sodium is reabsorbed and potassium, ammonia and hydrogen ions are secreted into it. Some water is passively lost from the urine at this site in the presence of antidiuretic hormone. The urine at this stage remains hypotonic to plasma. The urine then passes into the collecting tubule where much water is resorbed through the permeable epithelium in the presence of anti-diuretic hormone. The urine then passes into the ureter and thence into the urinary bladder where it is stored until micturition.

Normal kidney function depends critically on the maintenance of a normally high renal blood flow (renal perfusion), which is approximately 25% of cardiac output. Normal blood pressure must also be maintained. Normal glomerular filtration rate is 170 litres/day. Tubular reabsorption is very important as more than 99% of the glomerular filtrate is reabsorbed, bringing the normal urine volume to 1.5 L/day.

Disordered Renal Function

Functioning of the kidneys may be disordered through:

- congenital diseases;
- renal blood flow disorders and vascular disorders;
- tubular and interstitial disease;
- glomerular disease;
- obstruction of urine flow;
- hormonal dysfunction;
- tumours.

Investigation of disordered kidney function maybe carried out in the following ways:

- biochemical renal function tests on the blood and/or urine;
- microbiological examination of the urine;
- urine sediment examination under the microscope;
- biopsy of the kidney;
- autopsy examination of the urinary system (when all else fails!).

Urinary tract disease is manifested by a number of abnormalities. The most common clinically observed symptoms and signs of disordered renal function are:

- **proteinuria** — the presence of protein in the urine;

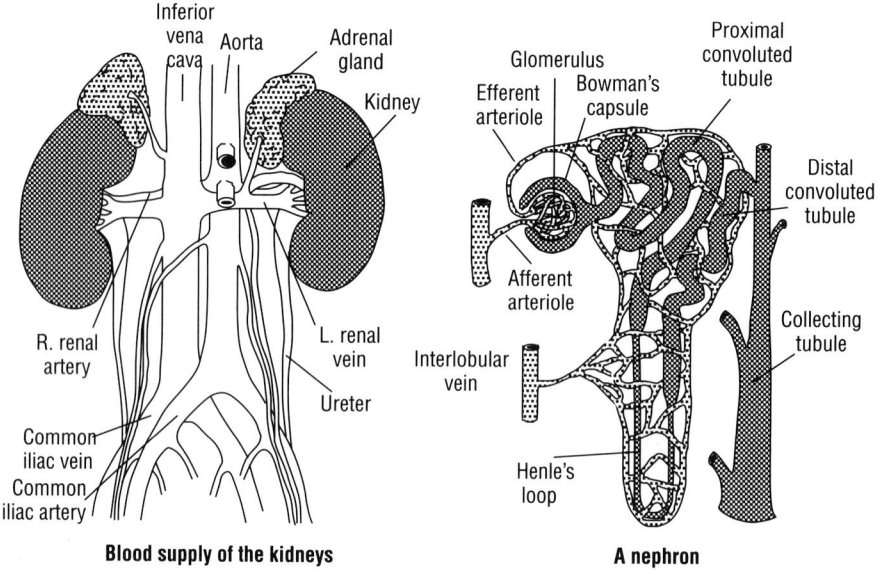

Figure 10.2 *The kidneys and nephron*

- **haematuria** — the presence of blood in the urine. This may be detectable by naked-eye inspection of a urine specimen or may only be detectable by microscopy;
- **bacteriuria** — the presence of bacteria in urine;
- **pyuria** — the presence of pus in the urine;
- **anuria** — failure of the kidneys to excrete urine;
- **oliguria** — the formation by the kidneys of very small amounts of urine;
- **diuresis** — an increase in the volume of urine excreted by the kidneys (polyuria);
- **renal failure** — develops when the kidneys are unable to clear the bloodstream of unwanted substances;
- **strangury** — great difficulty in producing urine, which is only passed in very small volumes and with pain, even though the urge for micturition may be present;
- **uraemia** — the terminal stage of renal failure. This causes an increase in the amount of urea in the blood and disturbance of water and electrolyte balance in the body.

Therefore, it is seen that the diagnosis of renal disease may be very complex as it often requires several widely different laboratory tests and procedures to be carried out. The interpretation of these tests may have to be carried out by several different specialists, such as biochemists, microbiologists, pathologists, radiologists and urologists.

Developmental Defects in the Kidneys

Variations in Number or Size

Congenital anomalies in the urinary system are commonly encountered, but very often these are only incidental findings, the variation being only a morphological anomaly that does not disrupt function or cause any disease. **Renal agenesis** occurs in one in 1000 individuals and in this case one of the kidneys has failed to form from its primordia. Unilateral renal agenesis is compatible with life and often the condition is only discovered incidentally later in life. Very rarely, the agenesis is bilateral and the condition in this case is incompatible with life, the foetus being stillborn.

Hypoplasia of the kidney is slightly commoner and is the condition resulting in one small kidney (or sometimes both kidneys may be affected). The hypoplasia may be asymptomatic, or in one form of the disorder patients present in adolescence with hypertension and renal insufficiency (**Ash-Upmark syndrome**). In 'duplex' kidneys there are two pelvi-calyceal systems in the kidney, often with separate draining ureters. This condition may be bilateral.

Abnormalities in Shape and Position

One kidney may show **ectopia** (situated in an abnormal position). Usually this condition arises unilaterally but more rarely both kidneys are affected. This results in the so-called **malascent kidneys**, which do not reach their normal position in the upper abdomen and are found in the pelvis or pelvic rim. Very rarely the kidneys may be found in the chest. Ectopic kidneys are often associated with other renal tract abnormalities. There may be, for example, failure of rotation of the calyces so that they may point anteriorly and/or medially instead of laterally, or the ureters may have strictures or kinks in them, greatly predisposing the individual to urinary tract infections.

Renal fusion is a common condition, occurring in 1 in 500 individuals and is known as **horse shoe kidney** (Figure 10.3). Over 90% of cases show fusion in the lower pole, the remainder being fused in the upper pole. This condition seldom leads to symptoms and signs or complications and is often an incidental finding at autopsy or investigation for other unrelated disease. Occasionally, renal fusion may be associated with other congenital anomalies in the kidney or ureters and thus may present in infancy (refer to Figure 10.4).

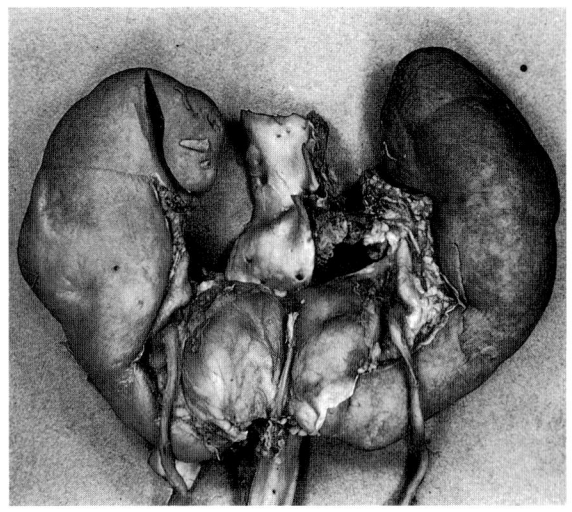

Figure 10.3 *'Horseshoe' deformity of the kidney. Incidental finding in an asymptomatic 30-year-old female*

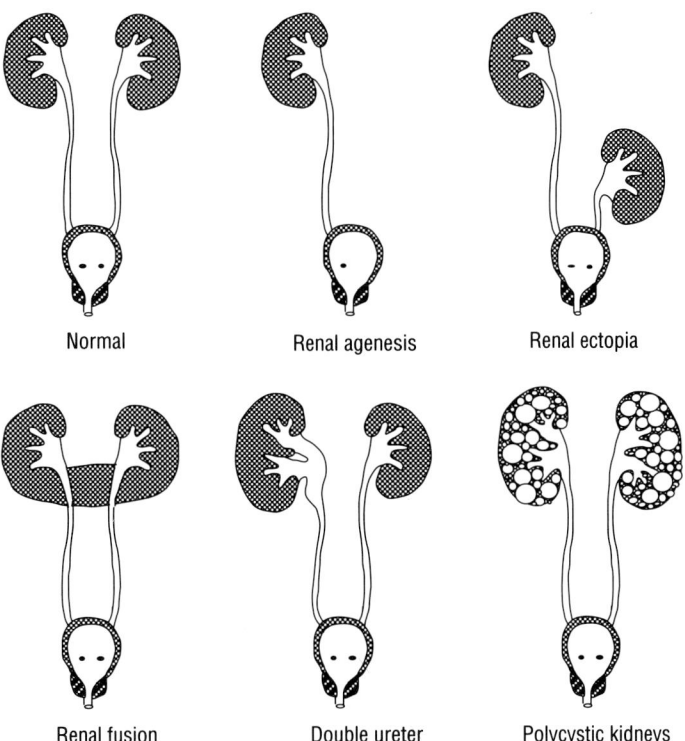

Figure 10.4 *Congenital diseases of the kidneys*

Vascular and Ureteric Anomalies

It is not uncommon for a kidney to have more than one renal artery and more than one renal vein. Multiple renal vessels are more common when the kidney is situated more caudally than normal. Usually, these accessory vessels do not cause any complications. The renal arteries may arise from the iliac arteries or the lower aorta rather than the upper abdominal aorta.

Ureteric abnormalities may be innocuous, such as a double ureter arising from a double renal pelvis. Alternatively, they may cause many complications as occurs with ureters that have strictures or are tortuous or kinked. These conditions may cause obstruction to urinary flow and the condition of **megaureter** and **hydronephrosis** may be seen in association with these congenital anomalies. Urinary tract infections occur commonly in these cases.

Polycystic Kidneys

This is an inherited disorder, either autosomal recessive, which is more severe causing multiple cysts in the foetal kidneys, thus is incompatible with life, or autosomal dominant, in which multiple cysts appear in the kidneys, usually when the patient is in the 30 to 40 age group (Figure 10.5). Most cases of the disease are in the adult onset group. Many patients die of renal failure by the age of 50 years, as the cysts gradually enlarge and destroy more and more renal tissue (the condition has already been discussed under 'Diseases of the Liver' in Chapter 9.)

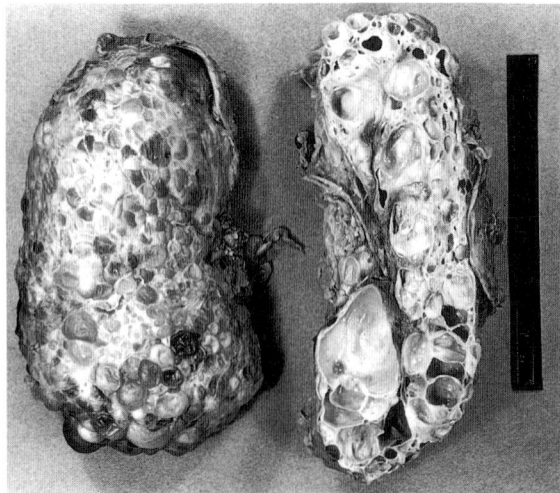

Figure 10.5 *Neonatal form of polycystic disease of the kidneys. The black bar is 25 cm in length*

The adult-onset form of the disease is characterised by the formation of cysts of varying size in the kidneys, sometimes in the liver, and also by the propensity to form **berry aneurysms** of the cerebral arteries (10% or more of the patients with polycystic disease of the kidney also have the aneurysms). The kidneys are enlarged and distorted by many smooth cysts of varying sizes with little renal parenchyma in between. The cysts may contain urine or a thick brown gelatinous material. Areas of infection or haemorrhage may occur. The disease remains symptomless for many years until hypertension, infection and renal failure occur.

Urinary Tract Infections

Haematogenous Infections

Pyaemia Involving the Kidney

Pyaemia is defined as the carriage of pyogenic organisms in the bloodstream. This condition is a frequent complication of localized infections by bacteria, for example an abscess caused by *Staphylococcus aureus*. In pyaemia, the kidney is often involved, multiple abscesses forming within the kidney substance. These are typical in their macroscopical and microscopical appearance, appearing as multiple, rounded, yellowish areas with numerous neutrophils within the abscess cavity, surrounded by inflamed tissue. They are caused by *Staphylococcus aureus*, enteric bacteria, streptococci and other bacteria, their sequelae being as for abscesses in other sites.

Carbuncle of the Kidney

This is a single, large abscess of the kidney exhibiting extensive destruction of renal tissue. It is usually caused by haematogenous spread of *Staphylococcus aureus*. The abscess may become multilocular and spread to involve the perirenal tissues. Usually, a great deal of destruction of renal parenchyma is involved and the scarring associated with healing may be extensive.

Perinephric Abscess

This is an abscess of the tissues surrounding the kidney, especially the perirenal fat. It may arise as a result of spread of infection from within the kidney substance or alternatively arise from a primary focus of infection within the perinephric tissues. Pus accumulates in very large deposits around the kidney and gradually involves the capsule. If the infection remains untreated, it may spread into the kidney parenchyma, with extensive involvement and tissue destruction. Perinephric abscesses may be very large and may respond poorly to antibiotics, requiring in some cases surgical treatment and drainage of the pus.

Pyelonephritis

This diffuse infection of the kidney parenchyma is rarely acquired haematogenously, most cases being ascending infections. The morphology is identical to pyelonephritis developing as an ascending infection (see below), despite the haematogenous pathogenesis.

Ascending Infections

As a group, ascending infections of the urinary tract represent the majority of infections encountered in the urinary tract. Generally, the term **urinary tract infection** (UTI) implies involvement of the urethra and urinary bladder (= **cystitis**), or of the ureters, renal pelvis and renal parenchyma (**pyelonephritis**). Cystitis may occur alone but very often the infection ascends via the ureters to involve the kidney also. Similarly, renal parenchymal infections are constantly seeding bladder infections. It is not surprising therefore that urinary tract infection is most frequently a cystitis associated with a pyelonephritis.

UTI is commoner in some groups of the population (see Figure 10.6). The very **young child** is likely to get a UTI as there may be a number of congenital defects associated with the urogenital tract. **Females of reproductive age** are the most commonly affected group, women being ten times more likely than males of the same age group to develop a UTI. This is due to various anatomical factors:

- the female urethra is shorter than that of the male;
- the urethral opening is much closer to the anus in the female;
- the vaginal opening and urethral opening are very close together;
- sexual intercourse predisposes to UTI in females because of the above factors;
- defective toilet hygiene is of more importance in the female as a predisposing factor to UTI;
- the female is more likely to undergo instrumentation procedures and trauma in the region;
- the gravid uterus may compress the ureters, leading to obstruction of urinary flow.

The **elderly individual** (especially the hospitalized one) is much more likely to develop a UTI, with one in five hospitalized adults succumbing to UTI. Several factors relate to this increased frequency of UTI:

- sphincter weakness associated with atrophic muscular changes of old age;
- obstructions associated with calculi;
- gynaecological problems (prolapsed uterus, vagina, etc.);
- andrological problems (especially prostatomegaly);
- turbulent urine flow and urethrovesical reflux (predisposed to by above factors);
- instrumentation procedures (especially catheterization in the hospitalized patient);
- stress incontinence.

In all UTI, the most commonly involved microorganisms are the enteric normal flora bacteria, especially *Escherichia coli*, *Proteus* spp., *Klebsiella pneumoniae*, *Streptococcus faecalis*, etc. Overall, approximately 80% of UTI are caused by *Escherichia coli*. It should be noted that the lower third of the length of the urethra has a normal flora that may include the above-mentioned organisms. However, the upper two-thirds of the urethra, the bladder, ureters and kidneys are normally sterile. In the female, the source of the organisms may also be the vaginal normal flora.

Cystitis

Most UTIs are confined to the urethra and urinary bladder, leading to a cystitis. Usually, in cystitis pathological changes are minimal and typical of an acute inflammatory response. Hyperaemic vessels are evident, with exudation and infiltration of the mucosa by neutrophils. Such changes are completely reversible, and in some cases resolution occurs spontaneously. However, in most cases without treatment the infection is progressive with increasing symptomatology. There may be dysuria, haematuria, frequency of micturition and pain. Especially in the case of untreated infections the ureters and renal parenchyma are involved, due to the reflux of contaminated urine.

Diagnosis of the infection is by sampling the urine and demonstrating significant bacteriuria (see the section on urinalysis). Once the laboratory has isolated the bacteria causing the infection and has performed an antibiotic sensitivity test, treatment with the appropriate antibiotic will lead to a rapid resolution of the infection.

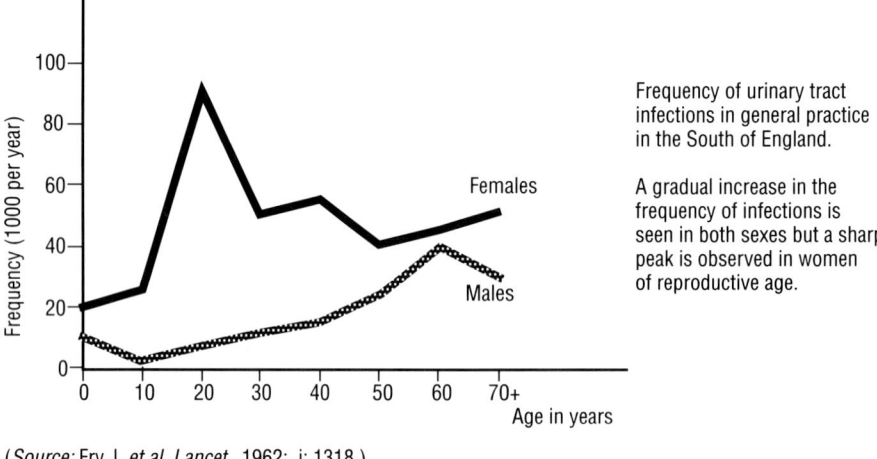

(*Source:* Fry J, *et al. Lancet* 1962; i: 1318.)

Figure 10.6 *Frequency of urinary tract infections*

Acute Pyelonephritis

Pyelonephritis is infection of the renal pelvis and kidney which is usually an ascending infection from the bladder and more liable to occur when there is urinary stasis. Very rarely, **pyelitis** (infection of the renal pelvis only) may occur. Pyelonephritis is most commonly seen in women of reproductive age, during pregnancy, and in elderly males. Pyelonephritis is seen commonly in diabetics with kidney disease and there is increased risk of infection in paraplegics and quadriplegics (neurogenic bladders) particularly due to indwelling catheters and chronic cystitis. Rarely, the infection may be haematogenous. The infection may be unilateral or bilateral.

In acute pyelonephritis the pelvis of the kidney is congested and hyperaemic. The whole kidney looks swollen with a tense capsule. Later, the inflammation is seen to spread upwards into the kidney parenchyma, purulent streaks being seen to run from the pelvis to the medulla and cortex. Initially, only the tubules of the kidney are involved and the glomeruli are spared. Small **abscesses** may develop and in severe cases they will coalesce to form large, ragged, pus-filled cavities. In some cases, there may be only focal involvement of the kidneys. On section, the kidney presents a picture of very severe acute inflammation. The condition may occasionally resolve, especially with long-term antibiotic therapy but sometimes, even with treatment, there is organization and scarring of the affected areas. **Pyonephrosis** may be seen in severe cases and this involves the accumulation of pus within the renal pel-

vis. Untreated cases of acute pyelonephritis quite often progress to chronic pyelonephritis.

Chronic Pyelonephritis

Chronic pyelonephritis is one of the commonest forms of fatal renal disease and is particularly prevalent amongst women. The condition results from persistence of acute pyelonephritis or recurrent acute infections with increasing tissue damage and fibrosis, making the kidney more likely to succumb to more infections. The condition is usually bilateral. The kidneys appear shrunken with a thickened adherent capsule over the pitted and scarred surface. On section, the cortex appears thinned, scarred and pale with the medulla contracted. The pelvis is dilated and the mucosa is thickened and inflamed.

Microscopically, there is evidence of widespread scarring and hyalinization of glomeruli (glomerulosclerosis, periglomerular fibrosis). The tubules are grossly dilated, their epithelium atrophic and the lumen contains protein casts, reminding one of thyroid tissue (the condition is sometimes termed '**thyroid kidney**'). An active, chronic inflammation is seen throughout the tissue with a diffuse infiltrate of lymphocytes, plasma cells and macrophages. Foci of neutrophils are present in some areas. The region around the pelvis may contain large cysts (a condition termed **pyelitis cystica**). The blood vessels are thickened and hyalinized, showing evidence of hypertensive changes.

The progressive loss of renal tissue observed appears similar to the renal changes seen in ischaemia, so the clinical diagnosis depends on history, microbiological examination of the urine and exclusion of other diseases. The disease may remain latent for many years, its course punctuated by episodes of acute inflammation where there may be symptoms and signs of acute urinary tract infection. Chronic pyelonephritis is very commonly associated with hypertension, which is triggered off by the destruction of renal tissue. The commonest complication of chronic pyelonephritis is renal failure that develops after many years (refer to Figure 10.7). The uraemia and hypertensive changes frequently cause the death of the patient. Treatment of chronic pyelonephritis is difficult and the development of the condition must be prevented in the patient who is likely to get multiple UTI by prompt antibiotic therapy to prevent renal tissue damage. Haemodialysis is necessary in the later stages of the disease and renal transplantation is the only recourse in very advanced cases.

Symptoms of Acute Urinary Tract Infections

It should be noted that acute kidney infections are very often involved with infections of the lower urinary tract and often it is not possible to differentiate between the two simply on the basis of clinical symptomatology. In mild cases, the patient may be asymptomatic, but significant bacteriuria will be demonstrated. Symptoms and signs generally related to UTI (upper or lower) are, in mild cases, the following:

- lower back pain, perineal pain;
- suprapubic discomfort, tenderness;
- low-grade fever;
- prostatitis in males with discomfort or pain in the region;
- frequency of micturition;
- dysuria.

In more severe cases, symptoms and signs are usually always present and in addition to those observed with mild infections the following changes and effects may also be seen:

- fever, chills;
- costovertebral angle pain;
- gastrointestinal tract symptoms (nausea, vomiting);
- renal papillary necrosis;
- acute renal failure, oedema;
- haematuria, pyuria.

In order to differentiate between upper and lower UTIs, in addition to microbiological examination of the urine, further more specific tests need to be carried out, for example intravenous pyelography and arteriography.

Renal Tuberculosis

Haematogenous spread of *Mycobacterium* spp. from the portal of entry (usually the lung) may involve the kidneys (Figure 10.8). A miliary tuberculosis may result bilaterally or, quite frequently, only one kidney is involved massively with the caseous necrotic material replacing all of the kidney tissue. The disease is less frequently seen nowadays but was very important in the past. Young adults present with renal tuberculosis as part of generalized tuberculosis. Typical tubercles

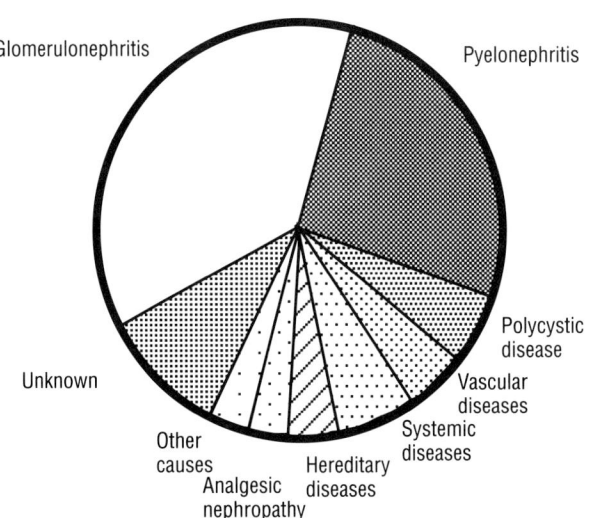

Causes of terminal renal failure that require haemodialysis or transplantation, in Europe. Figures in Australia and the United States are very similar to these.

Note the importance of glomerulonephritis and pyelonephritis.

Figure 10.7   *Causes of renal failure*

develop in the renal cortex and quickly coalesce to form large caseating and cavitating areas that involve the medulla. Glomerular involvement results in spread of the organism to the ureters, prostate and bladder and then to the seminal vesicles and epididymis (Figure 10.9). Eventually the kidneys may be entirely replaced by a mass of caseous necrosis.

The disease is often asymptomatic with no classical clinical presentation. The patient may present with generalized malaise, fatigue and low-grade, persistent pyrexia and night sweats. There may be a dull ache in the flank. The bladder may be swollen with vesical irritability. Dysuria, haematuria and proteinuria may occur. On examination of the urine a pyuria will be noted; however, culture of the urine on routine media will present normal numbers of organisms or a 'sterile' bladder urine. Culture of urine on Löwenstein-Jensen medium will grow *Mycobacterium* spp. Diagnosis is thus by specific culture, and a positive Mantoux test.

The results of the condition depend on the extent of involvement of kidney tissue and whether or not the condition is treated. In untreated, mild cases there may

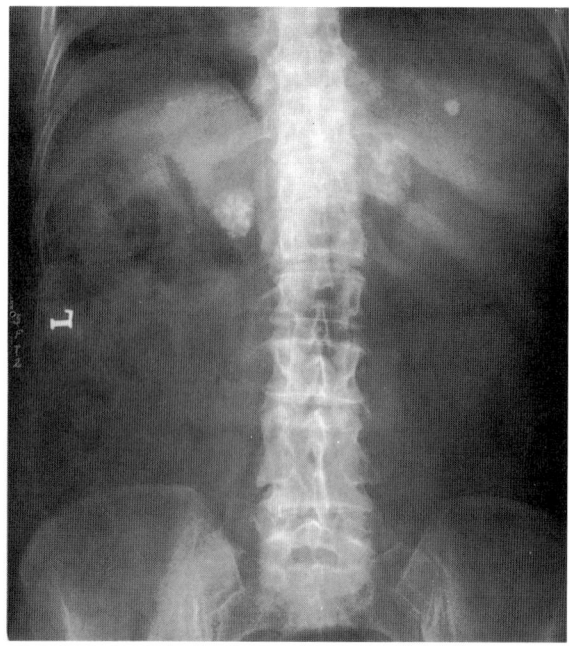

Figure 10.9 *Renal tuberculosis with subsequent spread to the spine and adrenals. Dystrophic calcification of the adrenals has then occurred (courtesy of Dr Thomas Molyneux, RMIT)*

be healing with fibrosis and calcification. Tuberculous pyonephrosis may occur, in which the caseous material initiates an acute inflammatory response in the pelvis and pus forms. Involvement of the whole kidney by caseous necrosis results in a '**putty kidney**', which will undergo an autonephrectomy. Spread of the infection to the lower urinary tract is extremely common, with cystitis, epididymitis and orchitis being common complications. Treated cases of the disease show fibrous healing of smaller lesions and scarring and calcification of the larger lesions. There is usually some loss of function of the affected tissue and complications may arise because of strictures and obstruction developing.

Renal Papillary Necrosis (Analgesic Nephropathy)

In renal papillary necrosis, the tips of the renal pyramids projecting into the minor calyces become necrotic and eventually become detached from the rest of the pyramid. Further damage may then be initiated in the remaining kidney parenchyma that often leads to renal

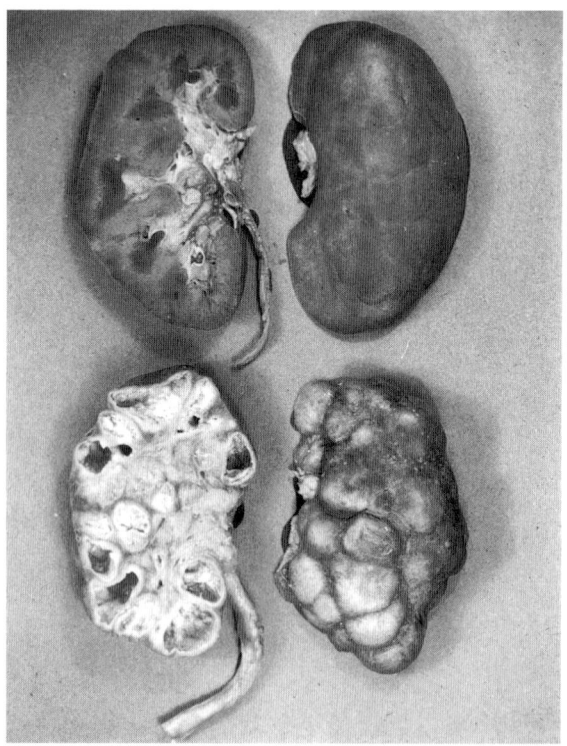

Figure 10.8 *Tuberculosis of the kidneys with numerous regions of caseation in a 51-year-old female*

failure. This disease is common in Australia (especially Queensland), Scandinavia and Switzerland but relatively uncommon in the United States. Middle to old aged people and particularly women are more commonly affected (especially those of a truculent, psychoneurotic personality).

Many cases of the disorder are associated with excessive intake of analgesics such as phenacetin, aspirin, indomethacin, phenylbutazone and mefenamic acid (in quantities of about 500 to 1000 g per year, over a period of 3–4 years). Such patients often have a history of chronic headaches and personality disorders. However, papillary necrosis may complicate other conditions, such as diabetes and severe pyelonephritis. A concentrated urine is associated with the pathogenesis of the disease and this may explain why the disease is seen in some geographical locations with hot climates. The necrosis of the papillae occurs first in response to direct toxic effects of substances in the urine, ischaemia, or a combination of the two. As ulceration of the necrotic papillae develops, dystrophic calcification and calculus formation usually occurs next, followed by infection, with pyelonephritis being seen in most cases associated with the disease.

Papillary necrosis is usually bilateral, involving several papillae. The distal part of the papillae is yellowish to white, indicative of coagulative necrosis. The adjacent tissue is red and congested with inflammation. Calcification, infection and ulceration may also be seen and the cortex is usually atrophic. Patients with this disease are predisposed to recurrent acute UTI, chronic pyelonephritis, renal failure, uraemia, transitional cell carcinoma, and very frequently the disease is fatal.

Vascular Lesions Affecting the Kidney

Renal Infarction

Due to its single blood supply, the arrangement of the arterial tree and the frequency of arterial disease at this site, infarcts of the kidney are very common (see Figure 10.10). Atherosclerosis affects the renal artery, especially at the aortic orifice, causing narrowing of the lumen with resulting ischaemia to the kidney. This causes gradual loss of kidney parenchyma and fibrosis, leading to hypertension. In advanced atherosclerosis, thrombotic emboli also commonly lodge in renal vessels, resulting in kidney infarcts.

More than 98% of renal infarcts are the result of arterial thromboembolism, while the remaining 2% are due to venous occlusion caused by renal thrombophlebitis. Renal infarcts are usually peripheral, involving a cone of the subcapsular cortex, thus presenting a wedge-shaped cross-section. They may be multiple and are typically pale infarcts, showing a yellowish white cut surface surrounded within 24 hours by a reddish rim of inflammation and hyperaemia. Microscopically, coagulative necrosis is seen, with numerous neutrophils surrounding the infarct. Granulation tissue formation and scarring of the infarcted area progressively occurs.

Most renal infarcts are asymptomatic as large areas of kidney tissue may be lost without ill effects. At autopsy, many scars due to past infarcts are frequently found in the kidneys. Occasionally, septic infarcts occur and abscesses will form in the tissue. Often,

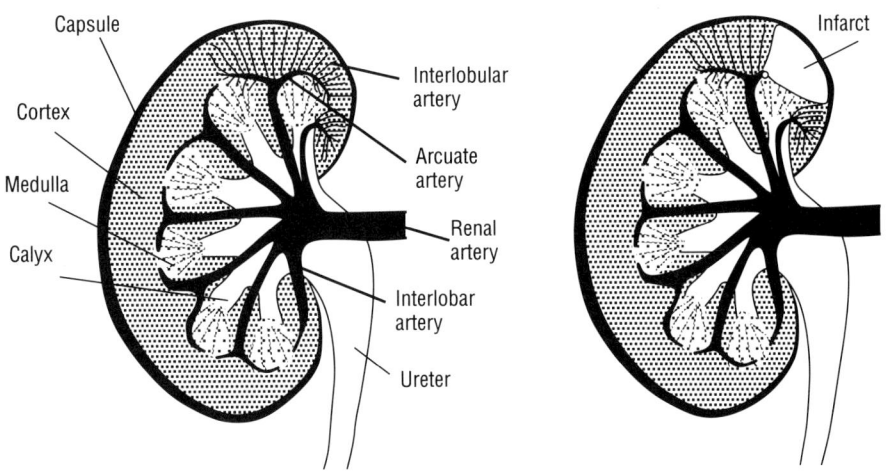

Figure 10.10 *Renal arterial blood supply and infarct of the kidney*

infarction in the kidney is an indication of the presence of other more important diseases in the body, for example hypertension, atherosclerosis of the aorta and thromboembolism.

Hypertension and the Kidney

Hypertension is defined as a persistent rise in systemic blood pressure, above 140/95 mmHg. Treatment is mandatory if the diastolic pressure reaches a value of 110 mmHg. Primary (idiopathic) hypertension accounts for 90% of cases of the disease and 95% of patients develop a slow rise in blood pressure over many years, called benign hypertension. Some patients display a very rapid rise in blood pressure over a relatively short time, termed malignant hypertension.

The kidney in **benign hypertension** shows evidence of benign nephrosclerosis and a group of changes develop in this tissue, often all described collectively as **chronic hypertensive renal disease**. This disease is very common, 75% of autopsies of people over 65 years showing its presence in their kidneys. In long-standing cases the kidneys become slightly reduced in size and granular on their subcapsular aspect. There is ischaemic atrophy and scarring throughout the renal substance, making the kidney look pitted and riddled with small haemorrhages, such an appearance being referred to as a 'flea-bitten' kidney. The cortex of the cut surface of the kidney is narrow, greyish, with loss of normal pattern, while the medulla is pale and decreased in thickness.

Microscopically the kidney in benign hypertension shows evidence of narrowing and arteriolosclerosis of the smaller arteries within the kidney substance. The afferent arterioles are affected especially and the change seen in the wall is **hyaline arteriolosclerosis**. There is progressive ischaemia to the glomeruli supplied by these arterioles and a **glomerulosclerosis** develops gradually. Atrophy of tubules is also seen. The larger arteries in the renal substance generally show evidence of atherosclerosis. The surviving nephrons undergo hypertrophy and renal function is usually maintained. As a result, not more than 5% of patients with benign hypertension die from renal failure, succumbing rather to cardiovascular system disorders such as hypertensive heart disease, myocardial infarction (MI) and cerebrovascular accidents (CVA).

The kidney in **malignant hypertension** shows evidence of malignant nephrosclerosis and the changes developing in this condition are referred to as **accelerated hypertensive renal disease**. The condition may arise *de novo* or supervene on benign hypertension. This disease occurs in about 5% of all patients with hypertension, arising *de novo* most usually in people of about 40 years of age, and is a sequela of benign hypertension in people around the age of 60 years.

The kidneys in malignant hypertension arising *de novo* are of normal size, with cortex and medulla of the normal thickness on section. The cortex may show some small haemorrhages. Microscopically, the characteristic lesion is reduplication of the elastic laminae of the small arteries (elastosis), with fibrinoid necrosis of the wall giving rise to the typical **'onion skinning' of arteries**. The lumen of the affected vessels is almost completely obliterated and microthrombi may be seen to occlude these vessels. Haemorrhages into the renal parenchyma may be seen in association with

Table 10.1 *Comparison of benign and malignant hypertension*

	Benign hypertension	Malignant hypertension
Incidence	95% of cases	5% of cases
Macroscopic findings	Granular, shrunken, contracted, scarred kidney, some haemorrhages	Grossly normal or slightly enlarged kidney with cortical haemorrhages
Microscopic findings	Hyaline arteriolosclerosis, glomerulosclerosis +++, glomerular hypertrophy, tubular atrophy, protein casts, atherosclerosis of larger vessels	Onion skinning of vessels, elastosis, haemorrhages, glomerular crescents, glomerulosclerosis +, protein casts in tubules
Results	5% die of renal failure. Most die of hypertensive heart disease, MI or CVA	>90% die of renal failure

damaged vessels. Some glomeruli appear normal but also many glomeruli show hypercellularity, occasional crescent-shaped accumulations of inflammatory and epithelial cells filling the Bowman's space and fibrinoid necrosis of the glomerular tuft. Generally, less glomerulosclerosis is seen than in benign hypertension. Despite these grossly normal findings in the kidney, over 90% of patients with malignant hypertension die of renal failure. The course of the disease in untreated cases is very rapid and death will ensue within about 12 months of the onset. The major features of benign versus malignant hypertension are compared in Table 10.1.

Glomerulonephritis

Glomerulonephritis (GN) is a general term embracing a wide group of disorders. The renal lesions in these disorders are primarily glomerular, some form of injury to the glomeruli initiating the disease process. All other lesions seen in GN are secondary to the disease in the glomeruli. Glomerular lesions developing after some other renal disease, as occurs, for example, in chronic pyelonephritis, are not included in the GN group. A large proportion of cases of GN is due to an immunological mechanism operating, especially related to deposition of immune complexes in the glomerulus. The destruction of glomerular tissue and acute inflammation are the primary contributors to the renal damage caused by the disease. In some types of GN, inflammation may not be very prominent. Characteristically, the following features are seen in glomerular disorders:

- proliferation, swelling of glomerular capillary endothelium;
- exudation and infiltration into the glomerular tuft;
- formation of hyaline material (fibrinoid necrosis);
- proliferation of capsular epithelium ('crescent formation');
- thickening of basement membranes;
- destruction of glomeruli;
- loss of glomerular function.

Acute, subacute or chronic GN may occur, the adjectives referring to the time course of the disease. However, with each of these forms there is associated a specific morphology and several different aetiologies; therefore, several different aetiologies may give rise to very similar appearances and clinical presentations. The classification of GN is difficult and several different systems of nomenclature and classification have resulted in many synonyms describing the same condition.

In order to understand the changes that occur in the kidney in GN, it is essential to be aware of the ultrastructure of the normal glomerulus (refer to Figure 10.11). A glomerulus is a tuft of fenestrated capillaries arising from the afferent arteriole. Each capillary is surrounded by a basement membrane that is produced and maintained by the mesangial cells that are close to the endothelium of the capillaries. External to the capillaries and basement membrane are the visceral Bowman's capsular epithelial cells, also called podocytes on account of the small foot-like processes that impinge on the basement membrane, interdigitating and surrounding the capillaries. The urinary space is external to these cells and the whole tuft of capillaries is surrounded by the parietal Bowman's capsular epithelial cells. The capillary tuft of the glomerulus drains into the efferent arteriole, which then leads to another capillary bed around the renal tubules. Filtration of the blood plasma is a passive process relying on hydrostatic pressure and the smaller luminal diameter of the efferent arteriole when compared to the afferent arteriole. The formed elements of the blood are retained within the glomerular capillary lumen as they are too big to pass through the fenestrations. The differential permeability of the basement membrane surrounding the capillary wall and the interdigitating foot processes of the podocytes ensure that only small molecules (i.e. solutes such as glucose and urea but not plasma proteins) pass into the urinary space.

Glomerular disease may cause the patient to present clinically with the **nephritic** or the **nephrotic syndromes**. It may also result in acute or chronic renal failure.

The Nephritic Syndrome

The nephritic syndrome is a collection of symptoms and signs seen in various forms of glomerular injury. It is often seen in association with the various forms of GN, typically following inflammatory disorders affecting the glomerular tuft. Depending on the aetiology, it may be divided into the acute nephritic syndrome (of acute onset and rapid resolution), or the chronic nephritic syndrome (of an insidious onset and leading to loss of renal function). A rapidly progressive nephritic syndrome is also sometimes described. Symptoms and signs associated with the nephritic syndrome include the following:

- Haematuria
- Red blood cell casts
- Mild proteinuria
- Hypertension
- Azotaemia
- Glomerular lesions
- Inflammation of glomeruli
- Casts in tubules
- Oliguria
- Oedema

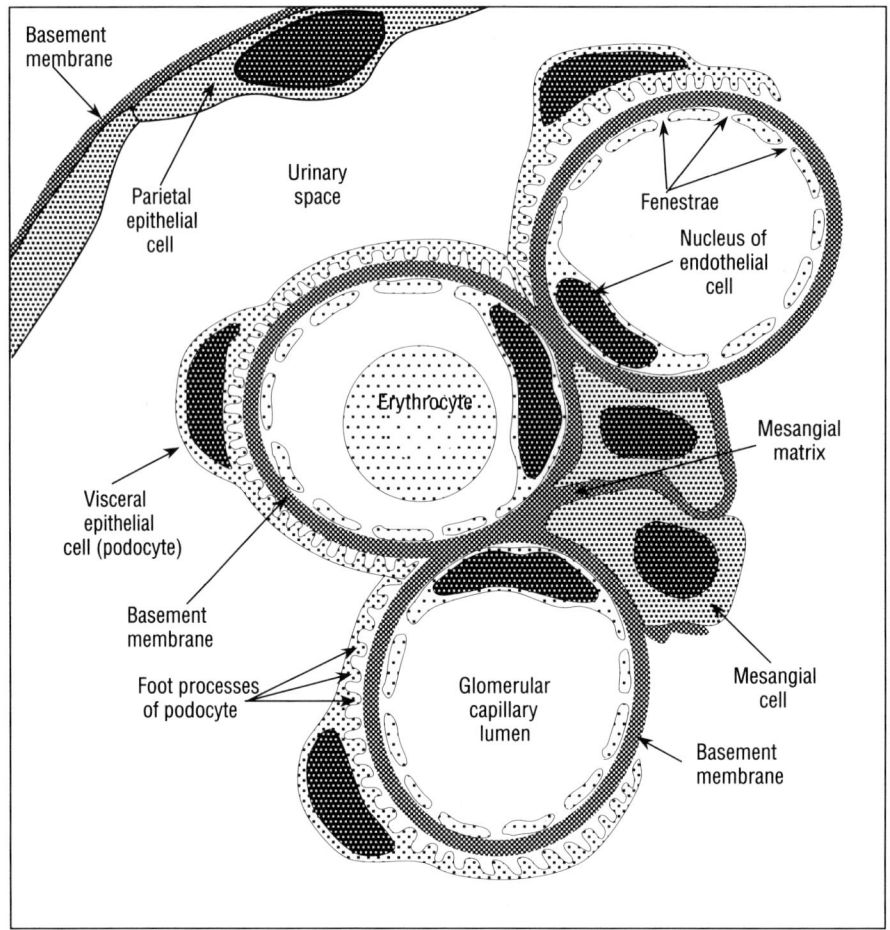

Figure 10.11 *A normal glomerular tuft*

The patient with the nephritic syndrome may recover completely or progress to a variety of sequelae as listed below:

- Resolution
- Nephrotic syndrome
- Renal failure (acute)
- 'End-stage' kidney disease and renal failure
- Death

The Nephrotic Syndrome

The nephrotic syndrome is a clinical state characterized by:

- Heavy proteinuria (1 to 10 g/day)
- Hypoalbuminaemia
- Generalized oedema (osmotic effects)
- Hyperlipidaemia

It follows a severe prolonged increase in glomerular permeability to protein. There are glomerular lesions, the tubules being usually intact. A whole variety of aetiologies are responsible for the syndrome but it is commonly associated with some types of GN. Other causes of the nephrotic syndrome are lipoid nephrosis, diabetes mellitus, focal segmental glomerulosclerosis and amyloidosis. Characteristics of the nephrotic syndrome are:

- Severe proteinuria
- Hypoalbuminaemia
- Oedema
- 'Foamy' urine
- Glomerular lesions
- Lipid infiltration of tubules
- Protein casts

Table 10.2 *Summary of factors initiating glomerular damage*

Ischaemia	Hypotension, shock
	Atherosclerosis
Diabetes mellitus	Glomerular lesions
	Nephrosclerosis (Kimmelstiel-Wilson bodies)
Immune damage	Post-infectious glomerulonephritis
	IgA nephropathy
	Mesangiocapillary glomerulonephritis
	Membranous glomerulonephritis
	Goodpasture's syndrome
Systemic diseases	Systemic lupus erythematosus (SLE)
	Polyarteritis nodosa
	Henoch-Schönlein purpura
Amyloidosis	Primary
	Secondary
	• Rheumatoid arthritis
	• TB
	• Chronic lung disease
	• Chronic pyelonephritis
Drugs/toxins	Gold salts
	Penicillamine
	Antibiotics
	Heavy metals

The results are:

• Resolution/remission
• Relapse
• Renal failure
• Death

It should be noted that the nephrotic syndrome is related to disorders affecting the integrity of glomerular capillary wall, especially the basement membrane. The nephritic syndrome is related to disorders evoking inflammatory and proliferative responses in the glomeruli.

Post-streptococcal Glomerulonephritis (Acute Diffuse Proliferative Glomerulonephritis)

Post-streptococcal GN is a typical, rapid-onset disease affecting the kidneys diffusely and usually resolving. It is one of the commonest of the glomerulonephritides, typically seen in childhood, but adults may also be affected. It is characteristic in its pathogenesis as immune mechanisms are largely responsible for the lesions developing in the glomeruli. Occasionally it may also be seen in association with other infections (e.g. staphylococci, viruses).

The disorder is seen to occur in susceptible individuals in association with infections by the 'nephritogenic' strains of β-haemolytic, group A streptococci. A sore throat or skin infection, usually trivial, develops first and may be treated successfully with antibiotics. The GN develops as an idiosyncratic response between one week to one month after these infections. The precise nature of the pathogenic antigen is not clearly established but it is suspected to be part of the bacterial cell that is released in large quantities into the bloodstream after it has been degraded by phagocytes. Antibodies combine with these antigens and circulating immune complexes form, eventually being filtered out in the glomeruli. Other nephrologists suggest that immune complex formation in situ within the glomerulus may be important in causation of the GN.

The kidneys in this disorder look normal or slightly

enlarged. Petechial haemorrhages may be seen on the surface and slight pallor of the organ may be apparent. There is diffuse glomerular hypercellularity with endothelial and mesangial cell proliferation, and neutrophilic and monocytic cell infiltrate. There may be occasional crescents of inflammatory and epithelial cells within the Bowman's space. With immunoelectron microscopy immune complexes can be demonstrated beneath the capillary wall, deposited in the subepithelial situations, trapped between capillary endothelium and basement membrane.

The effects of the disorder are variable depending on the age of the patient and the state of health prior to the onset of the disease. Typically, it is an acute-onset disorder, with usually the nephritic syndrome developing (or uncommonly, the nephrotic syndrome). Most children (about 95% of them) recover completely within 3 to 4 weeks. The remaining children develop rapidly

progressive GN or chronic renal disease. Adults are more likely to develop chronic renal disease than children are, with 15–50% of cases presenting in this manner. Children may die in the early stages of the disease from cardiac failure, while adults may die at a later stage from renal failure. The disease is important as no specific therapy is available. Generally, patients are put on a low-protein diet, their fluid and electrolyte balance is carefully monitored and the patient may have to be placed on haemodialysis.

Rapidly Progressive Glomerulonephritis (Subacute Crescentic Glomerulonephritis)

Rapidly progressive GN is a disorder characterized by rapid onset and quickly progressive loss of renal function. It is a clinical syndrome, not due to a specific

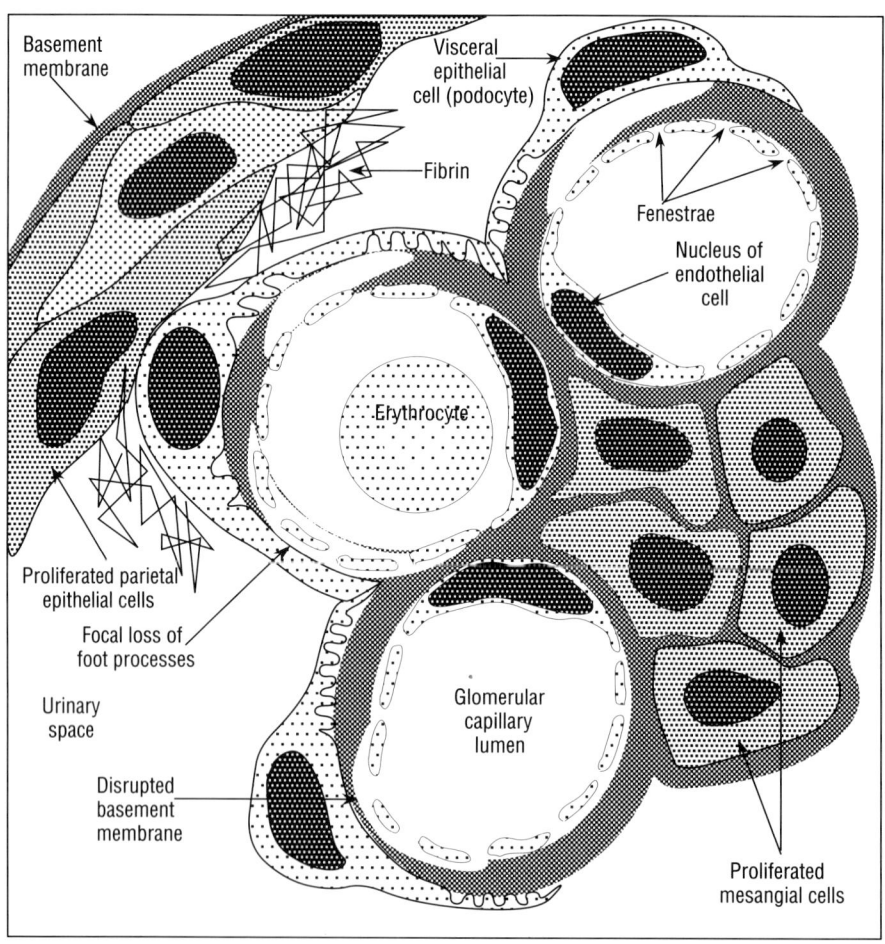

Figure 10.12   *Changes in the glomerular tuft brought about by crescentic GN*

aetiology. It is not very commonly seen and most usually occurs in association with systemic diseases. The following disorders may give rise to this type of GN:

* post-infectious (1–2% of cases of post-streptococcal GN);
* systemic lupus erythematosus;
* goodpasture's syndrome;
* Henoch-Schönlein purpura;
* other systemic diseases;
* antiglomerular membrane disease (autoimmune/ hypersensitivity pathogenesis);
* idiopathic.

The pathogenesis of the disorder has not been clearly elucidated, but immune mechanisms are thought to be important. Most of the systemic diseases with which this type of GN is associated are of an autoimmune nature. Fibrin deposits are seen in the glomerular tuft in active disease and therefore inflammation of the damaged glomerulus is important in the pathogenesis.

The condition causes the kidneys to appear enlarged and pale with cortical, petechial haemorrhages indicating glomerular damage. The glomeruli may show focal necrosis and hypercellularity but crescents are characteristic and occur diffusely throughout the kidney. The crescents are composed of Bowman's capsular parietal cells and of inflammatory cells, especially monocytes. Fibrin is present in the Bowman's space (see Figures 10.12 and 10.13). The crescents tend to heal by fibrosis, leading to fibroepithelial crescents or even complete destruction and fibrosis of the affected glomeruli. Tubular atrophy is seen with protein and red blood cell casts being present in the tubular lumen.

Rapid progressive loss of renal function is seen in this disorder and most patients present with severe oliguria and the nephritic syndrome. Renal failure may develop within a period of weeks to months. There is no time for the development of scarring or contraction of the kidney and at autopsy the kidney looks slightly swollen, pale and has multiple haemorrhages in the cortex. Untreated, the patients usually die in azotaemia. The only treatment is dialysis or transplantation.

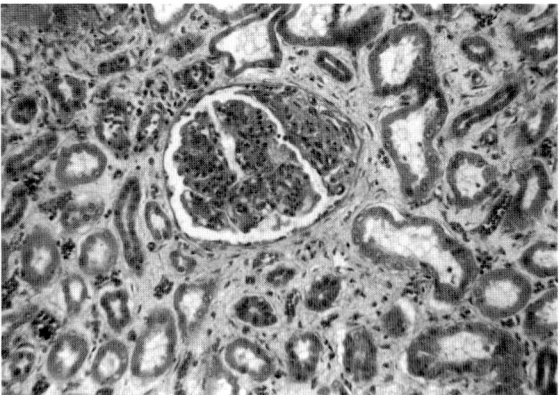

Figure 10.13 *Crescentic glomerulonephritis showing the prominent 'crescent' of cells after which the condition was named (×200)*

thus is often seen in arthritics). Studies have indicated that it is commoner in people with the HLA-DR3 antigen and other observed relevant features of this susceptible group of people is that they suffer from disrupted helper/suppressor T cell ratios. It also appears that complement dysfunction may be important in the pathogenesis of the disorder, the C5b-9 component of complement causing damage to glomerular cell membranes.

Under the light microscope, the glomeruli affected by the disorder show basement membrane thickening and with immunofluorescent labelling the deposits of immunoglobulin and complement in the basement membrane may be demonstrated. In addition, loss of podocyte processes is seen under the electron microscope (refer to Figure 10.14). The disease presents as an insidious developing nephrotic syndrome but the course of the disease varies greatly. Approximately 25% of patients develop renal failure, about 30% of them go into remission while the remainder have a persistent proteinuria and may get relapses of the condition. Overall, within about 20 years approximately half of the patients will develop renal failure.

Membranous Glomerulonephritis

Membranous GN is a slowly progressive disease of young adulthood to middle age. It involves deposition of immune complexes beneath the capillary endothelium of the glomerular capillaries with basement membrane thickening. It is associated with malignant tumours, hepatitis B, SLE, infections and drug administration (e.g. gold salts, mercurials, penicillamine —

Membranoproliferative Glomerulonephritis

Membranoproliferative GN is a disease that is frequently associated with a hypocomplementaemia brought about by consumption of complement components in the pathogenesis of the disease. The aetiology of the condition is thought to be a chronic immune complex type of reaction, where the C3 component of complement is acting as an autoantigen. The C3 nephritic factor activates the alternate complement fixation pathway, but how this produces the glomerular lesions is not known.

Microscopically, there is hypercellularity of glomeruli and thickening of the basement membrane with deposition of immune complexes subendothelially. The hypercellularity is mainly caused by mesangial cell proliferation. In addition to dividing, these cells elongate their cytoplasm and insert long processes between the endothelium and podocyte. Inflammatory cells also contribute to the cellularity (see Figure 10.15).

Further characterization of the disease may be carried out by close examination of the precise location of the immune complexes: type I disease shows subendothelial deposits, while type II disease shows deposits that are within the basement membrane. The nephrotic or nephritic syndrome develops in this type of GN, and roughly 40% of patients develop renal failure, about 30% of them show a renal insufficiency, the remainder having a persistent proteinuria with relapses of the condition. Type I disease has a marginally better prognosis than type II disease. If renal transplantation is carried out in type II patients, the condition will often recur in the transplanted kidney.

Focal Segmental Glomerulonephritis

Focal segmental GN affects only some of the glomeruli initially (i.e. it is focal) and in the affected tuft only some areas will be involved (i.e. it is segmental). Several types of this form of GN are known and in some countries this is the commonest of the idiopathic types of GN; in Australia, Japan, Singapore and some Euro-

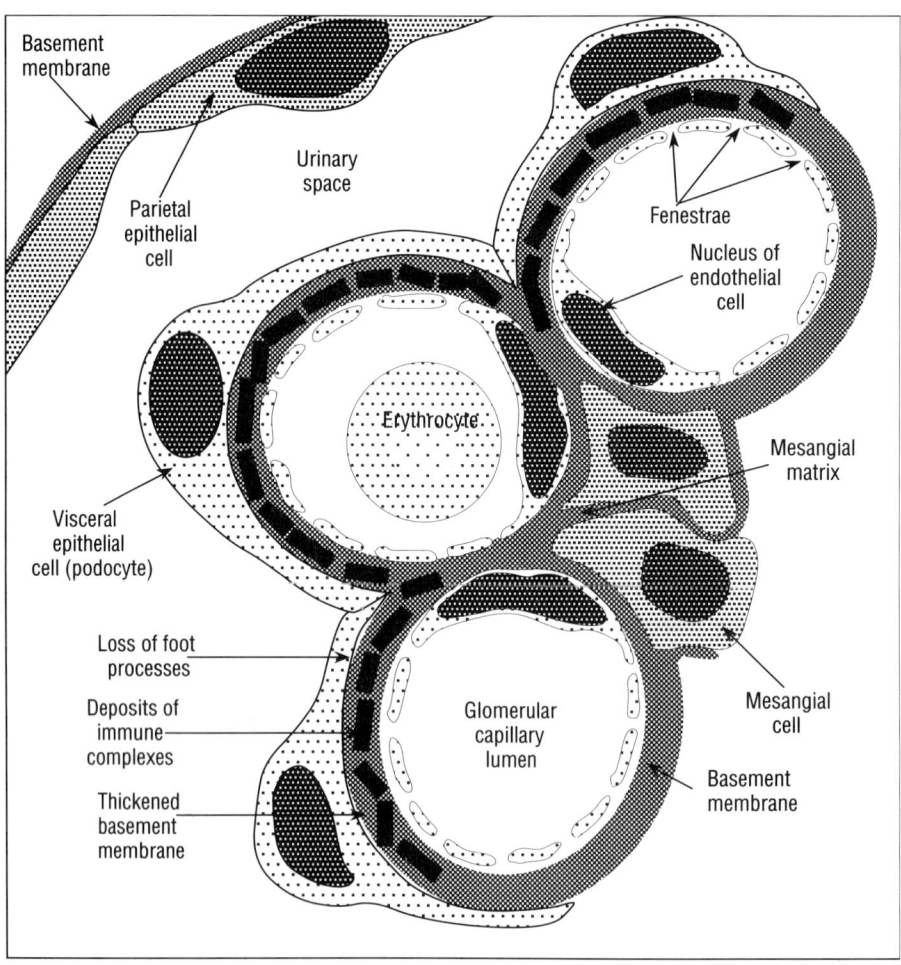

Figure 10.14 *Changes in the glomerular tuft caused by membranous GN*

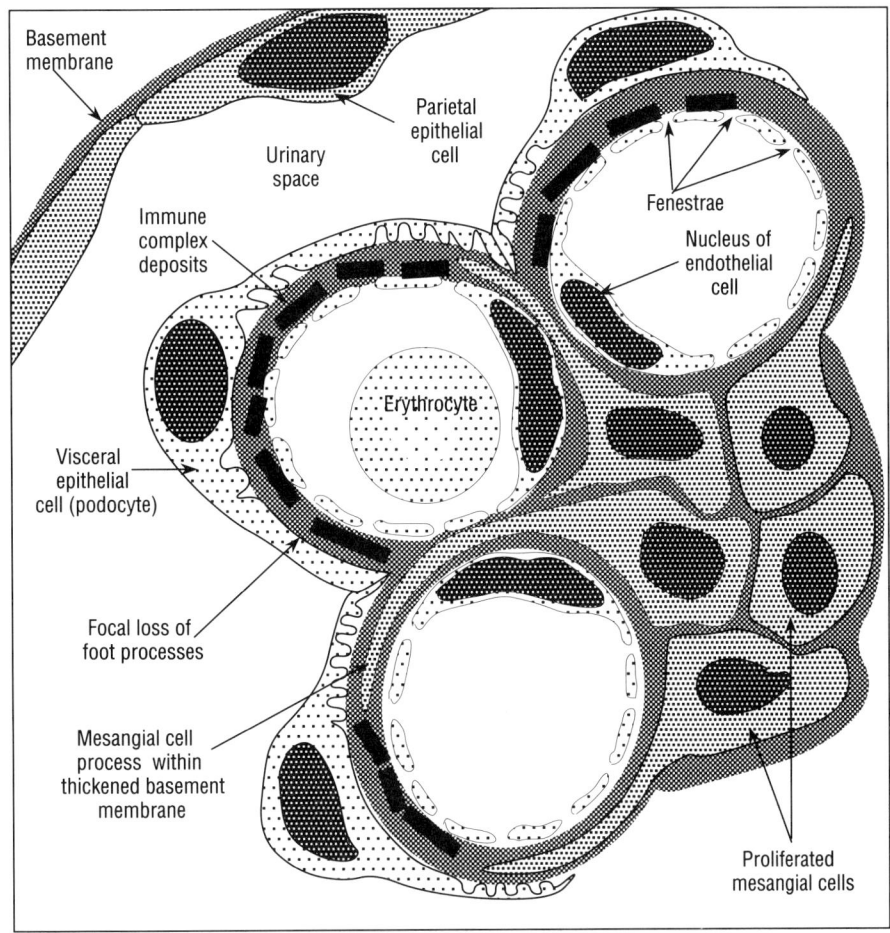

Figure 10.15 *Changes in the glomerular tuft caused by membranoproliferative GN*

pean countries it accounts for about 20% of cases of such diseases. Typically, this disease is seen in adolescents and young adults, men being more commonly affected than women. It is associated with systemic autoimmune disease such as Henoch-Schönlein purpura, SLE, Crohn's disease and Wegener's granulomatosis. An important subgroup of this type of GN is **Berger's disease** (IgA nephropathy), in which IgA antibodies and C3 components may be demonstrated within the affected glomerular tufts.

The glomeruli show segmental, or in later stages, global hyalinization, with IgA, IgG and/or IGM demonstrable in association with C3 components within the glomerular tuft. The disorder leads to a variety of presentations ranging from symptomless proteinuria to renal failure. The nephrotic syndrome may develop, followed by acute or chronic renal failure with malig-

nant hypertension. Generally, there is a poor prognosis with a quarter to half of the patients developing end-stage renal failure within 20 years.

Minimal Change 'Glomerulonephritis' (Lipoid Nephrosis)

Minimal change glomerular disease is the most frequent cause of the nephrotic syndrome in children, usually appearing between the ages of 2 and 3 years. However, older children and adults may also be involved, more males than females affected. The condition is not associated with inflammation in the glomeruli and changes in the glomeruli visible under the light microscope are minimal, the kidney often appearing totally normal. Hence, the condition is described as minimal change disease or a 'nephrosis'. The term 'lipoid' reflects the presence of fat within the renal tubular epithelial cells. Under the electron microscope, however, there is widespread loss of foot processes of the visceral epithelial cells in the glomeruli. This is the only change visible, which accounts for the relatively benign nature of the disorder (refer to Figure 10.16).

The loss of foot processes from the epithelial cell is thought to allow the loss of membrane polyanions with the permission of transmembrane passage of small plasma proteins (predominantly albumin) resulting in the proteinuria accompanying the disease. The aetiology and pathogenesis of the condition is unclear but it is suspected that it may be associated with a T cell dysfunction. In Hodgkin's disease where there is a T cell dysfunction, similar lesions to lipoid nephrosis may be found in the kidneys of patients. Some researchers suggest that a humoral component may be involved also, as circulating immune complexes may be demonstrated during exacerbations of the disease (however, these are non-complement-fixing complexes).

Clinically, the disease presents with proteinuria but with no loss of renal function, and no hypertension. Over 90% of cases respond well to steroid therapy, the proteinuria disappearing after eight weeks of treatment. If the steroids are discontinued, a relapse is noted, relapses being more likely the older the patient is. Progression to renal failure is very rare and many patients will go into permanent remission after steroid treatment. The good response to steroid therapy indicates the importance of immune mechanisms in the pathogenesis of the disease.

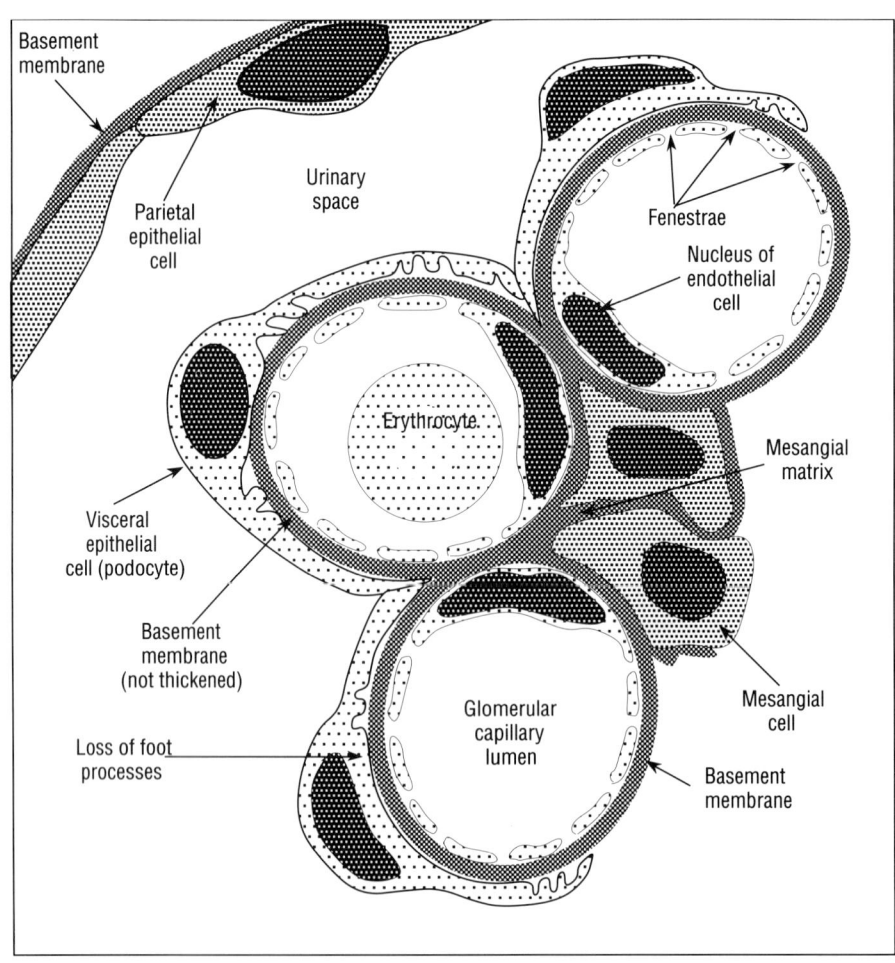

Figure 10.16   *Changes in the glomerular tuft in minimal change GN (lipoid nephrosis)*

Chronic Glomerulonephritis

Chronic GN is an outcome of chronic glomerular damage, the common end-stage effect of many renal diseases affecting the glomeruli and presenting as a chronic renal failure. More than half of patients requiring chronic haemodialysis or renal transplantation have this diagnosis, while 20% of these patients have no history of previous renal disease. Chronic GN is usually first noted in young and middle-aged adults.

The various disorders that may progress to chronic GN include:

* focal glomerulosclerosis, hypertension, diabetes;
* membranous and membranoproliferative GN;
* acute GN.

In all of the above diseases there is glomerular damage, nephrosclerosis, hyalinization and interstitial fibrosis with many vascular changes. Both kidneys are affected and are equally and greatly reduced in size. Their surface is reddish brown, uniformly irregular and granular. The kidneys resemble those of the end stage of benign hypertension. All degrees of glomerular hyalinization are present, with most glomeruli having been destroyed. The few surviving glomeruli will be found to be hypertrophied. There is marked tubular atrophy, interstitial fibrosis and the tubules contain protein and red blood cell casts. Focal accumulations of mononuclear cells are scattered throughout the kidney and hypertensive changes are seen in the arteries and arterioles. The larger arteries are found to have atherosclerosis.

The effects of chronic GN are quite severe and numerous. Clinically, the patient presents with the nephritic or nephrotic syndrome (hypertension, azotaemia, oedema, severe proteinuria). As a result of the considerable damage to both kidneys, chronic renal failure is usually inevitable, thus a poor prognosis is associated with the disorder, the patient usually progressing to uraemia and death within about 10 years of onset of symptoms if left untreated. Long-term haemodialysis is generally required to keep the patient alive longer and renal transplantation is the only effective treatment.

Nephrosis

Nephrosis is a clinical condition that may mimic the nephrotic syndrome and thus be misdiagnosed clinically as a form of GN. However, the lesions in nephrosis are in tubules and the glomeruli appear normal. There is albuminuria with protein casts visible in the tubules, the epithelium of which may be atrophic, show evidence of reactive changes or other damage.

The aetiology of nephrosis is complex and in many cases direct toxic effects on tubules may be important in the development of the lesions. Several causes of nephrosis are:

* **chemicals**: mercurials, potassium dichromate, CCl_4, uranium salts, etc.;
* **toxins**: diphtheria toxin, typhoid toxin, etc.,
* **diabetes mellitus**: deposition of glycogen in renal tubules;
* **bile**: obstructive jaundice causes nephrosis as bile pigments are deposited in the kidney;
* **tumours**: especially myeloma where there is infiltration of the kidney and Bence-Jones proteins are deposited in the kidney.

The prognosis of the condition is variable and depends on the degree of tubular damage sustained and whether or not the injurious or initiating agent can be removed.

Urinary Tract Obstruction

Urinary tract obstruction may occur anywhere along the length of the urinary tract and depending on the site obstructed different effects will be seen. The obstruction is commonly by congenital anomalies involving the ureter or urethra, stones, tumours, neurogenic causes, prostatic enlargement (benign or malignant), foreign body or stenosis. When the obstruction is below the insertion of the ureters into the bladder, the effects are bilateral. Dilatation occurs above the block, forming **hydroureter** and **hydronephrosis**, in which the kidney substance is reduced to a thin rim of cortical tissue with loss of renal papillae and gross dilatation of the pelvis and calyces (Figure 10.17). Widespread loss of tubules occurs although some fairly normal glomeruli may persist.

If the obstruction is sudden and complete (e.g. impaction of a necrotic papilla or inadvertent tying of a ureter in a surgical mishap), cessation of renal function and atrophy occurs in 2–3 weeks with little hydronephrotic change. If the change is unilateral it may be asymptomatic. If surgical decompression is impossible, unilateral nephrectomy is curative.

Hydronephrosis

Hydronephrosis may be unilateral or bilateral. Unilateral hydronephrosis is usually associated with ureteric obstruction and may be due to congenital stenosis of

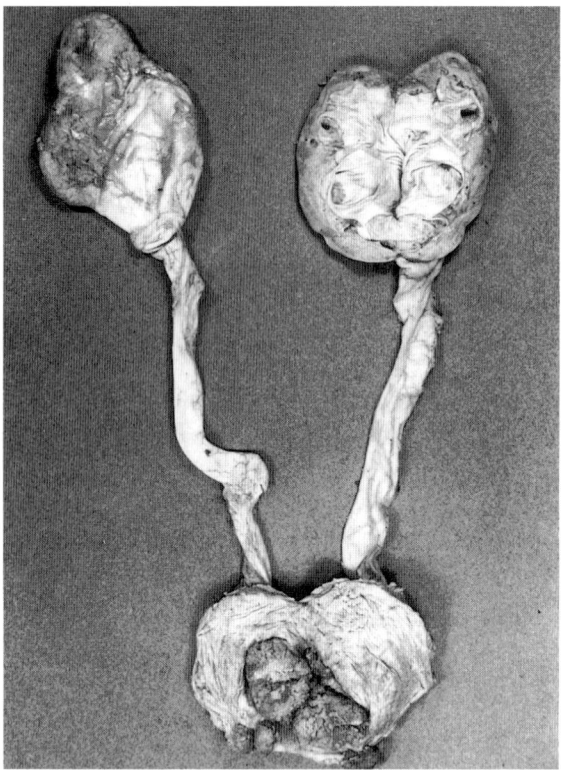

Figure 10.17 *Papillary carcinoma of the bladder causing obstruction of urinary outflow and hence bilateral hydroureter and hydronephrosis in an 85-year-old female*

the pelviureteric junction, or scarring of the surrounding tissues, a tumour in the wall or a calculus in the lumen. Bilateral hydronephrosis may be due to external pressure on the bladder, affecting both ureters, due to tumours of the bladder and obstruction of the bladder neck, as occurs, for example, with prostatic hyperplasia or stricture of the urethra (e.g. postgonococcal). Hydronephrosis may involve the pelvis primarily (extrarenal) or the calyces as well (renal hydronephrosis).

With progression of hydronephrosis, the renal parenchyma becomes increasingly stretched and the blood supply becomes obstructed, so that the renal tissue atrophies. There is less urine excretion with renal failure, hypertension and uraemia occurring. Hydronephrosis may be complicated by infection, which may result in **pyonephrosis** (accumulation of pus within the dilated pelvis).

Renal Calculi (Urolithiasis)

Renal calculi are very common, occurring mostly in middle to old age and are more commonly found in men than in women. Stones may be found anywhere along the length of the urinary tract, in the calyces, pelvis, ureters and bladder (Figure 10.18). The calculi consist of urinary salts bound by a colloid, proteinaceous matrix. The condition of urolithiasis is different from **nephrocalcinosis** in which calcium salts are deposited throughout the substance of the kidney but not in the large collecting passageways. Nephrocalcinosis may be considered as an example of metastatic calcification and is thus associated with disorders of calcium metabolism such as occur with hyperparathyroidism, sarcoidosis, multiple myeloma or multiple bone metastases.

Primary urinary calculi form in the absence of previous disease or inflammation and characteristically form in acid urine. Such calculi are often composed of uric acid, urates or calcium oxalate. **Secondary urinary calculi** form in association with another disorder, which may be inflammatory. The urine is usually alkaline and such stones are often composed of triple phosphates and ammonium urate (refer to Table 10.3).

Less than half of the patients with urolithiasis have predisposing defects. These may be:

- hypercalcaemia as occurs in the milk-alkali syndrome, hypervitaminosis D, hyperparathyroidism and sarcoidosis. In such cases, nephrocalcinosis may also be present (10 to 15% of cases);
- gout and myeloproliferative disorders, which lead to uric acid stones (6% of cases);
- cysteinuria and other metabolic defects that lead to cysteine or oxalate stones (1% of cases);
- chronic UTI with urea-splitting organisms (e.g. *Proteus*) that predispose to stones of magnesium

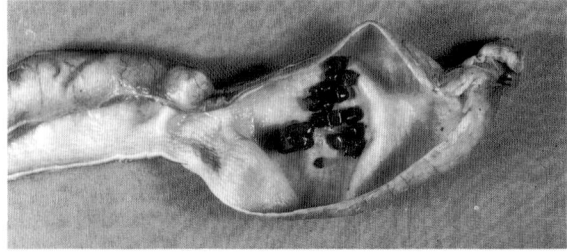

Figure 10.18 *Nephrolithiasis with multiple calculi found in the ureter. Note stricture and hydroureteric change*

Table 10.3 *Summary of correlations between urinary pH and stone constituents*

Acid pH (pH <5.5)	Acid pH (pH 5.5 to 6.0)	Alkaline pH (pH greater than 7.0)
Uric acid	Calcium oxalate	Magnesium ammonium phosphate
Cystine, xanthine	Apatite	Calcium phosphates (including apatite, calcium dihydrogen phosphate dihydrate, tricalcium phosphate

ammonium phosphate (= struvite stones, 15% of cases);
• vitamin A deficiency.

Oxalate stones are the most common, with calcium oxalate mixed with calcium phosphate accounting for approximately 70% of all calculi. The aetiology of such calculi is obscure and the calcium content does not imply that there is a generalized abnormality in calcium metabolism. Chronic production of concentrated urine may predispose to urolithiasis, and in many cases hypercalciuria is demonstrable in the absence of hypercalcaemia. Idiopathic hypercalciuria is thought to occur because of increased absorption of intestinal calcium with decreased proximal tubular reabsorption of the ion. Some sulphonamides precipitate in acid urine, acting as the nidus for calculus formation.

Renal stones vary greatly in size and appearance, their morphology dependent to a certain extent on their composition. They may be tiny (urinary 'gravel') or large solid masses that fill the calyces and pelvis (**stag-horn calculus** looking like the horns of a stag as it is a cast of the renal pelvis and calyces) (see Figure 10.19). Renal calculi exist in three common forms:

• uric acid calculi, being small, round, light or dark brown;
• calcium oxalate calculi, named 'mulberry' stones, as they are round with a prickly exterior;
• calcium phosphate calculi, being usually large, pale to white, chalky and friable.

Stones are often laminated on section and mixed with blood, giving them a brown colour. In some cases, the stones may be multiple and very small, giving rise to the so-called 'urinary sand'. Stones in the bladder are virtually confined to neurogenic bladders of spinal patients. Chronic cystitis is the probable cause. In some cases, bladder calculi may be associated with diverticulosis of the bladder as may occur with patients having a prostatomegaly.

Stones may lead to urinary tract obstruction through their lodgment in the ureter, ureterovesical junction, vesicourethral junction or in the urethra. In such cases, hydronephrosis may be the result, the condition being unilateral or bilateral depending on the site of lodgment. Often, the presence of the stone will cause irritation, ulceration and inflammation of the transitional epithelium and submucosa. Haemorrhage may be associated with the tissue damage and a clot may form in the ureter. Clinically, the patient may present with an acute, very severe pain in the flank termed **renal colic** or alternatively may complain of discomfort in the flank and often there may be an associated haematuria. In certain cases, infection may supervene and the patient presents with signs and symptoms of a UTI. Pyonephrosis and renal failure may be seen in severe, untreated cases of urolithiasis. In quite a number of cases nephrolithiasis is well tolerated by the patient and there is minimal clinical symptomatology associated with the presence of the stones.

Treatment of urolithiasis depends to a certain extent on the cause. For example, metabolic or hypercalcaemic causes may require treatment of the underlying disorder, as well as treatment for the calculi. In many cases a **lithotripter** is the preferred mode of treatment, where ultrasound is used to fragment the stones that are then passed with the urine. This is a relatively non-invasive technique and the patient's time in hospital is greatly reduced. However, it is only used with small stones. Larger calculi may often need to be removed surgically. The composition of the calculus may provide clues as to how further calculi may be prevented through, for example, dietary control or drug treatment.

Renal Failure

Urine formation is essential to life. **Anuria** is formation of no urine while **oliguria** is formation of little

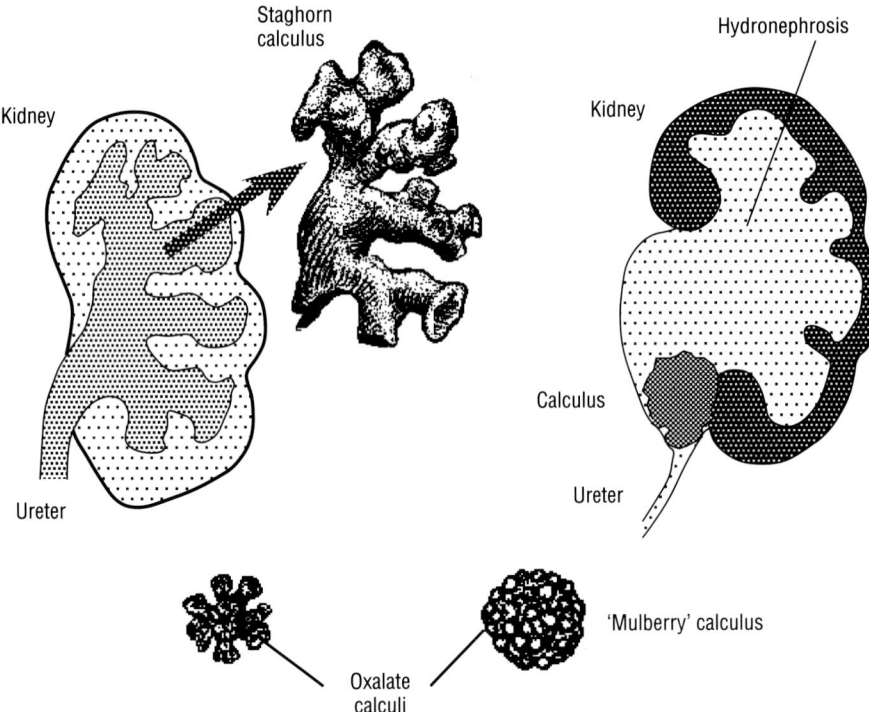

Figure 10.19 *Renal calculi*

urine (less than 400 mL in 24 hours). **Uraemia** means that excessive urea is present in the bloodstream and **azotaemia** means an elevated level of any kind of nitrogenous metabolites in the bloodstream. Renal failure is subdivided into acute and chronic renal failure.

Acute renal failure (renal failure occurring suddenly) is often due to:

• Severe trauma, burns
• Incompatible blood transfusion
• Severe acute hypotension (and ischaemia)
• Toxic agents, drugs
• Septicaemia
• Disseminated intravascular coagulation
• Some forms of glomerulonephritis

Chronic renal failure (occurs with progressive kidney disease over a longer time period) is often due to:

• Chronic glomerulonephritis
• Chronic pyelonephritis
• Hypertensive nephropathy
• Renal tubular syndromes, e.g. analgesic nephropathy
• Polycystic kidney disease

Common syndromes in which renal failure is often a prominent feature are discussed below.

Acute Tubular Necrosis

Acute renal failure is commonly the result of renal ischaemia. Pathologically this is expressed as acute tubular necrosis and acute diffuse cortical necrosis. The disorder follows a direct toxic action on renal tubules or major diminution of renal blood flow, as occurs in shock. Toxins may cause swelling of the kidneys with a pale cortex and irregular haemorrhagic areas. The major site of damage is the proximal convoluted tubule. In the ischaemic variety, pathological changes are most commonly seen in the distal convoluted tubules.

Clinically there is a period of oliguria or anuria, the urine often containing blood and haemoglobin. This stage may last from a few days to 2 months, during which time the patient is kept alive by maintaining an absolute balance between input and output of fluid and electrolytes, or may need to be put on dialysis. Regeneration of renal tubular cells occurs, leading to recovery, heralded by a brisk diuretic phase. A constant watch must be kept on serum potassium (normal range is 3.8–5.0 mmol/L) as sudden death due to cardiac arrest is an ever present danger at levels in excess of 9 mmol/L. Overall, the mortality of the condition varies, but is in the order of about 50%.

Diffuse Cortical Necrosis of the Kidney

This is less common than acute tubular necrosis but is almost always fatal. Disseminated intravascular coagulation associated with renal ischaemia is believed to be the major aetiology. The entire renal cortex becomes necrotic, the kidneys at autopsy being enlarged with sharply demarcated pale regions of necrotic cortex being seen. The glomeruli are involved, and unlike the tubules, do not regenerate. The disease is therefore fatal, dialysis serving only to postpone the outcome, renal transplantation providing the only hope of survival.

Chronic Renal Failure

In this disease there is gradual impairment of renal function over the years. Loss of concentrating ability of the kidney results in excretion of an increased volume of urine with a constant specific gravity. Failure of hydrogen ion excretion results in systemic acidosis. Impairment of calcium/phosphate metabolism results in generalised demineralization of bone, a change known as **renal osteodystrophy**. The disorder develops very similarly to osteomalacia and a secondary hyperparathyroidism with osteoclastic resorption of bone may be demonstrated. The mechanism behind this disorder involves:

- acidosis, which promotes resorption of bone and osteoporosis;
- failure to excrete phosphate which stimulates production of parathyroid hormone and accelerates demineralization;
- disturbances of vitamin D metabolism with reduction in the active form (1,12 dihydroxy cholecalciferol);
- increased excretion of calcium ions through the gut as a result of impaired activation of vitamin D.

Anaemia is invariably seen in chronic renal failure. Microangiopathic anaemia is caused by mechanical damage to circulating red blood cells due to altered renal vascular endothelium. There may also be hypoproliferative anaemia due to diminished production of active erythropoietin. Hypertension is almost invariably present. It results from chronic sodium retention and deranged renin/angiotensin mechanisms.

The onset of chronic renal failure is slow and insidious, at first only non-specific symptoms appearing, fatigue, weakness, anorexia and nausea being the most commonly observed ones. Pallor and breathlessness due to the anaemia may also develop. Cardiac failure and uraemic pericarditis then occur followed by peripheral neuritis, lethargy and coma. The patient is treated with regular dialysis sessions until renal transplantation can be performed. Not all patients are suitable for transplantation and their prognosis is grave.

Tumours of the Kidney

Benign tumours of the kidney are common but of little clinical significance, as most of them are small, very slow growing and produce no symptoms or signs. Large benign kidney tumours may undergo malignant transformation and thus are excised if diagnosed. Malignant kidney tumours are uncommon, accounting for approximately 1% of all primary cancers (see Table 10.4).

Adenoma of the Kidney

Adenoma of the kidney is the typical primary, benign tumour of the kidney.

Incidence. The incidence of the tumour increases with age, becoming more common over the age of 50 years. There is a slight male preponderance. Small adenomata are found in 10 to 20% of routine post-mortem examinations.

Sites affected. Usually these tumours arise in the cortex of the kidney and are often bilateral and multiple.

Table 10.4 *Renal tumours (commonest in italics)*

Benign tumours	Malignant tumours
Adenoma of the kidney	*Carcinoma of the kidney (Grawitz tumour)*
Haemangioma; angiomyolipoma	*Nephroblastoma (Wilms' tumour)*
Fibroma	Carcinoma of the renal pelvis
Leiomyoma	Fibrosarcoma

Aetiology. Most of the tumours are idiopathic, but it is suspected that some of them may arise in connection with chronic inflammation (e.g. pyelonephritis), diabetes mellitus and nephrosclerosis.

Macroscopic appearance. Adenomata are usually small, a few millimetres in diameter. They are greyish yellow tumours beneath the capsule or in the cortex of the kidney. Fibrous bands may be present within the masses, which may be solid or cystic. Single or multiple tumours may be present. If the tumour is 20 mm in diameter or greater, malignant transformation is likely.

Microscopic appearance. Typically, the tumours are papillary or tubular adenomata, with the tumour cells cuboidal to columnar, resembling the tubular epithelium. Fluid-filled cysts may be present in the tumour mass. The well-differentiated cells show no evidence of necrosis or invasion.

Signs and symptoms. If the tumours are 20 mm in diameter or less, they behave as typical benign neoplasms and are usually totally asymptomatic, discovered only as incidental findings in the course of other investigations or at autopsy. However, even these small tumours have an unpredictable long-term behaviour and at any stage may begin growing more quickly, reaching a critical size and undergoing malignant change. Larger tumours, greater than 20 mm in diameter, may be difficult to distinguish from a malignant tumour microscopically as they show evidence of invasion and loss of differentiation. Such large tumours will ultimately show a progression to clinical carcinoma. Metastases do not occur until the tumours reach a diameter of 25 mm or more.

Treatment. If adenomata are found in a biopsy it is difficult to determine their size and one is faced with a difficult decision as far as treatment is concerned. If the tumour is small and slow growing it may remain as such for the rest of the individual's life. However, it is also likely that the tumour may grow and undergo malignant change, where the only option is nephrectomy. Visualization of the mass by CT scanning or angiography is required to gain an idea of its size and therefore of its malignant potential. As malignant change has occurred or is likely to occur in larger tumours, a large mass even if it looks totally benign microscopically indicates nephrectomy.

Other Benign Tumours

All other benign tumours of the kidney are rare to very rare and they all tend to follow a benign course. There is little risk of malignancy occurring. Such tumours usually remain undiagnosed and appear as incidental findings at autopsy. Occasionally a **primary reninism** may be seen and is due to a hyperplasia or a benign tumour of the juxtaglomerular cells. This leads to increased levels of renin, resulting in hypertension, hyperkalaemia and hyperaldosteronism. The indication in this last-mentioned case is nephrectomy. The angiomyolipoma is a benign tumour of the kidney in adults that in up to 40% of cases is associated with tuberous sclerosis. In most cases the tumour is clinically silent although at autopsy it may be seen to be large and may resemble a renal carcinoma. On microscopy the tumour is seen to consist of masses of adipocytes, smooth muscle cells and thick-walled blood vessels.

Carcinoma of the Kidney

Carcinoma of the kidney is the typical, primary malignant tumour of the kidney and is also called **Grawitz tumour** and **hypernephroma**. It arises from the epithelium of proximal convoluted tubules and is thus in most cases a typical adenocarcinoma.

Incidence. Adenocarcinoma of the kidney accounts for 80% of primary kidney malignancies. It mostly affects individuals between 50 and 70 years, affecting males twice as commonly as females.

Sites. These are typically cortical tumours, most characteristically seen in the upper pole of the kidney. The left and right kidneys are affected equally (Figure 10.20).

Macroscopic appearance. Adenocarcinomata of the kidney are large tumours, 5 to 15 cm in diameter. They are well supplied with blood vessels, making them look very red. Often the masses are surrounded by a pseudocapsule and cystic spaces may be seen in the tumour. The tumours have a variegated cut surface, with yellowish regions of necrosis, reddish brown areas of haemorrhage, white, opaque regions of calcification and translucent, pale tracts of fibrosis. Often, even with the naked eye, invasion of the tumour into the renal vein may be seen.

Microscopic appearance. Several distinct patterns of growth are seen microscopically in kidney carcinoma. The typical appearance is termed **clear cell carcinoma** as the tumour cells are large and possess abundant, pale, foamy cytoplasm. This clear appearance of

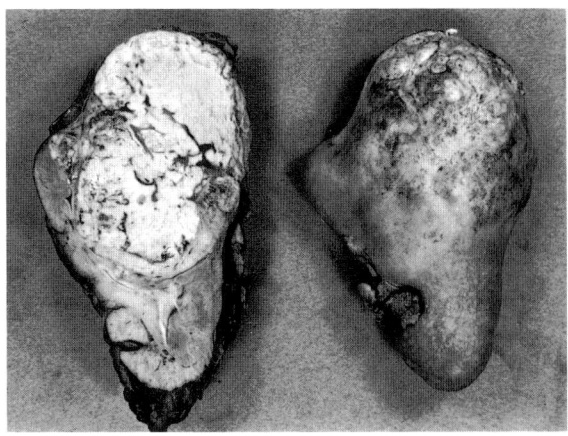

Figure 10.20 *Carcinoma of the kidney in a 60-year-old female*

the cytoplasm is due to the presence of large amounts of lipid, glycogen and cholesterol esters that are leached out of the tumour cells during processing of the section. These cells show variable degrees of acinar arrangement and papillary structure. The **granular cell carcinoma** is composed of cells that resemble normal tubular epithelial cells. These cells have a granular cytoplasm with small dark nuclei, and are arranged in papillary structures. **Mixed pattern tumours** show evidence of both clear cells and granular cells in regions of the tumour. Occasionally, tumours may show an **undifferentiated pattern**.

With all of the above microscopical subtypes of kidney tumours there are several common findings. Great numbers of thin-walled blood vessels are found within the tumours and often these vessels show evidence of invasion by the tumour cells. There are regions of haemorrhage and necrosis, around which there are many macrophages containing haemosiderin. There is calcification in many areas of the tumour.

Spread. Many of the tumours grow rather quickly and their rapid growth leads to compression of surrounding tissue to form a pseudocapsule around the tumour mass. However, microscopically one is able to see that direct spread is occurring around the tumour mass. Approximately 30% of cases will show lymphatic spread by the time the tumour is diagnosed. Haematogenous spread occurs early and is a characteristic feature of the tumour. Blood vessels within the tumour mass show evidence of invasion, and invasion of the renal vein usually occurs at an early stage. Direct spread of the tumour inside the renal vein, up the vena cava and into the right ventricle has been reported. Metastasis occurs to the lung, liver, bone and the brain.

Signs and symptoms. The tumour presents late, the commonest presenting symptoms being a painless **haematuria** ($\approx$ 50% of cases, but note that haematuria is not pathognomonic for this tumour — refer to Table 10.5) and **pyrexia of unknown origin** (PUO $\approx$ 20% of cases). A loin mass may be palpable. Later, the patients complain of pain ($\approx$ 50% of cases), there is weight loss, anaemia and weakness. Occasionally, **polycythaemia** may be detected due to over-production of erythropoietin by the tumour cells. Very severe flank pain or 'clot colic' occurs if haemorrhage from the tumour causes a clot to form within the ureter. Some patients may complain of costovertebral pain of a continuous, moderate nature. In males, **varicocoele** of the testis may be observed due to obstruction of the spermatic vein. Generally, the tumour may be associated with signs and symptoms mimicking other diseases, such as infection, anaemia and polycythaemia.

Treatment and prognosis. Treatment of the tumour is by **nephrectomy**, where the affected kidney is removed. In addition to nephrectomy patients may be treated with **radiotherapy**, but chemotherapy is generally ineffective with this tumour. The prognosis of the tumour is greatly variable but usually the extent of

Table 10.5 *Common causes of haematuria*

Site	Aetiology
Kidney	Neoplasm, infection, stone, trauma, hydronephrosis, polycystic kidney disease, glomerulonephritis
Ureter	Stone, neoplasm
Bladder	Infection, neoplasm, stone
Prostate	Hyperplasia or ectopic tissue, infection, neoplasm
Urethra	Stricture, stone

blood spread indicates the prognosis. If the renal vein has been invaded, the 5-year survival may be 30% or less. If the renal vein has not been involved, the 5-year survival is approximately 60%. Obviously, low-grade tumours confined to the kidney with no evidence of blood spread have the best prognosis.

Nephroblastoma

Nephroblastoma is a mixed tumour and is almost exclusively found in infants. It is also known as **Wilms' tumour** or **embryoma of the kidney**.

Incidence. Nephroblastoma accounts for approximately 8% of kidney malignancies and for 20% of all malignant, solid tumours of childhood. The average age of presentation is 3 years, the tumour being extremely rare after the age of 7 years.

Sites. The tumour arises in any part of the kidney with left and right organs affected equally. In approximately 4% of cases, the tumour is bilateral.

Appearance. Wilms' tumour is believed to arise from embryonal, mesodermal tissue that remains in the kidney in little, undifferentiated, rests. In its early stages, while the tumour is small it is surrounded by a capsule, but this is soon invaded by the growing mass. Usually when the tumour is detected, it is a solitary, rapidly growing, large mass. On section, it is of a homogeneous, pale-grey colour and of a firm consistency. Cystic areas and regions of haemorrhage may be present. The renal vein is often invaded. Microscopically, a mixed pattern is seen with tubular structures formed amongst a population of spindle cells. Primitive glomerular structures are often formed and are a characteristic feature of this tumour. In some cases, a variety of other tissues such as fat, cartilage and bone may be found within the tumour mass.

Spread. Direct involvement of the renal parenchyma and perinephric tissues occurs early. Lymphatic spread to involve the local lymph nodes has usually occurred by the time of diagnosis and blood spread is also commonly seen at an early stage. Metastases, especially to the lung, are common, with involvement of the brain and liver also seen.

Signs and symptoms. The infant presents with an abdominal mass that is usually painful. Wilms' tumours are large masses and may fill the abdomen at laparotomy. The general health of the child deterio-

rates progressively as the tumour grows. Haematuria is only observed in the later stages.

Treatment and prognosis. Nephrectomy is indicated if the tumour is diagnosed but as the tumour is highly sensitive to radiotherapy and chemotherapy, these treatment modalities are used in conjunction with surgery. If the tumour is removed early, about 75% of patients are cured. Otherwise, the clinical course is very rapid and death is almost inevitable very soon after diagnosis, with a 5-year survival of only 5%. Generally, the younger an infant is and the earlier the tumour is diagnosed and treated, the better the prognosis. Five-year survival figures of 95% or better have been reported for treated tumours in children of less than one year old.

Tumours of the Renal Pelvis, Ureters and Bladder

Tumours of the renal pelvis, ureters and bladder are all considered together as they have many features in common:

- all of these areas are lined by transitional epithelium;
- the same types of tumours are seen in all of these sites;
- most tumours are transitional cell carcinomata;
- aetiology for all of these tumours is similar;
- painless, profuse haematuria is the most common presenting symptom.

Incidence. Tumours of the renal pelvis and ureters are rare, accounting for approximately 0.2% of all primary malignancies. Tumours of the bladder are relatively common, causing about 4% of deaths from malignant disease. Men are more commonly affected by these tumours in the ratio of 3 to 1. The typical age range of presentation is between 60 and 70 years.

Sites. Right and left renal pelves and ureters are equally affected, with tumours of the ureters being rarer. In about 50% of cases, the tumours are bilateral and multiple. In the bladder, the base of the organ is mostly affected, most tumours arising within the trigone or in the ureteric orifices.

Benign tumours. Benign papillomata may occur at these sites and vary in size from 2 mm to 20 mm in diameter. The behaviour of these tumours varies according to their size. Tumours less than 10 mm in diameter are typically benign, non-invasive, non-recurrent if removed. Tumours above 10 mm in diameter are **atypical papillomata** and may show invasion, progression to obvious malignant tumours and recurrence if they are removed.

Carcinoma of the Urinary Bladder

As carcinoma of the bladder is the commonest tumour in the regions lined by transitional epithelium, it will be considered in detail, but it should be remembered that features of this tumour are shared by tumours of the renal pelvis and ureter.

Predisposing factors. A number of distinct aetiologies and predisposing factors have been associated quite clearly with these tumours by epidemiological data. These are:

* congenital anomalies in the region (e.g. ectopia vesicae);
* long-standing inflammation and tissue damage (e.g. associated with calculi);
* chronic infections (e.g. in Egypt where chronic infection with *Schistosoma haematobium*, a parasitic worm, is very common);
* disruptions to normal structure of bladder (e.g. diverticula of the bladder, leukoplakia, squamous metaplasia as seen in prostatic hyperplasia or chronic irritation);
* chemical carcinogen exposure (e.g. tumour is commoner in workers with aniline dyes in the rubber, printing and dying industries; the early use of β-naphthylamine in industry resulted in carcinoma of the bladder in 100% of workers exposed to it; cigarette smoking; excessive coffee drinking).

Macroscopical appearance. Bladder tumours characteristically occur in two major macroscopical types: **papillary carcinomata** are more common and grow into the lumen of the bladder as large, fronded masses with little or no invasion of the wall (Figure 10.21). **Solid carcinomata** are less common in occurrence, growing and invading within the wall of the bladder, with little projection of the mass into the lumen. Such tumours are often ulcerated with necrosis and haemorrhage being very prominent. The latter type is associated with a worse prognosis. In both types of tumour the adjacent mucosa shows various abnormalities, such as leukoplakia, squamous metaplasia and dysplasia.

Microscopical appearance. The majority of bladder tumours are well-differentiated transitional cell carci-

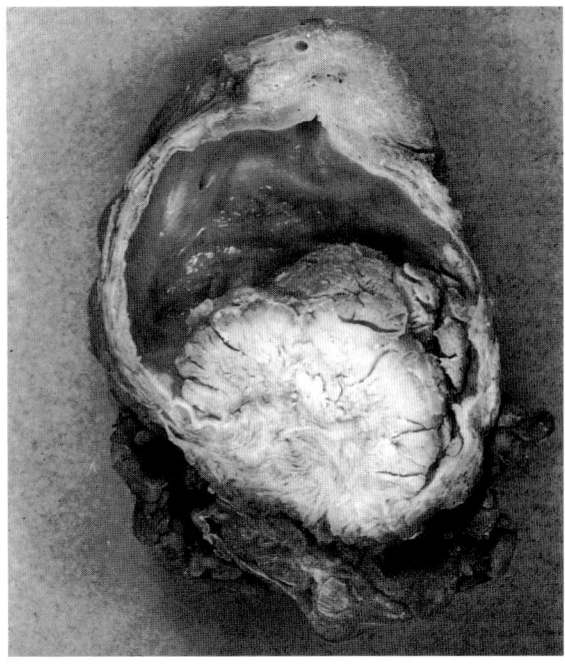

Figure 10.21 *Large fungating carcinoma in the bladder of a 57-year-old male*

nomata or undifferentiated transitional cell carcinomata. The tumour consists of sheets of large, polygonal cells with large nuclei and prominent nucleoli. Less frequently, typical squamous cell carcinomata will occur, and rarely, mucous-secreting adenocarcinomata are seen.

Spread. Spread of the tumour will depend on its macroscopical type, papillary carcinomata being less likely to spread early into the bladder wall while solid tumours invade into the wall very early on. Staging of the tumour reflects spread:

* **Stage A**: The tumour is confined to the mucosa, the cells showing atypia.
* **Stage B**: The tumour extends into the submucosa and muscle layers.
* **Stage C**: Invasion of perivesical tissues, but no lymph node involvement.
* **Stage D**: Involvement of lymph nodes, pelvic fixation and distant metastases.

Lymphatic spread has occurred in about 30% of fatal cases. Haematogenous spread usually occurs later in the disease with secondaries in the liver, lungs and bones commonly seen in these cases. Approximately 30% of fatal cases show blood spread.

Symptoms and signs. The most frequent symptom of transitional cell carcinoma is painless haematuria. Infections are common and are associated with varying degrees of obstruction to urine flow caused by the tumour. Dysuria, frequency of micturition, hypertrophy/hyperplasia of the bladder wall may be observed. Ureteric obstruction may lead to hydronephrosis and pyonephrosis with associated renal failure. Often, the spreading tumour will cause fistula formation into surrounding organs. Diagnosis of the tumour is by radiography and cystoscopy.

Treatment and prognosis. Treatment of carcinoma of the bladder is by cystectomy with anastomosis of the ureters into a segment of ileum. Radiotherapy may also be used. The prognosis will depend on the site, type of tumour and stage at diagnosis. For example, a well-differentiated carcinoma treated at an early stage is associated with a 5-year survival of 70%. On the other hand, a solid undifferentiated carcinoma may be associated with a 5-year survival of 30% or less.

Urinalysis

Normal Urine

Urine is an important body fluid which is excreted by the kidneys and which is formed continuously from birth till death. A normal individual excretes approximately 1 to 1.5 litres of urine daily. A wide variety of wastes formed by the body are excreted by the kidneys in the urine. Urine is an important fluid to evaluate in suspected diseases of many organ systems as changes in its composition may give a very accurate and early diagnosis of a serious disorder. It should be remembered, however, that the composition of normal urine varies considerably depending on which substances and how much of each substance the body needs to excrete at any given time. The normal, amber colour of urine is due to **urobilinogen**, a pigment derived from the metabolism of bile. It should be remembered that diet may influence the colour of urine (e.g. when beetroot has been eaten in large quantity), or the administration of drugs may be accompanied by spectacular changes in the colour of urine (e.g. sulphonamides change its colour to a rusty brown; see Table 10.9). Urine darkens on standing due to oxidation of the urobilinogen to urobilin. Stale urine which contains bilirubin may become green due to oxidation of bilirubin to biliverdin.

Normally, the urine should be clear, but not all turbid urines are abnormal. The pH of urine may vary considerably and either excessively acid or alkaline urine may cause precipitation of some normal urine components, causing turbidity. No blood or leukocytes should be normally present in urine, although both are frequently found in urine samples from females in which there has been contamination of the urine with vaginal secretion.

Urine Sampling for Analysis

A variety of methods are available for the collection of urine for analysis and the method chosen may depend on where and by whom the urine is collected, what test is to be performed on it and also on whether the patient is able to void urine normally. Basically, there are three methods for collection of a urine specimen.

The Midstream Sample of Urine (MSU)

This is the commonest method of collecting urine for analysis and if performed adequately yields a very useful urine specimen. The patients have a clean, sterile specimen container on hand when they are going to the toilet. They initiate voiding urine and allow the first few millilitres of urine to be discarded. Then **without stopping the flow of urine** they collect the middle portion of the urine they are voiding in the sterile vessel and then once again, without stopping the flow of urine, they do not collect the last portion of the urine they are voiding. This procedure greatly reduces the contamination of bladder urine by normal flora bacteria that inhabit the lower third of the urethra. The continuous voiding of urine during its collection is essential as this minimizes turbulence of the urinary stream and therefore prevents the dislodgment of bacteria from the lower urethral walls. A modification of this method of collection is the '**clean catch**' MSU which is used when collecting a specimen from a woman. In this case, a tampon is inserted into the vagina and the vulva is cleaned with sterile saline (no antiseptic), wiping once with a front to back movement. The urine is then collected as above in the standard MSU method. The 'clean-catch' method reduces greatly the possibility of vaginal secretions and menstrual blood contaminating the urine sample.

The Catheter Sample of Urine (CSU)

This method of collecting urine is performed usually in a hospital or clinic and occurs mostly in those cases where patients are unable to void urine normally (e.g. if an obstruction is present in the urethra or if there have been spinal injuries). A hollow tube (catheter) is inserted via the urethra into the bladder and the urine is collected into a sterile bag. Many patients in hospital may have an indwelling catheter in their bladder for very long periods of time (e.g. if they are in a coma). CSU is a good sample for urinalysis, but the disadvantages of the method are that catheterization is not a pleasant procedure for the patient and also there is the risk of introducing infection into a previously sterile bladder.

The Suprapubic Aspiration Sample (SPA)

This is another method of collecting urine which is performed in a hospital. What is done in this case is that the bladder urine is sampled directly percutaneously. The patient is examined to ensure that the bladder is full of urine and the area of skin just above the symphysis pubis is washed thoroughly with antiseptic. Using strict aseptic technique, a wide-bore needle with attached syringe is used to enter the bladder lumen through the skin and abdominal muscle and the bladder urine is aspirated directly into the sterile syringe. This is a very effective procedure and is no less uncomfortable than a standard venipuncture. Contamination of the bladder urine by the normal flora bacteria and introduction of infections are prevented.

Other Types of Urine Samples

Depending on the type of test that is to be performed on the urine, the sample may be collected at a specific time or a specific volume may be needed:

1. *Random or spot specimen:* This specimen refers to a sample of urine voided at any time of the day or night, collected by the MSU method.
2. *Fasting specimen:* This specimen is collected after a period of fasting. The patient is instructed to void urine four or more hours after having a meal and to discard all of that specimen. The patient then has nothing to eat and the next time urine is voided it is collected as an MSU sample.
3. *First morning specimen:* The patient voids urine before going to bed and discards the specimen. The first urine specimen voided the next morning is collected as an MSU.
4. *Post-prandial specimen:* The urine specimen which is voided 1–2 hours after a main meal is collected as an MSU. Note that the urine collected after a meal is often very cloudy ('alkaline tide').
5. *24-Hour collection specimen:* On arising in the

morning, the patient empties the bladder and discards the sample. The urine which is voided in the next 24 hours (day and night) is collected and the whole volume of the urine (i.e. not an MSU!) is placed in a large sterile bottle. Between collections the urine sample is refrigerated. Exactly 24 hours after first voiding, the last sample is collected and added to the bottle which is transferred to the laboratory immediately.

It should be noted that all urine samples are collected into clean, sterile containers, a procedure minimizing contamination, both chemical and bacterial. Urine which cannot be tested immediately may be refrigerated for a short period of time. Certain tests provide optimal results on a particular type of urine specimen collected in a particular way, for example glucose tests on post-prandial urine, protein tests on first morning specimens, bacteriological examination on MSU specimens, etc.

Testing Urine with the Multistix® System

The urine specimen is collected at the appropriate time by the MSU or 'clean catch' MSU method into a clean, sterile container. The specimen should at this stage be **split into two portions** and one of these should be refrigerated as a further test may be required and therefore analytical integrity of the sample is maintained. Remove a reagent strip from the bottle and replace cap immediately. Completely immerse all reagent areas on the strip in one portion of the urine and remove strip immediately to avoid leaching of reagents. Run edge of the strip against the rim of the urine container to remove excess moisture and hold the strip in the horizontal position to avoid mixing of chemicals from adjacent areas (tapping the strip sideways on a piece of absorbent paper may help). Compare the test areas to the corresponding colour chart on the bottle **at the time specified, holding the strip close to the bottle and matching carefully**! Colour changes that occur after 2 minutes are of no diagnostic value whatsoever.

Multistix® Tests, Normal Values and Major Disease Indications

It should be noted that although the Multistix® system is quite a useful means of routinely testing urine in the home, clinic, office and laboratory, it is only a rapid screening test and if any abnormal values are discovered, further investigations should be performed for definitive diagnosis. **As with all tests, definitive diag-**

nostic or therapeutic decisions should not be based on the results of any single procedure or test! Additional tests may be performed by you, the laboratory or the clinician, for example culturing the urine for bacteriuria, or Ictotest® tablets for bilirubin in the urine, etc. Note that blood tests may also have to be carried out for confirmation of a presumptive diagnosis based on urinalysis. There may also be indications for more extensive testing such as liver and pancreatic function tests.

Table 10.6 gives an indication of the normal values for the tests performed by Multistix® analysis and also shows the various abnormal values and the clinical disease states that they indicate. It should be noted that most abnormal results are elevations in the normal values.

Interfering Factors in Urinalysis with Multistix®

Glucose

False positives are caused by contaminants such as peroxides or bleach. These contaminants may have remained in improperly rinsed urine collection vessels.

False negatives are caused by high levels of ascorbic acid in the urine (question the patient about their intake of vitamin C supplements). Bacteriuria, with glucose being metabolized by the bacteria and high levels of ketones in the urine, will also cause reduced sensitivity of the glucose test.

Table 10.6 *Urine analysis with the Multistix® system*

Test substance	Readout time	Normal value	Raised value	Lowered value
Glucose	30 s	< 2 mmol/L	Diabetes	
Bilirubin	30 s	Nil	Liver disease — hepatitis, cirrhosis	
Ketones	40 s	Nil	Diabetic acidosis; starvation; COH deficient diet	
Specific gravity	45 s	1.016 to 1.022	Diabetes; concentrated urine; dietary	Dilute urine
Blood	50 s	Nil	Renal disease; cirrhosis; eclampsia; tumours of UT	
pH	60 s	5–9	UTI (NH_3) Dietary; respiratory disease	UTI (acid)
Protein	60 s	Nil	Renal diseases; multiple myeloma; SLE; eclampsia; renal tumours; stones	
Urobilinogen	60 s	3–16 µmol/L	Liver disease; haemolysis; chemical intoxications	
Nitrite	60 s	Nil	UTI (Gram-negative esp.)	
Leukocytes	2 min	Nil	UTI; tumours; TB; phenacetin nephritis	

Bilirubin

False positives are caused by high levels of chlorpromazine metabolites (e.g. Serenium®; Pyridium®) and high levels of indoxyl sulphate (Indican®).

False negatives are caused by high levels of ascorbic acid: in this case question the patient about their intake of vitamin C supplements. In order to detect low levels of bilirubin repeat the urine test using Ictotest® tablets.

Ketones

False positives are caused by high concentrations of L-dopa.

False negatives are caused by hydration of the test strip before testing the urine. A more sensitive test in the presence of low levels of ketones is the Ketostix® test, performed on urine which has been diluted 1 part in 10.

Specific Gravity

This test needs to be interpreted with care as it is of no value in isolation but needs to be considered in association with other test results. Sodium chloride and urea are the two principal solids in urine and thus influence the specific gravity the most. A large amount of urea in the urine indicates a protein-rich diet and a high NaCl content, a high-salt diet. Concentrated urines have a high specific gravity and look dark but the urine of a diabetic, which contains high glucose levels, has a high specific gravity and looks dilute. **False high values** may be caused by moderate to high (1–7.5 g/L) quantities of protein in the urine.

False low values may be caused by highly buffered, alkaline urines.

Blood

False positives may be caused by certain oxidizing contaminants (e.g. bleach) or by microbial peroxidase in bacteriuria. Menstruating females may contaminate the urine with blood and give a false positive result.

False negatives are caused by elevated ascorbic acid levels (question the patient about their intake of vitamin C supplements). Elevated specific gravity of urine or elevated protein content reduces the sensitivity of the test.

pH

The pH of the urine varies considerably in the normal individual between 5 and 9. Alkaline pH of the urine is usual in post-prandial specimens due to the 'alkaline tide' that is seen after meals. In most other situations collected urine should be slightly acid (pH 5–7). **False high (alkaline) pH** is caused by delay in testing the urine with the bacteria in it metabolizing urea to NH_3.

False low (acidic) pH is caused occasionally by bacterial activity in urine that has been left to stand around for too long before testing, due to bacterial action on urinary glucose converting it to acid. If inadequate care is taken during dipping the reagent stick in the urine there may be 'runover' of the acidic protein reagent onto the pH portion of the stick, causing it to indicate a very acid urine.

Protein

False positive results will be seen in highly buffered or alkaline urines. Contamination of urine with antiseptics such as quaternary ammonium compounds, chlorhexidine or some detergents may also give false positives.

False negatives occur if the reagent strip is held in the urine for too long, leading to leaching of the reagent. Also, the reagent is more sensitive to albumin than it is to the globulins (e.g. as in the Bence-Jones protein of multiple myeloma) or to mucoprotein. Thus a negative result does not rule these out and if these conditions are suspected this test system is not recommended.

Urobilinogen

False positives are caused by the presence of sulphonamides and para-aminosalicylic acid (PAS) in the urine.

False negatives are caused by contamination of the urine with formalin. Urobilinogen in urine is unstable and oxidises to urobilin. A fresh urine specimen must be used or a false negative may be obtained with a stale urine.

Nitrite

False positives occur only if the urine has been contaminated with nitrite.

False negatives are caused by high concentrations of ascorbic acid in the urine or if the urine has not been retained in the bladder for more than 3–4 hours. Nitrite negatives do not always indicate that bacteriuria is not present as some bacteria lack the reductase enzyme which converts NO_3 to NO_2. Also, if reductase-producing bacteria cause the UTI, the diet may be deficient in NO_3, and hence no NO_2 will be produced in the bladder. Sensitivity of the nitrite test is reduced if the urine has a high specific gravity.

Leukocytes

False positives are caused by vaginal discharge contaminating the urine specimen.

False negatives are caused by any drug which is highly coloured and colours the urine, thereby masking the colour of the reagent pad (e.g. nitrofurantoin).

Elevated glucose concentrations or high specific gravity may cause decreased test results. The presence of some antibiotics (e.g. cephalexin, cephalothin, tetracycline) or other substances (e.g. oxalic acid) may also decrease the sensitivity of the test and cause false negatives.

Microscopic Examination of the Urine

Examining the urine specimen under the microscope may give important diagnostic information. It should be kept in mind that a variety of sediments are normal (refer to Table 10.7). Usually the specimen is centrifuged and the sediment is then examined under conventional and phase contrast microscopy for the presence of the following:

Cells
Epithelial cells, red blood cells, white blood cells and micro-organisms may be seen. The presence of these may indicate, for example, the nephritic syndrome and hence glomerulonephritis, the presence of a UTI or even the presence of a neoplasm.

Casts
Protein casts ('hyaline' casts), white blood cell casts ('pus' casts) and red blood cell casts may be seen. The cellular casts on passage through the urinary tract will degenerate and give rise to 'granular' casts and 'waxy' casts. Protein casts and cellular casts generally indicate glomerulonephritis or pyelonephritis and in many cases may be taken as an indication of renal involvement in a UTI.

Crystals
The commonest crystals found are triple phosphate/calcium oxalate crystals, cystine, tyrosine, leucine crystals, cholesterol and uric acid crystals. The presence of crystals in the urine may be a routine finding in normal individuals or it may indicate nephrolithiasis or a metabolic disorder.

NB: Each of the these findings may give valuable diagnostic clues especially if combined with other urinalytic methods. Microscopy of the urine specimen is always requested when urine specimens are sent for analysis in the laboratory, the results of this procedure often being crucial in the diagnosis of a given disorder.

Microbiological Examination of the Urine

This is extremely important in diagnosing bacteriuria and hence UTI. It should be noted that the demonstration of bacteria in urine gives no indication of whether an upper or lower urinary tract infection is present. In order to determine whether cystitis or pyelonephritis is the cause of the symptoms, more specific tests need to be carried out (e.g. intravenous pyelography). The urine collected for bacteriological examination **must be collected in one of the three accepted methods and the specimen must be transported to the laboratory immediately**. If the urine specimen cannot be transported to the laboratory immediately, it may be refrigerated for a short period of time. The microbiological results differ, depending upon which of the three ways has been used to collect the urine.

Midstream and Clean-catch Urine
This method of urine collection has been considered above. Bacteriuria is diagnosed if 100 000 or more bacteria are present per mL of urine. This is the commonest method of urine collection and is about 80% effective in diagnosing a UTI.

Table 10.7 *Sediment in normal urine*

Sediment	Type or case where found
Blood cells	Erythrocytes or leukocytes (especially in females)
Casts	Hyaline, granular
Mucus	Especially in females
Epithelial cells	Renal tubular, transitional epithelial, squamous epithelial
Crystals	Type varies, depending on the pH of the urine
Micro-organisms	Especially bacteria, occasionally yeasts
Spermatozoa	Especially in males
Protein	In cases of asymptomatic proteinuria, after exercise or in high-protein diets

Catheterized Urine

A catheter is introduced into the bladder and the urine collected. Sometimes this is the most practicable way of collecting urine (e.g. in elderly men with considerable urinary obstruction caused by prostatomegaly). The complication of introducing infection into a previously sterile bladder is a problem. Bacteriuria is diagnosed if 10 000 or more bacteria are present per mL of catheterized urine.

Suprapubic Aspiration Urine

The bladder urine is sampled directly by aspirating the urine through skin and muscle from within the bladder. The method is 100% effective and the presence of any bacteria in the bladder urine indicates infection.

Useful Reference Tables in Uroscopy and Urinalysis

Table 10.8 *Protein excretion rates in various renal disorders*

Disease state	Protein excretion rate*			
	0.05–0.1 g 2/24 h	0.1–1.0 g 2/24 h	1.0–3.0 g 2/24 h	Over 3.0 g 2/24 h
Exercise proteinuria	+			
Febrile proteinuria	+			
Postural proteinuria	+	+		
Arteriosclerotic renal vascular disease	+	+		
Hypertension, arterial	+	+	+ (rare)	
Congestive heart failure		+	+	+
Pyelonephritis		+	+ (rare)	
Polycystic renal disease	+	+		
Acute glomerulonephritis	+	+	+	+
Membranous glomerulonephritis		+	+	+
Drug-induced, nephrotoxic agents (Hg, CCl₄, etc.)	+	+		
Nephrotic syndrome			+	+
Kimmelstiel–Wilson syndrome			+	+
Systemic lupus erythematosus	+	+	+	+
Polyarteritis nodosa	+	+	+ (rare)	
Multiple myeloma[†]	+	+	+	+

* Approximate ranges of daily protein excretion in some common diseases of the kidney should be taken as a guide, rather than as the absolute range of excretion in these diseases.

[†] Does not refer to Bence-Jones proteinuria but to more general proteinuria frequently seen in multiple myeloma.

(Adapted from Harvey A, *et al.* (eds.) *The Principles and Practice of Medicine*, 17th edition, Appleton-Century-Crofts, 1968.)

Table 10.9   *Substances that may 'discolour' urine*

Colour imparted to urine	Drugs, substances, conditions responsible
Amber	Normal; urobilin; bilirubin
Nearly colourless	Large fluid intake; reduction of perspiration; chronic nephritis; untreated diabetes mellitus; diabetes insipidus; alcohol ingestion; diuretic therapy; nervousness
Orange	Concentrated urine; restricted fluid intake; excess sweating; fever; urobilin; small quantitites of bile pigments; phenazopyridine and amidopyrine
Orange to orange-red	Ethoxazene (Serenium); phenazophridine (Pyridium)
Orange-red-brown	Rhubarb; senna; verdoglobin
Orange to purple-red	Chlorzoxazone (Paraflex)
Orange-yellow	Salicylazosulfapyridine (Azulfidine); anisindione (Miradon); phenindione (Hedulin; in alkaline urine)
Rusty yellow or brownish	Sulphonamides; nitrofurantoins (Furoxone, Furadantin and other related compounds)
Pink or red to red-brown	Diphenylhydantoin (Dilantin); phensuximide (Milontin); 1,8-dihydroxyanthraquinone (in Dorbantyl, Doxidan); Emodin in alkaline urine; phenolphthalein (in laxatives, etc.); phenothiazines (Thorazine, etc.)
Magenta	Phenolphthalein (in laxatives, etc.)
Red	Blood; amidopyrine (Pyramidon); phenazopyridine (Pyridium); neotropin; prontosil; aniline dyes; beetroot; porphyrins, haemoglobin; myoglobin, phenolsulphonephthalein; phenazopyridine
Purple-red	Phenol red and phenolphthalein in alkaline urine
Port wine	Porphyrin; mixture of methaemoglobin and oxyhaemoglobin
Dark brown	Altered blood (methaemoglobinuria); phenolic drugs (phenol, cresol); phenylhydrazine; porphyrins; melanin
Brown-black	Much haemoglobin; Iysol poisoning; melanin; iron–sorbitol–citric acid complex (Jectofer); homogentisic acid; cascara; rhubarb
Smoky	Red blood cells
Yellow	Riboflavin
Yellow foam	Bilirubin pigments
Green foam	Biliverdin
Green	Biliverdin and other bile pigments; methylene blue, indigo carmine; carbolic acid; guaiacol (in cough remedies); santonin; acriflavine (in bladder irrigants for presurgical skin preparation); methocarbamol (Robaxin) — urine standing a long time
Pale blue fluorescence	Triamterene (Dyrenium)
Blue	Methylene blue; indigo blue
Blue-green	Tolonium (Blutene); methylene blue; amitriptyline (Elavil)

Revision Questions and Case Studies

1. Discuss the symptomatology of acute kidney infections and correlate this with the pathology of acute pyelonephritis, indicating clearly why the condition is relevant to you in your future profession.

2. Write short notes on any four of the following topics:
   (a) Renal fusion
   (b) Renal cysts
   (c) Carbuncle of the kidney
   (d) Perinephric abscess
   (e) Pyaemia involving the kidney

3. What are the effects of systemic hypertension on the kidney?

4. Describe the characteristic changes observable in the kidney of a patient with untreated, primary, malignant hypertension of several months' duration.

5. Discuss the pathology of papillary necrosis of the kidney.

6. What are the characteristics of glomerulonephritis? Compare and contrast any two distinct types of glomerulonephritis.

7. What are the changes detectable in a kidney with chronic glomerulonephritis? Correlate these changes with the pathology of this condition, indicating two common aetiologies that may give rise to such a disorder in the kidney.

8. Discuss the pathology of post-streptococcal glomerulonephritis.

9. Write short notes on the following:
   (a) Nephritic syndrome
   (b) Nephrotic syndrome
   (c) Nephrosis

10. Compare and contrast nephritic and nephrotic syndromes, relating the differences observed to the glomerular lesions in each of the two syndromes.

11. What are the characteristics of carcinoma of the kidney? Include in your discussion incidence, predisposing factors, sites affected, morphology, symptoms/signs, spread, treatment and prognosis.

12. What is meant by the term 'renal failure'? Discuss the pathology of any two common conditions which frequently progress to renal failure.

13. Write notes on:
   (a) Urinary calculi
   (b) Hydronephrosis
   (c) Tumours of the renal pelvis

14. Discuss the pathology of carcinoma of the urinary bladder.

15. What are the characteristics of urolithiasis?

16. Discuss the pathology of cystitis.

17. Define the following terms:
   (a) Wilms' tumour
   (b) Staghorn calculus
   (c) Urinary bladder diverticulum

18. Discuss the significance of routine 'office' urinalysis in the diagnosis of renal disease.

Case study 1. A 68-year-old Caucasian woman presents with malaise, fatigue, generalized aches and pains and complains that she is finding it difficult to carry out her normal everyday activities at home. She is 1.70 m tall and 49 kg in weight, her blood pressure is 180/98 mmHg and her pulse rate is 82 per minute. Her temperature is 37.8°C. When questioned she admits to feeling a little 'flustered and hot' over the past 2 days. Physical examination showed largely normal abdominal findings with the exception of a palpable spleen tip, indicating enlargement. There is evidence of slight, generalized oedema. She says that she often 'has to go to the toilet during the night' and her embarrassment makes you suspect that she may also be incontinent. Your suspicions are shown to be justified when you question her directly and she admits to 'losing bladder control... once, earlier this week'. A Multistix® analysis of the urine shows the specific gravity to be 1.030, the pH is 9.1, the protein content is high and there are leukocytes and nitrite present. Questioning the woman further elicits the information that she has been treated in the past for 'kidney problems'.

(a) What is the diagnosis?
(b) What further tests need be done?
(c) How is the condition treated?
(d) What is the prognosis for the patient (given her treatment is purely medical)?

Case study 2. A 59-year-old Caucasian male, Sir Roger P. (he is a chemical engineer and was knighted last year for his services to industry), presents complaining of episodes of loin pain, which he describes as 'aching and deep'. There have been problems with micturition and last night he noticed some blood in his urine. The past week he has been feverish on a couple of occasions. Physical examination shows the following features: height, 1.80 m; weight, 63 kg; blood pressure, 155/90 mmHg (he is on antihypertensive medication); pulse rate, 80 per minute; temperature, 37.6°C; chest is normal but on palpation of the abdomen and flanks a mass is found around the right kidney. The patient is pale and appears weak. When questioned further he says that he has noticed that he has lost weight recently and attributes this to 'feeling full and having no appetite most of the time'.

(a) Give the differential diagnoses for haematuria as observed in this case.
(b) What investigations would be advisable?
(c) Given that infection and systemic diseases are ruled out by these investigations, what is the most likely diagnosis?
(d) List the features of this case study that influenced your decision in (c) above.

Case study 3. A man (27-year-old Caucasian single father) brings his 5-year-old daughter to your clinic because the girl has a mild fever which he initially did not treat too seriously as the girl often gets minor colds and often feels a little unwell. Besides, he says, his daughter was treated 2 weeks previously with penicillin for a throat infection and this infection resolved within a couple of days. The man became worried because the child became listless and weak, feverish and 'just went and crawled into bed without saying anything to anyone...'. The man has brought the child to you as he does not have confidence in the doctor who prescribed the antibiotics for the infection and is now seeking alternative treatments. Physical examination of the child shows a rather thin Caucasian girl, with a weight of 18 kg and a height of 1.2 m. There is oedema present around the ankles and in the face. The blood pressure is 135/94 mmHg and the pulse rate is 80 beats per minute. Her temperature is 37.9°C. Questioning the man and child it is determined that the volume of urine produced at micturition is reduced. Chest and abdomen are normal on auscultation and palpation. Multistix® analysis of a urine sample taken shows the following: glucose, a trace (5 mmol/L); bilirubin, negative; ketones, negative; specific gravity, 1.030; blood, large (200 cells/µL); pH, 6.3; protein, ++++ (>20 g/L); urobilinogen, normal; nitrites, negative; leukocytes, small (70 cells/µL).

(a) Give the most likely diagnosis for this child.
(b) What further tests would confirm the diagnosis?
(c) How is this disorder treated?
(d) What is the prognosis of this disorder?

Case study 4. A 19-year-old Caucasian female just returned from a week's holidays on the Gold Coast presents complaining of dysuria and frequency of micturition, often having to get up three to four times a night in order to pass urine. There is loin tenderness and itching around the vulva. Physical examination shows all normal findings except for an acutely inflamed urethral meatus. A midstream, clean-catch urine specimen is supplied by the woman and the results obtained after Multistix® analysis are as follows: glucose, negative; bilirubin, negative, ketones, negative;

specific gravity, 1.025; blood, trace (10 cells/µL); pH, 5.0; protein, +++ (1.0 g/L); urobilinogen, normal; nitrites, +/–; leukocytes, large (>500 cells/µL).

(a) What is the diagnosis?
(b) What further laboratory investigations should be carried out and why?
(c) How is this condition treated?

Case study 5. A 62-year-old Caucasian woman of German origin has her urine tested with the Multistix® test strip during a routine examination in your clinic. The following values are obtained: glucose, +ve (15 mmol/L); bilirubin, –ve; ketone, –ve; S.G., 1.025; blood, –ve; pH, 5; protein, +ve (0.3 g/L); urobilinogen, normal; nitrite, –ve; leukocytes, –ve. When questioned the woman tells you that she takes four 500 mg vitamin C tablets daily.

(a) What are the abnormal values in this urine?
(b) Would the vitamin C intake have influenced any of the results?
(c) What other tests should the woman be advised to have done?
(d) The woman's father died in his 70s from gangrene in his lower limb. What does this suggest about the diagnosis of the woman's condition?

Further Reading

Abel JA. 'Analgesic Nephropathy: A Review of the Literature, 1967–1970.' *Clin Pharmacol Therap* 1971; **12**: 583.

Andres G, *et al.* 'Biology of Disease: Formation of Immune Deposits and Disease.' *Lab Invest* 1989; **55**: 519.

Becker G. 'Urinary Tract Infection and Reflux Nephropathy in Adults.' *Med International* 1986; **2**(33): 1337.

Bennington JL. 'Cancer of the Kidney — Aetiology, Epidemiology and Pathology.' *Cancer* 1973; **32**: 1017.

Brenner BM. 'Haemodynamically Mediated Glomerular Injury and the Progressive Nature of Kidney Diseases.' *Kidney Int* 1983; **23**: 647.

Couser WG. 'Mediation of Immune Glomerular Injury.' *J Am Soc Nephrol* 1990; **1**: 13.

Davison AM (ed.). 'Nephrology.' 1988; Baillière-Tindall, London.

Fine LG. 'Preventing the Progression of Human Renal Disease: Have Rational Therapeutic Principles Emerged?' *Kidney Int* 1988; **33**: 116.

Gabow PA. 'Polycystic Kidney Disease: Clues to

Pathogenesis.' *Kidney Int* 1991; **40**: 989.

Kaysen GA. 'Hyperlipidaemia in the Nephrotic Syndrome.' *Kidney Int* 1991; **39** (Suppl 31): S8.

Kincaid-Smith P, Becker G. 'Reflux Nephropathy and Chronic Atrophic Pyelonephritis: A Review.' *J Inf Dis* 1978; **138**: 774.

Lutzeyer W, *et al.* 'Prognostic Parameters in Superficial Bladder Cancer, an Analysis of 315 Cases.' *J Urol* 1982; **127**: 250.

Mogensen CE. 'Prevention and Treatment of Renal Disease in Insulin Dependent Diabetes Mellitus.' *Semin Nephrol* 1990; **10**: 260.

Mostofi FK, Davis CJ. 'Tumours and Tumour-like Lesions of the Kidney.' *Curr Probl Cancer* 1986; **10**: 53.

Nissenson AR, *et al.* 'Poststreptococcal Acute Glomerulonephritis: Fact and Controversy.' *Ann Int Med* 1979; **91**: 76.

Oken DE. 'On the Differential Diagnosis of Acute Renal Failure.' *Am J Med* 1981; **71**: 916.

Peh SC, Lindop GBM. 'Chronic Pyelonephritis: The Significance of Renal Renin and the Vascular Changes in the Human Kidney.' *J Path* 1991; **163**: 343.

Sandler DP, *et al.* 'Analgesic Use and Chronic Renal Disease.' *New Engl J Med* 1989; **320**: 1238.

Smith LH, 'Calcium-Containing Renal Stones.' *Kidney Int* 1978; **13**: 383.

Tisher CC, Brenner BM (eds). *Renal Pathology*, 1989; Lippincott, Philadelphia.

Wallace DM. 'Occupational Urothelial Cancer.' *Br J Urol* 1988; **61**: 175.

11

Male Genital System Disorders

The Normal Male Genital System

Unlike the female urogenital system where the genital and urinary tracts are separate, in the male the genital and urinary tracts are fused into one distally, with one common conduit and orifice being present for the final passage of urine or semen into the exterior.

The normal urinary system of the male consists of the **kidneys**, **ureters**, **urinary bladder** and **urethra**. The genital system comprises the **testis**, **epididymis**, **vas deferens**, **seminal vesicle**, **prostate gland**, **penis** and **urethra** (see Figure 11.1). Spermatogenesis occurs in the testes, two glandular organs situated within the scrotum, suspended by the spermatic cords. Early in foetal life the testes are situated in the abdomen, behind the peritoneum. Just before or immediately after birth, the testes descend to the inguinal canal, through which they pass, with the spermatic cord descending into the scrotum via the external abdominal ring. In the process of their descent, they become invested by a number of coverings: tunica vaginalis, internal spermatic fascia, cremasteric fascia, external spermatic fascia, dartos and skin of the scrotum. The exocrine portion of the testis resides in the seminiferous tubules, whose function is to produce the male sex cells, the spermatozoa. The endocrine portion of the testis is contained between the seminiferous tubules, in the interstitial cells of Leydig, which produce testosterone.

The system of ducts beginning from each testis serves to convey the spermatozoa from this organ to the exterior. The epididymis is composed of a single, 6 m long, highly coiled duct that forms a small mass stretching along the posterior of the testis. The epithelium produces a viscid secretion that nourishes the spermatozoa during the 6-week trip through this tube. The epididymis allows the spermatozoa to develop fully and also acts as a storage organ for the spermatozoa. The duct of the epididymis enlarges into the vas deferens which straightens and courses though the inguinal canal, curving behind the peritoneum towards the urethra. The vas deferens is about 46 cm long. Within the testis and inguinal canal the vas deferens is contained in the spermatic cord together with the testicular artery, the pampiniform plexus of veins, lymph vessels and nerves. The vas deferens ends near

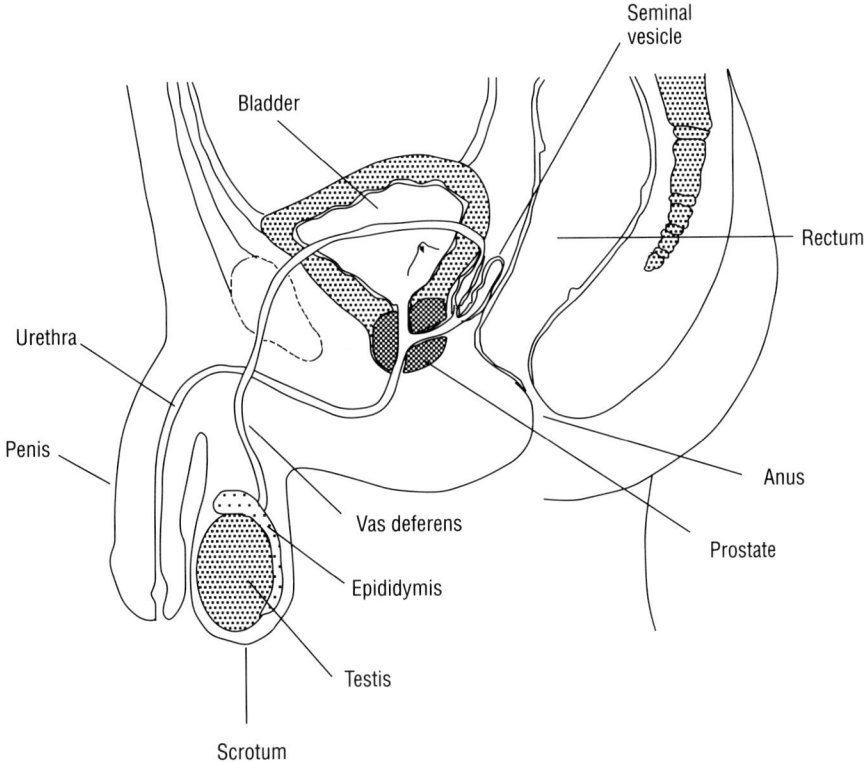

Figure 11.1 *The male genital system*

the posterior lobe of the prostate in the region of the ampulla, a dilated end portion of this duct, where there are also the diverticula from the lower vas deferens, the seminal vesicles. The seminal vesicles are elongated, saccular organs, placed between the base of the bladder and the rectum, serving as reservoirs for the semen and also secreting the viscid part of the seminal fluid, rich in fructose (this being a source of metabolic energy for the spermatozoa). The ejaculatory duct is formed, as it were, by the fusion of the ampulla and the seminal vesicle neck. The duct passes through the prostate gland and opens into the urethra on the urethral crest. The powerful contractions of the muscular wall of the epididymis, vas deferens and urethra forcibly expel the semen and contained spermatozoa (≈3 mL of fluid containing 250 000 000 spermatozoa) under the stimulus of sexual climax.

The prostate gland surrounds the urethra as it leaves the bladder and is composed of five lobes of glandular tissue supported by a fibromuscular stroma. It produces a thin, milky secretion, rich in citric acid and acid phosphatase. The prostatic secretion makes up about 75% of the seminal fluid and it helps in neutralizing the acidity of the urethra (acid conditions are detrimental to the spermatozoa), it dilutes the viscous semen and augments sperm motility. The prostatic secretion is said to be discharged first during ejaculation. The Cowper's glands (= bulbourethral glands) are paired organs lying behind the membranous urethra and produce a mucous secretion during sexual arousal, the mucus serving to lubricate the lumen of the urethra.

The penis is the male copulatory organ as well as the urinary outlet. It contains three cylindrical, fibrous compartments of erectile tissue. The paired corpora cavernosa are placed side by side along the upper part of the organ and the unpaired corpus spongiosum encloses the spongy portion of the urethra and is placed below. The extremity of the penis is the glans penis, an obtuse cone flattened from above downward. At its apex there is a vertical orifice, upon which is the urethral meatus. The three erectile cylinders are surrounded by skin and subcutaneous tissues, the skin terminating in a reduplicating fold, the prepuce (foreskin), which covers the glans penis. Erection of the penis is caused by parasympathetic nervous stimulation that produces relaxation of muscular tone in arterioles supplying the cavernous sinus of the erectile tissue, turgidity resulting because the constricting tunica albuginea compresses veins and limits venous return.

Diseases of the Prostate Gland

Prostatitis

Prostatitis is an inflammation or infection of the prostate gland. It is usually due to infections with pyogenic bacteria seen in association with obstruction in the urinary tract in elderly males with prostatic hyperplasia, and as a complication of urinary tract infection (UTI) or of sexually transmitted disease. Rarely, chronic prostatitis may occur in association with tuberculosis of the urinary tract or in cases of parasitic infestations. In some cases, prostatitis may result if there is some leakage of prostatic secretion into the stroma of the gland.

Acute non-specific prostatitis is rare and usually develops as a result of infection in the bladder or posterior urethra, or may follow surgery and instrumentation. **Acute suppurative prostatitis** is seen in pyogenic infections; a typical acute inflammatory infiltrate occurs and leads to abscess formation. In elderly males this type of prostatitis is more likely to be caused by *Escherichia coli, Enterococcus faecalis, Proteus* spp., and other bacteria commonly involved in UTI associated with prostatic hyperplasia and urinary obstruction. In younger males acute suppurative prostatitis is most often due to infection with *Neisseria gonorrhoeae* or *Mycoplasma* and *Chlamydia,* associated with sexually acquired infections of the genitourinary tract. Treatment of these types of suppurative prostatitis is with the appropriate antibiotic, but in the case of large abscesses, surgical drainage of the pus may be required. Untreated cases of the disease will rarely resolve, healing with scarring or progression to chronic prostatitis being the commonest outcomes.

Chronic prostatitis is also seen and leads to the formation of a hard, shrunken prostate, often containing a small number of calculi. This disorder may be the result of untreated or neglected gonococcal and coliform infections. Numerous lymphocytes and plasma cells infiltrate the gland and a fibrous scar leads to the shrinking and hardening of the tissue. Often, acute inflammatory episodes punctuate the course of the disease. Mild chronic prostatitis is seen quite commonly in association with prostatic hyperplasia and

may be caused by leakage of secretion into the glandular stroma. Granulomatous prostatitis may occasionally be seen as a complication of tuberculosis affecting the urinary tract. Treatment of chronic prostatitis may be difficult in view of the degree of scarring involved.

Prostatic Hyperplasia

Prostatic hyperplasia is a very common disorder characterized by enlargement of the prostate due to increase in cell number of both the glandular and stromal components, giving rise to large fairly discrete nodules, hence the synonym **nodular prostatic hyperplasia**. It should be noted that the term 'benign hypertrophy' is doubly incorrect as there is no malignant form of hypertrophy, and as proliferation of cells is evident in prostatic enlargement, hyperplasia rather than hypertrophy is the major pathological process. The condition is quite rare below the age of 45 to 50 years, but there is a progressive increase in incidence with increasing age, until 80% of men over the age of 80 years are affected.

Prostatic hyperplasia is caused mainly by hormonal imbalances and a canine experimental model has elucidated the precise nature of these imbalances. As men age, there are increased oestrogen levels of adrenal origin. These are seen in combination with decreasing testosterone levels associated with decreased testicular function. This may seem rather a paradoxical situation as the prostate depends on testosterone stimulation for growth. However, the paradox is resolved if one remembers that the increased oestrogen levels sensitize the prostate cells, making them more receptive to the effects of the androgenic hormones. Thus, even in the face of decreasing dihydrotestosterone levels, the underlying hormonal imbalance stimulates growth.

The prostate gland increases in weight and bulk as a function of age (see Figure 11.2). In hyperplasia, however, this enlargement may be quite marked, weights of 60 to 200 g being observed. The inner, periurethral zones of the lateral and median lobes are mainly affected, the anterior and posterior lobes showing minimal or no involvement. As the median lobe enlarges upwards, it may project into the urinary bladder, acting as a ball valve, causing obstruction to urine flow. The enlargement of the lateral lobes compresses the urethra laterally at the neck of bladder, further embarrassing urinary flow. The enlarged gland is nodular, firm and rubbery with discrete, encapsulated masses of tissue. Both the glandular part and fibromuscular stroma are involved in the hyperplasia and one or the other component may predominate. If the cut surface of the hyperplastic gland shows soft, yellow-pink tis-

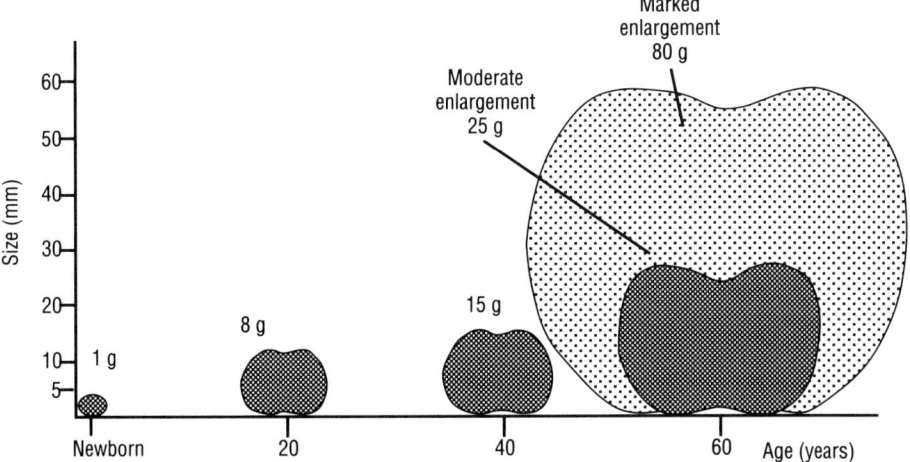

Figure 11.2 *Prostate gland size as a function of age*

sue with secretion, the hyperplasia mainly involves the glandular tissue. If the cut section shows tough, solid, grey nodules with no fluid, the hyperplasia is mainly stromal.

Microscopically, the hyperplasia of all three components of the gland is seen much more clearly. The glandular tissue, fibrous tissue and muscular tissue are involved, but to different extents. Adenomatous hyperplasia shows collections of large glands, irregular in size and shape with regular lining cells resting on an intact basement membrane. Frequently, folds or papillae of glandular tissue are seen to project into the enlarged lumina of the glands. This appearance is often referred to as a 'frond-like' growth pattern (Figure 11.3). Corpora amylacea are seen commonly in the enlarged gland lumina. There is often a lymphocytic infiltration around the hyperplastic tissue and sometimes squamous metaplasia of the epithelium lining the glands is observed.

In stromal hyperplasia the solid nodules are composed mainly of spindle-shaped, regular cells, fibroblasts and smooth muscle cells. Bundles of collagen fibres are also present and this fibromuscular tissue compresses the entrapped glands. It should be noted that mixed hyperplasia patterns are common with both the glandular and fibromuscular tissue being involved to the same extent. Cystic dysplasia may be seen, in this case the hyperplastic glands being greatly dilated to form large cystic spaces full of secretion. Secondary infection may be seen in the hyperplastic gland with an appearance typical of suppurative acute inflammation (liquefactive necrosis, neutrophils, abscesses, etc.).

The condition may remain symptomless for many

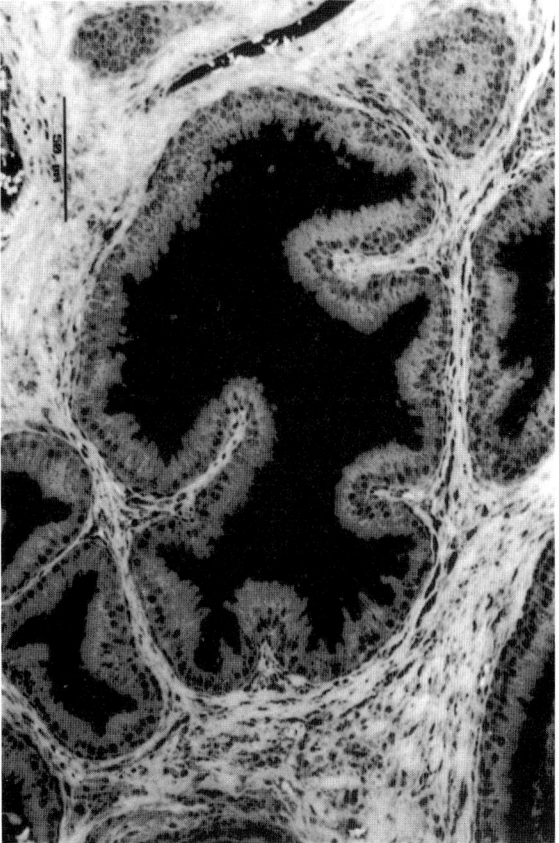

Figure 11.3 *Hyperplasia of the prostate gland showing the typical papillary projections of the hyperplastic epithelium into the lumen of the acini and ducts (scale bar is 50 μm)*

years while the gland enlarges, the manifestations of the disease only becoming apparent when the enlarging lobes start to cause obstruction to urinary flow. The affected man then begins to experience progressive difficulty in micturition, with difficulty in starting and stopping the urinary flow, poor urinary stream, all characteristics often referred to by the patient as 'dribbling' of urine. There is also frequency of micturition, nocturia, dysuria, chronic urine retention and incontinence. As obstruction of urinary flow and stasis of urine in the bladder develops, there is an increased incidence of UTI with all of its attendant complications.

The effects of nodular prostatic hyperplasia are manifold and include the following. In the urethra there is deformity and obstruction, leading to interference in the urine flow. In the bladder, obstruction to urine flow leads to hypertrophy of the smooth muscle in the bladder wall. As the bundles of smooth muscle increase in girth and length, they become very prominent, a change known as trabeculation. The increased pressure inside the bladder leads to the formation of diverticula in the weakened wall between the trabeculated bundles of smooth muscle. The urinary stasis predisposes to **cystitis** and **calculus formation**. Retained urine in the ureters leads to **hydroureter** and ascending infection. In the kidneys the increasing volume of retained urine causes **hydronephrosis**, **pyelonephritis**, **pyonephrosis** and eventually even **renal failure** (refer to Figure 11.4). It should be noted that hyperplasia of the prostate does not predispose to the development of carcinoma of the prostate, although both conditions may coexist in the same organ.

Treatment of the condition is by surgical resection of the redundant tissue. In most cases this is a simple surgical operation performed through the urethra. This is the **trans-urethral resection of the prostate** or TURP. An endoscope is passed up through the urethra to core out the enlarged lobes (usually the median and lateral lobes are involved, thus these are readily accessible). Approximately 10% of affected males are affected severely enough to require such treatment.

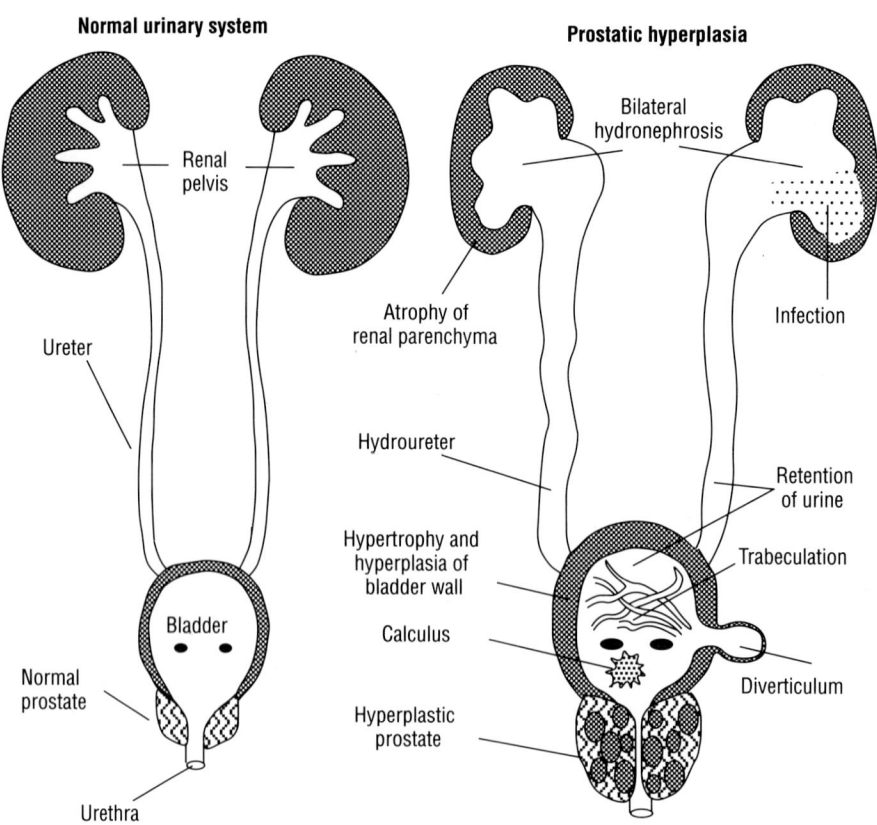

Figure 11.4   *Effects of prostate gland enlargement*

Carcinoma of the Prostate

This is a common malignancy of the glandular tissue of the prostate gland seen primarily in the elderly.

Incidence. Prostatic carcinoma accounts for 4% of all deaths from cancer. In males, death from prostatic cancer is the third most common cancer death (next to lung cancer and bowel cancer). Epidemiological studies have shown this tumour to cause 7% of clinically overt cancers in males. It has been shown, histologically, that up to 40% of males over the age of 50 years have carcinoma of the prostate, but it remains latent, only one-sixth of these males showing symptomatic disease. The frequency of this disease increases with age, such that between 50 to 60 years about 20% of prostates are cancerous; between 60 to 70 years approximately 35% of prostates are cancerous; between 70 to 80 years about 55% of prostates are cancerous and between 80 to 90 years about 80% of prostates are cancerous. The disease is rare below the age of 50 years. The death rate from this tumour is highest amongst blacks in USA (being of higher incidence than in African blacks); the tumour is of high incidence in Scandinavia, while the lowest death rate from this cancer is in Japan, with a very low incidence also in Mexico and Greece.

Aetiology. A number of aetiological factors have been associated with incidence of the tumour and several 'popular' beliefs about it have been laid to rest by epidemiologists (i.e. the tumour is not commoner in men who are excessively sexually active). Known predisposing factors in the causation of the cancer are:

- exposure to cadmium and its compounds (cadmium is a zinc competitor);
- hormonal disturbances — an excess of androgens and a relative deficiency of oestrogens;
- decline in immunological surveillance (an effect of increasing age).

Prostatic carcinoma does not seem to be related to nodular hyperplasia of the prostate, and the presence of hyperplasia does not predispose to the development of carcinoma.

Sites affected. Unlike hyperplasia of the prostate, the cancer affects primarily the posterior lobe of the gland, the lateral and median lobes being rarely affected. Approximately 85% of tumours are in the posterior lobe, 95% of them arising superficially, adjacent to the capsule.

Macroscopic appearance. It should be noted that although nodular prostatic hyperplasia does not predispose to the cancer, many of the cases of this tumour show concomitant hyperplasia of the gland. This is a finding consistent with the fluctuating hormonal levels that are seen in the body with ageing and is also due to the different responsiveness to oestrogen and testosterone of different parts of the gland. The tumour is a small, hard, pale area in the posterior lobe, posterior to the urethra or in the posterolateral aspect below the capsule, that is, in areas not affected by hyperplasia. Rectal examination detects the region of the carcinoma as a firm, nodular or craggy mass occupying all or part of the posterior lobe.

Microscopic appearance. Roughly 96% of the tumours are adenocarcinomata, showing typical tubular and acinar patterns. Less frequently, the tumour is composed of masses of irregular, spheroidal cells arranged in irregular clumps, and anaplastic tumours are quite rare. In about 4% of cases, the tumours are squamous cell carcinomata. The last-mentioned tumours arise in glands where the prostatic ducts have undergone squamous metaplasia.

Spread. The tumour first spreads by direct invasion, the posterior lobe being invaded by the tumour cells that also grow outwards to involve the capsule of the gland. In the later stages of the disease the other prostatic lobes are also involved through direct spread. Lymphatic spread commonly occurs with local lymph nodes being involved. However, it is the blood spread that is very important in the course of the disease, as 75% of cases show early metastasis of the cancer in bone, the vertebrae, pelvis, femora and ribs being predominantly affected. The metastatic bone tumours are osteosclerotic, with new bone formed around the metastases (Figure 11.5). The liver and lungs may also be invaded later in the course of the disease.

Signs and symptoms. The tumour usually remains asymptomatic for a long time, especially if it is a small carcinoma that grows slowly over a period of years. As it develops in the posterior lobe there will be no impingement on the urethra, and hence no urinary compression or obstruction. Raised acid phosphatase levels may be a feature of the disease, and a palpable mass on digital rectal examination will be discovered. Generalized symptoms and signs associated with widespread malignancy (e.g. fatigue, anaemia, cachexia) will be observed later on in the disease. It should be stressed that the local effects of the tumour are usually not severe (until very late in the disease when the tumour has spread to involve the lateral lobes of the

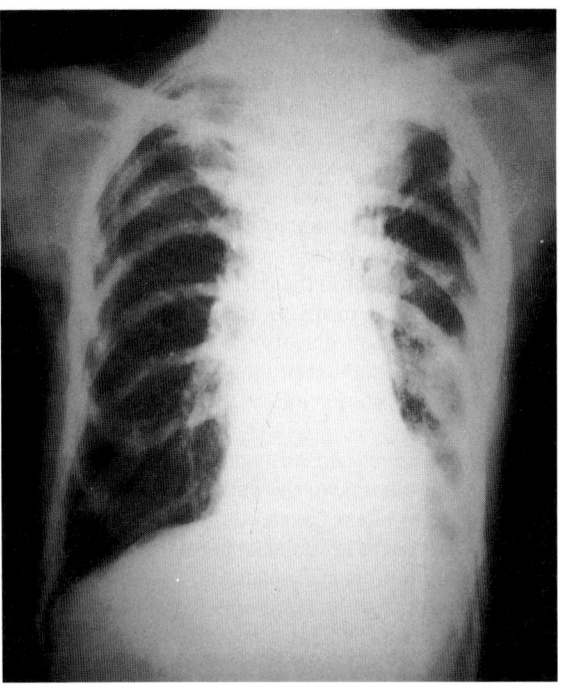

Figure 11.5 *Secondary carcinoma of the prostate, here shown involving the bones of the thoracic region; the patient also had metastases in the skull (courtesy of Dr Thomas Molyneux, RMIT)*

gland). Most effects of the tumour result from metastases and include bone lesions such as pathological fractures.

Diagnosis. Rectal examination of the gland will provide useful information as to the status of the prostatic tissue. Consistency of the gland, mobility, part affected, tenderness and symmetry of the enlargement are all important features that may aid in diagnosis (see Figure 11.6 and Table 11.1).

Differential diagnosis of a hard prostatic nodule should include the following as well as a carcinoma: localized nodule of hyperplasia; focus of non-specific chronic prostatitis, granulomatous prostatitis (including TB); prostatic calculus and prostatic infarct. Important in diagnosis may be the increased acid phosphatase levels that indicate prostatic activity and levels greater than 5 IU/100 mL should be investigated further. In the case of prostatic cancer metastases in bone, raised alkaline phosphatase levels may also be found, corresponding to the increased osteoblastic activity in the bone. Prostatic smears of the secretion obtained following massage of the prostate are examined by the cytologist who often will detect malignant cells present in the smear. Biopsy of prostatic enlargements may sometimes be used in diagnosis.

Treatment. Surgery of these tumours is only rarely possible because most of them are diagnosed in very late stages and metastases are already present. Also in many cases, the advanced age of the patient and other

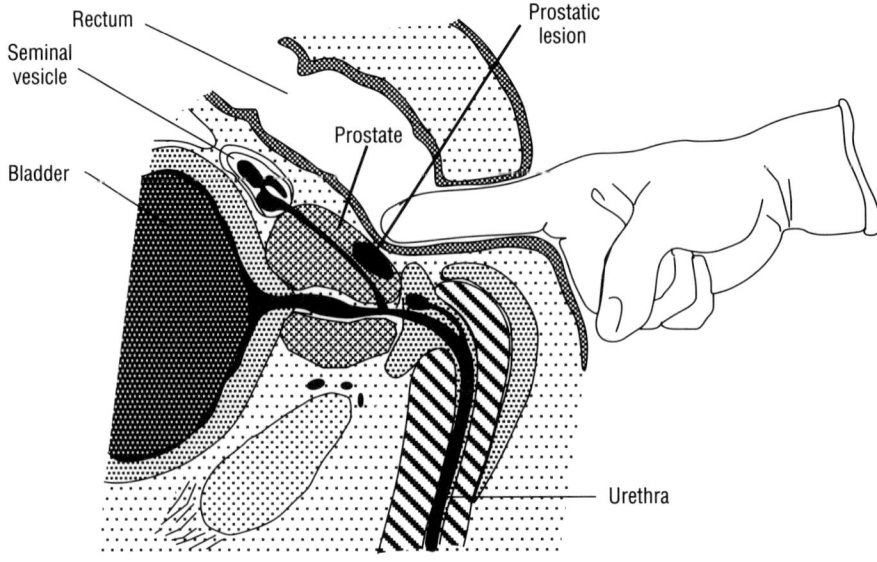

Figure 11.6 *Rectal examination of the prostate gland*

Table 11.1 *Palpatory findings of rectal examination of the prostate gland*

	Consistency	Symmetry	Tenderness	Mobility
Prostatitis	Boggy, soft	May be asymmetrical	Yes	Yes
Hyperplasia	Firm, rubbery	Usually symmetrical	No	Yes
Carcinoma	Hard nodule	Usually asymmetrical	No	No (later stages of the tumour)

unrelated health problems make the surgical procedure an undesirable option. Surgery is only attempted with small primary tumours in otherwise healthy men. In most cases, hormonal control of the tumour is quite effective in the short term and is the only option available in advanced cases. The patient is put on oestrogens and the androgen production is controlled chemically or by orchidectomy (castration). There follows a marked reduction in the size of both the primary and secondary tumours over a period of months (6 to 14 months usually). After this variable period the tumour loses its hormonal dependence and begins to grow rapidly again.

Staging and prognosis. The prognosis of the tumour depends largely on the stage at which it is diagnosed and treated.

• **Stage A**: The tumour is confined to the gland and the 5-year survival is greater than 80%.
• **Stage B**: The tumour is clinically manifest but remains intracapsular. The acid phosphatase levels may be normal and the 5-year survival is approximately 50%.
• **Stage C**: There is extracapsular invasion of the surrounding organs and lymph nodes. The acid phosphatase levels may be raised and the 5-year survival is approximately 35%.
• **Stage D**: Bone and extrapelvic metastases are present and the acid phosphatase is usually raised. The 5-year survival is approximately 20%.

The overall prognosis is poor, with an average survival figure for 5 years of 25%.

Disorders of the Penis

Epispadias and Hypospadias

Congenital disorders of the penis and the anatomy of the urethral meatus are associated usually with other malformations in the male urogenital system. In **hypospadias** and **epispadias**, the urethra opens on the dorsal or on the ventral surface of the penis, respectively. Both conditions are also associated with abnormalities of formation of the prepuce (Figure 11.7). **Chordee** may be present in hypospadias, and this is the ventral curvature of the penis, due to the presence of dense fibrous tissue instead of the normal connective tissue along the corpus spongiosum.

Depending on the degree of malformation and whether or not other abnormalities are present, the condition may be asymptomatic or may predispose to obstruction and infection or sterility. Plastic surgery may be required for allowing normal urinary and sexual function, and also for psychological reasons.

Phimosis and Paraphimosis

In **phimosis** of the penis, the orifice of the prepuce is too small to permit its retraction and exposure of the glans penis (refer to Figure 11.8). This may be a congenital lesion or it may follow infection and inflammation. The condition greatly predisposes to infection and there may be difficulty in sexual intercourse.

Often, the condition is complicated by a forcible retraction of the prepuce over the glans penis. This leads to an inflamed collar of prepuce over the coronal sulcus, resulting in constriction and swelling, a complication termed **paraphimosis**. In severe cases, this may lead to interference in venous return from the glans, and infarction. The condition is treated by circumcision.

Balanitis and Balanoposthitis

Balanitis is an inflammation or infection of the glans penis. If both the glans and prepuce are involved, the

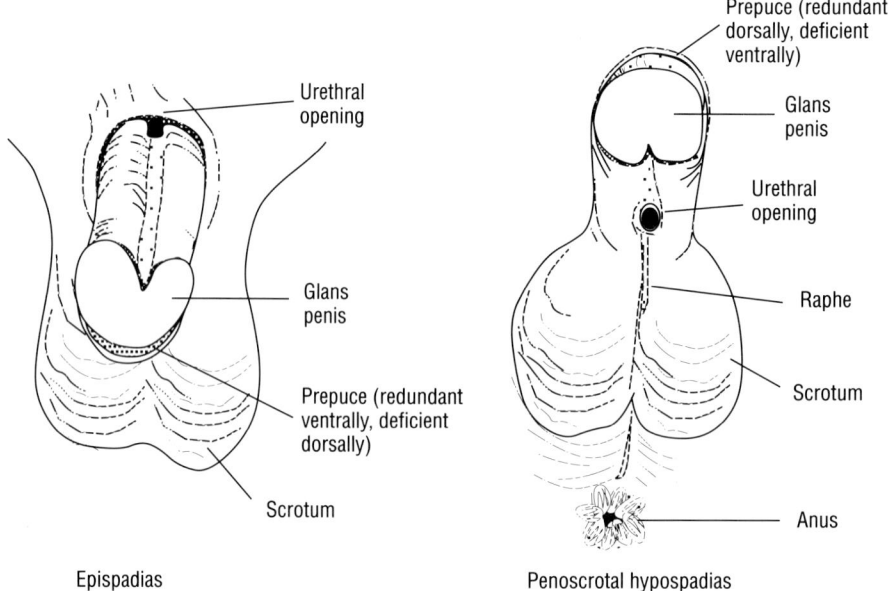

Figure 11.7   *Epispadias and hypospadias*

condition is termed a **balanoposthitis**. Staphylococci, streptococci, coliforms and gonococci are most often isolated from infectious causes of this condition. Phimosis or a large, redundant prepuce predispose to these conditions. Typical acute inflammatory changes are seen in the tissue, with congestion, oedema and exudation. If the condition remains untreated, ulceration, and scarring may result. If phimosis was not present previously, it may also complicate the untreated case in an uncircumcised man.

Premalignant Lesions of the Penis

Various dysplastic epithelial changes occur on the penis and may develop into carcinoma. In most cases these premalignant lesions develop idiopathically but in some cases they may be associated with the presence of a prepuce and poor hygiene. Both premalignant changes and carcinoma of the penis are rare in circumcised men. **Leukoplakia** is a premalignant lesion developing most commonly on the glans penis and presents a similar microscopic appearance to the lesion elsewhere in the body. It is a dysplastic change in the epithelium, with thickening, atypia, increased basophilia and disrupted architecture in the epithelial lining. If this condition is left untreated it is likely that a malignant change will occur eventually.

The remaining two changes are better considered as

lesions of **carcinoma** *in situ* as they both will inevitably progress to invasive carcinoma within a relatively short period of time if left untreated. **Erythroplasia of Queyrat** presents as raised, red, velvety or roughened plaques most frequently on the glans penis or prepuce. Microscopically, there is keratosis with all the cellular features of carcinoma seen, but the malignant cells do not invade past the basement membrane of the early lesion. A similar microscopic appearance is seen with **Bowen's disease**. Macroscopically, the latter appears as a raised, rough plaque of thickened epithelium.

Carcinoma of the Penis

Incidence. This is a tumour that is infrequent in Western countries, accounting for only approximately 0.5 to 1% of cancer deaths in males. In some countries, however, it is a much commoner tumour; in India and the East it may cause as many as 10% of male cancer deaths. It is a cancer seen usually from 50 to 70 years of age.

Aetiology. The most well documented predisposing factors and aetiologies of the tumour are inadequate hygiene, usually associated with the presence of a prepuce. The cancer is virtually unknown in societies where ritual circumcision is practised early in life (e.g. Jews). Chronic irritation of the penile tissue due to

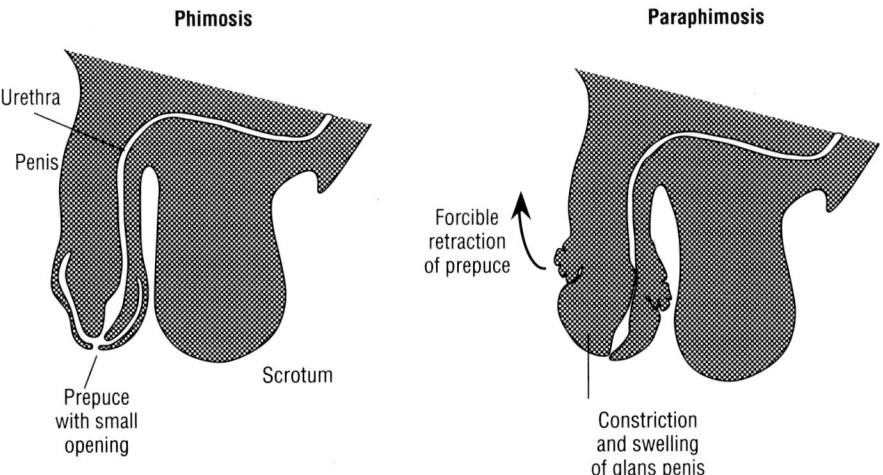

Figure 11.8 *Phimosis and paraphimosis*

accumulated smegma, a redundant prepuce and phimosis all predispose to the condition. The presence of premalignant lesions will greatly increase the risk of the carcinoma occurring.

Macroscopical appearance. The tumour usually develops on the dorsum of the glans or the inner aspect of the prepuce. It most commonly arises as a warty, fungating mass which usually ulcerates. On the periphery of the carcinoma there may be areas of leukoplakia.

Microscopical appearance. Most of the tumours are well-differentiated, squamous cell carcinomata. Rarely, an anaplastic tumour may be seen.

Spread. The tumour grows superficially as a papillary nodule. Direct growth and invasion along the shaft of the penis is the earliest way in which the tumour spreads. In neglected tumours there may be extensive destruction of tissue, deformity and urinary fistula formation. At the time of presentation as many as 30% of cases may have inguinal lymph node metastases. Haematogenous spread, however, is very rare and occurs very late in the disease.

Treatment and prognosis. The tumour is effectively treated by surgical amputation of the penis and block dissection of the groin if lymphatic spread has occurred. If no inguinal lymph node spread has occurred the 5-year survival, after treatment, is greater than 95%. With inguinal spread the 5-year survival is 50 to 70% with treatment.

Carcinoma of the Scrotum

Incidence. This is a rare tumour accounting for only approximately 0.25% of cancer deaths in males. It occurs more in industrialized regions than in rural regions. It usually afflicts individuals between 50 and 70 years of age.

Aetiology. The tumour is of historical interest as it was the first malignancy linked with chemical carcinogenesis due to occupational exposure. Sir Percival Pott, a London surgeon, in 1775 observed that this tumour, described as a 'soot wart' had a very high incidence in chimney sweeps. This accounts for the other name of the disease, 'chimney sweep's cancer'. Pott correctly attributed the development of the tumour to the poor hygiene in chimney sweeps at that time, that allowed soot and tar to accumulate in the rugal folds of the scrotal skin. Chronic irritation of the tissue by the carcinogenic substances present in soot and tar led to the development of the carcinoma after many years. Low standards of personal hygiene, even today, are associated with development of the tumour.

Macroscopical appearance. The tumour develops on any part of the scrotal skin, usually deep in a rugal fold. It arises as a warty mass that quickly ulcerates. Characteristically, this cancer has rolled edges, as occurs in squamous cell carcinomata in other parts of the skin.

Microscopical appearance. Most the tumours are well-differentiated, squamous cell carcinomata.

Spread. The tumour grows slowly and invades by direct extension radially and inwards to eventually involve the testes. Approximately 20% of cases have inguinal lymph node metastases. Haematogenous spread, however, is quite rare and seen in neglected, untreated tumours after many years.

Treatment and prognosis. The prognosis of this tumour is excellent if it is removed before it involves the testes. If the inguinal nodes have been involved and the testes invaded, the prognosis is poor, as there is subsequent spread internally to the abdominal lymph nodes and other organs.

Diseases of the Tunica Vaginalis

Hydrocoele

Hydrocoele is a collection of fluid within the tunica vaginalis and appears translucent macroscopically if the scrotum is transilluminated. The condition is a fairly common finding in male infants and sometimes in adults and is, in fact, the commonest form of testicular swelling (refer to Figure 11.9). In infants the accumulation of fluid is due to a patent or an incompletely obliterated processus vaginalis. In the adult, it may indicate trauma, infection or malignancy in the testis.

Initially, the fluid is contained in a smooth-walled chamber (sometimes the sac is loculated). As the condition progresses, adhesions form as organization of

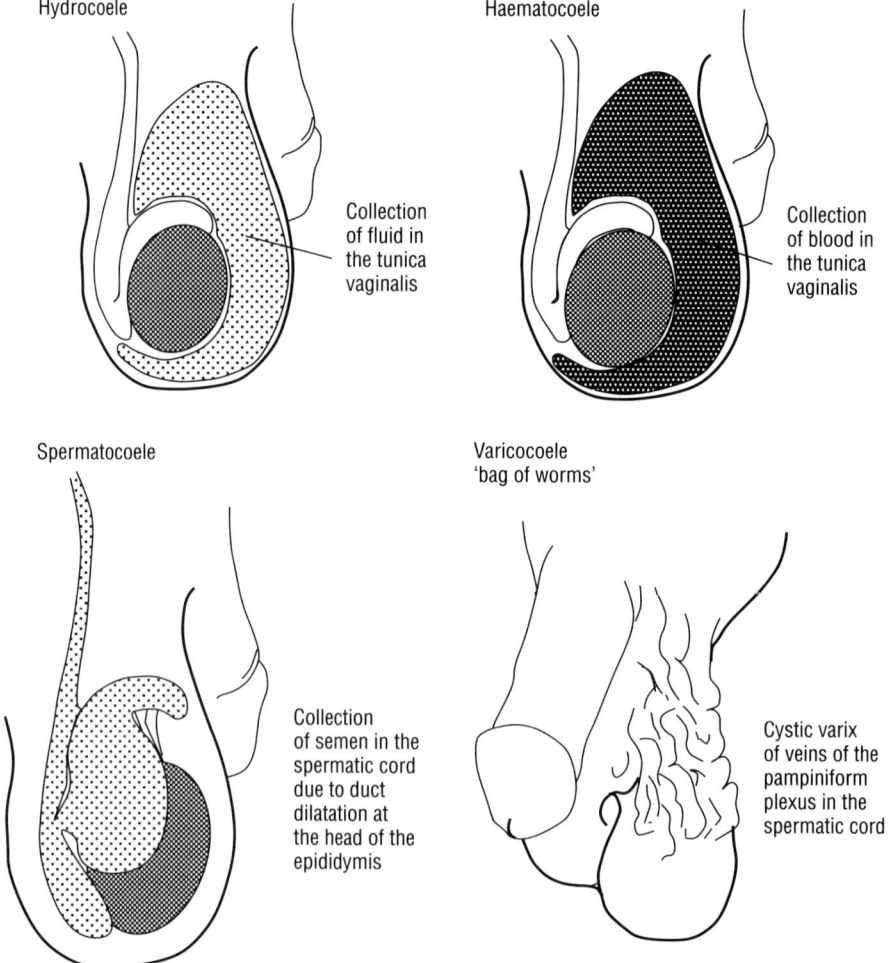

Figure 11.9   *Lesions of the tunica vaginalis*

the fluid occurs. There is considerable thickening of the walls due to the laying down of fibrous connective tissue. In the short term this condition may not cause any problem but in long-standing cases the constant pressure the fluid places on the testis may cause atrophy and sterility if bilateral. Infection of the fluid may also occur through extension from surrounding tissues or, rarely, following aspiration of the fluid.

Haematocoele

This is the condition where there is blood within the tunica vaginalis. Compared to hydrocoele, the condition is rather uncommon. It is often associated with trauma in the region, torsion of the testis and tumours that infiltrate through the tunica albuginea. The condition may also be seen as part of the generalized haemorrhages occurring in men with haemorrhagic diatheses. The presence of blood in this region initiates an inflammatory response with organization and fibrosis that may lead to testicular dysfunction through the compression effects of the scar.

Other Benign Testicular Swellings

Accumulation of lymph in the tunica albuginea is termed **chylocoele** and occurs whenever there is lymphatic obstruction in the region. A common aetiology of this condition is parasitic worm infestation (e.g. *Wuchereria bancroftii*) with resultant elephantiasis. The size of the scrotum may become enormous in these cases.

If semen accumulates in the spermatic cord due to dilatation of the ducts in the head of the epididymis or rete testis, the condition is termed **spermatocoele**. It arises in testes with congenital lesions or it may be acquired later in life. It is usually painless and in most cases it does not require any therapy.

Varicocoele is the term given to a condition where the pampiniform venous plexus in the spermatic cord becomes varicose such that a soft, elastic swelling forms and sometimes causes pain. The appearance and palpatory findings have given this condition the common name of 'bag of worms'. Varicocoele occurs most commonly in the left testis of males between the ages of 15 to 25 years. The condition may be caused by maldevelopment of the valves in the venous pampiniform plexi in which case it will be seen early in life. One other cause is carcinoma of the kidney, where the renal tumour invades the renal vein and compromises venous return from the testicular venous plexi. It is usually more pronounced and causes most discomfort when the affected man is in the standing position. Occasionally, the condition is complicated by thrombosis and surgical intervention is necessary. Varicocoele of long standing may increase the intrascrotal pressure considerably, compromising spermatogenesis and causing infertility.

Inguinal Hernia

This is a herniation in which a loop of the intestine enters the inguinal canal, sometimes filling the whole of the scrotal sac (see Figure 11.10). It may develop due to congenital lesions in which the vaginal process remains patent or is incompletely obliterated, and thus causes approximately 1% of paediatric disorders. In certain cases it develops later in life as the result of an opening of the obliterated vaginal process due to excessive stress being placed upon it, for example lifting of heavy weights, increased intra-abdominal pressure, or after surgical procedures in the region.

The condition is usually treated surgically, immediately after diagnosis, to prevent complications. The most important complication is strangulation of the herniating loop of bowel, with intestinal obstruction, compression of veins, infarction and gangrene.

Diseases of the Testis

Cryptorchidism

Cryptorchidism refers to cases of undescended or maldescended testes and may be unilateral or bilateral. The testes normally develop in the abdomen and descend to the pelvic brim in the third month of intrauterine life, a process termed internal descent. In the last 2 months of foetal life to very shortly after birth, passage of the testes into the scrotal position via the inguinal canal takes place, a process termed external descent. The testes need to be in the scrotum at puberty if effective spermatogenesis is to occur as the developing spermatozoa require a temperature that is 1.5 to 2°C lower than core temperature. Most boys with the condition are diagnosed and treated in infancy but the condition is found in 1% of school-age boys and 0.5% of men.

The cryptorchid testis may be situated in the abdomen or may be partially descended into the scrotum. If the testis is in the abdomen or anywhere along the length of the inguinal canal it is termed a maldescended testis. If the testis is found outside the inguinal canal but not in the scrotum it is termed an ectopic testis (refer to Figure 11.11).

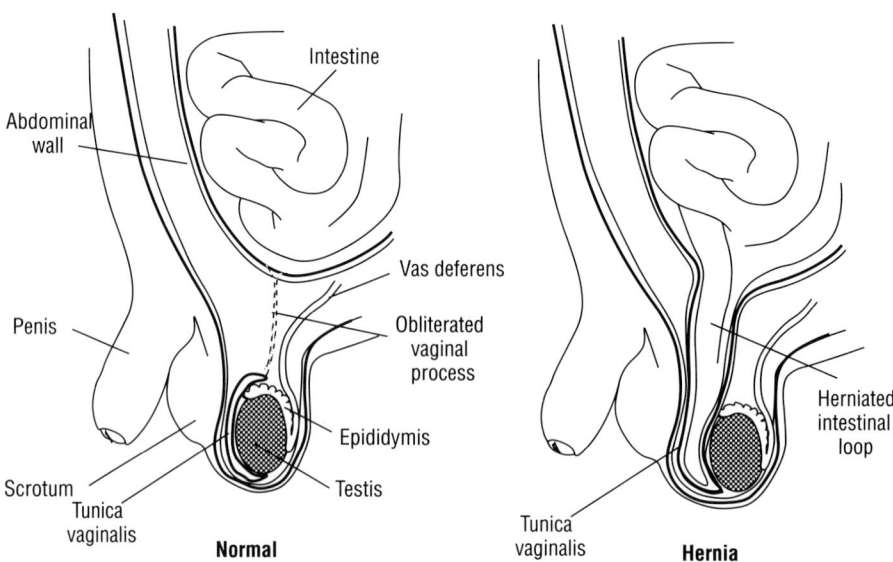

Figure 11.10   *Inguinal hernia*

Cryptorchidism must be treated early by **orchidopexy**, a surgical operation where the testis is put in its scrotal position and secured there, this procedure being best carried out before 2 years of age. If the condition is not treated by the age of puberty the testis will undergo atrophy and, if bilateral, may cause sterility owing to the elevated temperature inside the abdomen. Unilateral cryptorchidism very often will present as infertility. The affected testis is small and has a high fibrous tissue content. The seminiferous tubules are small and show no active spermatogenesis, the Sertoli cells being very prominent. Thickened basement membranes and increased numbers of interstitial cells of Leydig are also present, with hyperplasia of the connective tissue stroma. These changes are evident in a 5–6 year old boy with maldescended testes. The atrophic testis may also undergo malignant change later in life, cryptorchidism being associated with an increased incidence of seminoma. It should be noted that prompt orchidopexy not only ensures effective spermatogenesis but also protects against the development of carcinoma. Orchidopexy carried out later on in life does not preclude the development of carcinoma, nor will it treat the infertility if it is present.

Orchitis and Epididymoörchitis

Inflammation or infection of testis, termed orchitis, is rarely seen as an isolated entity, the inflammation most frequently also involving the epididymis. The condition is then termed an **epididymoörchitis**. Such disorders of the testis are associated with other infections in the genitourinary tract, such as cystitis, prostatitis, urethritis and sexually transmitted diseases. The organisms most commonly isolated from such cases are coliforms, Gram-positive cocci, gonococci and treponemes. In all of these cases a hot, severely painful, swollen testis results, which must be distinguished from torsion of the testis. Tuberculous orchitis may be rarely seen nowadays, in association with tuberculosis of the urinary tract. Among the viral causes of the condition, the most common and serious is **mumps orchitis** occurring approximately 7 days after salivary gland involvement in 20 to 25% of cases of the disease in adults.

Resolution rarely occurs in all cases of orchitis and epididymoörchitis, organization with variable amounts of scarring being the usual result. Suppuration may be seen rather uncommonly. Chronic inflammation, fibrosis and atrophy are the most commonly occurring sequelae of this condition. If both testes are affected, sterility is the expected aftermath, as commonly occurs in severe cases of mumps orchitis.

Torsion of the Testis

This is the condition where there is twisting of the testis about itself. Violent movements or trauma may cause it and thus it is often seen in sportsmen. Abnormalities of situation or attachment of the epididymis, a

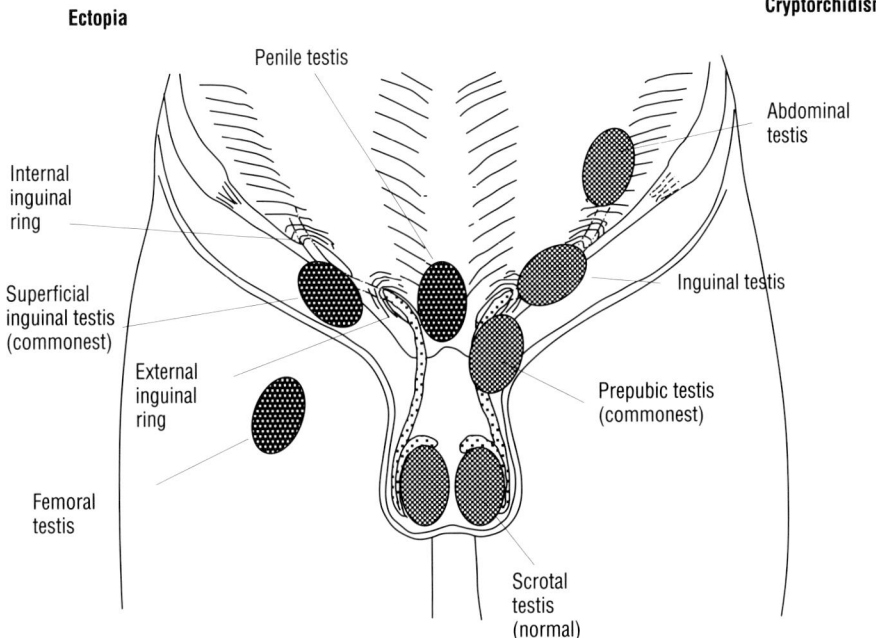

Figure 11.11 *Abnormalities in testicular descent*

long spermatic cord or testicular atrophy also predispose to it and in this second group of aetiologies the condition is commoner in infants and boys. As the testis rotates it causes twisting of the vessels and spermatic cord (see Figure 11.12).

The most serious effect of testicular torsion is obstruction to venous outflow from the testis (the artery having a thicker wall, thus being more difficult to obstruct). Venous obstruction causes red infarction of the testis as no adequate collateral venous drainage is present. Unless the condition is treated almost immediately, necrosis and total loss of function is seen in the affected testis. The tissue becomes necrotic, swollen and haemorrhagic, with enlargement of the affected testis. The condition is likely to recur in the other testis at a later date as the same anatomical or predisposing factors are present that caused the previous episode. Usually, surgical intervention is needed to anchor the testis securely in the scrotum.

Tumours of the Testis

Testicular tumours are rare, accounting for 0.5% of malignancies in males. However, the incidence is increasing slightly in recent years but there is no known, proven aetiological factor that may account for this. Some researchers have suggested that the wearing of tight clothing may contribute to the increase in incidence. The tumours are classified as shown in Table 11.2.

Incidence. Testicular tumours as a group cause approximately 0.2% of cancer deaths. Typically, they affect young and middle-aged men, between 16 and 36 years of age. Embryonal carcinoma and teratoma may be also seen in the first year of life.

Table 11.2 *Testicular tumours*

Germ cell origin (≈ 94%)	Stromal origin (≈ 6%)
Choriocarcinoma (1–2%)	Leydig cell tumour
Embryonal carcinoma (10–20%)	Sertoli cell tumour
Teratoma (10–15%)	Others
Seminoma (≈ 40%)	
Mixed tumours (≈ 40%)	
Others (≈ 1%)	

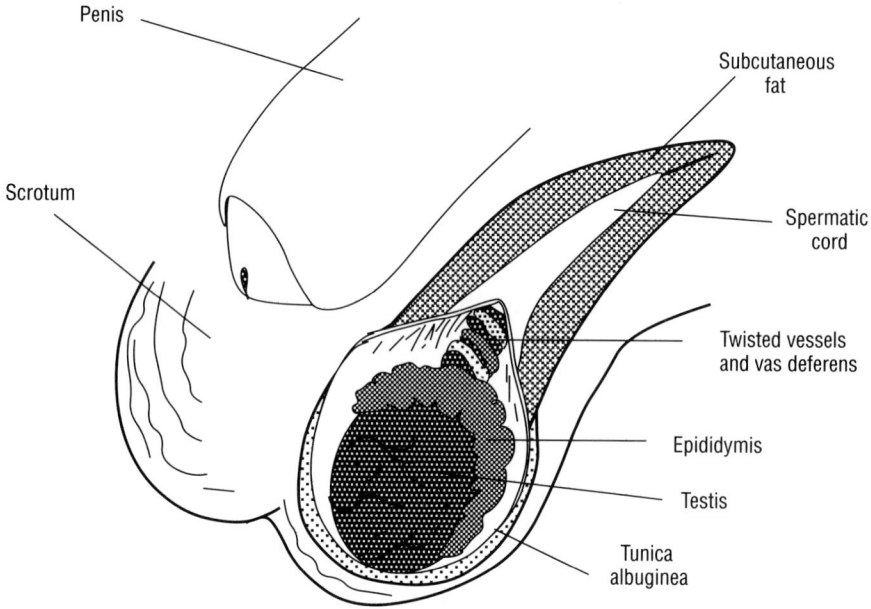

Figure 11.12   *Testicular torsion*

Sites. Mostly unilateral tumours occur, with an equal distribution in the left and right testes. Bilateral tumours are quite rare.

Aetiology. General factors relating to aetiology of all testicular tumours are:

- **Cryptorchidism**, with ≈10% of patients presenting with a testicular tumour having had a maldescended testis. Having an untreated maldescended testis increases a man's risk of developing this tumour 10 to 30 times. It should be noted that successful, early orchidopexy does confer immunity to the tumour.
- **Genetic factors** have been invoked to explain the occurrence of some of the tumours occurring in early life.
- **Racial and geographic factors** are important in some cases. African and USA black people have a lower incidence of the tumours when compared to white people, Jews in particular have a much higher incidence.
- **Hormonal effects** may be important as the tumours develop in the period of greatest sexual activity.

It should be noted that most tumours are idiopathic.

Seminoma of the Testis

Seminoma is a carcinoma of the seminiferous epithe-lium lining the testicular tubules. It is one of the commonest types of testicular tumours, accounting for approximately 40% of all testicular tumours. The typical patient is a young, otherwise healthy adult male who has noticed a painless enlargement of one of his testes.

Macroscopical appearance. Patients present with a uniformly enlarged, painless testis. On section, it is seen that there is diffuse replacement of testicular tissue with lobules of firm, homogeneous, pale pinkish grey masses of tumour. There may be paler, opaque areas of necrosis within the tumour. Characteristically, the tumour has a bulging cut surface.

Microscopical appearance. A very regular, uniform appearance is seen within the tumour mass, groups of regular polyhedral cells with dark nuclei and pale cytoplasm being present. The cells are arranged in lobules or in alveolar formation, no tubules as such seen (Figure 11.13). In about 10% of cases, giant cells may be detected within the tumour, containing human chorionic gonadotrophin (HCG). Usually, the tumour shows a marked lymphocytic infiltration corresponding to the tumour-associated immune response and necrosis may be another notable feature.

Signs and symptoms. Unilateral testicular enlargement

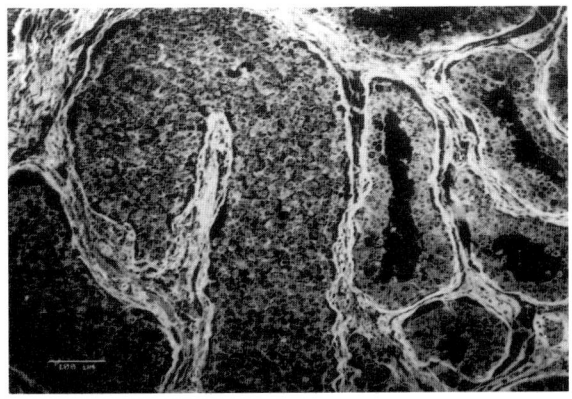

Figure 11.13 *Seminoma of the testis involving the two seminiferous tubules on the left of the micrograph, the remaining tubules being normal (scale bar is 100 μm)*

that is usually painless is the major clinical feature of the tumour, but other non-neoplastic testicular enlargements may also cause such a presentation (e.g. hydrocoele). Gynaecomastia may be seen if the tumour secretes chorionic gonadotrophins. Sometimes the patient complains of mild discomfort or pain if haemorrhage has occurred in the tumour. Metastatic spread is indicated by symptoms and signs referable to non-genital system sites. For example, spread to the lung and surrounding tissues is indicated by coughing and a supraclavicular mass, spread to bowel leads to obstruction and the presence of an abdominal mass. A retroperitoneal mass indicates involvement of the para-aortic lymph nodes. Generalized symptomatology indicative of malignant disease may be present and the patient may be anaemic, easily fatigued, anorexic and have a history of weight loss.

Spread. The tumour first spreads directly to involve the epididymis and spermatic cord. Lymphatic spread then occurs with the tumour invading the para-aortic lymph nodes, approximately 75% of fatal cases showing such involvement. Haematogenous spread occurs late in the course of the disease with metastasis to the lungs and liver, usually.

Treatment and prognosis. The tumour remains confined to the testis in the early stages, the tunica albuginea providing a stout barrier that limits its local spread. Orchidectomy and radiotherapy, therefore, is highly successful in these early stages. In addition, the tumour cells are very radiosensitive and good cure rates

are reported, even in cases where metastases are present. The average 5-year survival for seminoma is 85%.

Teratoma of the Testis

These are tumours showing a disorderly array of partially or completely recognizable foetal or adult tissues. They are thought to arise from dormant foci of embryonal pluripotential cells in the testis. Growth with equal rates of differentiation gives rise to the **organoid tumours**. Such tumours contain regions of recognizable tissues such as skin, thyroid, bone, cartilage, etc. A failure of differentiation results in anaplastic tumours that are very malignant. Teratomata show a range of clinical behaviours, from slowly growing, benign tumours to rapidly growing and metastasizing tumours. In the testis, most teratomata tend to be malignant. Teratoma of the testis is less common than seminoma, accounting for approximately 15% of all testicular tumours. The peak age of incidence is 30 years.

Macroscopical appearance. The tumours may be quite small so as not to produce enlargement of the affected testis. Often, the man may be totally unaware of the tumour until symptoms relating to secondary tumour masses force him to seek medical advice. The cut surface shows a variegated appearance, with regions of necrosis and haemorrhage. Often, cysts may be contained within the tumour mass.

Microscopical appearance. The histological appearance depends on the type of tumour and the degree of differentiation of the tissue cells. The more differentiated a teratoma is, the more benign it is in clinical behaviour. **Teratoma differentiated** (TD) refers to well-differentiated tumours of an organoid nature in which different adult tissues may be recognized. Thyroid, bone, skin, muscle, nervous tissue and cystic spaces may be found in such tumours. **Malignant teratoma intermediate** (MTI) contains incompletely differentiated adult tissues and there is evidence of invasion and infiltration with many cytological indications of malignancy. **Malignant teratoma anaplastic** (MTA) contains sheets of relatively undifferentiated cells with no recognizable adult tissues present, the tumour cells fulfilling all criteria of malignancy. **Malignant teratoma trophoblastic** (MTT) contains elements recognizable as cytotrophoblasts or syncytiotrophoblasts.

Spread. Differentiated teratoma grows initially by expansion and remains confined to the testis, in keeping with its benign clinical classification. Later in its development, after many years of growth, it may spread, even though the metastasis may not be clinically apparent for many years. Direct spread of the malignant forms of the tumour occurs early, with involvement of the testicular tissue, which is destroyed and replaced by tumour cells. Lymphatic spread is not commonly seen with this tumour and pelvic lymph nodes or para-aortic nodes are invaded only infrequently. There is, however, early blood spread with the more malignant types of teratoma, the liver and lungs being most commonly involved.

Treatment and prognosis. Orchidectomy and chemotherapy are the standard ways of dealing with the tumour, but in malignant tumours even early treatment is associated with a rather poor prognosis, an average 5-year survival of 25% to be expected. It should be noted that unlike seminoma, teratoma is not a radiosensitive tumour.

Mixed Tumour of the Testis

In mixed tumour of the testis, distinct areas of both seminomatous and teratomatous tissue exist. In some forms of the tumour, teratomatous and embryonal tumour tissue are admixed. It accounts for approximately 40% of all testicular tumours and it affects men between the ages of 15 to 30 years usually. The teratomatous component most frequently is the predominating tissue and may be of any of the histological types described with teratoma. The other component (seminomatous or embryonal tumour) is discovered only histologically. The treatment is similar to that described for teratoma, but the presence of seminomatous tissue improves the prognosis for the patient, the average 5-year survival being approximately 40%.

Embryonal Carcinoma

Embryonal carcinoma is a very small, highly malignant tumour of undifferentiated cells of the testicular epithelium. The tumours usually arise in infancy and they do not produce marked testicular enlargement. They consist of poorly demarcated, haemorrhagic, infiltrating masses; the cut surface is variegated, being greyish white with patches of dark haemorrhage. Microscopically there is great pleomorphism of cells with much mitotic activity in the flattened, dark cells with large nuclei. Often the cells are in cords, sheets or papillary forms. If the cancer is detected and removed

early, the prognosis is good. If not detected extremely early, survival beyond 1 to 2 years is unusual.

Choriocarcinoma

Choriocarcinoma occurs almost exclusively in men between 20 to 30 years of age but is a very rare disorder accounting for only about 1% of testicular tumours. It is a highly malignant tumour, not very radiosensitive, tending to invade extensively and spread early. Cytotrophoblast and syncytiotrophoblast-like cells are seen in the tumour without villus formation. There is a poor prognosis associated with the cancer.

Interstitial Cell Tumour (Leydig Cell Tumour)

The interstitial cell tumour of the testis is a cancer of the Leydig cells, which secrete androgens. It is a small, spherical, brown, encapsulated tumour. It is a mass composed mostly of well differentiated, functioning cells. The tumours produce hormone and follow a benign course. A very small proportion of tumours are malignant and may even metastasize. If the tumour arises in children, it may cause sexual precocity associated with excessive levels of testosterone production.

Diagnosis of Testicular Neoplasms

Symptoms and signs associated with testicular tumours are an enlargement or change in consistency of the testis, usually painless, although there may be a dull ache in the lower abdomen and groin together with a feeling of heaviness and dragging. Men in the high-risk group for testicular cancer are between the ages of 16 and 36 years and testicular tumours account for 12% of deaths due to cancer in this age group. Early detection of testicular cancer is vital and it is recommended that men perform a monthly, 3-minute **testicular self examination** (TSE, Figure 11.14). The best time for doing this is after a shower or bath when the scrotal skin is supple and most relaxed. If there are any suspicious findings, a doctor should be consulted promptly who will perform the testicular examination and also any other tests that may indicated. The TSE findings described, however, do not necessarily imply that a malignancy is present.

The patient's age may also give an indication as to which tumour is present. For example, an infant is more likely to suffer from embryonal carcinoma or

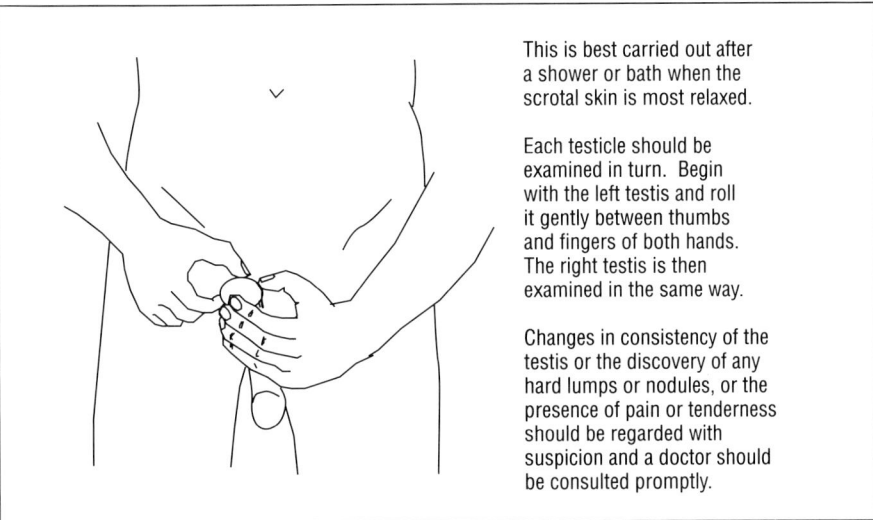

This is best carried out after a shower or bath when the scrotal skin is most relaxed.

Each testicle should be examined in turn. Begin with the left testis and roll it gently between thumbs and fingers of both hands. The right testis is then examined in the same way.

Changes in consistency of the testis or the discovery of any hard lumps or nodules, or the presence of pain or tenderness should be regarded with suspicion and a doctor should be consulted promptly.

Figure 11.14 *Testicular self-examination (TSE)*

teratoma rather than seminoma, which is more likely to be present in young adults. The most frequently seen tumours are seminomata and mixed tumours, which together account for approximately 80% of all testicular tumours, therefore the diagnosis of these tumours occurs more frequently. It was noted also that certain tumours may produce hormones that may lead to effects in the patients with tumours.

Certain researchers have identified elevated levels of tumour marker molecules, which if detected may be regarded as contributing to the diagnosis of testicular tumours. For example, it is known that 100% of choriocarcinomata are associated with raised levels of human chorionic gonadotrophin (HCG). All cases of yolk sac tumours are associated with raised levels of α-foetoprotein (AFP). As many as 90% of patients with embryonal carcinomata or with mixed tumours may have raised HCG or AFP levels. Half of the patients with teratoma have raised HCG or AFP levels. Only 10 to 15% of patients with seminoma, however, have raised HCG levels (Table 11.3).

Sexually Transmitted Diseases

The term 'sexually transmitted diseases' (STDs) has replaced the older term 'venereal diseases' and the euphemism 'social diseases', both of which were used commonly in the past. The common factor uniting all of these infections is that they are transmitted from one

Table 11.3 *Clinical features of testicular tumours*

Tumour	Frequency	Peak age	Markers	Prognosis
Seminoma	40%	16–36 years	10–15% ↑HCG	Excellent
Teratoma	7–10%	Any age	95% ↑HCG or AFP	Poor, better in children
Mixed tumour	40%	15–30 years	90% ↑HCG or AFP	Poor, better than teratoma alone
Embryonal carc.	10–20%	Infancy, 20–30 years	90% ↑HCG	Good in early stages
Choriocarcinoma	1%	20–30 years	100% ↑HCG	Poor if malignant
Yolk sac tumour	1%	3 years	100% ↑AFP	Good in early stages

individual to another during intimate contact. Sexual intercourse in all of its guises is the major way in which STDs are contracted, or alternatively such diseases may be transmitted from an infected mother to her baby as it is being born. It is unusual, although not impossible, for most STDs to be transmitted in ways not involving intimate, sexual contact. A large variety of STDs are known and they may be caused by any of the major groups of micro-organisms: bacteria, viruses, fungi and protozoa.

Bacterial Sexually Transmitted Diseases

Gonorrhoea

This is an infection caused by *Neisseria gonorrhoeae*, a Gram-negative diplococcus. The disease most commonly follows sexual intercourse with an infected person. Non-sexual transmission may be seen in young girls after contact with fomites (linen, towels, etc.). In babies delivered to infected mothers, **ophthalmia neonatorum**, a purulent eye infection due to this organism, often develops. The incubation period for gonorrhoea is 4 to 7 days. Symptoms are more prominent in males and they force the man to seek medical advice: dysuria, frequency of micturition, mucopurulent exudation from the urethra and inflammation of the glans penis are all common findings.

Females may show inflammation of the urethral meatus accompanied by a discharge and dysuria, but frequently the infection is totally asymptomatic. Where anal intercourse or oral sex are practised lesions occur in the rectal mucosa and throat. Left untreated, the disease spreads upwards to involve the genitourinary tract with much tissue destruction, fibrosis and strictures developing. Infertility is a common complication, especially in females. The organism may spread via the bloodstream or lymphatics to give systemic manifestations such as arthritis or mucocutaneous lesions. Diagnosis is based on laboratory culture of the organism, microscopical demonstration of the bacterium in discharge material and, recently, rapid serological tests.

The treatment of the disease is easily accomplished by a single large dose of antibiotics. In the past penicillin was very effective but the emergence of penicillinase-producing *N. gonorrhoeae* (PPNG) has necessitated the use of tetracyclines or erythromycin. Re-infection may be seen upon multiple occasions as little or no immunity is conferred to the individual after infection. Untreated infection in females may lead to the very serious pelvic inflammatory disease (PID, see below under 'Non-gonococcal Urethritis').

Syphilis

Syphilis is an infection caused by *Treponema pallidum*, a spirochaete. The disease is acquired by sexual contact, extremely rarely being contracted via non-sexual means. The organism is capable of crossing the placenta such that a baby may acquire the disease *in utero*. In 80% of cases the lesions are genital whereas in 20% of cases the first lesions are in extra-genital situations such as the anal canal, throat and breasts. The incubation period is 2 to 6 weeks and the disease typically occurs in the following three stages if left untreated.

Stage 1. The **chancre** develops, which is a shallow ulcer with a clean base and hard margins. There is no pain or discharge associated with it unless there is a secondary bacterial infection. The chancre persists for 4 to 6 weeks and then heals spontaneously. The first **latent period** lasts for 4 to 8 weeks, during which the patient shows no signs or symptoms.

Stage 2. This phase of the disease may last for a few weeks or months or up to 5 years. The manifestations of this stage are a coppery red, symmetrical, macular rash which may involve any part of the skin (including soles and palms); mucosal, shallow, painful ulcers with a white base that are teeming with spirochaetes (very infectious!); a generalized lymphadenopathy and an influenza-like syndrome of catarrhal inflammation of the upper respiratory tract. The organisms have by this stage spread all over the body. The **second latent period** then follows and may last for a few months or more, commonly for many years (up to 20). The patient gets less and less infectious with each passing year after the manifestations of the second stage.

Stage 3. The typical lesion of this stage is the **gumma**, a circumscribed, rubbery area of necrosis, firm, yellowish white, surrounded by inflammation and fibrosis. Hypersensitivity responses are important in its formation. Tertiary syphilis has a predilection for the CNS (10% of patients infected will develop neurosyphilis with dementia, etc.); for the cardiovascular system (11% will develop aortitis, dissecting aneurysms, carditis, etc.); with also many other organs being vulnerable (15% of syphilitics show skin, bone and visceral involvement). Only about 20% of untreated syphilitics will eventually recover.

Laboratory diagnosis of syphilis depends on clinical symptomatology, demonstration of the thin, spiral organism in exudates by dark-field illumination microscopy, and also by serology (VDRL, RPR,

Wasserman, Kline tests, etc.). Note that the organism cannot be cultured in the laboratory. The drug of choice in the treatment of syphilis is penicillin and up to 10 million units of penicillin are given over a period of 10 days in daily intramuscular injections. Other antibiotics such as tetracycline and erythromycin are used if allergy to penicillin is a problem.

Chancroid

Chancroid is caused by *Haemophilus ducreyi,* a Gram-negative coccobacillus. There is no relation to syphilis and the syphilitic chancre, other than the superficial resemblance of the primary lesions of the two infections. This infection is more commonly seen in males, especially the less hygienic, and itinerants such as seamen. An asymptomatic carrier state is thought to be possible in women. The incubation period is 3 to 5 days and the lesions develop on the glans and shaft of the penis, or the vulva, perineum, labia, urethra, vagina and cervix.

The typical lesion is a localized, painful, highly contagious genital ulceration with a grey base and undermined soft edges. If the infection is left untreated the organism spreads via the lymphatics to the inguinal lymph nodes, which greatly swell to form **buboes**. The buboes may suppurate, rupture and cause ragged ulceration in the inguinal region. Diagnosis is by demonstration of the organism in exudates, culture in the laboratory and also an intradermal hypersensitivity test may be used. Treatment is by oral administration of long-acting sulphonamides or tetracyclines for 4 to 5 days. Daily intramuscular injections of streptomycin may also be used.

Granuloma Inguinale

Granuloma inguinale is an infection caused by *Calymmatobacterium granulomatis* (*Donovania granulomatis*) a Gram-negative coccobacillus. The initial lesion develops 4 to 6 weeks after infection through sexual contact with another infected individual. It is a painless nodule which soon breaks down to form a sharply demarcated ulcer with a red, granulating base which bleeds easily. The lesions are chronic and may be found on the genitals and perianally. It has been suggested by researchers that the bacterium may be able to inhabit the gall bladder and alimentary tract of carriers and from there find its way to the perineal region and genital tract, thereby infecting sexual contacts.

The lesions are not as painful as those of chancroid

and initially they are small; however, the longer they are left untreated, the larger they become. Untreated cases will show spread of the bacteria to the viscera, granulomatosis and even death occurring. Diagnosis involves biopsy of the lesions under local anaesthesia and demonstration of typical 'Donovan bodies' (bacteria showing a safety-pin appearance within macrophages). The disease is treated with tetracyclines, chloramphenicol or streptomycin. Some degree of scarring will always be seen around the sites of the lesions, its extent determined by the length of time the disease was left untreated.

Lymphopathia Venereum

Lymphopathia venereum is caused by a Group A *Chlamydia*. It is an STD more common in the warmer, tropical climates. *Chlamydia* is a specialized bacterium being only able to grow within living cells. After an incubation period of 1 to 2 weeks, a primary lesion in the form of a small, superficial ulcer on the genitalia develops. This is seldom noticed as it is transient and heals quickly. Shortly afterwards, **buboes** form in the inguinal region as the organism spreads to the lymph nodes in the area. There is suppuration and softening in the bubo with the overlying skin becoming discoloured and adherent to the underlying tissue. Fistulae form and if the vagina and anal canal are involved there will be fibrosis and strictures developing. Elephantiasis of the genitals may occur because of impaired lymph drainage.

Diagnosis is largely by serology, rapid immunofluorescence techniques being used. However, the organism may also be cultured in the laboratory in cell culture, characteristic changes developing in the morphology of the cultured cells. Treatment of this infection is by the administration of sulphonamides or tetracyclines. Drainage of suppurating buboes by aspiration (never by incision) may be required. Ruptured buboes heal very slowly, with a great deal of scarring.

Non-gonococcal Urethritis

This condition is caused by *Chlamydia trachomatis* and the condition in the past was only diagnosed after exclusion of gonorrhoea, hence the term non-gonococcal urethritis (as *Chlamydia* was not known then, it was termed 'non-specific' urethritis). The organisms are spread by sexual contact and many cases remain asymptomatic for long periods of time, especially in females. In the male the infection may cause a urethritis with a serous discharge from the urethra, dysuria and frequency.

If asymptomatic infections in females are left untreated they will cause infections in the upper genital tract with cervicitis, salpingitis, oöphoritis and the spread of the infection into the pelvic peritoneal cavity being especially common, giving rise to **pelvic inflammatory disease** (PID). This complication of the disease is particularly serious as the pelvic abdominal cavity is infected in a chronic, low-grade infection that leads to chronic inflammation and widespread scarring in all of the surrounding tissues. PID is associated with abortions, stillbirths, infant prematurity, ectopic pregnancy, puerperal infections and sterility. Diagnosis is by laboratory culture of the organism or more frequently by serology. Treatment is by administration of tetracyclines.

Mycoplasmosis

This group of infections is another cause of non-gonococcal urethritis ('non-specific' urethritis), caused by T-strains of *Mycoplasma* (= *Ureaplasma*). The organisms are spread by sexual contact and they have a variable incubation period and many cases may remain asymptomatic for long periods of time, especially in females. In the male, the infections may cause a urethritis with a serous discharge from the urethra, dysuria and frequency.

The infection may spread to involve adjacent tissues but this is not usually seen in the male. Untreated cases in females will cause infections in the upper genital tract with salpingitis, oöphoritis and spread of the infection into the pelvic peritoneal cavity being especially common, giving rise to PID, with all the complications discussed above developing also with this infection. Diagnosis is by laboratory culture or by serology. Treatment is by administration of tetracyclines.

Fungal Sexually Transmitted Diseases

Candidiasis (= Moniliasis, 'Thrush')

Candidiasis is caused by *Candida albicans*, a yeast. This is a disease which affects primarily females, males not developing it unless they are immunosuppressed (e.g. AIDS or transplant patients). In the immunocompromised patient serious skin and systemic infections may develop. Although the disease may be sexually transmitted, in most cases the infection develops as a result of endogenous (opportunistic) infection since *Candida* is a member of the normal vaginal, intestinal and oral flora.

The disease will generally not occur unless certain conditions prevail, such as use of inappropriate vaginal douching preparations, administration of antibiotics, immunosuppression, etc., which have the effect of killing off the normal flora of the vagina, allowing the resistant *Candida* to overgrow and cause infection. Candidiasis may also occur in the oral cavity. It is characterized by a burning feeling, itching and discomfort and a white vaginal discharge with a characteristic 'beery' smell. On the vaginal wall or oral mucosa white pseudomembranes will form.

Untreated cases, especially in the debilitated or immunosuppressed, may be very serious as the organism may spread into the bloodstream (candidaemia) and cause systemic, life threatening infections. The disease is diagnosed through clinical symptomatology and laboratory culture of the organism. Treatment of the infection is with local nystatin ointment applications or systemic amphotericin B administration.

Protozoal Sexually Transmitted Diseases

Trichomoniasis

Trichomoniasis is caused by the flagellated protozoön *Trichomonas vaginalis*. This is one of the commonest causes of infection in the female genital tract. Males are also affected but they infrequently have symptoms, most males being asymptomatic carriers. The infection is spread by sexual contact but as the organism survives for considerable periods of time in fomites it may also be spread indirectly, through sharing of linen, towels, etc.

Symptoms in the female include itching, a burning feeling in the vaginal region, and a profuse, creamy yellow, frothy discharge with a penetrating, disagreeable odour. The organism colonizes the vagina, urethra, bladder and Bartholin's glands. In the male there may be urethritis, prostatitis and cystitis. Diagnosis is by clinical symptomatology and demonstration of the highly motile organism in the fresh discharge by dark-field microscopy. Treatment is by oral administration of tabrine HCl or metronidazole, both partners being treated simultaneously, even in the absence of symptoms in the male. As the infection may spread indirectly, other members of the household may be treated at the same time.

Amoebiasis and Gay Bowel Syndrome

Amoebiasis is an infection caused by *Entamoeba histolytica*, especially seen in male homosexuals or heterosexuals where anal intercourse is practised. Amoebiasis is part of the so-called 'gay bowel syndrome' in which amoebae and other intestinal flora organisms and pathogens are spread by anal sexual practices, causing gastroenteritis. Amoebiasis is particularly serious as dysentery develops and amoebic colitis with quite severe symptoms may ensue.

Diagnosis is by clinical symptomatology and patient history and also by demonstration of the organisms or their cysts in faecal material. Culture of faeces may be necessary in order to identify other bacterial pathogens such as *Shigella* or *Salmonella*. In male homosexuals who are infected with HIV there may be very serious intestinal infections causing severe diarrhoea and organisms such as the yeast *Candida* or the protozoön *Cryptosporidium* may be demonstrated.

Viral Sexually Transmitted Diseases

Herpes Genitalis

Genital herpes is an infection with the Herpes simplex virus, type II (HSV II). This infection is becoming increasingly more common and is important as it may also cause congenital and perinatal infections, as well as sexually transmitted disease. The incubation period is 3 to 7 days, symptoms beginning insidiously with a rash, minor itching and discomfort in the genital region. Clusters of blister-like vesicles then form which break open and ulcerate within 24 to 48 hours. The perianal skin, labia, vulva, vaginal and cervical mucosa are affected in females and in males the shaft and glans of the penis.

The lesions are exquisitely painful and usually force the patient to seek medical advice. Systemic manifestations such as headaches and malaise are not uncommon. In the first attack the lesions persist for 3 to 6 weeks with complete healing and no scarring seen afterwards. Subsequent attacks heal more rapidly and the lesions are not as painful as the first attack. The average patient has about four to five attacks in the first year of infection and two to three attacks in the subsequent years. During the period of latency, the virus is dormant and cannot be demonstrated as it ascends the nerve endings innervating the affected area. During the active phase of the disease, the infection is highly contagious and a woman may be unaware that she is infecting her partner as the lesions may be cervical and therefore not readily seen.

Although herpes is a disease without a permanent cure and affected people carry the virus for life, it may be treated symptomatically by analgesic preparations which minimize the pain and also with topical antivi-

ral preparations such as 'acyclovir' which reduce the extent of the lesions and promote a more rapid healing. Diagnosis is by clinical symptomatology and also by laboratory culture of the virus in cell cultures or embryonated eggs. In females, the infection has been linked with carcinoma of the cervix while in males no serious complications have been observed.

Molluscum Contagiosum

This is an infection caused by an unclassified member of the poxvirus group. Infections caused by this virus have been recorded as occurring through sexual transmission but also indirectly, the virus spreading by casual contact or by fomites. The infection is characterized by the development of small, wart-like papules which often have a central depression. The lesions are found on the genitals and perianal areas. They are removed by cauterization with phenol or carbon dioxide snow. Healing is rapid and no scarring occurs. In HIV-infected patients the lesion may be extensive and quite difficult to eradicate.

Condylomata Acuminata (= Genital Warts)

Genital warts are caused by strains of the same virus that causes warts elsewhere in the body (human papilloma virus — HPV). The virus is transmitted by sexual intercourse but it may also be spread by autoinoculation. The warts are pink to red in colour, moist and soft, and may be quite large in size with a diameter of several centimetres. Clusters of the warts may resemble cauliflower-like masses, which are very disfiguring, causing most patients to seek medical advice.

Genital warts are removed by application of 10 to 25% podophyllum resin tincture in benzoin or by other cauterization techniques. If left untreated, the warts may become necrotic and disappear, however, they may recur. Surgical removal may be performed in the case of large, complicated lesions. In females, the condition has been linked with carcinoma of the cervix.

Cytomegalovirus Infection

It is suspected that cytomegalovirus may be spread sexually as it is shed in semen and cervical secretions of infected persons. Infection with the virus produces an acute, febrile illness, not unlike infectious mononucleosis (glandular fever). Hepatitis and pneumonitis due to the virus may also be seen. Infection is followed by depression of the immune system, making patients susceptible to other infections. It causes very problematic congenital transplacental infections in infected mothers who pass the virus to the foetus, resulting in major malformations and defects in heart, brain and other organs. In the HIV-infected patient, cytomegalovirus superinfection is an almost invariable finding.

Hepatitis

Hepatitis caused by hepatitis B virus (HBV) may be a sexually transmitted disease in the cases where anal sexual practices are carried out, with damage to the anal mucosa and spread of the virus into the bloodstream, causing a serious hepatitis. The importance of carriers of the virus should be kept in mind as these people look well and have no symptoms but harbour the virus and may spread it to others. Hepatitis B is a potentially fatal disease, with cirrhosis and hepatocarcinoma being important complications (refer to the chapter on hepatobiliary disorders).

AIDS

AIDS is a disease caused by the human immunodeficiency virus (HIV) and this disorder has already been discussed (refer to the chapter on immune system disorders).

Are Sexually Transmitted Diseases Curable?

Except for genital herpes, AIDS and hepatitis B (carrier state), all venereal diseases are curable with antibiotics and treatments that are not painful or unpleasant. Free clinics for all patients with sexually transmitted diseases are situated in most major cities and towns. For example, in Melbourne, such a clinic is the *Melbourne Sexual Health Centre*, 580 Swanston Street, Carlton, Vic 3053 (telephone: (03) 347 0244).

No appointment or doctor's letter is necessary. All consultations are confidential. One may also go to any medical practitioner, or to the casualty section of any public hospital. If symptoms of any STD develop, or if a partner has symptoms, then

- stop sexual activity while either partner is possibly infectious;
- seek diagnosis and treatment; and
- inform partner(s), who should seek treatment.

In conclusion it should be noted that:

- prevention is better than cure of an STD;
- there is increased risk of infection associated with an increase in the number of partners;
- there is increased risk of infection if a new partner has had several partners previously;
- the chances of catching any of these conditions is greatly reduced by the use of condoms.

Therefore, it is important that **safe sex practices** should be carried out in all casual sexual encounters and during the early stages of new relationships. Condoms should be used even if the contraceptive pill is being used. A condom should be used whenever genital contact is likely to occur. Women who are sexually active should have regular genital system examinations and have Papanicolaou smears performed and evaluated.

Revision Questions and Case Studies

Male Genital System

1. Write an essay in which you compare and contrast the pathology of nodular prostatic hyperplasia and primary prostatic carcinoma.
2. Discuss the pathology of prostatitis.
3. What are the complications of prostatic carcinoma?
4. Nodular prostatic hyperplasia is a very common disease in Australia. Discuss its pathology under the following headings: incidence; sites affected; aetiological factors; pathogenesis; morphology; clinical features; complications; diagnosis; treatment and prognosis.
5. Discuss congenital disorders of the male genital system.
6. What are the commonest testicular neoplasms? Discuss the pathology of any two of these tumours.
7. Describe the procedure of testicular self-examination (TSE) and the significance of this procedure in early detection of testicular disorders.
8. What are the characteristics of penile carcinoma?
9. Write an essay on the pathology of seminoma.
10. Discuss the pathology of any three non-neoplastic testicular enlargements.
11. Discuss the complications of nodular prostatic hyperplasia with special reference to the urinary tract.
12. What is orchitis? What are the commonest causes of this condition? What are the sequelae and complications?

13. Compare and contrast:
    (a) Teratoma of the testis
    (b) Teratoma of the ovary
14. Differentiate between the different types of prostatic enlargement.
15. How may carcinoma of the prostate cause bone disease? Give the expected results of blood and plasma tests that are commonly carried out in conjunction with other examinations in the diagnosis of such disease.
16. Discuss the spread of carcinoma of the prostate and indicate treatment of the tumour in relation to its spread.
17. Discuss the symptoms and signs associated with nodular prostatic hyperplasia, explaining these in relation to the pathological changes in the gland and related tissues.
18. Write short notes on any four of the following:
    (a) Hypoplasia of the testis
    (b) Orchidopexy
    (c) Epispadias and hypospadias
    (d) Phimosis and paraphimosis
    (e) Peyronie's disease
19. What is erythroplasia of Queyrat?
20. Write brief notes on three, commonly occurring malignant tumours seen in the male.

Case study 1. A 22-year-old Caucasian man presents at his doctor's clinic complaining of 'feeling unwell and having slight abdominal pains and discomfort just like indigestion'. Lately, he has been sweating much at night, has suffered from headaches, feels tired a lot of the time and has suffered from diarrhoea for the past 2 weeks. Examination shows a rather thin, pale man, 1.82 m tall, weighing 60 kg. The blood pressure is 170/80 mmHg, pulse rate is 79 per minute. Physical examination shows lymphadenomegaly of the cervical and axillary nodes. The chest is normal and the abdomen shows a liver which is firm but not enlarged. There is jaundice evident, especially visible in the sclerae of his eyes. Liver tests are ordered and the laboratory report states:

Liver function test results:
Mr Rohan H. 6/1/93   Our Ref/N°: DF27857

Serum conjugated and unconjugated bilirubin: Elevated
Urine bilirubin: Elevated
Serum alkaline phosphatase: 1200 mmol/s/L
Serum 5'-nucleotidase: Elevated
Serum aspartate aminotransferase: 540 mmol/s/L
Serum alanine aminotransferase: 500 mmol/s/L

All other values well within normal range

On questioning the man further he says that he is homosexual, but has had a stable, monogamous relationship for the past year and he feels that he does not have to practice 'safe sex'. Neither the man nor his partner are drug users.

(a) What is the most likely diagnosis for the man's condition?
(b) What other diseases should be considered (differential diagnosis)?
(c) How are all of these diseases transmitted in relation to this case?
(d) What advice should be given to the man?

Case study 2. A 72-year-old Caucasian male presents at your clinic because he has had some problems with lower back pain which seems to be getting progressively worse over the past week. On questioning, he admits to suffer also from urinary frequency and dysuria. Lately, he tells you, he has had to get up two or three times a night 'to go and water the horses'. Asked about micturition he says that it's rather difficult to start and stop the urinary stream and lately, although he feels the urge to urinate, he fails to produce much urine once he goes to the toilet. Asked about joint and bone problems he tells that he has been diagnosed with 'ossyarthitis' in the knees and hip joints and this gives him some pain and discomfort, limiting his mobility and range of activities but he 'still manages to do a lot of gardening' (he used to be a gardener and he invites you to visit his garden at home, telling you 'it's the best garden in the street'). A rectal examination of the prostate gland yields the finding of an enlarged, elastic or rather rubbery gland, uniform in consistency.

(a) What are the differential diagnoses?
(b) What is the presumptive diagnosis if serum acid phosphatase levels are well within normal levels?
(c) What advice should be given to the man?
(e) What is the treatment of the condition and what is the prognosis?

Case study 3. A 73-year-old Caucasian male presents at his osteopath's clinic with persistent back pain which has been troubling him for the past 2 weeks. On examination he is seen to be 182 cm tall, weighing 71 kg. He appears a little pale and says that lately, it appears he gets tired very easily. When asked whether he has any trouble passing urine or whether he passes urine often, he remarks that 'the waterworks are A-OK, no trouble at all'. The man is married with five adult children, is a non-smoker but drinks about 2 bottles of beer per day. He is a retired iron foundry worker. Abdominal examination and chest examination show no abnormalities. A digital rectal examination shows a craggy mass in the area of the prostate with no evidence of the medial sulcus of the gland posteriorly. A plain film radiograph of the lumbar spine and pelves demonstrated multiple focal areas of osteoblastic lesions. Subsequently a blood sample tested for acid phosphatase levels yielded a value of 5.5 IU/L.

(a) What is the diagnosis?
(b) Explain the clinical presentation of the patient in relation to the pathological features of the condition.
(c) What are the predisposing factors for the development of this condition?
(d) Outline the various forms of treatment of this condition.
(e) What is the prognosis for this patient?

Case study 4. A 24-year-old Caucasian male visits his doctor's surgery as lately he has noticed that his left testis has enlarged appreciably and on palpation he can feel a firm mass within it. He mentions that there is no pain associated with the condition but in the last week he could elicit some tenderness on palpation. These observations are confirmed by the doctor's examination. The man is 195 cm tall, weighing 75 kg. He looks anaemic and says that for the past three months he is fatigued easily and 'has lost some weight'. When questioned about his enlarged testis, he says that he has been aware of the enlargement for the past six weeks but did not present earlier as he thought 'it was not serious because it was not painful'. Abdominal examination reveals small, palpable retroperitoneal masses, but otherwise normal findings while chest examination shows no abnormalities. The man lives in a *de facto* relationship and he has a 2-year-old daughter. On questioning, he reveals that he has been treated for a maldescended testis in his infancy, but he can provide no further details as both his parents perished in a house fire when he was 16 years old.

(a) What is the diagnosis?
(b) What are the predisposing factors for the development of this condition and how do they relate to the patient in this case?
(c) How is this patient treated?
(d) What is the prognosis for this patient?

Sexually Transmitted Diseases

1. Write a brief description of the gamut of changes occurring in the body in infection with *Treponema pallidum*. Assume that no treatment occurs at any stage of the disease.

2. Discuss the microbiology/pathology of gonorrhoea.
3. Discuss the various manifestations of the various congenital disorders that may be seen in association with the various sexually transmitted diseases.
4. Discuss the factors associated with cervical carcinoma with special reference to the sexually transmitted diseases that may be involved with the disease.
5. What are the complications of untreated chlamydial infections in the female?
6. Review the diagnosis and treatment procedures that are in use for any five, commonly occurring sexually transmitted diseases.
7. Define the following terms:
    (a) Donovan body
    (b) Bubo
    (c) Gumma
    (d) Fomite
    (e) Chancre
8. What is meant by the term 'gay bowel syndrome'?
9. Compare and contrast the conditions of granuloma inguinale and lymphopathia venereum.
10. Discuss genital herpes with special reference to the chronic nature of the infection and the underlying mechanisms associated with this.
11. Write short notes on any four of the following:
    (a) Rashes associated with sexually transmitted diseases
    (b) Vaginal thrush and its complications in the immunocompromised patient
    (c) Ulcers associated with sexually transmitted diseases
    (d) Systemic complications of sexually transmitted diseases
    (e) Important complications of sexually acquired hepatitis B infection
12. Can any of the sexually transmitted diseases also be transmitted by other means? If so, what are the diseases and what are the different modes of transmission?
13. Write brief notes on the three most commonly occurring sexually transmitted diseases seen in our society.
14. Give the name of the causative agent associated with the following infections and specify what type of microbe it is and how the infections are diagnosed.
    (a) Gonorrhoea
    (b) Syphilis
    (c) Candidiasis
    (d) Molluscum contagiosum infection
    (e) Non-gonococcal urethritis
    (f) Hepatitis

(g) Lymphopathia venereum

(h) Lymphogranuloma inguinale

15. List important complications of untreated syphilitic infections.

Case study 1. A 24-year-old Caucasian woman presents at her doctor's surgery with the following symptoms: dysuria, frequency of micturition and a feeling of urethral irritation. On examination it is observed that the urethral meatus is inflamed and that the inguinal lymph nodes are slightly enlarged and tender. There is no evidence of ulceration on the vulva, vagina or cervix. A serous exudate is expressed from the urethral meatus and this is sent to the laboratory for isolation of pathogens. The woman is not married but says that she has started a new relationship with a boyfriend, first seeing him 5 months ago. The laboratory request slip and report is shown on p. 440.

(a) What is the most likely causative agent of the woman's infection ?

(b) What are the complications of untreated infections in women?

(c) What steps need to be taken in treating this woman?

(d) What other steps need to be taken?

Case study 2. An 18-year-old Caucasian male presents at the sexually transmitted diseases clinic because he has had a sore throat and also dysuria during the past two days. Examination of the genitals revealed an inflamed glans penis but no exudate was apparent, nor could any be milked from the urethra. A shallow, painless ulcer with a red base approximately 1.0 cm in diameter was found in the perianal region and colonoscopy showed another similar ulceration in the posterior wall of the rectal mucosa. Examination of the mouth and throat showed the presence of a non-purulent pharyngitis and a shallow ulcer approximately 0.8 cm in diameter was found in the tonsillar region. The base of this tonsillar ulcer was covered by inflammatory debris and exudate, beneath which was a small collection of pus.

On questioning, the man says that he is a homosexual and he has been sexually active for the past 10 months. During that time he has had multiple sex partners and has practised 'unsafe sex' on many occasions.

(a) What is the presumptive diagnosis and which features of the case support your presumptions?

(b) What other sexually transmitted diseases should be considered as being present in a case like this?

(c) What laboratory investigations are to be ordered?

(d) What advice should be given to the man?

Case study 3. A 32-year-old Caucasian female presents at her doctor's surgery with extremely painful lesions on her vulva. Examination reveals several clusters of small, raised ulcers on the labia majora and some on the labia minora. Similar lesions are seen to be present on the cervical mucosa upon colposcopy. The woman is living in a *de facto* relationship with a man, whom she claims as her only sexual partner. She believes that the man is faithful to her.

(a) What is the diagnosis?

(b) Assuming that the woman is telling the truth what is the source of the infection?

(c) What is the treatment for the woman?

(d) What are the complications of this infection in women?

(e) How is the man treated?

Case study 4. A 26-year-old West Indian sailor is received into the Venereal Diseases Clinic in Little Lonsdale Street and is examined as he is suffering from a sexually transmitted disease. When the inguinal area is examined it is found that the inguinal lymph nodes on both sides have formed buboes and the superficial lower right node is showing softening with discolouration of the overlying skin. During the examination this bubo ruptures and discharges several millilitres of viscid pus which is taken for laboratory investigation. There are no lesions on the shaft or glans of the penis, but the testes appear to be oedematous and enlarged. No lesions are found in the perineal region and colonoscopy shows a normal rectal mucosa. Questioning the man it is ascertained that he is bisexual, with his last sexual contact being 3 weeks ago in Haiti, with a female prostitute. The man first became aware of his infection when the buboes appeared in his groin several days ago.

(a) What is the differential diagnosis?

(b) What is the most likely presumptive diagnosis and which features of the case prompted you to come to this conclusion?

(c) What is the causative agent and how does the laboratory identify this agent?

(d) What is the treatment for this infection?

Case study 5. A 23-year-old Caucasian woman and her husband present at their doctor's surgery, the woman complaining of itching, discomfort and a burning sensation in the vulva accompanied by a creamy yellow, foetid, viscid vaginal discharge. The husband is free from any symptoms and signs of sexually transmitted disease. The couple assure the doctor that they have not engaged in extramarital sex. They share a house with the woman's brother and his wife. Dark-ground

UNIT N°: WARD N°:	PATIENT'S ADMITTANCE N°: F 94/42
Preston Medical Centre	PATIENT'S NAME:
NATURE OF SPECIMEN: Urethral exudate	Ms C. Uren
TEST REQUIRED: Microscopy, Culture & abiogram	REQUIRED FOR: SURVEILLANCE: ☐ DIAGNOSIS: ✓	PATIENT'S SEX: MALE ☐ FEMALE ✓ PATIENT'S AGE: 24 years

DATE: 4·2·94	DATE AND TIME SPECIMEN WAS COLLECTED:
SIGNATURE: N Vau	4·2·94 9:30am

RELEVANT HISTORY (INCLUDE ANY MEDICATION PATIENT IS TAKING):

Dysuria, frequency for 2 days. Lymphadenomegaly of inguinal lymph nodes. Exudate non-purulent, milked from urethra

DO NOT WRITE BENEATH THIS LINE

MICROSCOPY OF SPECIMEN RESULTS:	CULTURE RESULTS:
Gram stain showed scanty polymorphs and a few Gram +ve rods and cocci. No erythrocytes were present.	Normal flora was isolated. ?Non-gonococcal urethritis? D. Mc

ANTIBIOGRAM RESULTS:

No antibiogram was performed

microscopy of the vaginal discharge reveals multiple, large, nucleated, flagellated, motile organisms.

(a) What is the diagnosis?
(b) What steps are taken in the treatment?
(c) Is there any way to prevent the infection from recurring?

Case study 6. A 26-year-old Aboriginal female just recovered from a serious respiratory infection complains to her doctor that she has a burning sensation upon micturition and itching in the genital region. She has also noticed a vaginal discharge. Examination of the genitals shows that the vulva is inflamed and that patches of a white, pseudomembrane have formed on the vaginal walls. The white material is quite thick in texture and has a distinctive, sour odour. The cervical area is inflamed, but no erosions or ulcers are seen on colposcopy.

(a) What is the aetiology and pathogenesis of the woman's infection?
(b) What are the complications of this infection if it is inadequately treated?
(c) How is the diagnosis confirmed by the laboratory?

Case study 7. A 22-year-old Caucasian female who is in the second trimester of her first pregnancy presents at her gynaecologist's surgery complaining of a sore throat and difficulty in swallowing. Examination of the throat reveals a pharyngitis with purulent exudate over the tonsillar areas, with the uvula greatly inflamed and swollen. No abnormal findings are seen in the vulva, vagina, cervix and anal region during the routine gynaecological examination. The woman is not aware of her husband engaging in extramarital sexual activity and he is described by the woman as 'perfectly healthy'. A throat swab is taken and a Gram stain of the purulent material shows many neutrophils with many intracellular Gram-negative diplococci, many free Gram-negative cocci and diplococci and a few Gram-positive streptococci. The woman is allergic to penicillin.

(a) What is the diagnosis?
(b) How is the diagnosis confirmed?
(c) What steps are to be taken in the treatment and how is the infection in the woman to be treated?

Further Reading

Aral SO, Holmes KK. 'Sexually Transmitted Diseases in the AIDS Era.' Sci Am 1991; February: 18.

Bartsch G, *et al.* 'Testicular Torsion: Late Results with Special Regard to Fertility and Endocrine Function.' *J Urol* 1980; **124**: 375.

Benditt J. 'The Syphilized World.' *Sci Am* 1989; March: 16.

Bostwick DG. *Pathology of the Prostate*, 1990; Churchill Livingstone, Edinburgh.

Chisholm GD. 'Benign Prostatic Hyperplasia: The Best Treatment.' *BMJ* 1989; **299**: 215.

Coffey DS, Walsh PC. 'Clinical and Experimental Sudies of Benign Prostatic Hyperplasia.' *Urol Clin N Am* 1990; **17**: 461.

Concato J, *et al.* 'Problems of Comorbidity in Mortality after Prostatectomy.' *J Am Med Assoc* 1992; **267**: 1077.

Cos LR, Cockett ATK. 'Genitourinary Tuberculosis Revisited.' *Urology* 1982; **20**: 111.

Davies J. 'The Genetics of Gonococcal Variation and Virulence.' *Today's Life Sci* 1990; **2**(1): 12.

Farram E, Mearns G, Smithyman A. 'Diagnosis of Chlamydia.' *Today's Life Sci* 1990; **2**(12): 24.

Fitzpatrick DR, Bielefeldt-Ohmann H, Gardner ID. 'Immune Responses to *Chlamydia trachomatis* Infections.' *Today's Life Sci* 1990; **2**(12): 18.

Gittes RF. 'Carcinoma of the Prostate.' *New Eng J Med* 1991; **324**: 236.

Guess HA. 'Vasectomy and Prostate Cancer.' *Am J Epidemiol* 1990; **132**: 1062.

Mills J, Masur H. 'AIDS-Related Infections.' *Sci Am* 1990; August: 32.

Richardson JD. 'Male Sexuality.' *Aust J Med* 1989; 155: 687.

Riley PA, Sutton PM. 'Why are Ovarian Teratomas Benign whilst Teratomas of the Testis Malignant?' *Lancet* 1975; **1**: 1360.

Rosenberg L, *et al.* 'Vasectomy and the Risk of Prostate Cancer.' *Am J Epidemiol* 1990; **132**: 1051.

Ross RK, *et al.* '5-alpha-reductase Activity and Risk of Prostate Cancer among Japanese and US White and Black Males.' *Lancet* 1992; **339**: 887.

Williams SD, *et al.* 'Disseminated Testicular Cancer: Current Chemotherapy Strategies.' *Sem Oncol* 1989; **16**(Suppl 6): 105.

12

Female Genital System Disorders

The Normal Female Genital System

The female genital tract is separate from the urinary system, and is more complex in its function and more dependent on changing hormonal stimulation than is the male system. The female genital tract undergoes complex cyclical changes during the reproductive years of the woman. Pregnancy also causes and is dependent upon various fluctuations of hormonal levels, initiated by fertilization and growth of the conceptus.

The normal female genital system comprises the **ovaries**, **Fallopian tubes**, **uterus** and **vagina** (see Figure 12.1). It is usual to also include the **female breast** in the genital system as profound changes occur in this tissue with pregnancy and parturition. However, it should be remembered that breast glands are modified sweat glands and therefore part of the skin. Disorders of pregnancy are also considered in the pathology of the female genital tract.

The ovaries lie on each side of the uterus on the lateral wall of the pelvic cavity. They are ovoid, exocrine and endocrine glands about 4 cm in length. The

surface of the ovary is a specialized layer of reflected peritoneum, termed the germinal epithelium. One margin of the ovary is attached to the mesoövarium, which in turn attaches to the broad ligament. The attached ovarian border is the hilus, where blood vessels enter and leave the organ. The cortex of the ovary contains the ova in follicles of various stages of development and different sizes. It also contains the remnants of discharged follicles, the corpora lutea (important hormone secretors of ovulation and pregnancy); degenerating remains of corpora lutea, which are the fibrous corpora albicantia, and also atretic follicles. The medulla is looser and more vascular than the cortex and communicates with the mesoövarium. Oestrogen is secreted by the theca interna cells surrounding the ovarian follicles, and also by the corpus luteum. Progesterone is secreted by the granulosa lutein cells of the corpus luteum. The ovary is dependent on pituitary gonadotrophic hormones for normal function.

The Fallopian tube, or oviduct, is the tube that conveys the ovum from the ovary to the uterine lumen. It courses from the ovary to the uterus in a fold of peritoneum. The mesosalpinx attaches the tube to the broad ligament. It is about 11 cm long and it does not attach

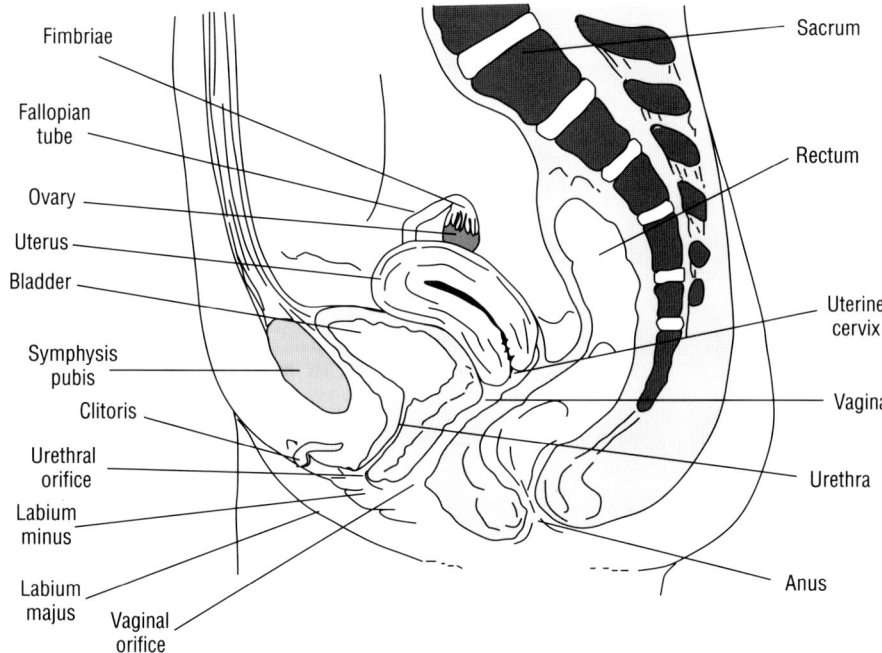

Fimbriae
Fallopian tube
Ovary
Uterus
Bladder
Symphysis pubis
Clitoris
Urethral orifice
Labium minus
Labium majus
Vaginal orifice
Sacrum
Rectum
Uterine cervix
Vagina
Urethra
Anus

Figure 12.1 *The normal female reproductive system*

to the ovary. The portion of the oviduct closest to the ovary, the infundibulum, has fringes, the fimbriae, that surround the ovary like the bell of a trumpet. The ampulla is the main part of the tube and the isthmus is the part that connects with the uterus and enters the myometrium to form the intramural portion of the tube. The Fallopian tube serves as the location for the meeting of the spermatozoa and ova and fertilization occurs in the ampulla of this organ. The infundibulum of the oviduct is open and is a potential portal of infection into the peritoneal cavity (e.g. PID).

The uterus occupies a site between the urinary bladder and rectum, and is retained in position by the round and broad ligaments on each side. It is a pear-shaped organ about 8 cm long with a thick smooth muscle wall, the myometrium, and a hollow lumen lined by the endometrium, a mucus-secreting epithelium. The serosa of the organ is termed the perimetrium. The uterus is divided into the fundus, corpus and cervix, the last-mentioned region opening into the vagina and projecting a short distance into it. The function of the uterus is to receive and rear the fertilized ovum within its lumen. It allows for nourishment and protection of the embryo while it is growing, and at the proper time will expel the fully developed foetus. The uterus undergoes changes during the life of a woman and these changes are dependent on many hormones and on whether or not pregnancy occurs.

Prepubertally, the uterus is small and covered by a thin, invariable mucosa. At the time of puberty, the increasing levels of ovarian oestrogen will cause enlargement of the organ and progesterone secretion will begin the functioning of the organ. The beginning of menstruation is termed **menarche** and in the last few decades menarche has been occurring at an earlier age that it has previously. The end of the woman's reproductive period is termed **menopause** and this may occur at any time after the woman is in her mid-forties. Menopause has also been delayed in the last few decades, women nowadays having a much longer reproductive life than they had at any period in the past. This is thought to be due to improved standards of living, better nutrition and public health.

The menstrual cycle occurs on average every 28 days, and anticipates the possibility of pregnancy once every month, serving to prepare the mucosa of the uterus as a suitable surface on which the fertilized ovum will implant (refer to Figure 12.2). The phases of proliferation seen in the uterine mucosa post-menstrually are orchestrated by the secretion of oestrogen. The secretory changes of the endometrium, seen in the post-ovulatory period, are directed by the luteal hormone, progesterone. If fertilization occurs and pregnancy follows, the egg implants at this fa-

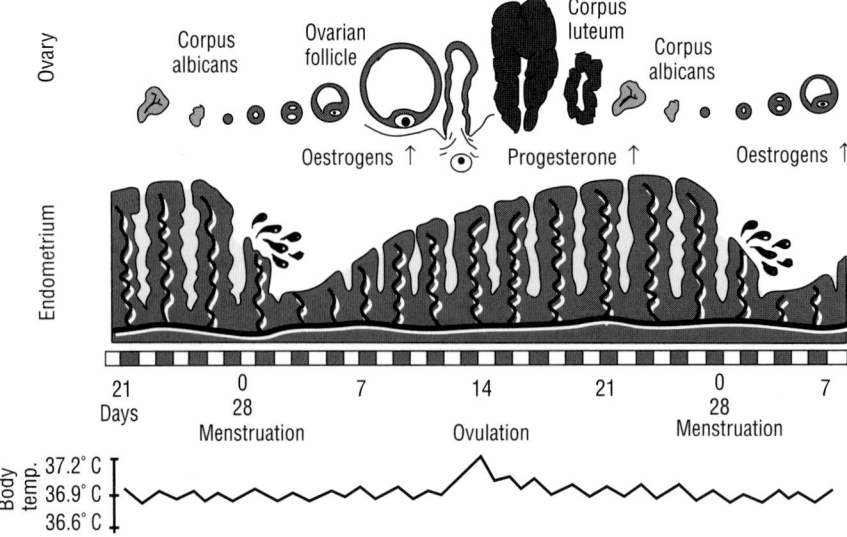

Figure 12.2 *The menstrual cycle*

vourable time of secretion, between days 15 to 27 of the cycle. If pregnancy does not occur, the corpus luteum begins to degenerate and does not secrete any hormone. The endometrium then begins to undergo ischaemia on the last day of the cycle and menstruation begins the cycle from days 1 to 4, as the endometrial functional layer, which has undergone ischaemic necrosis, is sloughed off.

In the face of continuing pregnancy the corpus luteum of pregnancy develops, growing in size and cell mass, continuing its secretion of hormone, which will continue to stimulate the endometrium. The hormone-stimulated mucosa of the uterus then becomes the thick decidua of pregnancy. Part of the decidua develops into the maternal portion of the placenta. The major portion of the placenta and all of the membranes surrounding the developing embryo are tissues that are embryonic in origin. The placenta is the organ responsible for functioning as a lung, food intake system and kidney for the foetus during intrauterine life. The trophoblasts of the placenta secrete chorionic gonadotrophin (whose presence in the urine is detected by several simple pregnancy test kits) while the syncytiotrophoblasts secrete oestrogen and progesterone. The placenta also functions as a barrier against micro-organisms, only a very few highly specialized microbes being able to cross it. Fat, blood proteins and other large molecular size substances need to be broken down into smaller fragments in order to cross the placental barrier. Certain small drug molecules can cross the placenta and influence adversely the devel-

oping embryo; their effects are termed **teratogenic**, as they cause congenital defects in the foetus. Such drugs are not administered during pregnancy.

The vagina is a fibromuscular sheath, lined by a folded mucosa, and functions as the copulatory organ in the female, being also the birth canal through which the baby is born. Its fundus is continuous with the uterine cervix while its lower end is bounded by the hymen, a transverse fold of the mucosa that is annular and separates the vagina from the vestibule. The vagina is lined by non-keratinized, stratified squamous epithelium. Mucus for the lubrication of the vagina is produced by the cervical glands as the vagina itself does not possess any. The epithelium in the postpubertal female contains variable amounts of glycogen, the amount depending on hormonal factors. The high oestrogen peak just before ovulation causes the glycogen concentration to be highest then. Glycogen is fermented to lactic acid by normal flora bacteria in the vagina and thus keeps the pH low, preventing infection by pathogens.

The external female genitalia comprising the clitoris, labia minora, labia majora and associated glands are known collectively as the vulva (refer to Figure 12.3). The vestibule in the female is a shallow urogenital sinus that corresponds to the male urethral meatus. The vestibule contains the urethral opening and the vaginal opening and is surrounded by the labia minora, forming two lateral walls consisting of a thin fold of mucosal membrane, devoid of hair or fat. The clitoris is an elongated ridge culminating in a small glans,

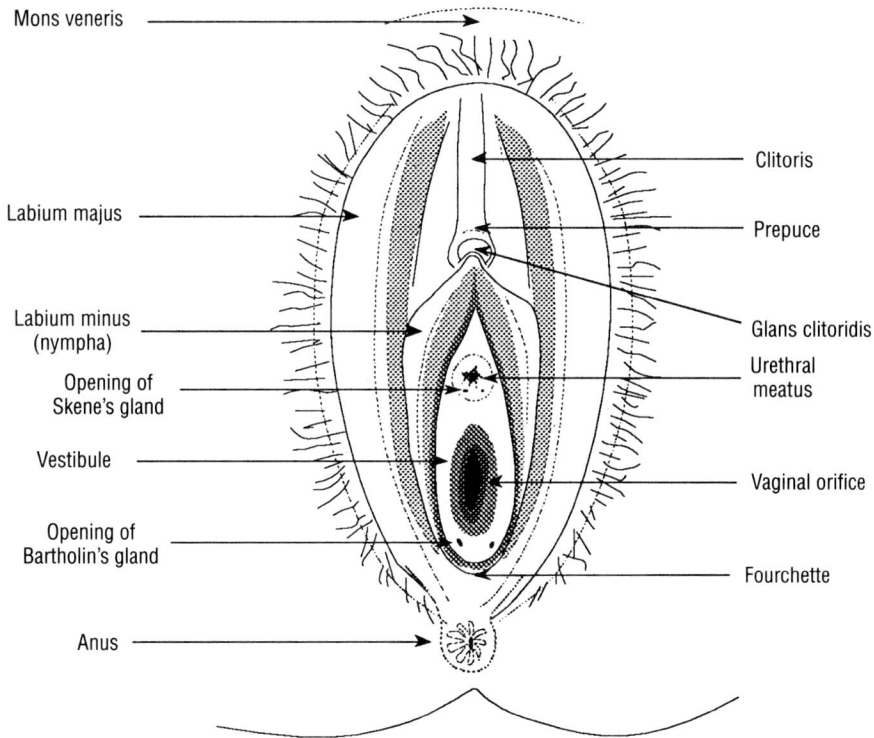

Figure 12.3 *The vulva*

partially concealed by the anterior commissures of the labia minora. It is a rudimentary and incomplete counterpart of the penis, having two erectile bodies and a glans. It is a highly sensitive receptor, having many specialized sensory nerve endings. The major vestibular glands (glands of Bartholin) are the female equivalent of the male's bulbourethral glands and are situated in the lateral walls of the vestibule. They produce a lubricative mucus upon stimulation.

After the menopause several degenerative and atrophic changes occur in the female genital system. In the ovary, in the later reproductive years, there is a gradually decreasing number of ovarian follicles. After the menopause, the follicles disappear completely, being replaced by a narrow zone of fibrocollagenous tissue. In the uterus after the menopause there is marked atrophy in all of its layers, the whole organ shrinking markedly. The endometrium ceases to undergo its cyclical changes and becomes a thin mucosal covering. The Fallopian tubes also atrophy, their muscular wall becoming thin and the internal folds of their mucosa atrophying and flattening out. Corresponding changes also occur in the vagina and the glycogen content of the cells greatly decreases with a rise in the vaginal

pH, as the lactobacilli numbers decrease dramatically. All of these changes described are a result of the oestrogen decline observed post-menopausally.

Diseases of the Uterus

Congenital Lesions

Congenital anomalies of the uterus do not occur often, but when present they are usually due to failure of Müllerian duct fusion resulting in such abnormalities as uterus bicornis, uterus septus and uterus unicornis (refer to Figure 12.4). In these and many other related conditions there are malformations in the structure of the uterine wall and lumen, resulting in a double uterus, a uterus with two lumina or a septate uterus. Very rarely, there is total absence of the uterus.

Hypoplasia of the uterus is more common than agenesis, and this disorder results in an organ that is smaller than normal. The canalization of the organ may be incomplete and **atresia** may thus occur in any part of the uterine tract. Atresia of the cervix is the most usual site of this disorder. All of these congenital

Pathology for the Health Sciences

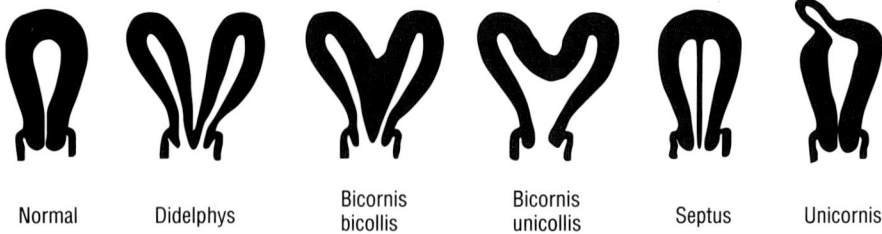

Normal   Didelphys   Bicornis bicollis   Bicornis unicollis   Septus   Unicornis

Figure 12.4 *Congenital uterine anomalies*

malformations are idiopathic and are associated with anomalies that may interfere with, or totally prevent, normal reproductive function. In some of these cases, plastic surgery may be effective in establishing normal structure and reproductive function.

Endometritis

Endometritis is an infection or inflammation of the endometrium, appearing almost exclusively as an acute disease. Chronic endometritis is unusual as the endometrium is shed monthly, and therefore, chronic endometritis will only be seen prepubertally and post-menopausally. Tuberculous infection is a rare cause of chronic granulomatous endometritis. In acute endometritis, bacterial causes are the most commonly encountered and the reaction is a typical suppurative acute inflammation. The uterine lumen may become filled with a collection of pus, a condition known as **pyometra**. By far, the commonest cause of endometritis is puerperal sepsis.

Puerperal Sepsis ('Childbirth Fever')

Puerperal sepsis is an infection of the endometrium and uterus following childbirth or miscarriage. Puerperal fever is defined as any febrile condition occurring within 21 days after childbirth or miscarriage, in which the woman's temperature is raised to 38°C or more for 24 hours or more. Puerperal disease is usually due to β-haemolytic streptococci, anaerobic streptococci, staphylococci, clostridia, coliforms or *Pseudomonas* spp. The sources of the infection are normal flora bacteria derived from the hands of the attendants at delivery and instruments poorly sterilized or contaminated by touching the perineum of the woman giving birth. Frequently, the infection is an autoinfection in which the skin or vagina of the woman is the source of bacteria. There may also be coloniza-

tion of the damaged endometrium and uterus by bacteria from a more distant site such as the mouth or respiratory tract. Blood-borne infection is another way in which the damaged uterine tissues may become involved.

Bacterial infection post-natally is less common nowadays in its severe form due to improved antisepsis and hygienic birthing. Antibiotic therapy has also limited the extent and spread of the infection once it does develop. Predisposing factors leading to puerperal sepsis are:

* prolonged, traumatic labour;
* retention of placenta requiring manual removal;
* retention of products of conception;
* requirement of instrumentation;
* septic abortions.

Bacteria enter at the sites of trauma, usually the lacerated cervix or the raw surface at the placental attachment site. They begin to multiply in the tissue and to spread locally and via the bloodstream. If the infection is untreated, there is a high fever, and the uterus is large and soft. The endometrium is ragged and sloughing, covered in foul-smelling, often purulent lochia. There is acute suppurative inflammation of the endometrium with extensive necrosis. Extension of the infection to involve the myometrium (myometritis) may occur and may lead to pelvic involvement. Extension to the Fallopian tubes (acute salpingitis), peritonitis, septic thrombophlebitis (infection and inflammation of uterine veins) may occur, leading to septic embolism with septicaemia and multiple metastatic abscesses developing. If the condition remains untreated or is neglected, it is very frequently fatal. Induced abortions ('back yard abortions') are particularly serious, as often clostridia are involved and may cause extensive, spreading necrosis of tissue. Septicaemia, toxaemia and shock are the commonest causes of death.

If the infection is treated early with the appropriate antibiotics, a resolution of the infection and inflammation occurs and the endometrium regenerates fully from surviving islands of tissue. Endometritis may also be seen in gonococcal infection. In some women, endometritis may be associated with an IUD. Obstruction of the cervical canal (e.g. due to tumours) may also result in endometrial infection and pyometra. In all of these cases treatment of the infection and removal of the predisposing factor will result in resolution.

Endometriosis

Endometriosis refers to the presence of endometrial tissue away from its normal position, as a lining of the uterus. It is thus a condition of ectopic endometrium. It is a very common condition, found in approximately 10 to 30% of all women. It has a high incidence in infertile women and most cases are diagnosed between the ages of 20 to 40 years, the condition being rare above the age of 50 years. There is a higher incidence in the higher socioeconomic groups, but this may be an artificial epidemiological observation as women in the lower socioeconomic groups may be more reluctant to seek medical advice about the condition (being less aware of it). It also appears that postponing the first pregnancy predisposes to the development of the condition and thus the disorder may genuinely occur to a lesser extent in the lower socioeconomic groups, as these women are more likely to have children at an earlier age. There are two subtypes of endometriosis: **adenomyosis** (endometriosis interna), where foci of endometrium are found deep in the wall of the uterus, and **endometriosis externa**, where there is ectopic endometrial tissue outside the uterine wall. Hence, this condition may be considered as a choristoma (normal tissue in an ectopic situation).

The sites for the ectopic endometrium in external endometriosis are widespread. The most common sites are the ovaries, Fallopian tubes, the rectovaginal septum, pelvic peritoneum, intestinal wall, abdominal wall, umbilicus, laparotomy scars and more rarely lymph nodes, lung and pleura. Endometrial tissue has even been found in more exotic sites such as the elbow skin and the eyelid, but these sites of occurrence are very rare.

As the endometrial tissue in the abnormal sites is completely normal in structure and function, it responds to hormonal changes in the woman's body and thus the normal cyclical changes of uterine endometrium will also occur in endometrium at ectopic sites. The shedding of degenerating endometrium gives rise to an inflammatory response in the tissue and if the deposit is extensive, cysts filled with necrotic, haemorrhagic material occur, known as '**chocolate cysts**' because of their dark-brown appearance. Such cysts are very commonly found in the ovary. Considerable fibrosis may occur at sites of endometriosis, with repeated inflammation and organization. This scarring gradually reduces the amount of endometrial tissue present.

Symptoms and signs associated with endometriosis vary greatly depending on the site affected and the amount of endometrial tissue present. In mild cases the condition may be asymptomatic or cause slight pain and discomfort during menstruation. In more severe cases, there may be:

- **dysmenorrhoea** (pain during ovulation or menstruation);
- **dyspareunia** (pain during sexual intercourse);
- **menorrhagia** (heavy menstrual bleeding);
- pain during defaecation or micturition;
- diarrhoea or constipation;
- bleeding from the bowel or haematuria;
- abdominal distension;
- premenstrual tension (PMT), depression, marked mood swings;
- insomnia, low energy levels, fatigue;
- infertility.

The main indicator of tissue with endometriosis is swelling (thus enlargement of the uterus may be palpated in adenomyosis and an enlarged ovary may be seen with ultrasonography in endometriosis of this tissue). Microscopically, there are deposits of typical endometrial glands found within the surrounding foreign tissue. Areas of haemorrhage and inflammation abound and large cystic spaces full of necrotic blood and surrounded by haemosiderin-laden macrophages may be seen where chocolate cysts have formed. Scarring is prominent and may cause stricture of tubular organs.

The aetiology and pathogenesis of endometriosis is not well understood but there are three theories attempting to explain the condition:

- **Implantation theory**: This theory invokes a reflux of shedding endometrium during menstruation, through the Fallopian tubes into the peritoneum, as the mechanism of implantation of the endometrium in the foreign sites (most commonly ovary and peritoneal wall). Ingrowth of endometrial tissue into the myometrium and subsequent isolation into islands explains the adenomyosis.
- **Metaplasia theory**: This theory assumes that the serosal cells lining the coelomic cavity (having the same embryonic origin as the endometrium) un-

dergo metaplasia into endometrial tissues. Why metaplasia should occur is not known, but deferment of pregnancy and the many menstrual cycles with their attendant hormonal changes that the nulliparous woman goes through may be instrumental in this (higher incidence of endometriosis in infertile women and women who have not borne children early).

- **Lymphatic or vascular embolism theory**: This theory indicates that some shedding endometrial tissue gains entry into the circulation or lymphatic system and, much like malignant tumour cells, embolizes in distant sites and grows there. This seems to be an unlikely occurrence, but it would explain unusual situations of endometriosis (e.g. lung and eyelid).

The condition may cause many complications, all related to the degree of fibrosis that occurs in association with the condition. Adhesions between abdominal organs may cause obstruction in the genital, urinary and gastrointestinal tracts. Such obstructions may lead to infertility, hydroureter, hydronephrosis and irregularity of bowel motions. Endometriosis may spontaneously regress, especially after a pregnancy. Often, hormonal treatment is given and in some cases may prove to be successful, but the condition may recur. Surgical excision of the ectopic tissue must be carried out in a majority of cases, especially where there are complications such as 'chocolate cyst' formation, fibrosis and strictures, or involvement of the ovary with destruction of the ovarian parenchyma.

Metropathia Haemorrhagica

Metropathia haemorrhagica is a hyperplastic condition of the endometrium resulting from excessive, unopposed oestrogen secretion by the ovaries, and causing dysfunctional uterine bleeding. The condition is not commonly seen and tends to occur at the extremes of reproductive life. Over 50% of cases are observed in women over 45 years of age, while about 20% of cases occur in adolescents.

In most cases the condition is associated with excessive endogenous oestrogen production by the ovaries. Tumours of the ovaries or cystic ovaries cause the hyperoestrinism, but in some cases the oestrogens may be secreted by a hyperplasia or tumour of the adrenal cortex. In a small number of cases therapeutic administration of oestrogens has been implicated in the aetiology of the disease.

The affected endometrium is greatly thickened and may show a highly vascular polypoid appearance.

Curettage of the uterus produces bulky and haemorrhagic scrapings. Microscopically the epithelium is hyperplastic and vascular with a non-secretory appearance. Both tubules and stroma are hyperplastic. There is a cystic dilatation of tubules, giving the mucosa a 'Swiss cheese' appearance. The ovaries in most cases contain follicular cysts but corpora lutea are not formed (i.e. progesterone is not produced).

The condition manifests itself as a menorrhagia and dysmenorrhoea with many menstrual cycle irregularities. The woman may be anaemic and is infertile. Complications of the condition include malignant change, with as many as 25 to 35% of cases of atypical hyperplasia developing carcinoma of the endometrium. Treatment of the condition depends on correcting the hormonal anomalies present, often simply through the removal of the ovarian cysts or benign tumours.

Fibroleiomyoma of the Uterus ('Fibroid')

Fibroleiomyomata are also termed fibromata and leiomyomata or referred to as 'fibroids' by the layperson. These are the commonest neoplasms of women, occurring in the myometrium. They are strongly oestrogen-dependent benign neoplasms of the smooth muscle cells and fibroblasts of the uterine wall. The tumour affects as many as one in four women, either asymptomatically (often the case, when they are extremely small), or commonly, symptomatically when they are large and multiple. They arise at a young age but are usually detected when the woman is between 30 to 40 years of age. They may occur in a younger age group if they are associated with hyperoestrinism.

The tumours arise anywhere in the myometrium and depending on their location they are termed subserosal, intramural or submucosal (refer to Figure 12.5). They are usually spherical or ovoid in shape and well demarcated due to a well-defined fibrous capsule. The subserosal and submucosal masses may be pedunculated and may project into the peritoneal cavity or into the lumen of the uterus. On cut section these masses are firm, white and show a typical whorled pattern of irregularly arranged muscle fibres. Large tumours show a red centre of degeneration and haemorrhage, a change known as **necrobiosis**. Microscopically, the tumours are composed of a little fibrous tissue and many smooth muscle cells in a whorling pattern (Figure 12.6).

The tumours are benign and require oestrogen for growth. After the menopause the masses begin to regress and gradually decrease in size. However, the tumours tend to grow very rapidly during pregnancy and may cause miscarriage. Fibroids are a common

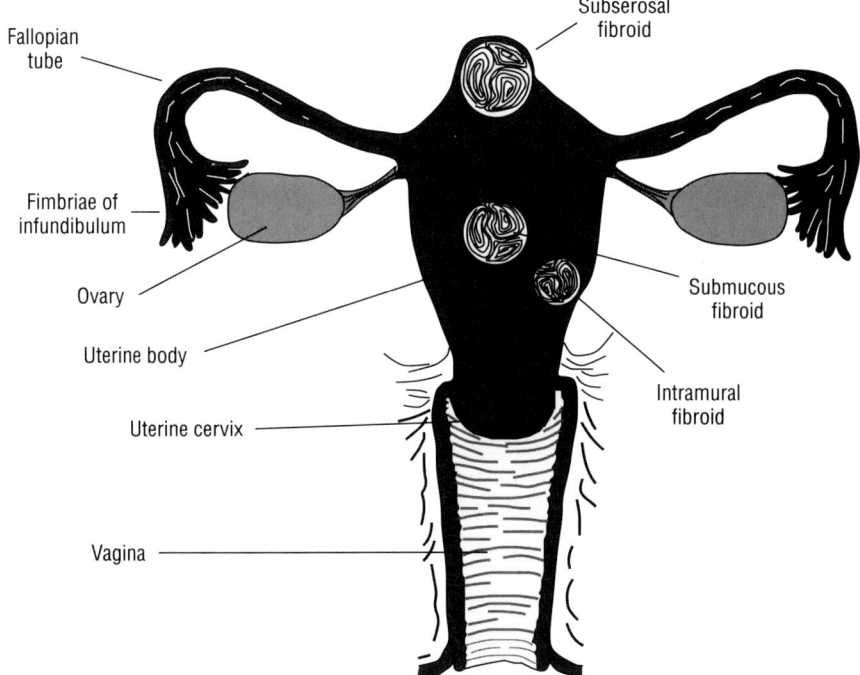

Fallopian tube

Subserosal fibroid

Fimbriae of infundibulum

Ovary

Uterine body

Uterine cervix

Vagina

Submucous fibroid

Intramural fibroid

Figure 12.5 *Fibroleiomyomata of the uterus*

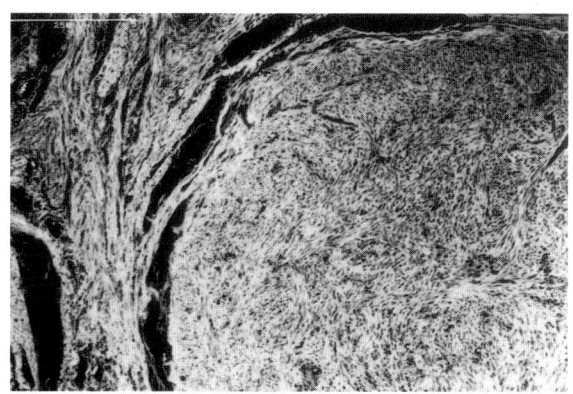

Figure 12.6 *A small fibroleiomyoma of the uterus showing the encapsulated nature of the lesion and the whorled pattern of the muscle and collagen fibres in its centre (scale bar is 250 μm)*

cause of infertility, especially if they are large and multiple. If an ovum is fertilized, it may lodge in the Fallopian tube, its entry into the uterine lumen being prevented by a fibroid, thus giving rise to an ectopic pregnancy. Although many of these tumours are microscopic and asymptomatic, some do cause many symptoms and complications, about 30% of admis-

sions into gynaecological hospitals being due to effects of fibroids. A woman may present with infertility, dysmenorrhoea, menorrhagia, discomfort, obstruction and pressure effects on adjacent organs such as bowel and bladder.

Degenerative changes in large fibroleiomyomata are common and include atrophy, hyaline degeneration, cystic change, mucoid change, fatty change, haemorrhage, fatty degeneration, calcification and ossification. Very rarely malignant change will supervene, with less than one in 1000 of the large tumours undergoing such a change. Fibroleiomyomata may remain untreated during a woman's life if they are small and cause no symptoms and signs. However, if the masses are large, they are surgically removed to prevent the complications mentioned above. The most frequently removed masses are those that occur in young women who wish to become pregnant and where the presence of the fibroids has prevented normal reproductive function.

Endometrial Carcinoma (Carcinoma Corpus Uteri)

Incidence. Carcinoma of the endometrium accounts for approximately 1% of all deaths from malignancy, and the incidence seems to be increasing. It occurs more commonly in childless women at an average age of 55 years (around the age of menopause, or slightly after).

Sites affected. The tumour is a typical carcinoma arising in the lining of the uterus, the endometrium. It usually originates in the endometrium lining the fundus of the organ.

Aetiology. Predisposing factors for the development of the tumour include endometrial hyperplasia or benign tumours of the endometrium associated with hormonal imbalances (high oestrogen levels). Other causes of endogenous hyperoestrinism such as obesity, ovarian neoplasms and infertility due to hormonal imbalance may predispose to the tumour. Exogenous hyperoestrinism, such as prolonged oestrogen therapy, is associated with a higher incidence of the tumour. The carcinoma is also associated with diabetes.

Appearance. Endometrial carcinoma may grow as a papillary or solid tumour in the cavity of the uterus or as a solid invasive tumour in the uterine wall. Ulceration, haemorrhage, necrosis and infection are common findings. Approximately 85% of the tumours are adenocarcinomata, usually well differentiated. The remainder of the tumours arise in metaplastic endometrium and are either adenoacanthomata or, rarely, typical squamous cell carcinomata.

Spread. The tumour spreads directly to involve the uterine wall, the Fallopian tubes, cervix, bladder, rectum and ovaries. The pelvic lymph nodes may be involved early, through lymphatic spread. Blood spread occurs in the late stages of the disease, usually producing metastases in the lungs.

Signs and symptoms. Pyometra occurs commonly due to obstruction of the cervical canal and secondary infection of the tumour. This leads to an enlarged, painful and tender uterus. Haemorrhage is a common feature of the tumour and post-menopausal bleeding *per vaginam* is a common presentation. Alternatively, leukorrhoea may cause the woman to seek medical advice.

Treatment and prognosis. The tumour is usually treated surgically, an extended hysterectomy being performed. This involves removal of the upper vagina, cervix, uterus, Fallopian tubes, ovaries and pelvic lymph nodes. With such a procedure the prognosis is very good, with an average 5-year survival of 80%.

Diseases of the Uterine Cervix

Cervicitis

This is a very commonly encountered inflammation of the cervix uteri, being acute or chronic in nature. It is often associated with infection, especially implicated being the sexually transmitted diseases (e.g. herpes, papilloma viruses, gonococci). It may also follow the trauma of childbirth or instrumentation in the region (e.g. hysteroscopy). It sometimes occurs in the absence of any demonstrable aetiological factor (nonspecific cervicitis). The condition is more likely to occur in the sexually active female.

The inflamed cervix shows evidence of redness, swelling, exudation, often with laceration and ulceration. Recurrent episodes of inflammation form an irregular, ulcerated surface with friable nodules visible on colposcopy. Occasionally, a frankly purulent cervicitis develops. Microscopically a typical acute inflammatory response is observed in acute cervicitis. With recurrent attacks of acute cervicitis or with chronic cervicitis, there is squamous metaplasia of the columnar cervical epithelium, a change known as **epidermalization**. Subsequent dysplastic changes are often seen. Cystic dilatation of the submucosal cervical glands is a common feature and these grossly dilated glands are known as **Nabothian cysts** (see Figure 12.6). Groups of chronic inflammatory cells may be found in the submucosa and the condition may progress to a follicular cervicitis.

Acute cervicitis may resolve, especially if the initiating stimulus was trivial or was promptly removed. More often than not, the injury persists and the acute inflammation progresses to active chronic inflammation. Chronic cervicitis may cause fibrosis and eversion of the cervix. Stenosis of the cervical canal region and the os will lead to great deformation in the region or complete blockage of the cervical canal. Compromise of mucus secretion and the presence of inflammatory debris generally produces an unfavourable environment for sperm and this, coupled with the deformation of the cervix, is often the cause of infertility in women with chronic cervicitis.

Symptoms and signs associated with cervicitis include **leukorrhoea** (a whitish vaginal secretion) that may progress to suppuration if bacterial infection becomes the major pathological process. Anomalies in menstrual blood flow may result when the cervical region becomes greatly scarred. The condition of chronic cervicitis is important, as the dysplasia in the region predisposes to carcinoma of the cervix. The Papanicolaou smear test may detect cervicitis and early

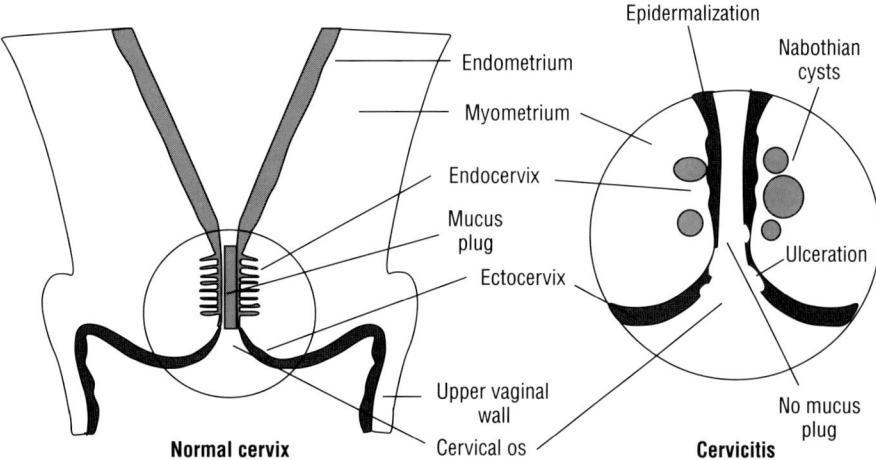

Figure 12.7 *Cervical changes in cervicitis*

dysplastic lesions (see section below on cervical carcinoma).

Carcinoma of the Cervix (Carcinoma Cervix Uteri)

Incidence. Carcinoma of the cervix is the most common pelvic gynaecological cancer which is increasing in its incidence. It accounts for only approximately 3% of cancer deaths; however, deaths from cervical cancer are decreasing because of earlier detection and treatment. The peak age of incidence is between 30 to 40 years, the average age of onset decreasing.

Sites affected. The tumour may occur in the ectocervix or endocervix, but typically it occurs at the squamocolumnar junction at the region of the cervical os. Such a site is readily accessible for view through a colposcope.

Aetiology. Cervical carcinoma is seen very rarely in virgins while it is very common in prostitutes, and is strongly linked with sexual activity. There is much evidence linking cervical carcinoma with:

- early age of first intercourse;
- early age of first pregnancy;
- multiparity (having more than one child);
- short interval between pregnancies.

It is also linked with:

- promiscuity (multiple sex partners);
- non-barrier contraceptive methods;
- lower socioeconomic class, poor hygiene.

All of these factors indicate that there is sexual transmission of a carcinogen and genetic studies on cells of cervical carcinoma have linked the cancer to herpes simplex virus type II (HSV II) infection ('genital herpes') and also human papilloma virus (HPV) infection, the cause of genital warts. The DNA of the cancer cells is found to contain viral DNA sequences in a very large number of cases.

The progression of changes which occur in the cervix usually spans a history of about 25 years, although 5% of cervical cancer patients have a history of less than 3 years. The malignancy commences in the metaplastic squamous epithelium that develops at the junction of cuboidal epithelium with squamous epithelium (junction of ectocervix and endocervix, near the external os). Such a change is often preceded by cervicitis. The metaplastic epithelium undergoes dysplastic change that eventually affects the full thickness of epithelium with hyperchromatic nuclei, pleomorphism and abnormal mitotic activity being seen. These severe dysplastic changes progress to carcinoma *in situ*, which is local and pre-invasive. Subsequently, the malignant cells proceed to invade the underlying tissues. Once invasion of the carcinoma progresses beyond 5 cm, metastasis is likely and the prognosis for the woman's cancer changes for the worse.

Appearance. The early stages of the cancer are not readily observable macroscopically with colposcopy. As the tumour grows, however, a nodular, polypoid or diffusely infiltrating mass may be seen. Frequently, the tumour ulcerates and secondary infection occurs. Microscopically, about 95% of cases are squamous cell carcinomata while the remainder are adenocarcinomata. All squamous cell tumours in the endocervix arise from metaplastic epithelium.

Diagnosis. Early diagnosis of the tumour has been greatly enhanced through the use of the Papanicolaou smear test ('Pap smear'). This is essentially a cytological test detecting abnormal cells in the region of the cervix (i.e. cells that show dysplasia and early neoplasia). A sample of the cervical epithelial cells is removed by gently scraping the cervical mucosa with a special spatula. The cells thus exfoliated are spread on a slide, fixed, stained and examined microscopically. A Pap smear properly carried out and interpreted by a competent cytologist can detect approximately 90% of cases of cervicitis, dysplasia, atypia and early neoplasia. The early diagnosis of cervical cancer by the Papanicolaou method has reduced the death rate of this cancer by about 50%. Women who are sexually active (especially women with multiple sex partners) are encouraged to have an annual Pap smear test. Currently, only approximately 50% of women do so.

Spread. Staging of the tumour indicates spread:
- **Stage 0**: Carcinoma *in situ*; the tumour is confined to the epithelium.
- **Stage 1**: Microinvasive carcinoma, confined to the cervix.
- **Stage 2:** Direct spread to involve the cervix, parametrium and upper vagina.
- **Stage 3:** Lymphatic spread with involvement of pelvic lymph nodes, upper uterus, lower vagina, pelvic wall.
- **Stage 4**: Haematogenous spread with distant metastases to the lungs, liver, brain. Lymphatic and direct spread to the rectum, bladder, etc.

Signs and symptoms. The tumour mass ulcerates and may cause vaginal bleeding, particularly postcoital. There is infiltration and invasion of the uterus, vagina, ureters, bladder and rectum, causing bowel obstruction and urinary tract obstruction with hydronephrosis, pyelonephritis and chronic renal failure. Rectovaginal fistula and vesicovaginal fistula may occur. Secondary infection of the mass may cause a vaginal discharge that may be frankly purulent.

Treatment. The Pap smear detects early dysplastic changes and further diagnosis can be made by punch or cone biopsy (**conization** where a cone of cervical tissue is removed), this containing the tumour mass. Such a procedure is often also curative. Alternatively, in the early stages treatment is by cauterization or now, more commonly, laser treatment. Hysterectomy and radiotherapy may be required if spread has occurred. In stage 4, chemotherapy is often given but this is not very successful, only 25 to 30% of tumours showing regression.

Prognosis of the tumour varies depending on the stage at which the tumour is treated. Overall prognosis is quite good with approximately 50% 5-year survival. However, many tumours are detected very early by yearly Pap smear examinations, giving 95% 10-year survival. If a stage 0 tumour is detected and treated, the 5-year survival is close to 100%. Treated stage 1 tumours have a 5-year survival of 90%; stage 2 tumours a 70% 5-year survival; stage 3 tumours a 35% 5-year survival and stage 4 tumours a 10% 5-year survival.

Diseases of the Vulva and Vagina

Inflammation and Infection

Vulvitis, vaginitis and vulvovaginitis are commonly observed entities and the precise aetiology differs, depending on the age of the female affected. The adult vagina is very resistant to infection due to the characteristic normal flora that utilizes the glycogen in the epithelium, converting it to lactic acid, lowering the pH significantly and making the environment unsuitable for the growth of most microbes. Usually, some predisposing factor such as debility, other diseases (e.g. diabetes) or drug therapy (antibiotics interfering with normal flora or cytotoxic drugs interfering with marrow function) predisposes to infection. Infections with *Candida albicans* (causing 'thrush'), *Gardnerella vaginalis* and *Trichomonas vaginalis* are very common. Most such infections present themselves as pruritus with a vaginal discharge that may be malodorous, viscid, ranging in colour from whitish to dark yellow.

At the extremes of age, premenstrually and post-menopausally, infections in the vulva and vagina may also occur due to the differences in vaginal physiology and normal flora. In both instances glycogen is not available and the lactobacilli that normally secrete the lactic acid keeping vaginal pH low are not present in large numbers as they are in women of reproductive age. The vagina is therefore more likely to become infected. In young girls, gonococcal vulvovaginitis is common, especially contracted through fomites. The adult vagina is very resistant to infection with *Neisseria gonorrhoeae*. In the post-menopausal woman, atrophic vaginitis is a common occurrence and many different organisms may be involved (see also the section on sexually transmitted diseases in Chapter 11).

Neoplasms

Benign tumours in this region are almost always **condylomata acuminata** (genital warts) caused by infection with the human papilloma virus. These are fleshy, soft, pinkish brown, pedunculated masses that are frequently multiple and fungating. Typically they occur around the vulva and affected women often show herpetic infection as well. The masses are removed for cosmetic purposes but also because they may undergo malignant transformation.

Squamous cell carcinoma is a rare tumour of the vulva and vagina. In the vulva it is associated with a range of premalignant conditions such as Paget's disease of the vulva, Bowen's disease of the vulva and other dysplastic lesions that may be associated with chronic infective or inflammatory changes in the tissue. In the vagina most such tumours arise idiopathically. In the vulva such tumours are usually detected and treated early with an average 5-year survival of 70%. In the vagina the tumour tends to be discovered and treated much later, the average 5-year survival being about 30%.

Diseases of the Fallopian Tubes

Salpingitis

Salpingitis is an infection or inflammation of the Fallopian tube. Such inflammations in the Fallopian tube are most often due to bacteria such as *Neisseria gonorrhoeae,* chlamydiae, mycoplasmata (PID), streptococci and staphylococci (especially post-partum) and coliforms. The route of infection is via the lumen of the uterus. The infection shows a typical acute inflammatory appearance that is usually suppurative. Resolution rarely occurs, healing with fibrosis being the usual sequela. **Pyosalpinx** (accumulation of pus inside the Fallopian tube) may result, a tubo-ovarian abscess often being a result of the pyogenic infection in this site. Chronic salpingitis is another sequela and in this condition extensive fibrosis of the tube may lead to infertility or ectopic pregnancy. Rarely, tuber-culous salpingitis is seen and in this case a typical granulomatous inflammation results.

Tumours of the Fallopian Tube

Primary tumours of the Fallopian tube are very rare. In carcinoma of the Fallopian tube, the tumour is not diagnosed until very late in the disease and metastases are usually present. Such tumours have a poor prognosis. Secondary tumours of the Fallopian tube are much more common than primary ones, arising in this site through direct spread from adjacent tissues, ovarian and uterine neoplasms being those most commonly involved.

Diseases of the Ovaries

Oöphoritis

Oöphoritis, the infection or inflammation of the ovaries is uncommon but can occur as an extension of salpingitis or PID. The ovaries become involved in an acute inflammatory response with, sometimes, suppuration and abscess formation. If the condition is bilateral and left untreated, it may progress to sterility. Alternatively, the condition may be associated with ectopic pregnancy. In a small number of cases, mumps in the adult female leads to an interstitial involvement of the ovarian tissue, with extensive damage to the organs, fibrosis and sterility resulting.

Ovarian Cysts

Cysts of the ovaries are very common. Simple cysts of the ovary are so common that they are considered as a physiological variant. Simple cysts account for over 80% of all ovarian swellings. These cysts are non-neoplastic and arise in Graäfian follicles or in corpora lutea. There may be single or multiple cysts, subserosal or cortical. Usually they are approximately 10 mm in diameter, but they reach sizes of up to 6 cm in diameter. They are filled with a clear fluid in which there is a high concentration of oestrogens.

Follicular ovarian cysts contain clear or blood-stained fluid and are lined by many layers of follicular epithelial cells. They are usually 1 to 3 cm in diameter, rarely greater than 10 cm in diameter (Figure 12.8). **Luteal ovarian cysts** usually contain blood-stained fluid and are lined by flattened cells. They are most

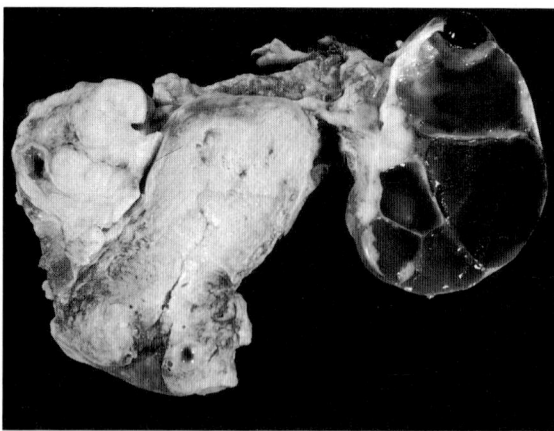

Figure 12.8 *Ovarian cysts causing a marked increase in the size of the affected ovary. They are filled with a blood-stained fluid*

often solitary, but occasionally may be multiple. They are usually less than 5 cm in diameter.

Both of these types of simple cysts represent unruptured, or ruptured and quickly resealed Graäfian follicles. As the cysts enlarge, the granulosa or luteal cells that line them may atrophy under the pressure of accumulating fluid. Cysts may rupture and bleed and are a cause of an 'acute abdomen' presentation with acute onset of severe abdominal pain.

The **Stein-Leventhal syndrome**, an uncommon syndrome, is characterized by the formation of multiple ovarian follicular cysts (i.e. **polycystic ovaries**) and oligomenorrhoea or amenorrhoea that reduces fertility. This syndrome seems to affect women who are obese, with hirsutism (excessive body hair). It presents in young women in the late teens to the 20 to 30 years age group. There is a defect in the hypothalamic pituitary axis resulting in continuous secretion of FSH leading to the growth of numerous ovarian follicles that fail to rupture, as there is no mid-cycle surge of LH. The anovulation seen in this condition may make the woman infertile and this is often why the woman first presents with the condition. Endometrial hyperplasia is often a feature in the disorder, but anovulation and the abnormal hormonal profile cause the oligomenorrhoea. The virilization that is often seen in association with the Stein-Leventhal syndrome is due to secretion of androstenedione. Exogenous hormone administration may correct the imbalance to the point where a normal pattern of ovarian follicle maturation and rupture occurs, with a normal pregnancy resulting.

Ovarian Tumours

Tumours of the ovary are important because of their diversity and their size. Classification of ovarian tumours is complex because of the diversity of precursor cell types that are present in the ovary, each cell type giving rise to highly characteristic tumours. Clinical behaviour of the tumours is also diverse, with typical benign and malignant tumours known, but also the more unusual intermediate tumours occurring. Some tumours of the ovary are extremely large and there are several well-documented cases where the tumour (serous or mucinous cystadenoma) weighed several kilograms. A well-known mnemonic regarding abdominal swellings in females runs: 'Fat, flatus, foetus, phantom pregnancy, football-sized ovarian tumours'!

There are three basic cell types in the ovary from which tumours may arise:

- Surface epithelium (coelomic):
  (a) serous secreting, ciliated columnar cells
  (b) simple columnar (non-ciliated) mucus-secreting cells
- Stromal cells:
  (a) Thecal; luteal or granulosa cells (sex cord cells)
  (b) Connective tissue
- Germ cells: totipotential cells (ova)

Tumours may be benign, malignant or intermediate in type making prediction of behaviour difficult if a mass is discovered when examination of the ovaries is carried out. Sometimes, the histogenesis of tumours is unclear due to anaplasia, although generally most anaplastic tumours tend to arise from the surface epithelium (refer to Table 12.1).

Despite the great variation in the histogenesis and behaviour of ovarian neoplasms, the basic clinical presentation of all tumours is rather similar. Unless the tumour is actively secreting hormones, it tends to present at a late stage, when it has reached a large size. When the tumour is large it produces signs and symptoms due to pressure effects and accidental complications:

- pain, discomfort;
- pressure atrophy of surrounding tissues;
- gastrointestinal complaints;
- urinary frequency;
- abdominal distension;
- torsion of the ovary, acute abdomen.

Generally, it may be said that early diagnosis of ovarian tumours is a rare occurrence. Ovarian cancer accounts for approximately 3% of cancer deaths and 6% of all cancers, and it is the fourth most common cancer in women. Ovarian cancer kills as many pa-

Table 12.1 *Ovarian tumours*

Histogenesis	Surface epithelium	Germ cells	Stromal cells	Secondary tumours
Age group	Adult women	Newborn to young females	Any age	Mainly middle aged women
Incidence	≈ 70% of all ovarian tumours	≈ 20% of all ovarian tumours	≈ 5–10% of all ovarian tumours	≈ 5% of all ovarian tumours
Types	• Serous tumours • Mucinous t. • Endometrioid t. • Clear cell t. • Brenner t. • Anaplastic t.	• Teratoma • Choriocarcinoma • Dysgerminoma • Endodermal sinus tumour	• Granulosa theca cell tumour • Sertoli-Leydig cell tumour • Fibroma	e.g. Krukenberg tumour (mainly from stomach)
Clinical behaviour (% of ovarian malignancies)	Mainly malignant (≈ 85%)	Mainly benign (≈ 4%)	Mainly benign (≈ 5%)	All malignant (≈ 6%)

tients as endometrial carcinoma and cervical carcinoma together. Almost all ovarian masses are diagnosed on routine pelvic examination. In order to make early diagnosis of such neoplasms a relatively easy exercise, there has been a widespread search for ovarian tumour markers. However, current markers are inadequate for routine screening as there are difficulties with specificity and sensitivity. Some markers that have been investigated are summarized in Table 12.2.

The predisposing factors for development of ovarian tumours are poorly documented and it is only in a small number of cases that there have been associations with specific aetiologies. A very small percentage of tumours arise because of a genetic or familial predisposition. Hormonal factors appear to have an important effect and it appears that neoplasms of the ovary are commoner in nulliparous women. A high level of unbalanced oestrogens seems to predispose to ovarian cancer, while the contraceptive pill appears to have a moderate protective effect.

Staging of malignant ovarian neoplasms is very similar for all types of these tumours, the following scheme being used:

• **Stage 1**: The tumour is confined to the ovary with or without ascites.
• **Stage 2**: The growth involves one or both ovaries with pelvic extensions.
• **Stage 3**: The tumour has intraperitoneal metastases outside the pelvis with or without growth in the retroperitoneal nodes.

• **Stage 4**: There are distant metastases present, the liver, lungs, etc. being involved.

Cancer of the ovary is treated with an elaborate protocol, including surgery, radiotherapy and chemotherapy, used alone or usually in combination. The surgical procedure in use for most of the malignant ovarian tumours is a bilateral salpingo-oöphorectomy and hysterectomy. With the intermediate and benign tumours a more conservative approach is taken in younger women in order to preserve fertility. Benign masses, for example, are often cured by local resection or a unilateral oöphorectomy. Supplementary chemotherapy in the case of malignant tumours may be systemic or intraperitoneal. It should be remembered that most epithelial tumours are diagnosed late, generally at stages 3 and 4, in which case treatment by radiotherapy and chemotherapy is the only option, and this type of treatment at these stages has only a palliative effect. The average 5-year survival therefore is rather poor, ranging from 30% to 35%.

Epithelial Tumours of the Ovary (70% of Tumours)
Serous tumours of the ovary. These are the most frequently seen of ovarian neoplasms. They are typically cystic masses, the spaces filled with a serous fluid (and varying amounts of mucus to a lesser degree), with or without haemorrhage. They have a range of clinical behaviours, 25% being benign cystadenomata, 65% being malignant cystadenocarcinomata, while 10% are intermediate in behaviour.

Table 12.2 *Ovarian tumour markers*

Tumour	Marker	Tumours + ve
Choriocarcinoma	Human chorionic gonadotrophin (HCG)	Most
Endodermal sinus tumour	α-foetoprotein	80–90%
Epithelial tumours	Common epithelial antigen	80%
Serous carcinoma	Carcinoembryonic antigen	50–70%
Mucinous carcinoma	Carcinoembryonic antigen	25–50%
Immature teratoma	α-foetoprotein	20–25%
Dysgerminoma	Human chorionic gonadotrophin (HCG)	5–35%

Cystadenomata occur in the 20 to 50 years age group, while the cystadenocarcinomata occur in the 30 to 60 years age group. Approximately a third of benign tumours are bilateral while two-thirds of the malignant tumours are bilateral. Most tumours grow to large sizes (up to 40 cm in diameter) but smaller (5 to 10 cm diameter) masses are also seen.

The benign tumours have a smooth and glistening serosal aspect. On section there may be many small solid regions separating large cystic spaces with thin walls and filled with a clear to yellowish thin, serous fluid. Some tumours have papillary growths into the lumen. Microscopically there is a single layer of epithelial cells lining the cyst. The epithelium is a secretory type comprising ciliated, columnar to flattened cells. Cystadenofibromata show an abundant stroma composed of dense collagenous tissue. The papillae of the tumour may show degenerating, calcifying foci called **psammoma bodies**. Invasion of the cyst wall by the epithelial cells and spread into the serosa implies that a malignant change is occurring. Benign tumours are slowly growing but produce clinical manifestations because of their large size. If diagnosed, these tumours are removed surgically as they may undergo malignant transformation at a later stage.

The malignant tumours have a rough serosal aspect, the exterior of the ovary appearing nodular and often showing evidence of penetration of tumour through the serosa. On section, the mass consists of a single cyst or it may be multilocular, the cysts containing clear serous fluid. The more malignant forms will often lose their cystic pattern and become more solid in appearance with polypoid or papillary projections into the cysts and infiltration through the cyst wall. The more exuberant the papillary growth the more malignant in behaviour the mass is. Microscopically the tumour is composed of undifferentiated cells, often in multilayered masses with nests of grossly pleomorphic or anaplastic cells in a connective tissue stroma. Haemorrhage and necrosis are common findings within the tumour masses.

Malignant serous tumours of the ovary first invade locally and then through the serosa of the organ and into the peritoneal cavity. Often the tumour forms secondary deposits throughout the peritoneum, numerous masses studding the mesentery, serosa of other organs and the peritoneum itself, in a condition that is termed **carcinomatosis peritonei**. Spread to regional lymph nodes has already occurred at the time of diagnosis in most cases and often there is also haematogenous spread to distant sites. Surgical excision of the tumour mass may be attempted if diagnosis occurs early in the history of the tumour, with radiotherapy and chemotherapy being used as adjunctive treatments. The average 10-year survival for these tumours is 13%, indicating that most tumours tend to be diagnosed late in the disease.

The intermediate tumours resemble the benign ones grossly, and they tend to grow slowly, but on section they are seen to invade the immediately adjacent tissue. They tend not to spread to distant sites, but they have all the histological criteria of malignancy. If left untreated for long periods they may transform into frankly malignant, metastasizing masses. Surgical excision of these tumours is usually curative and the average 10-year survival of treated patients is 85%.

Endometrioid tumours. These tumours contain tubular glands, resembling endometrial tissue, that line cystic spaces. Women between the ages of 35 to 50 years are most commonly affected. Approximately 30% of cases of this tumour are bilateral. Most tumours arise from the epithelial surface of the ovary but in a small number of cases the tumour has been known to develop in an area of ovarian endometriosis. In about 15 to 30% of patients with this carcinoma there is also a coexisting carcinoma in the endometrium. The relationship between the two separate primary tumours in the two sites is thought to be hormonal but the exact pathogenesis is unclear.

The ovarian lesion may be single or multiple, solid or cystic, often indistinguishable macroscopically from the cystadenocarcinomata. The tumour is sometimes seen in association with a chocolate cyst of endometriosis. Histologically the tumours are adenocarcinomata, resembling endometrial carcinomata. Foci of squamous cells may be found within the tumours, and also tumours showing the appearance of adenoacanthoma occur. A small proportion of these tumours become anaplastic. There is invasion of surrounding tissue and the serosa of the ovary, this being more marked with the less well differentiated tumours.

If the tumours are well differentiated and treated surgically early in their history, the 5-year survival is about 60%. If the tumours are more aggressive, anaplastic or if they are diagnosed later, the 5-year survival is approximately 20%. The overall 5-year survival for these tumours is around 40%.

Mucinous tumours of the ovary. These masses are similar to the serous epithelial forms but contain predominantly mucinous secretions. They tend to grow larger and are less likely to be malignant than are the serous tumours. Mucocystadenomata, the benign forms, constitute about 75% of these tumours; mucocystadenocarcinomata, the malignant counterparts, constitute 15%; while the intermediate forms make up the remaining 10%. The peak age of incidence of these tumours is between 30 and 40 years. About 5% of the benign tumours are bilateral, while 20% of the malignant ones are bilateral. All mucinous tumours of the ovary resemble their serous counterparts; however, they contain a mucinous secretion and tend to be larger and multilocular. Papillation is encountered less frequently in these tumours and usually its presence tends to indicate malignancy. Microscopically there are mixtures of tall ciliated and tall columnar cells lining the cysts. The latter cells often show apical vacuolation indicative of secretory events.

Benign tumours may produce clinical manifestations because of their very large size. The cysts of mucinous tumours may rupture, releasing copious mucinous secretion into the peritoneum, a condition termed **pseudomyxoma peritonei**. Malignant change in the benign and intermediate tumours is less likely to occur. The malignant tumours tend to invade the serosa of the ovary and metastasize widely, similar to their serous counterparts.

The mucinous tumours are surgically removed if diagnosed and in the case of the benign masses this is a curative procedure. If treated, intermediate tumours have a 10-year survival of 85%. The mucocystadenocarcinomata, with treatment, have a 10-year survival of 35%.

Clear cell carcinoma of the ovary. This is a rare tumour (about 2% of all ovarian tumours), occurring in women usually aged between 50 and 55 years. In about 5% of cases the tumours are bilateral. The masses develop from the surface epithelium of the ovary and are found in association with endometriosis in about a quarter of cases.

The tumours appear macroscopically as nodular or cystic masses difficult to distinguish from other epithelial tumours. Histologically, clear cell carcinoma of the ovary resembles clear cell carcinoma of the kidney, with large clear cells arranged in tubular, papillary or solid masses. The tumour cells appear clear because they contain abundant glycogen in their cytoplasm. The average 5-year survival for these tumours with treatment is 45%.

Brenner tumour. This is another rare, epithelial tumour of the ovary, accounting for 1 to 2% of all ovarian masses. On average, most patients present around the age of 50 years. The tumours are usually benign, but intermediate and malignant variants are also known. Solid, yellowish, firm encapsulated masses are typical of the tumour. Microscopically, a characteristic of the tumour is nests or cysts of transitional epithelium embedded in a fibrous stroma. The transitional cells are very similar to urothelial cells. Sometimes, nests of columnar, mucus-secreting cells occur in the tumour. Benign forms of the tumour have an excellent prognosis while malignant variants have an average 5-year survival of 50%, with treatment.

Germ Cell Tumours (20% of Tumours)
Teratoma of the ovary (ovarian dermoid cyst). Ovarian teratoma is typically a benign tumour of the ovarian germ cells (which embryonically arise in the yolk sac and are present in the organ at birth). Over 95% of these tumours are the so-called benign **mature teratomata** that are usually cystic. They are believed to arise from a single germ cell in which some error arose after the first meiotic division. Such tumours are extremely well differentiated and largely ectodermal in nature, a variety of tissue types forming in the tumour. Most of these tumours arise in girls and young women between the ages of 20 and 30 years. The right ovary is affected slightly more than the left, but in 10% of cases the tumour is bilateral.

The affected ovary is enlarged, heavy and hard with a smooth serosal aspect. The tumour is usually less than 10 cm in diameter and areas of calcification may be palpated. On section it is a cystic structure lined by normal-looking skin with appendages, a tuft of red hair usually being a prominent feature within the lumen. Often, a pultaceous or sebaceous material may fill the lumen. Nails, teeth and sebaceous glands may also be noted in the tumour. Tissues from other germ layers, usually bone and cartilage, are found in the mass, but any other tissue type may be present. Microscopically all components of the teratoma are well differentiated and functional (Figure 12.9).

Teratomata of the ovary are slowly growing masses, present at birth in the ovary and growing for decades thereafter. They may not give rise to clinical manifestations and they may be discovered in a routine pelvic examination. Signs and symptoms may arise if the enlarged ovary undergoes torsion and infarction (occurring in about 15% of cases and presenting as an acute abdomen) or if the mass causes pressure effects on surrounding tissues. Some tumours may have hormonal effects; for example, if the thyroid tissue in an ovarian teratoma predominates the condition is termed

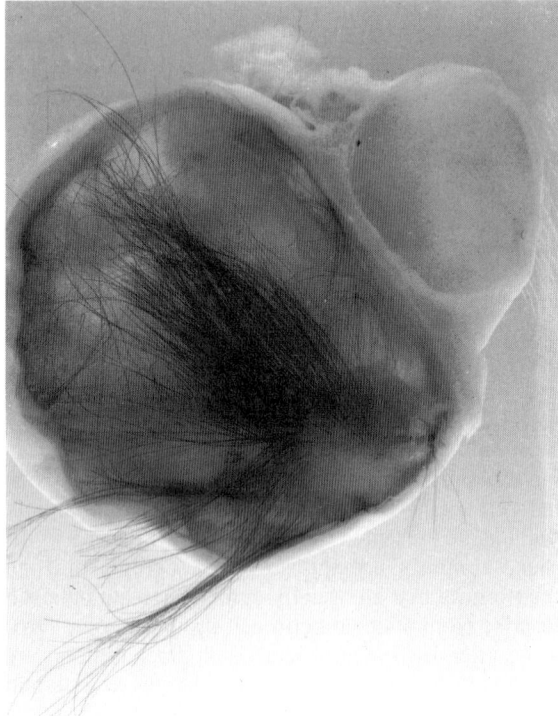

Figure 12.9 *Cystic teratoma of the ovary showing a prominent tuft of hair sprouting from the epithelial lining*

struma ovarii and the effect is essentially one of hyperthyroidism. Oöphorectomy of the affected ovary is curative for the differentiated type of teratoma. If the condition is bilateral it may be difficult to preserve the woman's fertility. In less than 2% of ovarian teratomata, one of the tissue types in the mass undergoes malignant transformation. It is usually the epithelial component forming a squamous cell carcinoma that behaves in a similar fashion to other tumours of this type in other situations in the body.

A very small proportion of teratomata of the ovary are the so-called **immature teratomata**, occurring in younger females (20 years old or younger). They are usually unilateral tumours that are composed of partially differentiated tissues, resembling a developing embryo. Neural tissue and cartilage are predominant tissue types present. This type of teratoma is malignant and is associated with a poor prognosis.

Malignant dysgerminoma. This is a type of germ cell tumour occurring primarily in children and young women under the age of 30 years. In about 15% of cases the tumours are bilateral. The tumour is large and fleshy, appearing encapsulated. On section, it is a pale to tan tumour with no necrosis or haemorrhage usually apparent. Microscopically the tumour resembles seminoma of the testis, consisting of large, polygonal, pale cells arranged in groups, with a prominent infiltrate of lymphocytes in the stroma. The tumour is highly radiosensitive and depending on the stage of the tumour at the time of diagnosis it has 5-year survivals ranging from 90% (unilateral tumours treated early) to 40% (bilateral or advanced stage tumours diagnosed late).

Endodermal sinus tumour (yolk sac tumour of the ovary). This is a rare ovarian tumour typified by the extremely rapid growth of an abdominal mass. It is seldom seen in women younger than 40 years of age and more than half of the patients have symptoms for one week or less when they present. The tumour is large (average diameter of about 15 cm), solid with a cut surface showing haemorrhage and necrosis. A very complex microscopic appearance is seen with several cell patterns forming highly characteristic structures (glomeruloid structures, reticular patterns, alveologlandular structures, etc.). Hyaline eosinophilic droplets are present in many of the tumour cells and these consist of α-foetoprotein. The tumour is highly malignant, with quite a poor prognosis and a very low 5-year survival.

Stromal Cell Tumours of the Ovary (10% of Tumours)
Granulosa cell tumours. These are the most commonly

occurring of the sex cord tumours and about half of them occur in post-menopausal women. They are tumours that secrete sex hormones and may have a virilizing effect. About 75% of the tumours secrete excessive oestrogens and are usually benign. Menstrual irregularity, endometrial hyperplasia, endometrial carcinoma and fibrocystic disease of the breast are often seen in association with the tumour. In young girls with the tumour, precocious puberty and menarche may be stimulated by the hyperoestrinism.

The tumours are solid and encapsulated, of varying sizes. Most tumours are slow growing and benign but if the tumour diameter is larger than 5 cm it is usually malignant. Microscopically several characteristic patterns are seen (e.g. micro- and macrofollicular, trabecular or diffuse). Benign tumours have a good prognosis but malignant ones have, on average a 5-year survival of 40%.

Thecoma and fibrothecoma. These masses consist of theca cells and fibroblasts. Usually they are unilateral and occur in young girls and women. They are almost always benign and are encapsulated yellowish masses. The theca cells are large, yellowish and round while the fibroblasts are elongated cells between the tumour cells. Such tumours elaborate oestrogens and produce a hyperoestrinism that causes precocious puberty and menarche in young girls and menstrual irregularity in women. Surgical removal of the mass is curative.

Other stromal cell tumours. Sertoli cell tumours and Leydig cell tumours of the ovary are very rare neoplasms that may be associated with hormonal irregularities. Excesses of androgens or oestrogens may be produced resulting in virilization or menstrual irregularities respectively. Signs and symptoms of virilization are hirsutism, amenorrhoea, clitoral enlargement and deepening of the voice. A small proportion of tumours is associated with Cushing's syndrome. Most such stromal tumours are benign and oöphorectomy is curative.

Secondary Tumours of the Ovary (5% of Tumours)
Krukenberg tumour. Krukenberg tumours are bilateral secondaries on the ovaries that contain mucus-secreting cells. These are usually from primary malignant tumours of the stomach that metastasize to the ovary through transcoelomic spread in the peritoneal cavity. Occasionally, other mucus-secreting primary tumours (e.g. colonic carcinoma) will spread to the ovary and lead to an appearance identical to Krukenberg tumours.

Others. Secondary tumours of the ovaries are fairly common and they are derived from primaries of the gastrointestinal tract and occasionally from the breast and genital tract.

Disorders of Pregnancy

Abortion

Spontaneous abortion occurs very commonly. Probably one in four pregnancies ends in abortion in the early stages. Most of these early pregnancies are not apparent, and the woman is not aware of the pregnancy or of the abortion. In some cases, the abortion is incomplete, with residual products of conception remaining behind in the uterus. In this case, infection of the uterus and pelvis is greatly predisposed to. In all cases of abortion there may be varying degrees and duration of haemorrhage and the woman may present with anaemia.

Septic abortion may particularly occur if the condition is self-induced or if the procedure is carried out by unqualified people in an unhygienic manner. In this case, severe infections of the uterus and pelvis may occur. Such infections, unless treated aggressively in the early stages, may result in a fatality.

Ectopic Pregnancy

Ectopic pregnancy implies that the fertilized ovum implants anywhere outside the normal uterine location. Ectopic pregnancy is not uncommon and occurs in approximately one in 120 pregnancies. About 95% of ectopic pregnancies are 'tubal pregnancies', that is, they occur in the Fallopian tube. The remaining 5% occur in the ovary, uterine portion of the Fallopian tube or in the abdominal cavity.

The condition occurs more commonly in association with any disorder that delays the passage of the ovum through the oviduct to the uterus. It may also occur when there is previous tubal damage, such as scarring resulting from chronic inflammation, PID or endometriosis. Intrauterine tumours (especially fibroids) or other tumours of the pelvis compressing the Fallopian tubes may cause ectopic pregnancy and the condition is also commoner in women with intrauterine devices (IUD). In approximately 50% of cases ectopic pregnancy is idiopathic.

In its early stages the embryo develops normally with formation of a placenta, amnion and decidual changes. Rarely, an intra-abdominal pregnancy is carried to full term and the baby is delivered by laparotomy. In tubal pregnancies, the embryo grows normally for 2 to 6 weeks following implantation and then as the

Fallopian tube enlarges greatly, it ruptures with a massive intraperitoneal haemorrhage. In rare cases, the embryo dies from poor placental attachment, with subsequent spontaneous proteolysis and absorption. In rarer cases the necrotic embryo may calcify through dystrophic calcification and remain *in situ* for many years, a condition known as a **lithopaedion**.

Macroscopically the Fallopian tube is seen to be distended by a haemorrhagic mass. The gestation sac containing the embryo may be visible. The tubal wall is thickened and haemorrhagic. In other areas the wall may be thinned and atrophic as a result of pressure atrophy and it is these sites that are likely to rupture. Microscopically the blood clot within the lumen of the Fallopian tube is seen to contain chorionic villi and decidual cells, with the embryo often seen in section.

Until rupture of the Fallopian tube occurs in ectopic pregnancy, the condition is indistinguishable from a normal pregnancy. Menstruation ceases, there is elevation of serum and urinary placental hormones (making pregnancy tests positive) and the uterus undergoes hypersecretory and decidual changes. Spotting, and cramping pain may be seen shortly after the first missed period. The amenorrhoea may last from 6 to 12 weeks. When the tube ruptures, at about 12 weeks gestation, intense abdominal pain results in a typical 'acute abdomen' presentation. The woman may go into shock associated with the massive internal and sometimes external (*per vaginam*) haemorrhages. Emergency surgical intervention is necessary to save the life of the woman. The risk of having a subsequent ectopic pregnancy is approximately 10%. Ectopic pregnancies may result in death from shock and disseminated intravascular coagulation. Approximately one in 800 ectopic pregnancies results in death.

Pre-eclampsia and Eclampsia of Pregnancy

This condition is also known as 'toxaemia' of pregnancy, and occurs in 5% of all pregnancies. It is an idiopathic clinical syndrome and it typically occurs in primigravidae, women who have hypertension also being more predisposed to it.

Pre-eclampsia is characterized by the triad of generalized oedema, hypertension and proteinuria. These changes develop from about week 20 of the pregnancy and continue until the end of the first week post partum. Pre-eclampsia is rarely fatal to the mother. If control of blood pressure fails and proteinuria appears, the preferred treatment is to deliver the foetus. Removal of the foetus and placenta improves the condition dramatically and the woman will recover completely shortly thereafter.

Eclampsia is seen less frequently and is characterized by the symptoms and signs outlined above for pre-eclampsia, as well as any, or all, of the following:

- epileptiform convulsions;
- coma;
- disseminated intravascular coagulation;
- kidney and liver failure;
- foetal death *in utero*.

In some cases, eclampsia develops suddenly with no preliminary signs. If the condition is untreated, there is high foetal and maternal mortality. Eclampsia may occur following delivery, usually immediately post partum.

Although both eclampsia and pre-eclampsia of pregnancy are idiopathic disorders, the improvement in the condition seen after the removal of the foetus and placenta from the uterus suggests that it may be a problem associated in part with an immune reaction to the foetal tissue. Eclampsia is more common in primigravidae, is associated with poor diet, excessive weight gains during the pregnancy, a large placenta, hydatidiform mole, Rh incompatibility, diabetes mellitus and multiple pregnancy. It is also more common in patients with pre-existing hypertension and renal disease.

If eclampsia is very severe there may be recurrent fits, coma and foetal death (the foetus dying in approximately a quarter of cases). Complications include an exceedingly high blood pressure, fever, tachycardia, cerebral haemorrhage, liver and kidney failure. Retinal haemorrhage may be a late sequela.

The kidneys show diffuse glomerular swelling and arteriolar wall oedema and degeneration. The liver, which is involved in 50% of cases of eclampsia, shows enlargement and softness with haemorrhage and necrosis in the periportal regions of the liver. The placenta is bulky, with prominent infarcts and degeneration of syncytiotrophoblasts in the chorionic villi. With pre-existing hypertension, the lesions described above are more pronounced and the disease will progress more quickly. The mother may die in approximately 10% of cases of eclampsia, usually of hepatic failure.

Congenital and Perinatal Infections

A large group of infectious agents can complicate a pregnancy or a delivery through infection of the baby while still *in utero,* while it is passing down an infected birth canal, or infecting the newborn soon after birth (refer to Figure 12.10). The normal placenta is quite resistant to infection and many agents cannot

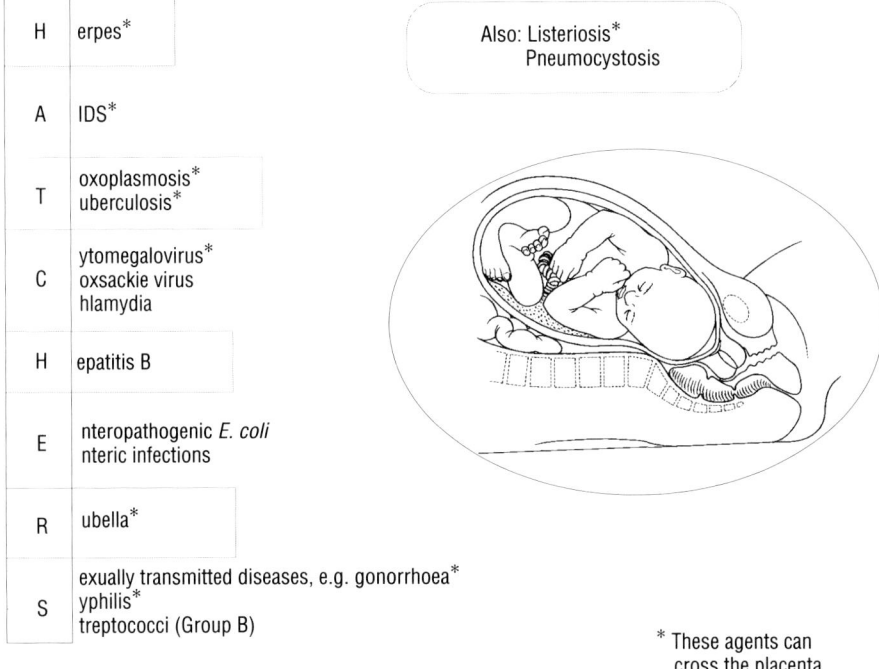

H	erpes*
A	IDS*
T	oxoplasmosis* uberculosis*
C	ytomegalovirus* oxsackie virus hlamydia
H	epatitis B
E	nteropathogenic *E. coli* nteric infections
R	ubella*
S	exually transmitted diseases, e.g. gonorrhoea* yphilis* treptococci (Group B)

Also: Listeriosis*
Pneumocystosis

* These agents can
cross the placenta

Figure 12.10 *Congenital and perinatal infections*

cross the placental barrier to infect the unborn baby. Usually two types of such infection are differentiated: those agents that have adapted to placental crossing or those agents that infect the newborn during passage through the birth canal cause infections that are termed **congenital infections**, implying that they are present at the time of birth. On the other hand if the infection is acquired through the usual routes of transfer from infected or carrier individuals or from the environment shortly after birth, the infections are termed **perinatal infections**.

The blood–foetal junction in the placenta is an important pathway for infection in the foetus. The number of cells separating maternal from foetal blood depends not only on the species of animal (compare four cell sheets in the horse to only one or two in humans), but also on the stage of pregnancy. The junction usually becomes thinner, often with fewer cell layers, in later pregnancy. There are regular mechanical leaks in the placenta late in most human pregnancies and up to 4 mL of blood is transferred across the placenta but this appears to be principally in one direction, from foetus to mother. There is little evidence for the passive carriage of micro-organisms across the placenta. Usually most micro-organisms are unable to cross the placenta.

Foetal infection takes place by either of two mechanisms:

- If a circulating micro-organism, free or cell associated, localizes on the maternal vessels it can multiply, produce toxins, locally interrupt the integrity of the junction and so infect the foetus (e.g. *Treponema pallidum, Toxoplasma gondii*).
- Alternatively, a circulating micro-organism can localize and grow across the placental junction (e.g. rubella and cytomegalovirus infections).

In both of these cases a placental lesion or focus of infection develops before the foetus is infected. Few micro-organisms can cause foetal infections and nearly always the foetus is protected from microbial as well as from biochemical and physical insults. The factors that localize micro-organisms to the placenta are not clearly understood, but blood flow is slow in placental vessels, giving maximal opportunity for localization. Once they are located in the placental vessels the micro-organisms' growth may be enhanced by particular substances present in the placenta. For example, erythritol promotes the growth of *Brucella abortus* and its presence in the bovine placenta makes this a target organ in infected cows (although *Brucella abortus* causes abortions in cows, it does not do so in humans because of the absence of erythritol in the human placenta).

Micro-organisms can damage the foetus without infecting its tissues. If they localize extensively in placental vessels and cause vascular damage there, this can lead to foetal anoxia, death and abortion. Also, the toxic products of microbial growth in the placenta (or elsewhere) can reach the foetus and cause damage. Once the micro-organisms have gained entry into the foetal tissues, they may have a variety of effects. Commonly, their presence in the developing organs of the foetus cause abortion or stillbirth. If the baby is not aborted, various malformations result, especially involving the cardiovascular and central nervous systems. Clinical disease typical of rubella and lung infection may be seen in the baby at birth, in association with the congenital lesions caused by the agent.

Rubella is an important infection because approximately a quarter of children born to mothers contracting rubella during the first four months of pregnancy have **congenital defects** (malformations). If the disease is contracted during the first four weeks of pregnancy then about 50% of children will be deformed (the total incidence of congenital rubella is about 17%).

From the mother's blood the rubella virus crosses the placenta into the tissues of the foetus where it can persist throughout gestation and into the neonatal period. The unborn child is infected at the same time as its mother and since the viral injury leads to irregularities of development of organs, malformations develop. Defects are common in the eyes (cataracts), ears (deafness), heart and brain. Many foetuses are stillborn or aborted after infection with rubella.

When infection with the virus persists after birth, the baby is born with congenital rubella, the manifestations of which may be mild or severe. These may be a single serious defect or multiple defects in a small undersized baby. The rubella syndrome indicates active infection in the newborn which is easily demonstrated by recovery of the virus from the nasopharynx, conjunctivae, urine and spinal fluid.

Serological tests confirm suspected rubella infections. Gamma globulin may be administered to infected mothers during the first or second trimester of pregnancy, but this has not proved to be a reliable treatment. The recommended treatment during the first trimester is therapeutic abortion to avoid the possibility of the rubella syndrome in the newborn (unless the mother is prepared to deal with a severely handicapped child). Girls should have natural rubella infections or be vaccinated against the infection before their childbearing years, and a pregnant mother should avoid at all costs exposure to the disease.

Congenital syphilis occurs because *Treponema pallidum* can cross the placenta and the disease is thus transferred to the foetus *in utero*. The treponemes are borne by the blood to the maternal side of the placenta and are deposited there. Syphilitic foci develop and the organisms then spread through to the foetal circulation. The shorter the time elapsing between infection of the mother and conception, the more likely it is that the unborn baby will be infected. If the mother is treated before the fifth month of pregnancy the child should be born free of the disease. Congenital syphilis usually appears at birth, within a few weeks of birth, or many years later. The child of a syphilitic mother may be:

- born dead;
- born alive with syphilis;
- born apparently healthy but showing signs of syphilis some time later;
- born entirely free of the disease.

In children stillborn, the lungs are very large, of a peculiar grey-white colour and incompletely developed. This is known as **pneumonia alba** and is pathognomonic of congenital syphilis. Congenital neurosyphilis simulates the acquired form and may appear early in life or be delayed until adolescence. Infants born with active syphilis are undersized and look like 'old people', greatly shrunken and wrinkled. A vesicular skin eruption and nasal discharge are common findings. The child may have linear scars at the angles of the mouth (**syphilitic rhagades**). Among the late manifestations of congenital syphilis are poorly developed, small, peg-shaped permanent teeth, the incisors being wedge-shaped and showing a central notch (**Hutchinson's teeth**).

Congenital syphilis is detected in the neonate with a modified fluoroserologic test detecting the presence of 19s macroglobulins formed by the baby against *Treponema pallidum* (these cannot cross the placenta as do the 7s globulins of the mother).

Gonorrhoea present in the mother during delivery of the baby leads to *Neisseria gonorrhoeae* infecting the eyes of the neonate, causing **ophthalmia neonatorum**, a gonorrhoeal conjunctivitis of newborn infants. The eyes are infected during birth through an infected birth canal and female babies may also acquire gonococcal vaginitis in this way. Similarly, ophthalmia and other perinatal infections may occur if the mother is infected with *Chlamydia trachomatis* or with *Mycoplasma* spp. Various forms of neonatal ophthalmia are routinely prevented through the instillation of tetracycline drops into the eyes of the newborn. In rare cases, gonorrhoea in a pregnant woman may infect the foetus, thus causing a congenital gonococcal infection in the newborn.

Toxoplasmosis is a disease caused by *Toxoplasma gondii*, a protozoon. It occurs in a wide range of mammalian and avian hosts as crescentic organisms about 6 μm long. It is an intracellular parasite that invades cells (mainly macrophages), multiplying within them until the cell is packed with organisms. Rupture of the cell releases the organisms to infect other cells. Proliferation occurs widely in the body but particularly in the CNS, muscles and lungs. In the chronic stage, infected cells may be up to 60 μm in diameter and contain thousands of parasites enclosed in a tough membrane, the cyst. The infection may proceed unnoticed for some time. The congenital form is acquired *in utero* from an infected mother. Stillbirth or abortion of the infected foetus are commonly the outcome, while in the babies that are born alive, the disease is characterized by CNS lesions which may lead to cerebral calcification, microcephaly, hydrocephaly and psychomotor disturbances. In congenital toxoplasmosis the newborn baby becomes very ill, develops a skin rash, turns yellow and may have convulsions. If it survives the damage done to the brain, mental retardation will result, and the chorioretinitis, which is also present, will lead to blindness.

The parasite is harboured in many animals and eating raw or undercooked meat may give rise to the infection. It has been detected in cat faeces and pregnant women should avoid handling cats, cats' faeces, etc. For the congenital form to develop the organisms must get into the bloodstream of the mother sometime after the first trimester of pregnancy. The organisms establish a focus of infection in the placenta that enables them to penetrate the foetal circulation and infect the foetus.

Listeriosis is an infection caused by *Listeria monocytogenes*, a small (≈ 2 μm long) Gram-positive, non-sporing, motile bacillus that infects humans, poultry and livestock. It causes a disease characterized by an increase in monocytes in the blood. The bacterium can continue to multiply in monocytes after it has been phagocytosed. In humans the microbe can cause purulent meningitis, conjunctivitis, endocarditis, urethritis and a type of infectious mononucleosis. It may cause asymptomatic infections. The number of human cases of the disease is small.

In pregnant women listeriosis is followed by abortion (usually in the fifth or sixth month), perinatal death or severe generalized infection of the neonate. Infection involving the surviving foetus and neonate is termed **granulomatosis infantiseptica**, which is an intrauterine *Listeria* infection associated with widespread necrosis of the internal organs (especially the spleen and liver) and haemorrhagic areas in the skin. The newborn infant usually dies within 2 to 3 days of delivery. The organism can be isolated in the laboratory and identified by means of biochemical tests.

Cytomegalic inclusion disease is an infection caused by the cytomegaloviruses (CMV). It may take on several clinical manifestations, the most important of which is the cytomegalic inclusion disease of the newborn. A mononucleosis-like disease is the usual result of infection with CMV and is most commonly seen after transfusions. The viruses have an affinity for the salivary glands and kidney where they produce highly characteristic lesions. Large, well-defined viral inclusions are seen in the nucleus and smaller ones in the cytoplasm of infected cells, which are greatly enlarged. In fatal cases, the inclusions are seen in the gastrointestinal tract, lung, liver, spleen and other organs. In non-fatal cases the infection is frequently asymptomatic.

In its overt form, CMV disease is seen in the newborn as a congenital infection acquired from the mother *in utero*. In the infected foetus CMV causes defects such as microcephaly, hydrocephaly, blindness and other lesions of the CNS. Malformed babies exhibit the viral inclusions in most organs, especially the kidney. Among the survivors, mental retardation due to microcephaly is usually evident, accompanied by chorioretinitis. Some children infected *in utero* or from the cervix uteri during birth do not show symptoms but may continue to excrete the virus in the urine over a period of years, despite the presence of circulating antibody. Chronic infections can occur in children and are associated with hepatosplenomegaly.

In a few instances it has been recorded that the **herpes virus** has crossed the placenta to produce generalized infection with malformations in the CNS and eyes. However, more commonly, herpes genitalis is known to infect babies during their passage through the infected birth canal. In 1 to 3 weeks after infection, the affected baby becomes gravely ill and usually dies, although many babies' lives have been saved through treatment with systemic antiviral agents such as iododeoxyuridine. Herpetic lesions in the infected infants can be found in all organs including the brain.

Hydatidiform Mole

This is a disorder of the chorionic tissue of the placenta where there is a mass of swollen or cystically dilated chorionic villi filling the uterine cavity. There is conversion of some or all of the chorionic villi into clear grape-like vesicular masses. In affected villi, blood vessels are absent, and the stroma is oedematous. Complete hydatidiform mole is the most frequently occurring form of the disease and this implies that an embryo is not present; whereas a partial mole, occurring less commonly, implies that an embryo is found amongst the abnormal villi.

The incidence of the condition in Western countries is approximately once in every 2000 pregnancies. However, in the Middle East the incidence increases to once in 300 pregnancies and in Asia it may be as high as once in every 100 pregnancies. The condition is idiopathic and is thought to represent a benign neo-plasm of the placenta beginning at conception. It is commoner in the extremes of reproductive life, more frequent when maternal age is less than 20 years or more than 40 years, and occurs more commonly with ectopic pregnancy.

The woman with hydatidiform mole presents with a uterus that is 'too large for the dates' and with no foetal heart sounds. There will be haemorrhage *per vaginam,* with passage of grape-like masses in some cases, usually at about 16 to 17 weeks after conception and spontaneous abortion of the hydatidiform mole by the 18th to the 20th week may occur. Frequently, there is associated **hyperemesis gravidarum** ('morning sick-ness'), and pre-eclampsia is more common with this condition. The hydatidiform mole secretes human chorionic gonadotrophin. In patients where hydatidiform mole is diagnosed, 80% of cases are successfully treated by curettage. In 15% of cases the condition is recognized as an invasive mole, better considered as a neoplasm of intermediate character between a benign and malignant one. These intermedi-ate lesions are termed **chorioadenoma destruens** and may require further treatment. In 5% of cases the mole may undergo malignant change to a **choriocarcinoma**.

Choriocarcinoma

This is a malignancy derived from the chorionic trophoblast. It may arise *de novo* or it may be a sequela of hydatidiform mole. It shows a very aggressive be-haviour and it must be remembered that it is a tumour derived from foetal tissue.

Incidence. It is an extremely rare carcinoma, occurring once in every 50 000 Caucasian pregnancies. How-ever, in Asians the condition is much commoner, oc-curring once in every 1000 pregnancies.

Aetiology. The condition is predisposed to by the fol-lowing factors:

- maternal age of less than 20 years or more than 40 years;
- pre-existing hydatidiform mole (50% of cases of the tumour);
- following abortions (25% of cases of the tumour);
- abnormal gestations (e.g. ectopic pregnancy);

- occurs in association with malignant teratoma of the ovary;
- occurs more frequently in certain racial/geographic groups.

Appearance. The tumour forms very haemorrhagic and necrotic masses in the uterus, often the whole of the primary neoplasm undergoing necrosis. The tu-mour is epithelial with masses of anaplastic cells, cuboidal cytotrophoblasts and syncytiotrophoblasts; however, no chorionic villi are formed.

Spread. The tumour is highly malignant, very aggres-sive and shows early haematogenous spread. At the time of diagnosis, 50% of the patients show pulmo-nary lesions with also the liver, brain and kidneys affected in many cases. The secondary masses are multiple, round and rapidly growing, known as 'can-non ball' metastases. Local spread to involve the vagi-nal wall occurs in about 35% of cases but lymphatic spread is unusual.

Signs and symptoms. The affected woman presents with bloody or brownish vaginal discharge after what has seemed a pregnancy. On abdominal examination there is absence of marked uterine enlargement and no embryo is present. There are grossly raised levels of HCG in both blood and urine.

Treatment and prognosis. Once, this condition was almost always fatal with 90 to 100% mortality. With the advent of chemotherapy, treatment with suitable cytotoxic drugs (e.g. methotrexate) have made the tu-mours curable. Cure rates of 100% have been reported for tumours that are confined to the uterus, vagina and lungs. For more disseminated tumours the cure rate is still 75%. This shows very well the sensitivity of the tumour to chemotherapeutic agents, but also the im-portance of the host immune response in fighting the tumour. As the tumour is of paternal/maternal origin (developing from embryonic tissue), the immune sys-tem recognizes the foreign cells and mounts an im-mune response against them, successfully eradicating the small groups of cancer cells that are still surviving following chemotherapy.

The Normal Breast

The normal breasts, or **mammae**, are typical exocrine glands which may be considered to be skin append-ages, modified sweat glands, found only in mammals. Breasts first appear on the mammary ridges ('milk lines') in the fifth week of intrauterine development.

These milk lines are bilateral ventral ectodermal thickenings running from axillae to ipsilateral groins. The caudal two-thirds of these lines disappears in the following 2 weeks. In a small number of cases, the breasts fail to develop and the condition, an example of agenesis, is termed **amastia**. In the seventh week there is thickening of the mammary ridge to form the precursor of the nipple. In humans only two nipples are normally formed but in lower mammals many nipples form. Not infrequently (5% of females, 1% of males), smaller accessory nipples may also be seen in humans as a congenital anomaly, a condition called **polythelia**. Between the twentieth and thirtieth week solid epidermal cords grow into the subcutaneous tissue and form 15 to 20 lobar ducts. At birth the nipple is formed by evagination of the epidermal pit and in both sexes breast enlargement and transitory secretion may be seen due to the action of maternal hormones. Further development of the breasts depends upon female sex hormone stimulation so the male breast remains infantile and rudimentary throughout life unless a hormonal disorder causes the male breasts to enlarge, a condition termed **gynaecomastia** (refer to Figure 12.11).

At puberty in the female, ovarian hormonal stimulation begins and causes an enlargement of the nipple, areola and the entire breast through a process of physiological hyperplasia. Adipose tissue is deposited in large amounts in the fibrocollagenous stroma. The lobar ducts elongate and subdivide, forming interlobular and intralobular ducts, lined by two to three cells. The breast then undergoes cyclical hyperplasia and involution during the menstrual cycle, but develops no further until the woman becomes pregnant. In rare cases, several well-developed breasts will be seen along the milk line, a condition termed **polymastia**.

In late pregnancy the intralobular ducts bud to form secretory acini that are lined by a single layer of epithelial cells. At delivery the acini secrete **colostrum** and in the puerperium lactation is seen, initiated by the pituitary and maintained by the suckling of the baby. During weaning there will be involution of the breast such that it shrinks back to almost pre-pregnancy size. At the menopause there will be parenchymal (lobular) involution and stromal sclerosis.

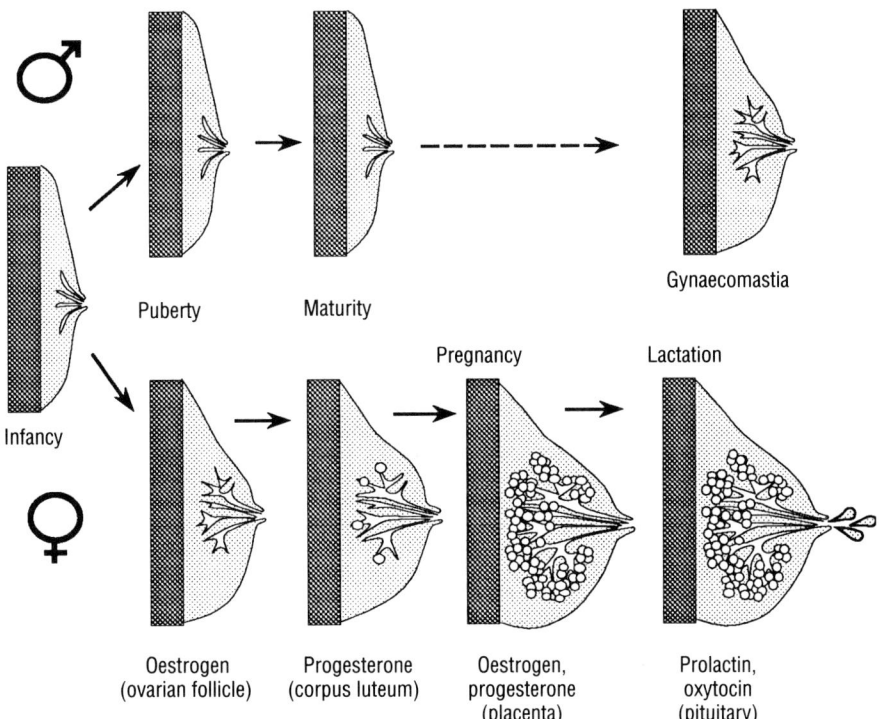

Figure 12.11 *Normal mammary gland development*

Diseases of the Female Breast

Inflammations and Infections

Mastitis

Inflammations of the breast are rather uncommon and most of these disorders are seen during the reproductive years and are associated with lactation and breast feeding when the infant may damage the nipple, allowing bacteria to gain entry. Pyogenic bacteria enter, via cracked or fissured nipples and cause an ascending infection of the breast ducts. The bacteria involved are most commonly *Staphylococcus aureus* and *Streptococcus* spp. Staphylococcal infections usually result in a single abscess or multiple abscesses while streptococcal infections cause a diffuse cellulitis.

The breast in mastitis is red, swollen, hot and painful. The nipple shows cracks, fissures, exudation or suppuration. Inspissation of secretions in the inflamed breast may lead to stoppage of milk flow. Untreated abscesses enlarge and eventually point through the skin, discharging pus. Antibiotic therapy usually controls the infection but drainage of large abscesses may also be required. Streptococcal infections usually resolve completely upon antibiotic therapy but staphylococcal infections heal by fibrosis, leaving residual foci of scar that are palpated as localized regions of induration ('lumps').

Syphilis

The primary lesions of syphilis, chancres, are common on the breast. These are painless ulcers caused by infection with *Treponema pallidum*. These lesions on the breast may be associated with syphilitic lesions on the genitals or cervix. The condition is treated by systemic antibiotic therapy and there is healing without scarring.

Traumatic Fat Necrosis

Fat necrosis of the breast may follow direct trauma to the breast (e.g. seat belt injury in a road accident, or a blow to the breast). The adipocytes in the breast stroma are damaged directly, release their fat and undergo necrosis. Inflammation and scarring follow. The condition results in a localized firm, fibrous mass frequently palpated as a hard lump by an alarmed woman. This lesion must be distinguished from a scirrhous carcinoma of the breast.

Fibrocystic Changes and Proliferative Changes

Fibrocystic changes of the breast are a wide variety of disorders ranging from the very innocuous, common lesions that are said to border on 'physiological variants', to the very rare, highly abnormal lesions that predispose to malignancy. A unifying feature of these disorders is the formation of breast 'lumps'. Within these lumps may be seen a variety of changes in various proportions:

- stromal fibrosis;
- stromal and epithelial hyperplasia;
- atypical epithelial hyperplasia;
- cystic changes (with microcyst and macrocyst development);
- cystic dysplasia.

It is accepted that many of these changes are an exaggeration and distortion of the normal cyclical changes that occur within the breast during the menstrual cycle. It has been observed that oestrogen therapy or the administration of the contraceptive pill does not increase the incidence of such lesions. Fibrocystic disease of the breast affects women of all ages, beginning during reproductive life but often persisting after the menopause. The aetiology of these various disorders is uncertain but excessive breast responsiveness to normal oestrogen levels is probably the underlying cause. Some degree of such changes is visible either macroscopically or microscopically in 60 to 90% of autopsies on women. With such a high incidence, one is prompted to ask if such changes constitute disease, especially as most of these changes are of no clinical significance (excepting the nodularity of the affected breast). A minority component is very important as it includes atypical epithelial hyperplasias and dysplastic lesions that are premalignant. It should be noted that more than one type of fibrocystic change may occur in the same breast. Four important alterations are seen in various combinations, as outlined below.

Fibrosis of the Breast

This is a totally benign proliferation of the stromal fibrous connective tissue, a hyperplasia of the fibroblasts with associated collagen deposition. Various degrees of epithelial hyperplasia may also be seen in this condition (**stromal-epithelial hyperplasia**). It should be noted that some degree of fibrosis is present in all forms of fibrocystic changes. Women between 30 and 40 years of age are most usually affected and the condition is common in incidence. Poorly defined solitary masses form in the breasts, 2 to 10 cm in diameter. They are of a rubbery consistency presenting as a tender or painful lump especially noticeable just before menstruation. A delimited area of induration is palpated but it is freely mobile and not attached to underlying tissues.

When the lump is removed at biopsy, it is seen to be a pale, firm lesion which on section shows a tough, greyish white, rubbery homogeneous connective tissue without any adipose tissue in it. Small regions of pinkish tissue may be present within the mass representing glands. Histologically, a mass of connective tissue will be seen, which sometimes encloses ducts, lobules and microcysts.

The condition does not predispose to carcinoma and is totally benign. However, as all breast lumps are considered to be malignant unless there is histological proof to the contrary, there is mandatory removal of such lesions at biopsy. Untreated lesions frequently regress after the menopause. Fibrosis of the breast is often described as a 'physiological aberration' rather than a true pathological condition.

Cystic Changes of the Breast

Cystic changes of the breast are a group of related disorders occurring in the breasts of women in the last half of their reproductive life. Cystic change implies the presence of **microcysts** (less than 1 mm in diameter) and **macrocysts** (greater than 1 mm in diameter) in the breast, formed by dilated, dysplastic tubules. They are examples of true cysts (fluid-filled spaces lined by epithelium). **Cystic disease** is said to be present if macrocysts larger than 3 mm in diameter are present, a finding observed in only 10% of cases of cystic change. The woman presenting with cystic change in the breast is usually between 40 and 55 years of age and has found a single or multiple lumps in her breasts. A solitary large cyst up to 5 cm in diameter may occasionally be present, but more commonly multiple smaller cysts are found in both breasts.

The aggregates of the cysts in this condition produce a large, irregular, multilobular mass. The cystic space is full of a thin turbid fluid and if a large cyst is close to the skin it may be detected as a bluish lump ('**blue dome cyst**'). Inspissation of secretion or haemorrhage in the cysts may occur and also there may be regions of epithelial thickening, fibrosis and calcification. Microscopically the prominent feature of the disorder is an epithelial hyperplasia involving the ducts

with cystic change and cystic dysplasia. Regions of stromal fibrosis are also commonly observed between the cysts. The cysts may be very large, in which case they are lined by a thinned, atrophic epithelium. Various metaplastic and dysplastic changes may be observed in the epithelium of the cystic ducts including **apocrine change** and **papillomatosis**.

Multiple bilateral cysts are easily distinguished from neoplastic conditions but a single cyst is more alarming. The presence of the cysts *per se* does not predispose to malignancy; however, there is a small risk of malignant change occurring in a breast where the cystic changes are accompanied by dysplasia, or if there is concomitant atypical epithelial hyperplasia, or if the woman has a history of breast cancer in her family. Cystic change is treated by drainage of cyst fluid from large cysts and biopsy to exclude atypical hyperplasias.

Adenosis and Intralobular Duct Proliferation

Adenosis implies a great increase in the glandular component of the breast, independent of normal lactation stimuli (see Figure 12.12). This condition therefore, is a pathological hyperplasia. This change is often accompanied by a diffuse increase in the stromal, fibrous tissue component, a change prompting some pathologists to classify the disease with the fibrocystic changes group as a **sclerosing adenosis**. Adenosis is usually seen in women of 35 to 45 years of age and presents as a unilateral, circumscribed lump of rubbery to hard consistency, most frequently in the upper, outer quadrant of the breast. The lump may be painful or tender, especially premenstrually.

Histologically there is an increase in the number and size of the acini which are only usually lined by a single (or at the most, double) layer of cells. Increased numbers of intralobular ducts (two to three cell layers) will also be observed. Increase in fibrous stroma that frequently accompanies this glandular proliferation will cause compression of the hyperplastic epithelium.

As adenosis and fibrosis occur in the same breast, both stromal and glandular elements will proliferate and often lead to widespread hardening of the affected breast, the condition being clinically difficult to differentiate from scirrhous carcinoma. It is treated by a 'lumpectomy', where the hyperplastic tissue is removed and examined for evidence of malignancy. Adenosis is not thought to carry an increased risk of malignant change.

Epitheliosis and Intraductal Epithelial Hyperplasia

This variant is similar to adenosis in that an epithelial hyperplasia occurs but there is also marked dysplasia in the hyperplastic epithelium. The surface epithelium of the acini and ducts becomes multilayered, and large ducts may become plugged with masses of cuboidal cells. There is variation in the size of the hyperplastic cells and the arrangement of the cells is abnormal. This condition is associated with an increased risk of malignant change. As it has an unpredictable behaviour it is widely excised at 'lumpectomy'.

Tumours of the Breast

Fibroadenoma

Fibroadenoma is the most common benign breast tumour (7% of lumps) seen typically in women between 25 and 35 years of age. It consists of a unilateral, encapsulated mass of proliferating ducts (adenoma) and fibrous stroma (fibroma) forming a well-defined, painless, mobile mass. It is usually approximately 3 cm in diameter, but may be larger, and is encapsulated. The cut surface of the tumour shows a firm, greyish white mass with areas of pinkish glandular tissue. Under the microscope the mass is composed of loose fibrous stroma containing duct-like epithelial structures of various forms and sizes. A variant of the tumour may also occur in adolescent girls and in this case the tumour is termed a **juvenile fibroadenoma**. Such tumours may attain great size. All types of fibroadenomata are thought to arise because of an increased sensitivity of the breast epithelial cells to oestrogens, and as such the tumours are seen to grow rapidly in pregnancy and to regress after the menopause.

Fibroadenomata are benign and seldom give rise to complications with little risk of malignant transformation. However, they are excised once diagnosed, 'just in case'. The removal of the breast lump is also of benefit to the woman involved, for her ease of mind. Such lumpectomy operations are very simple, leave little scarring and do not cause an unsightly appearance of the breast post-operatively.

Giant Fibroadenoma (Brodie's Tumour)

This is a variant of fibroadenoma that reaches a size of 10 to 15 cm and may cause a massive breast enlargement and distortion. It is usually seen in middle-aged to elderly women. Ulceration of the overlying skin and pressure effects, such as pressure necrosis, occur with the mass, but it is a benign lesion, frequently lobulated and quite clearly encapsulated. It may grow rather quickly and the lump that is palpated is often of a large size. Despite its alarming presentation, malignant transformation of the tumour is uncommon. Because of its rapid growth, pressure effects and the great anxiety that it causes the women presenting with it, the tumour is excised.

Papilloma

Papillomata of the breast are solitary, benign, papillary tumours which form in one of the main ducts or within a cyst. They develop most frequently in women aged between 20 and 30 years, becoming quite rare in women above the age of 50 years. Occasionally these tumours may protrude from the nipple if they form in the major secretory duct. As the tumour may haemorrhage into the lumen of the duct, a bloody discharge from the

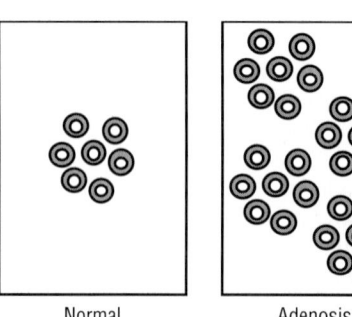

Normal
breast:
Ducts in stroma

Adenosis:
Excess
ducts in stroma

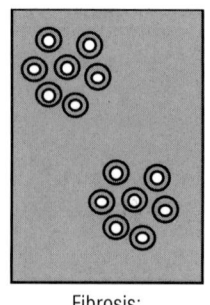

Fibrosis:
Ducts
in excess stroma

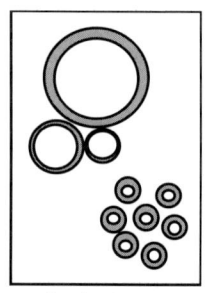

Cystic change:
Cystic ducts
in stroma

Figure 12.12 *Proliferative changes in breast tissue*

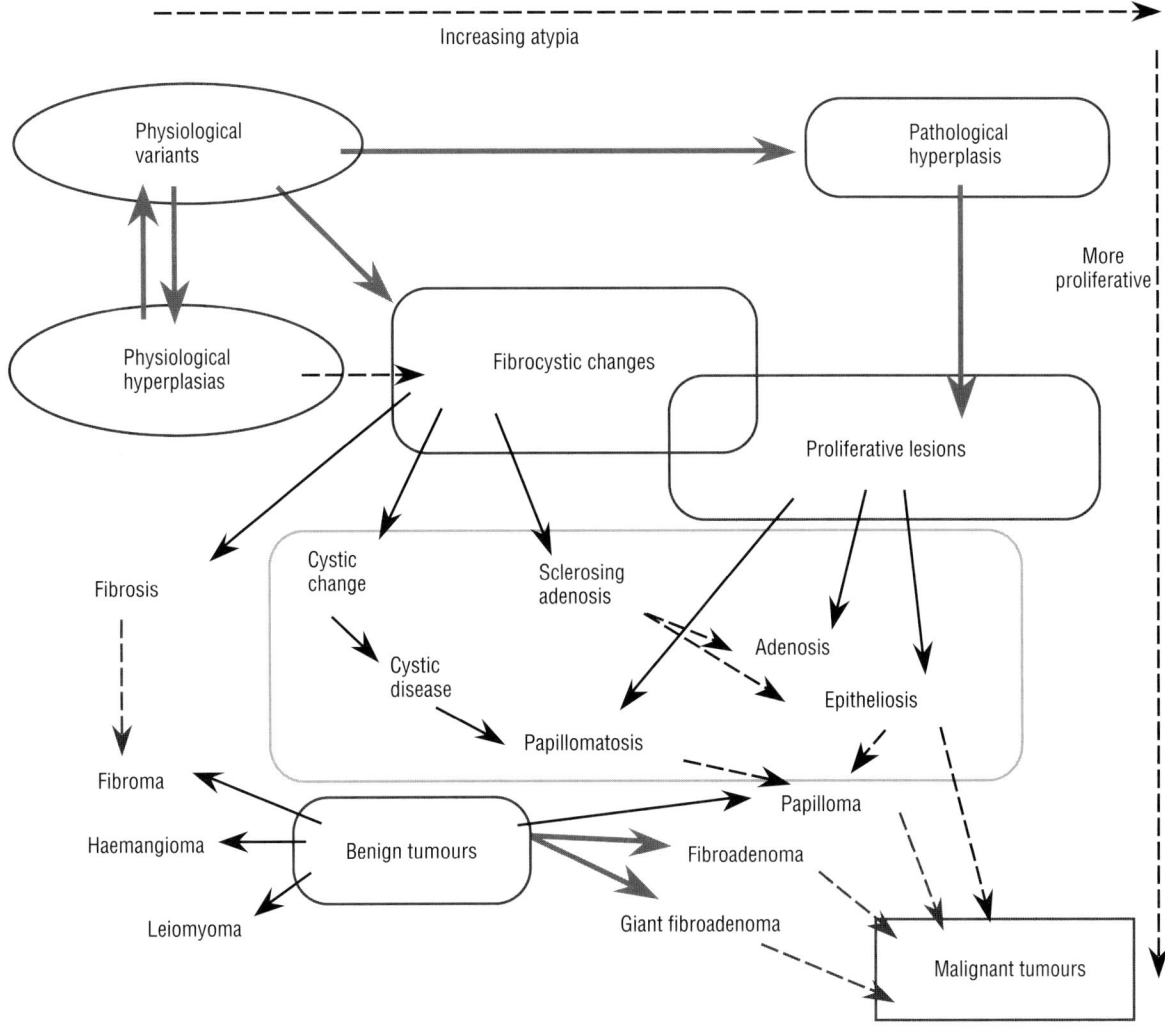

Figure 12.13 *Interrelationship of proliferative conditions in breast tissue (lightly shaded arrows indicate the commoner progressions)*

nipple will be observed in some cases. Microscopically these tumours are typical columnar cell papillomata composed of aggregates of regular cells growing as a mass with a narrow pedicle attached to the main duct or the cyst wall. The intraductal tumours may cause obstruction and dilatation of the ducts with cyst formation. Papillomata which are not excised may undergo malignant change if left *in situ* for many years (see Figure 12.13).

Carcinoma of the Breast

Incidence. Breast carcinoma is a malignant tumour derived from the epithelial component of the breast, ducts or acini. It is the major cause of cancer deaths in women (20% of all cancer deaths in women) and accounts for 16% of all cancer deaths. Most cases are in women over the age of 35 years, the majority of patients being perimenopausal. Breast cancer is more common in the Western world, being rare in countries such as Japan, Mexico and some Southeast Asian countries. It is almost exclusively a tumour of women, the sex ratio being 1:150, the males affected by the disease suffering from some endocrine disturbance and gynaecomastia.

Aetiology. The aetiological and predisposing factors as indicated by epidemiological studies are as follows:

- **Geographic/racial influences**: Breast cancer is five times more common in the USA and other Western countries than in Asia. It is possible that exogenous factors in the different regions play a role, such as diet and carcinogens in the environment, but also social factors such as parity may play a role.
- **Genetic predisposition**: The degree of risk is proportional to the number of close relatives with breast cancer. The younger the age incidence of breast cancer and the higher the incidence of bilateral breast cancer in close relatives, the greater the genetic predisposition. Occasionally there are seen 'high risk' families with apparent autosomal dominant transmission and familial association of breast and ovarian carcinomata.
- **Increasing age**: Breast cancer is uncommon before the age of 20, then there is a steady increase until menopause, and a slower rise through later life.
- **Exogenous oestrogen**: This is controversial, but some evidence shows moderately increased risk with high-dose oestrogen therapy of menopausal symptoms.
- **Endogenous oestrogens (hyperoestrinism)**: In conditions where there are high oestrogen levels in the body (e.g. ovarian or adrenal tumours) there is an increased risk.
- **Length of reproductive life**: The risk increases with early menarche and late menopause.
- **Parity**: It is more common in nulliparous than parous or multiparous women.
- **Age at which woman has her first child**: There is increased risk when a mother is over 30 years of age at the time of having her first child.
- **Obesity**: There is increased risk associated with the increased oestrogen synthesis in fat depots.
- **Fibrocystic changes**, **atypical epithelial hyperplasia** in the breast result in increased risk. The higher the degree of dysplastic change the higher the risk.
- **Carcinoma of the contralateral breast or endometrium** results in increased risk in the woman with these conditions.
- **Dietary factors**: Women with a high saturated fat diet and much red meat in the diet have a higher risk. These epidemiological data are supported by experiments in which the incidence of spontaneous breast carcinomata is observed to be much higher in mice that are fed on high saturated fat diets.

Pathogenesis. Breast carcinoma appears to be related, at least in part, to hyperoestrinism and is commoner in daughters and sisters of women with breast cancer. It is also more common in women with no or few pregnancies. Oestrogen receptors occur on breast cancer cells, and to a lesser extent in non-malignant tissues. It is thought that there is a genetic predisposition influencing the availability of hormone receptors in breast epithelial cells. This may explain the 'promoter' effects of high oestrogen levels (hyperoestrinism) on the breast, leading to breast carcinoma.

Some people still believe there may be viruses responsible for human breast cancer. This hypothesis is mainly derived from experimental data, as it has been discovered that certain viruses are 'inherited' in female mice from their mothers, the infection resulting in mammary tumours. However, no human virus has been to date linked with breast carcinoma or isolated from cancerous tissue. Other experimental data implicate various carcinogens which may have important links with diet. It is known that the polycyclic aromatic compound DMBA will cause breast tumours in animals under suitable conditions.

Sites affected. Carcinoma of the breast is usually unilateral, and occurs mostly in the upper, outer quadrant of the breast. In 4–10% of cases tumours develop bilaterally or a second tumour develops subsequently (see Figures 12.14 and 12.15).

Morphology. Carcinoma of the breast presents as various types of tumour with different macroscopic appearance. The majority of breast cancers (90% of carcinomata) arise from the duct epithelium, with only 10% from the lobular acini.

1. **Arising in the ducts**:
   Non-infiltrating: Intraductal (growing totally within the duct in the early stages). *Comedocarcinoma (5%, grows within the ducts and undergoes necrosis there, producing a pasty intraductal degenerate mass). Papillary carcinoma (~3%, large papillary masses in dilated ducts or in cysts within the affected breast).*
   Infiltrating: Extraductal (infiltrating and invading widely in the breast tissue). ***Scirrhous carcinoma (75%*** — scirrhous means hard, with a dense fibrous stroma, 'stony hard' on palpation). *Encephaloid carcinoma (= medullary carcinoma 5%* — soft, like brain in consistency, mostly glandular tissue, less stroma). *Colloid carcinoma (Mucinous carcinoma 2–3%* — 'gelatinous' type of tumour in which the cells produce mucin. *Paget's disease of the nipple*, involves the main excretory ducts of the nipple and shows large ring-like cells (Paget cells).

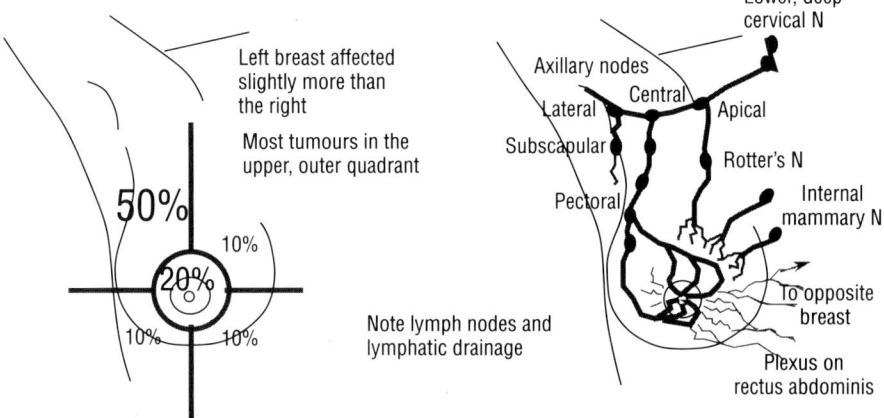

Figure 12.14   *Sites involved in breast carcinoma and relationship to lymph nodes*

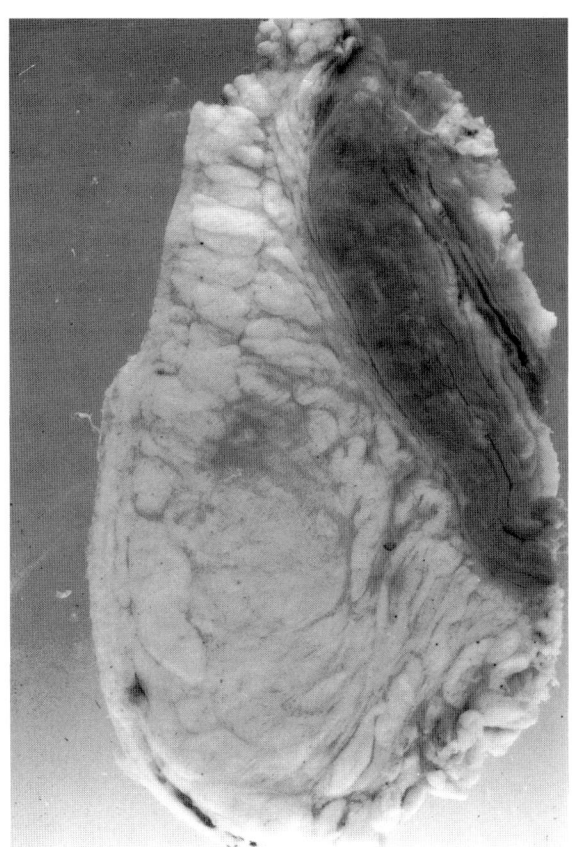

Figure 12.15   *Schirrous carcinoma of the breast, visible as a well-defined nodule in the centre of the breast tissue*

2.   **Arising in the lobules**:
   Non-infiltrating: *In-situ lobular carcinoma (≈ 4%, may be multicentric and bilateral).*
   Infiltrating: *Lobular carcinoma (~6%, often bilateral).*

In microscopic appearance, several distinct types also occur. **Adenocarcinomata** are well-differentiated, slow-growing breast carcinomata and they commonly occur in this tissue. **Spheroidal cell carcinomata** show some attempt to form ducts but are less well differentiated (Figure 12.16). **Anaplastic carcinomata** show pleomorphism, rapid growth and lack of differentiation (anaplasia). Uncommonly, **colloid carcinomata** occur and they produce a mucoid secretion which may form accumulations in cystic spaces within the tumour. **Squamous cell carcinoma** occurs in less than 1% of tumours. The **comedocarcinoma** shows tumour

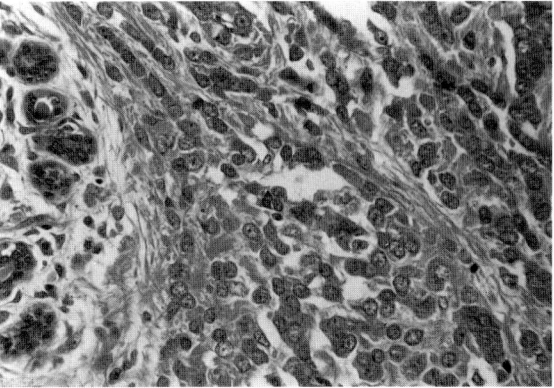

Figure 12.16   *Spheroidal carcinoma of the breast (×380)*

cells contained within the ducts and prominent necrosis of this intraductal tumour (Figure 12.17).

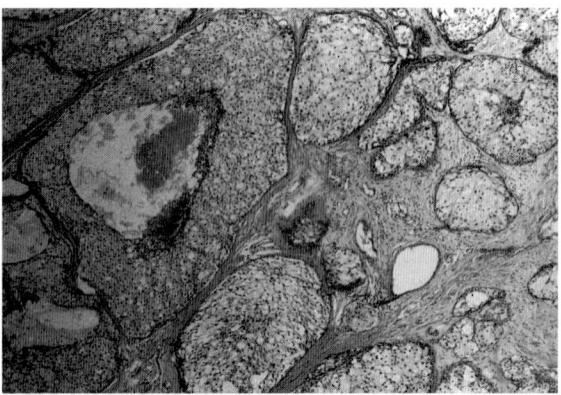

Figure 12.17   *Comedocarcinoma of the breast (×200)*

Spread. **Direct** spread occurs through the breast to involve pectoral muscles, skin and lymphatic vessels. **Lymphatic** spread occurs early (66% of cases show lymphatic involvement at the time of diagnosis). Tumours which arise in the upper, outer breast quadrant spread to the ipsilateral axilla, the number of axillary nodes involved correlating inversely with the prognosis. Breast cancer arising in the medial quadrants (especially the inner, lower quadrant) tend to spread to

the internal thoracic nodes (and to the liver; see Figure 12.14). They are associated with a poorer prognosis. **Haematogenous** spread occurs rather late but is very common and involves bone, the lungs, liver, brain, adrenals and sometimes ovaries.

Signs and symptoms. Certain features are common to all breast carcinomata and they are important diagnostically. The first indication that a breast tumour is developing in the breast is a **breast lump**, which the woman first palpates herself. It is important to note that most of the breast lumps that are palpated are due to benign disease or to no disease and only 10% of lumps palpated are due to malignant tumours (refer to Figure 12.18).

Fixation to deeper tissue occurs due to local spread of the cancer. It spreads to deep fascia and pectoralis muscle, thus fixing the cancer to the chest wall. This anchoring of the tumour to the underlying tissues will present with a typical palpatory finding of a 'fixed lump'.

Nipple retraction or deviation occurs as the tumour infiltrates and adheres to the overlying skin and nipple area. *'Peau d' orange'* (orange-peel-like skin) occurs due to the skin dimpling as the lymphatics of the skin are infiltrated by tumour cells. Dermal oedema associated with poor lymphatic drainage causes this appearance. **Acute inflammation** is often seen with breast cancer, associated with areas of necrosis (e.g. comedocarcinoma) or in some cases with secondary infection. The breast may be swollen, red and painful.

Calcification and microcalcification is seen in 60

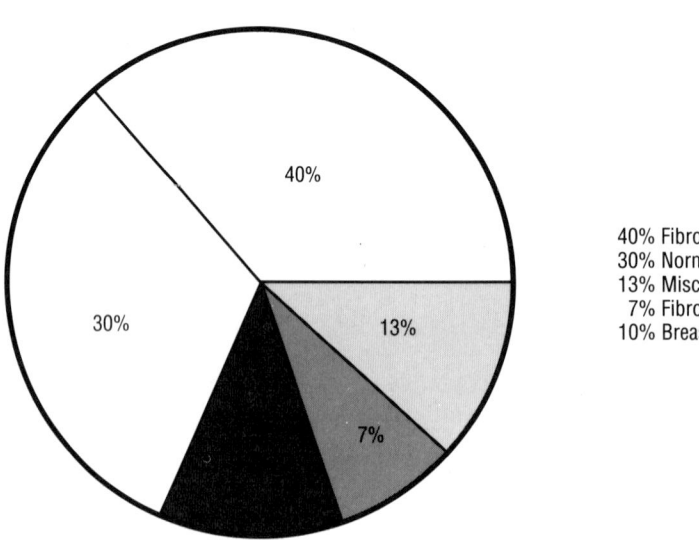

40% Fibrocystic changes
30% Normal breast
13% Miscellaneous benign
 7% Fibroadenoma
10% Breast cancer

Figure 12.18   *Identity of breast 'lumps'*

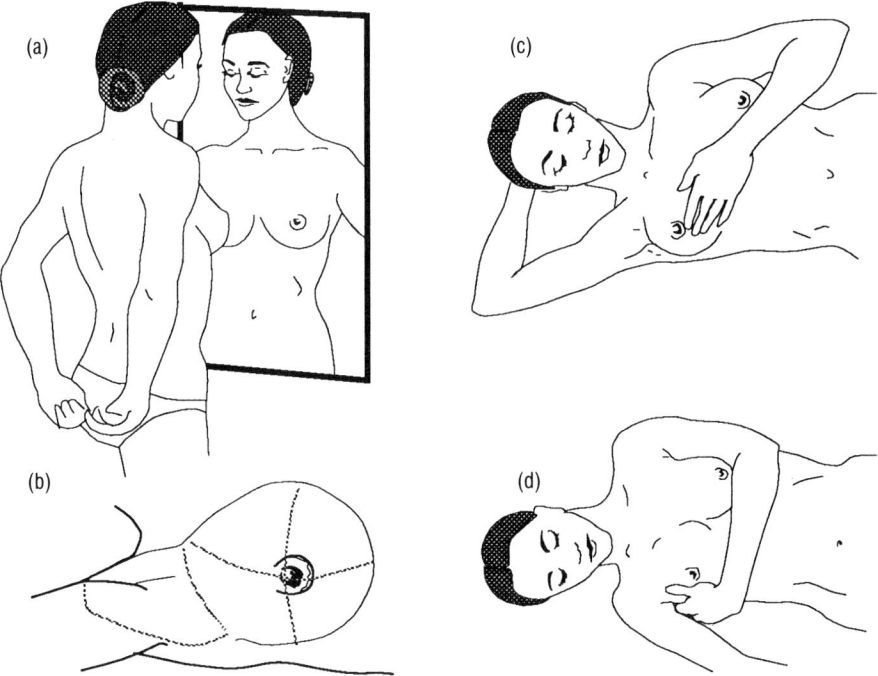

Figure 12.19 *Breast self-examination (BSE) (see text for explanation)*

to 80% of tumours, associated with degenerative lesions in the tumour, and this is an important, early radiographic finding.

Diagnosis. **Breast self-examination (BSE) or palpation** is carried out by the woman and her physician on a regular basis and will often allow detection of even small breast lumps. Figure 12.19 shows the way that BSE should be carried out. Cancer that produces a distinct lump is often invasive. The woman first stands in front of a mirror and inspects her breasts for any visible abnormalities (Figure 12.19a). This includes inspection of the nipple for deviation, inversion or discharge. The skin is examined for evidence of puckering or swelling, inflammation or depressions. The arms are put behind the back and also lifted above the head in order to facilitate inspection. The woman then lies down on her side and examines the breast on that side. The breast is examined in its four quadrants successively with the flat part of the palm, a gentle even pressure being used (Figure 12.19b). The axillary area is then examined for lumps or swellings (Figure 12.19c,d). The procedure is repeated for the other breast. The presence of any abnormality should be examined by the woman's doctor as soon as possible.

Radiological examination (mammography) will detect small lumps, and also regions of microcalcification, that are so often found in even small tumours. **Xerographic mammography** uses higher energy X-rays and provides a powerful tool to detect *in-situ* breast carcinoma which is not palpable and painless; however, because of the risk of inducing cancer in a normal breast, this is a technique not often used.

Thermography is being used increasingly as it is argued that any form of 'hard' radiation may be unsafe as a routine diagnostic tool. Thermography uses infra-red radiation detection from the region of the breast and is a perfectly safe alternative. It is known that breast cancer is associated with increased local heat and is thus detected. However, this technique will only detect relatively large tumours.

Biopsy is the definitive method of diagnosis and often it is a sufficient treatment for tumours diagnosed during their early stages of development. The diagnosis may be even made at the time of biopsy, on frozen section, and such a technique may be used close to the operating theatre, the surgeon being notified by the pathologist as to whether the lump removed is benign or malignant. Subsequent routine histological examination of the biopsy will determine whether the whole of the tumour was removed and what precise type of breast carcinoma it is.

Treatment and prognosis. **Surgery** is required to remove breast carcinoma. There may be a '**lumpectomy**' (segmental mastectomy) whereby the breast tumour with a sleeve of normal tissue around it is removed, or a **mastectomy**, in which there is removal of all of the breast tissue, preserving the pectoral muscles. A **modified radical mastectomy** is where all of the breast tissue is removed and the axillary lymph nodes are 'sampled' to check for involvement and may be further treated by radiation and or chemotherapy. A **radical mastectomy** involves removal of the entire breast, including pectoral muscles infiltrated by tumour and the axillary lymph nodes.

Radiotherapy and chemotherapy are frequently used in conjunction with surgery and greatly improve the prognosis of surgery alone with some types of tumours. In very advanced cases of carcinoma that prove inoperable at the time of diagnosis, chemotherapy and radiotherapy will prolong and improve the quality of the woman's life.

Hormone therapy may be used where there is hyperoestrinism. Tamoxifen, an oestrogen antagonist, is being administered and produces excellent results (one-third of breast cancers respond to anti-oestrogens). In some cases oöphorectomy, adrenalectomy and hypophysectomy may be carried out if the circumstances require it. Usually, if there is extensive metastatic spread of the tumour, hormone therapy and chemoradiotherapy are all that remain to be used.

Breast cancer is usually staged from 1 to 4 (or sometimes 1–5) and this depends on size and degree of spread of the tumour:

- **Stage 1**: Tumours are confined to the breast and immediate tissues and have the best prognosis.
- **Stage 2**: Tumours have spread to the draining lymph nodes and are also associated with a relatively good prognosis.
- **Stage 3**: Tumours have involved the deeper tissues such as the pectoral muscles and have become fixated and are associated with a poorer prognosis.
- **Stage 4 or 5**: Distant metastases have occurred and this is associated with the worse prognosis.

Stage 1 carcinoma (treated) has a 90% survival for 5 years, while stage 3 tumours (treated) have a 25% 5-year survival. Nowadays, with improved screening and treatment of breast carcinoma there is a good overall prognosis for breast cancer, the average 10-year survival being 60% (with treatment). This implies that many more women are aware of the condition and are presenting earlier with the tumour, mainly because of BSE procedures.

Other Breast Malignancies

Other malignant tumours seen in the breast are fibrosarcomata and liposarcomata but these tumours are extremely rare. A tumour termed **cystosarcoma phyllodes** is sometimes seen in the breast and this particular malignancy consists of both stromal and epithelial components undergoing neoplastic proliferation. Phyllodes tumours that are frankly malignant will metastasize via the bloodstream to distant locations rather than spreading by lymph to the axillary nodes. They are treated by wide local excision, if diagnosed early, and axillary dissection is not needed.

Sometimes a secondary tumour may be seen in breast tissue when there has been direct spread from a skin tumour in the skin overlying it but this is also uncommon. Secondary melanomata are rarely found in the breast and the commonest metastatic tumour of the breast is from a primary in the contralateral breast that has spread via lymphatic means.

Revision Questions and Case Studies

1. Discuss the pathology of any three conditions affecting the endometrium.
2. Discuss the pathology of the commonest neoplasm of women.
3. Write an essay on the pathology of carcinoma of the uterine cervix.
4. Discuss the pathology of ovarian tumours. Distinguish between benign and malignant ones and histogenesis of the tumours. Correlate clinically all types of ovarian tumours and indicate their significance as gynaecological disease in our country presently.
5. What are the commonest causes of ectopic pregnancy in Australia? What are the commonest sites affected? Discuss in detail the sequelae and complications of ectopic pregnancy.
6. Discuss pre-eclampsia and eclampsia of pregnancy, correlating pathological changes in tissues with clinically observed symptoms and signs.
7. Describe the characteristics of choriocarcinoma. What was the prognosis of this tumour 50 years ago and what is it now? Why is this so?
8. What is pyometra? What are the common causes of this condition?
9. Discuss the pathology of endometriosis.
10. Write short notes on any four of the following topics:

(a) Carcinoma of the endometrium (carcinoma corpus uteri)
(b) Puerperal sepsis
(c) Abortion
(d) Oöphoritis
(e) Krukenberg tumour of the ovary

11. Define the terms pelvic inflammatory disease (PID); endometritis; 'Pap' smear.
12. Discuss the pathology of any three sexually transmitted diseases that are commonly seen to affect females in this country.
13. Write short notes on all of the following:
    (a) Carcinoma of the vagina
    (b) Vaginitis
    (c) Dyspareunia
14. Discuss the pathology of the most commonly seen infectious diseases of the breast.
15. Discuss the fibrocystic changes that are seen in the female breast.
16. Discuss the pathology of benign breast tumours.
17. Carcinoma of the breast is an important medical problem in Australia currently. Discuss its pathology under the headings of: incidence; sites affected; predisposing factors; pathogenesis; morphology; routes of spread; clinical features; diagnosis; treatment and prognosis.
18. What is gynaecomastia? With what conditions is this disorder commonly associated? What are its complications?
19. Discuss the pathology of 'breast lumps' in women.
20. How may carcinoma of the breast result in bone disease?

Case study 1. Mrs Janice B., a 40-year-old Caucasian mother of three, presents with weakness and lassitude of several months' duration. For the last year or two she has noticed that her periods have become longer in duration and her menstrual blood flow is more profuse. For the last few months she has become aware of a dull, lower abdominal pain and backache, with a sensation of weight or of bearing down in that region. There has been no intermenstrual bleeding and no urinary tract or bowel symptoms. She has smoked 10–20 cigarettes daily for the last 20 years and does not drink alcohol to excess ('just the odd glass of wine with meals'). There is no relevant past medical history and she is on no medications. On examination she is a thin, pale woman (she has lost about 4 kg of weight in the last 3 months), with a pulse rate of 110 beats per minute. Her blood pressure is 135/78 mmHg and her temperature is 36.5°C. There are no abnormal findings in the chest. The breasts are rather lumpy but no obvi-

ous discrete mass is present. No hepatomegaly or splenomegaly is found, nor is there tenderness or rebound in the abdomen. Normal bowel sounds are auscultated. On palpation of the abdomen, the uterus is bulky and anteverted, non-tender, firm, smooth and readily movable. A large mass, approximately 5 cm in diameter, is palpated on the left side of the pelvic abdomen. A pregnancy test is found to be negative.

(a) What are the most likely diagnoses?
(b) What investigations should be performed?
(c) What is the management of cases such as this ?
(d) What is the link between her breast and uterine pathology?
(e) Explain the underlying causes for each sign and symptom.

Case study 2. Miss Eunice J., a 60-year-old nulliparous Caucasian female, presented with haemorrhage *per vaginam* and an offensive vaginal discharge. A vaginal and cervical swab are taken for microbiological examination and they show no bacterial pathogens, normal flora only having been detected. Cytology of the discharge shows numerous malignant cells consistent with an adenocarcinoma. No abnormal findings are observed in examinations of the chest and abdomen and laboratory values for blood tests are normal except for slight iron deficiency anaemia. After further tests, a hysterectomy is performed.

(a) What is the diagnosis?
(b) What do you know about the aetiology of this condition and how does this relate to the woman in this case?
(c) What were the 'further tests' which would have been done prior to the hysterectomy?
(d) What is the prognosis of this condition in this case?

Case study 3. Ms Cora S., a 29-year-old Caucasian female prostitute, presented with an offensive vaginal discharge. A vaginal and cervical swab were taken for microbiological examination and they showed no bacterial pathogens, normal flora only having been detected. A Pap smear performed at the time showed a Grade 1 cytology, with evidence of numerous bacteria and plentiful neutrophils but the cervical cells showed no evidence of dysplasia. The symptoms persisted for a week and broad-spectrum antibiotics prescribed resolved the infection. The woman was counselled and was encouraged to return 2 months later for a follow-up examination, but she came back a year later. The Pap smear is repeated and this shows mild dysplastic changes, typical of Grade 2 cytology. The woman is advised of the results and is told to refrain from sexual intercourse and to come back in a week to undergo further tests.

Nothing more is heard of her for some years. When she returns, she complains of vaginal bleeding after sexual intercourse. The cervix is inspected and a biopsy is taken. The biopsied tissue shows cervical metaplasia, severe dysplasia with evidence of ulceration and infection as there are numerous erythrocytes, lymphocytes and neutrophils on the surface of the cervical epithelium. The woman is lost to follow up for a further 2 years and eventually she returns, this time with more or less continuous vaginal bleeding and an offensive vaginal discharge. A large, ulcerated, haemorrhagic fungating mass arising from and obstructing the cervical os is seen on colposcopy.

(a) What is the diagnosis?
(b) What do you know about the aetiology of this condition and how does this relate to the woman in this case?
(c) What is the prognosis of this condition in its various stages?

Case study 4. Ms Deborah C., a 44-year-old Caucasian nulliparous woman presents at her doctor's clinic, as she has discovered a breast lump during BSE. The left breast is palpated by the doctor and he finds a mass, approximately 2.5 cm in diameter, in the left, lower, outer quadrant. The lump is of a rubbery consistency, freely mobile. Examination of the axillary area shows no abnormality and there are no changes in the appearance of the nipple or of the breast skin. There is some tenderness of the breast when the woman is menstruating, but no pain is associated with the lump. All other findings in the physical examination are within the normal range.

(a) What is the differential diagnosis?
(b) What is the most likely diagnosis given the woman's age, history and physical examination findings?
(c) What is the treatment in cases such as this?

Case study 5. Ms Christine R., a 35-year-old Caucasian nulliparous woman, is referred to a gynaecologist as she has been having considerable problems lately involving her genital tract. During the history taking it is found that Ms R. has had the following complaints. During the past year her menstrual periods have been becoming more painful, with the pain being particularly problematic in midcycle, around ovulation. There is menorrhagia and in the past 2 weeks she has suffered from dyspareunia. In the last 3 months she has

also suffered occasionally from pain during defaecation but has not noticed blood in the stools. There are no problems associated with the urinary tract. She admits that she has been worried over her condition, often lying awake at night thinking the worse, but her busy lifestyle (she is a buyer for a major department store and she frequently travels interstate and overseas) has left her no time to have a thorough medical examination. She is currently on long service leave and one of her other complaints is that she has not conceived even though she has made the decision to have a baby 3 years ago. Physical examination reveals a thin, pale woman 168 cm tall and weighing 52 kg. Chest findings are normal (she is a moderate smoker, smoking about 15 cigarettes a day), the breasts also normal. The abdomen is slightly distended (the woman is at day 20 of the cycle) and the uterus may be easily palpated as it is enlarged and slightly lobulated. The ovaries cannot be palpated and other abdominal findings are normal. A Pap smear is taken and at later examination shows no abnormality. The woman has been in a stable de facto relationship for the last 13 years. Further investigations are undertaken.

(a) What is the presumptive diagnosis?
(b) List features of the case study that have influenced your decision above.
(c) What 'further investigations' were undertaken?
(d) What is the treatment for this condition and what is the prognosis?

Case study 6. A 56-year-old Caucasian female presented with a thick, pale discharge from her nipple. She was very worried as her older sister was diagnosed with breast cancer 3 years ago. On examination, the breast was tender but no lump could be palpated and no lymphadenopathy could be detected. A mammogram showed a small, 0.5 cm diameter lesion with evidence of microcalcification situated in the central region of the breast in association with one of the main ducts. The woman was scheduled for biopsy.

(a) What is the presumptive diagnosis?
(b) What features of this case have influenced your decision above?
(c) What is the prognosis for this woman?

Further Reading

Ashman RB, Warmington JR. 'New Perpspectives on *Candida* and Candidiasis.' Today's Life Sci 1991: **3**(12): 22.
Berkel H, *et al.* 'Breast Augmentation: A Risk Factor

for Breast Cancer?' *New Engl J Med* 1992; **326**: 1649.

Carlson RW, Stockdale FE. 'The Clinical Biology of Breast Cancer.' *Annu Rev Med* 1988; **39**: 453.

Devor M, *et al.* 'Estrogen Replacement Therapy and the Risk of Venous Thrombosis.' *Am J Med* 1992; **92**: 275.

Fisher JC. 'The Silicone Controversy — When will Science Prevail?' *New Engl J Med* 1992; **326**: 1696.

Gardner JW, *et al.* 'Is Vaginal Douching Related to Cervical Carcinoma?' *Am J Epidemiol* 1991; **133**: 368.

Haines CJ, *et al.* 'Neonatal Outcome and its Relationship with Maternal Age.' *Aust NZ J Obs Gyn* 1991; **31**(3): 209.

Hendricks KM. 'Weaning Recommendations: The Scientific Basis.' *Nutr Rev* 1992; **50**(5): 125.

Jacobs HS, Loeffler FE. 'Postmenopausal Hormone Replacement Therapy.' *BMJ* 1992; **305**: 1403.

Kelsey JL. 'A Review of the Epidemiology of Human Breast Cancer.' *Epidemiol Rev* 1979; **1**: 47.

Lee HP, *et al.* 'Dietary Effects on Breast Cancer Risk in Singapore.' *Lancet* 1991; **337**: 1197.

Paul C, *et al.* 'Oral Contraceptives and Breast Cancer: A National Study.' *Br Med J* 1986; **293**: 723.

Rock JA, Markham SM. 'Pathogenesis of Endometriosis.' *Lancet* 1992; **340**: 1264.

Rose DP, Boyar AP, Wynder EL. 'International Comparisons of Mortality Rates for Cancer of the Breast, Ovary, Prostate and Colon, and *per capita* Food Consumption.' *Cancer* 1986; **58**: 2363.

Sattin RW, *et al.* 'Family History and the Risk of Breast Cancer.' *JAMA* 1985; 253: 1908.

Sauer MV, *et al.* 'Reversing the Natural Decline in Human Fertility.' *JAMA* 1992; **268**: 1275.

Sitruk-Ware R. 'Oestrogens and Menopause. An International Review.' *Curr Ther* 1990; **31**(8): 69.

Thomas EJ. 'Endometriosis Should not be Treated Just Because It's There.' *BMJ* 1993; **306**: 158.

UK National Case Control Study Group. 'Oral Contraceptive Use and Breast Cancer in Young Women.' *Lancet* 1989; **i**: 973.

Vessey MP, *et al.* 'Epidemiology of Endometriosis in Women Attending Family Planning Clinics.' *BMJ* 1993; 306: 182.

Wald NJ, *et al.* 'Antenatal Maternal Screening for Down's Syndrome: Results of a Demonstration Project.' *BMJ* 1992; **305**: 391.

13

Central Nervous System Disorders

The Normal Central Nervous System

The central nervous system comprises the brain and spinal cord, both of these organs being encased in the tough, membranous system of the **meninges**. Twelve pairs of cranial nerves arise from the brain and thirty-one pairs of spinal nerves arise from the spinal medulla, and together these form the peripheral nervous system. The brain, which is subdivided into the **cerebrum**, **cerebellum**, **midbrain**, **pons** and **medulla oblongata**, is an organ of great complexity (see Figure 13.1). It has the function of controlling and co-ordinating all of the normal functions of the body. This is done by conduction of electrical impulses and storage of information, functions carried out by the specialized cells known as **neurones**. The brain substance is composed of neurones embedded in a specialized supporting framework of **glial cells**, the astrocytes, oligodendrocytes, ependymal cells and microglia.

Neurones are pyramidal cells of the grey matter of the cerebral cortex containing a large nucleus, promi-

nent nucleolus and dark staining clumps of rough endoplasmic reticulum known as **Nissl substance**. From the nerve cell body emerge multiple cytoplasmic processes, the many **dendrites** and the single **axon**, which synapse with other neurones, their function being to conduct nerve impulses. A fundamental characteristic of neurones is excitability and conductivity; cell membrane polarizations and depolarizations with creation of travelling action potentials is the means whereby these two important processes are carried out. Neurones are very susceptible to any form of injury. For example, they are the most sensitive of all body cells to anoxia, undergoing reactive changes and necrosis within 3 to 5 minutes of anoxia. Neurones are also found in the cerebellum and spinal cord, where they are located in the grey matter, situated in the cortical part of the cerebellum and medullary portions of the spinal cord. The cerebellum also has some regions of grey matter in the medulla. Neurones in the adult have become such specialized cells that they have lost their ability to divide. All neuronal division stops shortly after birth (see Figure 13.2).

Astrocytes are the specialized supporting cells of

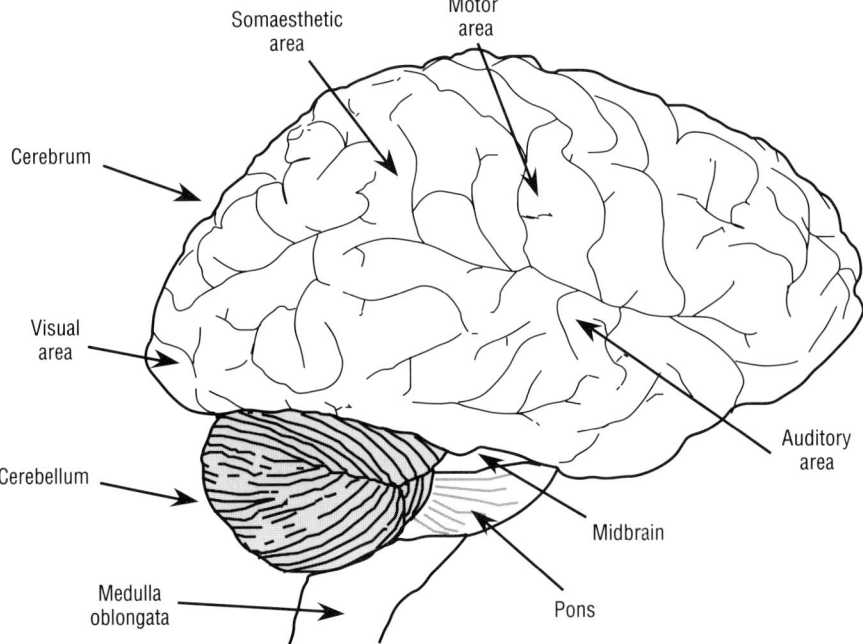

Figure 13.1   *The normal brain*

the CNS and are of two types: the **protoplasmic astrocytes** with many long cytoplasmic processes, found mostly in the grey matter, and the **fibrillar astrocytes** with few cytoplasmic processes, found mostly in the white matter. Both types of cells have cell bodies that are approximately 8 μm in diameter. Astrocytes help to insulate neurones and their electrically active processes, and help maintain the **blood–brain barrier**. This is a series of functional and anatomical barriers between the vascular and neurological components which regulates the entry of cells, fluids, electrolytes, small molecules and proteins. The blood–brain barrier is made up of three components: capillary endothelium with tight junctions, endothelial cell basement membrane, and the foot processes of astrocytes. There are very few places in the brain where neurones abut directly on capillaries (e.g. in parts of the hypothalamus); in most other situations capillaries are surrounded by the cytoplasm of glial cells so that diffusion of substances from the vascular system is regulated by the neuroglia. However, a diffusion barrier is also present at the capillary level, as the endothelium of vessels in the CNS is markedly impermeable to most macromolecules. It is important to note that the blood–brain barrier is incomplete in the foetus and newborn, and in certain discrete areas of the brain in the adult.

Astrocytes are cells that are important in **gliosis**, a repair process of the brain and spinal cord, equivalent to fibrosis in other tissues. In gliosis, glial cells proliferate following injury to the CNS where loss of neurones has occurred, with the proliferating supporting cells forming a glial 'scar' composed of a tangled mass of astrocytes with many interwoven fibrillary processes.

Oligodendrocytes have fewer processes than astrocytes and are found in both grey and white matter. In the grey matter they cluster around neurones and are called 'satellite cells'. They are smaller than astrocytes, their cell body being 6–7 μm in diameter, the nucleus often heterochromatic. These cells produce the myelin that surrounds the axons in the CNS, a single oligodendrocyte connecting with the sheath of several fibres.

Microglia are the CNS equivalent of the mononuclear phagocyte system. Unlike the previous two glial cells discussed, which have a neuroectodermal origin, microglia are derived from mesoderm. They are small cells in the cytoplasm of which are found lysosomes. Microglial cells are actively phagocytic and are stimulated in response to cerebral damage. In severe injury, blood monocytes are also recruited from the bloodstream to join forces with the local microglial cells to effect phagocytosis of debris.

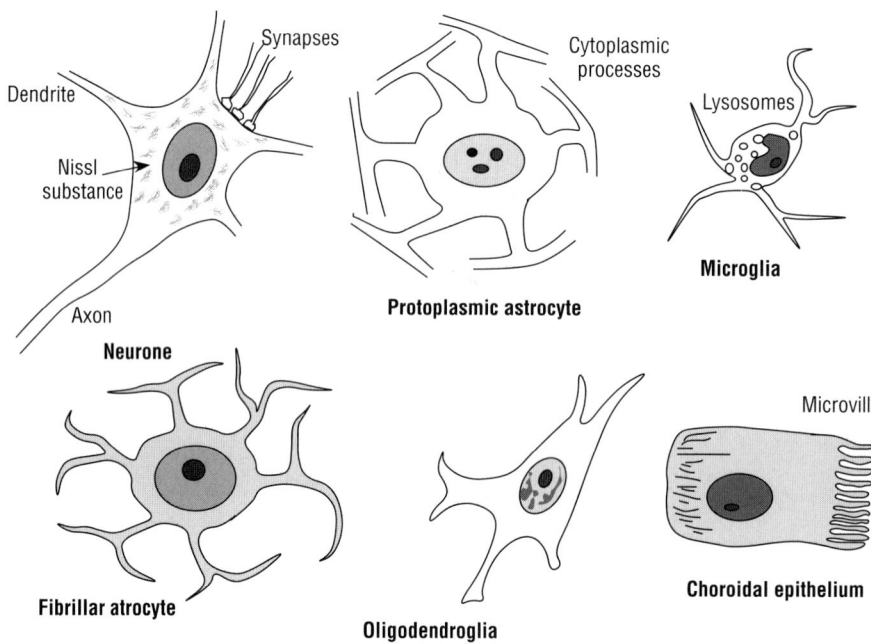

Figure 13.2   *Cells of the normal central nervous system*

Ependymal cells are the ciliated cuboidal cells that line the cerebral ventricles and central canal of the spinal cord. Numerous microvilli are found on the luminal aspect of these cells and between adjacent ependymal cells there are desmosomes and junctional complexes. In the roof of the third and fourth ventricles the ependymal epithelium forms the choroid plexus, a structure important in the formation of the cerebrospinal fluid.

The meningeal membranes consist of three layers: the outer, thick, fibrous **dura mater (pachymeninges)**, the thinner, middle layer, the **arachnoid mater** and subarachnoid space, and the inner, very thin, **pia mater**. The arachnoid mater, subarachnoid space and pia mater are termed the **leptomeninges**. Cerebrospinal fluid circulates in the subarachnoid space (refer to Figure 13.3).

Location and Nature of Injury in the Central Nervous System

The CNS is often thought of as a particularly specialized system which undergoes its own distinct types of pathological changes. However, when all things are considered it is seen that as in any other organ system of the body, there are congenital disorders, vascular disorders, infections, inflammations and tumours that affect this tissue. Often, it is found that the specific nature of the injury is not as important as its location. A small lesion in the frontal cortex may be asymptomatic, a similar lesion of the same size in the medulla oblongata may cause instant death. Deducing the location of a CNS lesion from the pattern of functional impairment is crucial to accurate diagnosis and an inevitable, essential exercise for many practitioners.

Another important factor that should be raised in relation to CNS disease is that for a long time the nervous system had been regarded as an immuno-privileged and protected site. It appeared to be inaccessible and unresponsive to many antigenic stimuli. These conclusions resulted from work earlier this century relating to intracerebral transplants of mouse sarcomata into a rat, which grew well in the CNS, whereas a subcutaneous graft of the same tumour was rejected by the animal. It was also observed that micro-organisms were found to proliferate more readily when inoculated directly into the brain than when given intravenously. These observations have been explained by the existence of certain anatomical characteristics of the nervous system, the most important of which are the existence of the blood–brain barrier and the lack of immunocompetent cells and lymphatic drainage in the brain. This absence of an organised lymphoid tissue in the CNS reflects the fact that the nervous system is not usually exposed to significant levels of antigenic

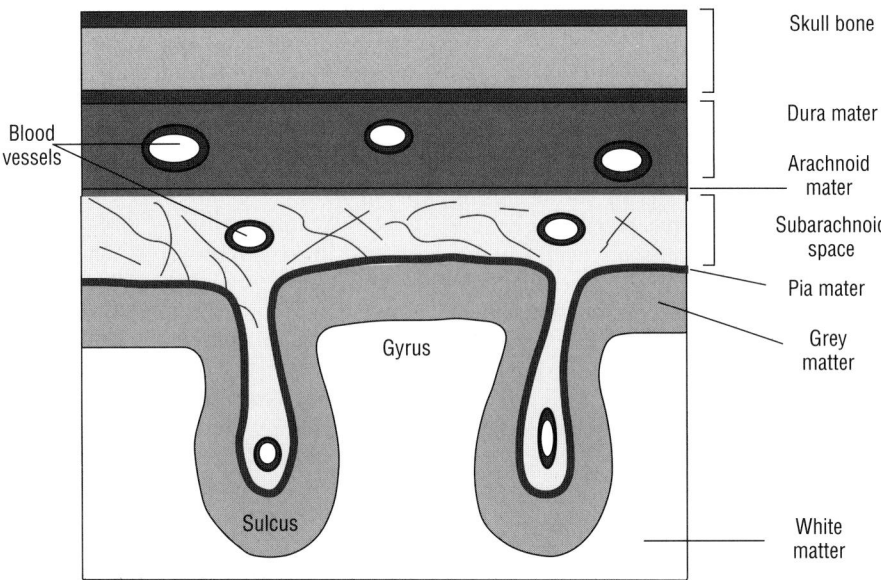

Figure 13.3 *The meningeal membranes*

stimuli, therefore it does not need to manufacture antibody or to mount immune responses.

Recent findings, however, have shown that an intracerebral immune response can occur. Tumours can be rejected, and in one experimental model, successful intracerebral transplanting of a tumour required administration of immunosuppressive drugs. There is also increasing evidence that the immune system is implicated in several neurological diseases, for example multiple sclerosis, Alzheimer's disease, Guillain-Barré syndrome, etc. Often in many of these disorders the exact pathogenesis of the disease process is not known but the data supporting the autoimmunity are incontrovertible.

Congenital Diseases

Agenesis, Hypoplasia of Brain

Both agenesis and hypoplasia may affect the brain, resulting in the first instance in anencephaly or in the second case in microcephaly. **Anencephaly** is a fatal condition resulting from the failure of the development of the brain and cranial bones, most marked in the frontal regions. It occurs in two out of every 1000 pregnancies. A depression is present in the skull and the affected babies are stillborn or die shortly after birth. Anencephaly may be diagnosed prenatally by amniocentesis through demonstration of high α-foetoprotein levels in the amniotic fluid. **Microcephaly** is a congenital smallness of the brain, causing a decreased head size of the baby and varying degrees of mental deficiency in the affected individual. Both disorders may be totally idiopathic congenital malformations or, especially in the case of microcephaly, may be associated with Mendelian defects, for example trisomy 13–15 and the 'cri du chat' syndrome.

Epiloia (Tuberose Sclerosis, Bourneville's Disease)

Epiloia is an autosomal dominant disorder where there are regions of glial cell proliferation in the brain (= sclerosis) occurring in multiple situations and associated with deformed neurones. Smooth nodules (= tubers) composed of glial cells, mainly malformed astrocytes, and nerve cells occur in the walls of the ventricles and cerebral gyri. The nodules grow slowly, producing pressure atrophy of the surrounding, relatively normal tissue. Affected people are mentally retarded and may have epileptic seizures. Other lesions found in this condition include adenoma sebaceum on the face and multiple hamartomata in various organs. Most commonly, the heart (rhabdomyomata), liver, kidney (angiomyolipomata) and pancreas are involved, with the disease having a rather poor prognosis. The patients are predisposed to the development of gliomata, especially astrocytomata.

Down's Syndrome (Mongolism)

This is the commonest of the autosomal, chromosomal disorders, occurring approximately in 16 out of 10 000 live births. The incidence of the disorder is markedly influenced by the maternal age at the time of conception, increasing maternal age carrying an increasing risk, until in women who become pregnant over the age of 45 years the risk of having a baby with Down's syndrome may be as high as 1 in 30. The condition arises most commonly through **non-disjunction**, where two chromosomes fail to separate at the first or second meiotic division of the ovum, leading to one daughter cell having 24 chromosomes, the other daughter cell 22. In Down's syndrome the affected chromosomes are the 21st pair. If the daughter cell with 24 chromosomes is fertilized by a sperm containing the normal number of 23 chromosomes, the resultant zygote has 47 chromosomes, leading to the condition of **trisomy 21**, where there are three copies of chromosome 21 in each cell of the developing embryo, and subsequently of the affected individual. More rarely, **translocations** will cause Down's syndrome. In this case there is exchange of one segment of a chromosome with a segment of a non-homologous chromosome. This occurs between chromosomes 15 and 21 or between chromosomes 21 and 22 in Down's syndrome.

The condition is characterized by mental retardation with a typical facial appearance where the eyes are slanted and have epicanthic folds, the neck is short and the occiput is flattened. The hands are broad and flat with short incurving fifth digits and abnormal dermatoglyphic patterns. There are associated visceral disorders with ventricular and atrial defects, oesophageal atresia, fistula formation and duodenal atresia. Most affected individuals die in childhood or young adulthood.

The disorder may be diagnosed while the embryo is still *in utero* and this is performed on high-risk mothers through the technique of **amniocentesis**. This involves taking a sample of amniotic fluid containing some of the embryonic cells suspended in it. The cells are grown in cell culture and a cytologist then examines them during mitotic divisions when the supernumerary chromosome may be demonstrated. The mother then has to make the decision of either proceeding with the pregnancy or terminating it through an abortion.

Spina Bifida

Spina bifida is a congenital disorder occurring in approximately 1 to 2% of births. It is a neural tube defect where there are varying degrees of failure of fusion of the neural tube and spinal canal. It may be a minor defect frequently remaining undiagnosed or it may be incompatible with life. A number of related variants also occur (see Figure 13.4).

Spina bifida occulta. This is a rather common but relatively minor defect of one or more spinal neural arches, most commonly in the lumbosacral region. Usually, this condition is only found incidentally through a radiological investigation for other disease. The spinal cord is normally formed, in a normal position and functions normally. There may be in some cases minor neurological defects such as enuresis.

Meningocoele. This is a fairly common type of spina bifida in which there is a simple herniation of the meninges through a defect in the neural arches, usually in the thoracolumbar region. Although the spinal cord is normal there is often an associated abnormality such as the Arnold-Chiari malformation. The condition carries with it the risk of infection and also there may be some neurological disability.

Meningomyelocoele. This variant of spina bifida shows herniation of the meninges and spinal cord through defects in the neural arches into a skin-covered sac, usually in the thoracolumbar region. The condition occurs in two out of every 1000 pregnancies. The nerve roots are abnormally situated and there is usually paralysis below the level of the defect. Infection is also common. Meningitis, which often complicates this condition, may cause further damage to the CNS.

Syringomyelocoele. This condition resembles meningomyelocoele in the position of the cord but is associated with severe defect of the neural arches and, in addition, there is extreme dilatation of the central canal of the spinal cord with associated considerable neurological deficits. The affected children die at a very young age with severe neurological disorders, infections and marked debilitation.

Rachischisis (myelocoele). This is the most severe congenital deformity associated with the error of fusion of the neural tube and spinal canal. The spinal cord is defective and malformed, lying exposed to the exterior in a groove running the length of the neural arches. The condition is incompatible with life. Extreme malformations associated with spina bifida may be diagnosed through amniocentesis by demonstrating higher than normal levels of α-foetoprotein in the amniotic fluid and also in the mother's blood. The solution offered in this case is aborting the pregnancy.

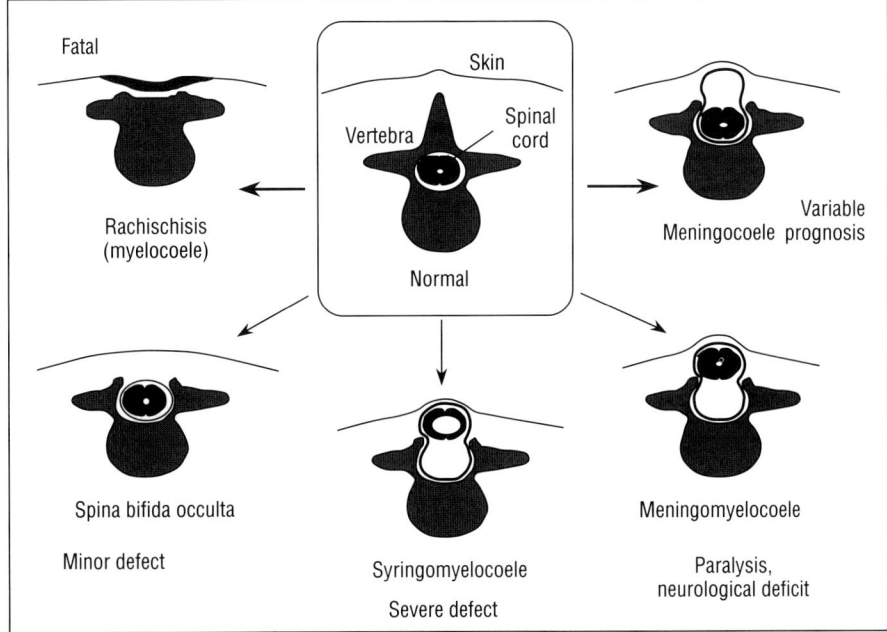

Figure 13.4 *Spina bifida*

Arnold-Chiari Malformation

This is a deformity commonly found in association with other congenital disorders of the brain and consists of a protrusion of the ventromedial portion of the cerebellum, fourth ventricle and medulla into the cervical spinal canal (see Figure 13.5). Often the tongue-like protruded portion of the cerebellum reaches the level of C3–C5. As can be expected, the herniated part shows evidence of pressure atrophy, especially in the neural tissue. A common associated disorder in this condition is a lumbosacral meningomyelocoele. Other neurological lesions observed associated with the Arnold-Chiari malformation are a deformation of the quadrigeminal plate to form a dorsal protrusion of the inferior colliculus, a flattening of the cerebellum, polymicrogyria of the brain surface and an S-shaped angulation of the upper cervical spinal cord.

Although the condition is present at birth it may not produce symptoms until later in life, or well into adulthood. If a patient is diagnosed with spina bifida, the presence of the Arnold-Chiari malformation must be considered also. The commonest associated complication of the Arnold-Chiari malformation is hydrocephalus and this is due to the obstruction of cerebrospinal fluid flow through the foramina of Magendie and Lutschka (see below).

Friedrich's Ataxia

This is a disease inherited as an autosomal recessive trait in some families and less commonly as an autosomal dominant in others. The disease that results is the same in both forms and presents at puberty, involving a degeneration of the spinal cord, kyphosis and optic atrophy. Especially the lower segments of the cord are markedly atrophied with degeneration of the posterior and lateral white columns. Glial cells proliferate and replace the lost nervous tissue and these regions of gliosis have a typical whorled pattern. The spinocerebellar tracts and posterior roots are also involved in the atrophy. Severe disability within a few years of onset develops and death is usually due to heart problems developing in association with a myocarditis that occurs due to necrosis of myocardial cells and resultant fibrosis.

Kinnier-Wilson's Disease (Hepatolenticular Degeneration)

Wilson's disease is an autosomal recessive disease associated with a biochemical anomaly of copper metabolism. The normal copper-carrying plasma protein **ceruloplasmin** is decreased in concentration, totally

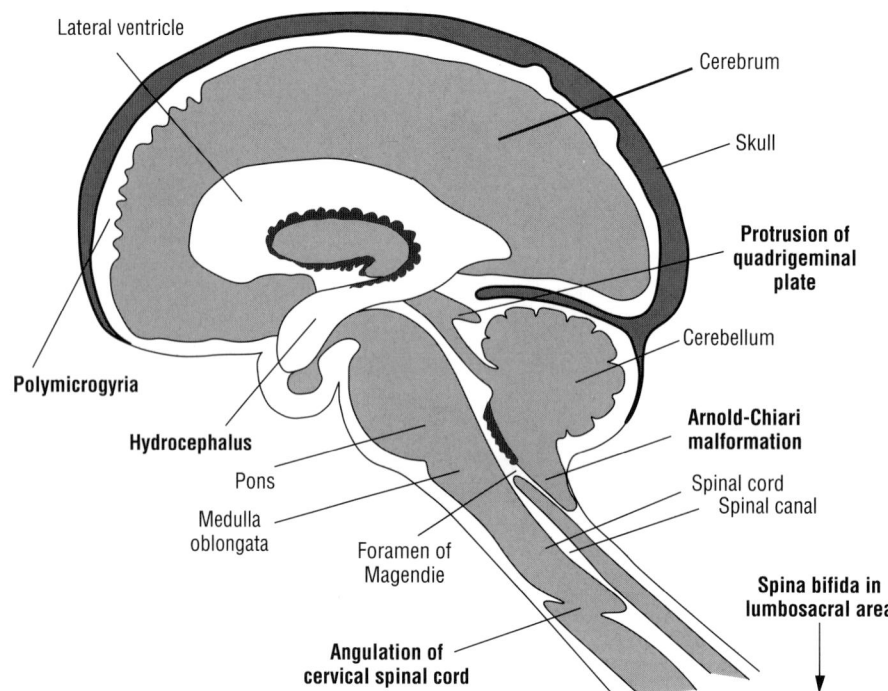

Figure 13.5   *The Arnold-Chiari malformation*

absent, or abnormal in its function. There is increased uptake of copper from the intestine and accumulation of copper in the liver, renal tubular epithelium, cerebral astrocytes and in the cornea. In the eye, the deposits of copper are visible as the **Kayser-Fleischer ring**, a greenish brown ring of pigmentation in Descemet's membrane. In the brain, the copper-containing pigment is deposited in the lenticular nucleus, especially the putamen, the tips of the frontal lobes, sometimes in the dentate and red nuclei. There is marked degeneration of nervous tissue and the surviving astrocytes in the affected regions contain great quantities of copper pigment. The glial cells show giant and multinucleated forms and there is degeneration of the nearby nerve roots. Cavitation of the affected regions develops in the advanced cases.

Typically, the disease begins in adolescence with disorders affecting the nervous system, causing aberrations of movement and co-ordination, rigidity and tremor, and liver dysfunction (see under the section on cirrhosis of the liver in Chapter 9). Treatment of the disorder with copper chelating agents has markedly improved the outlook, although an early death does occur, often associated with liver disease or intercurrent infections.

Tay-Sachs Disease (Amaurotic Familial Idiocy)

This is a congenital disorder inherited as a recessive trait in which there is a defect in the enzyme **hexominidase A**. Gangliosides accumulate in many organs but predominantly in the brain. The disease is most commonly seen in Ashkenazy Jews. The brain is atrophic and histologically the nerve cells are seen to be distended by accumulations of ganglioside, making the cells look foamy and vacuolated. Affected infants show mental retardation, blindness and die before the age of 3 years. Amniocentesis can detect the disorder in early pregnancy.

Diseases Associated with Defective Cerebrospinal Fluid Flow and Function

Normal Cerebrospinal Flow and Function

The cerebrospinal fluid (CSF) is secreted into the lateral ventricles of the brain by the choroid plexi, which are highly vascular accumulations of ependymal cells lining the surface of the tela chorioidea. It then passes through the foramen of Monro into the third ventricle, then through the aqueduct of Sylvius to the fourth ventricle and to the subarachnoid space via the median foramen of Magendie and lateral foramina of Lutschka (refer to Figure 13.6). CSF is also secreted into the subarachnoid space by the choroid plexi of the lateral recesses of the fourth ventricle. From there it passes through the median aperture and foramina of the lateral recesses of the fourth ventricle gaining entry into the subarachnoid. The fluid circulates around the spinal theca and also upwards over the brain surface, finally being reabsorbed by the arachnoid granulations, returning to the circulation via the large dural sinuses. The CSF supports and protects the delicate structure of the nervous tissue, maintaining a uniform pressure on them and acting as a 'buffer zone' between the nervous tissue and the surrounding membranes and bone. Thus, the CNS is bathed in a fluid that is quite different from blood plasma as it contains very few cells and 0.4 of the plasma protein concentration (see Table 13.1).

Samples of the CSF may be obtained through **lumbar puncture**, a procedure whereby a fine trochar and cannula are introduced between the laminae or spines of the third and fourth (or fourth and fifth) lumbar vertebrae, the meninges being punctured and the instrument introduced into the subarachnoid space below the lower end of the spinal medulla. When the trochar is removed, the fluid should normally escape at the rate of one drop per second. If the fluid is under pressure it may escape in a continuous stream. If a raised intracranial pressure is suspected, a manometer should be attached to the cannula, regulating the flow of fluid, lest the sudden fall in pressure that occurs lead to the impaction of the medulla oblongata into the foramen magnum, causing death.

Normal CSF is a crystal clear, slightly alkaline fluid with a specific gravity of about 1007. It contains in solution inorganic salts similar to those found in plasma and also traces of protein and glucose. A small number of lymphocytes (up to 5 per mL) are also found within the fluid. Examination of the CSF may yield valuable information as to various disease process occurring within the CNS. Usually this analysis is biochemical, but also direct microscopic, serological and microbiological examination may be undertaken, depending on the nature of the disorder suspected. For example, in order to diagnose neurosyphilis, the CSF is taken and examined biochemically, where an increased protein content is found; microbiologically, where it is found usually sterile; microscopically, where increased numbers of lymphocytes are found; and serologically, where the tests are positive for syphilis.

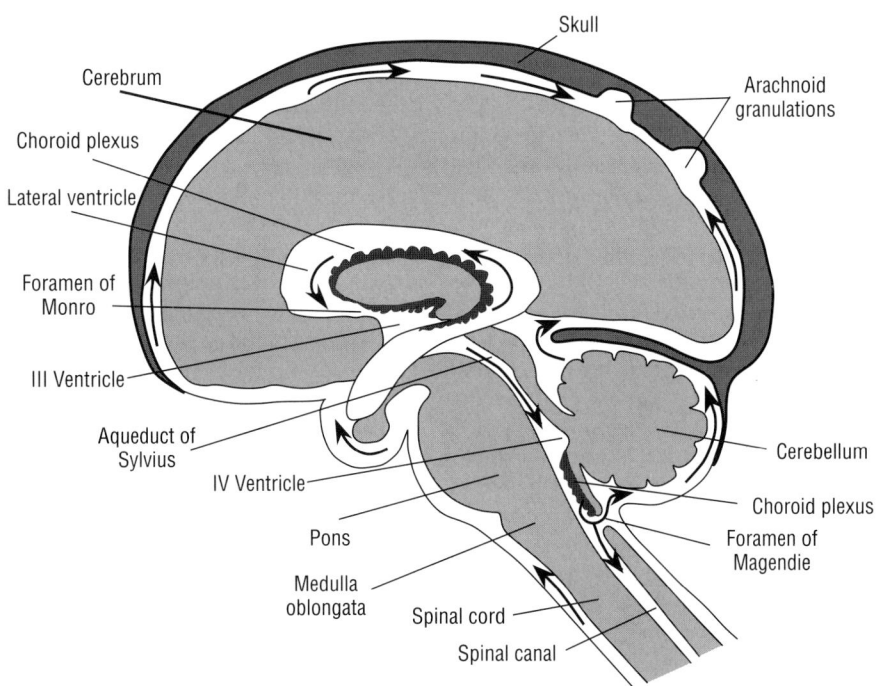

Figure 13.6   *Normal cerebrospinal fluid circulation*

Table 13.1 *Cerebrospinal fluid characteristics in various conditions*

Condition	Features of fluid	Cells per µL	Protein g/L	Glucose mmol/L
Normal	Clear	Up to 5 lymphocytes	0.15–0.45	2.75–4.40
Suppurative meningitis	Clear to turbid, bacteria on culture	200–3000 neutrophils	1–10 (↑↑↑)	0–2.5 (↓)
'Aseptic meningitis'	Clear to slightly turbid	50–200 lymphocytes	0.4–1.0 (↑)	Normal
Tuberculous meningitis	Clear to turbid, bacteria on culture	50–400 lymphocytes. A few neutrophils	0.6–4.0 (↑↑)	Normal
Neurosyphilis	Clear to turbid, positive serology	10–400 lymphocytes	0.6–1.0 (↑)	Normal
Paralytic polio	Slightly turbid	100–150 lymphocytes	0.45–1.0 (↑)	Normal
Encephalitis	Clear to slightly turbid	50–200 lymphocytes	0.40–1.0 (↑)	Normal
Multiple sclerosis	Clear	10–50 lymphocytes	0.2–1.0 (↑)	Normal
CNS tumour	Clear	Normal	0.4–1.0 (↑)	Normal

Hydrocephalus

Hydrocephalus is a condition where there is an increased amount of CSF in the nervous system. This results from an obstruction to CSF outflow either at the aqueduct of Sylvius or the foramina of Magendie or of Luschka. When there is no communication between the ventricles and the subarachnoid spaces the condition is termed **non-communicating hydrocephalus**. In non-communicating hydrocephalus if dye is injected into the ventricular spaces it will not gain access to the spinal theca and at lumbar puncture the CSF recovered will not be dyed. Sites of obstruction commonly seen are at the foramen of Monro, the aqueduct of Sylvius or at the roof of the fourth ventricle. If a communication remains between the ventricular system and the spinal theca, the condition is termed **communicating hydrocephalus**. Dye injected into the ventricles will stain fluid that is recovered at lumbar puncture. In this case, the obstruction is at the base of the brain and prevents fluid from reaching the arachnoid granulations and being resorbed there (refer to Figure 13.6).

In both cases of hydrocephalus there is an increase in CSF pressure somewhere, caused by the accumulation of excess fluid. There is usually ventricular distension, sometimes of enormous proportions, which may convert the cerebral cortex into an atrophic shell surrounding an enormous bag of fluid (compare hydronephrosis in the kidney). Hydrocephalus is also subdivided clinically into two groups, congenital **hydrocephalus**, if it presents at birth or in infancy, and **acquired hydrocephalus**, if it presents later in life in previously normal brains. This classification depends very much on the aetiology of the condition and the subsequent effects on the affected individual, effects dictated mainly by anatomical features relating to whether or not there is fusion of the bony sutures of the skull bones.

Congenital hydrocephalus commonly arises in association with various congenital anomalies of the nervous system, for example the Arnold-Chiari malformation, spina bifida and other anatomical defects, intrauterine infections and intracranial tumours of infancy. As the CSF accumulates in the spaces of the brain, there is dilatation of the ventricles with corresponding brain atrophy. As the bony sutures of the skull are not fused, this increased intracranial pressure will cause an enormous enlargement of the cranial vault if the condition remains untreated. The sutures are grossly separated and the fontanelles are large and tense. The brain is distended and may be reduced to only a thin rim of tissue lining the enlarged cranial vault. The neurological effects are variable depending on the amount of nervous tissue that has been destroyed. Surgical treatments of hydrocephalus involve placing indwelling drain tubes which shunt the excess CSF from the brain into the right atrium of the heart or into the jugular vein, and provided the condition is diagnosed and treated early the prognosis is good with minimal damage to nervous tissue.

Acquired hydrocephalus occurs in association with late clinical presentation of the Arnold-Chiari malformation; with CNS infections, especially meningitis; and with tumours of the CNS, especially those occurring in the brain stem. In the adult, the suture lines of the cranium are fused making the skull incapable of undergoing enlargement in response to the increased intracranial pressure. This causes rapid compression and pressure atrophy of the brain tissue. The ventricles become grossly enlarged proximal to the site of obstruction of CSF and the brain tissue often degenerates to only a thin rim abutting on the skull bones (refer to Figure 13.7).

Compensatory hydrocephalus is said to occur if there is increased CSF due to a decreased brain volume as may happen in some of the degenerations of the brain, for example Alzheimer's disease. Idiopathic hydrocephalus may be associated with CSF overproduction by the choroid plexi or under-resorption by the arachnoid granulations. Rarely, hydrocephalus develops in middle age without any anatomical anomaly and without increase in CSF pressure (normal pressure hydrocephalus). Similarly to other forms of hydrocephalus, this form subsides on CSF diversion via a ventriculojugular shunt.

Raised Intracranial Pressure

The brain is encased in a rigid, protective, bony shell, the calvarium. This situation becomes detrimental with any condition involving an increased volume of the brain, as the calvarium in the adult does not allow expansion of the brain substance. Thus, swelling of the brain results in mounting intracranial pressure. Such expansion may result from space-occupying lesions, for example tumours, abscesses, aneurysms, oedema of the brain, hydrocephalus or brain haemorrhages. **Cerebral oedema** may occur with any injury, and in contradistinction to oedema elsewhere, may be primarily intracellular or extracellular. Oedema in the brain also commonly accompanies brain tumours and most of the symptoms and signs associated with brain tumours are a result of the resultant brain swelling.

Clinically, increased intracranial pressure produces headache, vomiting (especially in the morning) and **papilloedema** (swelling of the optic disc due to oedema of the optic nerve papillae associated with congestion of the retinal veins). Later, coma and epileptic seizures may occur. If CSF pressure is increased unevenly, herniation of the brain through the tentorium cerebelli may occur. Compression of the midbrain causes loss of consciousness. The third nerve is also likely to become compressed, producing fixed, dilated pupils while compression of the aqueduct of Sylvius worsens the increased CSF pressure, setting up a vicious circle. If the cerebellar tonsils herniate through the foramen

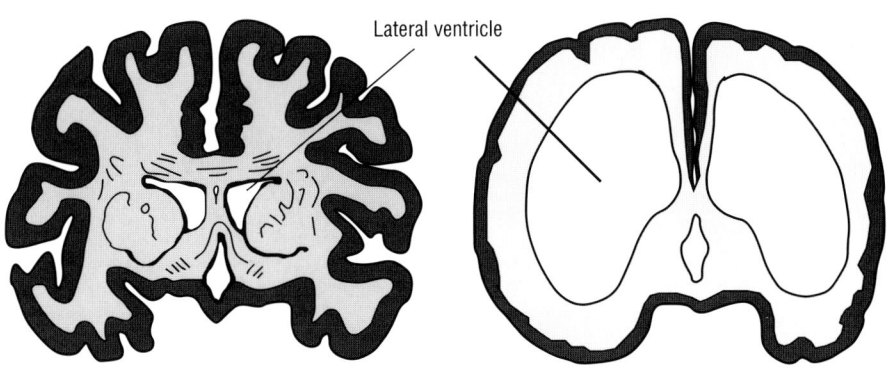

Lateral ventricle

Normal brain   Hydrocephalus

Figure 13.7 *Effects of hydrocephalus on the brain*

magnum, the medulla oblongata is compressed, causing instant death from failure of the cardiac and respiratory centres. With lateral herniation past the falx cerebri, the cingulate gyrus herniates across the midline, causing obtundation and perhaps shearing the anterior cerebral arteries (see Figure 13.8).

In all cases of raised intracranial pressure, the condition must be treated immediately, often by an emergency surgical procedure, as the disorder may be rapidly fatal, mainly through the effects of brain herniations.

Vascular Diseases

Intracranial Haemorrhage

The types of lesions that are encountered in intracranial haemorrhage depend on the anatomical partition that the haemorrhage develops in, the volume of blood involved and the rate at which the blood is lost from the circulation. A very important feature in all types of intracranial haemorrhage is that there is usually an accompanying rise in intracranial pressure as well as pressure atrophy of nervous tissue due to the accumu-lating blood in the haemorrhage. The four anatomical regions that are involved in intracranial haemorrhage are: the **epidural (= extradural) space**, the **subdural space**, the **subarachnoid space** and the **brain parenchyma** (including the ventricular spaces). Each of these regions has distinct aetiological and pathogenetic mechanisms involved with the haemorrhage.

Especially important in the aetiology of brain haemorrhages that occur in the meningeal spaces are factors often involved with **head and spinal trauma**. Traumatic injuries are usually caused by motor car accidents, but other common causes are falls, blows to the head and childbirth trauma. Head injuries may result in **meningeal haemorrhages**, **concussion**, **contusion** or **laceration** of the brain.

Concussion implies that the patient presents in a confused state or is unconscious following head trauma. There is usually some temporary impairment of the higher intellectual functions, but the condition rapidly resolves. In more severe cases the unconsciousness is more prolonged with hypotension, decreased pulse and respiration, flaccid muscles. Headache, vomiting and delirium upon return to consciousness are usually experienced, until the patient undergoes a complete

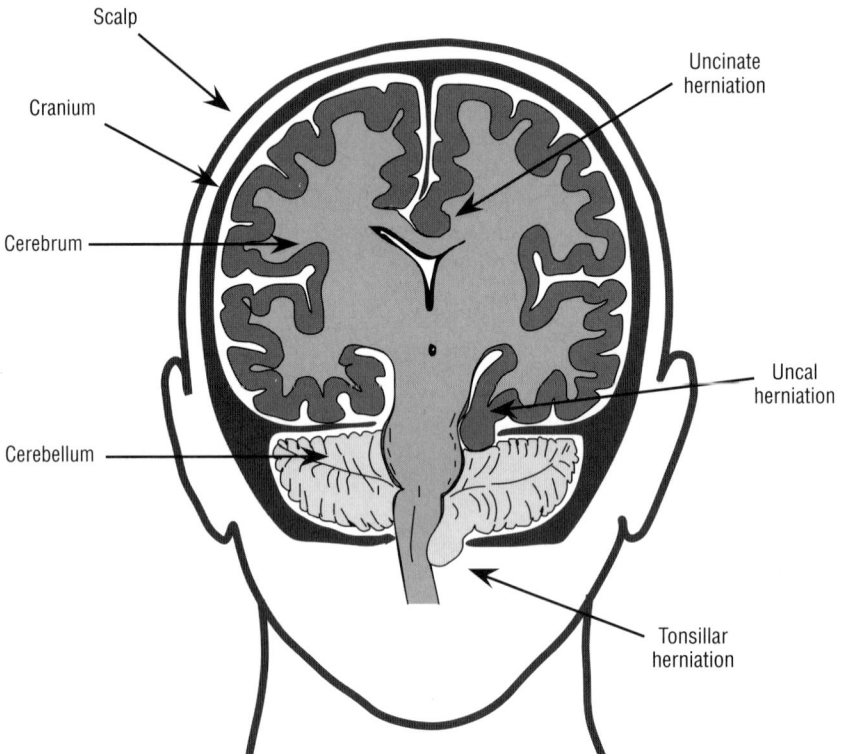

Figure 13.8 *Effects of raised intracranial pressure on the brain*

return to normal in a few hours. The exact pathogenesis of these changes in concussion is not known, but it is thought that they result from abnormal stresses acting on the delicate nervous tissue.

Contusion is a bruise developing on the brain associated with a blow to the head. There is some mild haemorrhage associated with these lesions, but it is only minor and occurs from damaged capillaries. Unconsciousness is the result of the injury and this may progress to coma and death if the bleeding is not arrested by haemostasis. The sites most commonly involved are the frontal and temporal lobes of the cerebrum, but it should be kept in mind that the contusion may not always develop beneath the region of impact but rather opposite it, since the brain may be jarred by the blow and a **contrecoup** may cause more damage to the opposite side of the brain. Regions of haemorrhage, oedema and brain necrosis may be seen in the areas affected. If the patient survives, gliosis will develop in the regions after there is resorption of the blood from the region. Usually there is no permanent neurological deficit in such cases.

Laceration of the brain develops when there are penetrating injuries to the head involving a fracture of the cranial bones. The exact sequelae of these injuries is variable depending on the degree of brain damage sustained and the amount of haemorrhage occurring. Prompt treatment of mild injury may lead to complete recovery. With more severe injury or damage to a more sensitive area of the brain, laceration proves rapidly fatal.

Epidural Haematoma (Extradural Haematoma)

In this case there is bleeding between the inner table of the skull and the dura (various types of brain haemorrhage are illustrated in Figure 13.9). It usually follows

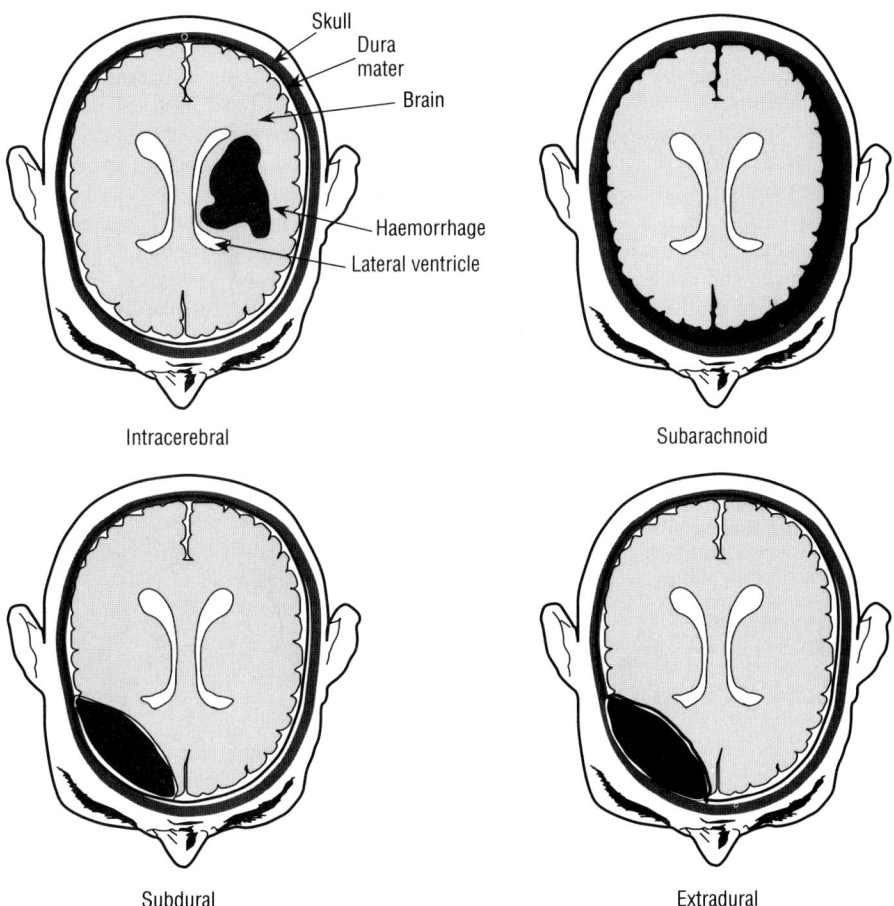

Figure 13.9 *Types of brain haemorrhages*

trauma to the temporal region or skull fracture with rupture of the middle meningeal artery or one of its branches. Blood accumulates relatively slowly in a localized area, stripping the dura away from the bone. Typically, such patients sustain concussion and lose consciousness for a time, then regain consciousness (termed the lucid interval), following which they progressively become comatose as the extradural haematoma collects and compresses the brain substance within the skull. Unless the haematoma is evacuated surgically, eventual brain herniation and death will be the outcome.

Subdural Haematoma

Subdural haematma refers to the formation of a collection of blood between the dura and the leptomeninges. Such haematomata may be acute (associated with an arachnoid tear, brain laceration or contusion), or chronic. Acute haematomata develop very rapidly when the cortical veins in the subdural space are ruptured and the brain, which is already damaged and oedematous, is further compressed by the rapidly expanding blood clot, leading to a very poor prognosis for such patients. The symptoms and signs are usually due to increased intracranial pressure and brain herniation. Often the patient is comatose and does not regain consciousness until death.

Chronic haematomata evolve insidiously in alcoholics and the demented who are especially liable to falls. Another typical presentation is following birth trauma, where the baby's head is injured during delivery. Brain haemorrhages of this type are caused by the tearing of the bridging cerebral veins between the pia mater and dura mater. Seepage of blood into the subdural space occurs very slowly and excites an inflammatory and fibroblastic response so that the haematoma becomes encapsulated in a meningeal scar. Signs and symptoms are greatly delayed, developing weeks to months after the traumatic event, and they include headache, increasing drowsiness, hemiparesis and seizures, with a deterioration of mental capacity. Eventually, brain herniation and death occur in most cases. Surgical treatment involving evacuation of the haematoma is life saving in these patients and leads to a dramatic and sometimes complete recovery, provided the lesion has not been present for a very long time. In rare cases some patients recover spontaneously and the blood is slowly removed by inflammation and organization.

Subarachnoid Haemorrhage and Berry Aneurysms

Although subarachnoid haemorrhage may sometimes be the result of head injuries, it is most often associated with other, more serious lesions. Generally, these lesions involve pathology of the brain vasculature and the clinical symptomatology is very similar for all of them, involving haemorrhage, compression of brain substance, raised intracranial pressure, neuronal destruction or brain herniation, seen alone or in any combination. The term **cerebrovascular accident (CVA)** is a blanket term covering all of these lesions

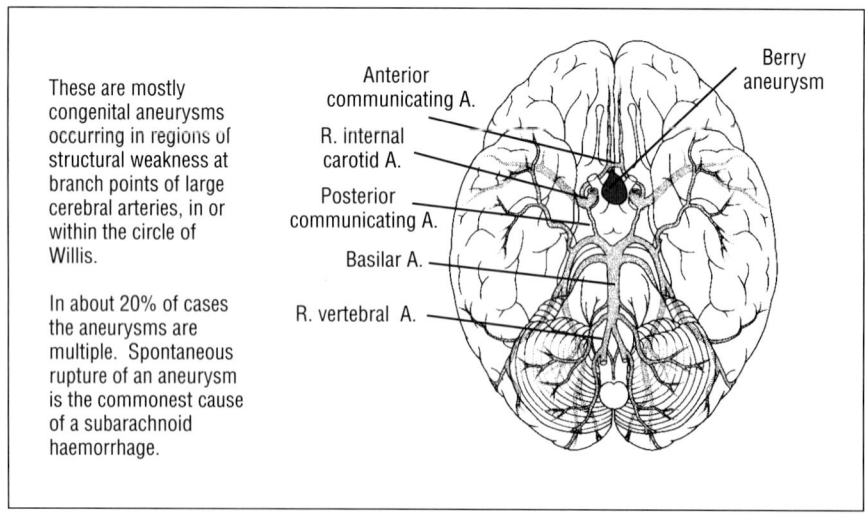

These are mostly congenital aneurysms occurring in regions of structural weakness at branch points of large cerebral arteries, in or within the circle of Willis.

In about 20% of cases the aneurysms are multiple. Spontaneous rupture of an aneurysm is the commonest cause of a subarachnoid haemorrhage.

Berry aneurysm
Anterior communicating A.
R. internal carotid A.
Posterior communicating A.
Basilar A.
R. vertebral A.

Figure 13.10 *Berry aneurysms*

affecting the brain and its vessels and typically such disorders include brain aneurysms, subarachnoid and intracerebral haemorrhages and brain infarcts.

Subarachnoid haemorrhage accounts for 5 to 13% of CVAs. Although trauma may cause a subarachnoid haemorrhage, by far the commonest cause is the rupture of a congenital saccular, berry aneurysm, usually at a bifurcation of the circle of Willis. Berry aneurysms are so called because of their resemblance to a berry fruit. More than 90% of such aneurysms occur within the carotid supply (see Figure 13.10). People with polycystic renal disease are predisposed to the formation of berry aneurysms and they are also hypertensive, rendering this group very vulnerable to subarachnoid haemorrhage. Hypertension, and therefore cigarette smoking, is largely responsible for both the enlargement of the aneurysm and its rupture. Physical or emotional exertion may precede the event. In some cases the aneurysm may rupture without any associated aetiology and be simply the result of a continuous enlargement of the lesion over a number of years.

As the aneurysm enlarges it may act as a space-occupying lesion, producing focal signs and palsies of the third nerve or, less commonly, of the fourth, fifth or sixth, as well as visual disturbances due to compression of the optic nerves or the optic chiasm. Sometimes, frank rupture is preceded by a series of small leaks producing transient headache and neck stiffness. More often, no warning is given. There is severe occipital headache, often with vomiting, followed by a loss of consciousness. The CSF is grossly bloody and under increased pressure. Meningeal signs (Kernig's, Brudzhinski's, and neck stiffness) are prominent, with nuchal rigidity being the hallmark. Focal signs are usually absent. Patients often show alterations in their mental status.

One-third of patients survive one month. If the patient survives two months, less than 19% will have a recurrent haemorrhage in the same site. Overall, subarachnoid haemorrhage has a very poor prognosis with 60% of patients dying after their first haemorrhage, 20% being permanently paralysed or crippled, the other 20% recovering. There is certainly a better prognosis if the patient is operated upon immediately after the aneurysm ruptures and most of these patients have a good long-term survival.

Intracerebral Haemorrhage

This constitutes 7–17% of CVAs, but is the form associated with the poorest prognosis and the most deaths. The incidence of this condition has fallen since the 1920s when it was the commonest form of CVA, largely because of control of hypertension and the increase in the incidence of atherosclerotic cerebral disease (causing more CVAs to be due to infarction). It is equally common in males and females. In 70% of cases the haemorrhage is cerebral, particularly in the putamen and claustrum (lateral basal ganglia) and the external capsule. These areas are supplied by the lenticulostriate branch of the middle cerebral artery ('artery of cerebral haemorrhage'). Another 15% are in the midbrain or pons, the remainder involving the cerebellum. Common causes precipitating massive intracerebral haemorrhages are:

- arterial disease and hypertensive crises;
- rupture of intracerebral vessel aneurysms;
- arteriovenous malformations;
- haemorrhage associated with neoplasms and leukaemia;
- haemorrhagic diathesis (congenital, acquired or iatrogenic);
- trauma.

Brain haemorrhages tend to expand rapidly, becoming massive lesions. Rupture into a ventricle often occurs, causing **intraventricular haemorrhage** and sudden death. Blood is usually present in the CSF if the haemorrhage involves the ventricles. Cerebral oedema is massive, in most cases leading to herniation of the brain. The clinical picture is catastrophic. Suddenly and dramatically, often following physical or emotional exertion, intense headache and vomiting develop, followed in minutes by loss of consciousness. The patient's head is thrown back with the face congested, and heavy, laboured breathing being apparent. There is usually total contralateral **hemiplegia** (paralysis down one side of the body), depending on the site of bleeding, and there may be faecal and urinary incontinence. Pontine haemorrhage produces pinpoint pupils and hyperpyrexia. If the haemorrhage occurs near the brain surface there may be convulsions. The coma may deepen with the passage of time and death usually follows in hours or days. One-month survival is only approximately 17%. If the patient survives, phagocytosis and gliosis occur, forming a cystic cavity. Within about 3 days the microglial cells begin to ingest the degenerating erythrocytes and within about a week haemosiderin deposits begin to become prominent. Within 3 to 6 weeks of the haemorrhage the central area is resorbed and a cystic space is left behind, surrounded by a peripheral sleeve of gliosis.

Multiple small haemorrhages within the brain may sometimes occur, instead of a massive haemorrhage. These **petechial haemorrhages** are commonly associated with infections (especially septicaemia, rickettsial and some viral diseases), anoxia and asphyxia (due to massive venous congestion, for example), trauma (common in boxers, especially in regions of contrecoup injury), haemorrhagic diathesis and vitamin B_{12} deficiency. Generally, the prognosis for this type of haemorrhage is much better than for the massive type.

Cerebrovascular Disease, Brain Infarct

Brain cells are extraordinarily sensitive to anoxia, and therefore, ischaemia. Although it represents only 2% of the body's weight, the brain consumes 20% of its oxygen and has no capacity to survive by anaerobic metabolism. Oxygen deprivation for only a few minutes leads to neuronal necrosis and, since there is virtually no functional reserve, even a very small infarct is usually symptomatic. By far, the most important aetiological factors are hypertension and atherosclerosis and both are linked to cigarette smoking. The ischaemia may be focal (cerebrovascular accident or stroke) or diffuse (anoxic encephalopathy).

Defences against infarction include the poorly understood capacity of cerebral vessels to dilate in the presence of hypoxia or hypercapnia, so that the brain maintains a near-normal circulation when other organs are so deprived of blood that they can no longer function. The brain shares this property only with the heart. The other defence lies in extensive collateral circulation, for example between the ophthalmic and external carotid arteries, which can thus substitute for the internal carotid, and by the circle of Willis. In addition, there are extensive corticomeningeal anastomoses. These defences are, however, inadequate if vascular occlusion is sudden. Pre-existing atherosclerotic disease modifies these processes and complicates the picture. For example, occlusion of the anterior cerebral artery may be adequately compensated for by collaterals

from the middle cerebral. Years later, stenosis of the middle cerebral by atherosclerosis may then produce an infarct in the territory supplied by the anterior cerebral arteries.

Brain infarcts account for 70% to 90% of CVAs (refer to Figure 13.11). The incidence increases steeply with age and above the age of 60 years this disorder becomes an important cause of death. The condition is commoner in women over the age 60 years than it is in men of the same age group (see Figure 13.12). Other important risk factors predisposing to its development are hypertension, diabetes, cigarette smoking and hyperlipidaemia. The most important aetiology is thrombosis of an atheromatous artery (44% to 75% of cases) and the patients who develop a brain infarct usually show advanced atherosclerotic disease in many other sites of the body. Such patients frequently have a history of myocardial infarction, and in fact cerebral infarction may occur very soon after a myocardial infarct as thrombosis commonly complicates a transmural or subendocardial myocardial infarct.

The commonest vessels involved in the aetiology of cerebral infarction are the cervical portion of the carotid artery and the vertebral, cerebral and basilar arteries. Occlusion frequently occurs fairly slowly, often allowing anastomotic collateral vessels to take over the blood supply of the region affected by the occluded vessel. If the collateral blood supply is inadequate, infarction occurs in the most distal branches of the vessel, along the border between the territories of the middle and anterior cerebrals ('watershed infarct'). In contrast, occlusion of the middle cerebral artery produces extensive proximal infarction, because it is distal to the circle of Willis and devoid of major collateral vessels (see Figure 13.13).

A **completed stroke** implies that an infarct has occurred and the signs and symptoms have developed rapidly afterwards, persisting for more than 24 hours.

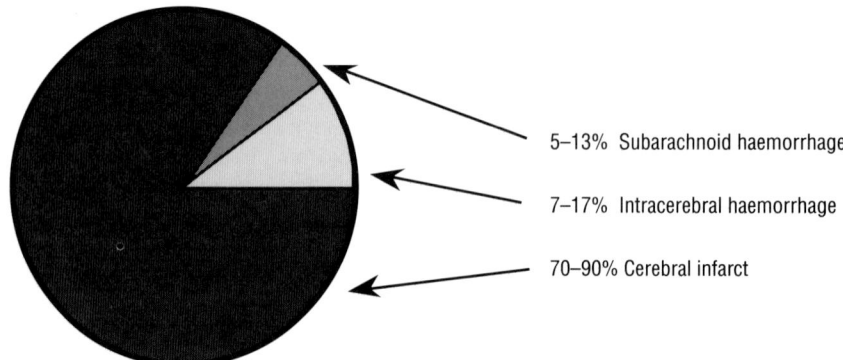

5–13% Subarachnoid haemorrhage

7–17% Intracerebral haemorrhage

70–90% Cerebral infarct

Figure 13.11 *The incidence of various types of cerebrovascular accidents*

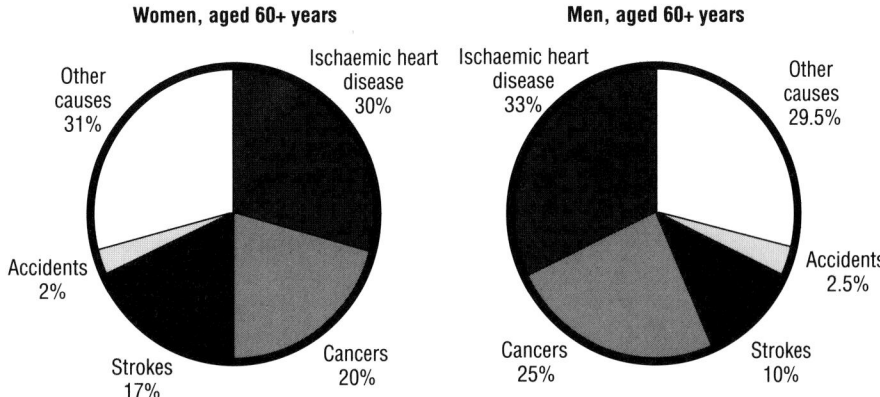

Figure 13.12 *Causes of death, Australia, 1984*

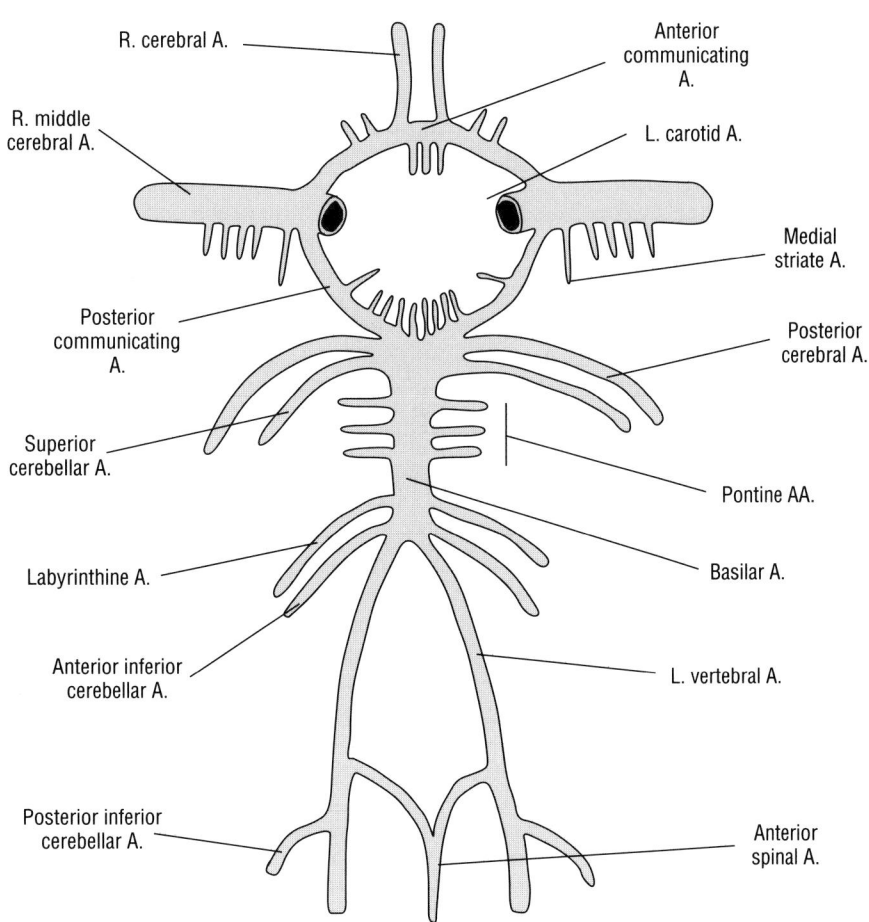

Figure 13.13 *Arteries of the base of the brain and the circle of Willis*

The symptoms of a cerebral infarct may develop over hours or days, usually over a period of 1 to 2 hours. The exact neurological symptomatology depends on the area of brain involved, but as the middle cerebral artery is commonly involved in the process, a **hemiplegia** is the commonest presentation and this affects the face and limbs on the side opposite the lesion. Loss of consciousness is rare while confusion and aphasia are common. Epileptic fits may be seen at the beginning or during the extension of a stroke, especially if it has been caused by an embolus. Severe headache is an unusual feature of infarcts. The CSF is usually normal.

Brain infarction due to embolism represents 3% to 14% of CVAs. The source of the embolus is the heart or the carotid arteries. Embolic occlusion is very sudden. Most commonly the middle cerebral artery is affected. If a large embolus impacts in one of the branches of the cerebral vessels an infarct may result very rapidly and the patient may become comatose or die almost instantly. Frequently, however, the emboli are very small and may give rise to a **transient ischaemic attack** (**TIA**). This is a commonly observed clinical presentation in patients with mild, or transient embolic occlusions of the brain vessels. By definition, manifestations of TIA must be over within 24 hours with complete recovery having occurred, otherwise the patient is described as having sustained a cerebral infarct.

Symptoms and signs associated with a TIA are variable depending on the site affected, but usually they include the following: transient loss of vision in one eye (**amaurosis fugax**), hemiparesis or sensory disturbances that indicate that the ischaemia involves the region supplied by the carotid artery on the contralateral side of the body affected. Consciousness is unimpaired in these cases. If the ischaemia affects the regions supplied by the basilar or vertebral arteries then vertigo, diplopia, hemiparesis or loss of consciousness may result. The signs and symptoms of TIA are usually over within a few minutes and if they persist for an hour or so, in most cases an infarct has occurred and complete recovery will not eventuate within 24 hours. TIA may be viewed as a warning of possible major strokes that will usually develop within a 6-month period.

A cerebral infarct softens quickly (colliquative necrosis) and eventually becomes cystic. Although the nerve cells will undergo necrosis within a few minutes of the interruption to the blood supply, there is only a slight discolouration in the region visible with the naked eye 6 to 12 hours following the infarct. The affected tissue at this stage shows reduced staining, swelling of cells, fragmentation of axons, loss of myelin and accumulating fluid. The softening and disintegration of the tissue become noticeable 48 to 72 hours after the infarct and the surrounding brain tissue is oedematous, so much so that herniations may occur. Surrounding the infarcted region are congested vessels and very few neutrophils, these cells quickly ceding their place to microglial cells and macrophages. The necrotic tissue is phagocytosed by these cells and the phagocyte response is maximal between 10 to 14 days after the infarct. The lipid-laden macrophages in the tissue are termed **compound granular cells** or **gitter cells**. Gliosis begins 7 to 12 days after the infarct has occurred and will become marked around the infarcted area with time. Brown staining due to haemosiderin deposition will become prominent following haemorrhage. Eventually, a cystic space forms surrounded by a margin of gliosis and this is known as an **apoplectic cyst**.

The diagnosis of cerebrovascular disease depends largely on clinical history and presenting symptomatology. It is important to differentiate between a completed stroke, a stroke in evolution, a TIA, a brain haemorrhage and other related disorders such as migraines, brain tumours and epilepsy (refer to Table 13.2). Computed tomography, EEG and cerebral angiography are all used in the diagnosis of such conditions. Treatment of a patient with stroke depends on the precipitating cause and the extent of the affected tissue and clinical symptomatology. Neurosurgery may be carried out, for example, in order to rapidly re-establish blood flow through a blocked carotid. Vasodilatory agents have been tried but their use has not been associated with improved prognosis for the patient. High doses of corticosteroids have also been used in acute stroke patients but although their use reduces the early death rate from severe strokes, there is no benefit in the long term. Anticoagulants are not used in completed strokes but they may be of some use in a stroke in evolution (although a cerebral haemorrhage must have been excluded!). Daily aspirin administration is used frequently in patients who have suffered TIA and this seems to reduce the incidence of future strokes in these patients.

The prognosis of patients who have suffered a stroke is much better than that of those who have had cerebral haemorrhages and the 30-day survival of stroke patients is approximately 70%. In the survivors, life expectancy is roughly halved and about 10% of these patients suffer a second stroke within the same year and 20% within 5 years of the original stroke. In addition, many of these patients succumb to myocardial infarction.

Table 13.2　*Cerebrospinal fluid findings in various vascular disorders of the brain*

Condition/ features	Intracerebral haemorrhage	Subarachnoid haemorrhage	Vascular anomalies	Thrombotic stroke	Embolic stroke
Clinical setting	Hypertension, heart disease	Trauma, hypertension	Young person, no hypertension	Prodromal TIA, atherosclerosis	Atherosclerosis, myocardial infarct
Onset	Usually during physical activity	Sudden, severe headache	Previous history, sudden headache	Gradual onset and progression	Sudden onset of symptoms
Symptoms	Headache if conscious, hemiplegia	Transient disturbance of consciousness	Paraesthesiae, eye pain, scotoma, focal epilepsy	Consciousness maintained, hemiplegia	Consciousness maintained, hemiplegia
Signs	Epileptic fit, papilloedema	Kernig's sign	Cranial bruits	Atherosclerosis related	Atherosclerosis related
Progression	Coma, death is the most usual outcome	Preretinal haemorrhage, aphasia, hemiparesis	Retinal angiomata, preretinal haemorrhage	Paralysis, dysphasia, coma, death or gradual improvement	Paralysis dysphasia, coma, occasionally improvement apparent
CSF	Often bloodstained	Often bloodstained	Often bloodstained	Clear	Clear
Prognosis	30-day survival is 20%	30-day survival is 35%	30-day survival is 35%	30-day survival is 65%	30-day survival is 70%

Central Nervous System Infections

Acute Suppurative Meningitis

Although acute suppurative meningitis may be caused by any pyogenic bacterium, the most commonly involved bacteria are *Neisseria meningitidis, Streptococcus pneumoniae* or *Haemophilus influenzae* in children and *E. coli* and other enteric organisms in neonates. *S. pneumoniae, Staphylococcus aureus* and *Candida albicans* can cause the disease in immunosuppressed patients. The disease has decreased dramatically in incidence in the last few decades since the advent of antibiotics but it still causes some deaths, especially in the paediatric setting. The organisms reach the CNS through the bloodstream, the primary involvement frequently being pneumonia, infective endocarditis or osteomyelitis. Infections of the face or throat (e.g. sinusitis or tonsillitis) or the ear (otitis media or mastoiditis) may lead to meningitis as may penetrating injuries or fracture of the base of the skull.

If pyogenic organisms cause the infection, there is a cloudy purulent exudate in the subarachnoid space. The pia and arachnoid mater (leptomeninges) become congested and opaque and the predominant cell in the CSF is the neutrophil. Later, the purulent CSF becomes fibrinous, may clot, and contains lymphocytes as well. Thrombophlebitis of the dural sinuses and bridging veins is frequent and may lead to venous infarction of the underlying cerebral cortex. Ultimately there is fibrosis with thickening of the meninges. Adhesions may form between the meninges and the brain, impinging on cranial nerves or blocking the flow of CSF from the ventricles, producing cranial nerve palsies and hydrocephalus.

The onset of the disease is sudden and dramatic with severe headache, fever, chills and neck stiffness. Delirium and coma rapidly ensue. With prompt treatment most patients survive, but approximately 20% will retain neurological impairment such as deafness, seizures, mental retardation, blindness, cranial nerve palsies or hydrocephalus. Some patients later develop brain abscesses.

Chronic Meningitis

This form of meningitis is caused mainly by the tubercle bacillus and *Cryptococcus neoformans*. In the former, tubercles form on the meninges; in the latter, a chronic inflammatory process occurs, typically at the base of the brain. The cryptococci may be demonstrated by Indian ink staining of CSF, while the tubercle bacilli may be visualized by Ziehl-Neelsen staining.

Tuberculous meningitis is usually metastatic from the lung or occurs with miliary TB; rarely, it is seen to complicate Pott's disease of the spine. The CSF is usually crystal clear. On standing, in TB, a fine clot like a cobweb forms within it. The cellular infiltrate is lymphocytic, and CSF pressure is elevated. Cryptococcal meningitis is seen following pulmonary infection, especially in people exposed to pigeon droppings or in patients who are already debilitated, for example those with Hodgkin's disease or AIDS.

With both of these infections there is gradual onset of non-specific symptoms such as headache, malaise, low-grade fever. Meningeal signs (neck stiffness, Kernig's sign) are present. Without treatment, tuberculous meningitis is fatal in weeks to months. Prompt therapy permits recovery, usually without residual damage. If treatment is delayed until focal signs or coma have appeared, recovery is 60% or less and survivors may be deaf, blind, epileptic or mentally deficient. In cryptococcal meningitis, treatment is difficult and many such patients succumb to the infection.

Viral Meningitis

Viral meningitis is still sometimes referred to as 'aseptic meningitis' since no bacteria will be isolated from the CSF. However, this term is a misnomer, as there are viruses present causing an infection. The causative organisms include echoviruses, Coxsackieviruses, mumps, measles and varicella viruses. Infectious mononucleosis may present as a meningitis. Most viruses reach the CNS from the gastrointestinal tract via a viraemia.

Clinically, there is sudden onset of disease with headache, fever and neck stiffness. CSF pressure is elevated and the predominant cell in the meninges is the lymphocyte (refer to Table 13.1). The disease is usually self-limited and ultimately full recovery within 1 to 2 weeks is the rule. Very rarely, complications may set in with the infection spreading to involve the nervous tissue, considerable inflammation and brain damage resulting from the encephalitis.

Neurosyphilis

Neurosyphilis may mimic any neurological disease, and symptoms are often puzzling. Some patients will develop the **meningovascular** form of the disease within 2–3 years of contracting the primary infection. In this type of syphilis, the CSF shows positive serology and lymphocytosis. The protein level is often raised due to increased gamma globulin. Treatment is with penicillin. In other cases, the infection remains asymptomatic for many years and **parenchymatous syphilis** (**general paralysis of the insane** and **tabes dorsalis**) involving the brain is a form of tertiary syphilis, occurring many years or decades after the primary infection. Relatively few of those who contract primary syphilis will develop parenchymatous syphilis even if they are left without treatment.

The disease manifestations are as follows.

Meningovascular syphilis. This is characterised by mononuclear cell infiltration of the leptomeninges and by syphilitic endarteritis and sometimes granuloma formation (gummata). It leads to cranial nerve palsies especially of the second, third and eighth nerves, headaches, fits and compression of the brain due to formation of space-occupying lesions (gummata). A cerebral endarteritis often occurs, leading to thrombosis and strokes. Involvement of the spine also complicates this form of the disease with pachymeningitis causing compression of posterior roots, leading to pain, or involving the anterior roots, causing muscular weakness (especially of the hands). Spinal thrombosis in spinal vessels with endarteritis causes transverse myelitis with interruption of the nerve tracts.

General paralysis of the insane. This is one of the manifestations of parenchymatous syphilis, with involvement of the brain substance in the disease process and degeneration of cortical neurones, leading to brain atrophy. The result is a dementia of insidious onset with slow progression to insanity and upper motor neurone paresis. The cortex of the brain becomes thinned and the line of demarcation between grey and white matter is obscured. The brain is shrunken with wide sulci and shrunken gyri. The meninges are opaque and adherent to the brain while the ventricles are dilated and show a granular lining. Very often this presentation is seen in association with tabes dorsalis.

Tabes dorsalis (locomotor ataxia). This is another manifestation of parenchymatous syphilis with atrophy of the posterior (sensory) roots in the lumbar region and thickening of the meninges overlying them, sometimes accompanied by atrophy of the optic nerves.

Paroxysms of severe lightning pains occur, most commonly in the legs. There is loss of normal pain sensation, vibration sense and deep reflexes. The Argyll-Robertson pupil (accommodates but does not react) is nearly always present. Ataxia is prominent, due to proprioceptive loss. Ulcers and Charcot-type joints occur. Very few cases of tertiary syphilis are now seen due to the treatment of the disease with antibiotics in its early (primary and secondary) stages.

Brain Abscess

Abscesses within the brain parenchyma are caused by pyogenic organisms reaching the brain by haematogenous spread, or by spreading directly into its substance as has already been considered for meningitis. Symptoms of the abscess develop over weeks to months and relate to the growth of the abscess and involvement of more and more nervous tissue. The patients present with the symptoms of raised intracranial pressure (headache, vomiting, papilloedema) and those of a space-occupying lesion. Diagnosis is by CT scan. Unless the abscess is surgically drained or controlled by antibiotics, death may follow from herniation of the brain as a result of elevated intracranial pressure. If the abscess ruptures into a ventricle, ventricular empyema results which is rapidly fatal.

Encephalitis

Encephalitis refers to the infection of brain substance, usually by viruses, hence the older name referring to these infections as 'aseptic encephalitides' as no bacteria could be isolated from cases of the disease. Murray Valley, Australian encephalitis and Ross River encephalitis are examples of this type of infection. Related diseases occur in other geographical locations, for example St Louis encephalitis, Japanese B encephalitis and Eastern equine encephalitis. A great many related viruses have been isolated from such diseases and they all share the feature of being arthropod borne (arboviruses). Very often, these brain infections occur in epidemic proportions and are associated with certain climactic conditions that cause migration of water birds carrying the viruses, and multiplication of the insects that spread the virus from fowl to humans.

In many cases the encephalitis causes fever, changes in the level of consciousness and very variable neurological signs, including tremors, rigidity and paralysis. The brain shows small haemorrhages and the conges-tion of small vessels, perivascular infiltrate by lymphocytes and monocytes. There may be neuronal degeneration and gliosis, especially in the basal ganglia, substantia nigra, pons and medulla. Depending on the specific virus and individual idiosyncratic factors, the encephalitis may cause minimal damage and complete recovery will occur (usually seen in the majority of cases), but in a few cases there may be widespread damage to the nervous tissue with spread of the infection to the spinal cord (**encephalomyelitis**), resulting in mental retardation, convulsions and other neurological deficits, occasionally with a fatal outcome.

Other viruses such as Coxsackieviruses, mumps virus, Epstein-Barr virus, polioviruses and rabies virus infect, and produce damage to, nervous tissue. Herpes simplex can produce encephalitis in the neonate and the elderly or immunocompromised patient. There is progressive degeneration and destruction of nerve cell bodies, with inclusion bodies in some cases, for example rabies. There is proliferation of microglial cells and blood vessels are surrounded by lymphocytes and plasma cells (perivascular cuffing). The disease may be mild or severe with serious residual effects. Meningeal signs may also be present (meningoencephalitis). Rabies is virtually always fatal after symptoms ensue, mumps encephalitis is nearly always benign. Measles encephalitis is rare but leaves children permanently and severely incapacitated. The incidence of this last-mentioned disorder has fallen dramatically since the introduction of measles vaccination.

Slow Virus Infections

Slow virus infections produce often fatal encephalitides that appear insidiously, after very long incubation periods (decades). They include progressive multifocal leukoencephalopathy (PML), Creutzfeldt-Jakob disease (caused by a member of the polyoma subgroup of Papovaviruses, which are oncogenic in experimental animals) and kuru.

Very atypical astrocytes are found in the lesions of PML. The virus probably only affects the immunocompromised. Approximately 69% of adults have circulating antibody to the virus. Creutzfeldt-Jakob disease occurs in middle age and produces dementia and myoclonus, leading to death within a year. Kuru was a disease of New Guinea cannibals. It was spread by eating the brains of affected individuals. It begins as cerebellar ataxia and then progresses to a general decortication. Death occurs within 6 months of onset of symptoms.

Demyelinating Diseases

Demyelinating diseases of the central nervous system have as a common factor a degeneration of the myelin sheath of neurones, the axons preserved until the later stages of the disease. The white matter is affected primarily and the necrosis of neurones and glial cells is a rare, delayed phenomenon. The aetiology of these diseases is unknown, although increasing evidence is pointing to an autoimmunne reaction causing these disorders. The trigger for the autoimmunity is unknown.

Multiple Sclerosis

This is a common progressive disease, mainly affecting young adults between the ages of 20 to 40 years, women more commonly affected than men. The aetiology is unknown although current thinking favours a viral aetiology complicated by T cell and B cell mediated immunological damage to myelin. The virus causing the autoimmunity is not known but it may be a common virus encountered during childhood or adolescence, and to this virus the affected individual is hypersensitive. It is thought that adverse immune reactions following exposure to this unknown virus are what cause the myelin destruction. The disease involves the brain and spinal cord in a random manner, forming plaques of demyelination with axon preservation. The disease has a long course over 5 to 20 years with numerous remissions and recrudescences.

The plaques of demyelination are characteristic of the disease and are found throughout the brain and spinal cord. They vary in size from a few millimetres to 6 cm in diameter. The early lesions are pinkish in colour, while later in the disease they become firmer and greyish. They are found predominantly in the paraventricular regions, the optic nerves, the cerebellar peduncles and the dorsal tracts of spinal cord and brain stem. The peripheral nerves tend to be uniformly spared. In the region of the plaques there is oedema, vascular congestion, microglial proliferation and perivascular astrocytosis, with infiltration by lymphocytes. The proliferating astrocytes lead to gliosis in the plaque region, causing the formation of the **sclerotic plaque**.

Clinically, the disease is extremely variable in its presentation, the individual cases showing a different neurological deficiency or compromise in function dictated by the region of nervous tissue affected. Remissions frequently occur, but these become less complete and more infrequent as more and more nervous tissue is involved. Typically, the disease is characterized by long chronicity and periods of relapses with exacerbations, showing new neurological signs that ultimately lead to progressive disability. Some patients live a normal life span, albeit with increasing disability. In others the disease may be fatal in a few months or years.

The disease onset may be sudden or slow with some of the early clinical presentations including paraesthesiae, retrobulbar neuritis, ocular disturbances, mild sensory or motor symptoms of a limb or cerebellar incoordination and mental changes. In later stages recovery during remission is incomplete. Not all patients become totally disabled, but many are confined to a wheelchair as the disease progresses. In the end there may be unsteady gait, incontinence and paralysis due to cerebral and spinal cord demyelination. Death is usually due to complicating infection, either pneumonia or extensive involvement of the urinary tract.

Subacute Combined Degeneration of the Cord

This neuropathy accompanies pernicious anaemia and is the result of vitamin B_{12} deficiency. The disease is characterised by degeneration of myelin in the spinal cord long tracts (dorsal and lateral columns). The grey matter is spared. Eventually, axon degeneration occurs as well as myelin degeneration. The brain stem, optic nerves and cerebral cortex may also contain foci of demyelination.

Paraesthesiae of the hands and feet are usually the first symptom, accompanied by loss of vibration sense and diminished deep tendon reflexes. Ataxia follows proprioceptive loss. Eventually spasticity and other upper motor neurone signs develop. Early treatment with cyanocobalamin is the treatment of choice. Therapy must be continued for life. Many patients eventually die of gastric carcinoma which is secondary to the associated atrophic gastritis.

Guillain-Barré Syndrome

This is an ascending paralysis that occurs days to weeks after a non-specific viral illness. It starts in the feet, ascends to the leg, affects the upper limbs and finally the muscles of respiration within hours or a day or two. The disease reaches a peak in a week, remains static for a fortnight then gradually subsides, usually leaving no sequelae. Artificial respiration for the duration of the illness is essential if respiration is affected.

Widespread segmental demyelination and lymphocytic infiltration is seen in the cord and CSF protein is raised.

Neurological Syndromes of the Basal Ganglia

This group of syndromes is a miscellaneous one and contains several diseases that will manifest themselves as dementia. Although some such diseases are treated here briefly, they are given in greater detail within the context of the dementias in the section on the pathology of dementia below.

Wilson's Disease

This is a genetic disease inherited as an autosomal recessive trait that has already been discussed in association with cirrhosis of the liver and congenital disorders of the CNS (see Chapter 9 and the beginning of this chapter). It is a defect of copper metabolism characterised by hepatic cirrhosis, the **Kayser-Fleischer** ring at the limbus of the cornea and degeneration of the putamen, globus pallidus, thalamus and cerebral cortex. Hepatic involvement usually precedes extrapyramidal symptoms. A low level of ceruloplasmin is diagnostic.

Huntington's Chorea

This is an autosomal dominant disorder in which symptoms usually become manifest at middle age although a juvenile form (Westphal variant) is known. Degeneration of the head of the caudate nucleus and putamen occurs. Neurone loss followed by gliosis may be so marked that almost total atrophy of the head of the caudate nucleus occurs. The affected areas are deficient in gamma-aminobutyric acid (GABA), a neurotransmitter substance. The disease is characterized by abnormal involuntary movements of the limbs and fingers (chorea). Choreiform movements are followed by dementia and both progress until over a period of 10 to 15 years the patient is totally incapacitated and bedridden.

Parkinson's Disease (Paralysis Agitans)

This disease may follow atherosclerosis and ischaemia of the basal ganglia, it may occur after encephalitis or be idiopathic. It may also follow reserpine or phenothiazine therapy and thus may be iatrogenic (drug-induced Parkinsonism). The disease is associated with a coarse pill-rolling tremor, paucity of movement (akinesia) and cog-wheel rigidity. Degeneration occurs in the substantia nigra, caudate putamen and globus pallidus. The disorder is characterized biochemically by loss of dopaminergic neurones. Symptoms are reversed by administration of L-dopa. The disease becomes manifest in middle or old age and is often, at first, unilateral (hemi-Parkinsonism).

Tremor is in many cases the first symptom, with akinesia and rigidity following this. Drooling of saliva is a common symptom and is due to akinesia of muscles of glutition. The mask-like expressionless face is due to akinesia of facial muscles. Despite a dramatic reversal of symptoms by drug administration, the disease progresses inexorably, the patient becoming demented.

Miscellaneous Disorders

There are several idiopathic degenerations of the spinal cord and cerebellum including amyotrophic lateral sclerosis, spinal muscular atrophy and progressive bulbar palsy. There is degeneration of muscle groups, altered Babinski reflexes, and, if the cerebellum is involved, ataxia and nystagmus. In some conditions cardiac anomalies also occur. The diseases are progressive and there is no known treatment. All lead to death after various times and some are familial.

Alzheimer's Disease

Alzheimer's disease is a common degenerative disease of the cerebrum which is idiopathic, though there may be a familial tendency. It is rare before the age of 50 years and more common after the age of 65 years.

Initially there is subtle impairment of the higher intellectual functions or increased emotional lability. During later stages there is progressive disorientation, loss of memory, language disorders and other severe cortical dysfunctions. In the final stages there is profound cortical dysfunction. The patient becomes mute, immobile and demented over the course of 5 to 10 years. Death occurs usually due to infections. The brain shows loss of cerebral cortical tissue with widened cerebral sulci (especially in the frontal and temporal regions) and there is compensatory ventricular enlargement. Microscopically, there are neurofibrillary tangles, senile plaques and granulovacuolar degeneration. Amyloid is found in senile plaques in later stages.

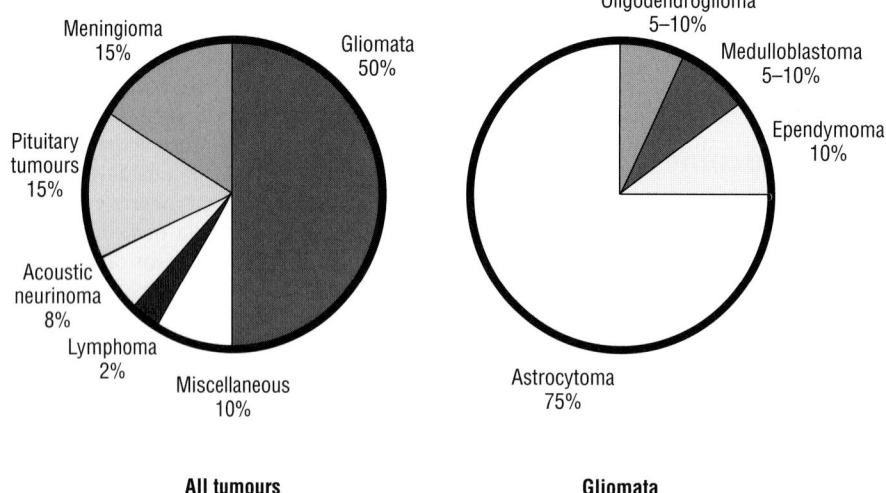

Figure 13.14 *Primary intracranial tumours*

Tumours of the Nervous System

This term includes all tumours within the cranium, including secondary tumours from outside the CNS, the tumours of the spinal cord and those of peripheral nerves. By far, the most important of all of these tumours are the intracranial tumours. Even those primary tumours that are histologically benign are likely to prove fatal because of their location and growth within a restricted space. Primary brain tumours account for approximately 2% of all cancer deaths while 20% of childhood cancers are brain tumours. In Australia, about 600 people die annually from primary gliomatous intracerebral tumours, while in the United States this figure is closer to 10 000 individuals annually. The majority of the primary neoplasms within the cranial cavity are totally idiopathic and no aetiological or pathogenetic factors have been associated with them. They occur anywhere between infancy and old age and their character ranges from the slowly growing 'benign' tumours to the rapidly expanding and quickly growing, highly malignant ones that may cause the patient's death within a few weeks.

Tissues of the CNS arise from the neuroectoderm and differentiate along two major lines, ultimately giving rise to the neuronal and neuroglial elements. In the adult, the neurones have lost their ability to divide and neuronal tumours are exceedingly rare. In the infant, the very rare tumours neuroblastoma and retinoblastoma are derived from primitive nerve cells. By far the commonest tumours in the CNS are derived from the glial cells, the **gliomata** which account for approxi-

mately 50% of primary intracranial tumours. Two other large groups are tumours derived from the meningeal fibroblast, the **meningioma**, and the pituitary tumours (refer to Figures 13.14 and 13.15).

Gliomata

Gliomata (40–50% of brain tumours) and meningioma (12–15% of brain tumours) make up the bulk of the intracranial neoplasms. Secondary tumours make up 25–30%. In adults, 70% of brain tumours arise above the tentorium, in children 70% are located below the tentorium.

Clinical features depend on the location and size of the tumour. Local effects are due to interruption or interference with neurological pathways (e.g. palsies) or irritative reactions (epilepsy). Thus a tumour arising in the parasagittal, posterior, frontal area will induce seizures beginning in the contralateral foot, while a similar neoplasm in the olfactory groove will induce unilateral anosmia. Oedema of the surrounding tissues may also contribute to the neurological signs. Generalized effects are due to increased intracranial pressure and the effects of haemorrhage into and about the tumour. Herniation of brain substance may occur.

Biological behaviour is variable even for the same tumour, and may depend on the tumour's location or age of the patient. Astrocytomata of the cerebrum in adults are very invasive and kill within a few years, while astrocytomata of the cerebellum in children behave much less aggressively. Brain tumours are frequently very well differentiated with no obvious mitotic figures, yet may be locally invasive and destructive. Glioblastoma multiforme is always very anaplastic, however, and shows pleomorphism, tumour giant cells and abundant mitoses. Gliomata include abundant neovascular proliferation, forming a good tumour circulation.

Metastases outside the CNS of tumours arising within the cranium are extremely rare. In a study of 18 000 brain tumours, only 35 metastasized systemically, nearly all of these being glioblastoma, and in nearly all these cases the metastasis followed surgical interference. Metastatic spread to other locations within the CNS, however, is the rule, including spread to the spinal cord. Spread is believed to be via the CSF circulation. Some astrocytomata do not form a discrete tumour mass but infiltrate diffusely throughout the white matter, causing hemispheric enlargement (gliomatosis cerebri). Five-year survival for the cerebral form of astrocytoma in adults is 25% following surgical resection and radiotherapy. Cerebellar astrocytomata have a peak incidence between 7 to 9 years and frequently regress, even after incomplete excision, allowing remission for decades. Cases are documented for degeneration of cerebellar astrocytomata into cystic lesions, apparently devoid of neoplasm after brain biopsy. Prognosis is far better than for the cerebral form. Glioblastoma multiforme and anaplastic astrocytomata (grade IV) are the commonest gliomata in adults. The anaplastic cells of these tumours grow rapidly and recur after treatment. Survival for more than 2 years after diagnosis of the tumour is exceptional.

Oligodendrogliomata grow slowly but appear to be able to dedifferentiate into astrocytomata, including glioblastoma multiforme. The tumours are often large and contain foci of calcification.

Ependymomata arise from the cells lining the ventricles of the brain, and the central canal of the spinal cord. Their peak incidence is in early childhood. They comprise over half of intraspinal gliomata. They are invasive tumours with a poor prognosis. Only tumours of the conus or filum terminale are sufficiently accessible to allow surgical curative resection.

Medulloblastoma

Peak incidence of this tumour is about the age of 10 years, although it may also arise in adults. The tumours are believed to arise from the embryonic cerebellum. In children they are usually midline in location and rapidly obstruct the fourth ventricle, causing massive hydrocephalus. Primitive cells may differentiate along both glial and neuronal lines. The tumour has a very poor prognosis and survival beyond 2 years is a rarity.

Meningioma

These tumours arise from cells at the junction of the arachnoid and dura mater and are uncommon in chil-

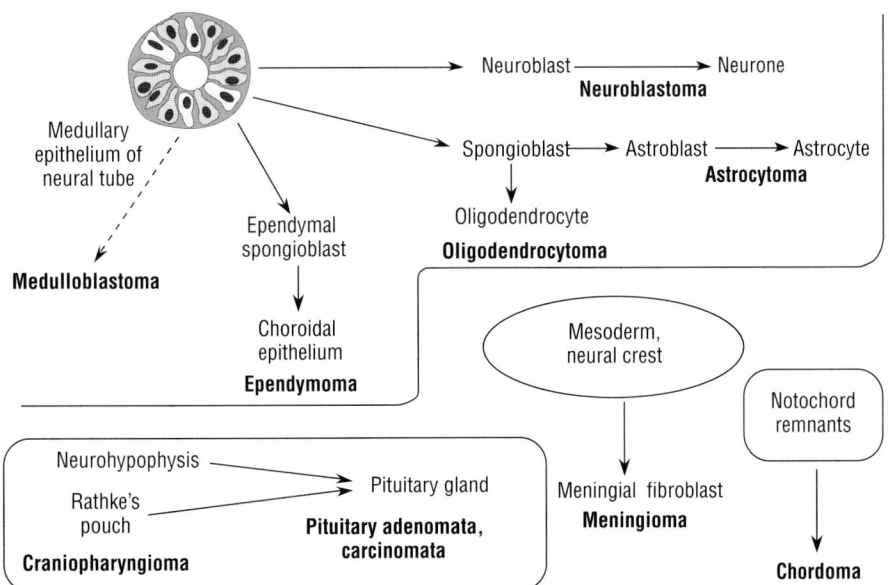

Figure 13.15 *Histogenesis of the primary intracranial tumours*

dren. They do not invade the brain substance, but by pressure may indent the brain and erode into the skull bones. Most can be surgically removed. A spectrum of differentiation is seen and controversy exists as to the presence of malignant behaviour; some experts recognise a malignant form, the so-called meningosarcoma, which is anaplastic and recurs after excision. The meningiomata are firm, white to grey, rubbery tumours with a cut surface showing whorling of the proliferating meningeal fibroblasts. A gritty, reddish, cut surface is also commonly seen. The cells of the tumour are very regular in appearance, elongated, with ovoid nuclei. Small clumps of tumour cells undergo necrosis and are subsequently calcified leading to the formation of small calcified masses called **psammoma bodies** ('brain sand').

Schwannoma

The commonest location of this tumour is in the acoustic nerve, typically at the cerebellopontine angle. The tumours are almost always benign. They are more frequent in patients with von Recklinghausen's disease. The tumours are almost always resectable. Acoustic neuromata produce tinnitus, deafness and ataxia or dizziness if they impinge on the cerebellum. Large tumours impinge on the fifth and seventh nerve, producing palsies. Tumours arising outside the CNS tend to be invasive and metastasize.

Neurofibromata, unlike schwannomata, arise within nerves from Schwann cells or fibroblasts in von Recklinghausen's disease (an autosomal dominant disorder). They occur in the CNS and peripherally and sometimes are very numerous. Café au lait pigmentation of the overlying skin is typical. Concomitant gliomata, meningiomata and schwannomata are sometimes seen. In 1 to 5% of cases malignant transformation occurs in one of the tumours.

Metastatic Tumours of the Central Nervous System

Most commonly these are carcinomata of breast, lung, gastrointestinal tract, kidney and malignant melanoma. These tumours may first present clinically due to symptoms caused by CNS metastases. The secondary deposits tend to occur at the junctions of white and grey matter. Multiple tumour masses are present, with massive involvement of the brain substance. The cerebrum tends to be involved more than the cerebellum and these secondary tumours have much the same effect on the patient as primary tumours, invariably ending in rapid death. Death may be preceded by many and varied neurological symptoms, which depend on the region of the brain involved. The histology of these secondary tumours is similar to that of the primary, unless anaplasia has occurred, in which case the primary tumour may not be identified.

Symptoms and Signs of Intracranial Neoplasms

All intracranial tumours, whether clinically benign or malignant, primary or secondary, tend to give rise to similar symptoms and signs. The clinical presentation is related to three major variables: Rise of intracranial pressure (rate and extent), location of the tumour (which part of the brain tissue it impinges on), and behaviour of the tumour (whether it irritates or destroys the nervous tissue it impinges on).

The presence of a growing tumour mass within the cranium and the associated oedema that almost invariably occurs with it cause a raised intracranial pressure which manifests itself as headache and vomiting. Herniations of the brain caused by the raised intracranial pressure may be fatal, especially the cerebellar (tonsilar) herniation as it causes compression of the respiratory and cardiac centres. A transtentorial herniation interferes with the circulatory dynamics of the midbrain and thus may cause a decreased level of consciousness. Compression of the third nerve may cause a palsy and a fixed dilated pupil. If there is midbrain necrosis or haemorrhage there is coma and death. Other features of raised intracranial pressure are generalized epileptic fits, dizziness, papilloedema with clouding or blurring of vision, progressive bradycardia and arterial hypertension.

The location of the tumour and its behaviour may give rise to a wide variety of clinical presentations. For example, lesions in the prefrontal lobes are associated with vague psychiatric signs in the early stages, while later the patients lose the ability to appreciate the consequences of their actions, becoming apathetic or demented. There is impairment of intellect and socially unacceptable behaviour becomes manifest (e.g. urinating in public). At the same time, there may be generalized convulsions and a grasp reflex is often found in the opposite hand. Lesions in the precentral gyrus cause Jacksonian epilepsy and there is a rapidly developing monoplegia and dysphasia is also present. Parietal lobe tumours may also cause Jacksonian epilepsy of a sensory type with disturbances in sensation. There may be spatial disorientation, apraxia, agnosia, dysphasia and hemianopia. Lesions in the occipital lobe may cause irritation and visual hallucinations such as flashing lights, or they may cause destruction with resultant hemianopia. The temporal lobe involved by neoplasms may react by becoming irritated, causing visual hallucinations of a more complicated type (colours and moving shapes, forms or pictures) and auditory, gustatory and olfactory hallucinations. Altered states of consciousness may also be experienced by the patient with temporal lobe tumours. Amnesiac periods, dream states, memory upsets and automatic behaviour are commonly seen.

Treatment and Prognosis of Intracranial Neoplasms

The mainstay of primary intracranial tumour therapy is surgery, although in some cases the tumour may be in such a situation (e.g. the brain stem or the dominant hemisphere) or in such an advanced stage that this may not be practicable. Medical management of the raised intracranial pressure may then be tried, as, for example, with administration of dexamethasone or mannitol. Palliation therapy with cytotoxic agents such as cyclophosphamide offer temporary relief.

In cases where surgery is possible, the objective is to remove the whole of the tumour while conserving as much as possible of the normal brain tissue around the tumour. Meningiomata and neuromata are the most accessible and easily treated of the intracranial tumours, although even their complete removal and failure to recur is marred by the propensity of some treated patients to develop recurrent fits. Craniopharyngiomata and pituitary tumours may be sometimes completely removed but if they are very close to the hypothalamus, an incomplete extirpation is the option available, with at least, prevention of further visual loss. Gliomata, generally, cannot be completely removed but the patient very frequently is operated upon as even partial removal of the tumour mass is associated in many cases (especially with the low-grade gliomata) with an increase in the patient's survival for a few years. In some cases, palliative surgery is carried out in an attempt to relieve raised intracranial pressure. The tumour mass or normal brain tissue in the frontal or temporal lobes may be removed for this purpose. Radiotherapy may be given in association with surgery or alone, especially in the case of some radiosensitive tumours such as medulloblastoma. However, acute or chronic radiation damage may cause many problems.

A new way of treating brain tumours is by surgery followed by photochemotherapy at the time of surgery. In this particular type of treatment the patient is given a photosensitizing drug which is selectively taken up by the tumour cells, and to date the only drug used is haematoporphyrin derivative. The tumour is then surgically excised and the cavity is irradiated by laser light of the specific wavelength needed to excite the photosensitizer in the tumour cells. This causes a series of photochemical reactions in the tumour cells which, hopefully, cause the destruction of the remaining tumour cells in the cavity. Clinically, patients who undergo such treatments have a much better prognosis and outlive patients who receive surgery alone. Research into new, more specific and more active photosensitizing agents is being carried out.

The prognosis of primary intracranial neoplasms is extremely poor and the majority of such tumours are invariably fatal within a short period of time. The average life expectancy following the diagnosis of a malignant brain tumour is usually less than 6 months. With the more benign growths (especially those that grow quickly) surgical extirpation is followed by some long-term survivals, especially if the tumour is accessible and is not in a vital part of the brain.

The Pathology of Dementia

Dementia literally means 'loss of mind', but this is an inadequate definition and the disorder may be more precisely defined as '**a global impairment of the intellect, memory and personality, without alteration of conscious level**'. Often the disease is described as a 'chronic brain failure', indicating that the condition is a prolonged state which affects the higher intellectual functions of the brain.

Incidence

The disorder affects approximately 5 to 10% of people over 65 years, but the incidence rises with age, such that no less than 20% of people are affected over the age of 80 years. Various studies in Britain have indicated that one person in 20 is affected by dementia by the age of 70 years and one person in five over the age of 80 years. Australian and American statistics are very similar to these. Some epidemiologists have suggested that these figures may be overestimates, often including in the dementia group patients presenting with other related disorders.

Features

Generally, the disorder is a progressive one, with an insidious course, often requiring several years to reach the profound state which is seen in some elderly patients. There may be a varied early presentation in terms of symptomatology, mainly contributed to by the patients' previous personality, age at onset, rate of progression and the cause of the disorder. However, in all cases the symptoms involve the intellect, memory, emotions and behaviour.

The earliest features of dementia are:

- loss of memory for recent events;
- global disruption of personality with the gradual development of abnormal behaviour;
- disinhibition of the patient, with noisy, antisocial, aggressive behaviour often being noted;
- often, insomnia with nocturnal restlessness.

As the disease progresses there will be:

- loss of long-term memory;
- confusion, disorientation, poor grasp of circumstances;
- restlessness, wandering, paranoia;
- incontinence, immobility, apathy;
- inability to converse;
- difficulty in engaging the patient's attention.

Related States

It is important to differentiate between dementia and several related states in which the patient may present with some features which could easily be misinterpreted as signs of dementia. These related states are often referred to as '**acute brain failure**'. It is important to diagnose these states early, as frequently they are treatable and the patients may recover. Acute brain failure is an acute confusional state or delirium, which is a dramatic and distressing state in which the patient becomes restless and agitated with episodes of clouding of consciousness and with misinterpretation of surroundings, visions or illusions alternating with episodes of lucidity. This condition of acute brain failure is not truly an organic mental illness but rather a common manifestation of physical disease which develops acutely. The causes of this disorder are quite varied and are summarized below (see Table 13.3). There may be intracranial and extracranial causes for acute brain failure and, unlike true dementia, the condition regresses when the disorder causing it is treated.

The clinical features of these acute confusional states are as follows. The patient typically shows a symptomatology which is of abrupt onset and which shows a marked variability, the patient showing episodes of lucidity. The consciousness is often clouded and recent memory is impaired. There is disorientation in place and time with delusions and hallucinations, fear, bewilderment and restlessness. Often, the patient also shows symptoms and signs of the underlying causes for the acute brain failure, for example respiratory distress, cyanosis and fever associated with a respiratory infection.

It should be noted that there is also the well-recognized syndrome of '**acute on chronic**' disorders in which acute brain failure is superimposed on a patient who is becoming demented. In this case, the diagnosis is often very difficult and the clinician is reliant on the information on the patient provided by relatives, friends or neighbours. Frequently, the diagnosis of acute and chronic brain failure is dependent on whether the condition is reversible (acute) or irreversible (chronic). In this context the term pseudodementia may also be used in order to describe the acute brain failure. **Confusion** is another term often used in this context but is a very vague term and may be applied to a variety of states. Usually, confusion is defined as the response of the ageing brain to stresses.

Table 13.3 *Causes of acute brain failure*

Intracranial causes of acute brain failute	Extracranial causes of acute brain failure
• Infarction ('silent' and often frontal)	• Infection (pulmonary, UTI)
• Infection (meningoencephalitis)	• Metabolic (hypoglycaemia, hypothermia fluid and electrolyte imbalances)
• Injury (head injury, falls, blows, etc.)	• Anoxia (cardiac or respiratory failure)
• Iatrogenic (drugs acting on CNS, e.g. for Parkinsonism, sedatives, steroids)	• Toxic (drugs with secondary effects on CNS)
• Alcohol intoxication	• Nutritional (Wernicke's encephalopathy)

Types of Dementia

In dealing with the true types of chronic brain failure, it is important to understand the causative and pathogenetic factors in the development of these disorders and the way in which they interact with the function of the brain in order to give rise to the multiplicity of mental symptoms. Despite the strong correlation of these disorders with increasing age, it should be stressed that dementia is not an inevitable consequence of ageing. There are two major varieties, the so-called '**senile dementia of the Alzheimer type**' (**SDAT or AD**) and the **multi-infarct dementia (MID)**. These two types of dementia account for approximately 50% and 30%, respectively, of all types of dementia. The remaining 20% of cases show a very diverse aetiology and are often referred to as 'mixed dementias' or as 'pre-senile dementias', depending on the age at which the patient first presents with them or on the underlying aetiology. Pre-senile dementia is a diagnosis usually reserved for patients who present with dementia before the age of 60 years.

The various types of dementias and their prevalence are given in Table 13.4. It can be seen that of all of these, the 'senile-type' dementia and the 'multi-infarct' dementia (which are more prevalent in the aged) are clearly the most important.

Another classification of the dementias subdivides them into two general groups, the **primary dementias** and the **secondary dementias**, depending on whether the condition is due to a primary neuronal degeneration in the absence of any other disorder or whether the neuronal degeneration is secondary to another state, the mechanism of which has been shown to cause the neuronal loss. In this scheme, Alzheimer's disease is a primary dementia while dementia following chronic drug administration is a secondary dementia. Generally, this classification is dependent very much on the aetiology of the dementia, and often the primary dementias are the ones in which the pathogenetic mechanism or aetiological factors responsible for the neuronal degeneration are unknown (see Table 13.5).

Table 13.4 *Types of dementia*

Commoner types of dementia	Rarer types of dementia
• Alzheimer's disease (50–60% of total)	• Chronic drug, alcohol abuse
	• Vitamin B_{12} deficiency
	• Neurosyphilis
	• Malignant disease (brain 1° or 2° tumours)
• Multi-infarct dementia (20% of total)	• Parkinson's disease
	• Pick's disease
	• Down's syndrome
• Mixed types of dementia ($\approx$20% of total)	• Huntington's chorea
	• Trauma to the brain
	• Normal pressure hydrocephalus

Table 13.5 *Aetiological classification of the dementias*

Idiopathic or miscellaneous	Nutritional or metabolic	Infections
• Alzheimer's disease(?)	• Niacin deficiency	• Neurosyphilis
• Pick's disease(?)	• Thiamine deficiency	• Tuberculosis
• Parkinson's disease(?)	• Electrolyte imbalance	• Abscesses
• Wilson's disease (gross copper overload — genetic)	• Hypothyroidism ('myxoedema madness')	• Viral infections (e.g. Creutzfeldt-Jakob disease)
• Huntington's chorea (genetic enzymatic defect)	• Vitamin B_{12} deficiency ('megaloblastic madness')	• Post-encephalitic dementia/ Parkinsonism

Vascular diseases	Toxic effects	Space-occupying lesions
• Vasculitis	• Arsenic and heavy metals	• Abscesses
• Cerebrovascular atheroma	• Alcohol	• Tumours (1° and 2°)
• Infarction	• Drugs (e.g. barbiturates)	• Brain haematomas

Aetiology of the Dementias

The general characteristic of the dementing disorders is a progressive and ineluctable loss of neurones from the grey matter of the cerebral cortex. With the different types of dementia, different regions of the brain may be involved (e.g. Pick's disease, *picks out* the frontal and temporal lobes whereas Alzheimer's disease eventually affects *all* of the brain; see Figure 13.16). However, with many of the dementias the precise aetiology for this progressive neuronal loss is not known. For example, for Alzheimer's disease much research in the area has suggested possible aetiologies, ranging from central nervous system viral infection to toxic effects of a variety of substances in the diet, for example aluminium. Various studies have tried to examine the chemical and biochemical changes that are occurring in the dementing brain and in this case some interesting data have emerged. For example, taking Alzheimer's disease again, it has been shown that in this type of dementia the brain is deficient in the enzyme choline **acetyl transferase**, which is necessary for the production of the neurotransmitter substance acetylcholine. This possibly reflects the neuronal loss in the cerebral cortex and in certain parts of the brainstem. Findings such as this have filled some people with hope, as it is thought that administration of these deficient chemicals to dementing patients may lead to improvement of the patient's condition, as was similarly observed in the case of treatment of Parkinson's disease with levodopa.

In the case of many of the primary dementias there may also be a familial/genetic component acting as often these disorders tend to 'run in some families'. No clear-cut Mendelian or hereditary association has been demonstrated but it is suspected that a polygenic effect may be involved, a particular 'assortment of genes' that is found to be inherited in a given family with a high incidence, making those individuals more likely to develop the condition. This mechanism does not exclude environmental factors and it is becoming apparent that the primary dementias are quite likely to be disorders with multifactorial aetiologies.

When the secondary dementias are examined, usually the mechanism of neuronal loss can be explained if one investigates the pathogenesis of the disease. It may be, for example, due to ischaemic effects, as occurs in the multi-infarct type of dementia where loss of blood supply to an area of cerebral cortex leads to destruction of nervous tissue, with permanent loss of neurones in the area. In the case of drugs or infections causing the dementia a similar effect may be seen, the offending agent causing a direct destruction of neurones.

As can be seen from Table 13.5, the aetiology of the dementias is varied but the majority of the conditions is in fact due to obscure aetiological factors (Alzheimer's disease) and it is with the rarer forms of

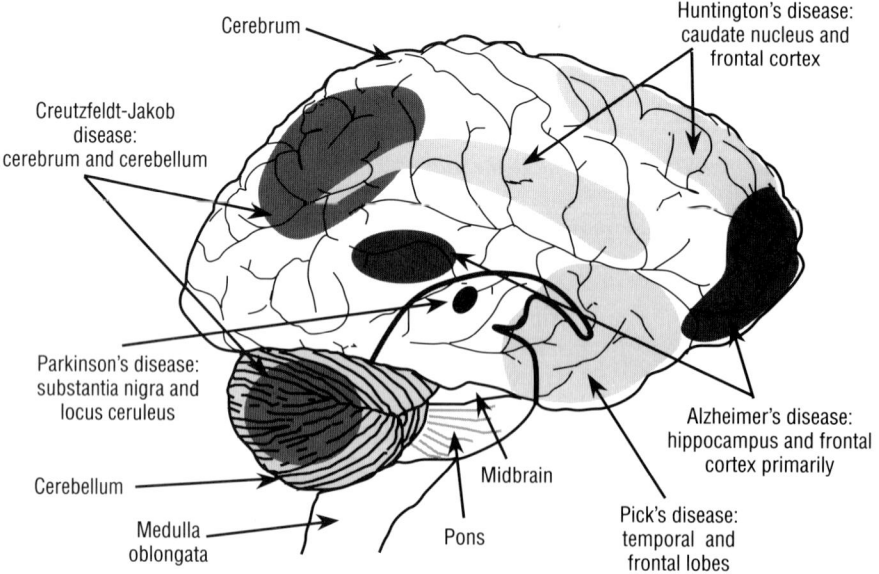

Figure 13.16 *The sites of degeneration of nervous tissue in various types of dementia*

the disease that we can, with certainty, outline the mechanism of the pathogenesis of the disorder.

Pathological Findings

Alzheimer's disease (AD)

This is the commonest cause of dementia in the elderly and it is attracting considerable interest in terms of research into causes, pathobiology, diagnosis and treatment. However, it is unfortunate that it is a disease we still know relatively little about. Although we may diagnose the condition with some accuracy and describe in detail the pathological findings of the disease when examining the brains of the patients at autopsy, we still do not have effective means of prevention and treatment of the disorder.

AD is a term which was initially used to describe the dementing disorder seen in people before the age of 60 years ('pre-senile dementia'). It then became associated with an indistinguishable disorder occurring in older people, known as senile dementia of the Alzheimer type (SDAT). In both disorders the pathological findings are identical and are often described as a grossly exaggerated form of the normal ageing process which is seen in the brain. The term 'Alzheimer's disease' now tends to be used generically for all disorders showing a similar pattern of pathological changes irrespective of the age of the patient.

The macroscopic changes that are apparent in the brain in AD are a marked atrophy of the cortical tissue. As much as 200 to 300 g of the brain substance may be lost over a period of 3 to 8 years. The loss is symmetrical and mainly involves the cortex of the frontal lobes and hippocampus. The temporal and parietal lobes are also involved rather frequently. Microscopically the brain shows loss of neurones and reactive gliosis as well as a characteristic triad of changes that are diagnostic of the condition when taken into consideration alongside macroscopic changes and clinical presentation (refer to Figure 13.17). These are:

1. **The senile or neuritic plaque**: This is a focal area, a few hundred microns in diameter, and is seen in vast numbers in the cortical grey matter. The plaque is composed of a centre of amyloid-like material (β-pleated fibrillar proteins) and surrounding this there are argyrophilic granules and filaments. The larger the number of plaques present in a brain, the more severe the form of the demen-

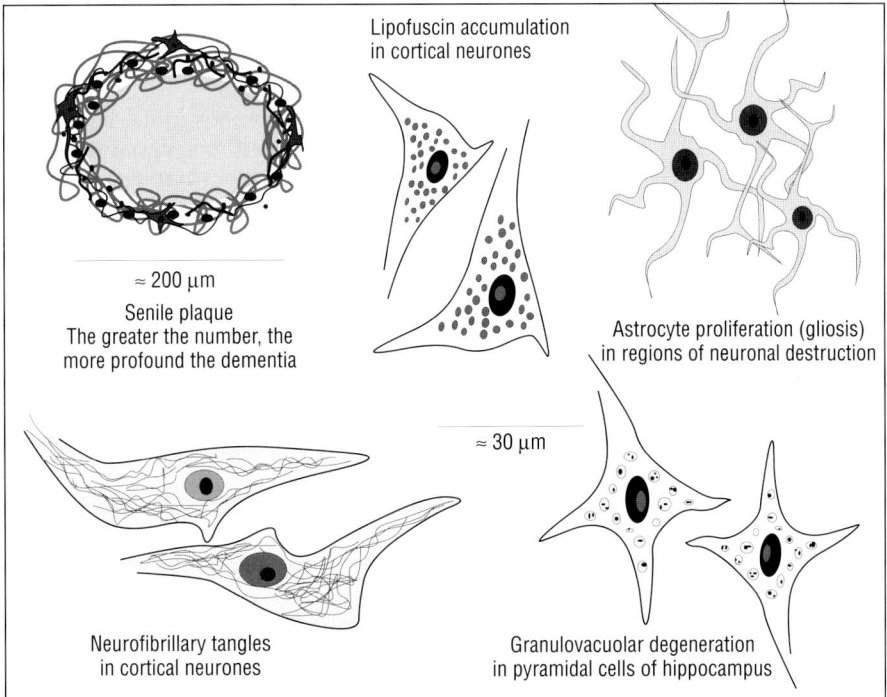

Figure 13.17 *The cerebral lesions characteristic of Alzheimer's disease*

tia. Amyloid material is also found in the arteries of the subarachnoid space and grey matter of the affected brains, but not the white matter. This change in the vessels is termed congophilic angiopathy.

2. **Neurofibrillary tangles**: These represent tangled masses of neurofibrils in many of the large neurones of the cortex. They are coarse, thick (10 nm) filaments twisted about in pairs in a helical fashion and occur within the cytoplasm of affected neurones.

3. **Granulovacuolar degeneration**: This change is confined mainly to the pyramidal cells of the hippocampus. Each cell showing such changes has multiple vacuoles in its cytoplasm, each vacuole containing one or more dense granules. Such cells do not often contain neurofibrillary tangles.

Several biochemical lesions have been identified in AD, most of these being reductions in specific nerve cell components, the most important one being a relatively severe loss in choline-acetyl transferase and acetylcholinetransferase, which implies a selective loss or dysfunction of the cholinergic neurones. Of the other decreased compounds, somatostatin has been shown to be important.

Many theories have been proposed for the aetiology and pathogenesis of AD, the major three being aluminium toxicity, the autoimmune theory and slow virus theory. It is known that aluminium is neurotoxic and experimental models suggest that aluminium toxicity may cause the formation of neurofibrillary changes in the brain. However, not all features of AD are seen in the experimental systems utilizing aluminium to induce these brain changes. In addition, the serum aluminium levels in patients with AD are normal and there is no history of environmental or occupational exposure to aluminium.

The autoimmune theory is based on the presence of brain-reactive antibodies in patients with AD, and also on the presence of amyloid material in the centre of the senile plaques. It is hypothesized that antigen–antibody complexes forming in the brain are broken down by phagocytes, leading to the deposition of antibody fragments as amyloid. The autoimmune reactions involving nervous tissue would be the cause of the neuronal loss.

The slow virus theory is a popular theory and implicates a group of viruses that have a long incubation period (2 to 30 years), therefore making transmission of the agents difficult to prove. It is known that cases of other proven viral encephalopathies (e.g. Creutzfeldt-Jakob disease) are characterized by changes that re-

semble the senile plaques of AD.

Other theories combine these three theories and postulate, for example, that a viral infection may trigger off an autoimmune or allergic reaction, which leads to the neuronal cell loss and formation of the senile plaques.

It should be kept in mind that a small number of cases of AD occur in a familial setting and also many patients with Down's syndrome develop changes that are characteristic of AD. The amyloid protein precursor found in the core of neuritic plaques is the β-amyloid precursor protein, which is a product of a gene found on chromosome 21. This is the chromosome involved in the genetic anomalies associated with Down's syndrome and also those cases of familial AD that have been observed. This genetic association of AD is currently being looked at with interest, although the exact pathogenetic mechanism remains obscure.

Pick's Disease of the Brain (PD)

This is much less common in incidence than AD. It is classified as a pre-senile dementia, slightly more common in women, which is caused by a destruction of neurones in the cortex of the frontal and temporal lobes with subsequent reactive gliosis in these regions. Symptoms of PD appear in mid-adulthood and progress over a period of 3 to 5 years, leading relentlessly to a typical presentation of dementia, clinically indistinguishable from AD.

Surviving neurones in the brains of these patients show a 'ballooned' cytoplasm which may contain intensely argyrophilic granules termed **Pick bodies**. These bodies are composed of dense aggregates of neurofibrils and are characteristic of PD (see Figure 13.18).

This disorder is an example of a typical idiopathic disease. Some cases show clustering in families but the case distributions do not conform to a hereditary pattern.

Multi-infarct Dementia

This form of dementia usually has a rapid and stepwise course and is the commonest of the secondary dementing disorders. In this type of dementia the typical patient is generally over 60 years of age, is hypertensive, has atherosclerosis in many arteries throughout the body and may be diabetic. In particular, the carotid and cerebral arteries are severely atheromatous, leading to many episodes of thrombosis, embolism and vascular occlusion, which precipitate ischaemia and

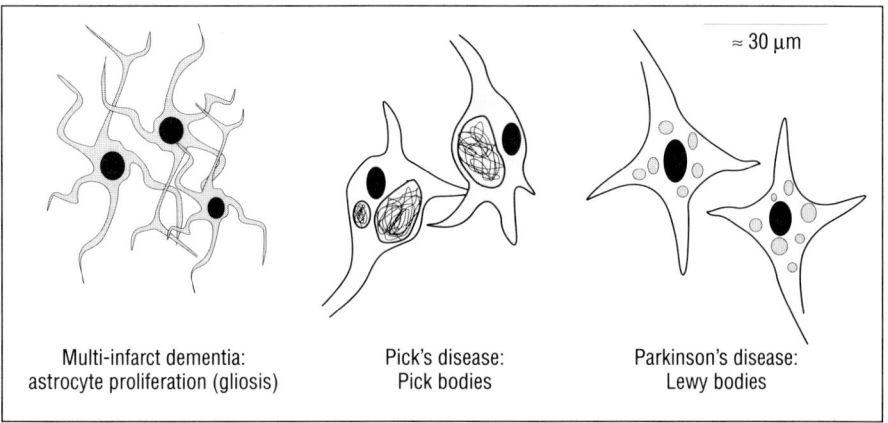

≈ 30 μm

Multi-infarct dementia:
astrocyte proliferation (gliosis)

Pick's disease:
Pick bodies

Parkinson's disease:
Lewy bodies

Figure 13.18 *Microscopic features of dementias other than Alzheimer's disease*

infarction, resulting in the loss of considerable quantities of cerebral substance. It appears that the development of the dementia does not correlate with the involvement of any one particular area of the brain but rather it is the quantity of brain substance that is lost that is of considerable importance. Overall, approximately 100 mL or more of brain substance must be lost in order for a dementing disorder to develop.

On examining these patients' brains at autopsy it is found that there are multiple small regions of infarction in both hemispheres, usually in the cortical area. The grey matter in these regions is collapsed and surrounded by regions of gliosis (see Figure 13.18). Cystic spaces may be seen, especially in the case of larger infarcts. The ventricles are usually enlarged symmetrically if both hemispheres show infarcts, or asymmetrically if any one hemisphere shows evidence of being affected by more infarcts.

In the case of cerebral infarction it often becomes necessary to distinguish the resulting clinical states that are caused by a true 'chronic brain failure' or dementia from what is often only an acute brain failure which is seen in the immediate post-infarction period. This acute brain failure is often the result of a variety of causes, quite commonly due to confusion, depression, disorientation, anger and other psychological factors associated with the patient's own ability in coping with 'taking the stroke'.

Parkinson's Disease (Paralysis Agitans, PA)

PA is an idiopathic, progressive, degenerative disorder of the brain which is incurable. The disease is quite prevalent in the elderly, 0.25% of people aged between 60 and 69 years being affected, the incidence rising to 2% of people over 80 years. With increasing years, PA becomes more severe. It is more commonly seen in males and very frequently is associated with other disorders of the ageing brain. Early PA has the following features:

- bradykinesia and rigidity;
- resting tremors, worse on stress, ceasing in sleep;
- impaired posture control.

Later in the course of the disease the patients show:

- a shuffling, hurrying (festinant) gait with frequent falls;
- weight loss, heartburn, dysphagia, constipation;
- dysphonia, drooling, dysarthria;
- mental depression, intellectual failure;
- muscle weakness and pain;
- micrographia.

Macroscopically there is loss of pigment in the substantia nigra and locus ceruleus of the brainstem, this tending to be more marked in severe cases. Microscopically such a change is seen to correspond with a degeneration of the pigmented neurones in these areas. As the neurones degenerate they release melanin pigment, which is found in macrophages and free within the brain parenchyma. The surviving nerve cells are atrophic and contain large intracytoplasmic inclusions which stain brightly with eosin and are known as **Lewy bodies** (see Figure 13.18).

The clinical symptomatology that is seen in PA is characteristic of loss of neurones in the extrapyramidal area and reflects a loss in the ability of the neurones to transmit and receive information through the secretion of dopamine. Substitution therapy in these patients with L-dopa in the early stages of the disease sometimes leads to quite spectacular remissions, with control of the symptoms. However, the neuronal loss continues and as more and more neurones become non-functional, the therapy becomes ineffective.

The diagnosis of PA in the elderly is often very difficult as the disorder may be associated with other diseases, notably mental depression, dementia and heart disease. Benign tremor may also be attributed to pathological states other than PA, for example depression, arthritis or hypothyroidism. It should be noted that PA may in some cases be drug induced as in the case of elderly patients who have been prescribed phenothiazines, butyrophenones and other anti-psychotics.

Huntington's Disease (Chorea)

This is a Mendelian genetic disorder which is inherited as an autosomal dominant trait. The defective gene is located on the short arm of chromosome 4. An important feature is that this defective gene remains clinically dormant until patients are in their fourth to fifth decade. The abnormal gene, when it is expressed, alters the metabolism of specific neurones in the extrapyramidal system, the caudate nuclei and the putamen being particularly affected. The neurones in these regions become progressively dysfunctional, atrophic and eventually, die becoming replaced by moderate amounts of glial tissue. The frontal cortex also shows some depletion of neurones, but this is a less marked loss. Biochemically, the disease is characterized by depletion of gamma-aminobutyric acid (GABA) levels and also a decreased level of glutamic acid decarboxylase in the brain. Increases in the iron levels are also seen.

The initial symptoms and signs of the disorder are athetoid movements which develop gradually. These movements are often described as choreiform ('dance-like') and occur bilaterally and symmetrically. As the disease progresses there is mental deterioration, eventually the patient becoming demented with loss of cognitive functions, often accompanied by paranoia and delusions. Death usually occurs approximately a decade after the onset of symptoms.

Creutzfeldt-Jakob Disease (CJD)

CJD is one of the slow virus infections of the brain, also called subacute spongiform encephalopathy. The specific virus associated with the disorder has not been conclusively identified but the infection may be transmitted from humans to primates by cell-free extracts from the brains of patients with the disease. The characteristics of CJD are the formation of small aggregates of microcysts in affected regions of the brain, mainly the cortical grey matter but also the basal ganglia, hypothalamus and cerebellum. As the neurones disappear from the affected areas, microcyst development and gliosis becomes more marked.

The predominant feature of CJD is a progressive dementia which is distinguishable clinically from AD as this disorder also involves the cerebellum, and is characterized by ataxia. Ataxia is not found in AD.

Diagnosis

The diagnosis of dementia is often quite difficult, especially in the elderly patient where multiple pathological states affecting the central nervous system may be present and will produce a variety of clinical symptomatologies. Thus, in the elderly patient a widely divergent and complex collection of factors will complicate the presentation of dementia and hinder its definitive diagnosis. Patients who have hearing impairments, who are depressed or drugged, or who suffer from acute brain failure may be misdiagnosed as being demented. A broad awareness of all related conditions is essential and often dementia may only be established as a final diagnosis through the process of elimination in a list of differential diagnoses.

Typically, the diagnosis of dementia depends on considering several important criteria, factors and procedures which are outlined below.

Physical examination. A complete physical examination is required and may disclose features attributable to other pathologies indicative of acute brain failure rather than dementia.

Listening to the patient. The patient may volunteer some important information which is often of diagnostic value. Memory loss, for example, is something that the patient admits to and this will often cause (or be the result of!) depression. Even dementing patients may show some remarkable insight into their condition and anything that the patient volunteers about their condition should be listened to carefully.

History evaluation. The previous medical history of the patient may furnish important details regarding the health status of the patient, which may be important as seen in the context of making a diagnostic decision (e.g. history of CVA, drugs being taken, Parkinsonism, etc.).

History taking. Questioning of relatives, friends and neighbours is invaluable in establishing the time course, extent and basic nature of the changes that were apparent to these people in the course of the patient's condition. This information provided by relatives in particular must be interpreted very critically as it may often be coloured by emotion or prejudice.

Critical evaluation of data collected. It should be remembered that certain features that may point towards a diagnosis of dementia or are most commonly seen with dementia may very frequently be also seen independently of it. For example, eccentricity of behaviour, a bizarre lifestyle and self-neglect are not always seen in connection with intellectual impairment. The **Diogenes syndrome** is a term applied to a variety of conditions in which an elderly patient is seen to live in squalor with an apparent lack of concern. Causative and contributory factors in its development that are independent of dementia are bereavement and isolation, poverty, alcohol and drug abuse, depression, disability, psychiatric disorders and so on.

Mental test scores. A mental test score should be given to the patient but not necessarily as soon as the patient is admitted as there may be considerable distress and confusion at the time of admission. Mental test score cards are easily constructed and a typical example is shown in Figure 13.19.

Other procedures. In certain circumstances other special procedures will be carried out and may be of considerable importance in either confirming or negating clinical findings. For example, computed tomography of the head (CT scans) may be performed, especially in the case of those patients with suspected pre-senile dementia. Tomography may also be used in the case of elderly patients where headaches and other physical symptoms relating to the head are the presenting features, where multi-infarct dementia is suspected and where the dementia appears to have developed acutely with a very rapid course. Occasionally, biopsy specimens of the brain are available for one reason or another and characteristic pathological findings in the brain substance are an important diagnostic feature. Finally, post-mortem examination may be the only certain way of diagnosing the cause of a dementia.

Treatment

Acute brain failure and pseudodementia states are often fully treatable and the patient may recover full lucidity after prompt treatment is instituted. Specific treatments for the chronic brain failure of dementia as typified by AD are unfortunately lacking and they still remain the geriatrician's hope. No wonder drugs are known, but some encouraging results have been reported in treatments with systemic cholinergic agents such as centrally acting anticholinesterases, in the case of AD.

In most cases of dementia, treatments centre around support and relief of the patients and their family. Often symptomatic relief may be necessary to control constipation, insomnia, agitation, hallucinations, etc. Counselling of the patients' family and friends is an important part of the support needed. Accurate information about the disease state and what may be expected to develop in the patient with the passage of time must be provided for the relatives and friends of the patient who has been diagnosed with any of the dementing disorders.

Patient's name: _____	
Patient's DOB and age: _____	
Date of test: _____	

Questions	Score (1 or 0)*
(1) What is your name?	
(2) What is (was) your occupation?	
(3) Are you married?	
(4) What is your address?	
(5) What is the date today? (day, month and year)	
(6) Where are you now? (If patient does not know, tell them) and ask again at the end of the test)	
(7) Ask patient to remember this address: 58 Arthurton Rd (Ask patient to repeat it to you immediately and to repeat it to you at the end of the test)	
(8) Who is the prime minister of Australia?	
(9) What is the name of the Queen of England?	
(10) Where is Darwin?	
(11) What disaster happened in Darwin in 1974?	
(12) Date of World War II (years)	
(13) Who was prime minister of Australia at the beginning of the war?	
(14) Who won the war?	

SCORE:

_____

(Score of 8 or less: Poor
12 of more: Good)

Other questions may be added or substituted: e.g. (1) Complete the proverbs:
A bird in the hand is.......
A stitch in time............
(2) Serial sevens:
Ask the patient to start from 100 and to then
subtract 7s serially (i.e. 100, 93, 86, 79...)

* (Note, one mark per question, no half marks allowed)

Figure 13.19   *An example of a typical mental test score card*

Revision Questions and Case Studies

1. Discuss the pathology of hydrocephalus, concentrating in particular on a common cause of this condition in an adult patient. Include in your discussion the various sequelae that may be seen in such a patient.
2. What is a 'berry' aneurysm? Why and where does it arise? What are its complications?
3. Brain haemorrhages are a common pathological condition. Discuss how such haemorrhages may arise and what their sequelae are.
4. Define the following terms:
   (a) Cerebrovascular accident (CVA)
   (b) Apoplectic cyst
   (c) Colliquative necrosis
   (d) Haematoma
5. Discuss the pathology of cerebral infarction with special reference to incidence, aetiology, morphology and sequelae.
6. What are the characteristics of multiple sclerosis?
7. Compare and contrast any two degenerative diseases of the cerebral cortex.
8. Discuss the pathology of Alzheimer's disease.
9. Define the following terms:
   (a) Dementia
   (b) Neurofibrillary tangles
   (c) Senile plaque
   (d) Argyrophilic body
10. Discuss the pathology of any two primary intracranial tumours.
11. What are the characteristics of astrocytomata?
12. Discuss the pathology of meningioma.
13. Write short notes on:
   (a) Wallerian degeneration
   (b) Polyneuritis
   (c) Neurofibromatosis
   (d) Segmental degeneration of nerves
14. Correlate the cardiovascular and central nervous system lesions that you would expect to find at autopsy in a 67-year-old male who had been a heavy smoker for most of his life and hypertensive for the last 10 years of his life.
15. What is an aneurysm? Discuss aneurysm formation in the cerebral vessels and indicate possible sequelae of these lesions.
16. Write short notes on all of the following:
   (a) Arnold-Chiari malformation
   (b) Arteriovenous malformation
   (c) Parkinson's disease
17. Discuss the pathology of tertiary syphilis in the central nervous system.

18. What are the characteristics of Huntington's chorea?

Case study 1. A 29-year-old Caucasian female patient presented with a history of a relapsing/remitting weakness of her lower limbs over a few months, 3 years ago. As the symptoms disappeared for a period of another few months, the patient did not seek medical advice. Over the last 2 months the symptoms returned and there were also bouts of facial pain and paraesthesiae affecting the limbs. The patient was admitted to hospital as she was developing diplopia, vertigo and ataxia. Treatment was initiated and the patient was discharged after a marginal improvement. She presented again 2 months later with depression, severe weakness and disability, frequency of micturition and tingling sensations down her back. The patient was readmitted to hospital for observation but over the next 3 months there was progressive, rapid deterioration with incontinence, impaired motor function and intercurrent infections, leading to her death.

(a) What is the diagnosis?
(b) Describe the characteristic lesions of this disease in the CNS.
(c) What is known about the aetiology of the disorder?

Case study 2. A 44-year-old Caucasian male patient had a history of headaches, temporary clouding of consciousness and less well defined 'changes in personality' over the past 5 months. In the last few weeks, the patient was said to be 'very flippant and morbidly facetious' with loss of appreciation of the consequences of his actions. His wife collected him from the police station one morning after the patient was arrested the previous night for urinating in public in a City hotel. He was admitted to hospital and over the last week deteriorated rapidly, finally hurling himself to his death from a fourth floor window.

(a) Given that the patient is suffering from a neoplastic disease, what is the most probable type of tumour that he had?
(b) Which region of the brain was involved?
(c) What is the behaviour of these tumours and what is the prognosis for patients presenting with them?

Case study 3. A 55-year-old Caucasian male patient presented with a history of episodic headaches and spatial disorientation. The patient also showed signs of apraxia, agnosia and receptive dysphasia. A 2.2 cm diameter rounded lesion was recovered attached to the meningeal membrane of the patient at surgery. The lesion was impinging on the brain substance. On cut section, the pale mass was found to consist of tightly coiled and whorled fibrous-like elements.

(a) Given that the patient is suffering from a neoplastic disease, what is the type of tumour that he had?
(b) Which region of the brain was involved?
(c) What is the behaviour of these tumours and what is the prognosis for patients presenting with them?

The following case studies present four typical elderly patients who may appear at first glance to all have features of dementia and may be used as illustrations of the importance of differential diagnosis. Notes should be made as to the possible cause of observed signs and symptoms and an interpretation of any laboratory or diagnostic test results should be attempted. The nature and aetiology of the patient's state should then be diagnosed in the context of the cases studies.

Case study 4. Mrs R. Gray, a 70-year-old Caucasian, was admitted to hospital at her doctor's request. He had been called to Mrs Gray's home, where she lives alone, by a concerned neighbour who had gone to visit her and who after repeated knocking at Mrs Gray's door had failed to get a response. After the door was opened by the caretaker, Mrs Gray was found in bed, rather disorientated, and she failed to recognize her neighbour. The patient has been living alone for the past 5 years and had last been seen about 5 days before her admission taking a walk. The doctor who examined her at home found her confused, with a clouding of consciousness and agitation. Two empty gin bottles were found in the kitchen.

After admission to hospital, the findings of disorientation, agitation and impaired consciousness were confirmed as they were still present. The patient's rectal temperature was 37.7°C, the peripheries cold and clammy. She was found to be cyanosed and her respiratory rate was 40 breaths a minute. The cardiac rhythm was atrial fibrillation at an apical rate of 118 beats a minute and a pulse deficit of 30 beats a minute. It was observed that there was pitting oedema in the ankles and sacrum. Chest expansion was diminished at the right base where the percussion note was dull and tactile vocal fremitus was increased. Examination of the central nervous system was limited by the patient's mental state. Blood cultures taken on three occasions grew Gram-positive, coagulase-positive cocci. There was a peripheral blood leukocytosis.

Case study 5. Mrs G. Collins, a 78-year-old Caucasian, was found wandering on the roadside verge of a highway near her cottage. She was unable to give her address to a motorist who stopped to assist her and when she was taken to a local police station she gave

incorrect personal details confusing dates of World War I with her birthdate, giving her age as 40 years and when asked for the names of her relatives she became tearful and asked to be taken home to her daughter. When Mrs Collins' daughter came to the police station to report her mother missing, Mrs Collins recognized her and the two women left together, the elderly woman appearing greatly relieved and pleased. This and other episodes occurred before the daughter was prompted to seek referral from the family doctor to a geriatric department in a nearby hospital. When questioned, the daughter said that she had noticed in the previous months that her mother was 'behaving oddly' at times but that she had attributed that to her 'mother's increasing years and idiosyncrasies of old age'. Examination of Mrs Collins showed her to be a frail, thin woman who showed some evidence of taking inadequate personal care. She gave her personal details correctly but repeated the year of her birth when asked for the dates of World War I. Serial sevens and retention of new information were poorly performed. At this point, Mrs Collins became greatly agitated, tearful and rather distressed, asking to go home.

Physical examination showed a slow atrial fibrillation but no other abnormalities. On asking the daughter whether her mother was on any medication, it was elicited that although the family doctor had prescribed a benzodiazepine hypnotic 5 months earlier, Mrs Collins had not taken it.

Case study 6. Mr G. Jones is a 70-year-old Caucasian who has recently suffered from a stroke, leaving him with a weakness in his right arm. He has returned from hospital to his home, where he lives with his wife, but during the past 2 weeks he has been very quiet, and when he talks he often has difficulty speaking, slurring his words and 'not making sense', according to his wife. Frequently he will attempt to get up from his chair, but when asked whether he wants anything, he does not appear to understand and ignores the questions that are put to him. When a district nurse comes to look in on how the old couple are coping, she finds their flat squalid and the wife of the patient distressed as she is having considerable difficulty looking after herself and her husband. Mr Jones appears withdrawn, not interested in his surroundings and not making any attempt to communicate. The nurse reassures the couple that she will get the doctor to visit them and suggests that the woman seeks assistance from a home help community group.

The very next day Mr Jones was found on the floor by his wife when she returned home from her shopping. He was confused and unable to move his right arm or leg. When he was admitted to hospital he was disorientated. The cranial nerves were normal other than bilateral, senile macular degeneration on fundoscopy. There was flaccid paralysis of the right arm and leg, but power and tone on the left side were normal.

The trachea was deviated to the left and air entry was reduced on the left side (he had suffered from TB in his youth). Apex rate was 85 per minute, the rhythm atrial fibrillation. Blood pressure was 168/95 mmHg supine. No pulses were palpated in the feet. Electrocardiography confirmed the atrial fibrillation. Within 24 hours, the right-sided weakness was still present but the patient remained disorientated and agitated.

Case study 7. A 62-year-old man presented 4 months ago with bradykinesia and rigidity. It was noticed on examination at a community health centre that he had a shuffling gait and impaired posture control. The patient is single and lives alone in a flat. Shortly after the examination he sustained a fracture of the tibia and fibula in the left leg. The patient was admitted to hospital and in the following months he developed a resting tremor, particularly in his arms and hands, he lost considerable weight, became depressed and increasingly dysphonic with drooling and dysphagia. There were times when the patient seemed confused. Muscle weakness and pain were also in evidence and the patient had considerable difficulties in writing.

Further Reading

Adams JH. 'Editorial: Cerebral Infarction — Its Pathogenesis and Interpretation.' *J Path* 1989; **157**: 281.

Agid Y. 'Parkinson's Disease: Pathophysiology.' *Lancet* 1991; **337**: 1321.

Chataway SJ. 'What's New in the Pathogenesis of Multiple Sclerosis? A Review.' *J Roy Soc Med* 1989; **82**: 159.

Colditz GA, *et al.* 'Cigarette Smoking and Risk of Stroke in Middle-Aged Women.' *N Eng J Med* 1988; **318**: 937.

Fishman RA. 'Brain Edema.' *N Eng J Med.* 1975; **293**: 706.

Gresham GE, *et al.* 'Residual Disability in Survivors of Stroke — The Framingham Study.' *N Eng J Med* 1975; **293**: 954.

Grotta JC. 'Current Medical and Surgical Therapy for Cerebrovascular Disease.' *N Eng J Med* 1987; **317**: 1505.

Joachim CL, *et al.* 'Clinically Diagnosed Alzheimer's Disease: Autopsy Results in 150 Cases.' *Ann Neurol* 1988; **24**: 50.

Katzman R. 'Alzheimer's Disease.' *N Eng J Med* 1986; **314**: 964.

Kawachi I, Pearce N. 'Aluminium in the Drinking Water — Is it Safe?' *Aust J Publ Health* 1991; **15**: 84.

Lees GJ. 'Common Threads in Neurodegenerative Disorders.' *Today's Life Sci* 1992; **4**(3): 24.

Main DM, Mennuti MT. 'Neural Tube Defects: Issues in Prenatal Diagnosis and Counselling.' *Obstet Gynecol* 1986; **67**: 1.

McFarlin DE. 'Treatment of Multiple Sclerosis.' N *Eng J Med* 1983; **308**: 215.

McFarlin DE, McFarland HF. 'Multiple Sclerosis (Parts 1 & 2).' *N Eng J Med* 1982; **307**: 1183; 1246.

Mendelsohn FAO. 'Brain Receptor Autoradiography: New Roles for Angiotensinogen.' *Today's Life Sci* 1990: **4**(4): 32.

Mozar HN, Bal Dg, Howard JT. 'Perspectives on the Aetiology of Alzheimer's Disease.' *JAMA* 1987; **257**: 1503.

Paul KS, *et al.* 'Arnold-Chiari Malformation: A Review of 71 Cases.' *J Neurosurg* 1983; **58**: 183.

Pearce JMS. 'Migraine: A Cerebral Disorder.' *Lancet* 1984; **2**: 86.

Portenoy RK, Lipton RB, Foley KM. 'Back Pain in the Cancer Patient: An Algorithm for Evaluation and Management.' *Neurology* 1987; **37**: 134.

Rumble BA, Beyreuther K, Masters CL. 'The Molecular Pathology of Alzheimer's Disease.' *Today's Life Sci* 1991: **3**(4): 24.

Sedgwick J. 'Immune Responses in the Central Nervous System.' *Today's Life Sci* 1992: **4**(7): 34.

Selcoe DJ. 'Amyloid Protein and Alzheimer's Disease' *Sci Am* 1991; November: 40.

Turner RD, Firgaira FA. 'Dicing with Dilemmas: Predictive Testing for Huntington Disease.' *Today's Life Sci* 1990: **2**(11): 4.

Walker AE, Robins M, Weinfeld FD. 'Epidemiology of Brain Tumors: The National Survey of Intracranial Neoplasms.' *Neurology* 1985; **35**: 219.

Wells CE (ed.). *Dementia. Contemporary Neurology Series*, second edition 1977; FA Davis Co, Philadelphia.

Zivin JA, Choi DW. 'Stroke Therapy.' *Sci Am* 1991; July: 56.

14

Muscular System Disorders

The Normal Muscular System

Striated muscle is the 'flesh' of the body and comprises the skeletal muscles and the cardiac muscles. Both of these tissues have cells showing prominent striations of the contractile elements in their cytoplasm. **Skeletal muscle** is the major part of the striated muscle group of tissues and like all other muscular tissues possesses the properties of conductivity and contractility. The movement of the body as a whole or of any of its parts is effected by the active contraction of a muscle or a group of muscles. Skeletal muscle is unique in that its action is able to be controlled by the will (unlike cardiac muscle and smooth muscle).

Each major body muscle is composed of many fascicles of myocytes, surrounded by connective tissue. Muscles differ widely in size, from the very substantial gastrocnemius that forms the major part of the calf of the leg to the stapedius, the tiny muscle of the middle ear whose length is only 2 to 3 mm. **Myocytes** are long thin cells 40 to 50 μm in diameter and up to 30 cm in length. They are syncytia containing many peripheral nuclei which are arranged around the cell membrane (this consisting largely of the myofibrils, actin and myosin filaments). The cytoplasm of myocytes is termed the **sarcoplasm** and the myocyte cell membrane is termed the **sarcolemma**. A myocyte is also called a muscle fibre because of its long and thread-like shape. Myocytes are surrounded by a thin connective tissue sheath, termed the endomysium. Between the muscle fibres are the **satellite cells**, which are relatively undifferentiated connective tissue cells. Groups of muscle fibres are aggregated into a fascicle and this is surrounded by the perimysium. The whole of the functional muscle is surrounded by the epimysium, which blends with the deep fascia. Lymphatics in muscles occur in the epimysium and perimysium.

The appreciation of the stretch in a muscle is mediated through the activity of the **muscle spindle**, a specialized neuromuscular aggregate found in muscles of posture predominantly. The motor activity of striated muscle is through the **motor end-plate**, a specialized termination of the motor neurone axon that ends in muscle. Each motor neurone axon that supplies a muscle repeatedly branches within that muscle and then each terminal twig from the axon supplies a muscle fibre, as many as 160 muscle fibres being supplied by a motor neurone. The nerve end-plate is a flattened structure that has lost its myelin sheath and closely approximates the sarcolemma, which is greatly folded. There is a minute gap between motor neurone end-plate and muscle cell. The nerve cell depolarization travelling down the axon causes the release of acetylcholine from storage vesicles inside the nerve terminal into the synaptic gap between nerve and muscle cells. The acetylcholine diffuses through to the muscle and changes the permeability of the sarcolemma to calcium ions, and thus the muscle cell contracts. Motor neurones exert a trophic action on muscles.

Tendons are white, fibrous cords of tissue, very often flattened and not at all elastic, although very strong and composed mainly of white collagenous fibrous tissue. They are supplied sparingly with blood vessels and within the larger tendons nerves are present (e.g. Achilles tendon). **Aponeuroses** are thinner than tendons and are ribbon-like in structure; they do not contain nerves and have only very few, small blood vessels. The tendons and aponeuroses are connected with the muscles on one side and movable structures such as bones, cartilages, ligaments or fibrous membranes on the other side. The **fasciae** are fibroareolar layers that invest softer and more delicate organs. They are subdivided into: the **superficial fascia**, immediately beneath the skin, investing the whole body and containing adipose tissue in varying quantities, and; the **deep fascia**, which is a dense, inelastic fibrous membrane that encloses and sheathes the muscles, forming intermuscular septa and investing major groups of nerves and vessels.

Disorders of cardiac muscle have been considered already. Skeletal muscle disorders are not very common in incidence and serious skeletal muscle disorders are most commonly of a congenital or of an autoimmune nature. The diagnosis of skeletal muscle diseases very frequently involves taking a muscle biopsy and examining the tissue under light and electron microscopy. The biopsy should be large enough to include blood vessels and nerves, transverse and longitudinal sections being examined. Usually, the quadriceps femoris or biceps brachii are biopsied and these muscles will indicate changes associated with most neuromuscular diseases. However, occasionally other muscles may need to be sampled as may occur with a disease which affects a specific group of muscles.

Necrotic and Degenerative Diseases

Ischaemia and Necrosis of Skeletal Muscle

Skeletal muscle has an extensive collateral circulation and infarction of this tissue is rare. However, extensive atherosclerosis of nutrient arteries will produce atrophy of the muscle with resultant dysfunction, including excessive fatiguability and weakness of the affected muscles. Ischaemic gangrene may develop in muscles in association with very severe atherosclerosis. Systemic or metabolic diseases such as diabetes mellitus predispose to it.

In normal muscles, ischaemic necrosis occurs in **Volkmann's ischaemic contracture** seen after elbow trauma (most often after a fracture around the elbow joint) and in this condition there is interference with the venous drainage from the muscles of the forearm, leading to necrosis and subsequent fibrosis. Multiple intramuscular thromboses such as those seen in polyarteritis nodosa may lead to necrosis and healing by fibrosis in muscle. Unaccustomed strenuous exercise may cause necrosis of the anterior tibial groups of muscles especially. In this last case it is the oedema associated with the hyperaemia induced by exercise which causes a great increase in pressure within the anterior tibial compartment of the lower leg which, in turn, causes the ischaemia and necrosis.

In all cases mentioned above, coagulative necrosis is seen followed by fibrosis. The laying down of collagenous scar tissue will often lead to a contracture developing and there may be serious compromise in the movement of the affected body part. Occasionally, patchy regeneration within the affected muscle may be observed (see below).

Zenker's Degeneration ('Toxic Necrosis')

This is a degenerative or necrotic change which develops in skeletal muscles when severe toxaemias, viral or bacterial infections are present. It is seen with typhoid fever, which affects the anterior abdominal muscles especially. In influenza epidemics, cases of Zenker's degeneration may be seen in the calf muscles of children, usually less than 10 years old. The disorder may also be seen in severe cases of pneumonia and diphtheria. The degeneration in muscle is a form of coagulative necrosis in which the coagulation of proteins has progressed to a lesser extent than is usual. The term 'hyaline degeneration' is often used to describe the appearance of the cells. The affected fibres look waxy and have a pale, eosinophilic hyaline ('glassy') appearance histologically. There is very little reaction to the necrosis with only mild inflammation. Blood vessels in the muscle are normal.

Rhabdomyolysis

Rhabdomyolysis is a diffuse lytic destruction of skeletal muscle fibres and may have many causes, most of them associated with obscure pathogenetic mechanisms. Some cases are associated with viral infections and may represent autoimmune or hypersensitivity manifestations (e.g. influenzal rhabdomyolysis). Other types may be due to unknown enzymatic or metabolic defects associated with the myocyte. It is believed that rhabdomyolysis which is seen even after relatively mild exercise may be an example of such a pathogenesis. With great exertion and strenuous exercise, rhabdomyolysis may be seen and this is thought to be associated with the toxic effects of metabolites accumulating in muscles, but also may be associated with the increased production of heat and dehydration that is seen in the exercising muscles. Heat stroke and malignant hyperthermia will stimulate a similar type of rhabdomyolysis. In some cases, alcohol intake or administration of anaesthetics such as halothane will trigger off an episode of rhabdomyolysis.

In an acute episode of rhabdomyolysis there is release of large quantities of sarcoplasmic contents into the circulation, with a resultant massive myoglobinaemia and myoglobinuria, the patient presenting with acute renal failure. The urine will be dark and the blood may be thickened to a molasses-like consistency. There may be lung, brain and liver damage. The muscles will be swollen and tender, the patient showing extreme weakness or collapse. Following acute episodes of the disorder, if the patient survives, the muscles may return to normal, presumably regeneration having occurred, or alternatively amputation of affected limbs will be needed, due to infection and gangrene supervening. Chronic rhabdomyolysis, for example that associated with alcohol intoxication, may lead to a milder disease with progressive destruction of muscle and a non-inflammatory myopathy developing. A few macrophages occur within the affected muscles and there may be only a little fibrosis.

Skeletal Muscle Regeneration

The capacity of myocytes to regenerate depends on the extent of damage within the muscle. If the basement membrane and the endomysium of the cells are destroyed there is no regeneration and the necrosis of the myocytes is followed by fibrosis. If, however, the basement membrane and endomysium are intact then there may be considerable regeneration. This latter case may occur after damage by a specific myotoxin which kills only the myocytes but leaves the connective tissue elements intact. In regeneration, the satellite stem cells around the myocytes proliferate and differentiate into mononuclear **myoblasts**. There is subsequent fusion of myoblasts to form syncytial myotubes. The nuclei migrate to the periphery of the cells and there is elongation and differentiation into an adult myocyte. This process is usually patchy and will not generally produce a fully functioning, perfectly normal muscle fibre.

Infections and Inflammations

Myositis

Inflammation in muscle, myositis, is encountered in a variety of clinical settings and there are many causative agents of muscle inflammation. Infection may be seen as a secondary involvement of muscle in the course of a systemic infection, or, less commonly, the muscle may be involved in the infective process primarily. Alternatively, many muscles around the body are inflamed in the course of non-infectious, autoimmune inflammatory conditions, generally specified by the term **polymyositis**.

Direct invasion by bacteria, viruses, fungi or parasites in the course of systemic infections may be seen in septicaemia or pyaemia which may result in multiple pyogenic abscesses scattered in muscles. Viral myositis is common in many viral infections, for example Coxsackievirus infection, and influenza. Influenzal infections may be quite severe with extensive necrosis, rhabdomyolysis and myoglobinuria. Tuberculosis may occasionally occur in muscle in the course of miliary disease or occasionally arise after the infection has spread to muscle from adjacent tissues, as occurs in Pott's disease of the spine with involvement of the psoas muscle and development of a 'cold abscess'.

A primary infection of muscle may also lead to myositis as is the case with necrosis and acute suppurative inflammation due to spread of infection from neighbouring (usually subcutaneous) tissues or due to wound infections. In **gas gangrene** there is a mixed infection with several species of *Clostridium*, which causes a rapidly spreading, necrotizing myositis. The bacteria produce gas from the breakdown of the tissue and this leads to a crackling sound (crepitus) from the festering, foul-smelling wound. Coxsackieviruses of the B group may produce pleurodynia (Bornholm disease), an infection of the muscles of the trunk and thorax. This is a very painful, acute illness with sudden onset of fever, pleuritic chest pain and abdominal pain with vomiting. The disease usually lasts 4 days and the affected muscles are very tender. Myocarditis is also very characteristically associated with Coxsackievirus infections of skeletal muscles. Parasitic infestations may also cause considerable damage and inflammation in muscle, especially *Trichinella spiralis* infestation, trichinosis. This is associated with the consumption of undercooked or raw infected meats, especially pork. The organism invades the muscle and the damage in the muscle is both mechanical as well as enzymatic as *Trichinella* is a tissue liquefier, secreting lytic enzymes that kill and lyse the myocytes.

Myositis due to infection may also occur if the infective organism is in a distant body site not within the muscle and in this case the damage to the muscle is due to circulating toxins or diffusion of toxins from adjacent sites. Mostly bacterial infections will cause toxaemias and muscle damage in this manner. For example, typhoid fever, pneumonia, diphtheria and botulism are involved with this type of muscle damage. The organisms in these cases are responsible for the secretion of a potent exotoxin that circulates around the body, causing damage in many body tissues, including muscle. Such involvement of muscle may be fatal, especially if the diaphragmatic muscle is involved, the result being asphyxia.

Myositis Ossificans

In its commonest form, **myositis ossificans circumscripta**, this is a condition in which muscle inflammation is followed by dystrophic calcification resulting in a hard area of calcium salts within the muscle. It is thought to result after fibroblasts undergo metaplasia to osteoblasts in these lesions. A frequent site in which it develops is the adductor insertion in the thigh, earning it the common name of 'rider's thigh'. It is also likely to develop if there has been haematoma formation in traumatized muscle near to bone. As the necrotic muscle is removed and fibrosis begins, osteogenic cells from adjacent periosteum migrate into the collagen, differentiate into chondroblasts and osteoblasts and begin to lay down cartilage and bone. Ossification of the lesion may be so perfect that within the normal bony tissue that develops at the site, a marrow space is present containing dividing bone marrow cells. The new bony mass thus formed in the muscle can be easily palpated or seen on X-rays. A much rarer disorder is **myositis ossificans progressiva** in which muscles, tendons and ligaments around the body ossify progressively. This disorder, occurring primarily in young males, is totally idiopathic.

Polymyositis–Dermatomyositis Complex

This is a group of disorders of largely uncertain cause where a chronic inflammatory myopathy with or without a skin rash is seen. If the skin is involved in the inflammation together with muscle tissue, the condition is termed a dermatomyositis (refer to Figure 14.1). If only muscles are involved in the inflammatory changes, the disorder is a polymyositis. Cardiac muscle is not involved in the inflammation but generally many of the skeletal muscles are. The disease may be subdivided into various clinical groups depending on

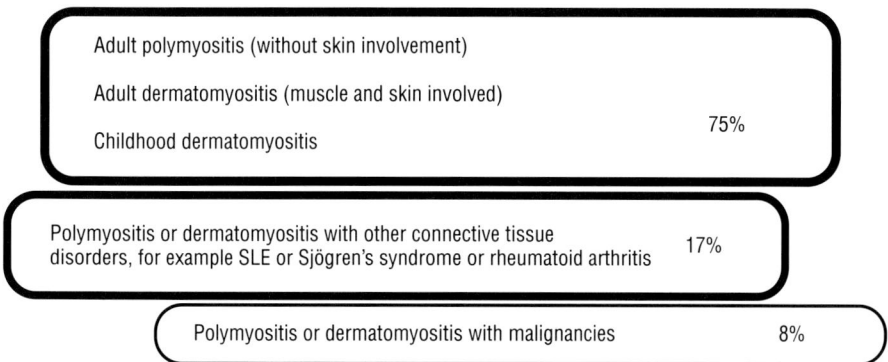

Figure 14.1 *Polymyositis–dermatomyositis complex*

the presentation of the patients. Skeletal muscle tissue may be inflamed quite specifically, or the inflammation may also involve other tissues, most commonly the skin and subcutis. Alternatively, the polymyositis may be involved with other systemic connective tissue diseases of an autoimmune nature.

The disorders are rather rare in incidence and show a bimodal age incidence, patients presenting between 5 and 25 years and between 50 and 60 years most commonly. Young women are particularly prone to developing the diseases. The older male patients with muscle disease are especially likely to also develop epithelial tumours, most commonly a carcinoma of the bronchus.

The disorders are suspected to be autoimmune in nature and certain immune system abnormalities have been demonstrated in patients. These include abnormal cell-mediated immunity with lymphotoxins and cytotoxic activity in the affected muscles being demonstrable. Some patients have autoantibodies to the MHC Jo-1 antigen. Some researchers in the field believe that the autoimmunity in some cases may be a manifestation of a hypersensitivity which is triggered off by viruses, Coxsackieviruses of the B group having been implicated.

There is atrophy, oedema and chronic inflammation of the affected muscles. Necrosis of myocytes may be apparent and a mononuclear cell infiltrate surrounds the areas of degeneration. There is great variation in size of myocytes in the lesions and in some cases the condition may not be distinguishable from a muscular dystrophy. If the skin is affected, there is dermal oedema, an infiltration by lymphocytes and plasma cells, vasculitis and some fibrinoid degeneration of the dermis.

The onset of the disease tends to be subacute and may follow disease of a viral type of presentation. Patients usually exhibit symmetrical, proximal muscle weakness and variable degrees of muscle pain, ache, swelling and atrophy. The commonest muscles involved are those of the upper arm, shoulder girdle, neck and upper thighs. Raynaud's disease and difficulty in swallowing may be seen with some patients. Other useful diagnostic features are, in some cases, elevated muscle enzymes in serum, for example increased levels of creatine phosphokinase. Electromyographic abnormalities and a raised erythrocyte sedimentation rate may be demonstrated in most patients. If skin involvement occurs, a typical 'heliotrope rash' around eyes, across the bridge of nose and over the dorsal aspect of the joints of hands will be observed.

The disease is characterized by remissions and exacerbations. Untreated cases will exhibit progressive weakness and atrophy of muscles with, eventually, a high mortality. Approximately 60% of patients recover with immunosuppression, a dramatic improvement seen after corticosteroid administration. If the steroids are discontinued there is usually a relapse, necessitating commencement of the treatment again. Patients that do not respond well to steroids will suffer from a slowly progressive disease with death after many years. Occasionally a patient may present with an acute episode of the disease where muscle destruction occurs and the disorder resembles an acute rhabdomyolysis.

Skeletal Muscle Atrophy

Skeletal muscle atrophy involves a progressive loss of bulk of muscles due to atrophic shrinkage, caused by apoptosis and progressive fibrosis. It may occur in a localized or generalized form. In both types, the affected muscles are smaller than normal, and are initially a yellowish brown colour due to accumulation of lipofuscin and later firm and grey as fibrosis occurs. Shrinkage of muscle fibres will be observed microscopically, the cells decreasing from 40–50 μm in diameter to less than 20 μm in diameter. There is prominence of sarcolemmal nuclei and increased lipofuscin deposition. Increasing fibrosis will be observed and degenerating nerve fibres may be seen. There will be muscle wasting and weakness leading to fatiguability, cramping, reluctance to move and tenderness, and as the atrophy progresses immobility will result with loss of ambulatory functions.

Generally, with most cases of skeletal muscle atrophy removal of the offending cause of atrophy or treatment of the primary condition will result in arrest of the atrophic changes in the muscle. Provided the disease has not progressed to extreme extents, the muscle cells will gradually undergo hypertrophy, regaining their initial size and function.

Localized Muscular Atrophy

In this form a whole muscle, fascicles of myocytes, or single neuromuscular unit may be affected. Disuse of specific muscles may lead to the disorder, as is commonly observed when a limb is encased in plaster for a length of time. Ischaemia seen in old age with advanced atheroma will also lead to progressive atrophy. This may be compounded by disuse of the muscles as often degenerative arthropathies will prevent the elderly from moving certain groups of muscles.

Interference with the motor innervation may also

produce atrophy of muscle and this is a typical example of neuropathic atrophy. Trauma may be followed by motor neurone damage and atrophy of the affected muscles. This is seen, for example, after car accidents with paraplegia and atrophy of the leg muscles. Neuromuscular disorders, such as poliomyelitis where viral damage to the motor neurones occurs, will also lead to a similar type of effect. Peripheral neuritides where peripheral nerves are damaged by various causes (e.g. alcohol, other toxins) and rare degenerative neuropathies will also cause the disease. The distribution and extent of the atrophy depends on the nerve involvement pattern.

Generalized Muscular Atrophy

This involves almost all skeletal muscles in the body and a typical example of this type of atrophy is seen in chronic malnutrition where the ingested protein is insufficient to maintain normal muscle mass, with atrophy of muscle occurring. Similar changes may be seen with panhypopituitarism, prolonged immobilization and senility, where there are generalized ischaemic and muscular disuse effects. With some systemic connective tissue diseases such as systemic lupus erythematosus or dermatomyositis, and with some metabolic disorders such as thyrotoxicosis, generalized muscle atrophy is observed.

Myopathies and Muscular Dystrophies

The term myopathy refers to a group of mostly congenital disorders affecting different groups of muscles, leading to progressive weakness and ultimately death. A characteristic feature of these pathological states is a disorder of normal neuromuscular function with resultant atrophic and degenerative changes occurring in the muscle. Accompanying inflammation may sometimes make it difficult to distinguish myopathies from polymyositis.

The muscular dystrophies are a group of genetically determined, myopathic diseases characterized by the progressive degeneration, atrophy and weakness of voluntary muscle. There is considerable variation in the rate and severity of the different forms. There are about 38 different types of myopathies and muscular dystrophies but most of these disorders are extremely rare.

Duchenne Muscular Dystrophy

Duchenne muscular dystrophy is a disorder transmitted as an X-linked recessive trait characterized by the onset of muscle weakness soon after birth, involving firstly the pelvic girdle and then the shoulder girdle. It is the commonest genetic myopathy, affecting 25 children per 100 000 births. The sex linkage of the trait implies that it is an almost exclusively male disease, females most commonly being carriers of the defective gene. The condition is manifest soon after birth and results in progressive disability as the child grows.

The gene defect causing the disorder has been identified and is one that leads to an abnormality in sarcolemmal permeability, causing excessive ingress of calcium within the sarcoplasm, eventually causing myocyte necrosis. Researchers have reported that nebulin, a protein necessary for the survival of muscle fibres, is missing in patients with the disease and this may have pathogenetic ramifications, as its absence may be an important factor in the degeneration and necrosis of the myocyte. This degeneration and necrosis begins patchily and is followed by hyalinization and fibrosis of the muscle. Breakdown of the sarcolemma leads to the release of sarcoplasm components, causing an increased level of creatine kinase in the plasma. In affected individuals of up to one year of age, biopsy shows hyaline and necrotic fibres with evidence of regeneration. In later years the regenerative capacity of muscle declines and necrotic fibres are replaced by fibrosis and adipose tissue. Serum creatine kinase levels, which are markedly increased in early years, fall progressively in the teens.

Affected children show winging of scapulae and scoliosis of the spine due to muscular weakness. There is pseudohypertrophy of the calves, which look quite muscular due to the extensive infiltration of fat tissue in the muscles which replaces the myocytes as they are destroyed (see Figure 14.2). Generally, affected boys present between birth and 5 years of age with delayed development of motor function. There is a characteristic waddling gait ('penguin gait') at presentation and an inability of the affected child to run. A weakness of the pelvic muscles causes difficulty in rising from the floor and the infant uses the arms to push the trunk to an upright position (this is the so-called **Gower's manoeuvre**). The majority of boys with Duchenne muscular dystrophy are confined to wheelchairs by the age of 13 years, and death in their late teens from respiratory failure is the usual outcome (this explains why this disease is so rare in females).

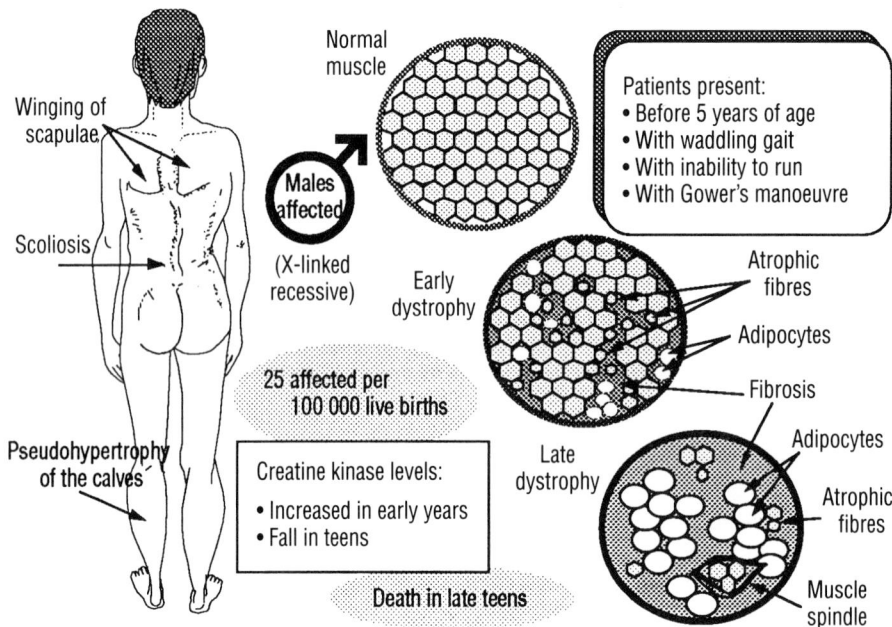

Figure 14.2 *Duchenne muscular dystrophy*

Becker Muscular Dystrophy

This is a related condition to Duchenne dystrophy but is a less severe disorder. It is thought to be transmitted as an autosomal recessive character. The age of onset is between 8 and 20 years. Similar changes in muscle to those in Duchenne dystrophy develop in Becker muscular dystrophy, but as the disease progresses more slowly, disability develops at a later stage and death usually occurs between 30 and 60 years. The pathophysiology of the disease is not understood.

Myasthenia Gravis

Myasthenia gravis is a relapsing, remitting neuromuscular disorder producing a generalized weakness and fatiguability of muscles, usually presenting as weakness in exercising muscles and recovery on resting. It is a rather uncommon disease with peak age of onset around 20 years, although a second, smaller group present in late adult life. In the younger age group the male to female ratio is 1:3, whereas in the older group there is a male preponderance. There is increased incidence of HLA-B8 antigen in young females with myasthenia gravis.

The disease is due to an autoimmune process (type V hypersensitivity) in which antibodies are formed against the acetylcholine receptors in muscle. IgG antibodies to acetylcholine receptors are found in over 85% of cases. The antibody attaches to these receptors at the neuromuscular junction and makes them unable to bind acetylcholine (see Figure 14.3). Complement-mediated lysis of post-synaptic membranes and cell-mediated immune mechanisms also play a role and what results is a disorder of neuromuscular transmission due to the severe reduction in acetylcholine receptors. Other autoimmune disorders may be found in these patients, for example pernicious anaemia, rheumatoid arthritis, thyroid diseases and systemic lupus erythematosus. Very rarely, myasthenia gravis develops congenitally due to a genetic defect of acetylcholine receptors on muscle cells and is unrelated to autoimmunity.

In 75% of patients myasthenia gravis is associated with abnormalities of the thymus gland, providing further evidence for the autoimmune nature of the disorder. Approximately 10 to 15% of patients have thymic tumours, such as thymoma (usually older males), while 60 to 65% have thymic hyperplasia (usually young females). The hyperplastic thymus has germinal centres in which B cells, specific for acetylcholine receptor autoantibody, are found. In the remaining patients the thymus may be atrophic or appear normal. It has been found that treatment by removal of the thymus may improve the disease.

Changes in the motor end-plates of muscles may be seen under electron microscopy but with light microscopy very little change is seen. Occasionally, small interstitial accumulations of lymphocytes are found in the affected muscles. In the thymus there may be hyperplasia with germinal centres developing or else thymic tumours (epithelial especially), both causing enlargement of the thymus.

There is great individual variation in the disease, making the course and the prognosis variable. In early disease, in most cases, the muscles of the patient appear normal both grossly and also under the light mi-

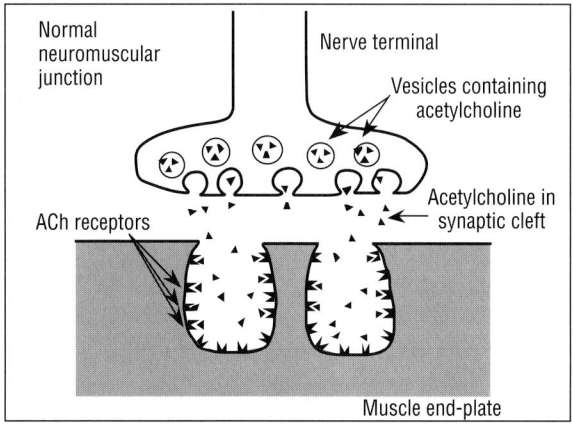

Normally, acetylcholine (ACh) is released into the synaptic cleft from the nerve terminal. It diffuses to the muscle end-plate and attaches to the ACh receptors, altering membrane permeabilities and initiating contraction of muscle.

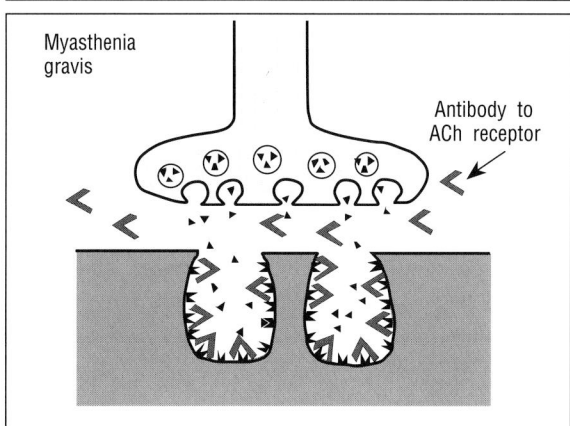

In myasthenia gravis, autoantibodies form to the ACh receptors. The Ab binds to these receptors, preventing the normal binding of ACh to the receptors. Although normal amounts of ACh are released from the nerve terminal, the muscle does not contract as quickly or as forcefully.

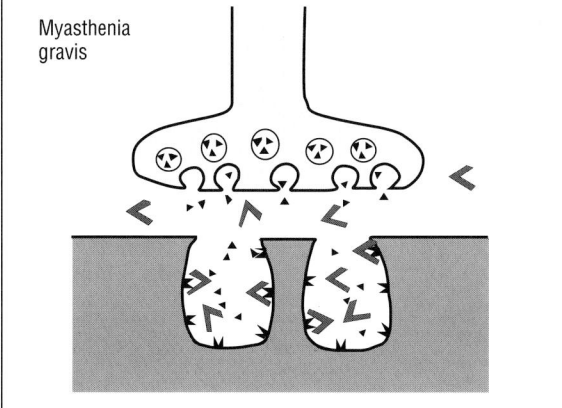

In long-standing myasthenia gravis, the autoantibodies destroy the receptors in association with complement- and cell-mediated immune mechanisms.

The ACh receptors are now much fewer in number and the autoantibody still attaches to what receptors are there.

There is profound muscle weakness and fatigue.

Figure 14.3 *Pathogenesis of myasthenia gravis*

croscope. In some cases the extrinsic ocular and facial muscles are involved early causing ptosis and diplopia. The patient may present with difficulty in speaking, chewing and swallowing. Later, there will be generalized muscle weakness and respiratory distress especially during exacerbations of the disease. A slowly progressive disease with exacerbations and remissions develops, with slow to rapidly mounting fatigue of skeletal muscles in most active use. Eventually, respiratory muscle involvement will cause respiratory distress, dyspnoea, aspiration pneumonias and asphyxia.

Treatment of the disease involves the use of anticholinesterase drugs (e.g. neostigmine) which delay the breakdown of acetylcholine in the neuromuscular junction, prolonging its activity. Immunosuppressive drugs and steroids may delay the course of the disorder in some people and are associated with an amelioration in the quality of life of the patient. Thymectomy is beneficial in a large proportion, especially if thymic anomalies are present. Plasmapheresis of the blood may be beneficial as it removes circulating acetylcholine receptor autoantibodies. Usually, combinations of these treatments mean that the patient can lead a near-normal life until the later stages of the disease.

Spinal Muscular Atrophy ('Neurogenic Muscular Weakness')

Progressive spinal muscular atrophy (SMA) refers to a group of childhood and adult diseases of varying severity. Most of these diseases are inherited and show varying patterns of inheritance. For example, juvenile SMA is inherited as an autosomal recessive. Others show sex-linked inheritance or are autosomal dominant traits and some occur sporadically. The pathogenesis is similar in all types of SMA and essentially this is because of an idiopathic loss of anterior horn cells in the spinal cord. A secondary atrophy of the muscle fibres in the motor units of the affected motor neurones develops and leads to muscle wasting and weakness eventually.

It should be noted that in a normal muscle, myocytes from different motor units are intermingled. Type I and type II muscle fibres, which develop different characteristics due to the differences in their innervation, may be identified histochemically by staining for oxidative enzyme. Type I fibres (or red muscle fibres) stain black and are capable of slow, prolonged contraction as they possess many mitochondria and many oxidative enzymes. Type II fibres (or white muscle fibres) stain a pale colour and are capable of fast contraction of short duration as they possess few mitochondria and oxidative enzymes, but much ATPase and glycogen. Normal muscle shows a random mosaic of type I and type II fibres on cross-section (illustrated in Figure 14.4).

Denervation of a motor unit resulting from death of a motor neurone will result in the atrophy of a group of myocytes of one type, scattered amongst normal myocytes. In response to the denervation, the atrophic fibres will develop more acetylcholine receptors on their membranes. Collateral sprouts from intact nerves will then annex the denervated, atrophic muscle cells which will then be reinnervated. However, the reinnervated atrophic fibres will take on the characteristics (either type I or type II) of the new nerve which has reinnervated them, irrespective of their original type. This will show up as a characteristic staining

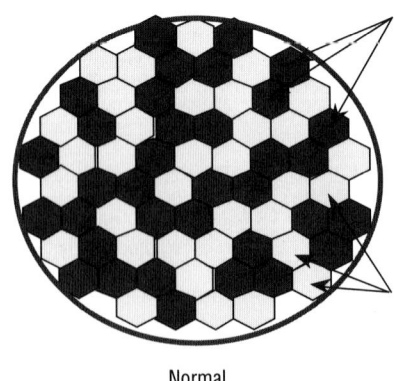

Type I fibres:
Dark, many oxidative enzymes, many mitochondria, little glycogen, ATPase, slow, prolonged contraction

The type of fibre, I or II, depends on the innervation

Type II fibres:
Light, few oxidative enzymes, few mitochondria, much glycogen, ATPase, fast, short-duration contraction

Normal muscle

Figure 14.4 *Muscle fibre types in a normal muscle*

non-random pattern of type I and type II fibres. With subsequent loss of more motor neurones, large regions of motor units will atrophy and as the muscle cells are unable to be reinnervated due to lack of viable neurones, the myocytes will degenerate (refer to Figure 14.5).

The various types of SMA are classified according to the rapidity of denervation and the completeness of reinnervation.

Acute Werdnig-Hoffman disease (progressive infantile SMA) exhibits a rapid denervation and an incomplete reinnervation. This generally implies that it has a short course, the affected infant dying at approximately 2 years of age.

Kukelberg-Welander syndrome (chronic childhood SMA) is one of the most common neuromuscular disorders of childhood. It is a comparatively mild form of SMA when compared to progressive infantile SMA. Its course shows a slowing denervation and a more complete reinnervation of affected muscles. The disease starts between the ages of 3 to 7 years and occurs more often in males than females. As the disease progresses, muscle weakness gradually spreads from hip and leg muscles to muscles of the shoulders and upper arms, and sometimes to the muscles of the neck and forearms. Typically, weakness advances slowly enough to permit a patient to walk, although with difficulty, for at least 10 years after symptoms are apparent. The disease is punctuated by remissions and exacerbations. Some time after a patient is confined to a wheelchair, skeletal deformities, especially curvature of the spine, may become pronounced. At the later stages, when sufferers are in their twenties, they are finally unable to carry out the simplest activities of

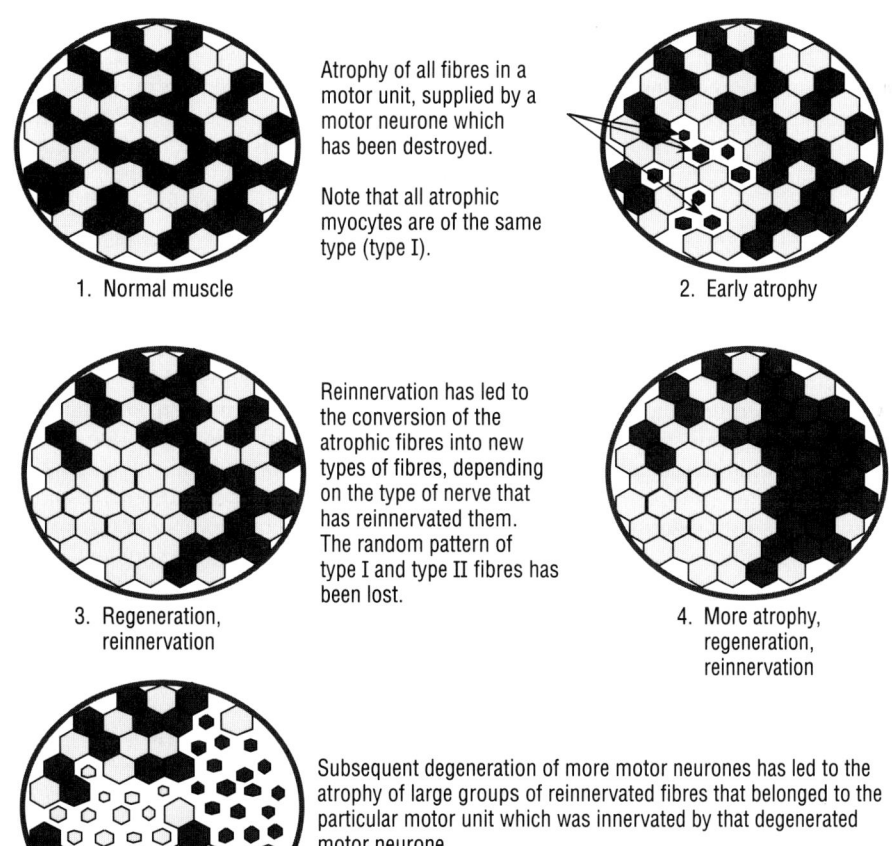

1. Normal muscle

Atrophy of all fibres in a motor unit, supplied by a motor neurone which has been destroyed.

Note that all atrophic myocytes are of the same type (type I).

2. Early atrophy

3. Regeneration, reinnervation

Reinnervation has led to the conversion of the atrophic fibres into new types of fibres, depending on the type of nerve that has reinnervated them. The random pattern of type I and type II fibres has been lost.

4. More atrophy, regeneration, reinnervation

5. Late atrophy

Subsequent degeneration of more motor neurones has led to the atrophy of large groups of reinnervated fibres that belonged to the particular motor unit which was innervated by that degenerated motor neurone.

Reinnervation after this stage is very patchy and the muscle shows progressively more shrinkage and weakness.

Figure 14.5 *Pathogenesis of spinal muscular atrophy*

everyday life and become totally dependent on others. They cannot combat intercurrent infections because of abnormal muscular function and related metabolic effects. Death usually results from respiratory disease, especially infections. Death may also be precipitated by atrophy of the heart muscle, where fibres are replaced by collagenous connective tissue.

Adolescent or adult onset SMA is the most benign as the denervation is very slow and the reinnervation very effective. It develops in older individuals and typically has quite a long course, the affected people often living almost normal life spans and showing the mildest symptoms and signs in the early stages of the disease. Long remissions are characteristic, as the effective reinnervation of the myocytes allows normal muscle function.

With the first two types of SMA, very early symptoms often go unrecognised because of their mildness. For example, the child may be slow in achieving the ability to sit, crawl, or walk, or may have trouble keeping up physically with others of the same age. Evidence of a problem becomes unmistakable when weakness in leg and hip turns the walk into a waddling gait, and makes falls frequent, climbing stairs and standing up difficult, and rising from the floor a problem.

Diagnosis of SMA depends on many criteria. Firstly, a genetic background may be available and there may be a history of SMA in the family. The clinical history and physical examination are important as their findings can indicate the type of SMA one is dealing with. Elevation of muscle enzymes (increased levels of creatine kinase in the serum) may be found and electromyographic studies often show abnormalities. Muscle biopsy and staining with special histochemical techniques are often required as this may provide the conclusive evidence for a firm diagnosis.

Treatment of SMA varies according to the degree of disability and severity of the disease type one is dealing with. Quinine, procaine amide, prednisolone and diphenylhydantoin are often prescribed in cases where myotonia is a problem. Adrenocorticosteroids are also being used to limit inflammation but the long-term use of steroids can induce steroid myopathy. Although vitamin E was once thought to help patients with SMA, clinical studies have proven this not to be the case. Doctors are now less likely to prescribe any drugs to combat the disease. Rather, appropriate medications are given for the treatment or prevention of complications, for example stool softeners to prevent constipation or antibiotics to combat infections. The use of orthopaedic braces, splinting and surgery are used in later stages of the disease. Ongoing physical therapy may be of use with active, passive and stretching exercises. The use of electrical stimulation combined with low-resistance weights have shown to be beneficial. The main focus is on increasing efficiency of functional activities of daily living. The use of hydrotherapy is also very beneficial for some patients.

Tumours of Skeletal Muscle

Rhabdomyoma

This is the benign tumour derived from striated muscle and is more likely to arise as a hamartoma congenitally, rather than as a true neoplasm later in life. It is an exceedingly rare (exotic!) lesion and is most commonly seen in the heart, seldom arising in skeletal muscles (Figures 14.6 and 14.7). It is often associated with tuberose sclerosis (epiloia), a disease in which sclerotic masses of proliferating glial cells occur in the brain. Mental deficiency is seen, as well as skin lesions and multiple hamartomata in many organs, including rhabdomyomata in the heart. Rhabdomyoma presents as a small nodular or lobulated mass composed of aggregates of myocytes. In the heart it may interfere with normal cardiac function and flow of blood through the chambers.

Rhabdomyosarcoma

Rhabdomyosarcoma is a highly malignant tumour of striated muscle occurring in skeletal muscle and occasionally the heart. It is a very rare tumour but is a true neoplasm arising from myocytes or their precursors. The tumours are entirely idiopathic and no aetiological or predisposing factors are known which are proven to be important in their development. As many of them develop in relatively young individuals, genetic factors may be of importance. Three main types are recognized. **Adult pleomorphic rhabdomyosarcoma** is an extremely rare tumour, affecting males and females equally. It usually occurs between the ages of 30 to 60 years. Characteristically, it is a very rapidly growing tumour often reaching a size of 25 cm or more in diameter. The muscles of the lower extremities are most commonly involved. The tumours are deeply situated in muscles and composed of soft, red to grey ('fish-flesh') tissue, with many regions of necrosis and haemorrhage within them. The tumours are very pleomorphic but usually contain a few cells that resemble striated myocytes. A tumour-associated immune response may be seen around the mass.

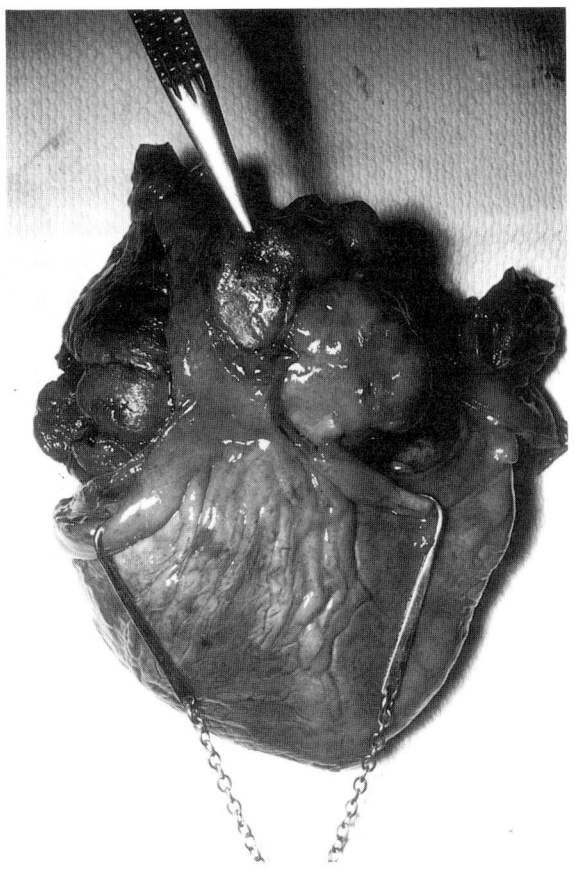

Figure 14.6 *Rhabdomyoma of the heart in a 12-month-old infant. The forceps are on the inferior vena cava*

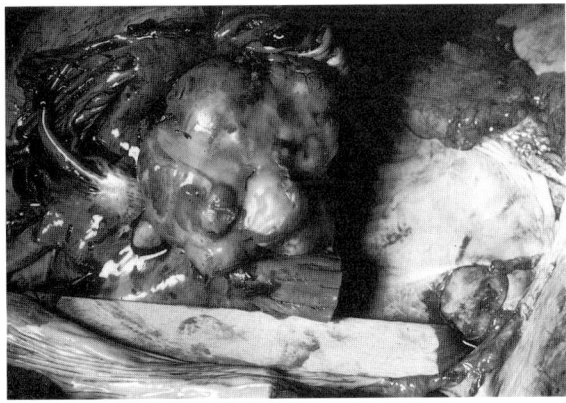

Figure 14.7 *Rhabdomyoma of the heart. Detail of the lesion in Figure 14.6*

Alveolar rhabdomyosarcoma is quite a rare tumour, although it is one of the commonest soft-tissue sarcomata in adolescents, most of these tumours occurring between 10 and 25 years of age. They are usually found in muscles of the upper or lower extremities but occasionally in the trunk. The tumours resemble the adult form grossly although they are not as large. Microscopically the tumour cells form rosettes or nests ('alveoli'). The neoplastic cells are small, round and undifferentiated, but occasionally multinucleate giant cells or striated cells may be found within the tumour.

Embryonal botryoidal rhabdomyosarcoma occurs in children and is often found in the genitourinary tract (e.g. vagina), biliary tract, the orbit and rarely in the extremities. They are 'grape-like' tumours forming large pedunculated, multilobate masses. Under the microscope, undifferentiated round or spindle-shaped tumour cells are found in a myxoid stroma.

Generally, rhabdomyosarcomata of all types are very aggressive tumours with widespread dissemination occurring very early in the history of the tumour. The embryonal type is less aggressive and may be involved with long-term survival if it is diagnosed and surgically excised. With the other types of tumour, the patients usually present late in the course of the disease, the tumour having spread via the bloodstream to involve the lungs. The 5-year survival of patients with pleomorphic and alveolar rhabdomyosarcomata is 10 to 30%.

Myoblastoma (Granular Cell Tumour)

Myoblastomata are uncommon tumours of uncertain histogenesis included here for convenience. They are typically benign but occasionally highly malignant variants may be seen. The commonest site of occurrence is the tongue or the gums. They may also arise in striated muscles, the retroperitoneum and subcutis. The cell of origin, initially thought to be a myoblast, is being debated and the likely cells from which the tumours are derived are thought to be Schwann cells, histiocytes or fibroblasts.

The neoplasm usually forms small circumscribed grey or yellowish tan masses. Microscopically they are composed of large, rounded cells with abundant granular eosinophilic cytoplasm. An interesting feature of the tumour is that it induces **pseudo-epitheliomatous hyperplasia** of the overlying epithelium, often this change being mistaken for a tumour of the epithelium. Local excision is curative for benign tumours but the malignant tumours spread early, causing death quickly.

Desmoid Tumour (Musculoaponeurotic Fibromatosis)

This is a connective tissue mass occurring at the aponeuroses (fibrous attachments) of muscles, usually in the anterior abdominal muscles of women, occurring commonly after pregnancy. It is not considered to be a true tumour despite the lack of a capsule and local infiltration into the surrounding structures. The lesion of this condition is a slowly growing and non-metastasizing mass. The cells in the mass are derived from the musculoaponeurotic white fibrous tissue and the disorder is thought to represent an atypical hyperplasia of this tissue. The lesions are small nodules approximately 2 cm in diameter, occasionally reaching a size of up to 15 cm in diameter. They resemble cellular scars and microscopically there are fibroblast-like cells among much collagen.

The exact aetiology is not known but it may be due to trauma or physical stress, or perhaps violent muscular contractions. Endocrinologic disturbances mediated by increased levels of oestrogens have also been suggested as a probable cause, in an attempt to explain the incidence in post-partum females.

Connective Tissue Disorders

Collagen comprises a third of the body's total protein. It is a structural protein and has important functions in healing, adaptation and remodelling. There are four major types of collagen with other, less important types also known. Collagen is synthesized by the fibroblasts that are present in connective tissues throughout the body. A third of the amino acids in collagen is glycine, in the pattern -GLY-X-X-GLY-X-X-, position X being occupied by either proline or lysine. If the collagen is to function normally the proline and lysine must be hydroxylated, with vitamin C and molecular oxygen being important in this step (thus, in scurvy, collagen is not formed normally). Collagen will not be secreted from the fibroblasts if it is not hydroxylated normally. The collagen fibre is a triple helix of three collagen fibrils twisted about one another. Interference with the polymerization step will interfere with the function of the molecule.

Collagen has a very slow turnover that is measured in months to years. It may be broken down by special enzymes, the collagenases, that are secreted by fibroblasts and macrophages. Thus, it is through this process that scars 'fade' and shrink with the passage of time. Collagenases are zinc-containing enzymes that require calcium to be active. Several inhibitors for their action are present in plasma and extracellular fluid.

The four major types of collagen are different in structure and function, the different collagen types being present in various situations in the body.

- **Type I collagen**: This is the major structural type of collagen in the body, found in skin, bone and tendon. It is very strong and is the predominant type in mature scars.
- **Type II collagen**: This is a very fine, fibrillar type of collagen found within cartilage, intervertebral discs and the notochord. The fibrils are glycosylated to a great extent and they are associated with the proteoglycans of the matrix in which they lie.
- **Type III collagen**: This type of collagen is also termed **reticulin**, is fibrillar in nature and is found in many visceral organs surrounding the parenchymal cells. For example, reticulin is found in the gut, kidney and liver, providing a fine support as reticular fibres. The dermal collagen is a mixture of types I and III. Reticulin is first laid down in scar tissue as a scaffold, upon which type III collagen will be deposited.
- **Type IV collagen**: This type of collagen is found only in basement membranes. It is associated with laminin and other components in the network that forms the anchoring structure of the basement membrane.

The term 'collagen disorders' was in the past commonly used to describe a heterogeneous group of disorders in which systemic involvement of the soft tissues and degenerating collagen (fibrinoid necrosis or hyalinization of collagen) were the common features. The group included such diverse diseases as rheumatic fever, dermatomyositis, hypertension, scleroderma, rheumatoid arthritis and many other diseases that were considered to be essentially idiopathic in nature. As more was learnt of the nature of these diseases it was discovered that most of them arose out of hypersensitivity or autoimmune reactions. Therefore, many of these diseases have been reclassified appropriately and they are considered within the context of the organ system which they affect most severely or most commonly. Some of the 'collagen disorders' that are not considered elsewhere in this text are covered for the sake of convenience here as connective tissue diseases.

Ehlers-Danlos Syndrome

The Ehlers-Danlos syndrome is a collection of nine related diseases all of which are uncommon genetic diseases and in all of which there are undefined defects in the structure and function of collagen. The transmission of the disorder varies from type to type, but in most cases the defect is transmitted as an autosomal dominant characteristic. Type I is the most severe of all forms of the disease and shows many features found in other types of the syndrome (see Table 14.1). Affected people have a very soft, velvety, distensible skin in infancy and youth. Large folds of the skin can be pulled out considerably and snap back in place when released ('India-rubber' people of the sideshows of yesteryear). As the person ages the skin becomes less elastic, is fragile, easily injured and often hangs in redundant folds. Wounds in the skin heal with large scars that are thin and paper-like. Large subcutaneous haemorrhages occur and the joints are easily dislocated or subluxated. Osteoarthritis develops at an early age because of repeated bone and joint injury. The mitral valve is often incompetent and varicose veins develop in many patients.

Marfan's Syndrome

Marfan's syndrome is a genetic disorder, inherited as an autosomal dominant trait with varying degrees of expressivity. In approximately one in five patients with the disorder the disease arises as a mutation. The incidence of the disease is one per 7000 people, men and women being affected equally. The disease affects sufferers variably, many patients showing only some features of the syndrome. One patient may only show the aortic changes, another may only show the skeletal changes, while still another may have all features of the disease.

The most striking feature of the disease is the general appearance of the patient. Affected people are tall and thin with long limbs and **arachnodactyly** (long, slender fingers). The chest shows evidence of **pectus carinatum** ('pigeon chest', protruding outwards), or of **pectus cavatum** ('funnel chest', hollowed inwards). The joints are very mobile ('double-jointed') or alter-

Table 14.1 *The Ehlers-Danlos Syndrome*

	Transmission	Skin features	Haemorrhages	Joint disease	Other features
Type I	Autosomal dominant	Very soft, fragile, hyperdistensible	In skin, up to 2 cm in diameter	Moderate	Mitral valve incompetent
Type II	Autosomal dominant	Moderately distensible	Bruising in skin	Mild	Generally a less severe disease than type I
Type III	Autosomal dominant	Little involved in disease	Not commonly	Severe	Osteoarthritis common
Type IV	Autosomal dominant or recessive	Thin, fragile, easily injured	Cerebral, skin, massive colonic haemorrhages	Mild (joints of digits only)	Collagen III is abnormal; spontaneous rupture of aorta or intestine
Type V	X-linked recessive	Mildly affected, not fragile	Not excessive	Moderate	Mitral valve abnormalities
Type VI	X-linked recessive	Moderately affected	Intramuscular	Moderate	Eyes abnormal, blue sclerae, less hydroxylysine in collagen
Type VII	Autosomal dominant or recessive	Moderately affected	Not commonly	Severe, multiple dislocations	Procollagen is abnormal in many patients
Type VIII	Autosomal dominant	Moderately affected	Not excessive	Moderate	Periodontitis is present
Type IX	X-linked recessive	Moderately distensible, not fragile	Bladder (haematuria)	Little affected	Diverticula of bladder, hernias, skeletal disease common

natively there may be contractures in the hands. The spine often shows kyphosis and scoliosis and there may be **striae** (streaky lines) on the buttocks and shoulders. Patients usually have an arched, high palate and the lens of the eye is dislocated upwards in most affected people.

The most important lesion in Marfan's syndrome occurs in the aorta. The media of this vessel begins to undergo a progressive degeneration and necrosis, beginning from infancy and advancing relentlessly throughout life. The abnormality causes a weakened upper aorta which often dilates and is prone to developing fatal dissecting aneurysms and massive haemorrhages. Aortic valve incompetence may occur due to dilatation and the mitral valve may have redundant cusps or show abnormal attachments to chordae tendinae (resulting in the 'floppy valve' syndrome). The pulmonary arteries in some patients also show medionecrosis.

The molecular defect in Marfan's syndrome has not been identified conclusively but various researchers have suggested that the syndrome may be caused by failure of cross-linkage of collagen, or abnormalities in elastin, or a defect in type II collagen chains. This results in a greatly weakened and dysfunctional connective tissue, and hence the systemic distribution of the disease.

Lupus Erythematosus

Lupus erythematosus refers to two related, autoimmune diseases that affect connective tissues in many organs and the skin. **Discoid lupus erythematosus** is a disease that primarily affects the skin, lesions in the viscera being very rare. In this type, the autoantibodies, if present, are present in low titre and various other serological abnormalities are present in half of the patients. In **systemic lupus erythematosus (SLE)**, as well as extensive involvement of the skin there are internal lesions in most of the viscera. High titres of autoantibodies are present and numerous serological abnormalities may be demonstrated. About 5% of patients with discoid lupus erythematosus will progress to SLE.

The lesions of discoid lupus are found most often on the nose and cheeks, but may also involve the scalp, arms, chest or the oral mucosa. The lesions are well-defined scaly red plaques that show oedema. With the progress of the disorder scarring occurs and if the disease is severe the ears and nose become deformed or totally destroyed. The skin is atrophic over the lesions, but at the margin it may be thickened and hyperkeratotic. Microscopically the lesions show a chronic inflammatory cell infiltrate, focal oedema and degenerative changes in the epidermal cells. Abnormalities in the basement membrane of the epidermis are linked with deposits of autoantibodies, complement components and fibrin. Discoid lupus is treated by topical corticosteroid application and systemic administration of chloroquine and most patients respond well to this treatment.

Systemic lupus erythematosus is a disease that primarily involves women, only one in 10 patients being male. The disease is first diagnosed between the ages of 15 and 35 years and approximately one in every 20 000 Caucasians has SLE. The disease has shown an increased incidence in the last few years, but this is thought to reflect better diagnosis and increased awareness of the condition.

The aetiology of SLE is autoimmune and numerous autoantibodies can be demonstrated in the serum of patients. In 99% of cases, antibodies directed against cell nuclear components are present. However, autoantibodies against blood cells, platelets, thyroid cells and rheumatoid factors are also present in many cases. The presence of antinuclear antibody (ANA) is one of the most reliable features of SLE. Individuals with SLE have a higher incidence of the HLA antigens DR2 and DR3 and one in 10 cases shows a familial association, another family member also having lupus. Abnormalities in complement may be present, especially involving the C2 component. The trigger for the autoimmunity is not known, but experimental studies with the New Zealand strain of laboratory mice show that these laboratory animals will develop an SLE-like disease if they are infected with a certain retrovirus. In some patients, retrovirus-like particles have been observed with the electron microscope in renal cells; however, the connection is tenuous. SLE can be seen to follow drug treatment, the substances implicated being hydralazine, chlorpromazine, isoniazid, d-penicillamine and others. Ultraviolet light may trigger off the formation of ANA in some patients and an SLE-like disease may develop. It is not unreasonable to suggest that in the presence of an underlying genetic predisposition, contact with a variety of largely unknown triggers will result in the autoimmune state that will progress to SLE in the affected individuals.

Clinically, the disease presents insidiously and then progresses over the years, characterized by remissions and exacerbations. The patient frequently presents with **polyarthralgia** (pains in many joints throughout the body) caused by a synovitis. **Myalgia** with weight loss and fatigue may also be present. There is a characteristic rash in exposed sites of the skin, especially the face, where a '**butterfly**' **rash** is seen across the bridge of the nose and cheeks. It is this malar rash that has given the disease its name. Lupus is the Latin word for wolf and the rash is a fancied resemblance to a wolf's malar markings. **Serositis** (inflammation of serous membranes) is present and this leads to cardiac murmurs and pleurisy that may progress to organization and painful adhesions. Renal disease leads to **proteinuria** and **haematuria**, while systemic inflammation and immune system factors often lead to a **fever**.

The organ changes in SLE are multiple and affect almost all major organ systems (see also Figure 14.8).

- **Joints**: About 90% of patients have a polyarthralgia with joint swelling, pain and an inflammatory synovitis. Usually the inflammation, although similar to rheumatoid arthritis in its early stages, is self-limiting with little permanent damage to the joints and no deformity.

- **Skin**: In as many as 85% of patients with SLE, the characteristic skin rash is seen, and microscopically there is a dermal lymphocytic infiltrate present, especially marked around blood vessels, with a focal degeneration of the epidermal basal layer.

- **Blood**: A characteristic feature of the disease in the blood upon suitable preparation is the so-called **lupus erythematosus cell** (LE cell). This is a neutrophil that has ingested degenerating cell nuclei, which are present as dark basophilic rounded masses within its cytoplasm and are termed **haematoxyphil bodies**. Similar bodies may be seen in many organs of the patient. The LE cell phenomenon occurs in about 80% of cases of SLE. It should be noted that a small number of patients with rheumatoid arthritis, scleroderma, dermatomyositis or allergic drug reactions will also show LE cells in their blood.

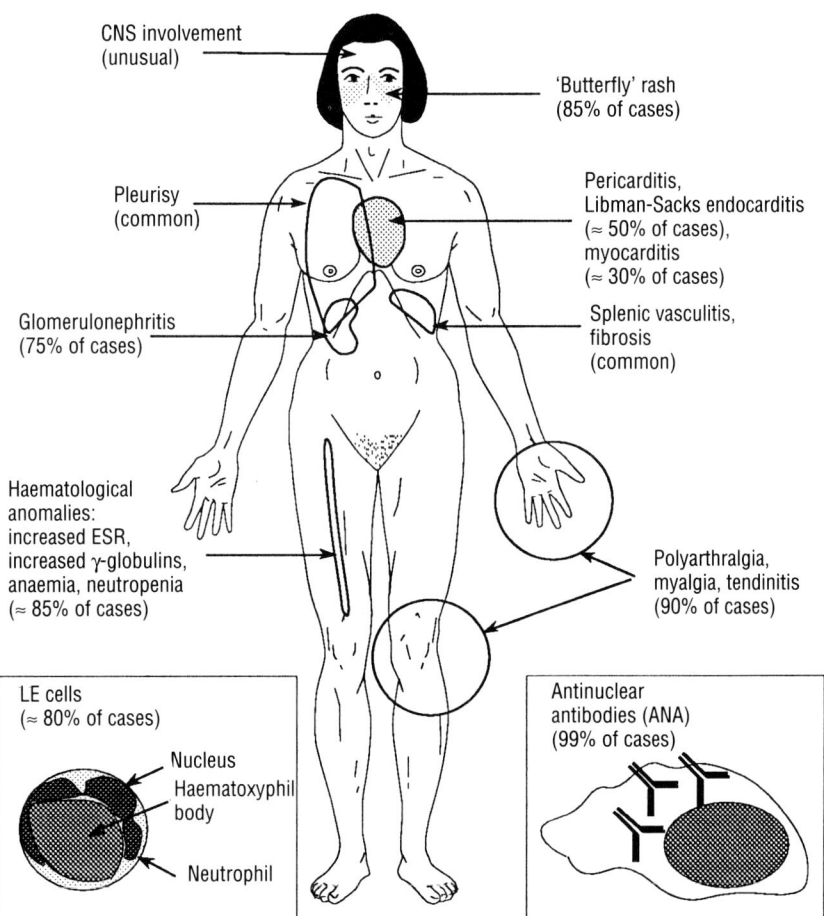

Figure 14.8 *The characteristics of SLE*

- **Kidneys**: The kidneys are very severely involved in about 75% of patients and the major process observed is glomerulonephritis. Typically, a diffuse, proliferative type of nephritis occurs, with epithelial crescents, hypercellularity and inflammation of the glomerular tuft, deposition of immune complexes and basement membrane changes. Another group of patients shows membranous glomerulonephritis with marked proteinuria. Other patients show less severe involvement of the glomeruli. Overall, about 15% of patients with SLE die of renal failure.
- **Serous membranes**: Approximately 70% of patients suffer from pericarditis, peritonitis and pleurisy. A typical exudative acute inflammatory response is seen in these tissues and the end result is focal organization with fibrous adhesions forming.
- **Heart**: Half of the patients with lupus show non-bacterial verrucous endocarditis, the so-called **Libman-Sacks endocarditis**. The tricuspid and mitral valves are involved but generally these lesions produce few clinical effects. About a third of patients will also show myocardial involvement and very rarely a congestive heart failure will result.
- **Other organs**: The **spleen** shows fibrosis and thickening of the penicilliary arteries with vasculitis. The **central nervous system** may be involved with vasculitis, haemorrhages and colliquative necrosis, these complications being particularly sinister. The **skeletal muscles** may show a myositis and vasculitis, causing pain and weakness. **Tendinitis** is common but tendon rupture, resorptive **arthropathy**, **osteonecrosis** and severe **myopathy** are all uncommon complications of the disease and in some cases have been associated with the steroid administration used to treat the disease.

The diagnosis of SLE is dependent on clinical presentation, the polyarthralgia and characteristic skin rash being suggestive of the disease. The LE cell, a very high erythrocyte sedimentation rate, raised gamma globulins in the plasma, anaemia and thrombocytopenia with neutropenia may all be demonstrated in the laboratory, further confirming the clinical diagnosis. Immunofluorescent techniques to demonstrate ANA in renal and skin biopsies may be used as a more conclusive means of diagnosis. The disease is treated by administration of corticosteroids. Renal dialysis may be required in cases showing severe renal lesions. Untreated, the disease progresses to death within about 5 years. Treatment and mild renal involvement markedly improves the prognosis for the patients.

Scleroderma (Progressive Systemic Sclerosis)

Scleroderma is an uncommon disease affecting about one person in 400 000. The disease is essentially an autoimmune disorder that tends to develop in patients who in 95% of cases show some chromosomal abnormality (deletions, translocations, chromatid breaks). This chromosomal defect is an acquired defect that develops because of some damaging plasma factor present in the patient's blood. People who are exposed to silica or vinyl chloride are more likely to develop scleroderma. The patients also have many immunological abnormalities:

- hyperactivity of B cells and hypergammaglobulinaemia;
- antinuclear antibodies are present (lower titre than in SLE);
- autoantibody to ScL-70, a nuclear protein, is highly specific for scleroderma;
- rheumatoid factor is often present;
- there are autoantibodies against collagen types I and IV;
- there are decreased T cell counts (inverted helper T/suppressor T ratio);
- T cells are sensitized to collagen.

Scleroderma is a disease characterized by the deposition of thick aggregates of collagen in many tissues throughout the body, especially the skin. The hands of the patient are usually affected first, then the arms, face, trunk and legs. The skin becomes thick, stiff and attached firmly to the subcutis; it eventually shrinks and the patients feel as though they are encased in an indistensible shell that is too small for them. The face is mask-like and impassive as it hardens and tightens, the hair thins, sweating is impaired and the skin is dry and leathery. Raynaud's phenomenon occurs in almost all patients with scleroderma and gangrene of the fingers is common as are ulcers, cyanosis and a burning or numbing feeling. The terminal phalanges may become resorbed and infections are often a complicating factor. **C**alcification of the subcutaneous tissues occurs in many cases and this together with **R**aynaud's phenomenon, o**E**sophageal abnormalities (dysphagia and anomalies of peristalsis), **S**clerodactyly, and **T**elangiectasia has given rise to the acronym **CREST syndrome** to describe a group of patients with this presentation. About half of the patients show changes in the joints that resemble early rheumatoid arthritis but in most cases this inflammation resolves away.

Other changes that may develop in scleroderma are the following:

- dyspnoea due to pulmonary interstitial fibrosis or pulmonary hypertension may occur in about 50% of patients;
- mild proteinuria in 50% of cases may progress suddenly to renal failure in a period of 3 to 4 years. Malignant hypertension may develop;
- Sjögren's syndrome develops in 20% of patients;
- a few patients develop abdominal pain or cramps with diarrhoea or constipation, malabsorption, diverticulosis of the colon and reduced intestinal motility;
- the heart may show left ventricular failure and right ventricular hypertrophy;
- rarely, some patients develop cirrhosis of the liver.

Microscopic findings of the disease include a marked intimal thickening of small and muscular arteries of the kidneys, lungs and often of the myocardium. There is focal oedema and telangiectasia. In the fibro-collagenous stroma of the skin, oesophagus, lungs, heart and intestine there is progressive fibrosis that begins patchily and then may become extensive. The fibroblasts produce normal collagen but about twice as much as they would produce normally, thought to be due to a defect in the regulation of collagen production.

The disease most commonly begins insidiously, the patient presenting with arthritis or with Raynaud's phenomenon or with thickening of the skin of the hands. The patient shows a slow progression over the years, the disorder sometimes showing remissions or remaining stationary but eventually it does tend to become more and more extensive. In a small number of people scleroderma follows a rapid course with severe systemic involvement within a period of months. Treatment of the disease is difficult and patients do not respond well to steroids or to immunosuppressive agents. Administration of D-penicillamine has helped some patients. The 10-year survival figure for scleroderma is 33%. If malignant hypertension complicates scleroderma the prognosis is very poor.

Revision Questions and Case Studies

1. Discuss briefly the pathology of the following conditions:
   (a) Skeletal muscle hypertrophy
   (b) Skeletal muscle atrophy
   (c) Ischaemic necrosis of skeletal muscle
   (d) Zenker's degeneration
2. Discuss the pathology of Duchenne muscular dystrophy.

3. What are the characteristics of myositis ossificans? How does this condition differ from dystrophic calcification of other tissues?
4. Differentiate between the different types of spinal muscular atrophy, indicating the pathogenesis responsible for the characteristic pathological features associated with each of these disorders.
5. Discuss the pathology of the polymyositis/dermatomyositis group of disorders.
6. What is the 'heliotrope rash'? Where would you see it and what would you consider as the most likely causes for it?
7. What are the pathological features of myasthenia gravis? Discuss in detail the aetiology and pathogenesis of this condition.
8. Write short notes on myoblastoma (granular cell tumour) and desmoid tumour.
9. Discuss the pathology of striated muscle tumours. Include primary and secondary tumours in your discussion.
10. Discuss the pathology of leiomyoma and leiomyosarcoma.
11. Define the following terms:
    (a) Zenker's degeneration
    (b) Satellite cell
    (c) Rhabdomyoma
    (d) Myositis and polymyositis
12. Write notes on the pathology of gas gangrene.
13. Discuss the pathology of hyperplasia, hypertrophy, atrophy and dystrophy, using as specific examples diseases affecting muscle tissue.
14. Write short notes on the pathology of rhabdomyosarcoma.
15. Discuss briefly the pathology of the following conditions:
    (a) Duchenne muscular dystrophy
    (b) Myasthenia gravis
16. What are the features of poliomyelitis, with special reference to the skeletal muscle effects of the disease?
17. Discuss the pathology of systemic lupus erythematosus (SLE), including incidence, aetiology and pathogenesis, characteristics of the disease, treatment and prognosis.
18. What is scleroderma? Why is the synonym 'progressive systemic sclerosis' a better name?
19. Compare Marfan's syndrome to the Ehlers-Danlos syndrome.
20. List the various diseases that may have muscle weakness and fatiguability as a feature.

Case study 1. A 17-year-old female patient presented with a history of a rapidly growing, lobulated mass in her calf. She first became aware of the mass in the left, proximal gastrocnemius muscle about a month ago. She lived on a farm close to Broken Hill and her transfer to Melbourne was delayed over 2 weeks. The patient deteriorated rapidly after admission to hospital, dying within a week. Disseminated tumour was found throughout the body at autopsy. The tumours consisted of soft, red to grey tissue that showed a resemblance to fish flesh. Many regions of necrosis and haemorrhage were found within the tumours, and under the microscope the cellular population was very pleomorphic with a marked tumour-associated immune response around the mass.

(a) What is the diagnosis?
(b) What is known about the aetiology of this condition?
(c) Is the patient a typical case of this disorder?

Case study 2. A 10-year-old boy presents with a history of swelling of the tongue and difficulty in mastication over the last 5 weeks. Examination of the tongue revealed a mass situated in the posterior, right part of the tongue growing rather superficially. A thickened and flattened mucosa overlaid the mass. Surgical removal of a small, firm, yellowish grey, encapsulated nodule associated with an overlying thickened mucosa was curative for this patient.

(a) What is the diagnosis?
(b) What is known about the histogenesis of such lesions?
(c) What other variant of this lesion is known?

Case study 3. A 5-year-old boy is brought into the family doctor as the mother has noticed that the boy is lately listless and complains of feeling tired all of the time. She has been surprised as William has always been an active child who never sits still. The boy does not run any more and on some occasions it appears that even walking is an arduous task. The child has often cried in the past 2 weeks as he is having trouble keeping up physically with his 7-year-old brother. The mother has noticed that when the boy attempts to run he walks with a strange waddling gait, and on three occasions this past week William has fallen over and, although he was not hurt at all, rising from the floor was a problem for him and he had to be helped up by his brother or mother. Examination of the child shows an alert, normal child except for some visible thinness and atrophy of his leg muscles. A biopsy of the quadriceps femoris muscle reveals atrophy of groups of myocytes, each group of one type, scattered amongst normal myocytes. There is some increased fibrous tissue between the myocytes.

(a) What are the differential diagnoses?
(b) What is the most likely diagnosis?
(c) How is the disorder likely to progress?
(d) Is the boy's brother likely to be involved by the same or similar diseases?
(e) Should additional information be sought from the mother? If yes, what would you ask her?

Case study 4. A 22-year-old Caucasian female university student presents at the university's optometry clinic a little concerned as she has lately noticed that she is having some trouble with her vision. When asked to describe what is wrong, she says: 'I have been tiring my eyes lately because I have been spending a great deal of time studying for my exams. One night last week I noticed that while I was reading, the page became blurry and I was seeing a double image. I stopped and went to bed but the problem kept recurring.' Examination of the patient shows slight ptosis of the left eyelid. The patient's vision is normal on examination and the optometrist refers the patient to a doctor. The next week when the woman presents at the Health Service, the doctor elicits the information that lately the patient has been having some difficulty in chewing and swallowing, but the patient attributes this to a 'cold or something' that has been troubling her and causing her breathing problems on exertion, and loss of appetite. The woman is a teetotaller and non-smoker.

(a) What is the diagnosis?
(b) The doctor who saw the patient ordered an investigation of the patient's thymus gland. Why was this? Would any other tests have been ordered at the same time?
(c) How is this disorder treated?
(d) What is the prognosis for this patient?

Case study 5. A 22-year old woman presents because during the past 2 months she has been suffering from worsening aches and pains in many of her joints. The small joints of the hands, the elbows, shoulders and knees are particularly affected and when questioned she also says that she has had muscle aches at various times. Initially, she thought that she had contracted the 'flu as she has been feverish on occasion, but as the aches and pains lingered she has sought medical advice. On examination, she is seen to be a thin Caucasian female, 1.7 m tall and weighing 57 kg. She is pale, except for a flushed, erythematous appearance especially marked over her cheekbones. Her temperature is 37.8°C and her pulse is measured at 78 beats per minute. Blood pressure is 120/80 mmHg. The abdomen and chest are normal, except for a pericardial friction rub that is auscultated. Questioned about her family, the woman says that her mother has dermatomyositis, otherwise all other family members are healthy. A urine sample is analysed with the Multistix® system but shows no abnormalities. A blood sample is taken for laboratory examination.

(a) What are the differential diagnoses?

(b) What is the most likely diagnosis?

(c) Explain the symptoms and signs the patient presented with inference to the pathological processes that are active in this disease.

(d) What tests will be performed by the laboratory on the patient's blood and what do you expect their results to show?

(e) What is the significance of the patient's mother suffering from dermatomyositis?

(f) Why is the urine examination normal (what does this imply about the disease stage)?

(g) How is this disorder treated, and what is the prognosis for the patient?

Further Reading

Agamanolis DP, Dasu S, Krill SE Jr. 'Tumors of Skeletal Muscle.' *Hum Pathol* 1986; **17**: 778.

Armbrustmacher VW. 'Pathology of the Muscular Dystrophies and the Congenital Nonprogressive Myopathies.' *Pathol Annu* 1980; **15**(1): 301.

Arnett FC. 'HLA and Genetic Predisposition to Lupus Erythematosus and Other Dermatologic Disorders.' *J Am Acad Dermatol* 1985; **13**: 472.

Bullough PG, Vigorita VJ. *Atlas of Orthopaedic Pathology with Clinical and Radiologic Correlations*, 1984; Butterworths, London; Gower Medical Publishing, New York.

Callen JP. 'Dermatomyositis.' *Neurol Clin* 1987; **5**: 379.

Callen JP (ed.). 'Lupus Erythematosus.' *Clin Dermatol* 1985; **3**(3): 1.

Cush JJ, Goldings EA. 'Drug-induced Lupus.' *Am J Med Sci* 1985; **290**: 36.

Drachman DB (ed.). 'Myasthenia Gravis: Biology and Treatment.' *Ann N Y Acad Sci* 1987; **505**: 1.

Harper PS. 'The Genetics of Muscular Dystrophies.' *Prog Med Genet* 1985; **6**: 53.

Kagen LJ. 'Dermatomyositis and Polymyositis.' *Clin Exp Rheumatol* 1984; **2**: 271.

Lenman, JARA. 'A Clinical and Experimental Study of the Effects of Exercise on Motor Weakness in Neurological Disease.' *J Neurol Neurosurg Psychiatry,* 1959; **22**: 182.

Mastaglia FL, Walton J. *Skeletal Muscle Pathology*, 1982; Churchill Livingstone, Edinburgh.

Miescher PA, Izui S, Huang YP. 'Immunopathogenesis of Systemic Lupus Erythematosus.' *Contribut Nephrol* 1984; **43**: 1.

Mimori T. 'Scleroderma–Polymyositis Overlap Syndrome.' *Int J Dermatol* 1987; **26**: 419.

Moser H. 'Duchenne Muscular Dystrophy: Pathogenetic Aspects and Genetic Prevention.' *Hum Genet* 1984; **66**: 17.

Nelson TE, Flewellen EH. 'The Malignant Hyperthermia Syndrome.' *N Eng J Med* 1983; **309**: 416.

Rosen G. 'Bone and Soft Part Sarcomas.' *Surg Annu* 1988; **28**: 121.

Rowland LP. 'Biochemistry of Muscle Membranes in Duchenne Muscular Dystrophy.' *Muscle Nerve* 1980; **3**: 3.

Ruyman FB. 'Rhabdomyosarcoma in Children and Adolescents.' *Hematol Oncol Clin North Am* 1987; **1**: 621.

Siegel IM. *107 Questions and Answers about Muscular Dystrophy*, 1987; Health Productions, Health Promotion Units, Health Department of Victoria (available from the Muscular Dystrophy Association, 208 Union Rd, Ascot Vale, Victoria 3032).

Seybold ME. 'Myasthenia Gravis: A Clinical and Basic Science Review.' *JAMA* 1983; **250**: 2516.

Sim FH. 'Musculoskeletal Oncology.' *Orthopedics* 1987; **10**: 1673.

Smith R, Triffit JT. 'Bones in Muscles: The Problem of Soft Tissue Ossification.' *Q J Med* 1986; **61**: 985.

Sternberg EM. 'Pathogenesis of Scleroderma.' *Surv Immunol Res* 1985; **4**: 69.

Symposium. 'Malignant Hyperthermia.' *Br J Anaesth* 1988; **60**: 251.

Vignos PJ Jr and Watkins MP. 'The Effect of Exercise in Muscular Dystrophy.' *JAMA* 1966; **97**(11).

Wallace DJ, Dubois EL (eds). *Lupus Erythematosus*, third edition 1987; Lea & Febiger, Philadelphia.

Walton J. *Disorders of Voluntary Muscle*, fourth edition, 1981; Churchill Livingstone, Edinburgh.

Walton J, Mastaglia FL (eds). 'The Muscular Dystrophies.' *Br Med Bull* 1980; **36**: 105.

Whitaker JN. 'Myasthenia Gravis and Autoimmunity.' *Adv Intern Med* 1981; **26**: 489.

15

Skeletal System Disorders

Normal Bone

Bone is derived from mesoderm and is a highly specialized connective tissue in that it possesses a calcified matrix. It is the building block of the skeleton and is one of the hardest tissues in the body. Normal bone is an active, dynamic tissue in a constant state of flux. Breakdown of old bone and remodelling constantly take place in order to replace the old tissue with newly formed tissue which is laid down along various planes, as directed by the muscles and weight-bearing stresses placed upon the bone. Normal bone is very strong and is almost as resistant to bending and twisting as is cast iron, at a third of the weight. A great force is thus required to break normal bone (a bending force greater than two tonnes per square centimetre is required to fracture bone).

The skeleton of the adult comprises 200 bones (not counting teeth, sesamoid bones and the ossicula auditus). The bones are divided into four groups, depending largely on their morphology:

- **the long bones**, such as the humerus or femur, are the bones of the limbs and serve as a system of levers supporting the weight of the trunk and being instrumental in locomotion;
- **the short bones**, such as the bones of the carpus and tarsus, are intended for slight and limited motion. They are in situations where strength and compactness are desired, as occurs in the hands and feet;
- **the flat bones**, such as the frontal bone or the scapula, are found in situations where there is a need for protection of delicate tissues such as the brain, or where there is a need for a broad surface on which muscular attachment may occur;
- **the irregular bones**, such as the vertebrae or temporal bone, are of an odd shape and cannot be placed in any of the other groups above.

Bone consists of two parts, the outer, compact bone **cortex** and the inner, spongy **medulla**. This is true for most bones in the body, except for the smallest ones that are all compact bone. The skull bones are said to consist of **outer** and **inner tables** of compact bone while the cancellous bone in between is termed the

diploë. Surrounding each bone is a fibrous **periosteum**, a loose connective tissue sheath richly supplied with vessels and nerves, which also contains osteogenic cells. In the adult, spongy bone in certain sites (chiefly the sternum, ribs, vertebrae and cranium) is filled with **red marrow**. This is the site for haemopoiesis. The spongy cavity of other bones in the adult is filled with adipocyte-rich, **yellow marrow** which is non-haemopoietic, but which may revert to haemopoietic marrow if there is need to. In children, all spongy marrow is haemopoietic.

The resting bone cells are the **osteocytes**, and it is they that are involved in bone substance maintenance. If new bone needs to be formed, as occurs in the process of remodelling, the synthetic form of cells, the **osteoblasts**, are responsible. It is these cells that form the bone matrix in which they become encased. If more osteoblasts are needed in bone there is a ready source in the bone marrow, periosteum and endosteum, in the form of the osteoprogenitor cells, which are spindle-shaped undifferentiated cells. The bone matrix consists of collagen fibres, a mucopolysaccharide substance rich in chondroitin sulphate and inorganic salts (mainly a complex calcium phosphate). Each osteocyte is an elongated cell shaped like a rockmelon seed, and has many, very long fine cytoplasmic processes that come out of its cytoplasm radially. Each bone cell is in a space within the matrix called a lacuna, and the cytoplasmic processes are contained within thin channels, the canaliculi. The osteocytes are arranged in concentric rings around blood vessels within the bone substance, making the bony lamellae that constitute the **Haversian systems** within the bone. Thus, even compact bone is very vascular, even if it is microscopically so. Bone is resorbed by the **osteoclast**, a multinucleated cell derived from the monocyte cell line, found on the surface of bones in small indentations known as Howship's lacunae.

There exist two types of bone, woven bone and lamellar bone, the difference being in the microscopic arrangement of cells and matrix. **Woven bone** has a rather irregularly arranged matrix of type I collagen fibres, in which are present large numbers of osteocytes of an irregular size. This type of bone is rapidly deposited and has a low inherent strength. Such bone is found in some bones of the developing foetus, healing bone fractures and bone tumours. However, its presence in the adult indicates some pathological process. **Lamellar bone** is more highly organized, containing Haversian systems and having a high tensile strength. Such bone is found in the normal adult skeleton. **Osteoid** represents either woven or lamellar bone whose matrix has not been mineralized. It usually indicates newly formed bone or alternatively bone that has become demineralized (e.g. as occurs in rickets or osteomalacia).

Most bones in the body are formed by **endochondral calcification**. Cartilage models of the bones are first laid down and the osteogenic cells that migrate there begin to lay down bone in regions of calcification that develop in the cartilage. These are what are known as primary centres of ossification and occur in central regions of the bone, the diaphysis (shaft) of long bones. Secondary centres of ossification develop in the epiphyseal regions (ends) of the bone. This process has as a result the formation of the bone, with two epiphyseal growth plates of cartilage where growth of the long bones occurs during childhood. The epiphyseal plates fuse in most bones at the end of puberty. Some bones are first laid down as woven bone and then become converted into lamellar bone (for example, the flat bones of the skull), a process called **intramembranous ossification**.

Because of the dynamic nature of bone tissue, injuries in bone tend to heal by tissue regeneration, where new bone tissue is laid down to replace tissue injured or lost. A prime example of this is the regeneration that is seen in bone following bone fracture.

Normal Cartilage

Cartilage is a tissue that does not contain blood vessels, lymphatics or nerves and its matrix is not heavily calcified as is bone. The matrix of cartilage is very different to that of bone, in that it is heavily hydrated, containing almost 80% of water. The solid components include type II collagen, proteoglycans and glycoproteins, the major component being chondroitin sulphates. Small amounts of calcium hydroxyapatite crystals may be found in cartilage. Similarly to bone, active cartilage cells are known as **chondroblasts**, while resting cells are known as **chondrocytes**. Damaged cartilage tends to heal by fibrosis.

Three types of cartilage are found in the body:

- **hyaline cartilage**, found in the articular cartilage of joints, in the airway walls, larynx and nasal cartilages, is the typical cartilaginous tissue. It is also found in healing fractures and some tumours of bone that form this type of cartilage;
- **fibrocartilage**, found in the intervertebral discs, symphysis pubis and menisci, is a hyaline cartilage that contains much type I collagen in its matrix, these fibres adding strength to this tissue;
- **elastic cartilage**, found in the ear, arytenoid laryngeal cartilage and the epiglottis, is a hyaline cartilage with much elastic tissue within it.

Normal Joints

A joint or articulation is formed where two or more bones in the skeleton come together. In the long bones it is the ends which usually form the joint while in the flat bones it is the edges which articulate. Functional considerations of the joint determine what type of articulating structure is formed. In certain positions (e.g. the skull) no movement of articulating bones is desired while in other parts (e.g. the limbs) a wide range of motion is highly desirable. Most of the joints in the body fall into the latter group and are the so-called **synovial joints**. These show definite characteristic features (see Figure 15.1).

- The contiguous bony surfaces are covered by an **articular hyaline cartilage** and are not attached to one another by bone. The bones of the joint are connected by a variable number of ligaments which are in addition to the fibrous capsule and usually superficial to it.
- There is a **joint cavity** containing a few millilitres of joint fluid.
- The joint is completely surrounded by an **articular fibrous capsule**, which is lined by a **synovial membrane**, this normally secreting the joint fluid.
- The synovial membrane lines the whole of the interior aspect of the articular capsule with the exception of the articular cartilage.
- All synovial joints are capable of **movement**.
- In some synovial joints there may be division (either complete or incomplete) by an **articular disc (meniscus)** consisting of fibrocartilage and being continuous with the joint capsule.

Two other types of joints exist, the **fibrous joints** (such as the **sutures** of the skull or **gomphoses** of the roots of teeth into the mandibles and maxillae) and the **cartilaginous joints** (such as the **symphysis pubis** or the joints between the vertebral bodies). These types of joints allow no movement or limited movement and are more important structurally than in locomotion.

Bone Diseases

Congenital Abnormalities

Achondroplasia (Dwarfism)

This is a congenital disorder of autosomal dominant inheritance that affects the long bones, the base of the skull and the pelvis. It is due to a dominant gene with a high mutation rate, most cases being due to a mutation occurring in one parent, whose chance of producing another affected child is the same as normal people's. Dwarfs with a normal spouse produce normal and affected children in equal numbers. The condition is due to a failure of endochondral ossification (intramembranous ossification being normal). It is present at birth and may even be diagnosed radiologically *in utero*. Approximately 80% of affected children are stillborn or die in the first year of life. Survivors are dwarfs. In these individuals there is failure of normal long bone growth and the achondroplastic adult will reach approximately 120 to 130 cm in height.

Achondroplastic dwarfs have normally developed trunks and skulls but short limbs, with growth of the

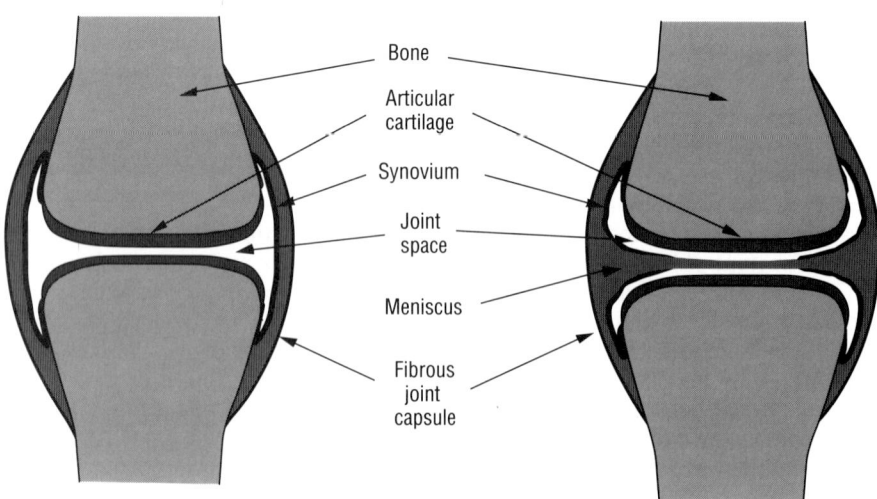

Figure 15.1 *A normal synovial joint*

soft tissues exceeding the growth of the bony tissues, leading to skin folds. The long bones are short and dumb-bell shaped, approximately two-thirds their normal length. The pelvis is reduced in all diameters. The spine shows lordosis and although the base of the skull is small the vault is normal with the forehead bulging, making the head appear large. There are 'trident' hands, that is, the hands are broad with fingers of equal length. Obesity is common with or without oedema.

The characteristic changes of achondroplasia are due to failure of bone formation in cartilage models. The major abnormality is at the epiphyseal line where the epiphyseal cartilage is narrowed due to the absence of a proliferating zone. Diminished growth in length results, with short shafts but with the epiphyseal bone being normally formed. The individuals with the disorder have normal intelligence and their life span is not shortened.

Dyschondroplasia (Enchondromatosis)

This is a condition in which there is hamartomatous proliferation of cartilage cells within the metaphysis of several bones, causing the thinning of the overlying cortex and distortion of bone growth in length. The disease has a familial tendency. There is persistence of epiphyseal cartilage into adulthood so that there are islands of cartilage within the bone, causing **enchondromata** to form; alternatively the hamartomata protrude towards the exterior as cartilaginous masses, forming **ecchondromata**. Some experts in the field consider both of these lesions to be bone tumours.

Enchondromata. These are single or multiple masses of cartilage in any bone but most commonly in the fingers (the condition in this case called **Ollier's disease**). The islands of cartilage may slowly ossify or become cystic by degeneration. Some grow to produce benign chondromata. They may also undergo malignant change forming chondrosarcomata. The lesions are removed surgically as soon as they are diagnosed to prevent these changes from occurring. A variant of the disease is **Mafucci's syndrome** where multiple enchondromata coexist with cavernous haemangiomata of the skin. This syndrome predisposes even more to malignant transformation within the cartilage islands and as many as half of the affected people may be expected to progress to chondrosarcoma.

Ecchondromata. These are cartilaginous nodules, frequently multiple, directed away from the epiphyseal line of origin. They are most commonly found ad-

jacent to the knee joint. Familial factors seem to be involved in their development. The cartilage ossifies from the base leaving a cap of cartilage covering cancellous bone, this also ossifying later.

The lesions produce protuberances, pain and deformity. A bursa may form, superficial to the mass. They are important clinically as they also may give rise to malignant lesions, the neoplasm arising out of any component of the ecchondroma: cartilage may give rise to chondrosarcoma; bone in the lesion may form osteosarcoma; and the overlying fibrous tissue may progress to a fibrosarcoma. Treatment of these lesions is by surgical excision and the prognosis is excellent provided they are treated early, before there has been malignant transformation.

Gargoylism (Lipochondrodystrophy)

This disease is also called Hurler's Syndrome and is a rare autosomal recessive trait in which there is a deficiency of the enzyme μ-L-iduronidase, resulting in a disturbance of glycosaminoglycan metabolism. It is characterized by gargoyle-like facies, dwarfism, severe skeletal changes, mental retardation, cloudy corneas, deafness, cardiovascular system defects, hepatosplenomegaly and joint contractures. Death usually occurs in the first decade.

The affected long bones show irregularities of endochondral ossification with variation in size and shape. There is kyphosis of the spine due to deformed vertebrae with posterior displacement. The accumulation of gangliosides and cerebrosides in the neurones of the brain causes mental retardation and convulsions. A similar lipid deposition is seen in the viscera.

Chondro-osteodystrophy (Morquio's Syndrome)

This is a rare example of one of the mucopolysaccharidoses. It is an autosomal recessive disease with no demonstrated enzyme deficiency. It affects predominantly the epiphyses and the spine. There is severe kyphosis due to wedge-shaped vertebrae. Irregular calcification and deformity of the epiphyseal cartilages results in enlargement of the ends of long bones.

Patients are dwarfs with normal intelligence, no facial abnormality or corneal clouding. The joints are lax rather than stiff. The kyphosis may cause spinal cord compression. Death occurs usually before 20 years of age from respiratory or cardiac problems.

Melorrheostosis

Melorrheostosis is a rare, congenital form of osteosclerosis characterized by cortical hyperostoses. It begins in childhood, slowly progressing as the patient ages. One or more bones of the limbs show thickened, flat, bony outgrowths from the cortex looking like wax gutters on a candle. The cause is unknown but sometimes the extracortical bone has a cartilaginous cap resembling ecchondromata.

Marfan's Syndrome

Marfan's syndrome is a rare, autosomal dominant disease affecting mesenchymal tissues, especially the skeleton, eyes and cardiovascular system. The basic defect is related to the metabolism of connective tissue, leading to abnormalities in collagen and elastin deposition, thus many tissues around the body are affected. Subluxations of the lens of the eye, retinal detachment and cataracts develop, with defects in the cardiac atrial septum and mitral valve. There is predisposition to medionecrosis of the aorta causing dissecting aneurysms.

Affected persons are tall and thin (**dolichomorphic**) with long and slender fingers (**arachnodactyly**) Patients generally die between the ages of 30 and 40 years, usually from complications of cardiovascular disease.

Osteopetrosis (Albers-Schönberg Disease)

Several forms of the disease exist, and a severe form is known, transmitted as an autosomal recessive trait, with a milder form occurring due to an autosomal dominant trait. The affected individuals suffer from increased density of all bones ossified from cartilage, especially the vertebrae, pelvic bones and ribs. The bones are very hard, dense and yet brittle so that pathological fractures are very common. The disorder develops due to defective osteoclast function and due to lack of bone remodelling.

The cortical compact bone extends into the medulla with no cancellous bone being present, the marrow having been displaced by the expanding, sclerotic cortex. As the blood-forming tissues are squeezed out of existence by the ingrowing bone **leukoerythroblastic anaemia** develops, both white and red blood cells being greatly depleted in the circulation. To compensate for the loss of haemopoiesis in the marrow, extramedullary haemopoiesis may be seen in the liver, spleen and lymph nodes, all of which are enlarged. As there is

progressive involvement of the skull the thickening of the bone may lead to compression of the cranial nerves with deafness and impairment of vision. Attempts to treat the condition have been made by transplanting compatible bone marrow into these individuals, in the hope that stem cells in the donor marrow may give rise to normally functioning osteoclasts.

Osteogenesis Imperfecta

This condition is also called the 'brittle bone syndrome'. It refers to a group of related disorders rather than a single entity and is characterized by heterogeneity, varying severity of pathological changes and many clinical presentations. In all forms there are abnormalities in the ossification of the skeleton. The bones are slender, with thin cortices, and very prone to pathological fracture. In severe cases multiple fractures occur *in utero*. During childhood, patients run the risk of fracturing bones on trivial trauma. The common factor in all forms of the disease is an abnormality of collagen metabolism, abnormal collagen being synthesized. As well as the skeletal disease, there are also problems in the skin, eyes, ears and teeth.

Type I is the commonest form of osteogenesis imperfecta, and is inherited as an autosomal dominant trait. This is a mild skeletal disease with the patients reaching normal height and having no severe deformities, their predisposition to fractures diminishing as they grow. However, 80% of affected people also show extraskeletal abnormalities, all related to a defect in the formation of type I collagen. They have bluish sclerae in their eyes (due to the thin sclera allowing the underlying pigmented choroid to show through), lax ligaments, thin skin, early-onset deafness (due to fusion of the ossicles), brownish, misshapen teeth and thin aortic valves.

Type II occurs as an autosomal recessive inherited disorder or it may arise sporadically out of mutations. At birth infants may show many fresh or healing fractures, short limbs and marked bone deformity. Most children die perinatally from intracranial haemorrhage due to a virtually unossified skull, or from respiratory failure due to multiple rib fractures. Very few survive past infancy. These few survivors join a heterogeneous group of severely affected infants and children of small stature with progressively worsening deformity and blue sclerae.

Type III is a heterogeneous group of children of small stature, with predisposition to fractures and progressively worsening deformity. It appears to be inherited as an autosomal recessive trait. The affected children are very liable to develop kyphoscoliosis. The sclerae tend to become white in the survivors and dental abnormalities occur commonly.

Type IV causes very severe disease and affected children are very deformed. This type is inherited as an autosomal dominant trait. The long bones are short and slender and many fractures occur including spine compression fractures. The shafts of the long bones are short and slender, the cortex is thin, there is little medullary bone and the epiphyses look very broad. Bowing of bones results from multiple fractures. The vertebrae show biconcave or wedge-shaped deformity as compression fractures are very common. The sclerae are bluish, with or without abnormalities in the teeth. The patients are treated with numerous orthopaedic devices and at adolescence the bones may in some cases show maturation of the cortex.

Histologically, in all of these disorders there are numerous, apparently active osteoblasts seen in the bone but little new, normal bone is being formed. Evidence of fracture healing is seen with attempts at repair, as well as ineffectual growth and abnormalities in ossification. Generally, because of the multiple disorders in the skeletal system most of these children die young.

Scoliosis and Kyphosis

Scoliosis is an abnormal, lateral curvature of the vertebral column, while kyphosis is an abnormal, increased convexity in the curvature of the thoracic spine when viewed from the side. Both conditions, if congenital, arise out of asymmetric growth of the vertebral bodies. Scoliosis is most commonly an idiopathic disease most often seen in adolescent girls. Alternatively acquired forms of the disease may be due to vertebral destruction by a variety of diseases (e.g. TB, osteomyelitis, rickets, bone tumours). The disorder is treated by treating the primary disorder if any is present and then by the use of orthopaedic devices such as braces or internal fixateurs in order to correct the wedge-shaped vertebral bodies. Untreated scoliosis will cause the spine to be an abnormal S-shape and may interfere with cardiopulmonary function and normal joint function (especially of the hip).

Kyphosis may develop congenitally, especially in association with the genetically determined skeletal diseases of Morquio's syndrome or gargoylism. The kyphosis very often produces a **gibbus** ('hump') due to the sharp angle formed by the protruding spine. Other, acquired forms of kyphosis result after neoplasms grow in the vertebrae, after crush fractures of vertebrae, in association with infection, or with any of the bone rarefactions such as osteoporosis, seen especially in elderly women (dowager's hump).

Bone Trauma, Malformations

Bone Fracture

The commonest type of bone disease is perhaps bone fracture, which is the breaking, cracking or loss of continuity of a bone. Healing of fractures resembles healing in soft tissues, but the major difference is that bone regeneration occurs, with complete reconstruction of the previous bony architecture. The age of the individual, adequate blood supply to the healing bone and the correct anatomical alignment of the broken bones are important factors in fracture healing. Also very important is whether or not a pre-existing disease is present in the bone, that is, if a pathological fracture has occurred. Provided the individual is relatively young and healthy and all the local factors are favourable, the bone will regenerate completely. The healing of bone fractures has been considered in full in Part I.

Osteochondritis Juvenilis (Osteochondrosis)

Osteochondritis juvenilis is a general term used to describe a number of disorders arising at the epiphyses of the bones of children. Usually there is a history of trauma at the affected site, thought to be a factor interfering with the blood supply. The term osteochondrosis is often used synonymously, but depending on the site of occurrence, the disease may also be given other names, for example **Perthe's disease**, when it affects the femoral head, or **Köhler's disease** if it affects the navicular bone.

The disease develops when there is interference with the epiphyseal blood supply, most usually the direct result of bone trauma. Avascular, ischaemic bone necrosis occurs and subsequent collapse of the necrotic bone results in deformity of the joint surface. Disabling secondary degenerative changes then occur around the joint, with evidence of haemorrhages and organization. Attempts at repair around the damaged region lead to areas of bone regeneration, sequestration and callus formation with further deformity.

The epiphyseal bone around the affected region is irregularly sclerotic and rarefied with fragmentation and deformity. In a weight-bearing site the deformity involves the articular cartilage, producing characteristic radiological changes. The condition results in pain and clinically it mimics joint tuberculosis. The affected individuals are greatly predisposed to osteoarthritis, especially at the hip. In some patients sarcomata may arise at the site, as multiple traumatic and repair episodes predispose to malignancy.

Drug-induced Phocomelia ('Seal Limbs')

Phocomelia is the incomplete development of limbs due to interference with limb-bud formation. **Amelia** is the complete, congenital absence of a limb. The most infamous example of these two disorders is that which occurred in the sixties after thalidomide administration during pregnancy. The drug was a sedative prescribed for morning sickness, which it relieved, but it also caused gross congenital abnormalities in the foetus, including amelia, phocomelia, defects in the pinna of the ear and the heart. Intelligence is normal in these affected children. Approximately 3000 affected children were born with these defects before the aetiology was linked with the drug, which was subsequently withdrawn from the market. Amelia or phocomelia are occasionally seen as spontaneously arising congenital malformations, affecting one in 5000 live babies.

Tetracycline-induced Bone Changes

When tetracyclines are administered to infants and young children they are found to accumulate in fast-growing bones and also in teeth with permanent staining of the tissues; some researchers also suggest that there may be interference with the normal growth of the tissue. Such effects are seen to occur also in the foetus if pregnant women are given these drugs. Because of the effects of tetracycline on calcified tissues, they are not used during pregnancy or in children under 8 years of age.

Inflammations, Infections and Degenerations of Bone

Osteitis and Osteomyelitis

Osteitis refers to infection or inflammation of compact bone, while osteomyelitis refers to inflammation of both compact and cancellous bone with involvement of the marrow cavity. Although an infection may start as an osteitis, it will in most cases develop into an osteomyelitis. Bone infection occurs most often following bacteraemia or less commonly trauma (compound fractures especially) or infection of the adjacent

tissues (e.g. abscesses due to pyogenic organisms infecting surrounding soft tissues). *Staphylococcus aureus* is most often responsible for acute or chronic osteomyelitis, while other organisms such as *Salmonella* spp., *Neisseria gonorrhoeae, Haemophilus influenzae* or *Escherichia coli* may also cause the infection. The affected region is most commonly the long bones adjacent to the knee joint, the ankle and hip. Children and young people are most likely to present with the condition. The infection causes great swelling and inflammation of overlying tissues, associated with severe pain and usually fever.

Infection in bone is characterized by suppuration within the bone and bone marrow, with destruction of bone. The destroyed, necrotic bone forms niches in which the bacteria lodge, making it difficult for phagocytes to ingest and destroy them and also shielding the microbes from the bloodstream, and thus from being reached by antibodies and administered antibiotics. These necrotic bone fragments which harbour micro-organisms are termed **sequestra**. Around the sequestra there is reactive bone formation to form a sheath of newly laid bone, called an **involucrum**. In chronic, untreated infections it is not uncommon for the pus to discharge to the exterior through the periosteum and skin via a sinus called a **cloaca**. It is of importance in the treatment of the disease to remove the sequestra and involucra and drain the pus in order to allow regeneration of the bone. Treatment is by antibiotic therapy and also surgical intervention to drain the abscess and remove necrotic bone.

Osteomyelitis may also be caused by *Salmonella typhi* and in this case is seen as a complication of typhoid fever. In tertiary syphilis there may be gummata developing in bones with associated destruction and deformity of the affected bones. Bone lesions may also be seen in tuberculosis with characteristic tubercles causing destruction of the bone. Tuberculous osteomyelitis of the spine was rather common in the past and caused the disease termed **Pott's disease of the spine**, which was an infection of the vertebral bodies (especially the thoracic ones) after haematogenous spread there. There is caseation and destruction of the affected vertebrae and commonly of the discs, with resultant kyphosis. The caseous necrotic material may be infiltrated by neutrophils and be partially liquefied, extending outside the bone to form collections anteriorly. These collections of caseous pus may be forced into the various fasciae and present as a 'cold abscess', implying that acute inflammation is not present around them. A cervical abscess and a retropharyngeal abscess are commonly seen, or a **psoas abscess** may form after the debris tracks down the spine along the spinal ligaments to the inguinal region where it points and drains. Pressure effects due to the accumulated caseous material around the spine and also effects due to vertebral collapse may cause paraplegia after cord damage.

Paget's Disease of Bone (Osteitis Deformans)

This is an idiopathic condition in which there is continuous destruction of bone with replacement by an abnormally soft, poorly mineralized matrix. It is a rather common disorder of bone found in 1 to 4% of elderly people. It is rare below 40 years of age and occurs in males slightly more than females, patients usually presenting over the age of 60 years. Many theories exist as to the aetiology of the disease and much research has been centred on finding evidence for implicating various agents or factors. It appears that there may are some familial and geographic factors involved, and a genetic disorder of connective tissues of undetermined nature has been suggested as the cause. The disease is more common in Britain and populations with a British origin in the USA, Australia, South Africa and Canada, while it is very rare in Asians, black people and South Americans. Other research has implicated some infectious cause and the most favoured agent is a virus. Experimental evidence which supports this is that paramyxovirus-like structures have been found in the nuclei of osteoclasts of lesions in patients with the disease and these structures are cross-reactive with the measles virus antibody. However, all attempts to isolate any virus have met with failure.

Paget's disease may be seen in polyostotic and monostotic forms. The **polyostotic form** is more uncommon and affects many bones in the body, the bones most often affected being those of the pelvis, the sacrum, skull, spine, tibia, humerus and scapula (in decreasing order of involvement). The **monostotic form** is the most commonly observed and it affects only one bone or a single portion of a bone, the most frequently affected bone being the tibia. Solitary lesions of the spine or pelvis are also seen.

Three phases are observed in the pathogenesis of the disorder. The first is the **osteolytic phase** in which there is intense bone resorption. Many osteoclasts, often of a bizarre form, each with as many as 100 nuclei are found in regions undergoing resorption. Replacement of bone by highly vascularized connective tissue occurs in association with the osteolysis (Figure 15.2).

The **mixed phase** then follows, in which osteolysis continues, but osteoblastic activity is also seen. La-

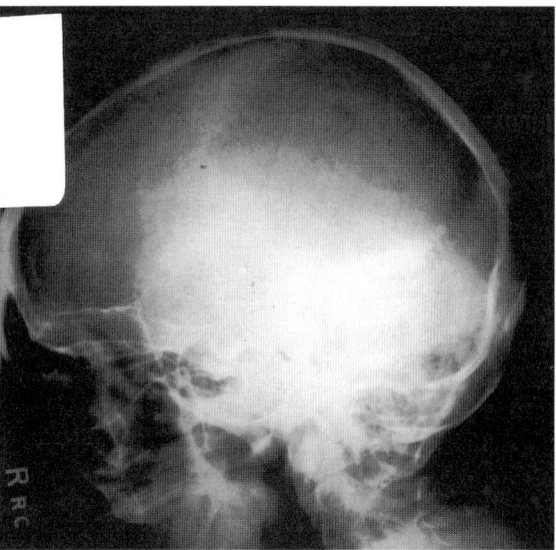

Figure 15.2 *Osteolytic phase of Paget's disease of the skull (osteoporosis circumscripta). Note the apparent thinning of the skull bone (courtesy of Dr Thomas Molyneux, RMIT)*

mellar bone replaces the connective tissue but mineralization of the newly formed osteoid lags behind and regions of osteoid and mineralized bone occur in a random pattern, characteristic of the disease. Histologically, the bones show increased osteoclastic and osteoblastic activity, so there is increased bone resorption of normal dense cortical bone and deposition of abnormal trabeculae of new bone. New bone is deposited irregularly causing a mosaic pattern of cement lines. There is no distinct layer between cortex and medulla. The medullary cavity is progressively replaced by a loose, highly vascular fibrous tissue.

The **sclerotic phase** develops only after the disease has progressed for some years. Osteoclastic activity wanes and osteoblastic activity predominates. Osteogenesis eventually increases bone thickness or size, but bone is laid down haphazardly, is poorly mineralized and soft, porous and lacking in strength. The affected bone is irregularly thickened, spongy, soft and vascular (Figure 15.3).

The effects of the disease vary and depend on the bones affected and severity of involvement. Some patients may be asymptomatic, evidence of Paget's disease being found at autopsy incidentally. Commonly, there may be pain and deformity of the affected bones. In the skull, enlargement of bones leads to **headaches** and pains in the face, due to compression of cranial nerves. **Deafness** and visual disturbances are often

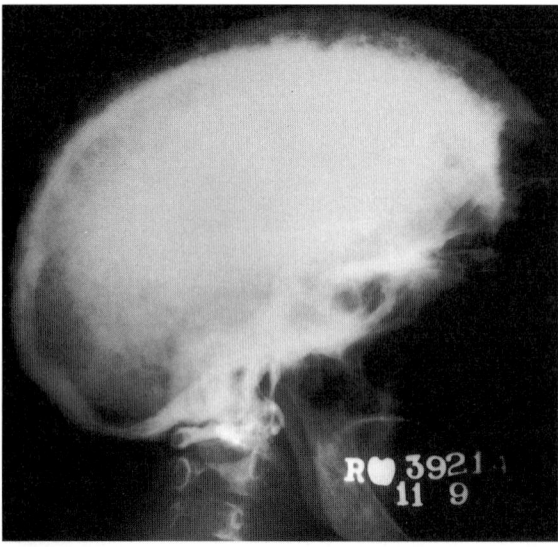

Figure 15.3 *Osteosclerotic phase of Paget's disease of the skull. The skull bones are now thickened but their extreme vascularity makes them appear as if there are 'cotton wool patches' on the bone (courtesy of Dr Thomas Molyneux, RMIT)*

noted as the corresponding nerves are squeezed by the expanding bone mass. Thickening of skull bones results in increased skull size, and in the past when wearing of hats was more widespread the patients often noticed that they had to increase their hat size. Extreme thickening of bones of the head produces the condition of **leontiasis ossea**, where the patient's face assumes a leonine likeness. Back pain due to compression of spinal roots and shortening of the trunk is seen commonly, with associated pathological compression fractures of the vertebrae. The heavy skull may, in particular, cause a compression of the C1 vertebra, producing **platybasia**. There is also thickening and softening of vertebrae, resulting in **kyphosis**. The long bones are affected by swelling, which causes changes in gait. The femur shows increased thickness and anterior bowing. The tibia shows anterior **bowing**, thickening and irregularity. The pelvis is thickened, especially in the iliac bones. There are thickened and prominent clavicles.

Radiologically, in the early stages there is **radiolucency** but later the bones become increasingly **radiodense**. The levels of calcium and phosphate in serum are normal since resorption and osteogenesis occurs almost simultaneously. There are increased levels of alkaline phosphatase as more new bone formation is seen.

The increased vascularity of the bones increases the volume of blood within them, and the cardiac output is increased, with diversion of much blood to affected bones; subsequent cardiomegaly is due to cardiac hypertrophy. Some patients may complain of **light-headedness**, thought to be caused by a diversion of cerebral blood from the internal carotids to the bone rather than the brain. **Cardiac failure** is often seen in elderly patients who also suffer from other disorders such as coronary heart disease and hypertension. **Pathological fracture** of the affected bones is very common, because although the bones are thickened, they are also more brittle and fragile. Osteosarcoma develops in 1 to 10% of cases of Paget's disease and represents 30% of all malignant primary bone tumours over the age of 50 years. The sites most commonly affected by the sarcomatous change are the pelvis, humerus and femur. Paget's disease is incurable and various treatments centre around dealing with the abnormal osteoclastic activity. Several drugs have been tried, with variable results, and they include calcitonin supplements, diphosphonates, sodium fluoride and mithramycin.

Albright's Disease (Fibrous Dysplasia of Bone)

This is an uncommon, idiopathic disease seen in young adults, usually not after 40 years of age. Some researchers have suggested that it is possibly due to developmental defects of mesenchymal tissue. However, it is unrelated to Paget's disease of bone or to hyperparathyroidism. The disorder exists in two major subtypes. In the complete syndrome, which is the rarest in occurrence, there is a triad of changes, seen predominantly in young girls: fibrous dysplasia of many bones, skin pigmentation ('café au lait spots') and precocious puberty. A large variety of endocrine disorders may accompany this disorder. There is bilateral jaw involvement but in the long bones the lesions are unilateral and multiple.

The second major subtype, the monostotic form, is more commonly seen and the ribs, femur, tibia, maxilla or mandible are affected in descending order, although any other bone may also be involved. The bone is expanded by firm, white fibrous tissue with palpable spicules of bone filling the medulla, associated with thinning of the cortex. The fibrous tissue replacing the bone is acellular and avascular with no inflammatory cells within it. A few fine trabeculae of bone may be seen to traverse the fibrous tissue. Pathological fractures are very common as are swellings and deformities of the affected bone. Fibrosarcomata may rarely arise in long-standing cases.

Diagnosis of the disease depends on clinical presentation and radiological findings. Laboratory investigations yield normal calcium and phosphate levels in plasma but alkaline phosphatase levels are raised. Commonly, the patient first presents with a pathological fracture.

Bone Rarefactions

Rarefaction implies a decrease in the density of bone (decreased calcium in the matrix) or in bone mass (decreased amount of bone), or both. These are changes evident radiologically and may arise from many pathologies, three different processes being the most important and most commonly encountered in this context:

• reduction in amount of bone, for example osteoporosis;
• defective mineralization, for example osteomalacia;
• resorption and fibrous change of bone, for example hyperparathyroidism.

Osteoporosis

In osteoporosis there is a pathological decrease in the amount of bone tissue in the body, but in the bone that remains the matrix is normally mineralized. The condition may result from decreased bone formation, increased bone resorption or, as commonly occurs, from both processes acting together.

The blood levels of calcium, phosphate and alkaline phosphatase are normal, while the urine levels of calcium are increased in the disorder. Osteoporotic bones are lighter in weight, less dense radiographically and show thinning of the cortex. There is an increased liability to pathological fractures as the affected bones possess an inherent weakness due to the reduced bone mass. The bony trabeculae are thinner and there may be a decreased number of osteoblasts, or an increased number of osteoclasts actively resorbing bone.

The condition is thought to arise from an initial episode of increased bone resorption, which is followed by an inadequate reactive bone deposition. A new equilibrium is reached where there are both resorption and deposition of bone but in this new state there is less bone overall. A variety of conditions and states may give rise to osteoporosis, for example immobilization, nutritional and endocrine causes and arthritis, but the majority of cases are the idiopathic, senile variety. Osteoporosis may be subdivided into localized and generalized forms (refer to Table 15.1).

Localized Osteoporosis (Disuse Osteoporosis)
This occurs in immobilized or paralyzed limbs and is associated with loss of muscle action and loss of normal weight-bearing stresses placed on bone. It may also be seen in association with malignant bone tumours and rheumatoid arthritis, both of which may prevent normal use of a limb because of associated pain. As many of the conditions precipitating localized osteoporosis are seen in the elderly, nutritional and endocrine factors may also contribute to the development of the disease process in the affected limb.

The affected bones show an increased radiolucency, and the trabeculae of cancellous bone become scantier and more slender (see Figure 15.4). The cortical bone is thinner and more porous due to the opening up of Haversian spaces on the endosteum, a process referred to as **cancellization**. Such changes are patchy and may be usually first recognized in the cancellous bone of the metaphysis. There is an initial increase in bone resorption, causing the osteoporosis, but later there is a return to equilibrium, with resorption and new bone deposition being approximately equal. As there is much bone resorption occurring initially (4% of the bone mass is resorbed per month) renal calculus formation may be seen in some patients, as the excess calcium is being excreted by the kidney (Figures 15.5 and 15.6).

If muscle activity is resumed or the underlying condition causing the osteoporosis is treated effectively, new bone is laid down and there is a slow return to normal. It is interesting to note that when astronauts

Table 15.1 *Osteoporosis types*

Localized osteoporosis	Generalized osteoporosis
Disuse osteoporosis (e.g. rheumatoid arthritis)	Endocrine disorders (e.g. Cushing's syndrome)
Neurogenic causes (e.g. poliomyelitis)	Dietary causes (e.g. scurvy)
Encasement of limbs in plaster	Drug caused (e.g. anticonvulsants, heparin)
Immobilization, etc.	Primary senile/post-menopausal osteoporosis

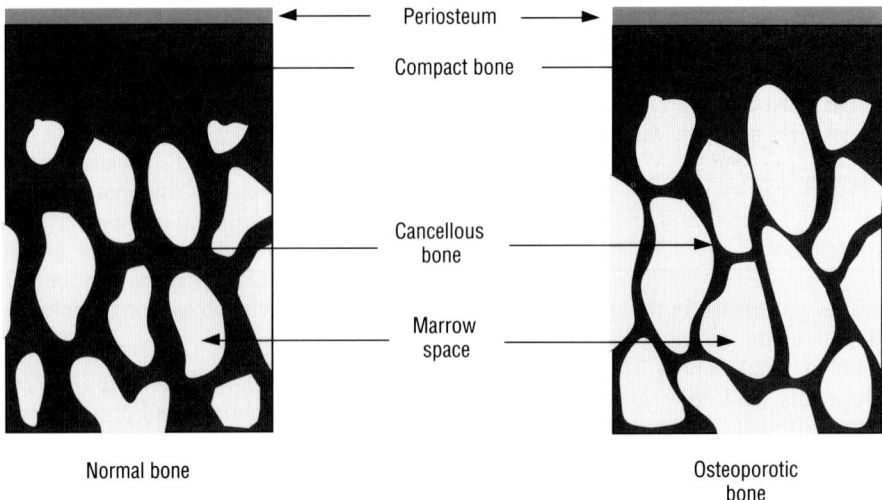

Figure 15.4 *Osteoporosis*

return to earth after prolonged excursions into space, they suffer from this type of osteoporosis in their weight-bearing bones, as the lack of gravity in space means that reduced stresses are experienced by their bones.

Generalized Osteoporosis

In generalized osteoporosis, there is involvement of many parts of the skeleton with the decrease in bone mass being evident almost right throughout the body. Various pathological states may lead to osteoporosis but generally all of these secondary cases of the disease account for only a small proportion of observed cases. The largest group of patients shows primary disease without demonstrable clear-cut aetiological or pathogenetic mechanisms for its development.

Secondary generalized osteoporosis (only a small proportion of cases). **Endocrine anomalies** will lead to this type of osteoporosis, for example **Cushing's syndrome**, where the excess of glucocorticoids will depress the activity of osteoblasts in bones around the body. It seems that the osteoclastic activity is also increased in this disease. The same type of disorder may be seen if excessive, prolonged administration of glucocorticoids is undertaken therapeutically.

Hyperthyroidism is associated with mild generalized osteoporosis due to the excess thyroxine levels stimulating osteoclastic activity and enhancing bone resorption.

Hypogonadism and **hypopituitarism** may lead to generalized osteoporosis mediated by lack of oestrogens or growth hormone.

Secondary generalized osteoporosis may be caused by diseases arising from dietary deficiencies, for example **scurvy**, which is caused by a lack of vitamin C due to dietary deficiency of fresh fruit and vegetables. Vitamin C is essential for collagen formation, osteoid tissue formation, production of intercellular cement substances and maintenance and integrity of blood vessels. In scurvy there is poor wound and fracture healing, lack of osteoid tissue and ground substance formation, bleeding, and osteoporosis which affects the whole skeleton.

The macroscopic appearance of bones in scurvy shows that calcification is normal in bones, with the zone of provisional calcification being a thick white line visible with the naked eye and also in X radiographs. Decreased osteoid formation and haemorrhages occur in the vascular metaphysis and in the subperiosteum and may be seen upon close examination. Microscopically, at the epiphysis the resting and proliferating zones are normal. The zone of provisional calcification is pronounced to form the **scorbutic lattice**. The osteoid deposition at the zone is deficient and a vascular, haemorrhagic, oedematous, myxomatous zone is seen.

Protein deficiency caused by inadequate dietary intake, by excessive loss of protein (e.g. nephrotic syndrome), or by a deficiency in production (e.g. cirrhosis of liver) results in osteoporosis due to the inability of the bone to form osteoid tissue in protein-deficient states.

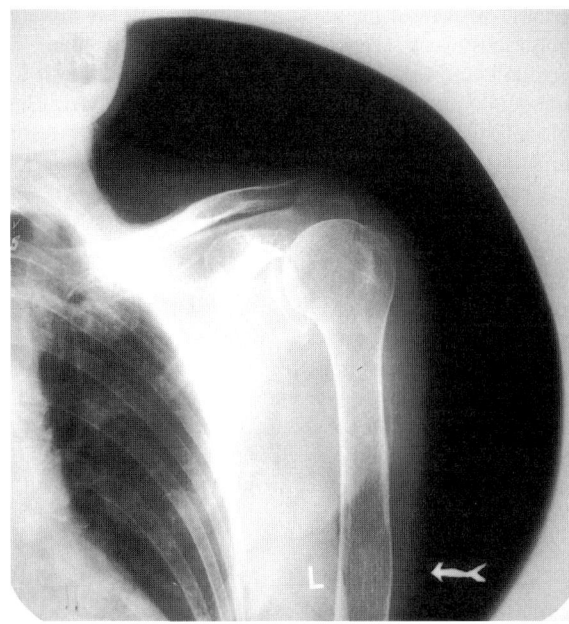

Figure 15.5 *Osteoporosis of the humerus (courtesy of Dr Thomas Molyneux, RMIT)*

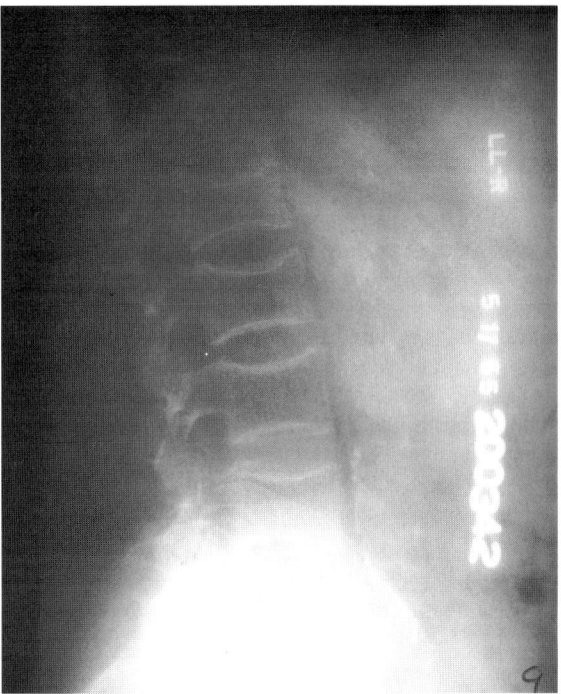

Figure 15.6 *Osteoporosis of the vertebral bodies (courtesy of Dr Thomas Molyneux, RMIT)*

Calcium deficiency and vitamin D deficiency are the most important factors which contribute to the development of osteoporosis as the lack of these compounds will interfere with osteogenesis.

Primary senile/post-menopausal generalized osteoporosis (the majority of cases). This is by far the most commonly seen type of osteoporosis and it is so termed because its aetiology is rather obscure and because it affects post-menopausal women and elderly men. It is thought to be related to ageing, generalized degenerative disease in the body, atrophy, decreased bone mass in the elderly, and genetic factors. It is most often seen in age groups of 50 years or more and is of quite common incidence in the community, 15 to 30% of women over 65 years being affected by it.

The pathogenesis of the disease is extremely complex and has only been correlated with a few specific aetiologies. It appears that several predisposing factors may contribute to the development of the disease. Calcium-deficient diets or inadequate absorption of calcium from the gut seems to be a central issue. Bone is the major reservoir of calcium in the body, 99% of this ion being found in bone. The blood level of calcium must be maintained within narrow limits, reduced levels especially causing muscular contractility problems, tetany, convulsions or even death. Normally,

calcium is absorbed from the gut through the mediation of vitamin D $(1,25(OH)_2D_3)$, activated in the proximal convoluted tubules of the kidney. The enzyme 1-α-hydroxylase activates vitamin D in the kidney and is in turn activated by parathormone. Thus, vitamin D and parathormone work together, parathormone especially being very important in raising plasma calcium. In the intestine the hormone controls the absorption of calcium through its kidney effect on vitamin D hydroxylation. In the kidney it minimizes calcium loss and in bone it initiates bone resorption.

The parathormone effect of osteoclast activation is potentiated by oestrogen deficiency, and thus the process is especially important post-menopausally. Women, who have a lesser skeletal mass than men, are therefore particularly prone to the effects of osteoporosis. It stands to reason that if in youth and young adulthood one has an adequate bone mass, the effects of osteoporosis in old age are not as marked as in an individual who in youth had a deficient bone mass to begin with. In the elderly, where calcium-deficient diets are often common, this, coupled with poor absorption from the gut due to vitamin D deficiency, leads to decreased levels of blood calcium. An increased mobilization of calcium from bone is effected under parathormone production. The low levels of oestrogen increase the sensitivity of bone osteoblasts to parathormone, thus increasing breakdown of bone.

All bones in the skeleton except the skull are affected in primary generalized osteoporosis but especially involved are the spine and upper femur. Generally, the changes are more marked where there is predominance of trabecular bone. The cortical bone is thinned and the cancellous bone is more fragile with thinner spicules, a change known as **osteopenia**. Vertebral changes are quite marked with bulging of intervertebral discs through weakened end plates, giving rise to **Schmorl's nodes**. There is a decrease in stature and thoracic kyphosis (known as 'dowager's hump'), lumbar lordosis and pain occurring quite commonly. The affected bones are prone to pathological fractures or they may collapse. Vertebral collapse with crush fractures of the spine and fractures at the hip are commonly seen. Microscopically what bone is there is normally mineralized but there is gross reduction in trabecular number. Osteoblasts show little activity. The blood calcium and phosphate levels are normal (refer to Table 15.2).

Osteoporosis is not a curable disorder. Treatments for osteoporosis are many and varied and often several regimes are used in combination. In post-menopausal women oestrogen and androgen administration, increased dietary calcium, vitamin D and vitamin C and increased exercise have all been tried with varying results. Whenever such treatments are attempted to combat osteoporosis one should always be aware of the various causes of the disease, and secondary osteoporosis should be ruled out (i.e. it is no use treating the osteoporosis due to multiple myeloma with vitamin D and calcium).

Table 15.2 *Comparison of osteoporosis and osteomalacia*

	Osteoporosis	Osteomalacia
Nature	Reduction in amount of bone but what is left is normally mineralized	Defective mineralization of bone, much osteoid is present in the affected bone
Age incidence	>50 years	>50 years
Sex incidence	Females affected more	Approximately equal
Sites affected	Spine, upper femur esp.	Peripheral skeleton esp.
Aetiology	Endocrine, dietary, idiopathic, genetic factors	Vitamin D deficiency, dietary factors
Features	Thin, fragile bones, Schmorl's nodcs, thoracic humping, lumbar lordosis	Decreased bone density, fragile bones, Looser's zones, 'penguin gait'
Biochemistry of blood		
Calcium	Normal	Normal or slightly lower
Phosphate	Normal	Decreased
Alkaline phosphatase	Normal	Raised
Biochemistry of urine		
Calcium	Normal or slightly raised	Decreased
Phosphate	Normal	Decreased
Complications	Pathological fractures, decrease in stature, spinal changes	Pathological fractures, severe deformities, secondary osteitis fibrosa cystica

Demineralizations

In these bone rarefactions the skeleton contains osteoid tissue, which is deficient in calcium. Usually there is lowered calcium and phosphate in the plasma and the alkaline phosphatase level is raised. The conditions arise most commonly when there is vitamin D and calcium deficiency in the diet. The disorders exist in two major forms, one occurring in children, **rickets**, and the other in adults, **osteomalacia**.

Rickets

This is a generalized bone disease seen in children and is due to a deficiency of vitamin D in the body. It usually results because of a dietary deficiency of vitamin D, failure of absorption of vitamin D, or low dietary intake of calcium or phosphate. Rickets is seen in young children and infants between 6 months and 2 years of age. It is rare in developed countries, but an important disease in developing countries.

As there is a lack of vitamin D, failure of mineralization of osteoid occurs and, most importantly, there is failure of mineralization of the epiphyseal growth plate. The plasma calcium levels are normal or slightly lowered and the phosphate level is lowered to half the normal values. Alkaline phosphatase levels are raised.

Enlarged epiphyseal lines are a hallmark of the condition and they appear as widened, lengthened irregular raised areas. This may be quite a marked change and visible through the skin as occurs in the ribs, giving rise to raised, protruding projections of the costal cartilages down the chest known as the '**ricketty rosary**'. There is softening of the bones and the skeleton becomes soft due to poor mineralization. Deformities occur because of the skeletal softening throughout the body and include:

- **coxa vara**, where the hip joints decrease in angle of inclination between the neck and shaft of the femur ('bow legs'), and a flattened pelvis;
- **scoliosis**, a lateral curvature of the spine;
- **pectus carinatum** (**pigeon chest**), collapse of the ribs, with protrusion of the sternum;
- **craniotabes**, a bossed appearance of the skull due to persistence of sutures and fontanelles and also a flattening of the skull due to the bone softening.

The condition results in stunted growth and delayed dentition. There is widespread muscular weakness and there is a distended abdomen because of abdominal muscle involvement. If rickets is severe and untreated it will cause deformities of the pelvis, important in females who will bear children. Diagnosis of advanced rickets is easy on clinical and radiological findings. The treatment is to correct the dietary deficiencies as early in the course of the disease as possible to prevent deformities and fractures from developing. The disease is rare in Australia even with lack of dietary vitamin D because sunlight allows the skin to form sufficient vitamin D to compensate for the dietary lack.

Osteomalacia ('Rickets in Adults')

In this condition there is a normal amount of osteoid but, due to lack of calcium, it is defectively calcified (refer to Figure 15.7). It is usually due to a low dietary intake of vitamin D combined with little exposure to sun. Old people, usually housebound and on restricted diets, are most affected by this disorder. It may also be seen in pregnancy where there is a drain of vitamin D and calcium to the foetus and a loss of calcium in breast milk. Occasionally it develops after gastrectomy, in malabsorption syndromes and in obstructive jaundice associated with poor absorption of calcium from the gut.

Vitamin D deficiency gives rise to failure of calcium absorption, but increased bone resorption maintains plasma calcium at a near-normal level. The initial hypocalcaemia that is seen in the disorder stimulates the parathyroid to secrete parathormone, resulting in bone resorption and reduction of calcium excretion by the kidney. The plasma phosphate is low and serum alkaline phosphatase is raised indicating increased osteoblastic activity. However, the osteoid that is formed is not being mineralized. As the bones are deficient in calcium and demineralized they are soft, leading to bowing and other deformities.

Patients with osteomalacia present with weakness, fatigue and a characteristic waddling, 'penguin gait'. They may complain of vague aches and pains relating to muscles, bones or joints. Another common presentation is that of pathological fractures with subsequent failure to form mineralized callus which may cause pseudoarthroses to form. **Pseudofractures** may also be seen radiographically in patients with osteomalacia. They form due to 'cracking' of the bone owing to lack of mineralization, and they are radiolucent lines, cutting the bone at right angles and affecting one cortex. They are termed **Looser's zones**, are found commonly on the concave sides of long bones, the medial side of the neck of the femur, the scapula and ribs, and are pathognomonic of the condition. Generalized decrease in bone density is especially noticeable in the peripheral skeleton. In severe cases, weakening and demineralization may lead to severe deformities. Some cases may show secondary osteitis fibrosa cystica due to secondary parathyroid hyperplasia caused by the low calcium level in the plasma (refer to Table 15.2).

The condition is rather difficult to treat, especially if

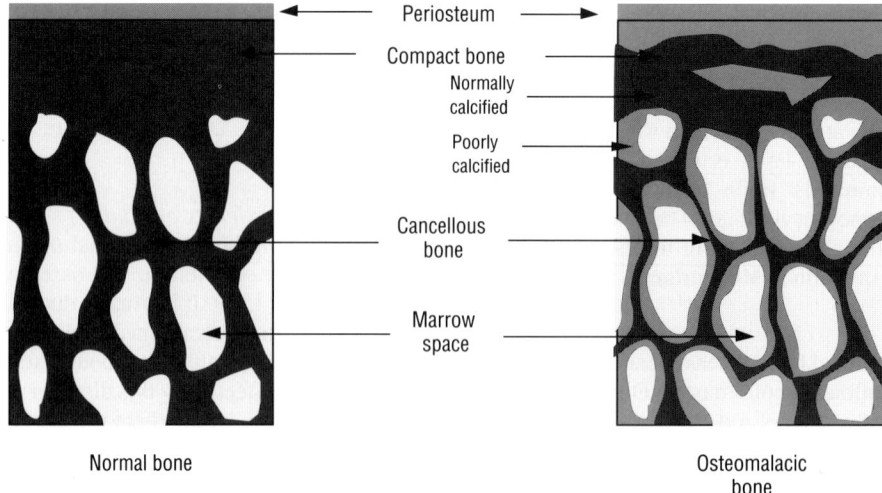

Figure 15.7 *Osteomalacia*

it is in the advanced stages. In females the condition may be precipitated by the reduced levels of oestrogens post-menopausally, therefore oestrogen supplementation is important in the prevention or early treatment of the disease. A balanced diet containing adequate levels of calcium and vitamin D is recommended as well as exercise which will keep the normal stresses on bone, promoting remodelling and osteogenesis.

Hyperparathyroidism

Hyperparathyroidism is also termed **osteitis fibrosa cystica generalisata** or Von Recklinghausen's disease. The disorder is associated with increased parathyroid function. Increased levels of parathormone are secreted and lead to bone rarefaction through activation of osteoclasts. Primary or secondary hyperparathyroidism may cause the rarefaction of bone that is characteristic of the disorder. Primary disease results mainly from neoplasms of the parathyroids, adenomata constituting 85% of cases and carcinomata 5% of cases. Hyperplasia of the glands accounts for 10% of cases of primary hyperparathyroidism. Secondary hyperparathyroidism is seen whenever there are prolonged states of calcium deficiency in the body such as occur in osteomalacia and rickets.

In both cases of hyperparathyroidism the effects are similar: increased levels of parathormone production lead to increased bone resorption in order to increase levels of calcium in the plasma, low plasma phosphate and phosphaturia leading to the formation of renal calculi. The high levels of plasma calcium mediate psychiatric depression, the patient often becoming dejected and mournful, and gastrointestinal anomalies, with bowel sounds often auscultated. In early, mild cases, primary hyperparathyroidism resembles osteomalacia. Later, where there is continued osteoclastic activity, fibrous replacement of the removed bone is characteristic. This change is also seen in the secondary form of the disease. Because of the above presentation the disease is often described as one leading to '**stones, moans, groans with bad bones**'.

Usually, the first skeletal manifestation of the disease is a cystic lesion in the jaw. The cysts are really soft tissue masses within bone and are visible on a radiograph as radiolucent 'cystic' areas. Often, these lesions are referred to by the morbid anatomist as 'brown tumours' because of their appearance (although they are non-neoplastic). Microscopically, they may resemble giant cell tumours of bone and the microscopist often refers to them as 'reparative giant cell granulomata'.

Correction of hyperparathyroidism may be undertaken by removing the tumour if one is present or, alternatively, by correcting the dietary deficiencies. This usually brings bone mineralization back to normal but the cystic lesions may persist.

Renal Osteodystrophy

Renal failure has widespread effects throughout the body, and bone is one of the tissues that is affected severely in this disorder. Renal dialysis that is used to treat renal failure also has serious effects on bone. The kidney is normally intimately involved in maintaining adequate levels of calcium, vitamin D and phosphate in the body. When the glomeruli are damaged in renal disease they will allow retention of phosphate in the plasma, leading to hyperphosphataemia. The tubular damage implies that there will be reduced levels of active vitamin D in the body, which will decrease the amount of dietary calcium absorbed in the gut. The resulting hypocalcaemia stimulates secretion of parathormone and secondary hyperparathyroidism will develop. This will lead effectively to osteomalacia as the parathormone will stimulate bone resorption in order to raise the plasma calcium. Aluminium salts that may sometimes contaminate dialysis machines, if taken into the body, will inhibit mineralization and contribute to osteomalacia.

Some patients on renal dialysis will paradoxically show osteosclerosis, especially in the spine. The mechanism underlying this is obscure, although the hyperphosphataemia seen in the disorder may be important. Metastatic calcification may be found in the arterial walls, eyes, skin and other sites. The treatment of the disease is through the correction of the plasma phosphate levels, control of the hypersecretion of parathormone and supplementation of the vitamin D levels in the body.

Primary Tumours of Bone and Associated Tissues

The general incidence of primary bone tumours is rare (1:100 000). Most primary bone tumours are malignant in the ratio of about three malignant to one benign. The malignant tumours only cause 0.6% of the total deaths from primary malignancies. However, as is often the case with rare diseases, many different types of primary bone tumours have been described. Primary tumours are mainly idiopathic and may arise in bone, cartilage, fibrous tissue and the marrow cavity. Some primary tumours have unknown cells of origin (refer to Figures 15.8, 15.9, 15.10).

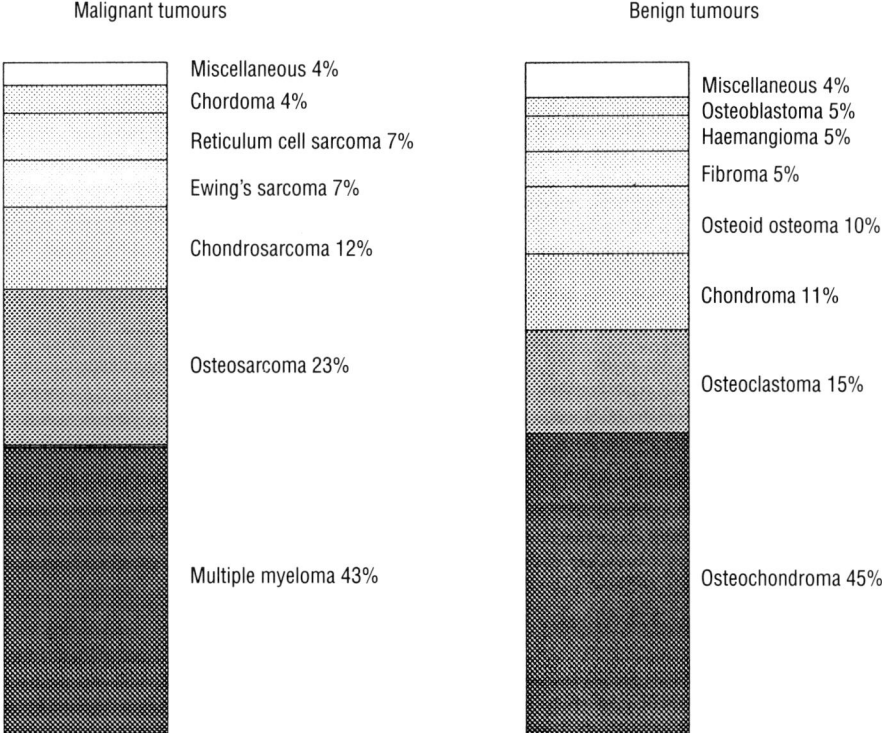

Figure 15.8 *Frequency of benign and malignant bone tumours*

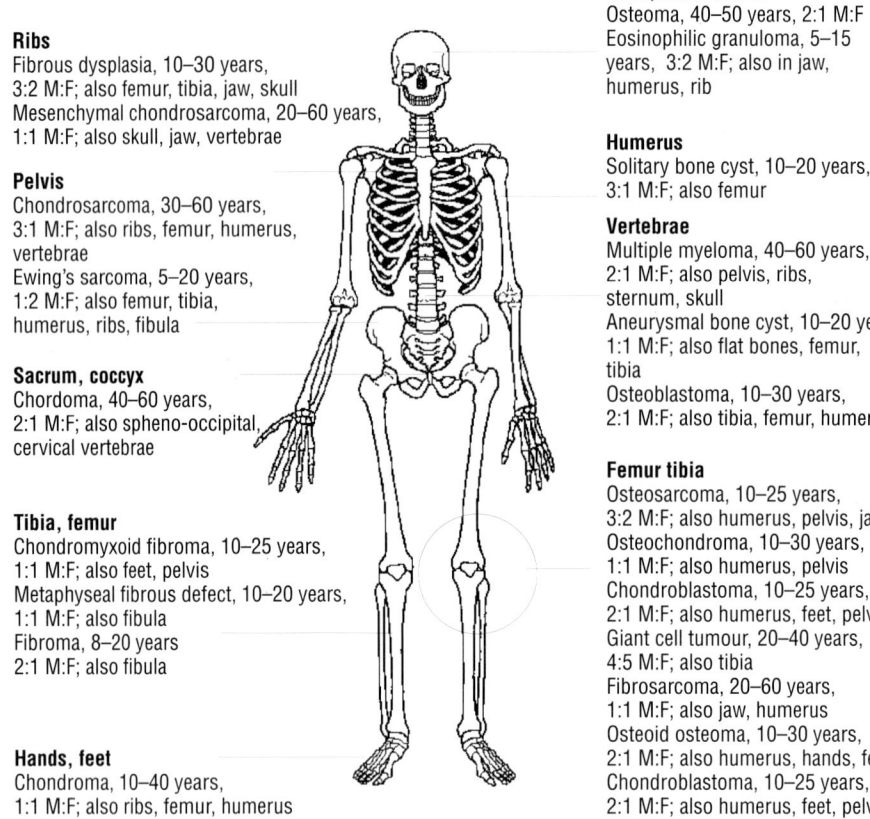

Ribs
Fibrous dysplasia, 10–30 years,
3:2 M:F; also femur, tibia, jaw, skull
Mesenchymal chondrosarcoma, 20–60 years,
1:1 M:F; also skull, jaw, vertebrae

Pelvis
Chondrosarcoma, 30–60 years,
3:1 M:F; also ribs, femur, humerus,
vertebrae
Ewing's sarcoma, 5–20 years,
1:2 M:F; also femur, tibia,
humerus, ribs, fibula

Sacrum, coccyx
Chordoma, 40–60 years,
2:1 M:F; also spheno-occipital,
cervical vertebrae

Tibia, femur
Chondromyxoid fibroma, 10–25 years,
1:1 M:F; also feet, pelvis
Metaphyseal fibrous defect, 10–20 years,
1:1 M:F; also fibula
Fibroma, 8–20 years
2:1 M:F; also fibula

Hands, feet
Chondroma, 10–40 years,
1:1 M:F; also ribs, femur, humerus

Skull, facial bones
Osteoma, 40–50 years, 2:1 M:F
Eosinophilic granuloma, 5–15
years, 3:2 M:F; also in jaw,
humerus, rib

Humerus
Solitary bone cyst, 10–20 years,
3:1 M:F; also femur

Vertebrae
Multiple myeloma, 40–60 years,
2:1 M:F; also pelvis, ribs,
sternum, skull
Aneurysmal bone cyst, 10–20 years,
1:1 M:F; also flat bones, femur,
tibia
Osteoblastoma, 10–30 years,
2:1 M:F; also tibia, femur, humerus

Femur tibia
Osteosarcoma, 10–25 years,
3:2 M:F; also humerus, pelvis, jaw
Osteochondroma, 10–30 years,
1:1 M:F; also humerus, pelvis
Chondroblastoma, 10–25 years,
2:1 M:F; also humerus, feet, pelvis
Giant cell tumour, 20–40 years,
4:5 M:F; also tibia
Fibrosarcoma, 20–60 years,
1:1 M:F; also jaw, humerus
Osteoid osteoma, 10–30 years,
2:1 M:F; also humerus, hands, feet
Chondroblastoma, 10–25 years,
2:1 M:F; also humerus, feet, pelvis

Figure 15.9 *Primary tumours and tumour-like conditions of bone*

Benign Tumours

Osteoma

This is a true, but rare, benign neoplasm of osteoid tissue in which there are areas of well-differentiated compact bone of lamellar structure. The aetiology is largely unknown but various predisposing factors have been suggested as possibilities, examples being former injury at the site, previously occurring osteochondromata or hamartomata. The tumour almost always occurs in the skull or facial bones and appears as a spheroid, dense mass which resembles ivory ('ivory osteoma'). Such tumours are most common in people between the ages of 40 to 50 years and there is a male preponderance.

The tumours are often asymptomatic. If they grow to a big enough size they may cause pressure effects in the cranial cavity or grow into the nasal sinuses and interfere with normal drainage. They may become in-

fected, in which case osteomyelitis will occur. Sometimes, osteomata are associated with Gardner's syndrome in which benign polypoid neoplasms are found in the colon. The diagnosis of an osteoma should immediately be followed by colonic examination and resection of the colorectal polyps, which are premalignant.

Osteomata are treated by excision and as there are usually no clinical effects except for pressure, these growths may often be removed for cosmetic purposes only. The lesions have an excellent prognosis with treatment.

Osteoid osteoma

This is a rare benign tumour of bone producing poorly mineralized bone. It occurs chiefly in the lower limb bones of young adults and adolescents, most tumours occurring between the ages of 10 and 30 years with

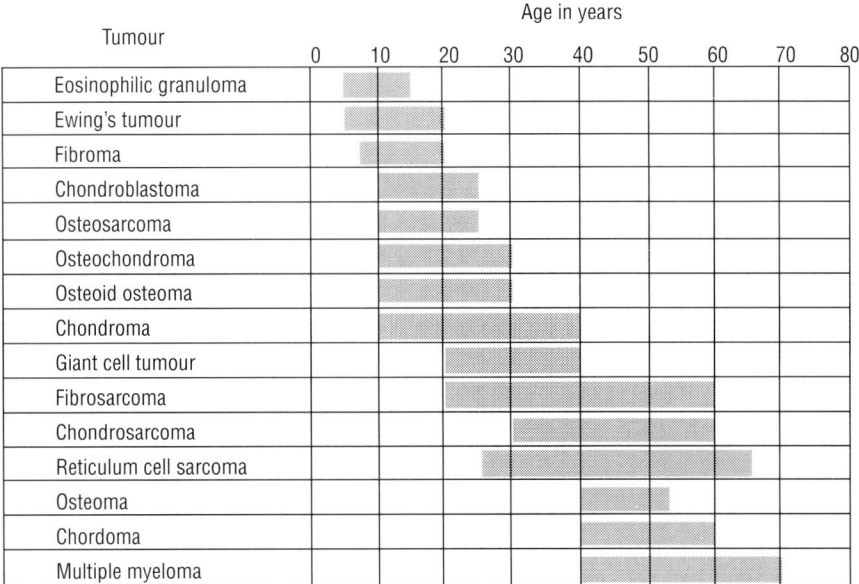

Figure 15.10 *Age distribution of primary tumours and tumour-like conditions of bone*

males being twice as likely as females to present with the tumour. It is one of the more common of bone neoplasms, constituting 11% of all benign tumours of bone.

Although the tumour may be located in any bone, the femur or tibia (or both) are most commonly affected. The lesion is located in the cortex where it erodes the underlying bone, appearing as a red-brown nodule, usually less than 1 cm in diameter. If the lesion is more than 1 cm in diameter it is known as an **osteoblastoma**. The lesion is surrounded by a zone of dense sclerotic bone arising because of reactive osteosclerosis of the surrounding bone in response to the presence of the tumour. Branching and anastomosing trabeculae of osteoid in the tumour are formed by active osteoblasts in a highly vascular connective tissue stroma. The tumour osteoid is patchily mineralized, and often a necrotic area in the centre of the lesion may be found and is known as a **nidus**.

Patients most often complain of a deep, aching pain of gradual onset which is especially severe at night. Local swelling is seen and if the tumour arises near a joint there is a decreased range of motion apparent and also gait disturbances. Patients often report that the pain is relieved by aspirin. When this lesion is of the osteoblastoma type, that is, larger than 1 cm in diameter, it is most commonly seen in the neural arches of the vertebrae. Expansion of a bony tumour of the vertebral arch may lead to compression of the cord and neurological symptoms. Surgical excision is the recommended treatment for these lesions and in the operation the tumour nodule is removed together with the surrounding sleeve of sclerotic bone. The pain that the patient was experiencing is relieved and recurrence of the tumour does not occur provided the whole of the lesion is removed.

Osteochondroma (Exostosis Cartilaginea)

This common neoplasm is due to localized overgrowth of bone, presenting as a bony exostosis projecting from the external surface of the bone covered by a hyalinized cartilaginous cap (Figure 15.11). While the skeleton is growing the osteochondroma will also increase in size, but this growth usually stops at about the age of puberty. Three types of osteochondromata are recognized. A single lesion in bone is called a **solitary osteochondroma**. If only two to three bones are involved, and there is no family history of such lesions, the tumours are referred to as **multiple osteochondromata**. When many tumours are found in many sites, there is usually a family history and the condition is termed **familial**, **multiple exostosis**.

Osteochondroma is the commonest benign bone tumour, accounting for 50% of benign tumours of bone and 10 to 15% of all bone tumours. The tumours are most commonly found in people between the ages of

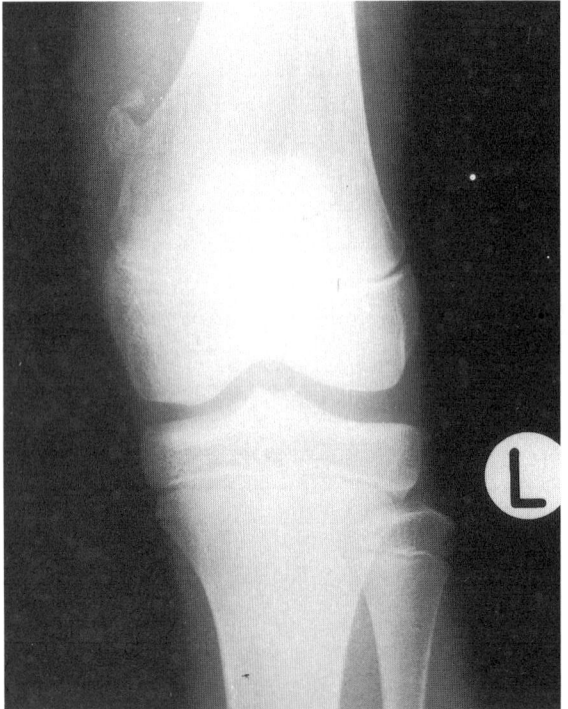

Figure 15.11 *Osteochondroma of the distal femur which shows a fracture. As the lesion protrudes from the bone it is predisposed to trauma and fracture (courtesy of Dr Thomas Molyneux, RMIT)*

10 and 30 years and 70% of the cases occur in patients less than 20 years old. The lesions are slightly more common in males than they are in females. The aetiology of the tumours is unknown but solitary osteochondromata are thought to arise from displaced growth plate cells, or possibly as a sequela to irradiation. In the familial condition genetic factors are operating, a hereditary bone dysplasia giving rise to multiple tumours.

The lesions may occur in any bone preformed in cartilage, but occur most commonly at the metaphyseal surface of long bones, mostly in the distal femur and proximal humerus; the tibia, pelvis, ribs and scapula are also involved commonly. The tumours appear as sessile or pedunculated exostoses arising from the metaphysis of a long bone. Pedunculated lesions are seen most commonly. A bony stalk merges with the normal bone and covering the tip of the lesion is a cap of cartilage. Lesions vary in size and may be up to 10 cm in diameter. Microscopically there is almost normal cartilage at the cap region and below this is a region of calcification giving rise to cancellous bone.

The lesions may be totally asymptomatic or more commonly they may produce a painless swelling on the part affected. Depending on the site involved and the size of the lesion, variable symptomatology will be seen. If the osteochondromata are found within or near a joint, or adjacent to nerves, spinal cord or blood vessels, they may produce decreased range of motion, pain, compression of tissue and sometimes bizarre neurological symptoms if the spinal cord is compressed.

Complications of the conditions include trauma and fracture with haemorrhage, but also 1% of solitary osteochondromata undergo malignant transformation to chondrosarcomata especially. In the familial form, 5 to 25% of these lesions will undergo malignant change. Solitary osteochrondromata may never be treated as they are often asymptomatic. With multiple, symptomatic or diagnosed lesions surgical excision is carried out.

Chondroma (Enchondroma and Ecchondroma)

These are benign cartilage tumours which may arise anywhere in the body where cartilage is found. Some pathologists consider these lesions to be examples of congenital malformations and refer to them as dyschondroplasia rather than chondromata, a term which implies that they are neoplasms. The lesions are divided into two types depending on their presentation.

Enchondroma. These lesions account for at least 10% of all benign bone tumours. They most frequently appear between the ages of 10 and 40 years, affecting males and females equally. They are often described as developmental lesions as they are thought to arise because of failure of normal endochondral ossification. This results in islands of cartilage left within the metaphysis as the growth plate grows upwards.

Tubular bones of the hands and feet are most commonly affected, but lesions may also be found in the humerus, femur, ribs and pelvis. The appearance of the masses is slightly lobulated, glassy, greyish and firm, the lesions encroaching on and eroding the overlying cortex. Reactive bone formation around the tumour occurs. Microscopically the tumour cells resemble normal chondrocytes and foci of calcification or ossification may be observed in the neoplasm. Approximately 80% of these tumours occur in the hands and involve the metacarpals and phalanges and the patient may complain of swelling or pathological fractures (as the lesions are erosive). The condition is often asymptomatic, pain being an uncommon finding.

Treatment of the condition includes curettage, cryosurgery and bone chip packing. The lesions are removed upon diagnosis as malignant transformation, although uncommon, is a possibility. It should be noted that the closer a lesion is to the axial skeleton the more the risk of malignant change.

Ecchondroma. Ecchondromata present as cartilaginous nodules, frequently multiple, which are directed away from the epiphyseal line of origin. They usually occur around the region of the knee joint. There appear to be inherited or familial factors involved in their formation. The lesion may resemble an osteochondroma as the protuberant mass of cartilage often ossifies partially. Three fates have been described for the condition: regression and disappearance; persistence of islands of cartilage and slow growth as a chondroma; and malignant change to form chondrosarcomata or osteosarcomata. The lesions are excised on diagnosis to prevent malignant transformation and accidental complications.

Fibroma of Bone

This is a rare lesion of bone accounting for only 5% of bone tumours, in which a well-defined area of fibrous tissue is seen within bone. Some authors regard it as an area of faulty ossification rather than a true tumour. It affects mainly young people between the ages of 8 and 20 years, occurring twice as commonly in males as it does in females. Sites commonly affected are the tibia, femur and fibula. It may lead to pathological fractures although some lesions are asymptomatic and often some may regress spontaneously.

Chondroblastoma and Chondromyxoid Fibroma

Both of these are exceedingly rare, benign tumours which affect young people of 10 to 25 years of age. They are most commonly found growing around the knee, but also in the humerus, the feet and occasionally the pelvis. They produce pain and local tenderness, swelling and discomfort. Chondroblastoma is found twice as commonly in males, whereas chondromyxoid fibroma is found in equal numbers in both sexes. Of the two, chondroblastoma is more sinister as it may sometimes undergo malignant transformation, Chondromyxoid fibroma is more likely to follow a totally benign course. Both of these tumours are treated by excision.

Haemangioma of Bone

Haemangiomata are benign, tumour-like conditions of bone that are found most frequently in the skull bones and vertebrae (predominantly in the lumbar area). They are usually solitary, microscopic lesions that remain asymptomatic throughout an individual's life and are most commonly discovered as a chance radiological finding. Rarely, the lesion is very large and may occupy most of the mass of the affected vertebral body.

Bone haemangiomata resemble such lesions elsewhere in the body and are composed of vascular spaces lined by endothelial cells, through which blood flows slowly, often undergoing thrombosis. The bone trabeculae are thickened between the vessels and tend to support the vertebra, collapse occurring only very rarely. Most lesions are totally asymptomatic although occasionally neurological symptoms will be seen because of cord compression by a bulging mass.

Tumours of Variable Behaviour

Giant Cell Tumours

The giant cell group represents a very broad variety of tumours and tumour-like conditions. Benign and malignant giant cell tumours are known, but generally all true giant cell tumours are locally invasive, some more aggressive than others. 'Giant cell variants' are also known and many of these are truly benign. True giant cell tumours constitute 15% of all benign bone tumours and 8% of all malignant ones. Twenty per cent of all giant cell tumours are overtly malignant, that is, they metastasize. The remaining 80% are of a benign or 'locally malignant' nature. They occur in young people between the ages of 20 to 40 years and females are slightly more affected, the sex ratio being 4:5. There are very few known predisposing factors to the condition, a very small number of cases arising in relation to Paget's disease. Radiation has also been quoted as an aetiological factor, but the evidence is not conclusive.

The exact histological origin of tumour cells is not known, but it is suspected that they are tumours of stromal cells that have the capability of differentiating into osteoclasts. Microscopically they are seen to be highly vascular tumours of spindle-shaped cells, with many interspersed giant cells resembling osteoclasts. The terms **osteoclastoma** and **osteoclastosarcoma** reflect the belief that they may arise out of osteoclast precursor cells, that is, the monocyte cell line. More correctly they should be termed tumours of 'non-bone-forming, primitive tissue cells of marrow' (Figure 15.12).

The lesions are found commonly around the knee

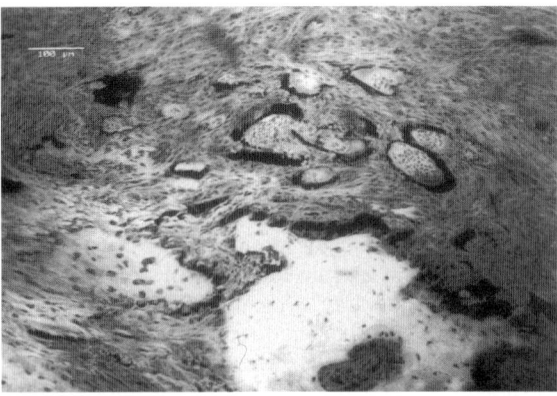

Figure 15.12   *Malignant giant cell tumour of bone actively destroying the bone substance (pale regions) and replacing it with tumour in which numerous giant cells are seen (scale bar is 100 μm)*

joint, with half of the tumours in the lower femur or upper tibia. They are also common in the lower radius and the sacrum. The tumour generally arises in the epiphysis and then spreads to the metaphysis. There is progressive enlargement of the affected region in the bone. The lesion is osteolytic but has a thin shell of bone covering it, the periosteum intact over it. The cut surface is red and fleshy, expanding the bone, with thinning of the cortex. Often the tumour extends into the neighbouring joint or soft tissues. Microscopically two types of cells are found in the tumours:

- typical 'sarcomatous' cells which are spindle-shaped and mononuclear with some round or oval forms also seen. Pleomorphism and mitosis may be noted in this population and it is this cell type which is the guide to the degree of malignancy in biopsies; and
- giant cells of the osteoclast type, with up to 250 nuclei. These cells are scattered throughout the tumour and are not considered to be the malignant element, although they may have been derived from the tumour cell precursor.

Patients present with pain of an intermittent, aching nature. There is swelling and tenderness of the affected area, and often the joint has a restricted range of motion. Because of the osteolytic nature of the tumour, pathological fractures are a common presenting feature. In the uncommon situation of a tumour occurring in the vertebral bodies, fracture and paraplegia may be seen.

All true giant cells tumours are locally malignant, implying that if they are left untreated they will invade and destroy the surrounding bone and joint and spread into the soft tissues around the affected region. About 20% of these tumours will eventually invade the blood vessels and metastasize haematogenously to the lungs.

If the tumour is treated conservatively with curettage there is almost always recurrence; therefore, wide surgical excision is preferred. Cryosurgery may be performed and bone chip packing or grafting is performed if a lot of bone is removed. Amputation is sometimes performed, especially if the tumour is seen on biopsy to be composed of a highly malignant, anaplastic cell population. Radiotherapy is given to patients with surgically inaccessible tumours and with metastases. The 5-year survival is on average 80%. About 33% of the tumours recur as osteosarcomata or fibrosarcomata. With the very malignant tumour variants, the 8-year survival is less than 10%.

Giant Cell Variants

All of these are benign conditions and the common factor is that they all show many giant cells on section. Most commonly, these conditions do not even represent neoplastic lesions but rather a miscellaneous group of disorders or malformations which happen to contain collections of giant cells within them. If a small amount of tissue is biopsied from patients who present with a mass or radiological evidence of a bone mass, the conditions may be confused with true giant cell tumours.

Simple bone cyst (unicameral bone cyst). This condition arises most frequently in young people of less than 20 years of age, the most usual presentation being pathological fractures. The aetiology of simple bone cysts is obscure and it is suggested that they are probably congenital disorders of bone. They appear as a cystic space within bone, easily detected on radiographs. There is a fibrous wall containing numerous giant cells of the osteoclast type. They are not a neoplasm and local excision is curative.

Aneurysmal bone cyst. These lesions are large and often rapidly expanding cysts of the long bones and vertebrae of young people. They are very vascular lesions filled with fibrous tissue and giant cells which contain much haemosiderin. The cells are thought to be macrophage-like and phagocytic rather than osteoclast-like and osteolytic. Aneurysmal bone cysts may greatly alarm both patient and clinician as they imitate malignancy because of their rapid growth. Pathological fractures may occur at the site and on presentation the lesions are treated by curettage which proves curative.

'*Brown tumours*'. These are lesions seen with osteitis fibrosa cystica (see under 'Inflammations, Infections and Degenerations of Bone' above). 'Brown tumours' of bone are composed of cystic, fibrous regions within bone, which on section show giant cells resembling osteoclasts. The condition is associated with an elevated serum calcium level, making their diagnosis slightly easier.

Other giant cell variants. Many other lesions containing giant cells may be seen in bone, for example **giant cell reparative granuloma of the jaw**, which is a benign tumour-like mass containing fibrous tissue and giant cells. **Benign chondroblastoma** often shows many giant cells within it and **non-osteogenic fibroma** often also contains many giant cells within it and may be confused with true giant cell tumours. Regions which show excessive osteoclastic activity may also resemble a giant cell tumour, for example a rarefying bone disease.

Eosinophilic Granuloma of Bone — Histiocytosis

Eosinophilic granuloma is a variant of the group of disorders known as **histiocytosis X**. The other two disorders in the group are **Hand-Schüller-Christian disease** and **Letterer-Siwe disease** In all of these idiopathic disorders there is the common factor of aggregates of histiocytes (= macrophages) laden with cholesterol accumulating within bones and soft tissues. Eosinophilic granuloma represents the localized form of histiocytosis most commonly seen in bone and the lung. It presents usually as one or two lytic lesions in the bones of the skull, jaw, humerus, rib or femur predominantly in children. The masses may cause slight pain, but usually are asymptomatic and are found in a routine X-ray examination. The condition derives its name from the many eosinophils that are scattered throughout the histiocytes. Diagnostic of the condition is the presence of **Birbeck granules** (racquet-shaped bodies seen with the electron microscope, similar to those found in the Langerhans cells of the skin) in the cytoplasm of the histiocytes. It is a benign condition and if treated surgically by excision it is curable.

Eosinophilic granuloma of the lung resembles the lesion in bone, although the condition usually occurs in young adults, presenting clinically as dyspnoea, pneumothorax or severe respiratory distress. It affects the upper lobes of the lung and causes large cystic spaces to form ('honeycomb lung'). In some patients with the lung disease the ribs are also involved. Most patients follow a benign stable course which may improve, but about 20% of cases will progressively worsen and patients may die in respiratory failure.

Hand-Schüller-Christian disease is also a disease of the young but it is widespread, with lesions in many sites of the body including the lungs, stalk of the hypothalamus, pituitary, skull and jaw bones, lymph nodes, skin, liver and spleen. The patients may present with diabetes insipidus, exophthalmos, deafness and lytic lesions in the affected bones. The patients often have a stunted appearance with reduced weight and height for their age. The disease is progressive and invariably fatal, the course being more rapid the younger the patient is.

Letterer-Siwe disease is a severe, systemic disease of infants, seen usually below the age of 2 years. There are tumour-like deposits of histiocytes, plasma cells and reticulum cells in bones, lymph nodes, liver, spleen, lungs and skin. There is progressive involvement of the bone marrow and lungs, leading to death within 2 months. In older patients the disease may have a slower course, taking up to a year to kill the patient.

Malignant Tumours

Although primary bone malignancies account for only 0.6% of deaths from malignancy, they are relatively common among sarcomata, especially in children. Typically, such malignancies are especially common in young people and no satisfactory explanation has emerged to account for this. Some researchers suggest that congenital malformations or inherited defects in bone may be important while other workers regard factors such as repeated trauma or radiation important in their causation. A smaller, second group of patients present later in life with these cancers, the predisposing factor in most cases being Paget's disease of bone.

Osteosarcoma (Osteogenic Sarcoma)
Incidence. Osteosarcoma is a highly malignant primary bone neoplasm and is one of the commonest ten malignancies of bone, accounting for 19% of all malignancies of bone. It is seen most commonly in youth, the affected people being 10 to 25 years of age, although there is a smaller peak of incidence in people 60 to 70 years of age. The condition is slightly more prevalent in males, the sex ratio being 3:2 (refer to Figures 15.9 and 15.10).

Aetiology. The aetiology of the tumour is essentially idiopathic although in a small number of cases tumours have been associated with a variety of factors and conditions which have been shown to be important statistically. Some of these are lised below.

- Greatly at risk are those who are exposed to **radioactive substances**. In the past this tumour afflicted with great regularity workers in clock factories who painted luminous watch dials with radioactive paint. These people used to ingest large quantities of radioactive compounds as they licked the tip of the brush with which they painted to obtain a fine point.
- **Irradiation of bone** has been shown by some studies to be important, but this needs to be a frequent occurrence or the bone has to be subjected to quite high doses of radiation.
- Several **premalignant lesions** are known in bone which predispose to the development of osteosarcomata and these include Paget's disease of bone (especially in flat bones), multiple osteochondromata, multiple ecchondromata and some other benign neoplasms of bone.
- Some tumours appear to be associated with **repeated previous trauma** in the bone site where the tumour arises, and children with osteochondritis juvenilis may present with tumour. It is important to realize that a single traumatic incident such as bone fracture does not predispose the bone to osteosarcoma.
- Some workers have suggested that perhaps **oncogenic viruses** may be involved in the pathogenesis of the tumour, but the evidence is very tenuous.

Sites affected. The tumour occurs primarily in the long bones of the extremities. Commonly affected sites include the femur, tibia and humerus, especially the distal end of the femur (42% of cases), the proximal tibia (16% of cases) and proximal humerus (15% of cases). It may also be seen in the skull (7% of cases), pelvis, mandible and fibula. The location of the tumour within the bone is often taken into account when naming the lesion, for example central osteosarcoma, multicentric osteosarcoma, parosteal osteosarcoma, etc. Juxtacortical osteosarcoma is a rare variant of this tumour and it is usually seen in females older than 25 years. It occurs in the periosteum of the bone, especially the lower femur, and grows outwards, sparing the bone (hence if treated by amputation the prognosis is good with a 5-year survival of 80%).

Morphology. Usually the tumours arise in metaphyseal cancellous bone and then grow into and replace the surrounding bone. The growing lesion then spreads and involves the cortex and soft tissues. As it extends through the cortex, it lifts the periosteum from the cortex and calcification between the raised periosteum and cortex then occurs. This gives rise to the characteristic appearance on radiographs known as **Codman's triangle** (a lesion, however, which is not pathognomonic for osteosarcoma as any condition raising the periosteum will result in this). The cut surface of the tumour shows a greyish white mass in the medulla, cortex and soft tissues, with areas of haemorrhage and cystic necrotic regions. Approximately half of the tumours are hard and gritty, implying that the tumour is laying down a mineralized osteoid; these tumours are termed **sclerosing osteosarcomata**. The others are found to be soft with little mineralization, and are termed **osteolytic osteosarcomata**. However, in all osteosarcomata there is evidence of osteoid formation by malignant cells microscopically as the cell of origin is a primitive osteoblast. If cartilage or collagen are present in large amounts, the tumour looks very pale and has a characteristic, pale, 'fish-flesh' appearance (Figure 15.13).

Microscopically the tumours show malignant elongated cells resembling osteoblasts laying down osteoid in patches and irregular masses which may or may not calcify. The cells are bizarre in size and shape, with pleomorphism, mitotic activity and, frequently, giant cells being observed. Cartilage and often haemorrhagic and necrotic areas may be seen in the tumour. Very

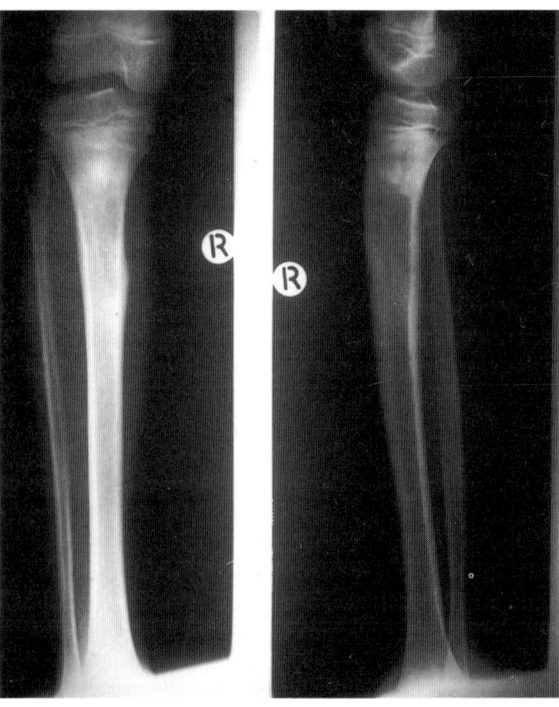

Figure 15.13 *Primary osteosarcoma of the proximal tibia (courtesy of Dr Thomas Molyneux, RMIT)*

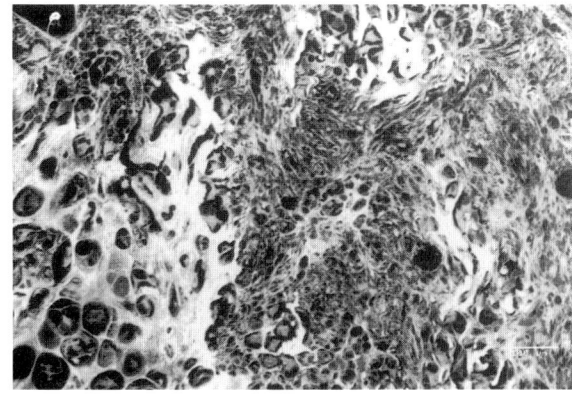

Figure 15.14 *Primary osteosarcoma showing deposition of osteoid and cartilage matrix by the malignant, spindle-shaped cells (scale bar is 100 μm)*

commonly vascular invasion will be detected at the microscopic level (Figure 15.14).

Spread. Spread of osteosarcoma occurs directly to involve the surrounding bony and soft tissues, often with extensive involvement of the joints nearby. Blood spread occurs very early in the tumour's history and is a characteristic feature. Almost always the secondary tumour deposits occur in the lungs. Other organs may also be involved, for example the liver. It is very unusual for this tumour to spread via the lymphatics.

Signs and symptoms. Pain is an early manifestation of the presence of tumour. A painful swelling on the bone appears and gradually increases in size, the pain progressively increasing. Pathological fracture may occur. Systemic signs such as weight loss and fever may be seen. If local swelling, redness and heat with fever and leukocytosis is seen, an infection of the tumour must be suspected.

Diagnosis. Diagnostic X-rays are taken and radiology is often all that is required for presumptive diagnosis of such tumours showing characteristic features. Codman's triangle is noted, and a mottled, permeative lesion with a poorly defined zone of transition is usually seen. The periosteal response is described as being of a '**sunburst**' or '**sunray appearance**' as periosteal new bone is laid down within the extracortical soft tissues and displays transverse spicules or radiating striations. Biopsy will confirm the diagnosis and histology will determine not only whether the tumour is truly malignant but what histological type it is and how well differentiated it is. Biochemistry is often a

diagnostic adjunct as patients characteristically show raised serum alkaline phosphatase levels, a direct result of the osteoblastic activity in the tumour.

Treatment and prognosis. The only effective treatment for osteosarcoma is surgical. Amputation of the affected limb and aggressive surgery of pulmonary metastases is generally the course treatment takes in the young and otherwise healthy patient. Surgical treatment is often complemented by chemotherapy with methotrexate commonly used in this context. Chemotherapy may be the only treatment available in cases where the tumour occurs in the elderly and debilitated, or in very advanced cases of the tumour. Generally, osteosarcoma is a tumour with an extremely poor prognosis because of early metastasis and extensive secondary deposits of tumour in the lungs at the time of diagnosis (Figure 15.15). Average 5-year survival figures of 5 to 25% are commonly quoted for the tumour. Recent combined treatments have yielded some cases with a more optimistic outlook, 5-year survival figures of 50% to 60% being reported. However, in the majority of cases, even with aggressive treatment, death

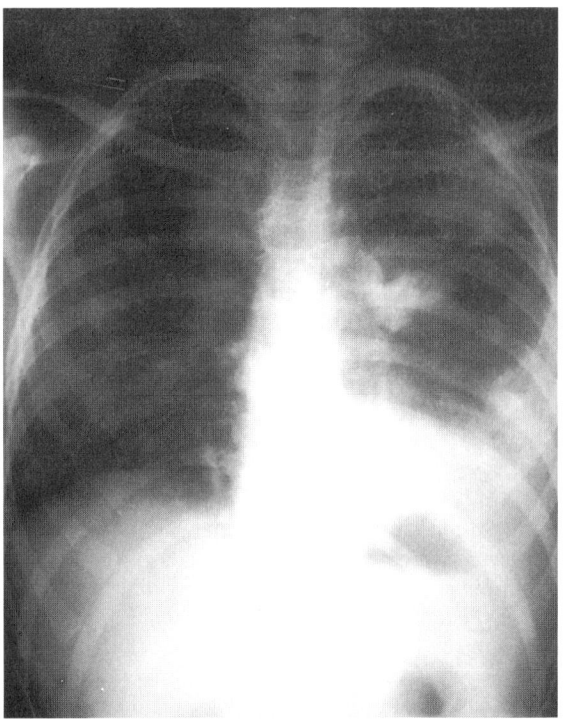

Figure 15.15 *Secondary osteosarcoma (primary in the tibia) of the lungs (courtesy of Dr Thomas Molyneux, RMIT)*

occurs within 6 months of diagnosis, an effect of the pulmonary metastases.

Chondrosarcoma

Incidence. Chondrosarcoma is another common malignancy of bone, accounting for 10% of all cancers of bone. It is seen later in life than osteosarcoma, the patients usually presenting between 30 and 60 years of age. The condition is more prevalent in males, the sex ratio being 3:1.

Aetiology. The aetiology of the tumour is idiopathic although in a small number of cases tumours have been associated with a variety of factors and conditions which resemble those discussed previously with osteosarcoma:

* exposure to **radioactive substances**;
* **irradiation of bone**;
* **premalignant lesions** including Paget's disease of bone, multiple osteochondromata, multiple ecchondromata and some other benign neoplasms of bone. Note that 10% of lesions arise from pre-existing benign chondromata in bone.

Sites affected. The tumour occurs in any bone preformed in cartilage. It commonly involves the pelvis and proximal femur (50% of cases), proximal humerus (10% of cases), ribs (15% of cases), distal femur and proximal tibia (7% of cases) and scapulae (6% of cases). It may arise in the medulla and spread outwards to involve the cortex and soft tissues, or alternatively it may arise from the outer margin of the bone and spread to involve the marrow space.

Morphology. This tumour remains cartilaginous throughout its evolution, producing collagen and cartilage matrix. It is a bulky, lobulated and translucent mass which may be totally within bone or frequently it may extend to the exterior, invading or impinging on soft tissues. White gritty areas of calcification are often seen, even with the naked eye. There may be necrosis and cystic degeneration. Microscopically the tumour consists of highly cellular, atypical cartilage with many pleomorphic tumour cells in the lacunae. Multiple nuclei, mitosis and hyperchromasia are evident in the tumour. Areas of calcification are commonly observed and the greater the degree of calcification the more aggressive the tumour is clinically. Occasionally a chondrosarcoma may be so well differentiated that it is difficult to distinguish it from normal cartilage.

Spread. Growth and spread of chondrosarcoma occurs at a slower rate and less progressively than osteo-

sarcoma. It first involves the surrounding tissues, compressing adjacent structures as it grows. It is not unusual for a chondrosarcoma to be present in a bone for 5 to 10 years, growing slowly and not metastasizing for that length of time. Direct invasion and blood spread occurs at a later stage. The tumour occasionally shows lymphatic spread. The lungs are most commonly involved in secondary tumour deposition.

Signs and symptoms. Pain and swelling of the affected region are noticed, although generally these are late symptoms. Early on, the tumours may be asymptomatic, especially in the peripheral skeleton. If the tumour arises in the pelvis, compression of the bladder, bowel and blood vessels may lead to severe pain. Pathological fractures are quite often the first indication that the tumour is present.

Diagnosis. Radiology and tumour biopsy will confirm the clinical diagnosis. No aberrant biochemical findings are usually noted.

Treatment and prognosis. Excision or amputation of the affected limb as indicated by the stage of the tumour and the extent of its direct spread are the recommended treatment regimes. Radical treatment is preferred because recurrence of conservatively treated tumours occurs and the new tumour is generally incurable. Early treatment has a given figure of 90% for the 5-year survival rate. In later stages and with tumours diagnosed late, 20 to 50% 5-year survivals are to be expected.

Multiple Myeloma (Plasmacytoma)

Multiple myeloma is a malignancy derived from the plasma cells, cells which normally produce immunoglobulins. Although the origin of this tumour is from the haemopoietic tissue of the bone marrow, it is most often included by convention with the primary malignancies of bone.

Incidence. Multiple myeloma constitutes 27% of biopsied tumours of bone and 46% of all malignancies of bone, accounting for approximately 1% of all types of malignant disease in the body. The commonest age group affected (75%) is people between the ages of 50 and 70 years with a male preponderance of 2:1.

Aetiology. The aetiology of the tumour is unknown although it has been postulated that prolonged antigenic stimulation in the body, chronic irritation or inflammation may be important in the causation of the tumour. It is thought that the prolonged antigenic stimulus interacting with plasma cells in inflamed sites may cause loss of growth control of plasmacytes and subsequent neoplastic transformation.

Sites affected. The tumour occurs in many sites around the body and the bones commonly involved are: the lower vertebral column, especially the lower thoracic and lumbar areas (66% of cases involved); the ribs (44% of cases involved); skull (41% of cases involved); pelvis (28% of cases involved); femur (24% of cases involved) and clavicle (10% of cases involved).

Morphology. Multiple myeloma produces 'punched out', soft, red or pink gelatinous areas of osteolysis within the marrow cavities of affected bones. As the tumour foci expand, they often coalesce and erode the cortical bone with destruction of the matrix (Figure 15.16). Pathological fractures are a common feature of the tumour-affected bones. Histologically, the tumour nodules are highly cellular and vascular. Most neoplasms comprise well-differentiated plasma cells with eccentric, 'clock-face' nuclei and basophilic cytoplasm due to the high RNA content. Often, cells with two or three nuclei are observed and many cells also show mitotic figures. Immature plasmablasts are seen in varying numbers.

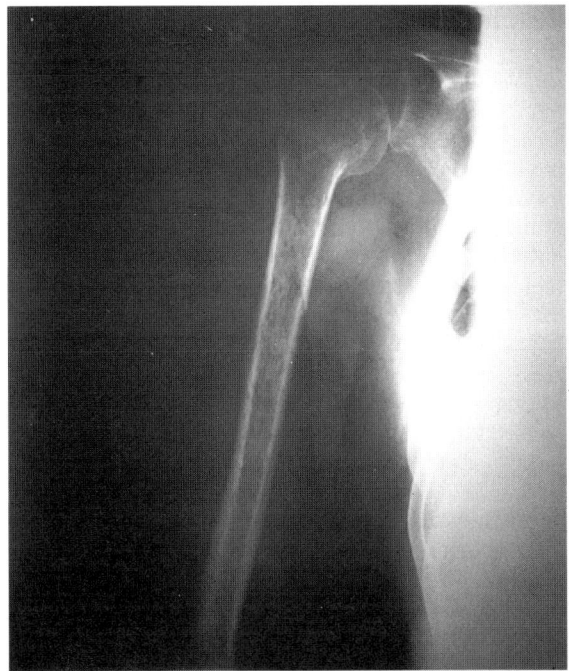

Figure 15.16 *Primary multiple myeloma of the humerus with dislocated humeral head (courtesy of Dr Thomas Molyneux, RMIT)*

Spread. Growth of multiple myeloma occurs in the multifocal sites of origin and subsequently there is spread to involve the surrounding tissues, with haematogenous spread such that the tumour may be found in the soft tissues. Rarely, in advanced cases of the disease there may be a plasma cell leukaemia with many of the malignant plasmacytes found in the circulation.

Signs and symptoms. Most of the afflicted patients first present with pain, often described as deep and exacerbated by activity, diminishing on resting. Weight loss and lethargy are common complaints, together with pathological fractures, soft tissue masses, infection or haemorrhage.

Diagnosis. Conventional radiography is the best means available for diagnosing the tumour, nuclear bone scans often giving a negative result. Early in the disease bone radiography may be normal although biopsy may be positive. A hallmark of the lesion as it develops is a 'punched out' pronounced, osteolytic defect in the bone which occurs multiply in the spine, skull and pelvis. Osteoblastic lesions are rarely seen. Laboratory and biochemical investigations are commonly used to confirm the diagnosis. Mild to severe anaemia is often found with a normal white cell count and raised erythrocyte sedimentation rate. About 30% of patients have a hypercalcaemia with normal phosphate levels due to the bone lysis. Approximately 60% of patients have raised plasma protein with a reversed albumin to globulin ratio caused by the excessive secretion of immunoglobulins by the tumour. In the urine, light chains of immunoglobulins will be found in about 40% of patients and these are termed the **Bence-Jones proteins**. Hyperuricaemia is often observed due to the accelerated nucleic acid metabolism.

Treament and prognosis. Chemotherapy is the most useful treatment regime for patients with multiple myeloma, although this is often combined with radiotherapy as the latter is of use in controlling pain. Excision of the tumour masses is impossible as they occur in multiple sites in the skeleton. Ambulation of the patient and adequate hydration are very important. Treatment of any other presenting features is undertaken, for example stabilization of pathological fractures and spinal cord decompression, requiring surgery. The prognosis of the tumour remains very poor despite advances in diagnosis and treatment. Over 90% of patients die within 3 years of diagnosis. Patients with good renal function have a better chance of long-term survival.

Fibrosarcoma

This is a very rare malignant tumour comprising 3% of bone tumours. It is a neoplasm in which fibro-collagenous-type tissue is seen, with no tendency of tumour cells to form osteoid or bone. It occurs mainly in young adults, most cases being seen between 20 to 60 years of age. The lesion affects males and females equally. Although the condition is idiopathic, several predisposing conditions are documented and include Paget's disease of bone, fibrous dysplasia, long-standing chronic osteomyelitis and irradiation of bone.

It frequently involves the ends of long bones, although occasionally it will occur in midshaft positions. Periosteal tumours are rarer and are found to arise in the periosteum, forming a dense white tumour invading the soft tissues more than the adjacent bone. Endosteal forms are commoner, giving rise to a firm white tumour mass in the medullary bone. As the tumour expands and grows it will destroy the bone, spreading outwards. Microscopically the tumour may be well differentiated and populated with tissue of a collagenous connective tissue appearance. Spindle-shaped cells surrounded by strands of collagen are seen. Pleomorphism, mitotic activity, invasion and other typical features of malignancy are readily observed in these tumours. Anaplastic forms may occur and the cells in these lesions are very pleomorphic, have multiple nuclei and show hyperchromasia. Regions of necrosis and haemorrhage are often found in the mass. Direct spread of the tumour occurs early and there is lymphatic and blood metastasis to involve the lungs and liver.

Symptoms and signs associated with fibrosarcomata include localized pain, swelling and pathological fractures. The tumour is treated by amputation of the affected limb, but generally most tumours present late and thus the average 5-year survival is approximately 30%, indicating a rather poor prognosis.

Ewing's Tumour of Bone

This is often also termed 'round cell tumour'. It was first described by Ewing in 1921. The exact cells of origin are not known but it is believed that the neoplasm arises from cells of the reticuloendothelial system in the bone marrow. It comprises 7% of all malignancies of bone and affects individuals between the ages of 5 and 20 years. Males appear to be slightly more affected than females. This tumour is most often encountered as a paediatric case.

Midshaft positions in the long bones, occasionally the pelvis and other flat bones are the sites favoured by the tumour. The tumour masses are fleshy and non-bony with a zone of reactive bone formation around them, causing a typical radiological finding called an '**onion skinning**' effect. Microscopically the tumour is composed of sheets of uniform, round or polyhedral cells with little cytoplasm and large hyperchromatic nuclei. Little or no stroma is seen. There is no bone, cartilage or fibrous tissue in the tumour. Haemorrhage and necrosis may be observed within the mass. Local direct spread of the tumour first occurs with destruction of surrounding bone and early invasion of blood vessels with secondary tumours developing in the lungs.

Patients present initially with dull pain which gradually becomes more severe as a palpable, soft tissue mass develops. These tumours are diagnosed radiologically and by biopsy. Differential diagnosis should include a **neuroblastoma** from the adrenals forming secondary deposits in bone, which may resemble Ewing's tumour histologically, but in this case there is a pronounced reticulin fibre network between the tumour cells. Radical operative procedures early in the history of Ewing's tumour have yielded a few long-term survivors but generally this is a rapidly fatal condition with an average 5-year survival of less than 5%.

Chordoma

Chordoma is a malignant tumour that arises from remnants of the notochord. Most of the cases occur between the ages of 40 and 60 years, although there is a smaller group presenting at about 35 years. The tumours most commonly arise in the sacrococcygeal area, but they may also arise in the base of the skull at the sphenoid and occipital areas, rarely at other sites in the vertebral column. The tumour is twice as common in males as it is in females.

Chordoma produces large, soft and gelatinous tumours that are locally destructive as they extend into the surrounding tissues, destroying the adjacent bones of the site they arise in. Haemorrhage, cystic areas and calcification are often present in the tumour. Microscopically the tumour cells are seen to be polyhedral, vacuolated and arranged in clumps and irregular groups. The stroma is mucoid and has scant fibrous elements.

The tumour grows slowly and invades actively into the surrounding tissues. It may present as a space-occupying lesion in the skull, cause spinal cord compression or be found as a pelvic mass, depending on the site of origin. The tumour has been found to invade lymphatics and spread to draining lymph nodes, but also spreads via the bloodstream to give rise to secondary tumours in the lungs and liver. At diagnosis, most chordomata are too advanced to treat surgically and therefore long-term survivors are few.

Reticulum Cell Sarcoma

Reticulum cell sarcoma of bone may be considered to be a solitary, anaplastic, lymphosarcoma that bears no relation to the more generalized types of lymphosarcomata. The tumour occurs between the ages of 30 and 60 years and affects the sexes equally. The tumour is discovered radiologically as a radiolucent mass usually midshaft in the long bones, the femur, tibia, humerus and ribs especially, but is also found in the pelvis, vertebrae and skull bones.

Microscopic examination of the tumours shows irregular masses of basophilic, rounded, reticulum cells that produce reticulin. The bone is invaded and replaced by the tumour. Reticulum cell sarcomata are radiosensitive and the prognosis is relatively good, as many as 50% of patients surviving for 5 years.

Secondary Tumours of Bone

Secondary tumours of bone, usually carcinomata, are much more common than primary malignant tumours of bone and will be found in 15 to 20% of all fatal cases of malignant disease. Secondary bone neoplasms account for about 70% of all tumours in bones. Primary bone tumours (benign and malignant) account for the remaining 30% of all tumours in bones. Certain carcinomata show a predilection for metastasizing to bone, for example tumours of the bronchus, breast, prostate, thyroid, stomach and kidney and also some lymphosarcomata.

Multiple tumour nodules are found in the affected bone, which is usually one containing red marrow. Common sites for the development of secondary bone tumours are the vertebrae, large long bones such as the femur, and the ribs (Figure 15.17). Most secondary bone tumours are **osteolytic**, causing local breakdown of the bone as they grow and invade it, or they may be **osteosclerotic**, especially neoplasms derived from the prostate, breast or Hodgkin's disease. This latter group of tumours cause the stimulation of osteoblasts in the adjacent bone with a subsequent increase in serum alkaline phosphatase levels detectable in the laboratory. In both cases the presence of tumour inside the bone causes it to become a great deal weaker, as the tumour tissue replaces the bony tissue. One of the commonest presentations of this type of disorder, therefore, is **pathological fracture** of the affected bone.

The tumours are detected by radiography or by nuclear bone scans which are indicated if a primary tumour is found in sites which commonly metastasize to bone. Treatment is usually limited to a combination of radiotherapy and chemotherapy, which relieves the symptoms. Generally, patients who present with tumour secondaries in bone have a very poor prognosis as these secondary deposits coexist with the primary tumours and often with multiple metastases in other parts of the body.

Joint Diseases

Metabolic Diseases

Gout

Gout is a group of inherited, metabolic diseases in which there is hyperuricaemia and deposition of urate crystals in and around joints. The affected patients (80 to 95% of them male) have a defect in the metabolism of protein and nitrogen with an excessive level of uric acid being formed and circulating in the bloodstream, in levels above 7 mg/dL. The disease has been known since ancient times and gout has been demonstrated in Egyptian mummies. The disorder is inherited as an autosomal dominant defect but other factors are important in its development such sex and hormones. Some enzymatic defects that lead to hyperuricaemia are X-linked. It was noted by Hippocrates that women did not present with gout until after the menopause. Most male patients present with the first attack of the disease between 35 and 50 years, whereas females present between the ages of 50 and 60 years. Incidence data from different countries vary between 2 and 20 per 1000 males and may be as high as 30 per 1000 males. Figures for females are generally lower (1 to 3 per 1000 females). In some groups there is even a higher incidence and in some Polynesian islands where the disease is common, familial factors are thought to be responsible. In Australia it is estimated that there are 75 000 sufferers from gout, 80% of whom are men mainly between the ages of 35 to 50 years.

The disease is divided into a primary and a secondary form, depending on whether a metabolic defect is present. **Primary gout** occurs if there is a congenital deficiency in hypoxanthine guanine phosphoribosyl transferase with an overactivity of 5-phosphoribosyl-1-pyrophosphate synthetase, both enzymes being X-linked. The genetic anomaly will lead to increased levels of uric acid in the plasma. **Secondary gout** may develop in the absence of the metabolic defect or family history of the disease if there is an overwhelming overproduction of uric acid in the body coupled with a reduced excretion, leading to a hyperuricaemia. This state may be brought about by various drugs acting on the kidney tubules, by dietary factors and by increased breakdown of body cells. Both primary and secondary gout develop whenever there are long-standing levels of high uric acid in the bloodstream.

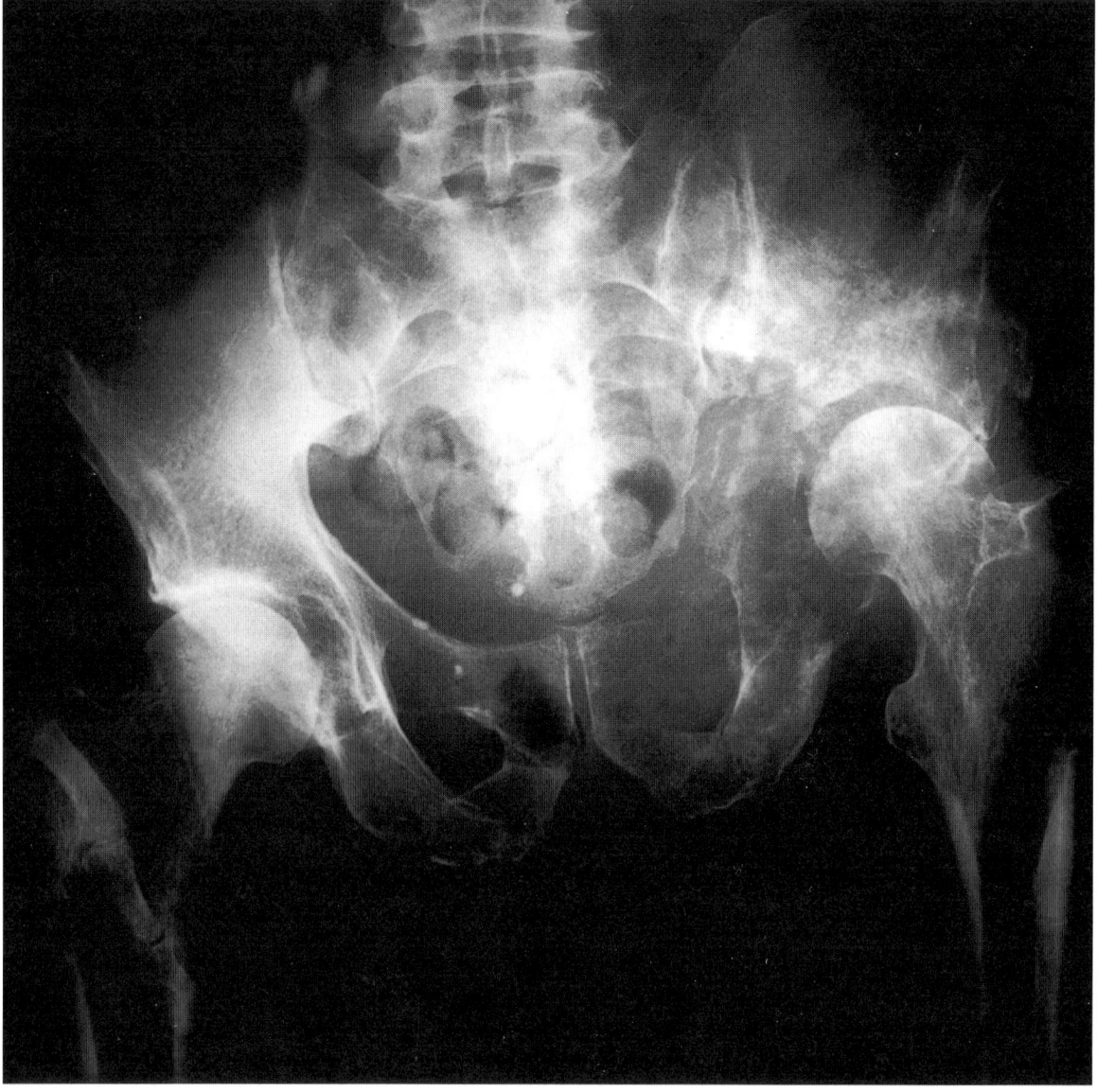

Figure 15.17   *Secondary lytic metastatic tumour deposits in the pelvis, the primary site of the tumour being unknown (courtesy of Dr Thomas Molyneux, RMIT)*

In about 80% of affected people the lesions first develop in the first metatarsophalangeal joint of the great toe, **podagra** being the term applied to this condition. The patient usually describes onset of acute pain, often at night or following trauma (either recent or old injury in that site). The disease may also develop following stress, alcoholic or dietary excesses. Systemic manifestations such as fever are very rare. Many patients recover from this first attack and are not affected by the disease for years or sometimes ever again.

Chronic gout is associated with long-standing hyperuricaemia, and generally poor treatment or patient non-compliance lead to it. Crystallization of uric acid and its salts occurs and there is deposition of the crystals in the soft tissues, where the needle-like crystals of sodium biurate set up a chronic inflammatory granulomatous reaction. The lesion so formed is known as a gouty **tophus**. Gouty tophi are found in cartilaginous sites such as the helix of the ear, around joint cartilage and in tendons but also in the kidney and rarely in heart, pleura and meninges. Tophi are discrete nodules and are associated with inflammation. If subcutaneous, the skin over them may become smooth and shiny, finally ulcerating with release of a chalky white material, representing the urates deposited in the tophus. Radiologically, tophi have a characteristic appearance, with the erosions in cartilage and bone of the joint overlaid by soft tissue swelling and secondary deposits of calcification.

Urates in the body largely result as an end product of purine metabolism from the breakdown of nucleoprotein. Foods high in purines, such as wheat, should be avoided by sufferers of gout. Weight reduction, avoidance of alcohol and increased urine output by consuming more non-alcoholic beverages may also be of use. Drug therapy for the condition involves several compounds which act to reduce the uric acid levels in the blood (e.g. allopurinol), anti-inflammatory drugs and analgesics (e.g. indomethacin) to manage acute gout, or even intra-articular steroids may become necessary for severe inflammation of the joints.

There are long-term complications in poorly managed gout. The production of excessive uric acid leads to its increased excretion via the kidneys, often causing renal calculi to form (urate stones). There is associated vascular disease and systemic hypertension due to unknown reasons, and renal failure due to nephritis may develop. In affected joints there is eventual destruction of articular cartilage and the condition may mimic osteoarthritis. Effective treatment of gout nowadays means that no patient should have to suffer from acute attacks. The kidney disease is no longer a common cause of death and most patients suffer ill effects from the vascular system complications. These may be controlled by antihypertensive medications and also by balanced diets low in saturated fats and high in fibre.

Infections

Infections of joints are not commonly seen primarily, and usually result after haematogenous spread of microbes to joints, or as some complication of an infection in adjacent sites of osteomyelitis or soft tissue infection. Infrequently, the infection may arise out of direct introduction of micro-organisms into the joint cavity as a result of penetrating injury or as a complication of a diagnostic or surgical procedure (arthroscopy being the most frequently performed nowadays).

Viral Arthritis

This type of arthritis results infrequently as a complication of the viraemic phase of viral infections that predominantly have localized elsewhere in the body. Examples of viruses which may occasionally cause an arthritic manifestation are hepatitis B virus, rubella virus and various arthropod-borne viruses such as the Ross River virus. This type of arthritis leads to swelling and inflammation of the joint with variable degrees of limitation of the range of motion of the joint. The condition usually resolves.

Bacterial Arthritis

The type of bacteria isolated from cases of bacterial arthritis depends on the age of the patient and health status. For example, in the neonate and young infant it is common to see *Staphylococcus aureus* or *Escherichia coli* causing joint infections. In slightly older infants up to 2 years of age, *Haemophilus influenzae* and *Staphylococcus aureus* are implicated. In the otherwise healthy adult *Staphylococcus aureus* may cause arthritis or the joint infection may complicate gonorrhoea, in which case *Neisseria gonorrhoeae* will be isolated from the affected joint. Young females are more likely to present with this latter type of arthritis. If the patient is debilitated, as occurs with the elderly, alcoholic or drug-addicted patient, many other bacteria may be isolated, for example *Streptococcus pneumoniae*, *Pseudomonas* spp. and *Serratia* spp.

In all of the cases mentioned above the infected joint shows the typical signs of acute inflammation, heat, pain, redness and swelling, with marked loss of function as manifested by immobility and decreased range of motion. Within the joint cavity will be found a purulent exudate which may lead to **pyoarthrosis** (a collection of frank pus within the joint capsule). Systemic manifestation of the infection such as leukocytosis and fever will also be present. Occasionally, tuberculous arthritis may be seen to complicate a case of pulmonary tuberculosis and in this case typical granulomata will form in the joint.

In recent times a new bacterial infection of joints has been characterized and this is termed **Lyme disease**, so designated as it was first described in the town of Lyme, Connecticut, eastern USA. The disease has now been reported in other American states, Europe and Australia. It is caused by a spiral bacterium, *Borrelia bungdorferi*, which is transmitted by the bite of infected body lice or ticks. The disease characteristically begins around the bitten site as a typical red skin lesion termed **erythema chronicum migrans**, with about half of cases also showing multiple, annular expanding secondary lesions.

The patient with Lyme disease complains of chills, fever, malaise, fatigue, general aches and regional lymphadenopathy. Arthritic manifestations then develop, commonly in the knee, other large joints and temporomandibular joints. The symptoms last 1 or 2 weeks and then recur at intervals over years. Neurological and cardiac complications may develop in untreated cases. Diagnosis depends largely on serology. Tetracyclines are the recommended drugs for treatment of Lyme disease and early treatment prevents joint involvement and the systemic complications.

Fungal Infection

Rarely, fungi may be isolated from a case of infective arthritis and in almost all instances these infections occur in severely debilitated or immunocompromised patients as a complication of blood-borne spread of such organisms as *Candida albicans* or *Aspergillus* spp.

Inflammation of Joints

Rheumatoid Arthritis

Rheumatoid arthritis (RA) is a non-suppurative, non-infectious, proliferative synovitis. Progressive destruction of articular cartilage is a characteristic of the disorder and the result is an increasingly disabling arthritis with deformity. Extra-articular involvement of other tissues makes it resemble systemic diseases such as SLE, scleroderma and other connective tissue diseases.

Incidence. The disease is seen predominantly in females, the sex ratio being 1:3. The incidence of the disease in the Australian population is approximately 3%. The onset of disease occurs usually in young adulthood but may occur anywhere between the ages of 30 to 60 years, with slow progression over many years or decades. It appears that the disease has a slightly higher incidence in urban populations compared to rural populations.

Aetiology. RA is a classical autoimmune disorder with self-perpetuating inflammation occurring in the joints resulting from immune reactions. The trigger setting off the autoimmunity is unknown but various agents have been speculated to cause it. They include various bacteria (especially some of the enteric bacteria), mycoplasmata, Epstein-Barr virus, etc. The precise triggering agent may not be a single organism but may vary from person to person. Genetic factors are extremely important in determining predisposition to development of the disease. RA patients possess the HLA antigens DW4 and DRW4 significantly more frequently than non-affected people. The percentage of patients with DW4 is 35 to 55% compared with controls without the disease where the incidence is 10 to 20%. About 50 to 80% of patients possess the antigen DRW4, compared with the normal people's incidence of 20 to 40%. As females are affected more than males, hormonal factors are thought to influence its development. Supporting evidence for this is that

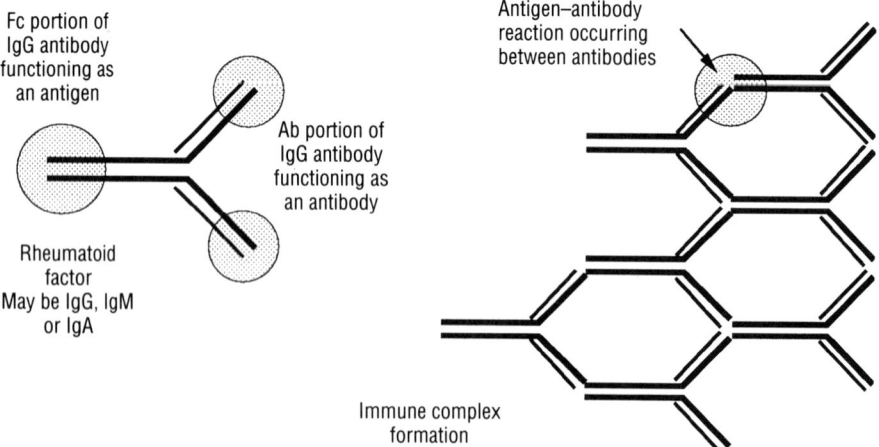

Figure 15.18 *Autoantibody in rheumatoid arthritis*

the disease tends to become quiescent during pregnancy. In summary it may be said that the joint damage of RA is autoimmune in nature, appearing in genetically predisposed individuals after exposure to an unknown trigger.

Pathogenesis. Immune mechanisms cause the lesions in the disease and both humoral and cell-mediated mechanisms are involved. Most RA patients have greatly increased levels of immunoglobulins in their bloodstream. The majority of patients have in their plasma an antibody called **rheumatoid factor** (RF) which is an autoantibody (see Figure 15.18). It is specifically directed against the Fc portion of autologous IgG. Rheumatoid factor is an immunoglobulin mainly of the IgM class but IgG and IgA antibodies may also function as rheumatoid factors. The IgM rheumatoid factor is not found in the affected joints but in the plasma and its level there is related to the severity of the disease the patient is experiencing. IgG is found in the affected joints and is thought to cause the articular damage. This intra-articular IgG functions both as the antigen and antibody, a situation leading to the formation of immune complexes. It should be noted that rheumatoid factor may be found in other diseases, such as Sjögren's syndrome, SLE, scleroderma, chronic active hepatitis, fibrosing alveolitis, pulmonary tuberculosis, syphilis, leprosy, and in normal elderly people and relatives of patients with RA.

A type III (Arthus-type) hypersensitivity develops at the site where the immune complexes form, usually this reaction taking place intra-articularly. The immune complexes lead to platelet aggregation and degranulation, with microthrombus formation and vasoactive amine release. Complement is activated and many neutrophils are attracted to the region, where they begin phagocytosing the complexes, degranulating and causing tissue damage. Other effects of complement fixation include anaphylatoxin and histamine release which increase the inflammation. The results of these processes within the joint are damage to the synovium and to the articular cartilage. The synovium is a very vascular tissue and there is widespread inflammation at this site with infiltration by neutrophils and plasma cells, the IgG rheumatoid factor being formed *in situ* (refer to Figure 15.19).

It is also important to realize that T cells and cell-mediated responses contribute to the tissue damage. Within the inflamed synovium and in the bloodstream the helper T4 cells are greatly in excess and it is believed that these mediate the type IV, delayed hypersensitivity reactions which contribute to the tissue damage. The activated T cells produce lymphokines, substances which attract and activate macrophages, promote the growth of fibroblasts and cause bone resorption. Activated macrophages produce a host of factors which cause bone and joint destruction and perpetuate inflammation.

The persistent inflammation leads to proliferative changes in the joint with the formation of the **pannus** (Latin for 'cloak') of RA. This is a granulation tissue forming in the synovium and eventually spreading within the joint cavity and covering the articular cartilage, like a cloak.

Sites affected. The disease is described classically as a symmetric polyarthritis. It affects the small joints of the hands, feet and ankles. Larger joints such as the

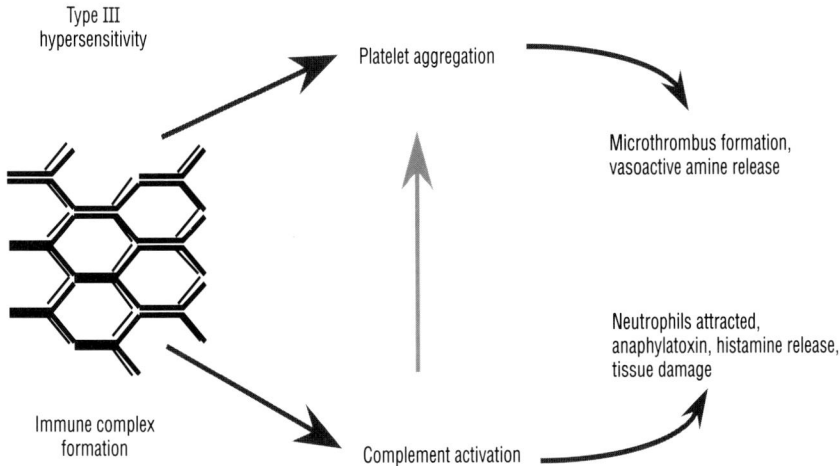

Figure 15.19   *Type III hypersensitivity in rheumatoid arthritis*

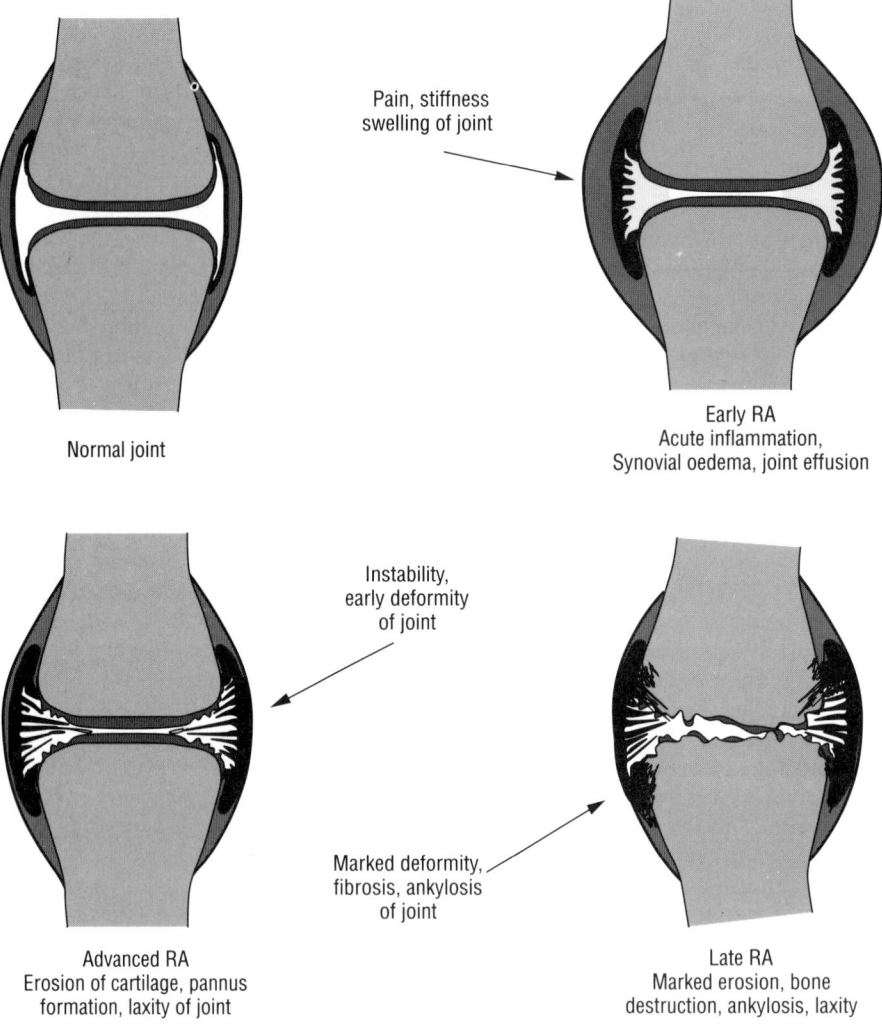

Pain, stiffness
swelling of joint

Normal joint

Early RA
Acute inflammation,
Synovial oedema, joint effusion

Instability,
early deformity
of joint

Marked deformity,
fibrosis, ankylosis
of joint

Advanced RA
Erosion of cartilage, pannus
formation, laxity of joint

Late RA
Marked erosion, bone
destruction, ankylosis, laxity

Figure 15.20   *Development of rheumatoid arthritis*

knees, wrists, elbows and shoulders may also be involved. The temporomandibular joints (TMJs) and the vertebral column are also involved in many patients. In the beginnings of the disease, multiple sites are affected in about 30% of cases. The joints of the hands, feet, knees, ankles and wrists are affected. In established disease, hand, foot, ankle, wrist, elbow, neck joints and TMJs are involved.

Morphology. The disease begins as a non-specific inflammation of the synovium, acute synovitis, with swelling, hypertrophy of the synoviocytes and hyperplasia of the connective tissue elements beneath. As the disease progresses, the proliferation of the

synovium becomes more marked with frond-like growths (**fimbriae**) projecting into the joint space. The synovium appears red and swollen and there are polymorphs and fibrin present. In later stages, macrophages and lymphocytes infiltrate the tissue, the lymphocytes and plasma cells forming follicles. Gross deformity of the connective tissue follows. Quiescent episodes may then cause a reduction of the inflammation and pain but there is always an infiltrate of lymphocytes and plasma cells within the joint capsule and synovium. Neutrophils will infiltrate the surface of the synovium during acute inflammatory episodes in exacerbations of the disease. As the inflammation continues, there is degeneration of connective tissue and necrosis. The **pannus** forms, and essentially this is a vascular connective tissue that grows into the joint space. There is destruction of articular cartilage and bone as the inflammation progresses, and the pannus eventually fills and obliterates the joint space (see Figure 15.20).

Fibrosis and calcification of the damaged joint may cause permanent **ankylosis**. Changes in the synovial fluid are also observed in RA as the disease progresses. There is an increased volume and turbidity of fluid, decreased mucin content and increased numbers of cells within it. Necrotic bone and cartilage fragments may float free in the joint cavity. Osteoarthrosis may supervene in these damaged joints. There is disuse atrophy of the bone and muscles working the affected joints, associated with the disuse of the joint.

Systemic manifestations. Rheumatoid subcutaneous nodules are present in about 25% of patients. They are most commonly found in the region of the elbow, but may also occur around the Achilles tendon, the back of the skull and the region of the tibia. Firm, non-tender, oval or round masses up to approximately 2 cm in diameter are seen to form in these sites. Microscopically, there is a focus of central fibrinoid necrosis surrounded by macrophages, lymphocytes, plasma cells and fibroblasts laying down collagen. This lesion is often described as a granuloma. Occasionally, these lesions may also be seen in the viscera especially the spleen, lungs and pericardium (Figure 15.21).

Other systemic manifestations include a necrotizing vasculitis in many sites around the body, Raynaud's phenomenon, a fibrinous pleurisy, progressive inter-stitial fibrosis of the lungs (**Caplan's syndrome**) and eye changes including uveitis and keratoconjunctivitis. Splenomegaly, lymphadenomegaly and anaemia may be seen combined with malaise, fatigue and depression (**Felty's syndrome** or **Still's disease** in children). Amyloidosis may also supervene in a significant number of patients (5 to 10% of cases).

Signs and symptoms. RA typically presents as a symmetric polyarthritis with weakness, malaise and low-grade fever (effects of interleukin-1 systemically). As the disease advances the joints become enlarged, painful and movement becomes limited. The hands may become immobilized in a claw-like position with ulnar deviation. The **carpal tunnel syndrome** may be seen in some patients and this develops when the median nerve becomes compressed as it passes through the carpal tunnel. The characteristic symptoms are tingling in the thumb, index and middle fingers, often waking the patient at night.

After approximately 10 years the disease stabilises or regresses in about half of the patients. The remaining 50% pursue a chronic, remitting–relapsing course. After 15 to 20 years about 10% of the patients become crippled, with gross deformity and **ankylosis** supervening. Approximately 5 to 10% of patients develop amyloidosis.

Diagnosis. Clinical findings are very important in the diagnosis of the disease. Often the patient presents with the classical findings, and these are enough to diagnose the condition very easily. Radiographic examinations of affected joints may then corroborate the diagnosis. Arthroscopic examination will provide a view of the interior of the joint and samples may be taken from the pannus or synovial fluid. Biochemical examination will detect changes in synovial fluid, with decreased mucin, increased cells and increased turbidity. Serological tests will detect rheumatoid factor in most patients, but the presence of this autoantibody is not pathognomonic, being found in other conditions also. Blood examination will often reveal an anaemia, raised erythrocyte sedimentation rate and raised plasma immunoglobulins.

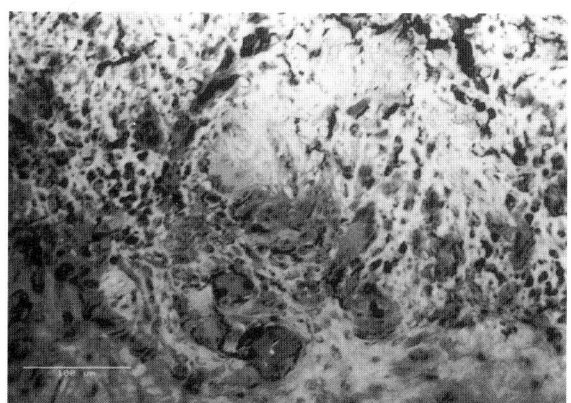

Figure 15.21 *Subcutaneous rheumatoid nodule showing the central fibrinoid necrotic area (pale region) surrounded by chronic inflammatory cells and giant cells (scale bar is 100 µm)*

Treatment and prognosis. RA has probably had more written it and more treatments tried than for most other diseases. This is because the condition is one which produces an unremitting joint pain which may make movement excruciating for the patients and their lives a misery, especially during exacerbations. Physical methods of treatment are often advised, rest coupled with moderate exercise such as swimming (hydrotherapy) or walking being recommended. Drug therapy regimes are complex and range in their relative activities, pharmacological actions and side effects. Analgesics and non-steroidal anti-inflammatory drugs provide the mainstay of treatment in many patients. Aspirin and its various derivatives remain one of the most popular and effective of treatments. Gold salts, antimalarials (such as chloroquinone) and D-penicillamine are also used in the more severe, recalcitrant cases and may prove effective with some of these patients. Corticosteroids and various immunosuppressive agents are used as a last resort, when other treatment regimes have been shown to be ineffective.

Orthopaedic surgery may be required for some complicated cases, or where deformity has resulted, and three basic types of procedures are carried out. **Synovectomy** is a procedure where as much of the inflamed synovium as possible is removed from a joint, the object being a reduction in the joint swelling, inflammation and pain. This procedure is being carried out less frequently nowadays, probably because of more effective medical treatments developing over the past few years. **Arthroplasty** is a procedure ranging from simple excision of damaged joint surfaces to prosthetic joint replacement surgery. **Arthrodesis** is fixation of a joint in a good, functional position, while at the same time removing pain and correcting instability, with prevention of some complications (for example, progressive pressure on the spinal cord).

The Seronegative Arthropathies

The seronegative arthropathies are a broad group of rheumatic-type disorders. Although they are clinically distinct entities, the synovial histology of the affected peripheral joints is indistinguishable from that of rheumatoid arthritis. In addition, rheumatoid factor is absent from the patients' bloodstream and affected joint spaces, hence the appellation 'seronegative'. Patients with these disorders have an increased incidence of the HLA antigen B27. A large number of these disorders have been characterized and they include the following:

- ankylosing spondylitis (0.5 to 2.0% incidence in the population);
- psoriatic arthritis and spondylitis (0.05% incidence in the population);
- Reiter's syndrome (0.02% incidence in the population);
- juvenile chronic arthritis (affects one in 4000 children).

Ankylosing Spondylitis

Ankylosing spondylitis (AS) is a chronic inflammatory arthritis affecting mainly the axial skeleton, but also commonly the shoulders and lower limb joints. Spinal movement becomes restricted and in advanced disease there may be complete rigidity from neck to sacrum. Patients with AS may show a wide variety of joint involvement and disease ranging greatly in severity. In mild disease periods of exacerbation with pain and stiffness are common manifestations, but there is little permanent limitation of spinal movement. In severely affected patients there will develop a relentless, marked and permanent spinal rigidity.

Incidence. The disease prevalence varies in different races and for Caucasians it has a prevalence of 0.5 to 2.0% in the population. It is more common in males and the sex ratio is 3:1. Most patients present in young adulthood, the age at onset being between 20 and 30 years. Often patients have a family history of the disease or associated disorders. Up to 7% of the patient's relatives may also have AS or other seronegative arthropathies.

Aetiology. The disorder is an idiopathic one but genetic factors are very important. The HLA antigen B27 is found in more than 95% of patients with AS, while only 7% of the normal population carry the gene for the antigen. Environmental factors are also important in the aetiology of the disease as studies have shown that identical twins may be discordant for AS. Some researchers have suggested that an infectious agent may be important in triggering autoimmunity and inflammation which lead to the changes observed in the disease. It is suspected that possibly, genitourinary or bowel infections may act as the trigger.

Sites affected. The disease often begins in the axial joints, in sites such as the sacroiliac, spinal apophyseal and costovertebral joints. The inflammation may later involve the vertebral column more extensively, with inflammation around the intervertebral discs and, more rarely, adjacent major joints such as the hip and shoulder. Tendinous insertions are also involved, especially around the ischial tuberosities, lesser and greater trochanters of the femur, the iliac crests, the Achilles tendon at the heel, the insertion of the patellar ligament into the tibial tuberosity and the insertion of the plantar fascia.

Morphology. In the peripheral joints, AS shows a synovitis identical to rheumatoid arthritis in appearance, the only exception being that the affected joint is more likely to progress to bony ankylosis. The characteristic feature of the disease occurs in the enthesis (the zone of ligamentous attachment to bone) and **enthesopathy** occurs (inflammation of the enthesis). Axial joints like the sacroiliac, spinal apophyseal and costovertebral show the above two processes occurring together, with progression to bony ankylosis of the joint periphery and central endochondral ossification.

The intervertebral discs are affected with enthesopathy at the insertion of the annulus fibrosus at the vertebral margin, progressing to calcification with the production of a bony bridge between the vertebral bodies known as a **syndesmophyte**. The earliest syndesmophytes occur at the thoracolumbar junction, followed in severe cases by their extensive development along the spine. This leads to a bony rigidity of the spine and a characteristic radiological appearance referred to as a '**bamboo spine**'. In advanced cases there may be a fixed kyphosis. If the costovertebral bodies are involved there may be difficulty in respiration and in severe cases patients may die from pulmonary disease. Some patients with ankylosing spondylitis show evidence of other autoimmune diseases such as iritis, ulcerative colitis and pulmonary fibrosis.

Signs and symptoms. The onset of AS is usually insidious and typically the patients present with low back pain and stiffness. Peripheral arthritis (usually of the lower limbs) is found in about 20% of presenting cases. In addition, patients may complain of systemic malaise, fatigue and weight loss less commonly. The pain the patient experiences is unrelieved by rest and is most troublesome at night and early morning, forcing patients to wake up and walk about to relieve the aching stiffness, which is often assuaged by this moderate activity. The pain tends to be episodic, lasting for several days or a few weeks and then gradually improving.

Early signs of the disorder include loss of normal lumbar lordosis due to muscle spasm and sacroiliac joint tenderness (a characteristic common to all seronegative arthropathies) due to sacroiliitis and restriction of movement in all three planes. Late signs are kyphosis, marked limitation of movement or complete rigidity of the spine and absence of sacroiliac joint tenderness, the patients having a bowed, rigid posture ('**poker-back**'). These changes are due to apophyseal joint fusion, syndesmophyte formation and calcification of the spinal ligaments.

Diagnosis. Clinical findings are very important in diagnosing the disorder as are the characteristic X-ray findings. Laboratory investigations provide confirmatory findings such as the demonstration of HLA B27, raised ESR and the presence of anaemia, but also absence of rheumatoid factor. Iritis is seen in approximately 25% of patients.

Treatment and Prognosis. The objectives in the treatment of the disorder are to relieve pain experienced by the patient and to prevent deformity in the long term. There are no specific therapies that alter the course of the disease. Drugs, mainly analgesics and non-steroidal anti-inflammatory agents, are used (e.g. indomethacin or phenylbutazone, aspirin not being very effective). Physical therapy such as a supervised exercise and mobility programme will minimize rigidity. Swimming is an excellent form of exercise in this respect. Advice with procedures that minimize back stress, promote deep breathing and avoid prolonged immobilization is very valuable for the patient. Weight reduction may prove of use in the obese patient. Surgery may be required in some complicated cases of the disease, but hip replacements which may relieve the presenting problem may be complicated by calcification and ankylosis around the prosthesis. In the past, X-irradiation was used to relieve the pain of the condition and was very effective in this. However, it no longer used because patients who undergo this treatment have ten times the risk of non-irradiated patients of developing leukaemia.

Psoriatic Arthritis

Psoriasis affects approximately 1% of the population and in 5% of psoriatic patients an associated arthritis manifests itself. Males and females are affected equally and the patients typically present between the ages of 30 and 50 years. There is a familial association and relatives of patients with psoriatic arthritis may suffer from psoriasis, psoriatic arthritis, sacroiliitis, ankylosing spondylitis or ulcerative colitis. An increased incidence of HLA antigens B13, B17, B27, B38, B39 and CW6 is seen in affected people.

Articular manifestations may accompany or follow the skin disease and usually there is no correlation between the severity of the skin and joint diseases. Distal interphalangeal joint involvement of the fingers is very characteristic of psoriatic arthritis, as is also asymmetrical oligoarticular arthritis in other joints. The joints resemble those affected by rheumatoid arthritis. Ankylosing spondylitis occurs in about 10% of people with this type of arthritis. Conjunctivitis, keratoconjunctivitis and iritis may also be seen in association with the arthritis and skin lesions. The prognosis of the disease is usually good and function of the affected joints is maintained.

Reiter's Syndrome

This is a disease comprising a combination of non-gonococcal urethritis, conjunctivitis and arthritis. It is a good example of a disease in which genetic predisposition coupled with an environmental trigger gives rise to the disorder. The disease is not uncommon and affects predominantly males. It may be associated with venereal infections, the urethritis being caused by *Chlamydia trachomatis* or *Ureaplasma urealyticum*, the male preponderance in this instance being 20:1. The disorder may also be seen following enteric infections, the triggers being particularly *Shigella flexneri, Yersinia enterocolitica* or *Salmonella* spp. The sex incidence in this latter case is 10 males to one female. Reiter's disease of childhood affects males and females in the ratio of 5:1. Predominantly the disease occurs between the ages of 16 and 35 years. There is usually a family history of psoriasis, spondylitis or sacroiliitis. The HLA antigen B27 is present in 60 to 80% of patients with Reiter's syndrome.

Patients may present with a dysuria, urethritis being the first symptom, with mild conjunctivitis accompanying it or shortly following it. The arthritis develops 1 to 3 weeks after the urethritis, and systemic malaise, fatigue, fever and weight loss are also common. The arthritis is usually polyarticular, involving the interphalangeal joint of hallux, tarsometatarsal joints and metatarsophalangeal joints. 'Sausage digits' caused by diffuse swelling of the whole digit, especially a toe, are characteristic of the disorder. Achilles tendinitis, plantar fasciitis, low back pain and sacroiliitis are also commonly seen. Approximately 10% of cases will develop ankylosing spondylitis. Skin lesions resembling psoriasis may be seen and patients may also have prostatitis, stomatitis and balanitis. Cardiac anomalies may also occur, including pericarditis, conduction defects and aortic incompetence. The disease is diagnosed easily in its classical form where conjunctivitis and arthritis follow urethritis or diarrhoea. Treatment of the urethritis or gastroenteritis with appropriate antibiotics resolves these conditions, but it does not influence the course of the arthritis or conjunctivitis. The disease is usually self-limiting but may recur in more than 50% of patients and about 30% of cases will progress to residual disability with painful, deformed feet, visual impairment, cardiac disease or spinal involvement.

A related, rarer disorder is **Behçet's syndrome** where there is oral and genital ulceration, uveitis, skin lesions, thrombophlebitis and arthritis with gastrointestinal and CNS involvement.

Juvenile Chronic Arthritis

This is a seronegative arthropathy affecting one in 4000 children, girls more than boys in the ratio of 9:1; the age of onset is around 5 years, although any age group can be affected. It is a polyarticular arthritis in which any joint in the body may be affected, although a symmetric and peripheral distribution is usual. The child usually presents with a limp, difficulty in handling objects, opening doors or turning taps on and off. Stiffness and pain in the joint is usually absent. Fever, especially in the afternoon or evening, is common, a rash often accompanying the fever, being seen on the trunk or limbs. The rash is often seen after a hot bath (**Koebner effect**). There is also lymphadenomegaly, splenomegaly and pericarditis, and sometimes cerebral symptoms and pleurisy.

An inflammatory arthritis develops resembling rheumatoid arthritis and rapidly causes muscle wasting, deformity and changes such as fixed contractures at the elbow, wrist, hips and knees. Ankylosis with calcium deposition is also frequent. There is growth impairment and eye involvement, typically a chronic uveitis which may cause blindness. Neutrophil leukocytosis is seen with white cell counts of 20 000 to 50 000 per μL, and thrombocytosis with a platelet count of over 500 000 per μL and a raised erythrocyte sedimentation rate also develop. Anaemia and hypergammaglobulinaemia are often features of the disease. The arthritis may persist for many years but is very severe in only a small proportion of cases. Treatment and management of the condition centre around prevention of deformity and muscle wasting with as little limitation of physical, educational and social development as possible. In many cases, the disease will ultimately become inactive and regresses as the child grows.

Degenerative Diseases of Joints

Osteoarthrosis

Osteoarthrosis (OA) is also termed osteoarthritis and degenerative joint disease. The major pathological change in the joint appears to be the degeneration of the articular cartilage and not inflammation hence osteoarthritis is not as correct a term as the other two. Osteoarthrosis has been classified into two types, the larger group being primary OA and associated with ageing. The aetiology of primary OA is unclear. Secondary OA may occur at any age, and is diagnosed when a known predisposing factor or aetiology is demonstrated.

Incidence. OA is the commonest form of joint disease and 16 to 17% of the population is affected by it to some degree. Most of the affected people (80% of them) are over 65 years of age. The peak age of onset for primary OA is 45 to 60 years. In the primary form, females are slightly more affected than males while in the secondary form males are slightly more affected.

Aetiology of primary osteoarthrosis. Primary OA is by far the commonest type of this disease and its aetiology is obscure. Several factors may contribute to its development but no clear-cut aetiological and pathogenetic mechanisms have been demonstrated. These factors are:

- **Ageing**: OA is more common in elderly people but this is not universal and it may also be seen in younger people. Therefore, it is not part of the 'normal' ageing process. Most researchers, however, agree that changes occurring in the tissues with age predispose to the development of the disorder.

- **Wear of cartilage**: In animal experiments, joints that are moved within the normal range fail to develop OA. Joints that are subjected to abnormal, shearing and impulsive forces exerted across the joint will rapidly lead to OA. In the normal individual the joint can cope with such forces to a reasonable extent as the forces are absorbed by reflex muscular joint flexion and extension. If such control mechanisms are impaired then cartilage destruction will ensue and OA will develop. This may be an important factor that predisposes the elderly to OA.

- **Wear of bone**: Bone immediately subjacent to articular cartilage has an important shock-absorbing role and a special structure to cope with this. If microfractures in subchondral bone develop, as is known to occur especially in association with the various bone rarefactions, the healing response will

Table 15.3 *Comparison of rheumatoid arthritis and degenerative joint disease*

Features	Rheumatoid arthritis	Osteoarthrosis
Age at onset	3rd or 4th decades	5th or 6th decades
Weight of patient	Normal or underweight	Often overweight
Sex incidence	Female preponderance	Male preponderance
Joints involved	Any joint (often bilateral, symmetrical, small joints, proximal interphalangeal)	Mainly knees, hips, spine, and distal interphalangeal joints
Appearance of joint	Soft tissue swelling	Bony swelling
Special deformities	Fusiform finger joints, ulnar deviation	Heberden's nodes, Bouchard's nodes
Subcutaneous nodules	Present in 20% of cases	Absent always
X-ray findings	Osteoporosis, erosions	Osteosclerosis, osteophytes
Joint fluid	Increased cell numbers, low mucin content	Few cells, good mucin content
Rheumatoid factors	Usually present	Usually absent
Blood count	Anaemia and leukocytosis	Normal
ESR	Markedly elevated	Normal
Disease course	Often progressive	Slow or stationary
Termination, sequelae	Ankylosis, deformity, amyloidosis	No ankylosis, no amyloidosis
Constitutional signs	Present	Absent
Symptoms	Pain or tenderness in the wrists, fingers, toes, or balls of feet, stiffness of joints, fatigue, low-grade fever	Aching, tenderness of joint, numbness, redness, swelling, difficulty in doing everyday tasks, 'unstable' joints

lead to loss of specialized structure and thus prevent the normal shock-absorbing function of this bone, leading to further damage if force is applied to the joint.

- **Obesity**: The role of this factor is unclear, especially as the ankle joints seem to be spared in obese people with OA in other joints. However, it stands to reason that increased weight will put greater stresses on joints and thus contribute to OA.
- **Diet**: This is generally considered not to be relevant to the development of OA. However, in osteoporosis and osteomalacia where there is weakening of bone, a dietary component may be implicated in some cases of OA seen in association with these disorders.
- **Genetic and hormonal**: Familial forms of primary, generalized OA are known and these occur slightly more commonly in females. Different patterns of inheritance have been reported.

Aetiology of secondary osteoarthrosis. Secondary OA develops after some other disorder has caused damage to the joint, especially such conditions that injure the articular cartilage. Common disorders that progress to secondary OA are:

- **Trauma**: Any injury which results in the weakening or damage of the joint will predispose greatly to OA. Fractures, repeated traumatic injury, malalignment and constant strong forces on the bone are likely to cause microfractures and articular cartilage damage. In this last-mentioned group various occupational factors are involved in the development of the disease as with some occupations great stresses are placed on joints almost daily. It is known, for example, that secondary OA develops more frequently and at a younger age in footballers, ballet dancers, wrestlers, jack hammer operators, and so on.
- **Genetic diseases**: Some genetic disorders of connective tissue make it more likely for OA to supervene as they are associated with poor connective tissue structure and function. Examples of such disorders are Marfan's syndrome, Ehlers-Danlos syndrome, osteochondrosis, cartilage and bone dysplasias.
- **Post-inflammatory**: After various inflammatory conditions of joints such as septic arthritis, gout or haemorrhagic arthritis (as seen in haemophilia) there will be destruction of joint structures and initiation of the process of OA.
- **Others**: Hyperparathyroidism, Paget's disease, haemochromatosis, Charcot's neuropathy, ochronosis and many other miscellaneous disorders may

lead to an increased predisposition to damage to the articular cartilage and subchondral bone and therefore the development of OA.

Sites affected. Classically, the large weight-bearing joints and the spine are affected by this disorder. It is typical of patients to present with involvement of the cervical and lumbar regions of the spine, the hips, knees and shoulders. However, small joints may also be affected, for example the hands, especially the distal interphalangeal joints and the carpometacarpal joint of the thumb, and the wrists (see Figure 15.22). Involvement may be monoarticular or polyarticular.

Morphology. The major change in OA is a degeneration of the articular cartilage. There is fissuring and splitting of the cartilage due to loss of proteoglycans and water from the matrix, a change termed **fibrillation**. The cartilage loses its lustre and takes on a velvety appearance due to the fibrillation. This change then progresses to focal cartilaginous erosions which denude the bone underlying them. Articular cartilage cannot regenerate and once it is damaged it is permanently lost. The surface of the joint and remaining cartilage become compressed, worn and smooth. **Eburnation** of the bone is then apparent on the surface of the bones in immediate contact with each other in the joint. This change describes the smooth and very dense appearance of the bone surface which becomes thickened and 'burnished' due to reactive osteosclerosis as the two bony surfaces rub against one another. **Subchondral cysts** form which are full of fluid due to synovial fluid being forced into remaining islands of cartilage through fissured, exposed surfaces. This contributes to the degeneration of the cartilage.

Bony outgrowths from the lateral aspects of the bone in the joint then begin to form around the joint margin and are called **osteophytes**. Their formation is another manifestation of reactive osteogenesis. The osteocytes rub against one another and cause pain, bony swelling and limit the range of motion of the joint. Osteophytes may break off and float free within the joint space causing more pain, and limiting of joint motion. These broken pieces of bone are often referred to as 'joint mice'.

Symptoms and signs. The patient with OA experiences pain of gradual onset, more common at night or after activity. Morning stiffness of joints for 5 to 15 minutes after rising is described and is due to the joint 'locking up' during the relative inactivity of the night. As the person begins to move and blood flow is restored to the joint, the stiffness eases. Functional impairment of the affected joints results because of the destruction of

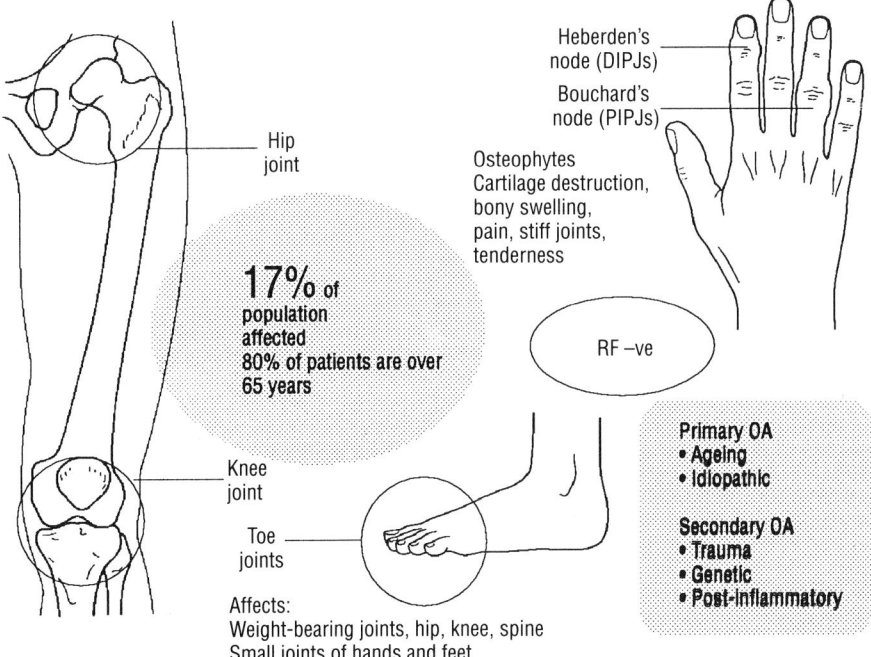

Heberden's node (DIPJs)

Bouchard's node (PIPJs)

Osteophytes
Cartilage destruction,
bony swelling,
pain, stiff joints,
tenderness

Hip joint

17% of population affected
80% of patients are over 65 years

RF −ve

Knee joint

Toe joints

Primary OA
• Ageing
• Idiopathic

Secondary OA
• Trauma
• Genetic
• Post-inflammatory

Affects:
Weight-bearing joints, hip, knee, spine
Small joints of hands and feet

Figure 15.22 *Summary of the occurrence and effects of osteoarthrosis (also called osteoarthritis and degenerative joint disease)*

cartilage, the bony swelling due to osteophytes and effusions. Muscle wasting around the affected joint occurs and is due to the relative immobility of the joint and disuse of the muscles (an effect of pain). Tenderness of the joints is seen especially during acute exacerbations where there may be episodes of synovial inflammation. **Heberden's nodes** are small bony projections on the fingers, developing in the distal interphalangeal joints (DIPJs). **Bouchard's nodes** are similar lesions on the proximal interphalangeal joints (PIPJs). There is no ankylosis in OA, although eventually deformity of the joint and laxity will develop with considerable loss of function and severe pain.

Diagnosis. Clinical symptomatology in association with typical radiological findings will result in a diagnosis. This may be made more conclusively if laboratory tests show normal values for haemoglobin, erythrocyte sedimentation rate and white cell count. Rheumatoid factor should be absent, unless the condition coexists with rheumatoid arthritis or another rheumatic condition. The biochemical profile is normal and the joint fluid is clear and straw coloured with high viscosity, with white cell counts of 1000 to 2000 per mL.

Treatment and prognosis. The disease is not one which is readily amenable to treatment and so management of the condition is more important. Patient education about their condition is an important factor. The sufferers should have explained to them that the disease is a degenerative one and that overuse and excessive stresses on joints should be avoided, but at the same time they should exercise sensibly to maintain muscle function. Advice regarding suitable forms of exercise should be given. Any correctable conditions causing secondary osteoarthrosis should be treated and this includes weight loss in obese patients. Drug therapy will often be resorted to, such that the inflammation is reduced, the drugs of choice being the non-steroidal anti-inflammatory agents with analgesics being of secondary importance. Corticosteroids systemically, gold salts and penicillamine are not used in OA.

Physical and occupational forms of therapy are quite important in the management of the disease as also are various appliances and aids that may help the patient in carrying out simple everyday tasks with ease and without much pain. Orthopaedic surgery is indicated if the disease is very severe and leads to complications such as joint instability or severe limitation of movement and pain. Different types of operative procedures are offered and they may involve **arthrotomies** in order to realign joints, **arthrodesis** to stabilize joints and, commonly, **arthroplasty** to regain joint mobility.

The course of the disease is slowly progressive over the years, the disease being quiescent for long periods of time. Stepwise deterioration is seen with exacerbations and remissions occurring over many years. Crippling disease due to OA is rarely seen nowadays and is confined to those people in whom surgery is contraindicated or has failed.

Tumours of Joints

'Synovioma' (Pigmented Villonodular Synovitis)
Synoviomata are not true tumours but rather, localized proliferative/hyperplastic lesions arising in sites that show a reactive inflammatory process. The lesions develop in the fingers, toes, knee or hip joints and give rise to a swollen, painful joint. The condition occurs most typically around the age of 30 years. The synovium is swollen, forming a fronded, brown-coloured or yellow, lobulated mass, poorly encapsulated. Extension into surrounding tissues may be seen. Microscopically the mass is composed of villi and frond-like outgrowths covered by synovial cells, with a core of macrophages and giant cells full of haemosiderin. The condition is totally benign and quite often spontaneously regresses, although it may recur in approximately 20% of cases. If surgical resection is carried out on symptomatic grounds, the lesion is excised widely and this prevents its recurrence.

Synoviosarcoma
This is a primary malignancy of joints arising from the synovium. It is a rare tumour, most often seen in people of an average age of 35 years. It occurs in the knee and hip joints mainly. Synoviosarcomata are pale tumours arising from the synovium and spreading locally to involve the joint, bone and soft tissues immediately adjacent to them. Microscopically the tumour is composed of cuboidal to fusiform cells lining clefts in the tumour, attempting to form structures similar to joint spaces. Early haematogenous spread is seen with less differentiated forms which gives rise to secondary deposits in the lungs. Such tumours have a very poor prognosis, a 5% 5-year survival to be expected. Well-differentiated tumours grow more slowly and a local excision may be curative.

Revision Questions and Case Studies

1. Discuss the pathology of the following conditions:
   (a) Achondroplasia
   (b) Dyschondroplasia
   (c) Gargoylism (lipochondrodystrophy)
   (d) Chondro-osteodystrophy (Morquio's syndrome)
2. What are the characterizing features of osteogenesis imperfecta?
3. Explain the clinical features observed in osteopetrosis (Albers-Schönberg disease) by referring to the pathological changes occurring in the tissues of such patients.
4. Define the following terms:
   (a) Arachnodactyly
   (b) Ecchondroma
   (c) Melorrheostosis
   (d) Avulsion fracture
   (e) Phocomelia
5. What are the major pathological features of osteochondritis juvenilis?
6. What are the major factors that delay the healing of bone fractures?
7. Compare and contrast osteoporosis and osteomalacia.
8. What are the characteristic pathological features of rickets?
9. Define the following terms:
   (a) Scurvy
   (b) Von Recklinghausen's disease
   (c) Dystrophic calcification
   (d) Metastatic calcification
   (e) Psammoma body
10. Discuss the pathology of osteitis deformans (Paget's disease of bone).
11. What are the characterizing features of Albright's disease (fibrous dysplasia of bone)?
12. Compare and contrast osteosarcoma and chondrosarcoma.
13. Write short notes on all of the following conditions:
    (a) Osteoma
    (b) Chondroma
    (c) Osteoclastoma
    (d) Osteoclastosarcoma
14. Discuss the pathology of secondary bone neoplasms.

15. Discuss the pathology of Ewing's sarcoma of bone.
16. What are the characterizing features of multiple myeloma?
17. Define the following terms:
    (a) Ulnar deviation
    (b) Gout
    (c) Ectopic bone formation
    (d) Osteomyelitis
    (e) Schmorl's nodes
18. Discuss the pathology of any three of the most commonly occurring primary malignant bone neoplasms.
19. Some carcinomata frequently metastasize to bone. Discuss the pathology of any three of these primary tumours and indicate the effects that secondary growths of these tumours may have in bone.
20. A 75-year-old male presents with lower back pain. Upon rectal examination he is found to have a palpable, nodular enlargement of the posterior lobe of his prostate gland. Indicate the possible nature of his complaint and discuss the pathology of the condition(s) he is most likely to be suffering from.
21. Discuss the pathology of any three bone diseases which may cause localized areas of osteolysis as seen in an X-ray film.
22. What are the characteristic bone changes seen in a patient with hyperparathyroidism? What are the causes of this condition and how is it treated?
23. A 68-year-old woman complains of vague aches and pains in her bones, of fatigue and weakness and is seen to have a waddling gait when she walks. Upon examination, it is found that she has a degree of lumbar lordosis; she says that her back is often painful. She lives alone and admits to not going out often and not looking after her diet properly. What pathology is consistent with such a presentation? Discuss the aetiology and pathogenesis of this disorder.
24. Define the following terms:
    (a) Looser's zones
    (b) Coxa vara
    (c) Cancellization
    (d) Pseudoarthrosis
25. Compare and contrast Paget's disease of bone and Albright's disease.
26. Discuss briefly any three of the following conditions:
    (a) Dyschondroplasia
    (b) Skeletal changes in Cushing's syndrome
    (c) Ewing's sarcoma
    (d) Synovioma
    (e) Fibrosarcoma of bone

27. Compare and contrast the pathologies of rheumatoid arthritis and osteoarthrosis (degenerative joint disease, DJD).
28. What are the characteristic pathological features of ankylosing spondylitis?
29. Discuss the pathology of degenerative bone disease (DJD, osteoarthrosis).
30. Discuss the pathology of the seronegative arthritides.
31. What are the characterizing features of synoviosarcoma?
32. Define the following terms:
    (a) Pannus
    (b) Osteophyte
    (c) Exostosis
    (d) Arthroplasty
    (e) Ankylosis

Case study 1. A 67-year-old male patient with a recent history of bone pain in the left lower leg presents at his chiropractor's clinic. Upon examination, the left tibia shows some bowing and a radiograph of the bone shows it to have been thickened considerably through deposition of cortical and cancellous bone, making the bone look enlarged. Upon further examination, symptoms of hearing loss are discovered, which were not present on the patient's previous visit a year ago. When asked if any other bones in his body are affected by any symptoms, the man says that his 'arms ache now and then', and that often he has to sit down because he feels 'very tired and light-headed'. He also admits to suffering from the 'odd headache now and then'. The man had suffered a heart attack 5 years previously and is on antihypertensive medication. He has modified his lifestyle and diet after his heart attack and he now no longer smokes (he used to smoke about 15 cigarettes a day before his MI); he has become a vegetarian and he also swims regularly, and has had no further problems with his heart since then. The man is 1.8 m tall and weighs 80 kg. His blood pressure is 150/94 and other physical examination findings are normal except for a slight deformity of the skull in the frontal and occipital regions, and a problem with the man's dentures, which seem not to fit properly and tend to fall out (the man says that he is to visit his dentist that afternoon).

(a) What is the presumptive diagnosis?
(b) Explain the signs and symptoms that the patient presents with by reference to the pathological changes wrought by the disease.
(c) What are the major complications of this disorder?

(d) What is the treatment for this patient and what is his prognosis?

Case study 2. A 15-year-old boy is taken to the family doctor with a history of joint pain, swelling and tenderness about the left knee region for the past 2 months. The boy is a keen footballer and often suffers trauma on the playing field, so aching bones and injuries are not uncommon. The current problem has been different, in that the pain has worsened instead of getting better and a visible lump has become apparent on the outer aspect of the proximal left tibia. The boy has also lost weight in the past month and he is seen to be pale and thin on examination. He had to miss the last football game as he felt too tired and unwell. Physical examination reveals normal results except for the knee problem.

(a) If infection has been ruled out what is the most likely diagnosis for this patient?
(b) What are the predisposing factors for the condition? Do any of these relate to this case?
(c) What is the course of treatment?
(d) What is the prognosis for this patient?

Case study 3. Mr John F., a 69-year-old man, is hospitalized as he has fractured his first and second lumbar vertebrae and his left fourth and fifth ribs presumably after he fell while getting out of bed in the nursing home where he lives. The man has had a viral respiratory infection for the past 2 weeks and he has been on antibiotics for the past week. The man has been complaining of deep bone and joint pain that is worse when he has been active but diminishes on resting for the past few months. A radiograph of his vertebral column taken 6 months ago showed no remarkable findings. When questioned, the nursing staff has said that Mr F. has been sleeping a lot lately and while normally he is quite 'chirpy', in the last few weeks he has seemed depressed and easily tired. Physical examination shows a thin, frail man who has several haematomata associated with the areas of his fractures. The man is taken in for X-rays and radiography which reveals many pronounced, 'punched out', osteolytic defects in the bone of the spine, skull, pelvis and ribs, especially in association with his fractures.

Laboratory and biochemical investigations are carried out and he is shown to have a severe anaemia, a normal white cell count and raised erythrocyte sedimentation rate. A hypercalcaemia with normal phosphate levels is found and also a raised plasma protein with a reversed albumin/globulin ratio. The man is also hyperuricaemic and proteinuric.

(a) What is the diagnosis?
(b) What is the incidence of this disorder?
(c) Explain the presentation in terms of the pathological changes occurring in the tissues.
(d) What is the nature of the protein found in the urine?
(e) What causes the hypercalcaemia with normal phosphate levels?
(f) How is the disease treated and what is the prognosis for the patient?

Case study 4. A 38-year-old male football coach and ex-player has a history of joint swelling, tenderness and pain affecting the right knee and both hip joints, occurring episodically over the past 3 years. The man attributes his symptoms to the rather harsh treatment he deals out to his body during training. Lately, the pain in the knee joint has become very intense and almost constant and the man has a slight but noticeable limp. Palpation of the knee reveals a firm and tender swelling and there is limitation in the range of motion with much pain if the joint is moved to extremes of rotation. Blood examination shows that he is negative for rheumatoid factor, has a normal ESR, is not anaemic and has a normal white cell count and morphology. Arthroscopic examination of the knee showed several erosions in the articular cartilages, and yielded two small necrotic bone fragments and a biopsy specimen of a fronded, brownish, seaweed-like tissue which was within the joint space.

(a) What is the diagnosis?
(b) What is the pathogenesis of the disorder in this patient?
(c) How is the disease managed?
(d) Is the man predisposed to malignancy because of his condition?

Case study 5. A 36-year-old female patient with a history of rheumatoid arthritis over the past 9 years presents as she feels that some subcutaneous nodules at the region of the olecranon process of the left arm are unsightly and she wants them removed for cosmetic reasons. The lesions are non-tender, firm nodules, one approximately 2 cm in diameter and a smaller, 0.7 cm nodule adjacent to it. The nodules are removed without any complication.

(a) Describe the microscopic structure of the nodules removed.
(b) What other non-articular manifestations of her disease could the woman have presented with?
(c) What laboratory tests are performed in order to aid in the diagnosis of this condition?
(d) What can the woman expect as far as progression

of her disease is concerned? What sequelae should she be made aware of?

Case study 6. A 13-year-old girl presents with pronounced swelling, redness and pain in the right ankle joint which has developed in the last 2 to 3 days and has quickly produced a great compromise in the function of the joint. The girl was seen to be limping about 5 to 6 days previously after she had sustained an injury in her right ankle about a week ago in a hockey game but the pain associated with the injury subsided within a couple of days and the limp improved. The girl can now walk only with difficulty because of the pain and tenderness at the site. Physical examination shows no abnormal findings except for the swollen, tender and painful ankle and a fever (38.2°C). The girl also has rather severe acne on her face.

(a) What is the presumptive diagnosis?
(b) What investigations are mandatory?
(c) Attempt to explain the pathogenesis of the condition in this patient.
(d) How is this condition treated?

Further Reading

Angus RM, Eisman JA. 'Osteoporosis: The Role of Calcium Intake and Supplementation.' *Med J Aust* 1988; **148**: 630.

Altman RD. 'Paget's Disease of Bone.' *Bull Rheum Dis* 1984; **34**(3): 1.

Arnett FC. 'Seronegative Spondyloarthropathies.' *Bull Rheum Dis* 1987; **37**: 1.

Avioli LV. 'Paget's Disease.' *Clin Ther* 1987; **9**: 567.

Benson DR. 'Idiopathic Scoliosis.' *Orthopedics* 1987; **10**: 1691.

Brandt KD. 'Osteoarthritis.' *Clin Geriatr Med* 1988; **4**: 279.

Bullough PG, Vigorita VJ. *Atlas of Orthopaedic Pathology with Clinical and Radiologic Correlations*, 1984; Butterworths, London; Gower Medical Publishing, New York.

Calin A. 'Ankylosing Spondylitis.' *Clin Rheumat Dis* 1985; **11**: 41.

Carette S, *et al*. 'A Controlled Trial of Corticosteroid Injections into Facet Joints for Chronic Low Back Pain.' *New Engl J Med* 1991; **325**: 1002.

Collins DH. *Pathology of Bone,* 1966; Butterworths, London.

Courtenay BG, Bowers DM. 'Stress Fractures: Clinical Features and Investigation.' *Med J Aust* 1990; **153**: 155.

Dahlin DC, Unni KK. *Bone Tumours*, fourth edition,

1986; Thomas, Springfield.

Eckardt JJ, Grogan TJ. 'Giant Cell Tumour of Bone.' *Clin Orthop* 1986; **204**: 45.

Editorial. 'Chiropractors and Low Back Pain.' *Lancet* 1990; **336**: 220.

Editorial. 'Osteoporosis and Cardiovascular Disease in Women: Converging Paths?' *Lancet* 1990; **336**: 1121.

Espinoza LR. 'Rheumatoid Arthritis: Etiopathologic Considerations.' *Clin Lab Med* 1986; **6**: 27.

Evans HL. 'Synovial Sarcoma.' *Pathol Annu* 1980; **15**(2): 309.

Fong S, *et al*. 'Rheumatoid Factor in Human Autoimmune Disease.' *Pathol Immunopathol Res* 1986; **5**: 305.

Frost HM. 'Osteogenesis Imperfecta.' *Clin Orthop* 1987; **216**: 280.

Frost HM. 'The Pathomechanics of Osteoporosis.' *Clin Orthop* 1985; **200**: 198.

Garrington GE, Collet WK. 'Chondrosarcoma.' *J Oral Pathol* 1988; **17**: 1.

German DC, Holmes EW. 'Hyperuricaemia and Gout.' *Med Clin North Am* 1986; **70**: 419.

Goorin AM, Abelson HT, Frei E. 'III: Osteosarcoma.' *New Engl J Med* 1985; **313**: 1637.

Green NE, Edwards K. 'Bone and Joint Infections in Children.' *Orthop Clin North Am* 1987; **18**: 555.

Gruber HE, Singer FR. 'The Spectrum of Pathology of Osteomalacia.' *Appl Pathol* 1987; **5**: 160.

Healey LA. 'Rheumatoid Arthritis in the Elderly.' *Clin Rheum Dis* 1986; **12**: 173.

Husby G. 'Amyloidosis and Rheumatoid Arthritis.' *Clin Exp Rheumatol* 1985; **3**: 173.

Huvos AG. 'Surgical Pathology of Bone Sarcomas.' *World J Surg* 1988; **12**: 284.

Karlin JM. 'Osteomyelitis in Children.' *Clin Podiatr Med Surg* 1987; **4**: 37.

Kelley WN, Harris ED Jr, Ruddy S, Sledge CB. *Textbook of Rheumatology*, second edition, 1985; WB Saunders, Philadelphia.

Kessler E, Brandt-Rauf PW. 'Occupational Cancers of Brain and Bone.' *State Art Rev Occup Med* 1987; **2**: 155.

Kouri T. 'Etiology of Rheumatoid Arthritis.' *Experientia* 1985; **41**: 434.

Lane JM, Vigorita VJ. 'Osteoporosis.' *Orthop Clin North Am* 1984; **15**: 711.

Law MR, *et al*. 'Strategies for Prevention of Osteoporosis and Hip Fracture.' *BMJ* 1991; **303**: 453.

Levinson AI, Martin J. 'Rheumatoid Factor: Dr Jekyll or Mr Hyde?' *Br J Rheumatol* 1988; **27**: 83.

Lewis MM, *et al*. 'Benign and Malignant Cartilage Tumors.' *Instr Course Lect* 1987; **36**: 87.

McCarty XX (ed.). 'Crystalline Deposit Diseases.' *Rheum Dis Clin North Am* 1988; **14**: 253.

Meade TW, *et al.* 'Low Back Pain of Mechanical Origin: A Randomized Comparison of Chiropractic and Hospital Outpatient Treatment.' *BMJ* 1990; **300**: 1431.

Meyers PA. 'Malignant Bone Tumors in Children: Osteosarcoma.' *Hematol Oncol Clin North Am* 1987; **1**: 655.

Meyers PA. 'Malignant Bone Tumors in Children: Ewing's Tumor.' *Hematol Oncol Clin North Am* 1987; **1**: 667.

Midtvedt T. 'Intestinal Bacteria and Rheumatic Disease.' *Scand J Rheumatol* 1986; Suppl 64: 49.

Osband ME. 'Histiocytosis X.' *Hematol Oncol Clin North Am* 1987; **1**: 737.

Panush RS, Brown DG. 'Exercise and Arthritis.' *Sports Med* 1987; **4**: 54.

Paterson AH. 'Bone Metastases in Breast Cancer, Prostate Cancer and Myeloma.' *Bone* 1987; **8**(Suppl 1): S17.

Phillips PE. 'Evidence Involving Infectious Agents in Rheumatoid Arthritis and Juvenile Rheumatoid Arthritis.' *Clin Exp Rheumatol* 1988; **6**: 87.

Rashad S, *et al.* 'Effect of Non-steroidal Anti-inflammatory Drugs on the Course of Osteoarthritis.' *Lancet* 1989; **ii**: 519.

Revell PA. 'Examination of Synovial Fluid.' *Curr Top Pathol* 1982; **71**: 1.

Revell PA. *Pathology of Bone*, 1985; Springer Verlag, Berlin.

Rodysill KJ. 'Postmenopausal Osteoporosis.' *Chronic Dis* 1987; **40**: 743.

Schorr-Lesnick B, Brandt LJ. 'Selected Rheumatologic and Dermatologic Manifestations of Inflammatory Bowel Disease.' *Am J Gastroenterol* 1988; **83**: 216.

Sherrard DJ. 'Renal Osteodystrophy.' *Semin Nephrol* 1986; **6**: 56.

Silman AJ. 'Musculoskeletal Disorders in Childhood.' *Br Med Bull* 1986; **42**: 196.

Smith GE. 'Fluoride, Teeth and Bone.' *Med J Aust* 1985; **143**: 283.

Stevenson JC, *et al.* 'Determinants of Bone Density in Normal Women: Risk Factors for Future Osteoporosis?' *BMJ* 1989; **298**: 924.

Thomson GH, Salter RB. 'Legg-Calvé-Perthes Disease.' *Clin Symp* 1986; **38**(3): 1.

Unni KK (ed.). 'Bone Tumors.' *Cont Issues Surg Pathol* 1988; **11**: 1.

Unni KK, McLeod RA, Dahlin DC. 'Conditions that Simulate Primary Neoplasms of Bone.' *Pathol Annu* 1980; **15**(1): 91.

Vick KE, Johnson CA. 'Aluminum-related Osteomalacia in Renal Failure Patients.' *Clin Pharmacol* 1985; **4**: 434.

Younai F, Eisenbud L, Sciubba JJ. 'Osteopetrosis.' *Oral Surg* 1988; **65**: 214.

16

Integumentary System Disorders

The Normal Integumentary System

Integument is the term applied to the skin, nails, hair and some specialized glands associated with these structures. The normal skin is the largest organ in the body, weighing approximately 4 kg and with an area of 1.7 m. It is a very resilient, waterproof, tough, covering which protects the underlying tissues from various environmental agents. It is divided into the epidermis and the dermis. The **epidermis**, at the free surface, comprises the following layers:

- stratum corneum (upper fully keratinized layer);
- stratum lucidum (upper keratinized layer);
- stratum granulosum (middle keratinizing layer);
- stratum spinosum (prickle cell layer);
- stratum basale (basal proliferating layer).

The **dermis**, the subjacent layer, comprises the:

- reticular dermis (with skin appendages such as sweat glands and sebaceous glands); and
- subcutaneous fat.

The keratinocytes are the specialized parenchymal cells of the skin and they are found in the epidermis in layers, comprising the stratified squames of the epidermis. The basal cells are the germinative elements of the skin, the stem cells from which upper layers are derived. A basal cell takes 4 to 14 weeks (depending on skin thickness) to reach the surface of the skin and desquamate. Mitosis occurs in the basal region of the epidermis mainly during sleep. Cells are securely attached to one another through desmosomes, and when skin tissue is fixed for histology the cells shrink slightly with only the desmosomes remaining in contact with one another and being seen as the 'prickles' of the stratum spinosum. As the cells move upwards they flatten and synthesize more and more granules of keratohyalin, a protein. The keratohyalin almost completely fills the cells in the upper stratum granulosum and it is this change that gives rise to the keratin squames in the stratum corneum.

Some specialized cells are also found in the epidermis: **Langerhans cells** are small cells possessing long processes and numerous racquet-shaped inclusions

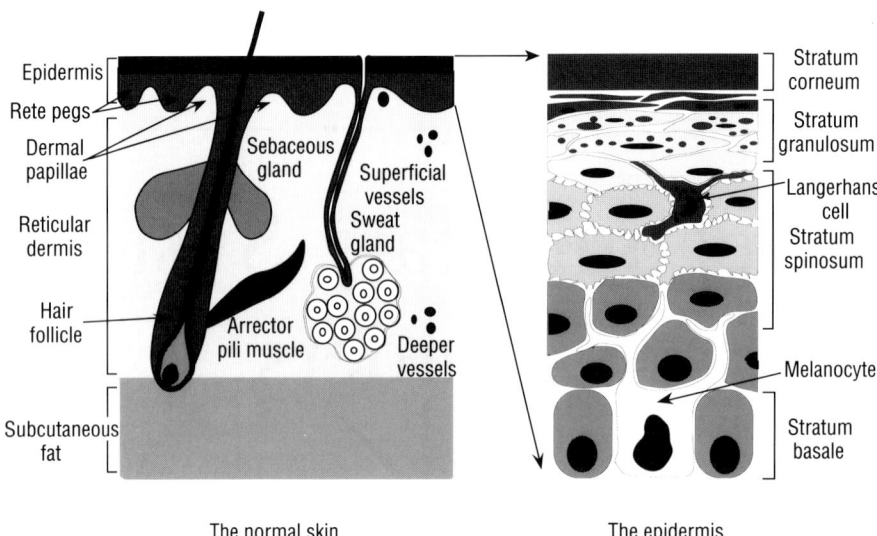

Figure 16.1   *The normal skin*

(Birbeck granules) in their cytoplasm. Their function is to recognize and process antigens that are contacted through the skin. The Birbeck granules may be related to antigen processing. **Melanocytes** are cells derived from neuroectoderm. In the foetus they migrate from the neural crest to the skin, squamous mucosae, leptomeninges, choroid and adrenals. In the skin they are found in the junction between epidermis and dermis, appearing as the lightly staining cells in the stratum basale. They produce melanin pigment that they pass on to the keratinocytes and the function of this is to protect the body from the effects of ultraviolet radiation. **Merkel cells** are found in the stratum basale of the epidermis and are small polyhedral cells present in only certain sites of the skin (the lips, oral cavity, fingertips, hair follicles). They are connected to keratinocytes via desmosomes and at their base Merkel cells are attached to a short unmyelinated axon that in turn connects to a myelinated axon. In their cytoplasm these cells possess characteristic Merkel granules. The function of these cells is tactile mechanoreception.

The dermis underlies the thin basement membrane on which the epidermis rests. It is a dense connective tissue layer that interlocks with the epidermis through a system of ridges and papillae. It has numerous blood vessels and nerves that serve to nourish both layers of the skin (the epidermis not possessing blood vessels). The dermis also contains epidermal downgrowths that are termed skin appendages and these include hair follicles, sweat glands and nails.

Apart from its function as a protective outer wrapping, the skin also has other important functions in homeostasis (temperature regulation), sensory perception, protection from ultraviolet light and antigen recognition.

Important Terms Used to Describe Skin Lesions

Many pathological states of the skin will lead to very similar appearances in the morphological structure of the tissue both macroscopically and microscopically. Some conventional terms are used to describe these lesions and serve as a form of 'shorthand' when dermatologists describe the findings of a given pathological condition. The commonest of these are listed below.

Microscopical Descriptive Terms

Dermatologists use the following terms when describing histopathological features of skin lesions (the appearance of the changes the terms describe are shown in Figures 16.2 and 16.3):

- **Acantholysis** refers to a loss of cohesion between keratinocytes, and formation of intraepidermal spaces containing fluid and rounded, degenerating cells.
- **Acanthosis** is a thickening of the epidermis either focally or diffusely.

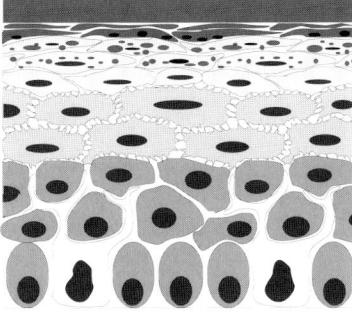

Normal epidermis

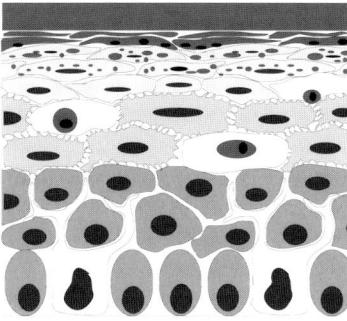

Acanthosis

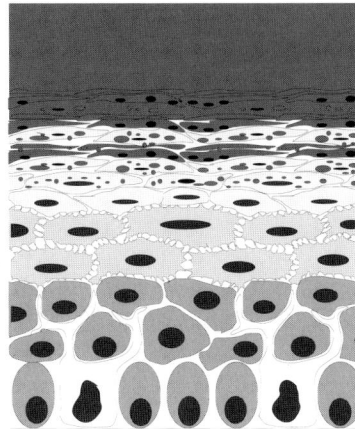

Hyperkeratosis

Acantholysis

Figure 16.2 *Microscopic skin lesions*

- **Dyskeratosis** is the premature or abnormal keratinization of keratinocytes. The cells lose their prickles and become spherical, with pyknotic nuclei, while still deep in the epidermis.
- **Hyperkeratosis** is a thickening of the stratum corneum and stratum granulosum.
- **Pigmentary incontinence** is loss of melanin pigment from damaged basal cells in the epidermis. There is accumulation of melanin in macrophages in the upper dermis.
- **Parakeratosis** is an abnormal but orderly keratinization of cells. The stratum corneum consists of nucleated keratinized cells instead of anucleated keratin squames.
- **Spongiosis** is intercellular oedema, with formation of large spaces between epidermal cells. If it is severe, large vesicles may form.
- **Vacuolar degeneration** is a severe degeneration of the stratum basale associated with pigmentary incompetence.

Macroscopical Descriptive Terms

The following terms are commonly used to describe skin lesions visible with the naked eye (refer also to Figure 16.4):

- An **abscess** is a localized collection of pus in an artificial cavity created by tissue necrosis, and results after infection with pyogenic bacteria.
- A **furuncle** is a large, unilocular abscess with a single discharging point (a 'boil').
- A **carbuncle** is a very large, multilocular abscess that has several discharging points on the skin surface.
- A **vesicle** is a blister (less than 1 cm diameter). It consists of a bleb within the skin filled with fluid. Vesicles may be **subepidermal**, where the fluid collects between epidermis and dermis, **intraepidermal**, where the fluid collects between epidermal cells, or **subcorneal**, where the fluid accumulates immediately beneath the stratum corneum.

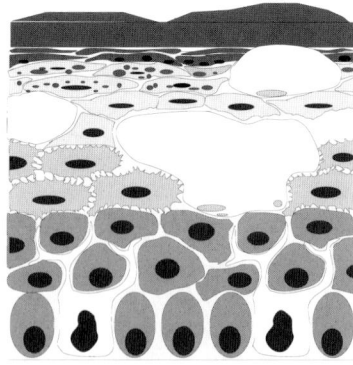

Spongiosis

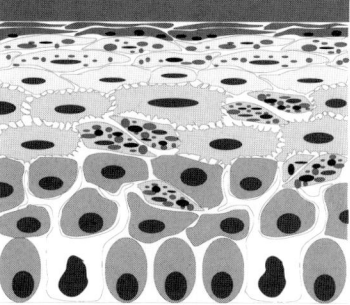

Dyskeratosis

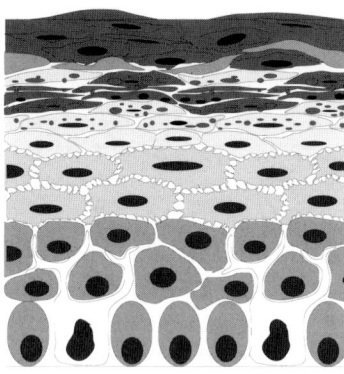

Parakeratosis

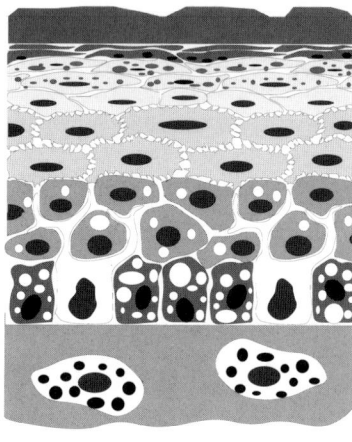

Vacuolar degeneration
pigmentary incontinence

Figure 16.3 *Microscopic skin lesions*

- A **bulla** is a large vesicle (more than 1 cm in diameter).
- A **papule** is a small, circumscribed, solid, elevated lesion of the skin — a small nodule.
- An **abrasion** is a superficial removal of epidermal cells.
- A **crust** is a localized region of solid matter formed by the drying of a body fluid, exudate or secretion.
- A **cyst** is a closed and epithelial-lined cavity containing fluid.
- A **fissure** is a crack or split in the epidermis.
- **Lichenification** is an irregular thickening of the skin with exaggeration of skin markings.
- A **macule** refers to a circumscribed, spot-like lesion that lies flat on the skin.
- A **nodule** is a localized tumour-like mass, a swelling.

- A **petechia** is a small spot-like haemorrhage.
- A **pustule** is a vesicle filled with purulent fluid.
- A **rash** is a reddening of the skin, localized or diffuse; a skin eruption.
- A **scale** refers to a thickened, epidermal area where there is marked keratinization with excessive desquamation of the cornified layer.
- An **ulcer** is an erosion of the epidermis, with exposure of the dermis.

Frequently, the above terms may be combined to describe more complex lesions or lesions that tend to evolve in particular ways. For example, an erythematous macular rash may be described, or one may speak of a papulovesicular eruption.

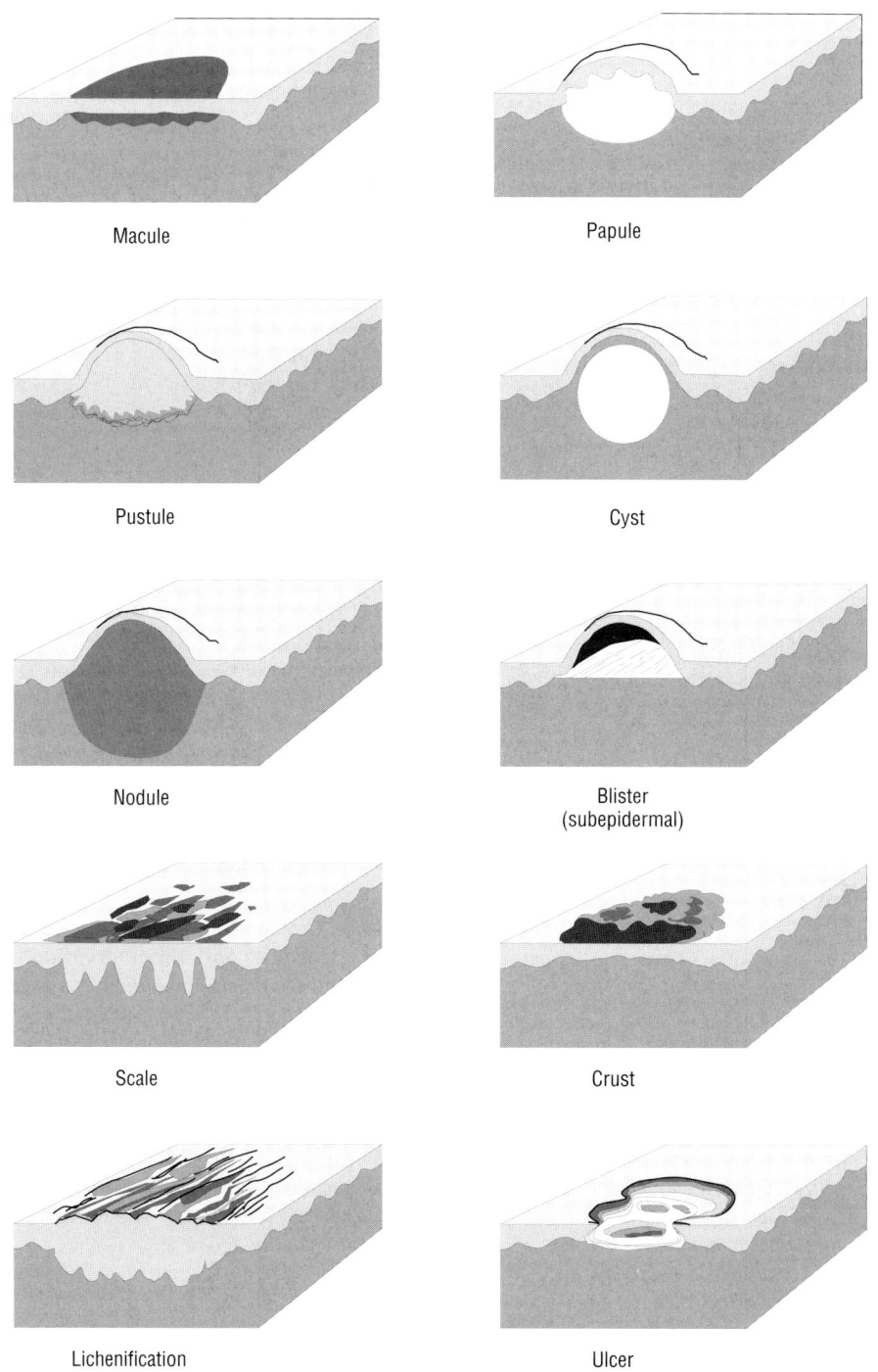

Figure 16.4 *Macroscopic skin lesions*

Congenital Diseases of the Skin

Xeroderma Pigmentosum

This is an autosomal recessive disorder in which there is hypersensitivity to ultraviolet light, such that lesions are maximal on the exposed skin. There is reddening, scaling and patchy pigmentation of the skin. The condition is made worse by exposure to sunlight and affected people must shield themselves from the sun. It is a premalignant condition. In the later stages warty excrescences form which may eventually form squamous cell carcinoma, basal cell carcinoma or malignant melanoma. A person with xeroderma pigmentosum has a thousand times the risk of a normal person of developing these cancers.

The fundamental defect in this disorder is an abnormality in the repair of ultraviolet-light-damaged DNA following exposure to sunlight. In the normal person, endonucleases and replicases excise and repair damaged DNA regions following exposure to ultraviolet radiation. As a consequence of these repair mechanisms, skin cancers in the normal individual are rather rare before the age of 50 years, whereas in the individual with xeroderma skin cancers develop from 8 years of age onwards.

Ichthyosis

Ichthyosis is a term describing a large variety of skin diseases in which there is a marked increase in the stratum corneum with very prominent hyperkeratosis. The afflicted individual shows dry, rough 'fish-scale' skin which is maximal on the extensor surfaces, very rarely affecting the flexural surfaces. There are four major forms of ichthyosis: **ichthyosis vulgaris, lamellar ichthyosis, ichthyosiform erythroderma** (all of these showing autosomal inheritance) and **sex-linked ichthyosis** (X-linked disorder). Some rarer forms have also been described and in these there may also be abnormalities in lipid metabolism, bone disease and nervous system disease. In all major forms, except ichthyosis vulgaris, the lesions are present at birth while in ichthyosis vulgaris the disease develops in infancy. In congenital ichthyosis, the baby may be born with a thick, brown, shiny membrane covering the skin all over the body ('**collodion baby**'). Several days later this membrane develops into large, polygonal scales, making the surface of the skin resemble that of a reptile (= 'ichthyosis sauroderma'). All congenital varieties of ichthyosis tend to improve somewhat with age.

In some of the ichthyoses enzymatic defects have been identified (e.g. deficiency of steroid sulphatase and aryl sulphatase-C in sex-linked ichthyosis), while in others the defects are more subtle and are linked with abnormal differentiation of the keratinocytes as they ascend through the layers of the epidermis. The stratum granulosum and the stratum corneum are particularly affected, with vesicles and bullae forming, atrophy of the stratum spinosum, marked hyperkeratosis and keratin plugs in hair follicles (follicular plugging).

Treatment for this disorder depends on the application of various medicated ointments and lotions. The condition often responds to treatment with 40 to 60% aqueous propylene glycol, 5% α-hydroxy acids (e.g. lactic acid) in hydrophilic ointment, or topical retinoic acid cream.

Hydroa

Hydroa describes a group of congenital conditions in which there is photosensitivity, especially during the time of the year when sun exposure is more likely to occur (i.e. summer). **Hydroa vacciniforme** is a relatively rare, papulovesicular eruption usually seen in boys during the summer months and associated with photosensitivity and congenital porphyria. Intraepidermal vesicles form and are associated with marked dermal inflammation, vascular thrombosis, dermal necrosis and scarring. Bullae may also form and the condition is often accompanied by pruritus and lichenification. This form is the most severe and persists throughout life, resulting in extensive fibrous dermal scars. Anti-inflammatory agents may be used with varying success and the individual is prescribed sunscreening preparations and is advised to avoid exposure to sunlight.

Hydroa aestivale is a milder form, and is the more common of the two types. It typically occurs after exposure to sunlight. The vesicles that form are smaller and the dermal inflammation is not marked. The condition disappears at puberty, rarely recurring afterwards and does not produce dermal scarring. Use of sunscreens and avoidance of sunlight are usually advised.

Porphyria

Porphyria refers to a group of inherited disorders (a dominant trait in most cases) in which there is an increased production of porphyrins in the body. This occurs mainly because of inadequate enzymatic production of haeme, and an overproduction of porphyrins instead. As these substances are deposited in many tissues including the skin, there is photosensitivity, abdominal pain and neuropathy. In some cases, porphyria may be acquired, especially after ingestion of some drugs or toxins (e.g. alcohol, barbiturates, arsenicals, phosphorus and sulphonamides). It is suspected, however, that in this case the drug is merely precipitating the porphyria in an individual who was already showing subclinical, congenital porphyria. Two main subgroups of porphyria occur, the erythropoietic porphyrias, where the failure of haeme production occurs in the erythrocytes, and the hepatic porphyrias, where the main defect is failure of haeme production in the liver.

Porphyrins are iron-free pyrrole derivatives and are normally found in the plasma and urine in minute amounts. In the urine they are excreted as coproporphyrins. In porphyria, many milligrams of porphyrins will be excreted in the urine per day, which upon several hours standing will become discoloured to a burgundy-red colour. Red-brown discolouration may also be noted in the teeth and in bones. Photosensitivity in the skin may manifest itself as hydroa.

Congenital porphyria does not present until several years after birth while another form, acute idiopathic porphyria (also inherited), occurs primarily in females and together with dark-coloured urine these patients show abdominal colic, vomiting and later on in the course of the disease, skin lesions, neuritis, liver damage, paralysis and mental symptoms (confusion and emotional lability). The diseases are treated by avoiding sunlight and using barrier creams, consuming increased amounts of β-carotene, large doses of glucose, high-protein, high-carbohydrate diets or administration of haematin depending on the type of porphyria.

Inflammatory Diseases

Eczematous Disorders

These are inflammatory reactions in the skin usually due to idiopathic causes or in some cases due to hypersensitivities to a large variety of substances. The allergens may be externally and locally applied or may be more distant in origin as manifestations of a generalized hypersensitivity reaction. Often eczematous reactions are also described by the term dermatitis. There are many types of eczematous lesions which may be acute or chronic. The superficial dermatitis resulting in eczematous disorders may cause in the early stages pruritic, erythematous, papulovesicular, oedematous and weeping lesions, but eventually the affected areas may become thickened and lichenified, crusted and scaly. It should be noted that eczema is not a specific disease entity, but rather a term applied to a large variety of skin disorders of similar presentation in which pruritus and inflammation of the skin due to ill-defined causes are the primary characteristics.

Acute eczema is a common condition and a typical example of this is **contact dermatitis**, in which there is a variable rash of macules, papules and vesicles, later coalescing to produce a diffuse red rash. The disease has an allergic basis and develops as a typical type IV hypersensitivity reaction when the allergen is contacted through the skin. Often the offending allergen may be identified, but in other cases the disease remains totally idiopathic and the eczema is treated by anti-inflammatory preparations rather than by avoidance of known allergens. Typical allergens implicated in contact dermatitis include chemicals encountered in occupational situations, cosmetics and perfumes, items of clothing and footwear that contain the offending substance and jewellery worn in contact with the skin. Eczema may also be seen to follow systemic exposure to the allergen and often such patients may also suffer from asthma and urticaria. Various drugs and foods are implicated in these disorders.

Chronic eczema is a more severe, long-standing inflammation, as occurs, for example, in **neurodermatitis**, where the skin thickens and there are mixtures of scaling, oozing, crusting and fissure formation. Neurodermatitis is a condition developing mainly in people who are overly anxious or nervous and it is believed that the skin condition is exacerbated by the patient's psychological condition. Regions of lichenification and excoriation are found on the patient's forearms and forehead especially. This condition is often confused with atopic dermatitis.

Counselling of the patients in these cases is very important and combined with anti-inflammatory drug treatments and emollient lotions and creams the condition may regress.

Atopic Dermatitis

This is an inflammatory condition of the skin that appears to have a familial component in its causation and occurs in about 2% of the population. It is a relapsing, intensely pruritic dermatitis in which red, excoriated, oozing patches develop acutely. These lesions may develop into hyperpigmented, lichenified plaques. Often the condition is seen to begin at an early age (2 months to 2 years) as acute eczema on the cheeks and extensor extremities. In childhood and adolescence the chronic lesions are common in the antecubital and popliteal fossae and the sides of the neck. In some patients severe disease leads to the generalization of the lesions. The skin of these patients, even in unaffected regions, looks and feels dry.

Patients with atopic dermatitis or their immediate family members often have a history of asthma, allergic rhinitis or other skin disorders. The condition may be aggravated by excessive bathing, skin infections, rough or woollen clothing worn directly over the skin, exposure to irritating chemicals, overwarming and sweating or stress and anxiety. There are no useful diagnostic histological or laboratory findings and the disease must be diagnosed from its clinical and historical features. High levels of IgE may be found in the plasma of these patients and there are immune system abnormalities, mainly associated with a decreased suppressor T cell number.

Atopic dermatitis is treated by firstly avoiding all known triggering factors. Often the disease may improve or disappear with increasing age, but a considerable proportion of patients will continue to suffer from it episodically throughout their life. Emollient soaps and balneotherapy (bathing in medicated water) may be used, antibacterial topical preparations will control secondary infections of acute lesions and topical corticosteroids are often important in the initial clearing of acute lesions. Antihistamines are useful for their antipruritic and mild sedative effects, especially in children. Systemic corticosteroids and antibiotics are limited to patients suffering from very severe disease.

Exfoliative Dermatitis

Exfoliative dermatitis, also known as exfoliative erythroderma, is a condition of generalized epidermal peeling in which a rapidly developing generalized skin erythema is followed by fine scaling or marked desquamation of thick sheets of the epidermis. The condition is idiopathic in about half of the cases and the other half is due to a severe drug hypersensitivity reaction following penicillin, sulphonamides, etc., scarlet fever, leukaemia, lymphoma, generalized dermatitis, atopic dermatitis or psoriasis.

The generalized exfoliation of the epidermis results in extensive weeping, reddened and raw inflamed areas with associated widespread lymphadenomegaly, hepatosplenomegaly and low-grade fever. Chills are typical as heat is radiated away from the vasodilated, erythematous lesions. Severe fluid loss may occur from the weeping areas and the condition is occasionally fatal as there may be severe hypothermia, hypovolaemic shock and cardiac failure as the blood is diverted to the skin.

Hospitalization of patients with the condition is advisable and diagnostic tests to rule out systemic disorders such as lymphoma must be carried out. The patient is kept in a warm room, may be encouraged to bathe frequently in medicated water (colloidal balneotherapy) and treated with low-potency, topical, corticosteroid preparations.

Staphylococcal Scalded Skin Syndrome

The scalded skin syndrome is a dermatitis caused by *Staphylococcus aureus*, typically in infants less than 5 years of age. It is caused by the release of an exfoliative toxin from certain strains of the bacterium. This toxin splits the epidermis, without causing necrosis or much inflammation in the deeper layers. The infection usually localizes in mucosal sites (causing pharyngitis, otitis media and conjunctivitis), where the organism elaborates the toxin, which enters the bloodstream and affects the skin. The face, neck, axillae and groin are primarily involved and the first indication of disease is a faint, reddened, tender eruption which within 24 to 48 hours develops into confluent vesicopustules. These rupture and cause patches of exfoliation to appear with denuded, oozing, raw skin exposed. The condition is treated with antibiotics, electrolyte and fluid balance and supportive care.

Impetigo Contagiosa

Impetigo or 'school sores' is a childhood infection which *Staphylococcus aureus* or *Streptococcus pyogenes* or both bacteria may cause. The infection begins as erythema and progresses to vesicles which provoke intense pruritus. The lesions erode and form into honey-coloured crusts. Uncommonly, acute glomerulonephritis may complicate the disease. Impetigo typically occurs on the face and exposed portions of the body. The lesions and their discharge teem with the bacteria and the disease is highly contagious. Treatment is by administration of systemic penicillin or erythromycin, and isolation of the affected child to prevent spread.

Tinea

Tinea or 'ringworm' is a superficial fungal infection of the skin caused by many species of dermatophytic fungi belonging to three main genera: *Trichophyton*, *Epidermophyton* and *Microsporum*. Depending on the region of skin affected, tinea may be specified by an appropriate adjective, for example **tinea corporis** (of the body), **tinea capitis** (of the head), **tinea unguium** (of the nails), **tinea cruris** (of the groin), **tinea pedis** (of the foot — 'athlete's foot') and **tinea barbae** (of the beard region). All types of tinea produce similar lesions with reddened, pruritic, scaling and sometimes painful lesions. The lesion may start as a small reddened patch and gradually enlarge, the margin being slightly raised and erythematous (as though a worm were burrowing under the skin, hence 'ringworm'). In the head the condition leads to alopecia (generally temporary, non-scarring, patchy hair loss) and in some severe cases may lead to formation of **kerion**, a raised, boggy nodule with extensive inflammation and tissue destruction leading to scarring and permanent hair loss. Kerion is formed because of an exaggerated host response to the presence of the fungi, indicating possibly a hypersensitivity to the fungal antigens.

The lesions of tinea are usually quite characteristic and the diagnosis may be confirmed by demonstrating bright green fluorescence of affected regions under **Wood's lamp** (an ultraviolet light lamp under whose light only *some* fungi will fluoresce) and more conclusively by culturing the causative agent from infected specimens in a microbiology laboratory.

Treatment of tinea is with topical and systemic antifungal drugs (e.g. griseofulvin), and the family pet or other members of the family may also need treatment. Treatment is for long time periods and hair regrowth may be very slow. Generally, the condition of tinea is mild and easily amenable to treatment and cure.

Acne Vulgaris

Acne is an extremely common condition, usually maximal in adolescence, and affecting young males more commonly than young females. Occasionally, acne may be seen in the neonate and in this case is due to maternal androgens entering the baby's circulation and causing the disorder. Neonatal acne resolves without therapy by about 4 months of age. Acne affects predominantly the face, upper chest, back and neck. The precise aetiology is unknown, but the sebaceous glands are predominantly involved in the disease process and the following factors may be contributory:

- **Hormonal**: Androgens, in particular dihydrotestosterone, cause hyperplasia of the sebaceous glands, and oestrogens result in their atrophy. Conversely, acne may be controlled by large doses of oestrogen. Also, some patients on cortisone in high doses develop acne.
- **Familial tendency**: Acne seems to be more common in some families, so that there may be an hereditary overproduction of keratin, plugging hair follicles.
- **Dietary**: The role of diet in acne is obscure but some people with acne find that certain foodstuffs (e.g. chocolate, dairy foods) may exacerbate the condition.
- **Vitamins**: Deficiency of vitamin A may produce hyperkeratosis and follicular plugging, thus promoting acne. It should be noted, however, that most people with acne do not have vitamin A deficiency.
- **Emotional stress**, **cutaneous friction**, **heavy make-up**, **oily hair products** and **manipulation of the affected skin area** may all further aggravate the problem.

The lesion of acne begins as an obstruction of the pilosebaceous gland by keratin, and inspissation of the sebum. This is thought to be related to androgen-dependent hypersecretion of viscous sebum with poor drainage. The plugged follicle produces a **comedo**, a 'whitehead' or 'blackhead'. The pigmentation develops only in the more superficially plugged skin pores where the epithelium is heavily pigmented with melanin and thus pigments the plug. Later, as the sebum escapes into the dermis through overdistention of the comedo and bacterial action, a folliculitis and perifolliculitis develops, forming a papule. Secondary bacterial infection by *Propionibacterium acnes* and/or *Staphylococcus* spp. results in suppuration with typical pustules developing ('pimples'). Enzymatic destruction of the sebum by bacterial enzymes results in the formation of highly inflammatory by-products. Granuloma formation may result in response to the tissue breakdown products and released sebum. Healing of the damaged regions is by fibrosis and the scarring may be severe and disfiguring (refer to Figure 16.5).

Treatment of the condition relies heavily on patient education, especially in the matter of avoiding the different aggravating factors that are important in the various cases. Picking, squeezing and otherwise manipulating the lesions must be strenuously discouraged. Adequate hygiene of the skin with superficial desquamation diminishes follicular plugging by removing excessive keratin scales and plugs that may be forming in association with hair follicles. This may be achieved by chemical or physical peeling agents (e.g. benzoyl peroxide creams, retinoic acid 2.5 to 10%, lotions containing sulphur, salicylic acid and/or resorcinol, abrasive soaps and exposure to ultraviolet light). Anti-inflammatory preparations may be beneficial and topical corticosteroid preparations may be used. Antibiotics applied topically or administered

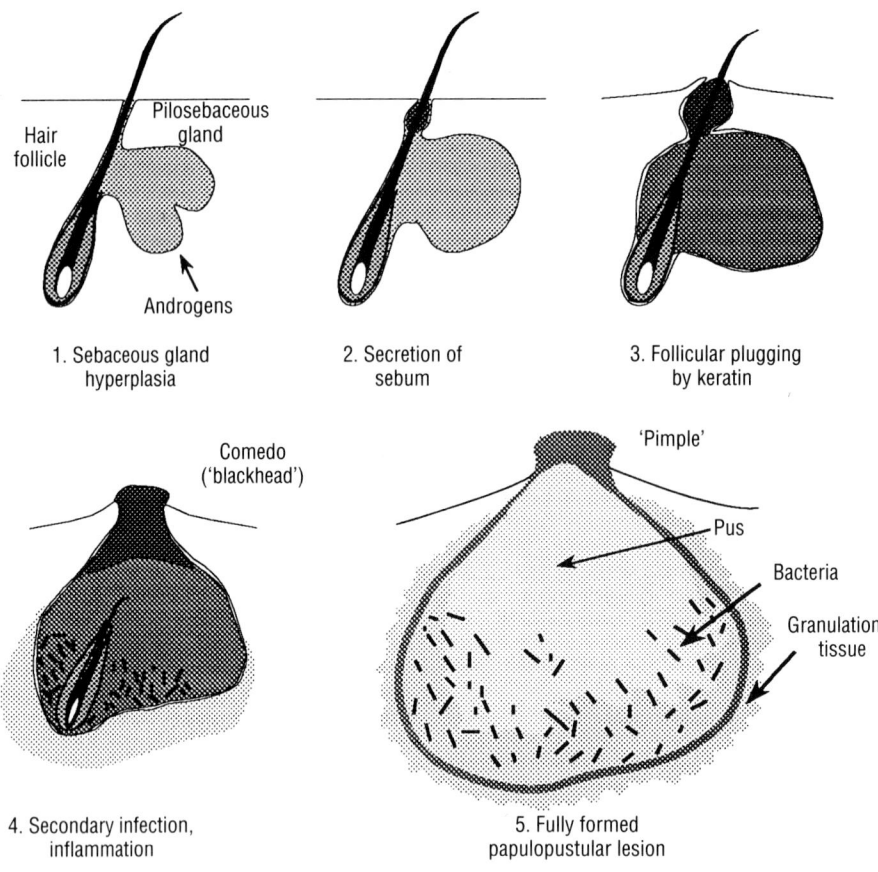

Figure 16.5 *Acne vulgaris*

systemically over a long period may limit the degree of secondary infection, prevent suppuration, damage and scarring. Tetracyclines, erythromycin or clindamycin are usually the antibiotics of choice. Oestrogen-rich oral contraceptives may prove beneficial to a female patient's acne.

It should be noted that allergic contact dermatitis may develop in the patient with acne in association with the various agents that are applied topically for treatment. After improvement of the condition occurs, the therapy is eased off, not abruptly discontinued, thus preventing flare ups. Residual acne scars may be treated by local excision and closure, dermabrasion, deep chemical peel or by cutaneous collagen implants.

Seborrhoeic Dermatitis

This is an extremely common condition in its mild form of seborrhoea or 'dandruff'. The scales of dan-druff are desquamated keratin matted together by sebaceous material. Seborrhoea results from excessive epithelial proliferation and formation of large quantities of keratin scales. Areas with a large number of sebaceous glands are favoured and the condition is primarily seen in the scalp, eyebrows, nasolabial folds, moustache and beard, upper central chest and perineal areas.

In the more florid form a dermatitis is present also. Seborrhoeic dermatitis manifests itself as raised reddened plaques with greasy yellow scales overlying them. Microscopically the appearance is not diagnostic and resembles other forms of chronic dermatitis with hyperkeratosis and parakeratosis, acanthosis, mild spongiosis and mild chronic inflammation of the dermis. There appears to be a familial predisposition to the disorder but it may also be aggravated by poor hygiene, emotional stress, immobility and debilitating illness. Often, if a patient is hospitalized for an unrelated disorder, seborrhoeic dermatitis will develop or become much worse. The condition tends to be chronic and recurrent with therapy often required for many years.

The treatment regime involves the use of medicated shampoos (selenium sulphide, zinc pyrithione and sulphur/salicylic acid types) that prevent rapid epithelial proliferation and hence scale formation. If very severe scaling is present, overnight applications of keratolytic agents (keralyt gel) are advised and the patient wears a shower cap during the night, which keeps the medication in place. Topical lotions and creams containing mild corticosteroid preparations will limit the inflammation and may cause the condition to regress. Often, stress management and relaxation classes will be of benefit in the treatment of the disorder.

Miscellaneous Diseases

Pemphigus Vulgaris

Pemphigus vulgaris is an uncommon serious disorder of the skin and mucous membranes. It is a bullous eruption which affects any skin surface, but especially the chest, scalp, groin, axilla and mouth. Although the disease is described as idiopathic, there is mounting evidence that it is an autoimmune state where there is autoimmune destruction of epidermal structures. Autoantibodies against the epithelial basement membrane may be demonstrated in 90% of patients. It appears between the ages of 40 and 60 years, affects males and females equally, is more common in Jews and follows a life-long course.

Microscopically there are numerous areas in the skin showing marked acantholysis with contained acantholytic cells. These regions enlarge to form flaccid bullae within the epidermis that are often several centimetres in diameter. If the fluid within the bulla is sampled and a smear made, the degenerate acantholytic cells can be identified readily, forming the basis of the **Tzanck test**. There is dermal oedema and marked inflammation with neutrophils and some eosinophils apparent. The bullae enlarge and rupture, leaving a raw skin surface that is inflamed and becomes easily infected. In half of the patients, similar lesions in the oral cavity and other mucous membranes develop up to a year before the skin lesions do.

The patient loses weight, becomes weak and is subject to major systemic infections. This is a very severe condition which was often fatal before cortisone therapy was available. The disease may be confused with less serious disorders such as contact dermatitis, but it must be diagnosed rapidly as it may cause the patient's death (even with hospitalization the mortality remains considerable, death occurring owing to toxaemia, shock or infection). Diagnosis is by skin biopsy, serology and the Tzanck test. Treatment of the condition is by systemic corticosteroid administration, but other immunosuppressives such as methotrexate, cyclophosphamide and azathioprine may all be helpful, leading to a controlled disease and a near-normal life.

Pemphigus Vegetans

This is a disorder similar to pemphigus vulgaris, but the bullae that develop are followed by the formation of warty excrescences and by pustules. Abscesses filled with eosinophils are present in the epithelium of skin and mucous membranes affected. The disease has a similar course and prognosis to pemphigus vulgaris. Some other uncommon forms of pemphigus also occur, namely **pemphigus foliaceus** and **pemphigus erythematosus**, both of which affect the skin only, the former being more likely to be extensive, the latter more likely to be confined to the face. Both of these disorders are milder than pemphigus vulgaris and will frequently resolve after several years, even in the absence of treatment.

Pemphigoid

Pemphigoid is a self-limited disorder in which large, tense bullae form on inflamed skin. The bullae are subepidermal and are not found in the mouth and mucosae. No acantholysis is present and the Tzanck test is negative, although often pemphigoid is confused with pemphigus clinically. Microscopically there is inflammation in the dermis associated with the bullae and there may be large collections of eosinophils in these regions. The condition has a predilection for the elderly and occurs typically in intertriginous areas, but usually remits 2 to 6 years after onset. It is treated similarly to pemphigus and the disease often resolves spontaneously.

Psoriasis

Psoriasis is a common, often familial, chronic progressive dermatitis of uncertain aetiology. Approximately 3% of the population suffer from this condition in varying severity. About 10% of cases of psoriasis develop before the age of 10 years and in this presentation the condition may be associated with acute respiratory infections. Although the majority of cases are idiopathic, some cases of psoriasis may be drug-induced and in this instance resemble more a drug-associated rash with scaling than the typical lesions of psoriasis. Some cases of psoriasis are brought about by traumatic injury to the skin and underlying tissues (**Köbner's phenomenon**); the disease thus often develops around surgical incisions, abrasions, cuts, sunburn or other sites of physical and chemical injury. In about 10% of patients with psoriasis, an arthritis also occurs and affects particularly the distal, small joints. This suggests possibly an autoimmune component being important in the pathogenesis of both skin and joint disease.

Psoriasis presents as lesions primarily on extensor surfaces, bony prominences, the scalp, ears, genitalia and perianal area, although any other part of the skin may also be involved. Typical lesions are dry, irregular, sharply demarcated plaques of reddening covered by many layers of silvery scales. On scraping, the scales are removed to expose fine, multiple bleeding points. In about half of the patients with psoriasis the nails are involved, with pitting, separation of nail from nail bed, thickening of the nail, and accumulation of keratin scales under the nail. The disease is often confused with tinea unguium and this must be excluded by microbiological examination. The lesions of psoriasis are generally not associated with pruritus and display bilateral symmetry. Microscopically there is acanthosis, parakeratosis and hyperkeratosis. There is prolongation of the rete pegs and the dermal papillae protrude upward into the epidermis, becoming very superficial. The blood vessels in these dermal upgrowths give rise to the multiple bleeding points when the lesions are scraped. Foci of inflammatory cells may occur in the epidermis and dermis, microabscesses thus forming (**microabscesses of Munro**).

Up to 20% of cases of exfoliative dermatitis are due to psoriasis, and destructive lesions in the joints may be seen in patients who also have the arthritis. The disease is a chronic one and tends to remit and relapse. Although the disease is not 'curable', it may be very adequately controlled with appropriate treatment. Several treatment regimes are possible and they may be used in isolation or in combination. Ultraviolet light alone or in combination with coal tar derivatives may be used in the hospital to initiate an intensive treatment that has clearing of extensive lesions as an objective. **Psoralens** are photosensitizing chemicals that are natural or synthetic and react on exposure to ultraviolet light to increase melanin production in the skin. Psoralens and ultraviolet light treatment (PUVA) combines an orally administered psoralen with long-wave ultraviolet light exposure of the skin. Topical corticosteroid preparations may improve greatly many cases of psoriasis, and other immunosuppressive agents such as methotrexate or hydroxyurea may be administered systemically, being useful in refractory cases of severe disease. Intralesional injections of corticosteroids may be used in treating nails affected by psoriasis but this is a painful treatment and recurrences are common.

Pityriasis Rosea

This is thought to be a viral infection but to date the causative agent has not been identified. It tends to occur in the autumn and spring, predominantly in adolescents and young adults, having a benign course, although it may cause a great deal of alarm for the patient. The disease begins with a large, ovoid, reddish, scaly lesion known as the **herald patch**. Two to ten days later the chest and back, mainly, become filled with numerous, small, rounded, scaling maculopapular lesions. The patient may experience mild malaise and pruritus. The condition may be confused with secondary syphilis, but in pityriasis rosea the palms and soles are not affected and the mucous membranes show no lesions. Spontaneous recovery will occur in approximately 4 to 14 weeks and the patient is not considered contagious during this period. Sunlight exposure may hasten recovery and application of a mild, topical, corticosteroid lotion will decrease pruritus.

Skin Tumours and Tumour-like Diseases

Verrucae (Warts)

Warts are virally induced lesions caused when there is an infection with the Human Papilloma Virus (HPV) in the skin. **Verruca vulgaris** is the common wart, showing a papillomatous appearance. **Verruca plantaris** is the plantar wart, where the effect of pressure forces the lesion into the underlying dermis of the sole of the foot. **Verruca plana juvenilis** is the flat wart occurring in children and is usually multiple, especially on the hands and face. **Condyloma acuminatum** is the sexually transmitted or genital wart. It is a fleshier, softer, sometimes pedunculated excrescence on the genitalia and perianal region. Multiple genital warts are commonly seen.

Warts tend to be elevated, tan or flesh-coloured papillomatous lesions with an irregular rough or smooth surface. Genital warts tend to be larger and fleshier.

Microscopically all warts show gross papillary overgrowth of the epidermis with hyperkeratosis, acanthosis, spongiosis and vacuolation of the epidermal cells, the cells often showing viral inclusion bodies. The basal layer of the epidermis is intact and the dermis shows an inflammatory infiltrate.

Warts may spontaneously disappear but there is a high recurrence rate. Treatment regimes include local excision or liquid nitrogen cryotherapy of isolated warts, electrodesiccation and curettage, intralesional cytotoxic agents (e.g. bleomycin), or applications of 6% salicylic acid gel. Venereal warts if less than 0.5 cm in diameter respond to applications of podophyllin in tincture of benzoin. Larger venereal warts need to be excised surgically, which is especially important as these warts may undergo malignant transformation.

Callus (Corn)

Corns are horny thickenings of the epidermis with a broad base on the skin surface and an apex in the dermis. They occur usually on the feet in association with ill-fitting or tight shoes, or they may occur at any point of long, continued pressure. Microscopically there is hyperkeratosis, the compressed mass of keratin producing atrophy of the adjacent epidermis and indenting the underlying dermis in which there is an inflammatory cell reaction. Corns may be surgically or chemically removed.

Keratoacanthoma (Molluscum Sebaceum)

Keratoacanthoma is a rapidly enlarging lesion which typically occurs on the face of elderly people. Alternatively, it may be seen in other parts of the body and frequently occurs after irritation, for example after a rose thorn has entered the skin on the hands. The lesion presents as a raised plaque with a central keratin plug. The lesion grows rapidly, thus mimicking a malignant tumour and yet the vast majority of these lesions are self-healing within a few months. Microscopically there is a central core of keratin which is laminated, surrounded by squamous epithelium extending deeply downwards. It is a 'horny' outgrowth which is quite firm and may reach a size of several millimetres. It either drops off or is easily excised.

The lesion should not be confused with **molluscum contagiosum** which is due to a viral infection and presents as a papillary, hyperkeratotic mass, resembling a wart with a central depression or dimple. This lesion is due to a Poxvirus infection and may be found on, or near, the genitals of adults, or most commonly the face and trunk of children. The lesions resolve spontaneously within 6 to 12 months but resolution may be hastened by cryotherapy, excision or electrodesiccation.

Squamous Cell Papilloma

This is a fronded, pigmented or non-pigmented, hyperkeratotic, papillary lesion. If hyperkeratosis is excessive it may form a cutaneous 'horn'. Microscopically there is papillary overgrowth of the squamous epithelium which is regular and forms an excess of keratin on the surface. The squamous cells may show melanin pigmentation and there is frequently an inflammatory cell infiltration at the base. The lesion is totally benign and shows no invasion, but it is generally excised for, if nothing else, cosmetic reasons.

Keratotic Lesions

Senile keratosis is a very common condition appearing on the exposed skin surfaces of elderly people, as small, hard, often scaly lesions astride a red base. They consist of regions of acanthosis and hyperkeratosis and dyskeratosis with prolongation of the rete pegs. Mitotic activity may be seen in the prickle cell layer and there may be dysplasia present. This lesion can be described as the response of ageing skin to continued damage by ultraviolet radiation. Some of these lesions may progress to squamous cells carcinoma.

Actinic keratosis is similar to senile keratosis but may develop in younger individuals if they have exposed themselves excessively to ultraviolet radiation. These lesions typically occur on the face, ears and forearms, presenting as rough-surfaced, keratotic papules. They slowly develop into invasive squamous cell carcinoma.

Seborrhoeic keratosis is a benign surface lesion, usually pigmented and multiple, appearing from about the age of 30 years and becoming more common with increasing age. These lesions are also known as **seborrhoeic warts**, **verruca senilis** and **basal cell papillomata**. They occur typically on the trunk, face and arms, often appearing symmetrically, and they may show a familial tendency in their development. They are sharply circumscribed, pigmented, rough and raised lesions appearing as though they had been 'stuck on', varying in size from a few millimetres to a few centimetres in diameter. The lesions are usually treated by electrodesiccation or cryotherapy under local anaesthesia.

Leukoplakia

Leukoplakia may occur on mucous membranes (e.g. mouth, vulva) and on the skin where it presents as thickened, white, fissured plaques. Microscopically there is hyperkeratosis, acanthosis, and prominence of rete pegs, which form atypical downgrowths into the chronically inflamed dermis. This is a premalignant condition and a high percentage of untreated cases will progress to squamous cell carcinoma. On the skin, leukoplakia may be seen in regions of chronic irritation, especially where there is prolonged injury or contact with irritating substances. Some of the chronic skin inflammatory conditions may progress to leukoplakia.

Bowen's Disease (Carcinoma in situ of the Skin)

This is a condition presenting as a slightly thickened, scaly or brown lesion, usually solitary, which slowly grows and extends outwards. It may be seen in sites that had previously been involved in leukoplakia or it may arise spontaneously, after prolonged contact with carcinogenic chemicals, for example arsenic. While this is a malignant condition, there is an intact basement membrane, justifying the term carcinoma *in situ*. However, if the condition is left untreated, evolution into a typical, invasive squamous cell carcinoma will occur. Microscopically there is hyperkeratosis, parakeratosis, spongiosis and dyskeratosis. The prickle cells appear very atypical and show all the hallmarks of malignancy. The basal cell layer appears intact.

A similar condition to Bowen's disease of the skin is **erythroplasia of Queyrat** occurring on the glans penis and prepuce. This presents as single or multiple, flat, red patches which may be crusted. There is marked dysplasia and atypical appearance of the epidermis with keratosis. Although the all hallmarks of malignancy may be observed in the cells, there is no invasion. If the condition is left untreated, it will progress to typical carcinoma.

Squamous Cell Carcinoma (SCC)

Incidence. SCC is the characteristic tumour of squamous epithelia and squamous mucosae. It accounts for approximately 10% of all malignant tumours, and over 1% of all cancer deaths. It is seen especially in the elderly (older than 50 years of age) but may be seen in younger people following irradiation. It affects males more often than females (M:F = 3:1).

Aetiology. Predisposing factors associated with the tumour include the following:

- It is more common in fair-skinned, fair-haired individuals who work outdoors.
- SCC occurs more often in people with premalignant skin lesions and other skin diseases, such as leukoplakia, senile keratosis, Bowen's disease, xeroderma pigmentosum, etc.
- Sunlight exposure predisposes to it as excessive UV radiation causes DNA damage in the skin cells (an additive effect may be demonstrated). Irradiation by X-rays, etc. also predisposes to SCC. These are the so-called **actinic cancers**.
- Exposure to carcinogenic hydrocarbons is predisposing and workers contacting pitch, tar, paraffin, creosote and soot may, after many years, develop skin cancer.
- Arsenic, after prolonged contact, produces an arsenical keratosis which may be followed by squamous cell or basal cell carcinoma. This may be an occupational cancer occurring in workers handling arsenical compounds.
- Chronic inflammations and thermal injuries may predispose to SCC and it may arise in burn scars, chronic ulcers, varicose ulcers, etc.

Sites affected. Typically SCC occurs on exposed skin surfaces such as the face, neck and hands but it is also the primary malignancy associated with squamous mucosae such as the mouth, tongue, oesophagus and vagina. It is also found in mucocutaneous junctions such as the lips, anus, glans penis and vulva. Squamous metaplasia may lead to the tumour in unexpected or unusual sites as occurs with some tumours of the bronchus, endocervix, bowel and gall bladder.

Morphology. Typically, SCC first appears as a small raised papule or papillary lesion. The majority of lesions then progress to form indolent ulcers with a central scab. The edges are raised and rolled outwards (everted), and scaling may be seen. There is invasion of underlying tissue with local fixation and surrounding induration. Histologically 80% of the tumours are well differentiated. They arise from adjacent epithelium and are seen as nodular, sheet-like accumulations under the epithelium, invading the dermis or mucosa. The tumour cells are keratinocytes with prickle cell forms seen; also, active keratin formation in the centre of the nodules occurs, these central laminated aggregates of keratin being known as **keratin pearls**. Approximately 20% of the tumours show varying loss of differentiation, some being totally anaplastic. Surrounding the invading tongues of tumour, which may be found deep in the dermis, is a tumour-associated immune response with numerous lymphocytes and some plasma cells and macrophages. Neutrophils of acute inflammation and exudate may be seen in infected tumours.

Spread. The spread of the tumour depends on the differentiation. Well-differentiated tumours grow more slowly and are less aggressive in their spread. There is local infiltration with attachment to the underlying dermis. Lymphatic and blood invasion then occurs. Distant metastases may be seen. Distant spread is more frequent with poorly differentiated tumours.

Signs and symptoms. These skin lesions tend to be discovered while still small and less than 5% of patients have lymph node involvement at the time of diagnosis. Most patients notice the region of induration or ulceration and usually present because of the cosmetic effects. Some tumours may become secondarily infected and there is pain and exudation or suppuration. Elderly patients, in particular, may neglect the tumour and at the time of presentation there may be a very large mass present with extensive ulceration.

Diagnosis. The tumour has a characteristic appearance and usually naked eye examination is sufficient to diagnose a malignant tumour of this type. Histological examination of the excised mass confirms the diagnosis and indicates the grade of tumour, the degree of differentiation, whether or not lymphatic invasion has occurred and if the draining lymph nodes have also been involved.

Treatment and prognosis. Treatment of SCC is by excision of the tumour and removal of regional lymph nodes if this is indicated. Squamous cell carcinoma of the skin tends to be discovered while still small and the tumour in most cases is still confined to the site of origin. Excision is then curative with 5-year survivals of 90% or greater. Half of the SCC in mucosae have metastasized to the regional draining lymph nodes by the time of diagnosis and the prognosis depends on the extent of the spread and completeness of excision. Most SCC of the bronchus have an extremely poor prognosis because of early spread via the lymph and blood. Radiotherapy may be used where spread has occurred and this is usually only a palliative treatment. Overall, the average 5-year survival for skin SCC is approximately 80%.

Basal Cell Carcinoma (BCC, Rodent Ulcer)

Incidence. BCC is a tumour of basal cells of the epidermis, although the precise cell of origin or stage of development of the cell undergoing neoplastic change is still debatable. It is also known as the 'rodent ulcer' as it tends to erode or ulcerate, destroying the skin site in which it arises, spreading locally only. It occurs most commonly between 60 and 80 years of age, affecting males twice as often as females (M:F = 2:1). This is the commonest malignant neoplasm in Caucasians, approximately 15 to 18% of all malignancies being of this type.

Predisposing factors. BCC is predisposed to by excessive sunlight, ultraviolet light, previous radiation therapy (e.g. deep X-rays) and prolonged contact with arsenic. It tends to affect more the fair-haired, fair-skinned individuals who spend much of their time outdoors.

Sites affected. BCC may be found anywhere on the skin except the palms of the hands and soles of the feet. The majority occur on the face above a line joining the angle of the mouth to the ear. It is common in the nasolabial folds, around the eyes and the scalp. About three-quarters of the tumours arise on the nose or cheeks.

Morphology. The tumour begins as a slowly growing, pearly, flattened nodule. The centre soon breaks down and a central ulcer and scab develop. The periphery forms a smooth, slightly raised margin, which as it spreads forms characteristically a 'rolled edge' which is undermined. Histologically, the tumour begins as groups of small, dark, basal-like cells apparently sprouting from the undersurface of the intact epidermis, or rarely from a hair follicle. The cell groups enlarge and spread downwards to invade the dermis. Clumps form, composed of sheets of cells with a characteristic **palisaded margin**, where the cells lining the periphery of the nodules are arranged side by side very regularly, like the palings of a palisade fence. Many mitoses are seen and in typical BCC no keratin or prickle cells are observed. Sometimes, **cystic variants** of BCC are seen and in this case numerous cysts are present within the tumour mass, lined by tumour cells and filled with fluid.

Spread. Spread of BCC is local only. Invasion of blood vessels or lymphatics virtually never occurs, hence there are no metastases. It must be remembered that these tumours are still malignant tumours and if they are neglected they may cause the death of the patient

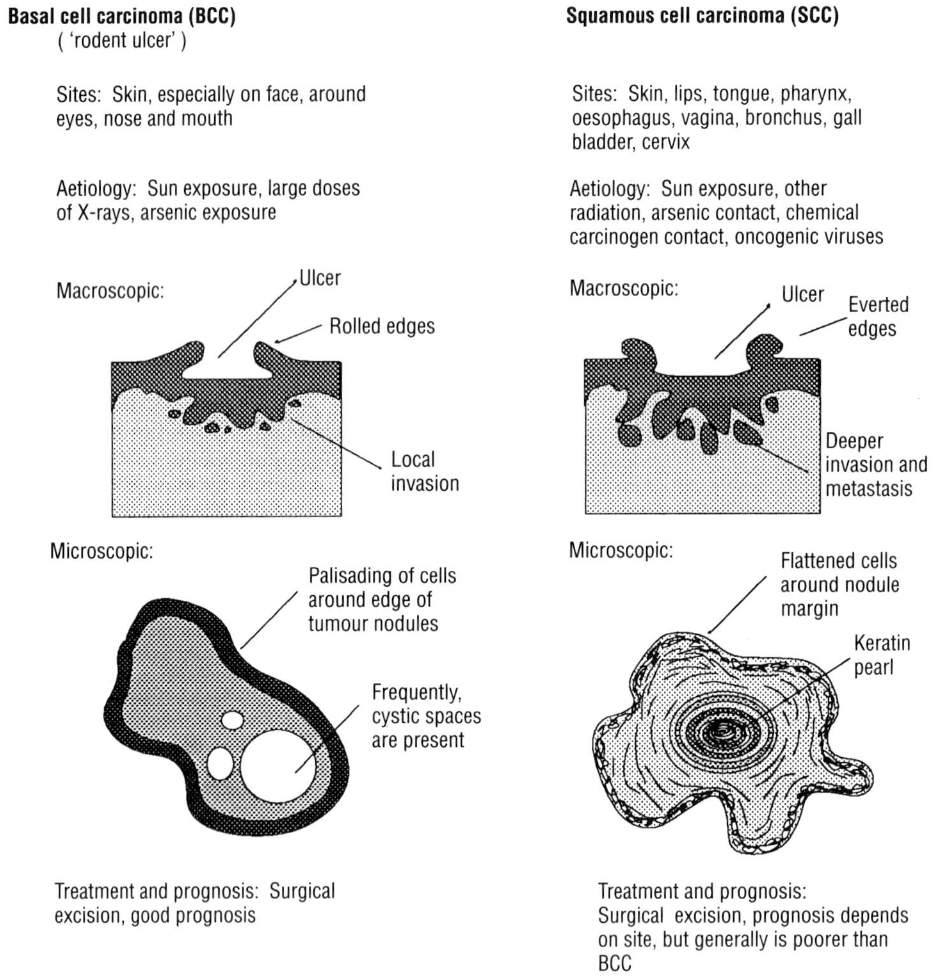

Basal cell carcinoma (BCC)
('rodent ulcer')

Sites: Skin, especially on face, around eyes, nose and mouth

Aetiology: Sun exposure, large doses of X-rays, arsenic exposure

Macroscopic: — Ulcer — Rolled edges — Local invasion

Microscopic: — Palisading of cells around edge of tumour nodules — Frequently, cystic spaces are present

Treatment and prognosis: Surgical excision, good prognosis

Squamous cell carcinoma (SCC)

Sites: Skin, lips, tongue, pharynx, oesophagus, vagina, bronchus, gall bladder, cervix

Aetiology: Sun exposure, other radiation, arsenic contact, chemical carcinogen contact, oncogenic viruses

Macroscopic: — Ulcer — Everted edges — Deeper invasion and metastasis

Microscopic: — Flattened cells around nodule margin — Keratin pearl

Treatment and prognosis: Surgical excision, prognosis depends on site, but generally is poorer than BCC

Figure 16.6 *Comparison of basal and squamous cell carcinomata*

simply because of local invasion effects. For example, a basal cell carcinoma occurring near the eye may invade into the eye, destroy it and replace it eventually invading into the brain and causing the death of the patient. However, this situation rarely occurs and most of the tumours are treated early.

Signs, symptoms and diagnosis. As for SCC.

Treatment and prognosis. Following excision, the prognosis is excellent with a 95% or better 5-year survival. The tumour may recur in 15% of cases but excision once again checks its progress. If BCC is left untreated it may cause death due to local invasion.

Basosquamous Carcinoma

Basosquamous carcinoma is a variant of BCC which is a predominantly typical BCC in appearance, containing regions which appear more like SCC, even containing prickle cells and keratin pearls. The behaviour of these tumours is still typical of BCC and they have a similar prognosis.

Lesions of Melanocytes

Melanocytes are the melanin-producing cells of the body and have a neuroectodermal origin. Early in foetal life they migrate from the neural crest to the skin, squamous mucosae, leptomeninges, choroid and adrenals. Most lesions of the melanocytes occur in the skin. Melanocytes are DOPA-positive cells since they possess the enzyme tyrosinase. Cells containing this enzyme may be identified by allowing them to react with DOPA, a colourless compound, which is converted to a black oxidized compound by the tyrosinase in the DOPA-positive cells.

dihydroxyphenylalanine $\rightarrow$ tyrosinase $\rightarrow$ blackened
(DOPA)   oxidation   DOPA

Normal skin has melanocytes on the basal layer in ratios of one melanocyte to ten basal cells (in most of the skin surface) and one melanocyte to five basal cells (in deeply pigmented skin such as the areola of the breast) depending on the site. The number of melanocytes per unit area of skin is the same irrespective of race or skin colour. During infancy the balance between the normal ratio of melanocytes to basal cells is upset at a few or many sites, resulting in formation of hamartomata ('birthmarks'). A pigmented **naevus** or 'mole' is the most common hamartoma. The average Caucasian has between 10 and 40 of these throughout the body.

Another common skin blemish encountered is the **ephelis** (plural ephelides, 'freckles'). These macules occur in regions where there is a normal number of melanocytes that produce an increased quantity of melanin focally. Exposure to sunlight will often give rise to ephelides in genetically predisposed people. Freckles will usually be seen to be prominent in the summer months, fading away or completely disappearing in winter.

Hyperpigmentation of the skin is seen most commonly in people who expose themselves to ultraviolet radiation and is what is termed a 'suntan'. In this case there is no increase in the number of melanocytes in the skin, but simply an increased production of melanin in response to increased secretion of MSH. There are some states where hyperpigmentation of the skin is an associated symptom and these include endocrine disorders (e.g. Addison's disease), inherited metabolic disorders (e.g. haemochromatosis, porphyria, Wilson's disease) or even some normal states such as pregnancy or taking the contraceptive pill where the oestrogens cause increased melanin production. **Chloasma** of pregnancy (= melasma or 'pregnancy mask') is an irregular, blotchy pigmentation of the face that develops because of the increased circulating oestrogens. Increased pigmentation of the nipples and genitalia may also be seen in these cases. Two other disorders involving hyperpigmentation ought to be mentioned and these are the Peutz-Jeghers syndrome and Von Recklinghausen's disease. In both of these disorders there are hyperpigmented spots on the skin caused by a localized overproduction of melanin by a normal number of melanocytes.

Proliferation of melanocytes can produce a large variety of black blemishes on the skin, most of these being quite benign and commonly observed. **Lentigo** is a proliferation of melanocytes replacing the basal layer of the skin or producing a flat, brown to black blemish on the skin. Most of these lesions appear in elderly people, usually on exposed parts of the skin and the majority of them remain benign. Sometimes, there are epidermal downgrowths into the dermis and in a small number cases the lesions will continue to grow and show increasing atypical morphology of melanocytes and if left untreated may progress to malignant melanoma.

A **junctional naevus** is a proliferation of melanocytes at the dermoepidermal junction which gives rise to nests of cells, macroscopically appearing as a flat, dark blemish similar to lentigo. During puberty some of these junctional naevi may enlarge and show 'junctional activity', which is a benign occurrence. If the junctional activity occurs later in life in a junctional naevus it is indicative of malignant change and such junctional naevi may progress to malignant melanoma.

Intradermal naevi consist of nests of naevus cells in the dermis and represent the commonest type of naevus found in the body. The lesions may be flat or raised, varying in colour from light tan to almost black; they may be scaly, hairy or inflamed. Small hairy naevi in adults are not premalignant and most intradermal naevi follow a totally benign existence throughout life, although people with many such naevi (>30–40) on their skin are more likely to present with malignant melanoma. In intradermal naevi the melanocytes are found in nests of cells deep within the dermis and the overlying epidermis does not contain increased numbers of melanocytes.

A **compound naevus** is a raised lesion which contains nests of melanocytes both in the dermis and epidermis. Such naevi are very commonly seen in childhood. Frequently they are hairy moles that may undergo malignant change. A variant seen in childhood especially is the so-called '**giant hairy naevus**' (often occurring in the sacral area, reaching a size of several centimetres in diameter and often associated with spina bifida). Such giant hairy naevi may undergo malignant change.

A **spitz naevus** or 'juvenile melanoma' (an unwarranted misnomer as the lesion is characteristically totally benign!) is a variant of the compound naevus which appears in children as a fleshy, pink papule. It is composed of nests of large, spindle-shaped melanocytes and epithelial cells in groups.

A **blue naevus** is a bluish or blue-brown lesion that

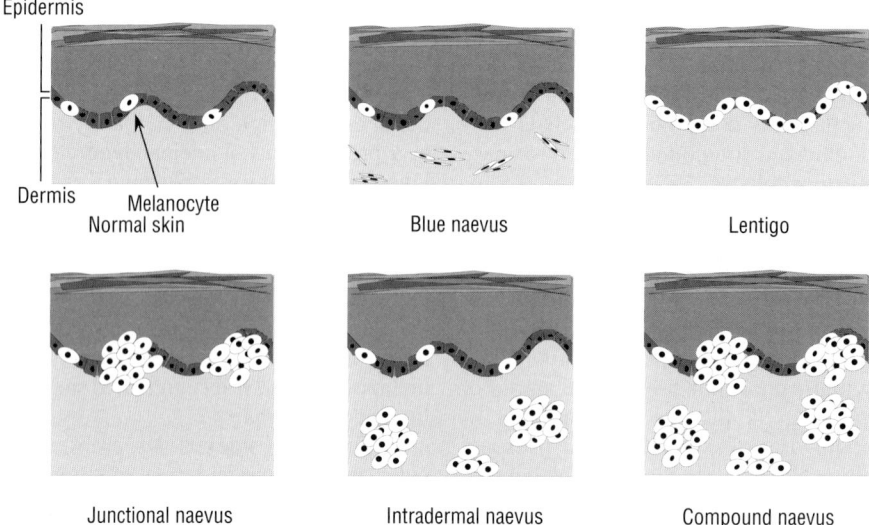

Figure 16.7 *Benign lesions of melanocytes*

appears as a nodule located in the dermis, causing a palpable thickening there. It is seen most often in children and young adults. Microscopically the epidermis is normal and in the dermis there are aggregates of melanin-containing phagocytes called **melanophores**, giving rise to a brownish colour if situated close to the epidermis or a bluish colour if situated deep in the dermis. These lesions are totally benign, contain no melanocytes and are generally removed for cosmetic reasons.

Hypopigmentation of the skin may also occur in some states, the condition being especially striking in the dark-skinned races, but decreases in the melanin content of the skin are generally less common than increases. Hypopigmentation may be seen in various endocrine disorders (e.g. in hypopituitarism, or even in Addison's disease where there may be foci of depigmentation in the darkened skin of the patient). Kwashiorkor in Africa leads to hypopigmentation and the normally black hair of the affected children turns a rusty red, this being a manifestation of the severe nutritional deficiencies in this disease. In phenylketonuria there is a disorder in melanin production and the affected individuals have brown or sandy coloured hair and a pale skin. Some infections such as leprosy and pinta may produce focal depigmentation in the skin.

Albinism is an autosomal recessive disorder, two variants of which are known, and in both the number of melanocytes in the epidermis is normal but the cells cannot produce melanin normally. The affected people

therefore have pink skin, pink irides and white hair. The disorder may be seen in dark-skinned races as well as the pale-skinned ones. In one of the variants of albinism the melanocytes do not possess tyrosinase and hence cannot produce melanin. In the other variant the melanocytes possess tyrosinase and form melanosomes, and are able to make a little melanin but not enough. Albinos are very prone to developing various skin cancers and must keep out of the sun as much as possible, wearing protective garments and sunscreen whenever they need to go out.

Vitiligo is a disorder of pigmentation in which melanin is lost from irregular, patchy regions of the skin as melanocytes in such areas degenerate and disappear. The lesions tend to enlarge with time and often they are surrounded by hyperpigmented margins. The disease is idiopathic, although an autoimmune pathogenesis is suspected. A small number of cases of this condition have occurred after viral meningitis and this further supports the autoimmune hypothesis.

Malignant Melanoma

Incidence. Malignant melanoma is a very aggressive malignant tumour of the melanocytes which tends to spread early. It is most commonly seen in the skin. Australia has the highest incidence of skin cancer and melanoma in the world, and Queensland has the highest incidence of malignant melanoma in Australia. The incidence of malignant melanoma has doubled in

Queensland in the last 20 years with 16 Caucasians out of every 100 000 developing the tumour. The tumour is rarely seen in childhood (except in association with hairy naevi) and is most often seen between 30 and 50 years of age. There is a slight male preponderance. Malignant melanomata account for approximately 4% of skin cancers.

Aetiology. The following aetiological and predisposing factors have been identified in connection with malignant melanoma.

- There is increased risk with **increasing age**.
- There is increased risk with prolonged **exposure to sunlight**. The further north one lives in Australia the greater the risk of developing the tumour.
- **Genetic factors** are very important and racial factors in this context are extremely important. People with red hair, freckles and fair skin ('Celtic type') are more at risk. On the other hand Aborigines and other black-skinned people, with their darkly pigmented skin, are protected. There is a higher risk with a family history of melanoma.
- Most melanomata arise from **pre-existing naevi**, especially junctional naevi and lentigo. There is also a risk with compound naevi, dysplastic naevi and traumatized naevi.
- **Solar keratoses** or 'sunspots', indicating skin damage caused by ultraviolet radiation, also predispose to the tumour.

Sites affected. Any part of the skin may be affected, including the palms of the hands and soles of the feet. It is most common on the backs of men and on the legs of women. Exposed areas commonly affected are the face, neck, hands and arms. Malignant melanoma may also occur at other sites where melanocytes are normally found, such as the vagina, meninges, locus ceruleus, basal ganglia in the brain and also in the eye and adrenal gland. However, extracutaneous malignant melanoma is very rare.

Morphology. Malignant melanomata are usually pigmented lesions, brown, deep brown or black in colour. In rare cases they may be unpigmented, the so-

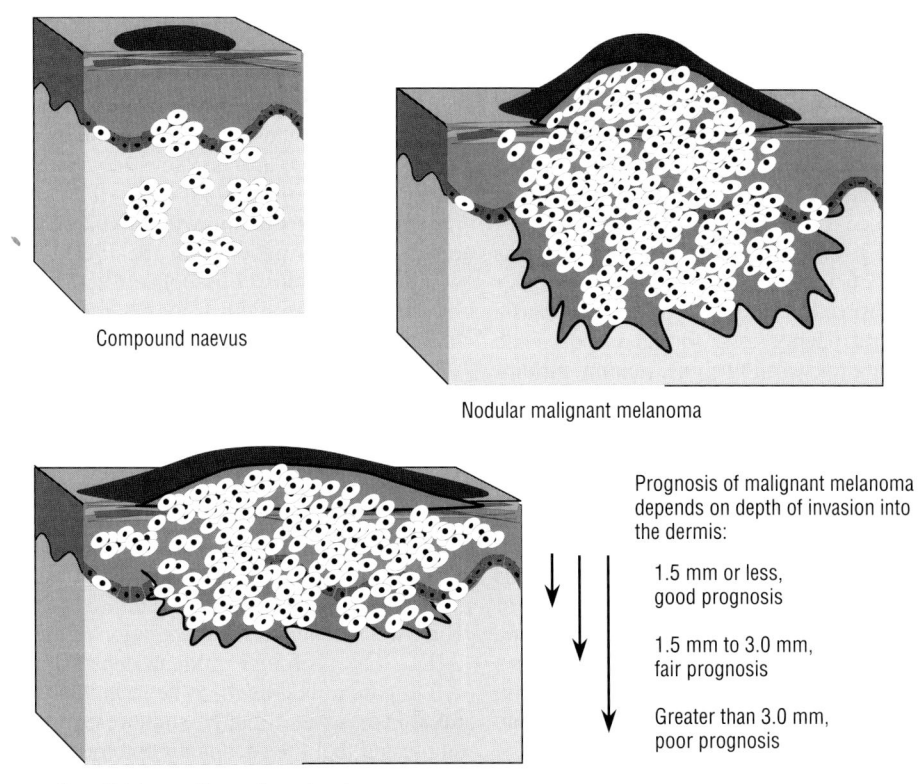

Compound naevus

Nodular malignant melanoma

Superficial spreading malignant melanoma

Prognosis of malignant melanoma depends on depth of invasion into the dermis:

1.5 mm or less, good prognosis

1.5 mm to 3.0 mm, fair prognosis

Greater than 3.0 mm, poor prognosis

Figure 16.8 *Malignant melanoma types*

called **amelanotic melanoma**. In the latter case they still contain DOPA-positive cells and the tumours may be identified as melanomata by the DOPA reaction. The tumours form rapidly growing flat or raised lesions and they are of two basic macroscopic types. The **superficially spreading melanoma** forms a flattened lesion which initially grows horizontally along the skin and may show satellite lesions, which are smaller masses of tumour, around the central, larger mass. The **nodular melanoma** forms a raised lesion that grows vertically, projecting from the skin surface, but also invading deeper into the dermis at an early stage. Both types of lesions may ulcerate or haemorrhage. The histological appearance of melanoma is diverse. The majority of tumours are well differentiated, the cells being large, polyhedral, pale staining, with large nuclei and prominent nucleoli. Melanomata most commonly show pigment production, with numerous granules of melanin within the tumour cells and also extracellularly. Melanin granules in the keratinized cell layer of the epidermis is usually an ominous sign. Pleomorphism, giant cell forms, many mitoses and irregularity of pigment distribution are often noted, and in some tumours there may be anaplasia.

Signs and symptoms. The warning signs of malignant melanoma are increase in size, change in shape and/or colour of a pre-existing naevus. The appearance of ulceration, haemorrhage and satellite lesions around a naevus is also commonly observed and should be immediately investigated further. It should be kept in mind that naevi occurring in sites liable to be chronically irritated (e.g. around the waist where there is constant rubbing of waistbands against the naevus, or along the bra strap line) are likely to show dysplasia over the long term. Hence, one should inspect such naevi often looking for warning signs. Itching, inflammation and a diameter larger than 5 mm are also signs worthy of further investigation.

Spread. Local spread is rapid, producing an enlarging, more extensive lesion. The tumour can spread in a superficial area rapidly or may grow vertically as a nodular type. In many cases lymphatic spread has often already occurred by the time of diagnosis of melanoma. The regional lymph nodes are seen to be affected, and tumour cells are found in lymphatics between the primary mass and the affected lymph nodes. Haematogenous spread also occurs early and metastases may be found in almost any organ of the body but especially in the liver, lungs and brain.

Treatment and prognosis. Treatment must be by excision of the malignant melanoma and removal of in-vaded regional lymph nodes. The depth of invasion is related to the prognosis. If the tumour has grown down into the dermis to a depth greater than 3 mm from the dermoepidermal junction, the prognosis is poor; if the tumour cells are found to have invaded to a depth of 1.5 to 3 mm, the prognosis is fair; and if the tumour is confined to a depth of 1.5 mm or less, the prognosis is good. Early recognition and treatment of melanoma is therefore essential. If the tumour is treated early, the 5-year survival is 80% or better. However, the average 5-year survival is approximately 25%, indicating that many of the tumours which may appear very small to the naked eye have already spread quite deeply and extensively by the time the patient presents. The very aggressive, anaplastic tumours show very early spread and highly destructive secondaries.

Kaposi's Sarcoma

Prior to the 1970s Kaposi's sarcoma was an extremely rare malignancy of vascular tissue of the skin. There was a slightly higher incidence of the lesion in southern Europe (especially in Italy) among Ashkenazy Jews and also in Africa. It was seen to occur primarily on the legs and feet of men (M:F is 10:1) between the ages of 65 and 70 years. It appeared as purplish, painful nodules and patches on the skin. It has recently been demonstrated that in certain parts of Africa the incidence is high and accounts for about 5 to 10% of all tumours. In the 1970s, cases of this tumour were reported in association with immunosuppression in renal transplant patients. In the 1980s, Kaposi's sarcoma became mostly associated with HIV infection. In AIDS, patients with Kaposi's sarcoma are characteristically young males.

It is clear from the epidemiological data that are available that the tumour is associated with states where the immune system is depressed. In old age, in renal transplant patients receiving immunosuppressive drugs and in the African population where there are numerous chronic infections undermining the immune defences, decreased immunosurveillance may be invoked to explain why these tumours arise. Perhaps the best evidence for immune depression leading to Kaposi's sarcoma is the association of the tumour with AIDS. The profound immune depression seen in the AIDS patient is thought to be sufficient reason for the tumour to arise, although some researchers have also suggested that the secondary cytomegalovirus (CMV) infections that are seen in the majority of AIDS patients may also contribute to the pathogenesis of AIDS-associated Kaposi's sarcoma.

In AIDS-associated tumours of this type (by far the

commonest type of Kaposi's sarcoma that is seen in Western countries), the skin and the mucosae, especially in the mouth, are the most frequent sites involved. The tumour is usually multiple, with many plaques developing in many sites throughout the body. Initially, the tumour appears as well-demarcated flattened plaques of a brownish or purplish colour, which represent regions where the neoplastic vascular endothelium is proliferating. The vascular spaces that form initially in the tumour may not be grossly atypical and around them are found regions of lymphocytes and proliferating fibroblasts. The plaques grow into firmer, elevated nodules which may show haemorrhage. The skin lesions in later stages may be quite florid and fungating, involving the lymph nodes. Histologically, bizarre vascular spaces are seen in the dermis with infiltrating and invading spindle cell populations that resemble vascular pericytes.

Three major subgroups of progression and prognosis are seen in relation to Kaposi's sarcoma and these are related to the three major forms of the tumour:

1. **Sporadic form** (not associated with HIV infection): The tumour is typically of low-grade malignancy, mostly occurring in elderly males. It is easily controlled by chemotherapy and the patients do not usually die as a result of this condition.
2. **Endemic form** (seen in Africa): The tumour is typically malignant and invades many tissues. It is thought that this tumour arises in association with viral infections (including HIV II infection) that are widespread in certain parts of Africa and therefore this subtype of tumour is of a higher inherent malignancy. This is because it occurs in the context of a generalized immunosuppression that is more marked than that observed in the sporadic form. These tumours may be controlled by chemotherapy but the prognosis is worse.
3. **Epidemic form** (seen with AIDS): The tumour is highly malignant and is associated with HIV infection, and in most cases CMV superinfection, thus occurring in patients with extreme immunodeficiency. Such tumours are multiple, quite extensive, liable to spread early and more difficult to control chemotherapeutically. Many AIDS patients die as a result of this malignancy, even if they have been treated rather aggressively for this tumour from an early stage.

Haemangioma

Haemangioma is a hamartomatous developmental anomaly of vascular tissues, rather than a true tumour, but it is included here for convenience. These lesions are also known as '**strawberry marks**', '**birthmarks**' and '**port wine stains**'. Three major types of haemangioma are distinguished.

Capillary haemangioma. This is so designated as it is composed of numerous blood vessels of a very small diameter. Any organ or tissue may contain these lesions but they most commonly occur on the skin, subcutis or mucous membranes. All such lesions are well demarcated but non-encapsulated. They are small, flattened or slightly elevated lesions, bright red or bluish in colour. Rarely, they may be very large, with an irregular, map-like margin situated on the face or upper trunk. Histologically they are seen to be composed of closely packed capillary-like vascular spaces, in some of the lumina of which may be found organized thrombi. Clinically, the lesions are totally benign and it is only rarely that they ulcerate and become secondarily infected. Transformation into neoplasms is very rare, if it ever occurs. The lesions may be removed by a plastic surgeon for cosmetic considerations.

Cavernous haemangioma. This type of haemangioma is characterized by the formation of an aggregate of large, cavernous, vascular spaces in continuity with the normal circulation and consequently filled with blood. The lesions occur in the skin and mucosae but are also quite common in many internal organs, for example the liver, spleen, pancreas and brain. In **Lindau von Hippel disease**, cavernous haemangiomata are found within the brain stem, pancreas and liver. Grossly, cavernous haemangiomata are reddish blue, spongy masses, 1 to 2 cm in diameter. On section, the lesion is well demarcated but not encapsulated; it is compressible and blood may exude from it. Rarely, giant forms occur, especially on the face, upper trunk and in other body sites. Histologically the mass comprises large vascular spaces partly or completely filled with fluid blood, separated by scanty amounts of connective tissue. The haemangioma remains in most cases subclinical but in certain situations it may lead to serious or fatal complications, mainly due to thrombosis or haemorrhage (e.g. a footballer receiving a blow to the abdomen causing his undiagnosed haemangioma of the liver to burst and haemorrhage intraperitoneally).

Sclerosing haemangioma (dermatofibroma; histiocytoma). This type of haemangioma is believed to arise out of a capillary haemangioma that becomes transformed into a solid tumour by the progressive proliferation of endothelial cells and the connective tissue stroma between the vessels. This change occurs over a period of many years and although the capillary haemangioma is present at birth, the sclerosing mass will not be well defined until young to middle adult life. The lesion presents as a firm, reddish or tan nodule that rarely causes any clinical manifestations. It may be excised for cosmetic considerations.

Other Skin Tumours

Other tumours which may affect the skin or subcutaneous tissues are lipoma and liposarcoma, which are tumours of adipose tissue; fibroma and fibrosarcoma, which are tumours of fibrocytes of connective tissue; and lymphangioma and lymphangiosarcoma, which are tumours of lymphatic vessels. Most of these are rather rare tumours and are seldom encountered in clinical situations. Tumours of the skin appendages are also sometimes seen, for example **hidradenoma**, a benign tumour of the apocrine sweat glands, **syringoma**, a benign tumour of the sweat glands, and **hibernoma**, a benign tumour of the brown fat adipocytes, a tumour arising out of the 'mulberry' cells of the foetus. The benign tumours are easily cured by local excision and this is often performed for cosmetic purposes by plastic surgeons. The malignant counterparts tend to be very invasive and spread early, therefore the prognosis is generally poor unless the tumours have been diagnosed very early and treated by wide excision. Some of these tumours are considered briefly below.

Lipoma. This is the commonest of the tumours referred to above and is an encapsulated, well-differentiated mass that grows slowly. It is a yellow nodule found most commonly in the subcutaneous tissues of the back of the neck, the shoulders and buttocks. The tumour may also be found in the periosteum, submucosal and retroperitoneal tissues. Most of these tumours follow a totally benign course, but, rarely, malignant change may occur. Lipomata are often excised for cosmetic reasons.

Liposarcoma. This is a very rare tumour that may arise *de novo* or from a pre-existing lipoma, especially in the retroperitoneal tissues. It is a soft, yellow, non-encapsulated mass containing atypical adipocytes and some spindle-shaped, undifferentiated cells. The tumour invades early and has a poor prognosis unless it is diagnosed and treated early.

Fibroma. This is a benign tumour derived from the fibroblast and is especially common in subcutaneous tissue, fascial planes, gastrointestinal mucosa, breast and ovary. It is subdivided clinically into the hard and soft types, relating to either more or less collagenous, stromal elements within the tumour mass. The soft form contains many tumour cells within a scanty fibrous stroma and it is this cellular type of tumour that may undergo malignant change. Often, these soft fibromata are misdiagnosed for fibrosarcomata.

Fibrosarcoma. This arises in the same sites as fibromata and forms large, firm, pale infiltrating masses. The tumour often possesses a pseudocapsule as it grows very rapidly and compresses the surrounding stroma. Histologically the malignant cells are elongated and spindle-shaped with pleomorphism, basophilia and varying degrees of collagen formation. It tends to have a poor prognosis.

Lymphangioma. This benign tumour of lymphatic vessels often occurs in the oral cavity, neck, axillae or groin. It consists of well-differentiated lymphatic vessels that may be cystic. Superficial lesions are sharply demarcated, greyish pink in colour, compressible and slightly raised from the surrounding tissue. Several histological variants are known.

Lymphangiosarcoma. This very rare malignant counterpart of the lymphoma may occasionally arise out of a pre-existing benign lesion or it may arise in a limb with chronic lymphoedema. The tumour invades and destroys surrounding structures, eventually spreading widely.

Revision Questions and Case Studies

1. Discuss the pathology of dysplastic changes occurring in the skin and other covering epithelia. Describe the microscopic features of such changes and the sequelae observed.
2. What are the characterizing features of xeroderma pigmentosum?
3. Explain the clinical features observed in eczematous skin eruptions and relate these to the pathological features of these disorders.
4. Define the following terms:
   (a) Hydroa
   (b) Ichthyosis
   (c) Acanthosis
   (d) Carbuncle
   (e) Bulla

5. Discuss briefly any three of the following conditions:
   (a) Exfoliative dermatitis
   (b) Pemphigus vulgaris
   (c) Psoriasis
   (d) Seborrhoeic dermatitis
6. Discuss the pathology of the benign neoplastic and hamartomatous masses that may be found on the skin. Begin your discussion by defining neoplasm and hamartoma.
7. Compare and contrast basal cell carcinoma and squamous cell carcinoma of the skin.
8. Write brief notes on all of the following:
   (a) Squamous cell carcinoma
   (b) Verrucae
   (c) Corns
   (d) Keratoacanthoma
   (e) Leukoplakia
9. What are the characteristics of benign naevi?
10. Discuss the pathology of squamous cell carcinoma of the skin and contrast this disorder with squamous cell carcinoma of the bronchus and oesophagus.
11. Define the following terms:
    (a) Keratin pearls
    (b) Bowen's disease
    (c) 'Rodent ulcer'
    (d) Basosquamous carcinoma
12. Discuss in detail the pathology of malignant melanoma.
13. Discuss the pathology of Kaposi's sarcoma.
14. Write brief notes on any three of the following topics:
    (a) Lipoma
    (b) Fibrosarcoma of the subcutaneous tissues
    (c) Haemangioma
    (d) Fibroma
15. Write short notes on the following:
    (a) Systemic lupus erythematosus
    (b) Scleroderma

Case study 1. A skin lesion was removed from the face of a 70-year-old Caucasian male patient after his family doctor referred him to a dermatologist. The man is a retired gardener living in a coastal town of northern New South Wales, who presented with the lesion on his left temple. The lesion was an indolent ulcer, about 1.5 cm in diameter, with a central scab and raised, rolled and everted, non-pigmented edges. The mass was firmly fixed to the underlying tissues and was rather hard and tender on palpation. The man is fair and has a deep tan (he is a keen swimmer) and on several areas of his face and arms he has lesions of solar keratosis. A few naevi that are found on his skin

are normal in appearance. The lesion on the temple was removed surgically and the man also underwent adjunctive therapy.

(a) What is the presumptive diagnosis?
(b) What predisposing and aetiological factors are present in this case that are consistent with the development of the lesion on the temple that the man presented with?
(c) Describe the characteristic histological feature of the lesion.
(d) What may have been the 'adjunctive treatment' that the man received?
(e) What is the prognosis for the patient?

Case study 2. A 46-year-old Caucasian male patient, who works as a builders' labourer, presented with a lesion on the left side of his back, at the level of the third thoracic vertebra. The lesion was a flattened deeply pigmented, almost black, mass approximately 1.6 cm in diameter, with several, smaller, flatter, outlying brownish pigmented macules that were in contact with the central larger lesion. In the past week there was some bleeding from the mass, which forced the man to seek medical advice. On the skin of the back there are several darkly pigmented naevi and the man says that he likes to work without a shirt and hat, as he has a dark complexion and has always tanned well, not being easily sunburnt. The patient was immediately admitted into hospital where the back lesion and the draining lymph nodes from the site were removed surgically.

(a) What are the differential diagnoses?
(b) What is the presumptive diagnosis?
(c) Describe the characteristic histological feature of the lesion.
(d) What is the connexion between the pigmented naevi and the lesion for which the man required treatment?
(e) What is the prognosis for the patient?

Case study 3. A 68-year-old Caucasian female patient presented with a lesion on the skin between the bridge of her nose and her left eye. An ulcer was present in the centre of a slightly raised mass, 0.9 cm in diameter. The centre of the lesion had a small amount of haemorrhage associated with it and the edges were raised and inverted. The lesion was removed by local excision, no other treatment being required. Histology of the lesion showed masses of malignant cells around an ulcer that extended into the superficial dermis. The sheets of tumour cells were invading into the dermis and had a characteristic 'palisaded' margin.

(a) What is the diagnosis?
(b) What do you know of the incidence of this condition?
(c) What is the behaviour of this tumour if it is left untreated?
(d) What is the prognosis of the woman in this case?

Case study 4. A 24-year-old Caucasian woman presents at her doctor's surgery with annoying, scaling lesions that have developed over her elbows over the past few months. Recently, the woman has noticed that she has a dandruff-like condition on her scalp and that lesions similar to those on her elbows have also begun to develop on her knees. She has tried using various skin creams and proprietary anti-dandruff preparations but these did not help her condition. The lesions on her elbows are irregular, raised plaques, ranging in size from 0.5 to 2.5 cm and are sharply demarcated from the surrounding skin. The margins of the lesions are hard and raised and covered by scales, which when rubbed off are fine and silvery, disclosing a reddened surface on the lesion on which multiple small bleeding points appear. When questioned about her joints, the woman says that they have not been troubling her at all, but that her mother suffers from rheumatoid arthritis.

(a) What is the presumptive diagnosis?
(b) What are the characteristic microscopic findings of this disorder?
(c) Why did the physician ask the woman about her joints and what is the significance of the woman's mother suffering from arthritis?
(d) Describe the various forms of treatment for this disorder.

Case study 5. A 23-year-old Caucasian female patient presented with a painful and inflamed lesion on the skin of the right side of the back of the neck, at the margin of hair growth. She says that she has had the lesion ever since she can remember and had always had to warn the hairdresser of its presence so that it would not be lopped off during a trim. The lesion has not troubled her greatly in the past but recently when she had her hair cut shorter she found that the lesion often became irritated when she combed her hair. She presented at her doctor's surgery after she managed to injure the lesion while she was combing her hair. The pigmented and irritated lesion was excised under local anaesthesia. It was a 0.5 cm diameter, brown, papillomatous lesion from which several hairs were sprouting. The woman works as a night shift nurse and says that she seldom gets out in the sun; even when she is on holiday she tends to cover up well and uses

sunscreen. She is dark haired and has an olive complexion. She does not have many pigmented naevi on her skin.

(a) What is the presumptive diagnosis?
(b) Of what general pathological group of disorders is this lesion an example?
(c) What are the characteristic microscopic features of this lesion?
(d) Is this woman a candidate for malignancies of the skin? Justify your answer.

Case study 6. An HIV-positive Caucasian male, 36 years old, presents at his doctor's surgery for one of his regular check-ups greatly alarmed as he has noticed some dark plaques in his mouth. On examination, the doctor sees several sharply demarcated, flat plaques of a purplish colour, approximately 1 cm in diameter. They were present on the palate, soft palate and pharyngeal mucosa. When the doctor asks the man whether any similar lesions have developed on his skin, he replies that he has not seen any, and upon examination she confirms this. The man is currently on zidovudine and is also being treated with antibiotics for a lung infection. He is also seeing a naturopath who has prescribed various vitamin supplements, megadoses of vitamin C and has advised on a healthy diet and exercise plan.

(a) What are the dark plaques that have developed in his mouth?
(b) What is the pathogenesis of these lesions?
(c) What is the prognosis for the patient?

Further Reading

Ancona AA. 'Occupational Acne.' *State Art Rev Occup Med* 1986; **1**: 229.

Bos JD. 'The Pathomechanisms of Psoriasis.' *Br J Dermatol* 1988; **118**: 141.

Breathnach SM. 'Immunologic Aspects of Contact Dermatitis.' *Hum Pathol* 1986; **4**: 5.

Breslow A. 'Thickness, Cross-sectional Areas and Depth of Invasion in the Prognosis of Cutaneous Melanoma.' *Am Surg* 1970; **172**: 902.

Clark WH Jr, *et al.* 'A Study of Tumour Progression: The Precursor Lesions of Superficial and Spreading Malignant Melanoma.' *Hum Pathol* 1984; **15**: 1147.

Cohen SR. 'Skin Diseases in Health Care Workers.' *Occup Med* 1987; **2**(3): 565.

DeSwarte RD. 'Drug Allergy.' *Clin Rev Allergy* 1986; **4:** 143.

Dyall-Smith D, Varigos G. 'Human Papillomaviruses and Cancer.' *Australas J Dermatol* 1985; **26**: 102.

Emmett EA. 'Occupational Skin Cancers.' *State Art Rev Occup Med* 1987; **2**: 165.

Epstein WL. 'Plant-induced Dermatitis.' *Ann Emerg Med* 1987; **16**: 950.

Gill PG. 'Malignant Melanoma: A Clinical Perspective.' *Med J Aust* 1988; **148**: 638.

Gottlieb AB. 'Immunologic Mechanisms in Psoriasis.' *J Am Acad Dermatol* 1988; **18**: 1379.

Guin JD, Beaman JH (eds). 'Plant Dermatitis.' *Clin Dermatol* 1986; **4**(2): 1.

Halliday G, Cavanagh L, Barnetson R StC. 'Regulation of the Skin Immune System by Local Antigen Presenting Cells.' *Today's Life Sci* 1990: **2**(11): 26.

Herlyn M, *et al.* 'Biology of Tumour Progression in Human Melanocytes.' *Lab Invest* 1987; **56**: 461.

Kaplan AP, Buckley RH, Mathews KP. 'Allergic Skin Disorders.' *JAMA* 1987; **258**: 2900.

Kernohan NM. 'Editorial: Cutaneous Melanoma: A Fresh Outlook.' *J Path* 1991; **163**: 283.

Klinesmith D'AM, Perricone NV. 'Common Skin Problems in the Elderly.' *Dermatol Clin* 1986; **4**: 485.

Kraemer KH, Lee MM, Scotto J. 'Xeroderma Pigmentosum.' *Arch Dermatol* 1987; **123**: 241.

Kripkie ML. 'Impact of Ozone Depletion on Skin Cancers.' *J Dermato Surg Oncol* 1988; **14**: 835.

Laurent MR. 'Psoriatic Arthritis.' *Clin Rheum Dis* 1985; **11**: 61.

Lee JA. 'Melanoma and Exposure to Sunlight.' *Epidemiol Rev* 1982; **4**: 110.

Lin AN, Carter DM. 'Skin Cancer in the Elderly.' *Dermatol Clin* 1986; **4**: 467.

McGavran MH. 'Cutaneous Pigmentation.' *Clin Plast Surg* 1987; **14**: 301.

McKee PH. 'Pathology of the Skin.' 1989; Lippincott, Philadelphia.

Nordlund JJ (ed.). 'Pigmentation Disorders.' *Dermatol Clin* 1988; **6**: 161.

Parsons JM. 'Pityriasis Rosea Update: 1986.' *J Am Acad Dermatol* 1986; **15**: 159.

Reeves JRT, Maibach H. *Clinical Dermatology Illustrated. A Regional Approach*, second edition, 1991; MacLennan & Petty, Sydney.

Rhodes AR, *et al.* 'Risk Factors for Cutaneous Melanoma.' *J Am Med Ass* 1987; **258**: 3145.

Steele K. 'Wart Charming Practices Among Patients Attending Wart Clinics.' *BJ Med Prac* 1990; December: 517.

Stegman SJ. 'Basal Cell Carcinoma and Squamous Cell Carcinoma.' *Med Clin North Am* 1986; **70**: 95.

Stevens A, Wheater PR, Lowe JS. *Clinical Dermatopathology*, 1989; Churchill Livingstone, Edinburgh.

Tuazon CV. 'Skin and Skin Structure Infections in the Patient at Risk.' *Am J Med* 1984; **76**(5A): 166.

Wickboldt LG, Fenske NA. 'Streptococcal and Staphylococcal Infections of the Skin.' *Hosp Pract* 1986; **21**(3A): 41.

Williams ML. 'A New Look at the Ichthyoses.' *Pediatr Dermatol* 1986; **3**: 476.

17

Haematological Disorders

Normal Blood and Blood Cell Production

Haematology is the branch of pathology concerned with the study of the blood. In the adult, the blood cells are produced in the bone marrow and lymphoid organs. The process of blood cell formation, **haemopoiesis**, involves the production and destruction of 2.5 million cells per minute in a normal adult. The blood is a dynamic tissue which exemplifies the process of homeostasis in the body. The favoured theory of haemopoiesis is the so-called **unitarian theory**, which states that all blood cells arise from a common precursor stem cell which is pluripotential and can give rise to all the different blood cell types, both red and white. This stem cell is called the **haemocytoblast.** It constantly divides and some of the daughter cells are identical to it and help to keep the number of stem cells in the bone marrow at a constant reserve level. The remaining daughter cells differentiate along different pathways to become the mature blood cells.

There are four major pathways of differentiation of stem cells (also refer to Figure 17.1):

- the erythroid line, which gives rise to erythrocytes;
- the lymphocytic line, which gives rise to lymphocytes (T or B after further processing in the thymus or bursa);
- the megakaryocytic line, which gives rise to mega-karyocytes (producing platelets);
- the myelomonocytic line, producing monocytes, macrophages, neutrophils, eosinophils and basophils.

Blood is a rather atypical connective tissue in that under physiological conditions it is a liquid. The **plasma** is the liquid ground substance in which the blood cells are suspended. It should be noted that although there are no fibres present in blood normally these make their appearance in the blood when it clots: a soluble protein **fibrinogen** is converted into an insoluble fibrillar network of the protein **fibrin**. When blood clots and all the clotting factors, fibrin and cells have been removed, the clear, yellowish fluid that remains is

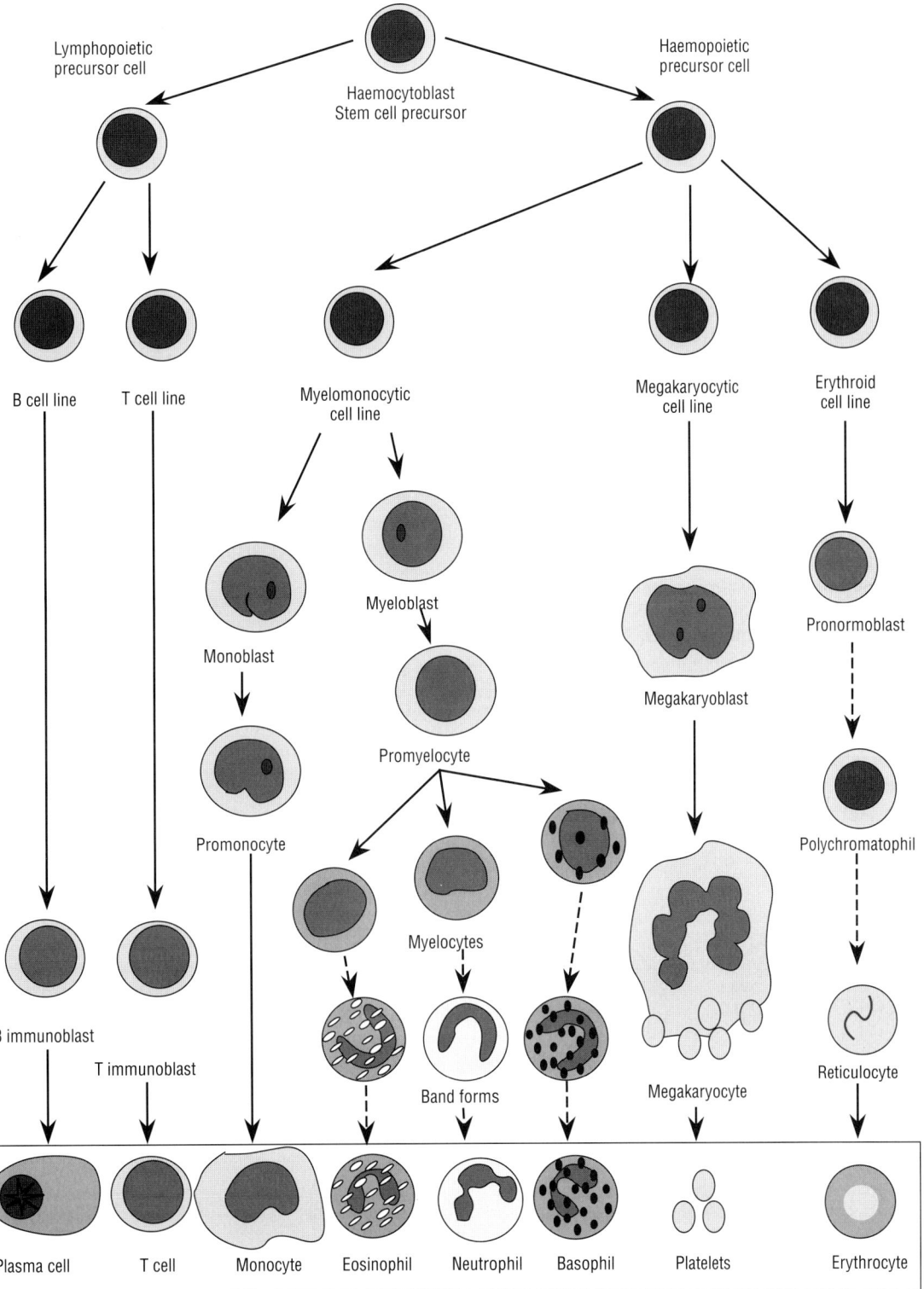

Figure 17.1 *Blood cell development*

called **serum**, which differs greatly in composition from plasma.

Cells of two main types are found in the bloodstream, the red blood cells, **erythrocytes**, and the white blood cells, **leukocytes**. There are also the **platelets**, which are anucleate cell fragments of the giant bone marrow cell the **megakaryocyte**.

Blood has a respiratory function in that erythrocytes (which are the most numerous of the cells) are full of the pigment **haemoglobin**, which has a strong affinity for oxygen. When the blood reaches the lungs the haemoglobin combines reversibly with oxygen to form **oxyhaemoglobin** which upon reaching the tissues releases the bound oxygen for consumption by the cells.

The leukocytes are thought to be rather inactive in the bloodstream, having their most important function when they enter the extravascular tissues. They enter these tissues when the tissue becomes inflamed or when the immune response requires them to do so. The leukocytes may be divided into three groups, granular cells, agranular cells and blood platelets (see Figure 17.2).

The **granular cells** are the **neutrophils, eosinophils** and **basophils**. When the basophils migrate into the tissues they become the **mast cells**. All of the granular cells are active in **phagocytosis**, but the neutrophils are especially active. Eosinophils are important in parasitic infections but they are also thought to control the inflammatory response, some of their granular contents counteracting the effects of the mediators of the inflammatory response. The mast cells are important in the release of inflammatory mediators.

The **agranular cells** are the **lymphocytes** and the **monocytes**. The monocytes upon migrating into the extravascular tissues differentiate into the **macrophages**, which as well as being actively phagocytic have a very important role in immune system reactions. The lymphocytes are divided into the **T cells** and the **B cells** both of which are very important in immunity; the latter differentiate into the **plasma cells** when they enter the extravascular tissues and thereafter are important in synthesizing the **antibodies**.

The **blood platelets**, or **thrombocytes**, are important in the process of blood clotting and also in the agglutination around injured portions of blood vessels, helping in plugging leaks and covering injured spots.

Blood is a very complex tissue with many functions, which are dependent not only on the blood cells and plasma proteins but also on the other components present in it. If we consider blood as a whole, viewing it as the complex tissue that it is, we may then review its major functions. These are:

- **respiratory**: carrying oxygen and carbon dioxide to and from tissues;
- **transport**: carrying nutrients and metabolites to and from tissues. Helping in the absorption of nutrients from the gut. Carrying hormones to their site of action;
- **reparatory**: clotting and agglutination of platelets to areas of injury;
- **immune**: carrying cells to sites of damage or invasion by foreign particles; carrying the substances that neutralize these foreign compounds to the sites where they are needed;
- **regulatory**: maintaining fluid and electrolyte balance throughout the body. Maintaining a constant body temperature.

Haemopoiesis is a very complex process, controlled in part by genetic factors and in part by hormonal

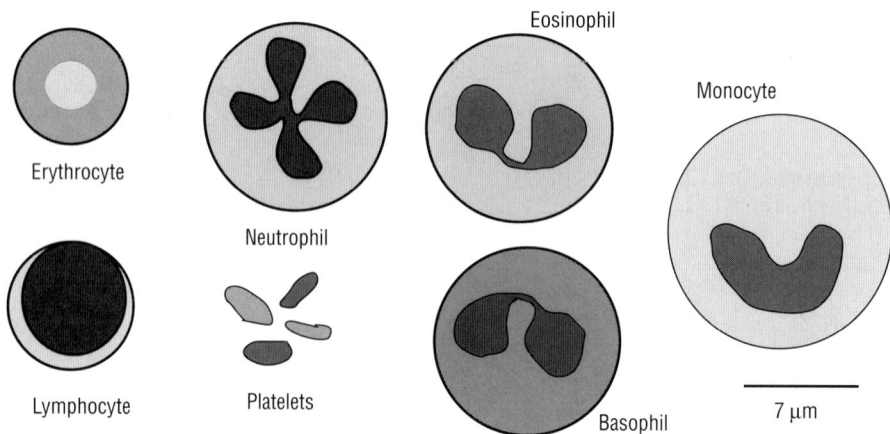

Figure 17.2 *The normal blood cells*

factors (haemopoietins) and environmental influences (e.g. oxygen tension in inspired air). The equilibrium of haemopoiesis may be upset in many ways and blood disorders develop as a result of many disease processes, giving rise to an abnormally constituted blood in which any blood cell may be present in abnormally high or low numbers, and/or have an abnormal structure and function (see Table 17.1). Such anomalies in the blood may arise because of the following aetiologies:

- inherited/congenital factors (e.g. sickle cell anaemia);
- physical agents (e.g. X-irradiation causing leukopenia);
- chemical agents (e.g. benzene exposure causing leukaemias);
- infectious agents (e.g. HTLV I causing leukaemia);
- immunological factors (e.g. thrombocytopenia caused by autoimmune diseases);
- dietary factors (e.g. iron deficiency anaemia);
- iatrogenic factors (e.g. agranulocytosis caused by phenylbutazone administration);
- idiopathic factors (e.g. polycythaemia rubra vera).

Any cell in the bloodstream may be affected by a disease process and the affected cell may be at any stage of its differentiation process. The disease most commonly affects the bone marrow, but the blood cells in the peripheral blood will usually reflect the disease process as it occurs in the marrow, both blood and marrow best considered as a single organ. Examination of a peripheral blood smear (**PBS**) may be all that is required to diagnose the disease process that affects the marrow and bloodstream

Erythrocyte Diseases

The Anaemias

Anaemia is the state in which there is reduction of haemoglobin in the blood below the normal for the patient's age and sex. The World Health Organization (WHO) defines as anaemic anyone whose haemoglobin is below 13 g/dL (males) and 12 g/dL (females). The condition may also be defined in relation to the haematocrit: if this falls below 40% in men or below 37% in women, anaemia is present. About 7% of the population are anaemic when WHO criteria for anaemia are used. Most of the anaemics in the population have the condition in a mild, subclinical form and the majority of affected people are women. Anaemia can be due to a very wide variety of aetiologies, ranging from genetic diseases which affect the haemoglobin

Table 17.1 *Disorders of the blood cells*

	Decreases in number of cells	Increases in number of cells
Erythrocytes	Anaemias	Polycythaemias
Platelets	Thrombocytopenias	Thrombocythaemias
Leucocytes	Leukopenias	Leukocytoses (benign)
		Leukaemias (malignant)

molecule itself, or are due to inherited enzymatic function, to acquired diseases with a variety of causes and effects. Acquired anaemia may often be the consequence of diseases in non-related body systems (e.g. as an effect of malignancy or chronic systemic diseases).

A wide variety of changes in erythrocyte morphology are seen with the various types of anaemias. Haematologists use a set of terms to describe these changes in the erythrocytes that are shown in Figure 17.3. Cells that are biconcave discs, between 7 and 8.5 μm in diameter and with a cell volume of approximately 87 fL are called **normocytes**, and are the majority of red blood cells in the circulation of a normal healthy person. Erythrocytes that are smaller than 7 μm in diameter with a cell volume of less than 80 fL are called **microcytes**. Erythrocytes that are larger than 8.5 μm in diameter with a cell volume of more than 95 fL are called **macrocytes**. Erythrocyte precursors that have nuclei and are larger than normal are termed **megaloblasts**. These changes are easily appreciated when a suitably prepared PBS is stained and examined under the microscope.

If the erythrocyte contains less haemoglobin than normal (i.e. below 19 mmol/L = 31 g/dL), the cells look pale in a PBS and are said to be **hypochromic**. If the cells contain normal quantities of haemoglobin (i.e. above 19 mmol/L) they look a normal reddish colour in a PBS and are said to be **normochromic**. If in the PBS the erythrocytes are found to vary considerably in **size**, the film is said to exhibit **anisocytosis** (unequal cell size). If in the PBS the erythrocytes are found to vary considerably in **shape**, the film is said to exhibit **poikilocytosis** (variable cell shape). Various inclusions may be seen in erythrocytes. Reticulocytes are young erythrocytes that contain a basophilic, stippled reticulum of RNA fragments (Figure 17.4). The **Howell-Jolly body** represents nuclear remnants that are seen in the periphery of the erythrocyte as dark particles. **Heinz bodies** are peripheral, rounded, dark

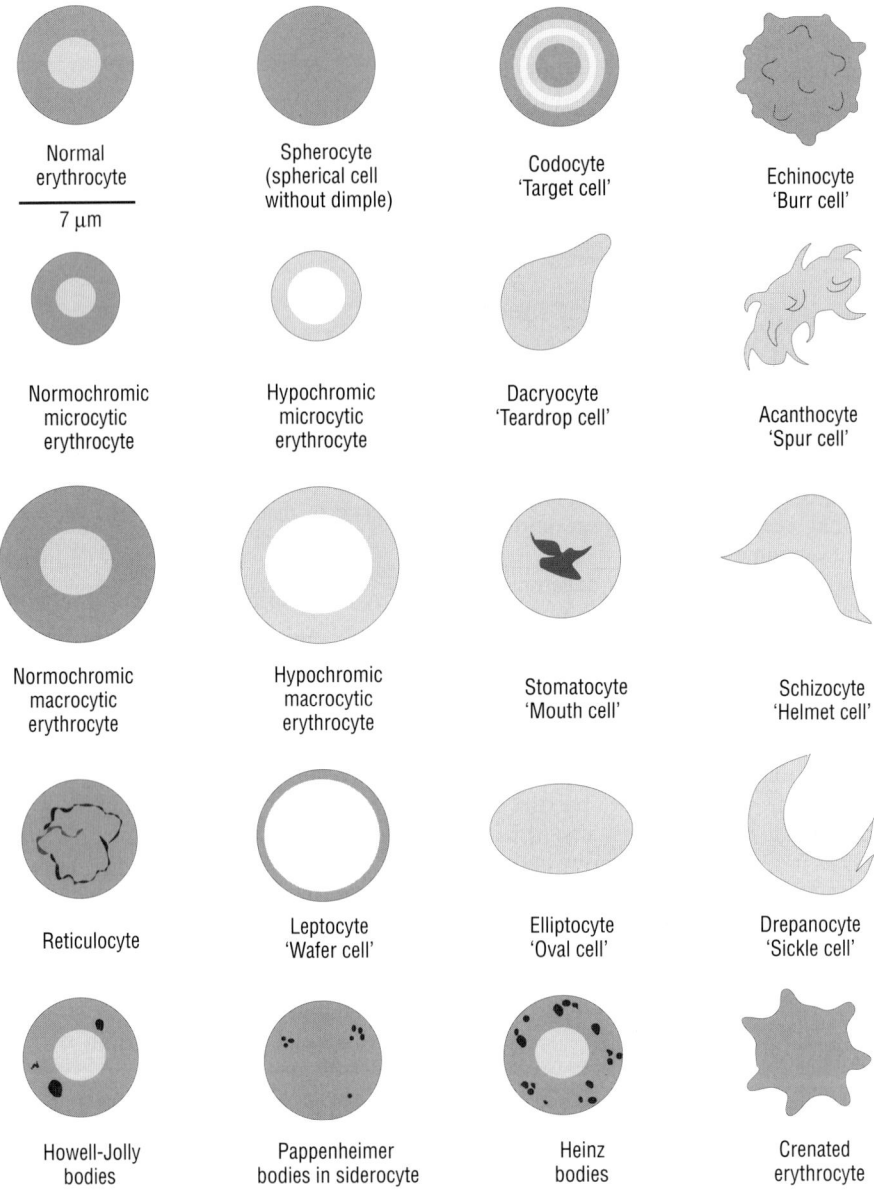

Figure 17.3 *Variations in erythrocyte size and morphology*

blue specks representing denatured globin. **Pappenheimer bodies** are iron-containing granules in erythrocytes that contain iron not associated with haemoglobin (these cells are called **siderocytes**; Figure 17.5). Occasionally in a PBS **crenated erythrocytes** will be seen and these represent cells that have lost water by osmosis, caused by suspension in a hypertonic solution.

Whatever the type of anaemia that a patient presents with, the major problem is that the oxygen-carrying capacity of the blood is compromised. This is the result of the decreased amount of haemoglobin that is present in the blood of an anaemic person. Oxygen content of the blood is directly proportional to the amount of haemoglobin, and in an anaemic subject there is a tendency for hypoxia in the body. Symptoms and signs in anaemia reflect this hypoxia, but also the compensatory mechanisms initiated by the body in

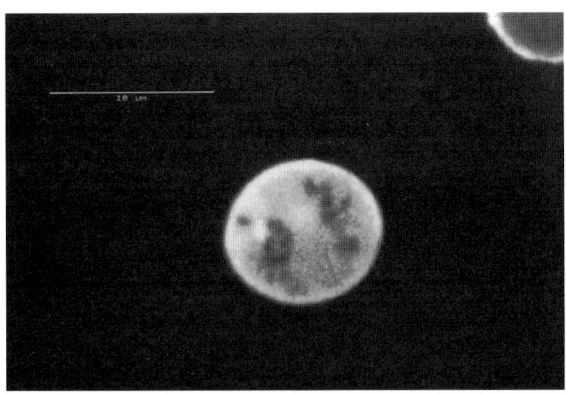

Figure 17.4 *A reticulocyte seen in the peripheral blood smear of a patient with haemolytic anaemia (scale bar is 10 μm)*

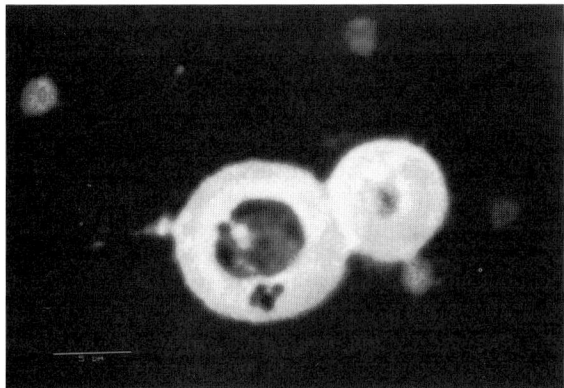

Figure 17.5 *Pappenheimer bodies seen in an erythrocyte in the peripheral blood of a patient with splenic atrophy and the malabsorption syndrome (scale bar is 5 μm)*

order to correct the hypoxia. The clinical presentation of the patient with anaemia is rather similar for all types of anaemias, but in many cases depends very much on whether the condition develops quickly or slowly. Even in severe anaemia, if the disorder has progressed slowly, adaptation may be very effective and the patients recognize the debilitating effects of the anaemia only when treatment commences, which makes them feel so much better. Rapid onset of anaemia may produce very serious symptoms. Generally, clinically observed effects of anaemia are:

- increased heart rate at rest or on exertion (palpitations, breathlessness);

- fatigue, almost constant weakness, feebleness (hypoxia);
- headaches, giddiness, 'roaring or buzzing' in the head, spots before the eyes;
- pallor of the skin (not easily seen in tanned or dark-skinned people) and pallor of mucosae, nail beds and conjunctivae (more reliable indicators);
- mild fever (below 38.5°C);
- mild proteinuria (reduced kidney blood flow, blood flow to brain and muscles maintained);
- koilonychia, gastritis, glossitis, etc., depending on the type of anaemia.

Depending very much on the state of health of the patients with anaemia and their age, various other symptoms and signs may be observed. For example, in the elderly who have a compromised cardiopulmonary function, anaemia may cause angina pectoris or congestive heart failure.

Anaemias are classified on whether they are **acquired** or **inherited**. A very large group of inherited anaemias is known and these are due to abnormal haemoglobins, defects in porphyrin and haeme synthesis, abnormalities in the erythrocyte cell membrane or enzymatic deficiencies. The acquired anaemias may result because of dietary deficiencies, bone marrow dysfunction, excessive loss of blood, autoimmune destruction of erythrocytes, mechanical damage to erythrocytes or as a result of multiple or idiopathic mechanisms.

Both acquired and inherited anaemias may be classified into three major groups depending on what the pathogenesis of the anaemia is:

- **haemorrhagic anaemias**, due to excessive blood loss;
- **dyshaemopoietic anaemias**, resulting from defective production of erythrocytes;
- **haemolytic anaemias**, associated with excessive destruction of erythrocytes.

Haemorragic Anaemias

Acute Haemorrhagic Anaemia

Acute haemorrhagic anaemia is due to an acute blood loss resulting from wounding that has caused a severing or rupture of blood vessels. The blood loss may be external (blood lost to the environment, which would include blood loss into the gastrointestinal tract) or internal (blood released into one of the body cavities or intercellularly within tissues). In healthy individuals, up to 600 mL of blood may be lost with few symptoms. The homeostatic mechanisms act quickly to replenish blood volume and the bone marrow will generate more blood cells to take the place of those lost. If the volume of blood lost is up to 1200 mL, there will be few symptoms if the patient is lying down, but weakness or fainting will be experienced on standing or on activity. Up to 1500 mL of blood lost within 24 hours is tolerated well and the symptoms the patient experiences in the short term disappear as vasoconstriction increases peripheral resistance and raises blood pressure, and as the blood volume is replenished. Plasma volume, in this case, is fully restored within a day and the normal erythrocyte count restored within 2 to 5 weeks. If 1500 to 2000 mL of blood are lost within 24 hours, the loss may prove fatal unless the patient is treated with plasma volume expanders or with a blood transfusion.

The excessive loss of blood within a short period of time causes its harmful effects mainly through the reduction of blood volume. A dramatic fall in blood pressure, prostration, thirst, a rapid pulse rate and rapid shallow breathing are observed. The patient is cold, pale and sweating, showing all of the symptoms and signs of hypovolaemic shock.

The treatment of acute haemorrhagic anaemia, in all cases, consists of firstly arresting the haemorrhage. Depending on the amount of blood lost and whether or not the patient is exhibiting signs of shock, further treatment regimes include the transfusion of blood or reconstitution of the blood volume by plasma, or dextran/plasma expander infusions. The iron lost must also be replenished if plasma expanders are used and if the haemorrhage was external, as for every 500 mL of blood lost to the exterior of the body, 300 mg of iron is lost as well. Generally, acute haemorrhagic anaemia has a good prognosis if treated adequately.

Chronic Haemorrhagic Anaemia

This is due to small, repeated or constant blood losses to the exterior of the body. The haemorrhage may not be immediately obvious to the patient or the examining person. Causes of this type of anaemia include haemorrhage from chronic peptic ulcers, haemorrhoids, hiatus hernia, ulcerative colitis, malignant tumours or primary haemorrhagic disorders (e.g. purpura, haemophilia), and also the blood loss of menstruation and menstruation disorders. Because one of the commonest causes of occult blood loss in men or post-menopausal women is carcinoma of the large bowel, anaemia due to occult blood loss from such a tumour is a condition that needs to be carefully considered first and excluded conclusively in a differential diagnosis for chronic haemorrhagic anaemia.

Combinations of symptoms will be seen due to the primary condition as well as due to the anaemia itself. If it is possible, the primary condition is treated first, and then the anaemia and its effects. In some cases (e.g. with advanced malignant neoplastic disease), only palliative treatment can be given for both conditions.

Dyshaemopoietic Anaemias

Iron Deficiency

The total amount of body iron is 3.0 g to 4.5 g, and two-thirds of it occurs in the blood in the form of haemoglobin, in myoglobin and iron-containing enzymes. The remaining third represents stored iron, present in the form of soluble ferritin and insoluble haemosiderin. Iron in various forms (mainly ferric ions) is ingested in food and is converted to the ionic form in the stomach by hydrochloric acid. In the intestine, ferrous ions form (a process assisted by vitamin C and hence in scurvy iron deficiency may be a complication) and pass into the mucosa. In the intestinal cells iron is stored in the form of **ferritin**. When iron is required it is released bound to a β-globulin in plasma (**transferrin**), which distributes the iron all around the body. When the body content of iron is high, most of the iron remains in the intestinal cells and as they are shed the iron is lost also. If there is an iron deficit, the intestinal cells do not store the iron intracytoplasmically, but rather bind it to transferrin and shunt it directly into the bloodstream. The normal daily intake of iron is approximately 20 mg, of which only 1 to 2 mg is absorbed, mainly in the duodenum. An equivalent amount of iron to that absorbed is lost daily in desquamated cells (refer to Figure 17.6).

Deficiency of iron is one of the commonest medical problems in many countries throughout the world. There are many causes of decreased levels of iron in the body. **Deficient dietary intake** is commonly encountered in milk-fed infants and old people on poor diets who do not receive iron supplementation. **Defective iron absorption** is often seen in various gastrointestinal diseases, for example achlorhydria, coeliac disease, infections or following intestinal surgery. **Increased loss of iron** from the body is encountered in chronic haemorrhagic diseases, in parasitic infections (e.g. malaria, hookworm infestation, trypanosomiasis), haemoglobinuria, exfoliative dermatitis and especially commonly in various menstrual disorders.

Clinical symptoms of iron deficiency anaemias are pallor, weakness, dyspnoea on exertion, fainting, anorexia and koilonychia. Epithelial changes are also

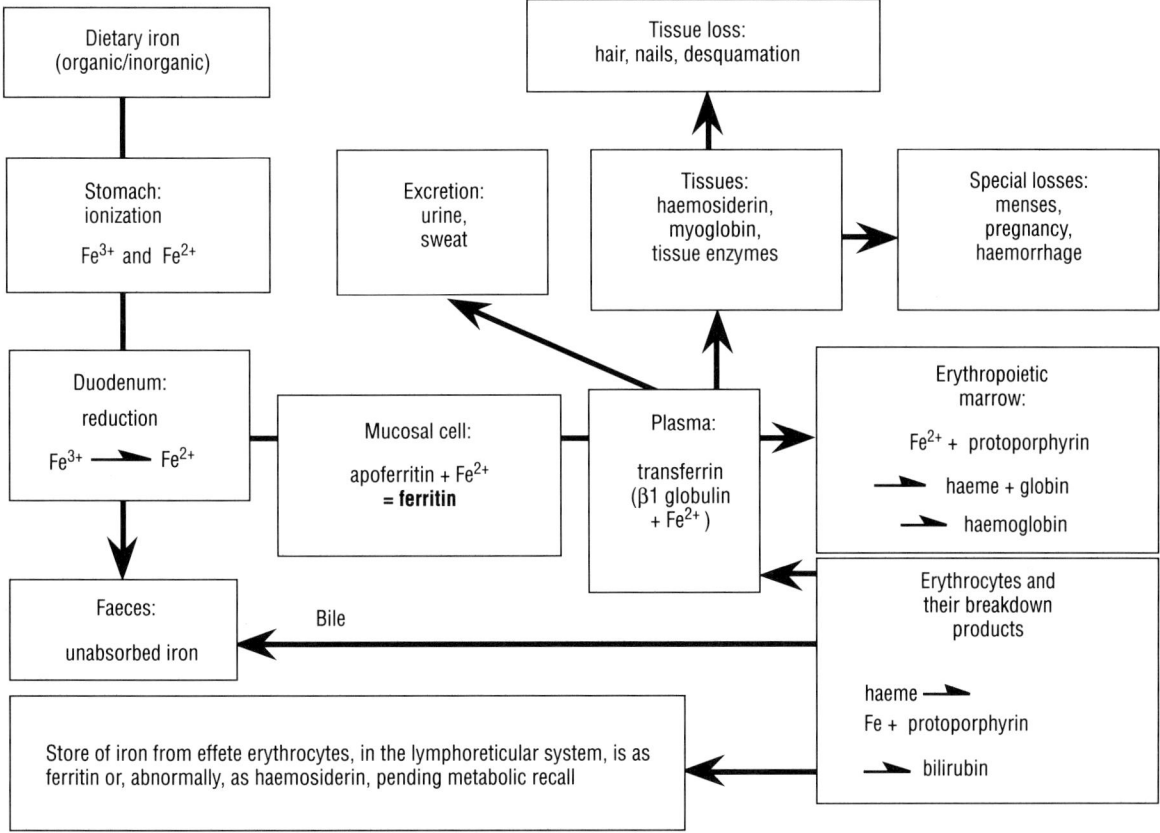

Figure 17.6 *Iron metabolism*

seen commonly, as an expression of decreased intracellular enzymes that contain iron. Glossitis with atrophy, and angular stomatitis are two such manifestations. In severe iron deficiency anaemia, **pica** (craving to eat unusual foods or substances) will be observed.

In this form of anaemia PBS examination will reveal a normal number of erythrocytes but the haemoglobin within each cell will be reduced. Under the microscope the cells display hypochromia, erythrocytes looking paler, with only a thin, peripheral rim of haemoglobin. Microcytosis, anisocytosis and poikilocytosis are also observed. The bone marrow shows a marked decrease in the haemosiderin iron content of macrophages and an absence of ferritin in the developing erythrocytes.

The deficiency is corrected by either administering dietary supplements (provided absorption is normal) or by administering iron parenterally. The latter treatment provides rapid results and is also used in the case of compromised intestinal absorption.

Vitamin B$_{12}$ Deficiency (Megaloblastic Anaemia)

The normal daily requirement of vitamin B$_{12}$ (= cyanocobalamin) is 1 to 2 μg. The vitamin is only synthesized by certain microbes and humans depend for their source of the vitamin on foods of mainly animal origin, such as milk, eggs, liver, meat and seafood. Thus, dietary deficiency of vitamin B$_{12}$ is seen most commonly in strict vegans (vegetarians who eat no dairy products or eggs). Normally, the vitamin is absorbed in the terminal ileum, the process requiring **intrinsic factor** which is secreted by the stomach mucosa. Deficiency of vitamin B$_{12}$ is due to:

- **inadequate dietary intake** (lack of animal proteins, eggs, milk, etc., this being an uncommon cause);
- **defective absorption** (common cause) because of (a) lack of intrinsic factor (inherited and acquired stomach mucosal diseases) and (b) disorders of the small intestine (e.g. Crohn's disease);

- **increased requirements**, as occurs in pregnancy, parasitic infections, etc. (common cause).

Of the three, the lack of secretion of intrinsic factor is most important as it produces a very severe disease, termed **pernicious anaemia** (= Addison's anaemia). The name pernicious anaemia is only given to those disorders that are caused by congenital lack of intrinsic factor production or those cases of an autoimmune aetiology. Other cases of anaemia caused by vitamin B_{12} deficiency are not called pernicious anaemia.

Pernicious Anaemia (Addisonian Anaemia)

Pernicious anaemia is due to either **congenital causes** or **acquired causes** of severe or total lack of intrinsic factor secretion by the gastric mucosa. This type of anaemia derived its name (pernicious = tending to a fatal result) before the days of adequate treatment when it always used to have a rapid fatal result. The rare congenital form is inherited as an autosomal recessive trait and appears within the first few months of life, while the 'classical', acquired form is unusual before 30 years of age and maximal between 50 and 70 years of age. Pernicious anaemia is a rather rare disease, with 16 people per million suffering from it, i.e. about 250 cases annually in Australia. Classical pernicious anaemia has a complex aetiology. Its incidence is higher in people with blood group A, it is found more frequently in the Northern European races and their descendants and it tends to run in some families. In Scandinavia, one person in every 800 has the disease. Autoimmunity is important in the pathogenesis of the disease and at least 85% of patients have autoantibodies to the gastric parietal cells and about 50% of them have autoantibodies to intrinsic factor.

The disease is associated with gastric atrophy, hypochlorhydria or achlorhydria. Pepsin production is also greatly decreased, and the volume of gastric secretion is only about 10% of the normal. Before modern treatments for pernicious anaemia were undertaken, almost all patients showed evidence of CNS disease, often with dementia setting in and giving the disorder the name of 'megaloblastic madness'. Nowadays, only about a third of cases have minor neurological symptoms that are not correlated with the severity of anaemia the patient is showing. About 5% of treated patients have spinal cord abnormalities, the commonest being subacute combined degeneration of the cord where demyelination of axons occurs, being most severe in the mid-thoracic part of the cord. The lesions are patchy, although they may become confluent with time, and the posterior columns are affected first, followed by the lateral columns. The peripheral nerves may show similar changes.

In the congenital form there is evidence of severe anaemia a few weeks after birth, the stomach appearing normal. In the classical form, there is pallor, jaundice, weakness, paraesthesiae, stiffness of limbs, glossitis, weight loss, anorexia, achlorhydria and atrophy of the mucosa of the stomach.

In a PBS there is a decreased number of erythrocytes (approximately half of the normal number). There is evidence of normochromic macrocytosis, anisocytosis, poikilocytosis and reticulocytosis. The more severe the condition, the larger and more abnormal looking the erythrocytes (Figure 17.7). Howell-Jolly bodies may be present in the erythrocytes. There is neutropenia with abnormal cells present, the neutrophils being larger than normal, their nuclei being hypersegmented with six to eight lobes ('giant neutrophils'). The platelets are reduced in number. In the bone marrow, which is hyperplastic, deep red and jelly-like, the fat content is decreased. The erythrocyte precursors are megaloblastic, with large prominent nuclei. There are increased numbers of white cell precursors, some of them as large as 30 μm in diameter. Although there is hyperactivity of the marrow, the cells that are produced are abnormal and hence are destroyed before they reach the circulation, making **pancytopenia** (decreased numbers of all blood cells in the peripheral blood) a hallmark of the megaloblastic anaemias. The megakaryocytes are decreased in number but show a normal morphology. The decreased quantities of the vitamin in the body causes abnormal DNA synthesis which is especially marked in the rapidly dividing cells of the bone marrow.

The prognosis is poor in untreated cases of per-

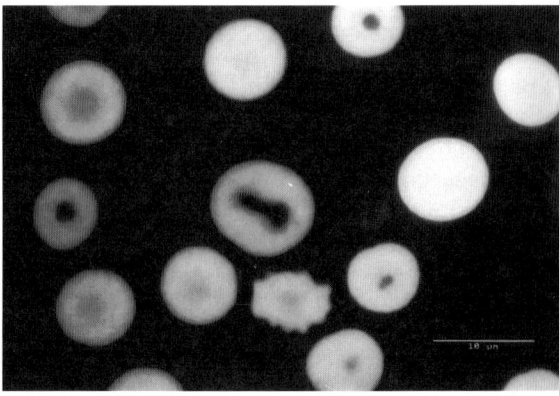

Figure 17.7 *Anisocytosis, macrocytosis and stomatocyte in vitamin B_{12} deficiency anaemia (scale bar is 10 μm)*

nicious anaemia, the patient usually dying between 1 month and 3 years after onset of symptoms. Treatment of pernicious anaemia is by administration of intrinsic factor orally or of vitamin B_{12} parenterally for the rest of the individual's life. Antibodies to the administered intrinsic factor limit the usefulness of this treatment. The neurological disease is arrested by treatment and the lesions heal by gliosis. It is not possible to treat the stomach lesions and incidence of carcinoma of the stomach, diabetes mellitus and myxoedema (with or without goitre) is higher in these patients than in the general population. There is also a higher incidence of autoimmune diseases such as Hashimoto's disease of the thyroid.

Anaemia of Folic Acid Deficiency (Megaloblastic Anaemia)

The daily requirement of folic acid of about 50 µg is absorbed in the jejunum, with no special factor required for its absorption. The coenzyme is present in eggs, meat and leafy vegetables, but it is heat labile and therefore easily denatured by prolonged cooking. However, the body stores are in the region of 5 mg, sufficient for about 5 months, even if no folic acid is consumed. The deficiency of folic acid has similar causes to vitamin B_{12} deficiency, that is:

- **inadequate dietary intake** (lack of meat, eggs or leafy vegetables, or overcooking of food, an uncommon cause);
- **defective absorption** as occurs in the malabsorption syndrome, coeliac disease, tropical sprue, alcoholism, etc. (common causes);
- **increased requirements**, as occurs in pregnancy, malignancy, for example lymphomata and leukaemias, and haemolytic anaemia and tuberculosis (common causes);
- **decreased utilization of folate** when there is drug interference, for example methotrexate, anticonvulsants (e.g. dilantin).

This condition has a similar clinical presentation to pernicious anaemia, although neurological manifestations are uncommon. The blood and bone marrow picture is almost identical to that seen in pernicious anaemia. When folate is not present in the body in sufficient quantities, DNA synthesis is compromised and there is accumulation of an abnormal by-product of histidine metabolism, formiminoglutamic acid (FIGlu), which is present in the urine. Therefore, diagnosis of folate deficiency depends on laboratory demonstration of decreased folate in the serum and of increased urinary levels of FIGlu.

Folate deficiency is managed by treatment of the primary condition which is often associated with the disorder. For example, low-gluten diets are prescribed for some enteropathies, treatment of alcoholism is instituted, or the patient is put on a low-fat, low-carbohydrate and high-protein diet for malabsorption. Dietary folate is then increased, to about 10 mg or so daily, while in many cases supplementation of vitamin B_{12} and iron may be needed also. Most cases of folate deficiency respond well to treatment.

Toxic Dyshaemopoietic Anaemias

This is a large group of anaemias due to impaired formation of erythrocytes caused by a variety of aetiological factors. These are:

- **Infections**: For example, kala-azar, pneumonia, osteomyelitis, etc. In most cases the anaemia results indirectly from multiple toxic and marrow depressive effects of the infection. In addition, there is reduction in the life span of the erythrocytes and decreased efficiency in the utilization of iron.
- **Chronic diseases**: Many chronic diseases, especially autoimmune diseases such as rheumatoid arthritis, SLE and polyarteritis nodosa, are often associated with anaemia. The condition in these cases results from shortened erythrocyte life span, inadequate response of the marrow to erythropoietic stimuli and abnormal macrophage function, resulting in impaired release of stored iron from these cells.
- **Neoplasia**: The anaemia in this case is due to many causes, haemorrhage, infection of tumour, bone marrow involvement, liver invasion and liver disease, kidney involvement, therapy with radiation or cytotoxic drugs.

Leukoerythroblastic Anaemia (Myelophthisic Anaemia)

Leukoerythroblastic anaemia is associated with space-occupying lesions of the bone marrow that have as a result the depressed synthesis of all blood cells, both erythrocytes and leukocytes. Usually the change occurs in multiple sites within the blood-forming marrow. The commonest aetiologies of this condition have been considered previously and are:

- marble bone disease (Albers-Schönberg disease);
- Paget's disease (especially the polyostotic form);
- lipid storage disease (e.g. Gaucher's disease);

- primary bone tumours (e.g. multiple myeloma);
- secondary bone tumours (commonest cause).

The clinical picture is one of anaemia as well as one of neutropenia and lymphopenia. In the PBS the erythrocytes are decreased in number and invariably there are many nucleated erythrocytes present. There is also reticulocytosis, anisocytosis and marked poikilocytosis with many dacryocytes. There is moderate normocytic and normochromic anaemia. Leukocyte and platelet numbers may be lowered, normal or raised but the differential white cell count will show that there is an increased number of granulocytes and their precursors. The platelets may be very large in size.

The patient often displays the extreme weakness and debilitation of anaemia but also the immunodepression and increased susceptibility to infection that is the result of neutropenia and lymphopenia. There is hepatosplenomegaly present because of extramedullary haemopoiesis. The treatment of the condition is difficult and the prognosis for the patient depends very much on the primary condition that is the cause of this anaemia. In most cases the prognosis is very poor.

Aplastic Anaemia

Aplasia or severe hypoplasia of bone marrow will lead to this condition in which there may be severe depression in the formation of blood cells. **Pancytopenia** refers to a dramatic drop in the numbers of all blood cells (i.e. anaemia, leukopenia and thrombocytopenia) in the peripheral blood and indicates a failure of the bone marrow to produce enough cells to replace those lost in the peripheral blood. Both red and white blood cells are involved. The bone marrow looks hypocellular and the blood-forming elements are replaced by adipose tissue. This type of anaemia may rarely be the result of congenital causes or more commonly be an acquired disease.

Primary aplastic anaemia is an idiopathic, very rare condition, also termed **Fanconi's syndrome**, which manifests itself in children between the ages of 5 and 10 years. It is suspected that the disease is caused by an autosomal recessive gene but chromosomal abnormalities are also often seen in the blood-forming cells of the marrow. The proportion of foetal haemoglobin in the erythrocytes is increased. In addition, many children show congenital malformations such as skeletal deformities (abnormal numbers of digits, lack of thumbs or hypoplastic thumbs and radii, dwarfism), hypoplasia of the kidneys or spleen, microcephaly and microphthalmia. Mental retardation is also common in these patients. The prognosis is poor even after treatment with androgens and corticosteroids, most patients dying before they reach the age of 20 years. There is a high incidence of leukaemia and other malignancies in many cases contributing to the death of the patient, while infection and haemorrhage are the commonest causes of death.

Secondary aplastic anaemia is much commoner, affecting about one person per 150 000 annually. There are various aetiologies associated with it, all of them in some way interfering with normal red marrow, causing disrupted haemopoiesis. Common causes of the disorder are:

- **physical agents**, for example radiation, exposure to radioactive material, radium, ^{32}P;
- **drugs and chemicals**: cancer treatment agents (e.g. cyclophosphamide, methotrexate, busulphan, vinblastine, 6-mercaptopurine), antibiotics and other chemotherapeutics (e.g. doxorubicin, chloramphenicol, streptomycin, mepacrine, paradione, tridione), anti-rheumatics (e.g. gold, phenylbutazone, indomethacin, gold salts) and industrial chemicals such as CCl_4, trinitrotoluene, benzole and benzene;
- **infections**, for example TB of bone marrow, typhoid fever, hepatitis and dengue fever;
- **other disease**, for example paroxysmal nocturnal haemoglobinuria;
- **idiopathic** in approximately half of all cases.

The disease develops insidiously and features of anaemia may be seen together with symptoms of leukopenia and thrombocytopenia. Weakness, fatigue, pallor, increased incidence of infection, bruising and haemorrhages are all commonly observed. As the bone marrow shows increasing involvement, the symptoms worsen and widespread infection may become life threatening or cerebral haemorrhages may cause death acutely.

The blood examination in this condition shows reduced haemoglobin content, sometimes as low as 3 g/dL, and greatly reduced erythrocyte numbers but the erythrocytes have a normocytic and normochromic appearance. The leukocyte numbers are also greatly decreased, sometimes to numbers as low as 500 cells/µL, the platelets also falling greatly, to numbers as low as 10 000 per µL.

In determining the course of treatment for this type of anaemia, it is important to be aware of the cause. If the patient is on any drug that is suspected of being involved with the condition, the drug is withdrawn and never administered to that person again. Chloramphenicol is a drug which causes aplastic anaemia in about one in every 50 000 people and is an example of a drug where individual idiosyncratic factors are important in the causation of the disease. On the other hand, benzene causes aplastic anaemia in all cases if the dose administered is large enough (the precise dose differing between individuals). Administration of androgens and corticosteroids may help in the recovery of the patient as these agents can cause a stimulation in the mitotic activity of the marrow. In some patients immunosuppression is of help, while in other patients the only option is bone marrow transplantation (a procedure that is successful in about 60% of cases of severe aplastic anaemia). Untreated, severe aplastic anaemia is fatal in a few months.

Haemolytic Anaemias

Haemolytic anaemias are caused by a pathological destruction of erythrocytes. There are both inherited and acquired forms of these types of anaemias, the clinical and haematological pictures varying depending on the rate and quantity of erythrocyte destruction and the ability of the marrow to undergo compensatory hyperplasia. Secondary effects caused by increased erythrocyte destruction may also be important, for example haemoglobinuria and jaundice. The haemolysis may occur in the circulation or within the reticulo-endothelial system, in the latter case no haemoglobinuria being seen.

Inherited Haemolytic Anaemias

In congenital haemolytic anaemias the defect that causes the lysis of erythrocytes resides within the red blood cell itself and may be due to abnormal haemoglobins, enzymatic defects, or a defective erythrocyte stroma or cell membrane. The life span of the erythrocyte is reduced from its normal 120 days to much lower values, differing with each type of anaemia. If erythrocytes from a normal person are transfused into the patient, they function normally and survive for the normal length of time. The bone marrow can increase its production of red blood cells up to about eight times the normal, but if the rate of erythrocyte destruction is great, this compensatory activity of the marrow is in vain and symptoms of haemolytic anaemia will develop.

The normal haemoglobin molecule is made up of a porphyrin, iron-containing ring, the **haeme** portion, and four protein chains, the **globin** portion. Globin consists of two identical halves, each half comprising two peptide chains of approximately 300 amino acids. The normal adult has two α chains and two β chains, the normal adult haemoglobin being designated as $\alpha_2\beta_2$ or **HbA**. A different form of adult haemoglobin found in a small number of people (about 3% of the population) is known as HbA$_2$, the place of the β chain being taken by a different form, the δ chain, making the formula of HbA$_2$ $\alpha_2\delta_2$. In the foetus haemoglobin is made up differently again, the foetal haemoglobin, **HbF**, containing two α chains and two γ chains, thus having the formula $\alpha_2\gamma_2$. It is known that the different globin chains are under the control of different genes and thus genetic disorders affecting each of the different globin chains are known, the haeme portion of the haemoglobin molecule in all of these disorders being normal.

There are approximately 550 different kinds of abnormal haemoglobins known and this number is increasing. The nomenclature of these abnormal haemoglobins initially started as an alphabetic enumeration, but when the large numbers of abnormal forms became known the naming of the abnormal chains was changed to the place where the abnormal haemoglobin was first described, for example haemoglobin Christchurch, haemoglobin Wien, haemoglobin Alexandria. In some cases, the place name is preceded by a letter prefix, for example haemoglobin G Philadelphia, which indicates that this haemoglobin is similar in character to the abnormal haemoglobin G which was discovered previously. Some abnormal haemoglobins retain the original letter nomenclature and these are: **haemoglobin S** (the sickle cell haemoglobin found predominantly in Africa, the Americas where African blacks have migrated, and around the Mediterranean); **haemoglobin C** (found predominantly in Africa); **haemoglobin D Punjab** (found predominantly in India and Iran); **haemoglobin E** (found predominantly in China and Indonesia); and **haemoglobin H** (found predominantly in Africa).

Sickle Cell Anaemia

Sickle cell disease develops in people who have HbS instead of HbA in their erythrocytes. This presupposes that they are homozygotes for the sickle cell gene and the formula for their haemoglobin is $\alpha_2\beta_{s2}$. The sickle cell gene is allelic for the HbA gene and homozygotes have no normal haemoglobin in their erythrocytes. Heterozygotes for the sickle cell gene are said to show the **sickle cell trait**, and their erythrocytes contain a mixture of HbS and HbA. The global distribution of the sickle cell gene is shown in Figure 17.8 and if this figure is compared with Figure 17.16, will it be seen that the sickle cell gene is prevalent in areas where malaria is a problem. This observation suggests that HbS confers some protective effect against malaria, especially that caused by *Plasmodium falciparum*. Studies in Africa have shown that there is an inverse relationship between the frequency of cases

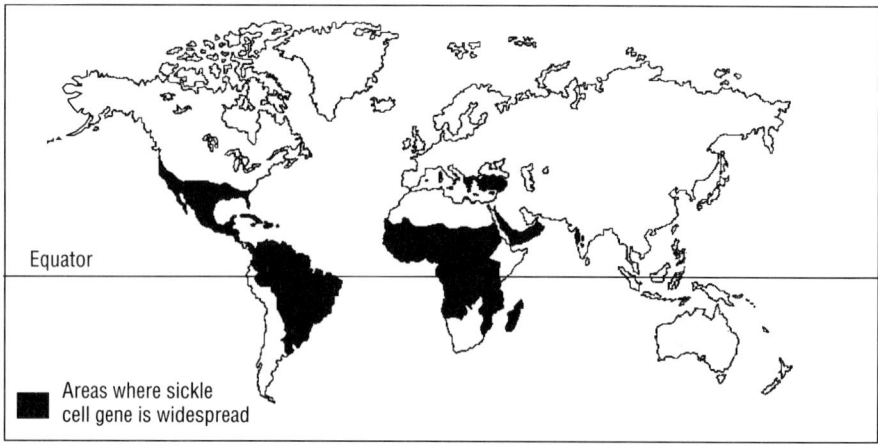

Figure 17.8   *The global distribution of the sickle cell gene (also see Figure 17.16)*

of falciparum malaria and the frequency of the sickle cell gene.

The name of the disease is derived from the characteristic 'sickle-shaped' drepanocytic erythrocytes that develop when the blood of the patient is mixed with a reducing agent in the laboratory. This sickling is seen only in the homozygotes. In the heterozygotes that have the sickle cell trait a similar treatment of the blood gives rise to 'holly-leaf' deformation of the erythrocytes (see Figure 17.9).

The sickle cell gene involves a point mutation in DNA that causes a single amino acid substitution in the globin molecule, which is sufficient to cause the disease (valine is substituted for glutamic acid as the sixth amino acid from the N terminal of the β globin chain). The substitution affects the surface of the haemoglobin molecule and the resultant HbS polymerizes when it is unoxygenated, in conditions of low oxygen tension, forming long, rod-like aggregates called **tactoids**; it is these that cause the abnormal sickle cell shape. If oxygen tension rises the tactoids dissolve and the cell returns to its normal shape. While in the circulation a sickle cell may undergo many cycles of sickling and unsickling. This causes the cell to lose some of its cytoplasm, as long tactoids deform the membrane. These damaged cells will remain sickled and their life span is reduced to 20 to 30 days. These cells are removed by the spleen, are phagocytosed by macrophages or their fragments often block small blood vessels in many organs.

Sickle cell disease first becomes evident during the first few months of life. It must be noted that the presence of HbF in the bloodstream of the neonate protects against sickling and it is only as the HbF is slowly replaced over the first 6 to 9 months of life by HbS that the sickling of the erythrocytes begins, with haemolysis and anaemia becoming evident. As the child becomes older, **crises** develop and these may be caused by either episodes of widespread haemolysis or by episodes of venous occlusion. The veno-occlusive crises may be delayed until later in life and they affect bones, joints, the lungs, gut, brain, skin and liver. There may be infarcts developing in any of these organs, with deformity in the long bones, arthritis, increased risk of osteomyelitis (especially commonly caused by *Salmonella* spp.). Perthes' disease of the femora may occur because of repeated fractures of the damaged bone (Figures 17.10 and 17.11). There may be pain in the chest and dyspnoea associated with lung involvement and also a high risk of respiratory infections. In the gut, blockage of vessels by sickled cells causes acute abdominal pain that may persist for a few days. Cerebral ischaemia may be very marked with hemiplegia, convulsions, aphasia and altered states of consciousness. The spleen enlarges during infancy because of the increased destruction of red blood cells, but later in life it shrinks and becomes very fibrotic, until in adulthood it may weigh only 30 g. The kidneys are often involved in the disease with small infarcts and interstitial fibrosis present. Some patients develop membranoproliferative glomerulonephritis and the nephrotic syndrome. The heart undergoes hypertrophy, haemosiderosis and some patients may experience heart failure. The vessels of the skin may become blocked, with leg and foot ulcers developing, while eye problems may also occur because of the blockage of eye vessels. It should be noted that the sickle cell trait rarely causes any clinical symptomatology or any

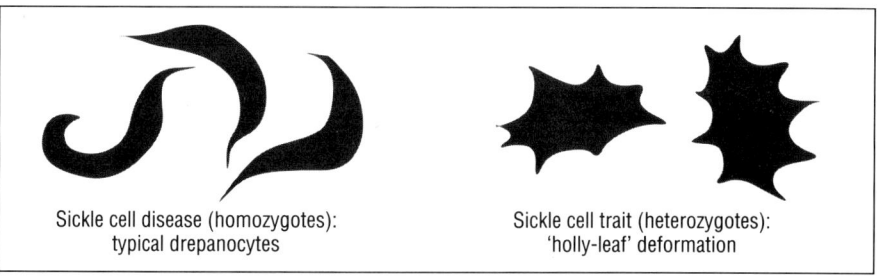

Figure 17.9 *Erythrocyte changes due to the sickle cell gene*

serious organ disease in most of the patients. In a very few patients intermittent sickling in kidney vessels will cause some renal problems, including infarction and papillary necrosis. Such patients are cautioned to avoid being exposed to low oxygen tension.

The PBS shows few abnormal cells if the blood sample was well oxygenated; however, upon the addition of sodium metabisulphite to the sample, numerous sickle cells develop. Reticulocytes may be seen, and also some erythrocytes will contain Howell-Jolly bodies or Heinz bodies. The haemoglobin content of the blood is lowered to values as low as 6 g/dL and hyperbilirubinaemia may also be observed. The ESR is lowered.

Treatment of the disease involves management of the complications as they develop, since no cure is known and there is no way to prevent the sickling of

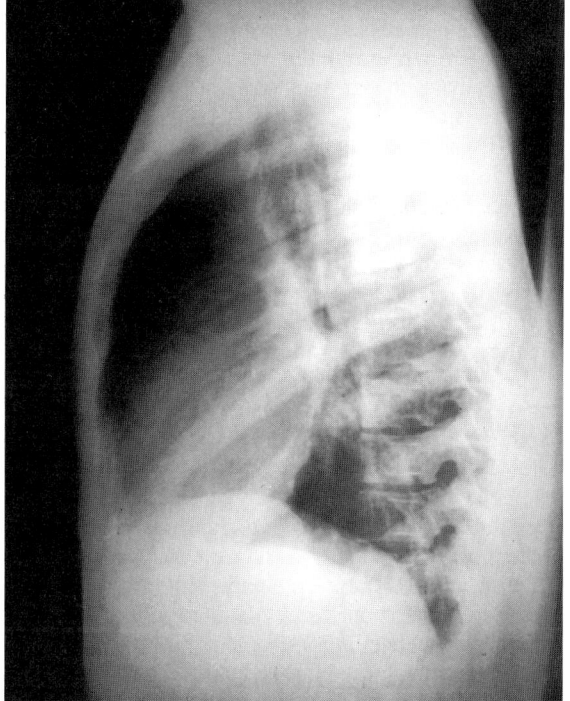

Figure 17.10 *Sickle cell anaemia causing spinal changes known as the Reynold's phenomenon, a step defect in the vertebral body. It is due to multiple central vertebral body infarcts. Only the secondary ring epiphyses increase the size of the vertebrae around their periphery, leading to the defect (courtesy of Dr Thomas Molyneux, RMIT)*

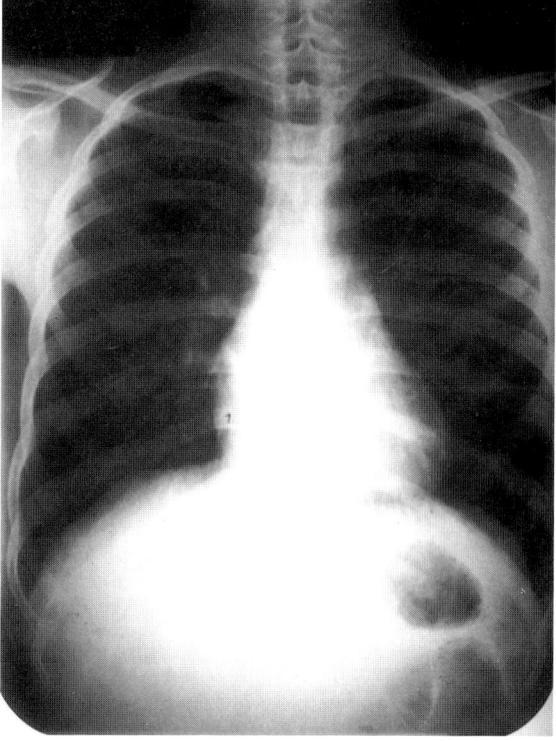

Figure 17.11 *Sickle cell anaemia causing spinal changes known as the Reynold's phenomenon (courtesy of Dr Thomas Molyneux, RMIT)*

the cells. If the spleen is excessively large, splenectomy may help the patient. Several drugs (e.g. blood alkalinizers, carbonic anhydrase inhibitors, etc.) have been tried in order to prevent sickle cells from forming, but none of these has been shown to be highly effective. In most African countries, children who are homozygous for the gene rarely survive into their teens. In the USA the prognosis is better and only about a fifth of patients die in childhood. Most children die of infections and most adults of renal failure.

Other Haemoglobinopathies

In certain African countries, especially northern Ghana, West Africa and South Africa, **HbC** has a high incidence in the population. The homozygotes for the gene causing this disorder have a mild, haemolytic anaemia. Most of the cells in the circulation are codocytes, with a few spherocytes. The heterozygotes for the gene suffer no disease.

About 10%, frequently more, of the populations of Thailand, Cambodia and Burma and lesser proportions of the populations in the Philippines, Malaysia and India possess the gene which results in the presence of **HbE** in the erythrocytes. This abnormal haemoglobin has lysine substituted for glutamic acid as the sixth amino acid from the N terminal of the β globin chain. Homozygotes for the gene suffer from a mild haemolytic anaemia. In the PBS many target cells are seen. The heterozygotes suffer no ill effects.

An abnormal haemoglobin affecting either the α or β chain is **HbD**, the commonest variant of which is **haemoglobin D Punjab (HbD$_β$ Punjab)**. The gene for this disorder is commonest in its occurrence in India, Iran, Turkey, Africa and Spain. In this case, glutamine is substituted for glutamic acid as the 121st amino acid from the N terminal of the β globin chain. The majority of homozygotes suffer from mild haemolytic anaemia, more serious in a few cases. The heterozygotes suffer from no disability.

Foetal haemoglobin, **HbF**, is normal in the foetus but sometimes it may appear in adults with haemolytic anaemias and very rarely as an hereditary abnormality.

β Chain Thalassaemia (Mediterranean Anaemia, Cooley's Anaemia)

Thalassaemia is from the Greek word for 'sea' and this term is given to the disease because it has a high incidence in the countries around the Mediterranean Sea. It is mostly seen in Sardinia, Sicily, southern Italy, Greece, Cyprus and Turkey, where up to 20% of the population may carry the gene. However, the disease is also commonly seen in some South East Asian countries (Cambodia, Burma), in southern China, Iran, India and Pakistan and also to a lesser extent in other European countries and Africa (see Figure 17.12). Thalassaemia is a genetic disease in which there is an abnormality in the formation or function of messenger RNA coding for the production of the β globin chains. This results in deficient HbA synthesis and the erythrocytes may also contain other forms of haemoglobin, such as HbF and HbA$_2$.

The heterozygous form of the disease is termed **thalassaemia minor** and causes little disease, while the homozygous form is called **thalassaemia major** and is the one associated with severe anaemia. In addition, some patients with thalassaemia form abnormal haemoglobins. The abnormal haemoglobin may be the one that is synthesized deficiently, or alternatively the person may be a double heterozygote, one gene coding for underproduction of a normal haemoglobin while the other gene codes for abnormal haemoglobin. There are many variations in the combinations of haemoglobins that are seen in thalassaemia, β$^+$ thalassaemia denoting reduced synthesis of the β chain while β^0 thalassaemia denotes its complete absence.

Clinically, thalassaemia major manifests itself when the baby is a few months old. In the PBS there is poikilocytosis and anisocytosis, microcytosis, hypochromia and reticulocytosis and there are many codocytes present (Figure 17.13). Many of the erythrocytes are nucleated (erythroblastosis) and the white blood cell numbers are increased, mainly neutrophils being present in excess. The haemoglobin content of the blood is decreased to levels as low as 3 g/dL, the packed cell volume being 20% or lower and the osmotic fragility of the erythrocytes is decreased (i.e. they will not lyse if put into distilled water).

The affected children often have a Mongoloid appearance because of the extreme enlargement and distortion of the cranial and facial bones caused by the marrow hyperplasia. A characteristic radiological appearance of the skull is seen in this condition, with inner and outer tables having trabeculation perpendicular to their surfaces, giving the skull a 'hair-on-end' appearance. There is hepatosplenomegaly caused by the increased erythrocyte destruction and the extramedullary haemopoiesis. Haemosiderosis is seen in many organs, including the heart, and is due to the iron overload caused by the massive destruction of erythrocytes.

The only effective treatment for thalassaemia major is blood transfusions that raise the haemoglobin content of the blood and hence systemic oxygenation. Iron chelating agents may also be administered. Some patients need a splenectomy, especially if there is gross splenomegaly. In this case the need for frequent transfusions decreases. Most patients with the disease die in

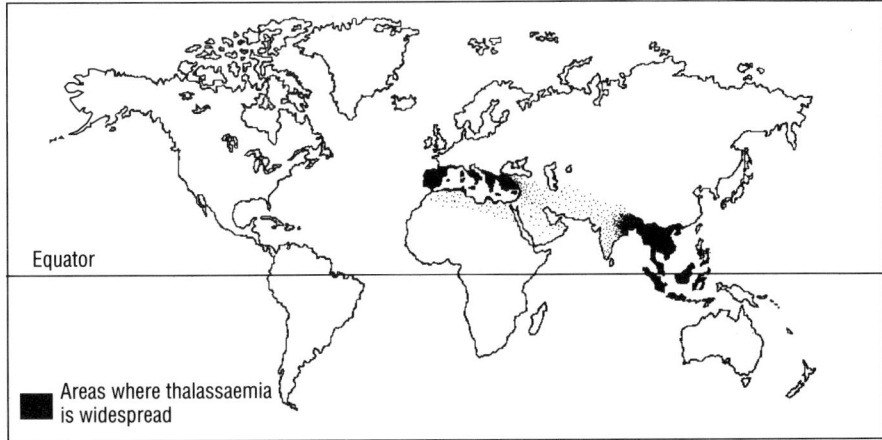

Figure 17.12 *The global distribution of thalassaemia*

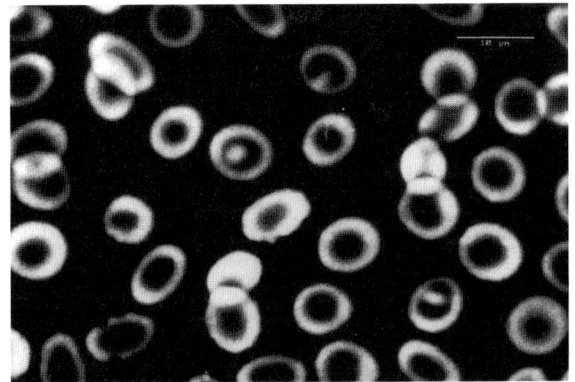

Figure 17.13 *Thalassaemia major showing several prominent codocytes or 'target cells' (scale bar is 10 μm)*

childhood from infections or heart failure, few patients surviving into young adulthood.

Thalassaemia minor is a mild disease, the haemoglobin concentration in the blood being slightly reduced to levels of 12 g/dL in men and 11 g/dL in women. There is microcytosis, anisocytosis, poikilocytosis and codocytosis, and there are no nucleated erythrocytes in the peripheral blood. The organ changes that are seen in thalassaemia major are absent, and the marrow is only mildly hyperplastic. Such patients usually live a normal life and their life span is not appreciably decreased. **Thalassaemia minima** is a form of the disease in which patients are totally normal in their haematological profile and organ findings, but if the reticulocytes from their blood are cultured it can be demonstrated that they produce fewer β globin chains than α globin chains.

α Chain Thalassaemia

The α chain thalassaemias are prevalent in southern China and South East Asia and it is estimated that in Thailand about 225 000 people are affected by the disorder. It is also seen in the Middle East, West Africa and some Mediterranean countries. The disease may occur in major and minor forms as is the case with β chain thalassaemia. People who are termed carriers of this disease usually show no abnormality at all, DNA studies or construction of pedigree charts being required in adulthood to demonstrate the defective genes. These people have three loci on chromosome 16 for the α chain instead of four loci (refer to Figure 17.14). The people with α chain thalassaemia minor have only two active loci on chromosome 16 for the α chain and have minor or no symptoms of anaemia. In most cases the defect is found when the blood is examined routinely or in the course of another investigation. The erythrocytes are microcytic and the PBS shows anisocytosis, poikilocytosis and hypochromia.

Haemoglobin H disease results when there is only one active locus on chromosome 16 for the α chain. Patients develop anaemia in infancy, there is hepatosplenomegaly and the PBS shows microcytosis, hypochromia and codocytosis. At birth about a third of the haemoglobin is haemoglobin Bart's (formula γ_4) but this disappears progressively over a few months, being replaced by haemoglobin H (formula β_4), which persists in the adult to levels of about 12%. The rest of the haemoglobin in these patients is HbA.

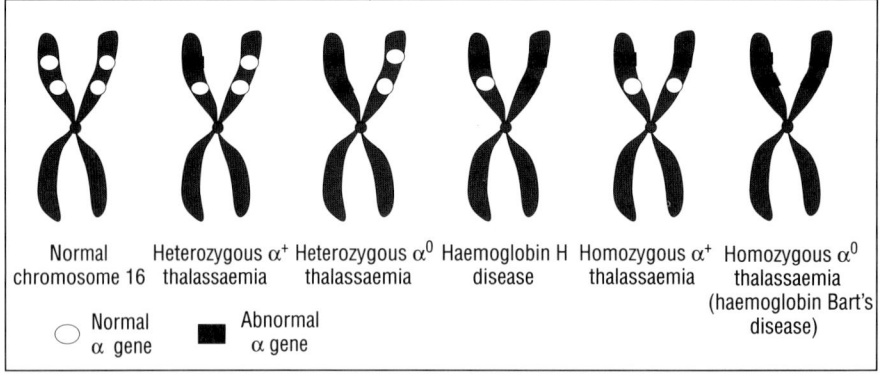

Figure 17.14   *The genetics of α thalassaemia*

The major form of the disease is termed **haemoglobin Bart's disease** and in this case no α chain loci are active on chromosome 16 and no α chain globin is produced at all. This is a condition that is incompatible with life as the α chain is required for the formation of foetal haemoglobin. The affected foetus dies *in utero*, between the 28th and 40th week of pregnancy. If the baby is born alive it is bloated and pale (hydrops foetalis) and usually dies within a few hours of delivery. About 80% of the haemoglobin in the erythrocytes is haemoglobin Bart's, which does not function as an oxygen carrier. The rest of the haemoglobin is haemoglobin Portland (formula $\zeta_2\gamma_2$) and haemoglobin H. Haemoglobin Bart's disease is a common cause of foetal death in South East Asia and Cyprus. The blood shows severe poikilocytosis, anisocytosis and erythroblastosis and the haemoglobin content is low.

Hereditary Spherocytosis
Hereditary spherocytosis is an uncommon genetic disorder that is transmitted as an autosomal dominant character with varying degrees of penetrance and expressivity, affecting males and females equally. The gene involved is on chromosome 8 or 12. Spherocytosis is the commonest form of inherited haemolytic disorder in the Northern European races and their descendants. The lesion in this condition resides in the erythrocyte membrane, its lipid content being low and the membrane proteins being abnormal. This causes the cells to become spherocytes and they are also very fragile, especially in the absence of glucose. The spherocytes have a markedly decreased life span.

Usually the disease is diagnosed in childhood, the clinical hallmarks of the condition being **acholuric jaundice** (no bile in the urine), **anaemia** and **splenomegaly**. Gall stones may form because of the increased bile pigment metabolism and the bones may show abnormalities because of bone marrow hyperplasia. The anaemia in this condition is usually moderate to mild, the concentration of haemoglobin being 11 to 14 g/dL in adults and 9 g/dL in children. Often the anaemia is only apparent when the patient has a haemolytic crisis. In a PBS there is evidence of spherocytosis, reticulocytosis, microcytosis and polychromasia.

The disease is treated by splenectomy, a procedure that prevents excessive haemolysis, gall stone formation and raises blood haemoglobin. The hyperplastic bone marrow returns to normal and although there are still spherocytes in the blood the condition may be considered to be controlled effectively. As splenectomy increases the risk of infection in the young child, the procedure is usually carried out in adolescence unless the disease is very severe earlier on.

Hereditary Elliptocytosis (Ovalocytosis)
This is another Mendelian disorder, the trait being transmitted as an autosomal dominant, the gene segregating together with those controlling Rh blood group. Approximately 40 people per 100 000 suffer from this disorder in which up to 90% of the circulating erythrocytes are elliptocytes (Figure 17.15). This is a mild disease, most patients presenting with no clinical disease, the elliptocytes being discovered in a routine full blood examination. The affected cells have a normal life span and they are not excessively fragile. It is only in some cases of the disease that a mild haemolytic anaemia develops, a severe anaemia being rare with this disorder. In these last-mentioned cases the clinical presentation resembles hereditary spherocytosis. Splenectomy is indicated in these patients.

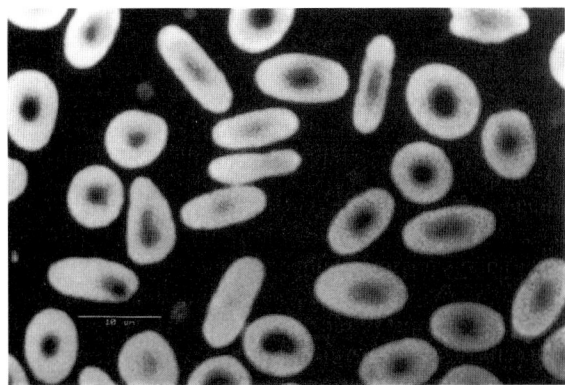

Figure 17.15 *Hereditary ovalocytosis (scale bar is 10 mm)*

Stomatocytosis and Acanthocytosis

Stomatocytosis is present to a small degree in the blood of alcoholics. **Hereditary stomatocytosis** is transmitted as an autosomal dominant character and the condition causes a very mild anaemia. It is suspected that there are membrane defects in the erythrocyte, causing it to be bowl-shaped and to show the characteristic mouth-like central pale region. The haemoglobin content of the blood is around 8 g/dL. The abnormal cells are fragile and have a slightly shortened life span. Rarely, the anaemia developing in this condition is severe, with haemoglobin as low as 4 g/dL. Splenectomy does not help in the treatment of the disease.

Acanthocytosis is seen usually with the genetic disorder **abetalipoproteinaemia**. In this disease there is lack of β lipoproteins, hypocholesterolaemia, progressive ataxic neuropathy, malabsorption syndrome and retinitis. Acanthocytosis also develops in cirrhosis of the liver. In both cases the erythrocytes are thought to be affected by disturbances in lipid metabolism that cause abnormalities in the red blood cell membrane. A few patients suffer from haemolytic crises but most cases of the disorder are only a striking finding in a PBS, without much clinical haematological disease.

Enzymatic Defects

There are various deficiencies known in the enzymes that erythrocytes need for normal metabolism. The two most common of these enzymatic defects are deficiencies in glucose-6-phosphate-dehydrogenase and in pyruvate kinase.

Glucose-6-phosphate-dehydrogenase deficiency is rather common in incidence and many people in the population have less than a quarter of the normal activity of the enzyme in their erythrocytes. The disorder is transmitted as an X-linked trait and hence is commoner in males. The incidence of the gene is common in areas where malaria was common (i.e. Mediterranean area, Africa, Middle East, South East Asia) as the deficiency is thought to protect against malaria. In Sardinia approximately a third of the population in some areas has the defect, while in Northern Europe only 0.1% of men have the defect. Numerous variants of the enzyme are known and these have been named alphabetically and also by the name of the place where the variant was first described (e.g. G6PD B is the normal enzyme, common variants being G6PD A, G6PD Mediterranean and G6PD Corinth).

The disease results in paroxysms of haemolysis that are linked to administration of a drug, or occur after an infection or after consumption of a certain foodstuff. Various drugs implicated are anti-malarials, aspirin, streptomycin, sulphonamides and chloramphenicol. Infections causing the disorder are hepatitis, respiratory infections (bacterial and viral) and candidiasis. Foodstuffs implicated are fava beans (broad beans), peas and some types of mushrooms. Even the pollen of the broad bean flowers is enough to cause an attack. Pythagoras, aware of favism, in 500 BC barred his followers from eating fava beans or even walking through fields where they were growing as he decreed it 'unhealthy'. However, the anaemia does not result every time these offending foodstuffs are consumed, so unknown co-factors are also involved.

The haemolysis caused by this enzyme deficiency is intravascular and the haemoglobin content of blood during a crisis can fall to about 4 g/dL. Haemoglobinuria follows and jaundice is common. Symptoms of anaemia ensue and persist until the bone marrow is able to compensate for the loss of erythrocytes. In the first few days of the anaemic state, numerous erythrocytes contain within them Heinz bodies, which are denatured globin molecules aggregating together and adhering to the cell membrane. The Heinz bodies are removed from the erythrocytes when they pass through the spleen. In Mediterranean countries, Thailand and China, babies with the enzyme defect will show jaundice soon after birth. An exchange transfusion may be needed in cases where the hyperbilirubinaemia is severe in order to prevent kernicterus.

The disease is usually not severe enough to cause serious problems, but if any drug or condition is found to bring on an attack this agent should be avoided and the offending drugs or other substances should not be administered again. In some patients diabetes mellitus or infections bring on attacks and these states should be fully treated or controlled in order to limit the anaemia. Splenectomy is of no help in this condition.

Pyruvate kinase deficiency is an uncommon disorder inherited as an autosomal recessive trait and is more common in Northern European races. The anaemia usually manifests itself in childhood and is moderately severe. The haemoglobin concentration is reduced to as low as 6 g/dL and the PBS shows evidence of polychromasia, macrocytosis, poikilocytosis and acanthocytosis, and there may be a few nucleated erythrocytes present in the film.

The disease is caused by deficiency of the enzyme which is needed to regenerate ATP from ADP in the erythrocyte. It is thought that inadequate levels of ATP in the erythrocyte may be the cause of membrane instability that makes for an increased liability to lysis. The erythrocytes are lysed predominantly in the spleen, the reticulocytes and younger red blood cells being more likely to be sequestrated and lysed. Splenomegaly is often noted in patients and there may be jaundice, biliary calculi and haemolytic crises. The disorder is treated by splenectomy which may benefit the patient suffering from severe haemolysis and gross splenomegaly; however, the haemolysis still continues after the procedure, although at a reduced rate.

Acquired Haemolytic Anaemias

Malaria

Malaria is a parasitic disease of mainly tropical and subtropical areas, and according to WHO it is the world's major health problem, causing more disease and deaths than any other disease in the world. Several tens of millions of cases of malaria are believed to exist presently, and each year about a million people die of this disease globally. The infection occurs in developing nations mostly where it is a problem among the poor living in the countryside, children, the elderly, the debilitated and the malnourished. It is suspected that even though many people in the endemic areas may not show clinical signs of disease, they still harbour the parasites. The disease is transmitted by female mosquitoes of the genus *Anopheles* and malaria is seen in warm, wet regions where the mosquitoes transmitting the parasite may breed (refer to Figure 17.16).

The disease is caused by infection with one or any combination of the four species of the malaria parasite: *Plasmodium vivax, P. falciparum, P. ovale* and *P. malariae*. The last two are now infrequently encountered. There are another three species of malarial parasites but they are considered to be 'benign'. Of all the malarial parasites, *P. falciparum* is the most sinister as it can kill a patient acutely. This is because it may infect erythrocytes of any age, causing them to become 'sticky', leading to microthrombus formation in small blood vessels with resultant microinfarcts.

The malarial parasites have two stages of development, one taking place in the mosquito, the other in the human. In the mosquito the sexual reproductive phase (called **sporogony**) of the parasite occurs and this takes 7 to 12 days. When an infected mosquito bites a human the parasites enter the blood through the infected saliva of the mosquito. The asexual life cycle (called **schizogony**) occurs in the liver where parasite merozoites develop in the hepatocytes (about 7 days); the merozoites are then released into the bloodstream where they infect erythrocytes. In the red blood cells the trophozoites develop and, depending on the species of *Plasmodium*, the erythrocytic phase lasts between 36 and 72 hours. Once inside the erythrocytes the trophozoites develop into schizonts which divide

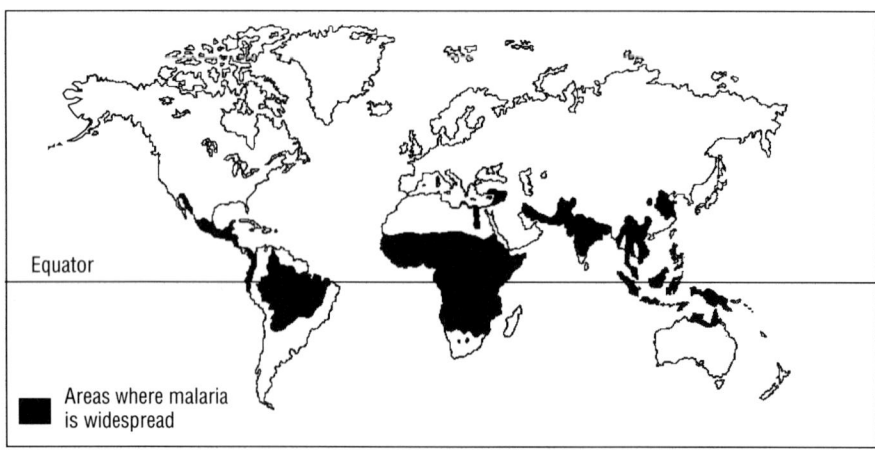

Figure 17.16 *The global distribution of malaria*

to form merozoites (Figure 17.17). The merozoites are released from the damaged erythrocyte and they can then infect more erythrocytes, the cycle being repeated five or six times. The merozoites then change into male and female gametocytes which may infect a mosquito when it bites a human (see Figure 17.18).

The symptoms and signs of a malarial infection are characteristic cyclic bouts of fever and chills with anaemia and hepatosplenomegaly. The bouts of fever are caused by the release of new crops of merozoites from the ruptured erythrocytes. Different species of *Plasmodium* are characterized by different intervals between the pyrexia (see also Table 17.2):

- *Plasmodium falciparum:* 'malignant' malaria, fever every 36 hours;
- *Plasmodium vivax* and *Plasmodium ovale:* 'tertian' malaria, fever every 48 hours;
- *Plasmodium malariae:* 'quartan' malaria, fever every 72 hours.

The reticuloendothelial system is involved in the phagocytosis of the parasite, erythrocyte pigments and debris that are released when infected erythrocytes rupture. There is enlargement of the spleen, liver and lymph nodes. The spleen, in particular, is grossly enlarged and in the acute phase of the disease may be haemorrhagic and soft. In the chronic stages the enlarged spleen becomes almost black in colour, is very firm and contains fibrous regions. In *P. falciparum* malaria, the brain and heart show congestion of small blood vessels, microinfarcts and, with time, numerous areas of gliosis and fibrosis respectively (these are

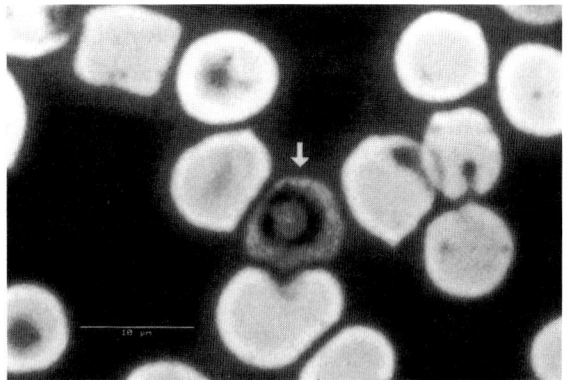

Figure 17.17   *Malaria due to* Plasmodium vivax *infection. A ring form of the organism is seen in this erythrocyte (scale bar is 10 μm)*

often referred to as **malarial 'granulomata'**). Sudden rupture of enormous numbers of infected erythrocytes around the body in falciparum malaria will release large amounts of haemoglobin, leading to jaundice, haemoglobinuria, kidney damage, oliguria and the passage of very dark urine, a presentation known as **'blackwater fever'**. The liver shows enlargement and under the microscope, in the acute stages, there will be pigment and parasite-laden Kupffer cells. Similar changes will be seen in the bone marrow and lymph nodes.

The diagnosis of malaria is made by demonstrating

Table 17.2   *Characteristics of the various types of malaria*

Organism	Malaria type	Frequency of fever (hours)	Severity of disease	Features in PBS
P. malariae	Quartan	72	Mild to moderate (untreated disease lasts many years)	No dots or granules in RBC
P. ovale	Tertian	48	Mild (untreated disease lasts for 2 to 3 years)	Schüffner's dots
P. vivax	Tertian	48	Mild (untreated disease lasts for 2 to 3 years)	Schüffner's dots, active movement of trophozoites in RBC
P. falciparum	Malignant	36 to 48 (irregular)	Often fatal if untreated	Crescentic gametocytes

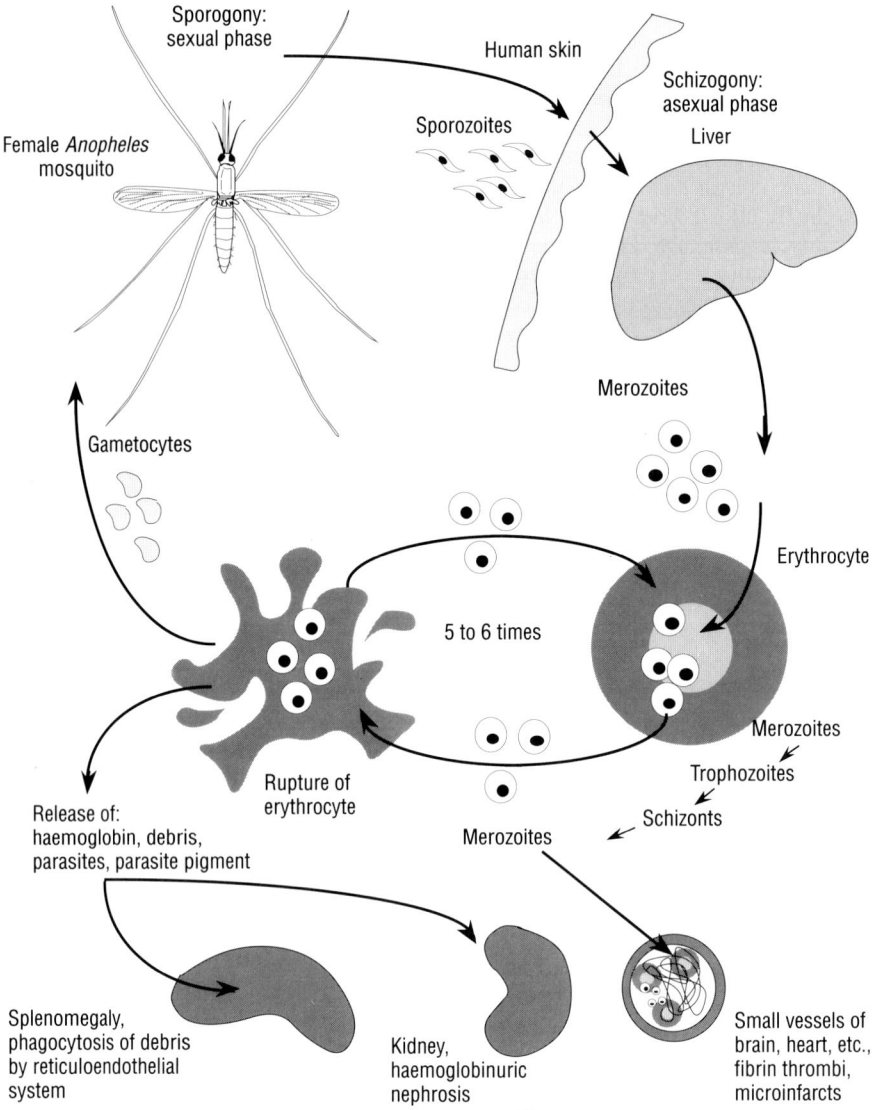

Figure 17.18 *The life cycle of the malaria parasite*

the specific and characteristic inclusions each type of malaria parasite causes to be present in the erythrocytes in a thick PBS prepared from the patient. Clinical presentation, physical examination and tests for anaemia will also help in the diagnosis. Malaria in Australia is mainly seen in returning overseas visitors who have not taken adequate precautions against malarial infection while travelling in endemic areas; therefore history of the patient's travel may also help in diagnosis. The prophylaxis of malaria involves taking drugs that prevent the multiplication of the parasite in the bloodstream. These have traditionally centred around chloroquine administration, but in several parts of the world where malaria is prevalent chloroquine-resistant strains have developed, and additional drugs need to be taken. It is important for travellers to be aware of malaria and to avoid being bitten by mosquitoes by taking adequate precautions. Several mosquito eradication programmes have been initiated in certain countries. Treatment of malarial infection is also by the administration of the appropriate chemotherapeutic agents, but because of developing resistance to these agents it is not unusual for patients to die, especially in the case of falciparum malaria.

Autoimmune Anaemias

In the large group of autoimmune anaemias the common factor is that antibodies against a component of the erythrocyte membrane attach to that component and bring about lysis of the cell. These types of anaemias must be distinguished from the transfusion reactions and haemolytic disease of the newborn in which the antibodies causing the lysis are normal antibodies present in the plasma. The lysis in these cases occurs because of mismatching and transfer of foreign antibodies or erythrocytes into the body of the patient (both of the conditions have been considered already). Autoimmune haemolytic anaemias may be divided into two major groups, the primary and secondary diseases. The **primary form** is an idiopathic and uncommon disorder. The **secondary form** is seen in association with various precipitating causes:

- **malignancy** (e.g. leukaemia);
- **other autoimmune disease** (e.g. rheumatoid arthritis, SLE);
- **infections**, especially viral (e.g. pneumonias, glandular fever);
- **drug administration** (commonly) [e.g. penicillin, insulin, streptomycin (all of which function as haptens), phenacetin, quinine, anti-TB drugs, sulphonamides (functioning as immune complexing agents) and levodopa, α-methyldopa and mefenamic acid (giving rise to a classical autoimmune type of lysis)].

The autoimmune anaemias have been subdivided into the **cold-antibody** type and the **warm-antibody** type depending on the temperature at which the autoantibodies have maximal activity. In the warm-antibody type the haemolysis is seen at 37°C, IgG being the majority of the antibody class involved, while in the cold-antibody type the haemolysis is best observed at temperatures below 31°C (for example, in the extremities and skin *in vivo*), IgM being the majority of the antibody class involved. The warm-antibody type of autoimmune anaemias cause approximately 85% of cases of the disease. In the classical autoimmune type of anaemia an association with the HLA B7 antigen has been noted. Complement-mediated lysis is important in the pathogenesis of both types of autoimmune anaemia. However, it should also be noted that antibody-coated erythrocytes will be selectively sequestered in the liver and spleen to be destroyed by reticuloendothelial cells in these organs. Cell-mediated lysis is another important mechanism of haemolysis and macrophages are particularly important in this type of lysis. The **Coombs' test** is a laboratory test used to detect erythrocytes with attached antibodies on their surface, and is of use in diagnosing these disorders.

Clinically, the anaemia may develop acutely if it is due to an infection or administration of a drug, while in other cases symptoms due to anaemia will develop insidiously. In a PBS, macrocytes may be seen, spherocytes are present and many reticulocytes are observed, sometimes the reticulocyte count being up to 50% of all red blood cells. Haemoglobin content is reduced to levels as low as 6 g/dL. The haemolysis may bring about haemoglobinuria, renal injury and often clotting and thrombotic abnormalities because of associated platelet involvement. Treatment of these types of anaemias involves withdrawal of the offending drug that has brought about the condition, treatment of the infection if possible, and in other precipitating conditions corticosteroid therapy may be of benefit, while treatment of the primary condition may also curb the anaemia.

Toxic Anaemias

Snake and spider venoms induce anaemia by causing direct damage to the erythrocytes. In many cases this is due to the action of lecithinase in the toxin, which is an enzyme converting lecithin to lysolecithin, an agent capable of haemolysis. The haemolysis induced by these toxins may be very severe or fatal. **Bacterial exotoxins** may also cause haemolysis, as occurs, for example, in *Clostridium perfringens* infection, where a very powerful haemolysin is secreted by the bacteria. Some **chemicals and drugs** may cause haemolysis directly, as, for example, occurs with benzene, naphthalene, toluene, aniline, nitrofurantoin, para-aminosalicylic acid and sulfoxone. All of these agents are thought to interfere with redox reactions in the erythrocytes, thus causing lysis. Entry of **water** into the circulation will cause haemolysis through osmotic effects.

Lead, **copper**, **arsenic** and a number of other metals will cause anaemia in cases where chronic ingestion is the case. The metals alter the metabolism of the erythrocyte and may even interfere with the incorporation of iron into haeme. Sideroblasts may be seen in the marrow and there may be porphyriuria. Symptoms and signs of poisoning will coexist with those due to the anaemia.

Paroxysmal Nocturnal Haemoglobinuria (Marchiafava-Micheli Syndrome)

Paroxysmal nocturnal haemoglobinuria is a rare disease that affects adults around the age of 35 years, both sexes being affected equally. There are no familial or genetic influences involved in the aetiology. The patients have in the blood a mixture of normal and abnormal erythrocytes, the abnormal ones being more easily lysed by complement. The severity of the disease differs according to the proportion of highly sensitive erythrocytes patients have in their bloodstream. If less than 20% of the red blood cells are abnormal, the disease is mild and episodic, while in cases where more than 50% of cells are abnormal, there is constant haemoglobinuria due to haemolysis of these erythrocytes by complement (the normal erythrocytes are not lysed). There appears to be a defect in the erythrocyte membrane that makes these cells more liable to complement-mediated lysis. The disease is termed nocturnal as the lysis is more likely to occur during sleep; this may be due to the fall in pH that occurs in some organs during sleep (if the patient sleeps during the day, the lysis will occur during that period).

Clinically, the patient will show haemoglobinuria in the first morning specimen of urine and this may be of variable severity. Some patients have haemosiderinuria instead of haemoglobinuria. The haemoglobinuria may be precipitated by infections, stress, menstruation, inoculations or as is often the case it may occur spontaneously. Aplastic anaemia may be seen in some patients, thrombosis is very common in the leg veins, portal venous system and cerebral veins, and infections may also be seen commonly in these patients. The haemoglobin content of the blood may be as low as 5 g/dL and the PBS will show anisocytosis, polychromasia, thrombocytopenia and leukopenia. Occasional nucleated cells will be seen. **Ham's test** is used in diagnosis of this disorder and consists of incubating erythrocytes in an acid environment, which in this anaemia causes haemolysis (positive).

Treatment of the condition involves blood transfusions, anticoagulants (coumarin type, not heparin), corticosteroids, androgens and bone marrow transplants, but all of these have not been very successful and no cure is known. Splenectomy is not carried out. Oral iron may be needed to replenish that lost in the haemoglobinuria. In some patients the disease spontaneously remits, but in about half of the cases death ensues 10 to 15 years after the onset of the disease due to thrombosis or aplastic anaemia, a minority of the patients also developing leukaemia.

March Haemoglobinuria
The condition of march haemoglobinuria is usually seen in soldiers who march excessively but may be seen after any strenuous exercise where running on hard ground with inappropriate footwear is undertaken. The injury is a mechanical one caused by the pounding of feet against ground, which damages the vessels (and hence erythrocytes contained therein) of the soles. The haemoglobinuria lasts for a few hours after the exercise. Running on soft ground while wearing running shoes does not cause the disease. The same mechanical damage to vessels and resulting haemoglobinuria may occur on the palms of the hands of energetic, passionate Congo drum players!

Polycythaemia (Erythrocytosis)

Polycythaemia or erythrocytosis refers to an increased mass of erythrocytes in the circulation. The erythrocyte numbers, haemoglobin and the packed cell volume are increased also. The most common type of this condition is secondary polycythaemia, which is the result of some other state or disease in the body. The most usual stimulus for secondary polycythaemia is a decreased oxygen delivery to the tissues, which in turn stimulates increased haemopoiesis in the bone marrow. Primary polycythaemia (polycythaemia rubra vera) is very rare.

Secondary Polycythaemia

Secondary polycythaemia may occur physiologically or pathologically. It is most commonly seen physiologically in people who live in high altitudes and breathe air with a lower partial pressure of oxygen. This causes a lowered saturation of the arterial blood with oxygen and the increase in the number of erythrocytes that is seen in the circulation is an example of compensatory hyperplasia in the bone marrow. The condition is seen in people who live in altitudes greater than 1800 m above sea level, and the higher the altitude the more marked the polycythaemia. For example, people who live at an altitude of 4500 m above sea level have 7.5 million erythrocytes per µL of blood. There are raised levels of erythropoietin in the blood, the marrow responding to its presence by producing increased erythrocyte numbers. The spleen is not enlarged and patients are not hypertensive. When the polycythaemic person descends to lower altitudes the erythrocyte numbers return to normal levels.

In certain pathological situations where there is compromise of oxygenation of the blood, polycythaemia will develop secondarily. The commonest causes are cardiovascular and pulmonary diseases. For example, in Fallot's tetralogy secondary polycythaemia is seen. In emphysema, other cases of COAD and chronic bronchitis secondary polycythaemia will result as a response to decreased arterial oxygen saturation. Polycythaemia may also occur in certain renal diseases (e.g. carcinoma of the kidney, infections, renal cysts and polycystic disease), in some endocrine disorders (e.g. Cushing's disease), CNS diseases (e.g. brain stem lesions and haemangioma of the cerebellum), hepatocarcinoma and in women with massive uterine fibroids.

In all cases of secondary polycythaemia there is an increased erythrocyte mass while the leukocyte count remains normal. The marrow shows erythroid hyperplasia. Pathological secondary polycythaemia is treated by therapy of the primary condition that has caused the disease. For example, surgical removal of tumours or surgery for congenital heart lesions.

Polycythaemia Rubra Vera (Primary Polycythaemia)

Polycythaemia rubra vera (**erythraemia** or primary polycythaemia) is a rare idiopathic disease that is seen more commonly in men than women, with a ratio of occurrence of 3:2. Most patients are over the age of 40 years when diagnosed with the disorder and it is commoner in Jews and Caucasians and rare in black people. Most haematologists regard this condition as a neoplasm of cells of the erythroid line in the bone marrow. An abnormal clone of erythroid cell precursors may be demonstrated in the marrow in about 10% of patients, the commonest disorder being a trisomy 9. These abnormal erythroid cells divide continuously and inappropriately, without regard to the body's needs, and do not depend on erythropoietin stimulation (erythropoietin levels are normal in this condition). Other experts in the field regard polycythaemia rubra vera as an abnormality in the sensitivity of a clone of the erythroid cell precursors to erythropoietin.

The erythrocyte count in primary polycythaemia ranges between 7 and 10 million per μL, often being as high as 12 million per μL. The concentration of haemoglobin in the blood also increases, with values between 18 to 24 g/dL. The packed red blood cell volume rises to 0.8 L/L (80%) or more. Often there are increased numbers of leukocytes and platelets in the peripheral blood, their numbers being about 12 000 per μL and 800 000 per μL respectively. The morphology of both erythrocytes and leukocytes is normal, unless iron deficiency develops (often the case) resulting in the red blood cells becoming microcytic and hypochromic. The viscosity of the blood increases dramatically in the disorder, and it is difficult for blood to go through small vessels. The skin is congested and red, the eyes bloodshot and frequently there are nose bleeds and gum haemorrhages. Thrombosis is common with infarction resulting in the heart, brain, lungs, gut and legs. The spleen is enlarged in about 75% of

cases and half the patients are hypertensive. One in ten patients has a peptic ulcer.

Clinically, the disease develops slowly and insidiously. Most patients seek advice after the disease has been present for some years. The symptoms and signs result from the increased blood volume and hyperviscosity of the blood. Headache is common, dizziness and visual disturbances are also usual. Severe pruritus is often experienced (especially after hot baths), and weakness, loss of weight, sweating, dyspnoea on exertion, arthralgia and paraesthesiae are other features of the disorder.

If the disease is untreated most patients will die within 2 years of developing symptoms, the commonest causes of death being thrombosis and infarction, less commonly haemorrhage or leukaemia. A small proportion of patients may live for 10 years or more, the polycythaemia changing to myelofibrosis and acute or chronic myeloid leukaemia supervening. Venesection, which reduces the blood volume and circulating excess erythrocytes, provides immediate relief and in many patients this lasts for months. In such cases removal of about 500 to 1000 mL of blood every few months may be sufficient treatment. In other cases radiation and cytotoxic therapy may be required. With treatment, the 10-year survival is 50% or better.

Platelet Diseases

Decreases in Numbers (Thrombocytopenias)

Thrombocytopenia is said to occur if the platelet count falls below 100 000 per μL. If the count falls below 60 000 per μL there is the danger of spontaneous bleeding occurring. **Purpura** is the condition in which small haemorrhages occur from capillaries throughout the body, resulting in small areas of haemorrhage, called **petechiae**, in the skin, mucous and serous membranes. The mechanism by which thrombocytopenia induces purpura is not known but it is thought that low platelet numbers cause an abnormal capillary fragility, so that what in the normal person is trivial trauma to capillary endothelium in the thrombocytopenic patient causes severe damage which is not stopped up by a platelet plug, resulting in persistent bleeding leading to purpuric petechiae.

Purpura may also be due to non-thrombocytopenic causes in which the platelet count is normal. In this case purpura may be caused by toxic damage to capillaries, may be drug associated (e.g. sulphonamides), or may be the result of direct damage to capillaries or congenitally poor supportive tissues. Henoch-Schönlein purpura and anaphylactoid purpura may occur with immune anomalies. Also, if the platelets are normal in number but abnormal in structure and function, **thrombasthenic** purpura may occur.

Thrombocytopenia may be caused by a variety of disorders. The megakaryocytes in the bone marrow may be involved leading to decreased platelet numbers in the circulation or alternatively the circulating platelets may be destroyed at an excessive rate leading to a drop in the numbers.

Reduced Numbers of Megakaryocytes

This occurs after therapy with marrow-depressive drugs such as cytotoxic agents, gold or chlorpropamide. Ingestion of certain poisons also has the same effect. When the bone marrow is infiltrated by tumours such as carcinomatous metastases or in the acute leukaemias, the megakaryocyte numbers are also decreased leading to thrombocytopenia. Occasionally, the marrow may undergo a spontaneous, idiopathic hypoplasia where all elements are reduced in number.

Inhibition of Megakaryocyte Maturation

Inhibition of megakaryocyte maturation occurs in a variety of bacterial and viral infections and their sequelae, for example typhoid fever, TB, influenza, hepatitis and bacterial septicaemia. The condition also occurs in renal failure and in the megaloblastic anaemias where there is ineffective haemopoiesis.

Excessive Destruction of Circulating Platelets

Drugs, for example quinine, sulphonamides, barbiturates, tolbutamide, ethanol and gold salts, may cause destruction of platelets in the circulation. The drug or one of its metabolites in many cases acts as a hapten by binding to the platelet and in the hypersensitive person this leads to the formation of an antibody to the drug–platelet complex with subsequent destruction of the platelet, leading to thrombocytopenia. This is not a very common occurrence with most drugs, but in a few it can be a frequent complication of the treatment (for example, one person in every 100 treated with gold salts will develop thrombocytopenia). In other cases the drug will cause direct toxic damage to the platelet (e.g. ristocetin). Ethanol taken in large quanti-

ties will not only decrease production of platelets but will also increase the rate of their destruction.

Hypersplenism, in which the spleen is hyperactive and destroys a much greater number of platelets that it normally would, leads to thrombocytopenia.

Immune thrombocytopenia, which is an autoimmune disease, causes a massive drop in the numbers of circulating platelets. Antibodies to platelets are demonstrable in 50% of cases. There are two forms: a juvenile, acute and self-limiting disease, and an adult form, a more chronic and difficult to treat disorder. In the adult this immune thrombocytopenia is often linked to SLE. The antibody reacts with the platelets so that their life span is reduced, with excessive sequestration and destruction of platelets in the spleen.

Certain **infective states** will reduce the number of circulating platelets. It is known, for example, that during the viraemic phase of rubella and influenza, the viruses infect the circulating platelets and destroy them. In glandular fever the number of circulating platelets falls because antibodies to platelets are produced.

In all of these conditions the numbers of megakaryocytes in the bone marrow may be increased in an attempt to compensate for the excessive platelet loss in the circulation. However, it should be remembered that in many cases the bone marrow production of platelets is also affected by the same agent that is causing the thrombocytopenia.

Disseminated Intravascular Coagulation (DIC)

In DIC there is the generalized formation of thrombi in the body, using up much fibrinogen and very large numbers of platelets, which leads to a thrombocytopenia and tendency to bleed. The condition occurs after the release into the bloodstream of various thromboplastic substances in complications of pregnancy such as intrauterine death, amniotic fluid embolism, eclampsia and septic abortion. Various infections may cause the condition (e.g. meningococcaemia), as may severe trauma. Several haematological conditions may be complicated by DIC, especially the leukaemias, incompatible transfusion reactions and paroxysmal nocturnal haemoglobinuria.

Clinically, DIC presents acutely with haemorrhages that are usually severe and follow the various aetiologies of DIC listed above. On the skin, purpura and ecchymoses may be seen and the patient also bleeds from the gums, nose, respiratory tract, gut and urinary tract. Renal failure, hepatic failure and adrenal failure may result in association with massive haemorrhages in these sites. Cerebral infarcts and haemorrhages may be very important in the clinical setting. A PBS will show dramatic decreases in platelet numbers and also, in many patients, the presence of schistocytes.

Treatment of the condition consists of relieving any primary disease that has led to DIC, if this is practicable. Transfusions to reconstitute the blood may be needed and heparin administration will often break the cycle of repeated coagulation, fibrinolysis and haemorrhage. In about half of the cases of DIC the condition is fatal due to the effects of thrombosis or haemorrhage.

Increases in Numbers (Thrombocytosis)

Thrombocytosis implies an increase in the number of circulating platelets. The condition may be subdivided into the primary and secondary forms. The primary form is a neoplastic condition resembling polycythaemia rubra vera and it is usually termed thrombocythaemia. Secondary forms of the disease are usually termed thrombocytoses and they do not involve neoplastic disease of the megakaryocyte. In a number of cases the thrombocytosis or thrombocythaemia is combined with **thrombasthenia**, in which case the platelets are abnormal in function.

Essential Thrombocythaemia (Primary Thrombocytosis)

In this disease there is a sustained rise in platelet numbers, which may be as high as 1×10^7 platelets per μL. The disorder occurs in middle age or in the elderly, males and females being affected equally. There are a variety of abnormalities in the bone marrow of the patients. Megakaryocytes are increased in number and look pleomorphic, being excessively large in size, with some looking malformed and often clumping together in sheets. The other blood-forming elements in the marrow may be undergoing hyperplasia and some patients will show chromosomal defects in some of the marrow cells; in other patients viruses have been demonstrated in the haematopoietic cells with electron microscopy. In the PBS platelets are much larger than normal, have a very granular cytoplasm and are of unusual shapes. Some patients may show a slightly increased number of erythrocytes and an increased number of leukocytes (mainly neutrophilia) in the blood.

The patients present with a history of spontaneous bleeding from the gastrointestinal tract or nose and even small injuries may cause profuse haemorrhage. Thrombosis may occur in some patients and this may cause infarcts. The spleen is enlarged in the first stages of the disease but as the disease progresses the organ shrinks because of thrombosis and infarcts. Extramedullary haemopoiesis may be detected in the spleen and liver.

The disease often goes into spontaneous remissions that may last for months to years, during which time the patient shows no symptoms. The disease does persist for many years and may require treatment at some stage. Platelet numbers are decreased with cytotoxic drug therapy, which is effective in a short course and does not need to be repeated for many years. Splenectomy is not carried out as this may cause an increase of platelet numbers to enormous proportions, with fatal results. Atrophy of the spleen seen in the late stages of the disease may also have the same effect. In the acute emergency situation, treatment is with thrombocytopheresis (removal of platelets from the blood), which relieves the symptoms of the crisis.

Secondary Thrombocytosis

This is a common disease where there is a transient increase in the circulating platelet numbers. It is usually a self-limiting disorder and seldom needs treatment. Platelet numbers generally do not exceed 1×10^6 per μL. Secondary thrombocytosis is seen after injury, haemorrhage or removal of the spleen. It also accompanies some other disruptions in the blood cell numbers, for example neutrophil leukocytosis, polycythaemia rubra vera or multiple myeloma. The platelets are normal in structure and function and their increased numbers increase the risk of thrombosis. This is especially true of patients who are already predisposed to thrombosis, for example cardiac patients.

Hereditary Thrombasthenias

An inherited form of thrombasthenia, also called **Glanzmann's disease**, is inherited as an autosomal recessive trait. The platelet count is normal and the platelets look normal and react with collagen and thrombin as do the normal cells. However, the defect is in their failure to interact with fibrinogen and to aggregate when they are exposed to ADP. The defect resides in the platelet cell membrane. Bleeding time is protracted and clot retraction is impaired. Haemorrhages, purpura and haemorrhagic anaemia are common in these patients. The disease cannot be treated effectively.

Another type of thrombasthenia inherited as an autosomal recessive characteristic is the **Bernard-Soulier syndrome**. The PBS in these patients shows striking giant platelets, often as large as 8 μm in diameter, and slight thrombocytopenia. There is a tendency for severe haemorrhages to occur in homozygotes and mild haemorrhages in heterozygotes. Once again, the platelet cell membrane is abnormal and the platelet cannot bind the von Willebrand factor and fails to attach normally to exposed collagen. The bleeding time is prolonged while clot retraction is normal. This disease is not treated with any degree of success.

Leukocyte Diseases

The Leukopenias

Leukopenia implies a decrease in the numbers of circulating white cells to below 4 000 per μL. Leukopenias may be **primary** due to a decreased production of white cells in the bone marrow or they may be **secondary** due to other diseases. Any or all types of the white cells may be affected and depending on the cell component affected there is a more or less severe disease. Failure of the bone marrow to produce adequate blood cell numbers is due to many causes, the most important of which are summarized below:

- **Marrow aplasia/hypoplasia**: Radiation, drugs and infections, leading to decreased haemopoiesis.
- **Severe anaemia**: Abnormal haemopoiesis.
- **Primary bone tumours, secondary bone tumours and leukaemia/myeloma**: Replace normal tissue, leading to failure of normal haemopoiesis.

Alternatively, the bone marrow may be producing adequate, normal numbers of cells but there may be excessive peripheral destruction or consumption of these cells in the blood and tissues, especially the spleen.

Secondary leukopenia is seen to occur in typhoid fever, influenza and many other viral infections, malaria and in many haematological disorders. Overwhelming infections such as disseminated tuberculosis and advanced septicaemia will also lead to the condition. Bacterial toxins are involved in both depression of the marrow and destruction of leukocytes.

Another important way in which leukocytes are reduced in number is by their excessive destruction by antileukocyte antibodies. In this case drugs are usually involved and in the hypersensitive individual the drug acts as a **hapten**. By itself, and in the normal person, the drug cannot generate an immune response with the formation of antibody against it. In these individuals, however, the drug binds to the white blood cells, forming an antigenic complex stimulating the production of antibody. The resulting antibodies have the capability of destroying or damaging the circulating leukocytes and their mature precursors in the bone marrow. Examples of such drugs are amidopyrine, phenylbutazone and sulphonamides.

When the leukopenia affects only the granular cells in the blood the resulting state is called an **agranulocytosis**. The most numerous granulocyte in the blood is the neutrophil and this is the type of cell that is usually decreased in numbers in agranulocytosis. **Neutrophil agranulocytosis** or **neutropenia** is the term given to the condition. Severe neutropenia has a high mortality, especially when the neutrophil number falls below 500 per μL. There is an increased likelihood of major infection by pathogenic organisms but also of serious infection by organisms that are normally innocuous (opportunistic infections).

Pure eosinophilic agranulocytosis or **eosinopenia** is seen as a response to increased secretion or therapeutic administration of adrenocorticotrophic hormone and adrenal glucocorticoids. It is not associated with severe clinical disease states, but renders the individual more prone to develop parasitic infections. No basophil leukopenia has been characterized.

Lymphopenia is a decrease in the number of circulating lymphocytes which occurs irregularly in various miscellaneous conditions. In infancy it is seen as a feature of some hereditary immunological deficiency syndromes: Bruton-type agammaglobulinaemia (B cell absence); Di-George syndrome (T cell absence); and Swiss-type deficiency (B and T cells absent with virtually no circulating lymphocytes). In these cases the near absence of lymphocytes from blood and lymphoid tissues is associated with fatal deficiencies of the immune system. Lymphopenia of a secondary type occurs as a result of X-irradiation and after the administration of immunosuppressive drugs or in the treatment of neoplasia. AIDS is also another important cause of secondary lymphopenia (immune deficiencies resulting from the primary and secondary lymphopenias have already been covered in Chapter 5).

Myelofibrosis is a rare, idiopathic disease that results in leukopenia as the bone marrow of the patients becomes increasingly fibrotic, leading to increased extramedullary haemopoiesis. About one person in every 50 000 has the disorder and it appears most commonly in elderly Caucasians, men and women being affected equally. As the disease progresses fibrosis occurs in the bone marrow, replacing the blood-forming elements. In about half of the cases of the disease osteosclerosis develops also. Chromosomal abnormalities in the haemopoietic cells are found in about half of the patients and this suggests that the condition may be a neoplastic disorder of the haemopoietic cell precursors. In the PBS, anaemia will be observed with anisocytosis, poikilocytosis and many dacryocytes. The white blood cell count in most patients is increased to levels as high as 50 000 per μL, while in others it is reduced to levels as low as 2000 per μL. The platelet count is firstly increased and then reduced to the level of thrombocytopenia. There is hepatosplenomegaly with haemopoiesis not only active in these tissues but also observable in the lymph nodes, adrenals and kidneys.

The disorder develops insidiously over a number of years and the patient may become aware of symptoms of anaemia, feel discomfort due to the hepatosplenomegaly or occasionally develop gout because of the hyperuricaemia induced by the high turnover of marrow cells. The prognosis for the disorder is rather poor, most patients dying within 5 years of diagnosis, although some long-term survivors are known. Some patients die as a result of infection, others of haemorrhagic complications and in a small proportion of patients leukaemia will develop. Treatment of the disorder is with cytotoxic agents such as busulfan, by splenectomy and by administration of androgens that may increase the erythrocyte numbers in the blood.

Defects of Neutrophil Structure and Function

Chronic Granulomatous Disease of Childhood

Chronic granulomatous disease of childhood is a disease affecting both neutrophils and macrophages, these phagocytes being unable to destroy phagocytosed bacteria. It is usually inherited as an X-linked genetic disorder, more rarely as an autosomal recessive character. Most patients are boys who have no normal phagocytes. Girls who are heterozygous for the X-linked trait have two populations of phagocytes, one normal and one abnormal. Generally girls tend to show little evidence of disease, whereas boys are severely affected by infections caused by catalase-positive organisms such as staphylococci, *Candida*, and Gram-negative organisms. The defect in the phagocytic cells is in the mitochondria and also in

the production of hydrogen peroxide and superoxide in the phagosomes.

Patients with the disease begin to develop serious infections in infancy, most commonly recurrent respiratory system infections, abscesses in the liver, spleen and lungs, enteric infections, suppurative lymphadenitis, osteomyelitis and skin infections. Although normal acute inflammation is seen in the infected tissue, with numerous normal-looking neutrophils and macrophages present, these cells are unable to destroy phagocytosed bacteria, which continue to multiply intracytoplasmically. As the infection in the tissue persists, the inflammation becomes chronic and severe fibrosis occurs.

Treatment of the disease is difficult and prevention of infection is one of the goals. If infections do occur, antibiotic treatment is given; however, often the bacteria are not destroyed by the chemotherapeutics administered as they are protected within cells. Rifampin may be taken and is more effective than other drugs as it may kill bacteria intracytoplasmically. The prognosis for the patients depends very much on how severely they are affected by the disease. Girls who are heterozygous for the X-linked trait live a normal life while boys with the X-linked trait (being homozygous for the gene) suffer from a severe form of the disease and usually die in childhood. In some patients with the autosomal disease there are long remissions that may last for several years.

Chediak-Higashi Syndrome

The Chediak-Higashi syndrome is a genetic disorder transmitted as an autosomal recessive trait. The neutrophils are affected and they contain in their cytoplasm only a few, abnormal, enlarged lysosomes (refer to Figure 17.19). Similar large lysosomes may be found in a few of the other granulocytes and macrophages. The babies born with this disorder have an associated disorder of pigmentation and are silver haired, pale skinned and have hypopigmented retinas. The blood contains only about half the normal numbers of neutrophils. There are several abnormalities in the patients' neutrophils: microtubules in the cells are abnormal, causing impaired chemotaxis; the lysosomes do not fuse with the phagosomes containing the ingested bacteria, thus the organisms are not killed; and the lysosomes do not contain adequate amounts of myeloperoxidase and are grossly deficient in elastase, both of these enzymes being important in the destruction of intracellular microbes.

The children affected develop serious infections repeatedly. Staphyloccocal infections of the respiratory tract, skin and internal organs are particularly troublesome. Even if the child survives the infections, anaemia, thrombocytopenia and lymphoma develop, all of which tend to make the condition one with a poor prognosis, most affected children dying very young.

Lazy Leukocyte Syndrome

The lazy leukocyte syndrome describes a disorder in which there is a poorly defined defect in the motility of leukocytes, the bactericidal ability of the neutrophils also being impaired in some cases of the disease. The defect leads to poor chemotaxis and failure of the cells to localize in the sites where they are needed. Hence, bacteria and other microbes which in the normal individual would cause trivial or undetected infections will in patients with the disorder cause life threatening infections as the organisms proliferate unchecked.

Pelger-Huët Abnormality

This is a condition inherited as an autosomal dominant trait and it affects about one in 5000 people. It causes an abnormality in the structure of the neutrophil nuclei, but function of the cell is unimpaired. In heterozygotes over 60% of neutrophils observed in a PBS have a bilobed or oval nucleus instead of the three- to five-lobed nucleus that normal cells have. In homozygotes all neutrophils have the abnormal nuclear morphology, most of the cells having an oval nucleus. It should be stressed that these cells function normally.

Myeloperoxidase Deficiency

This is a genetic disorder transmitted as an autosomal recessive character in which there is a lack of the bactericidal myeloperoxidase in neutrophils. The individuals affected respond normally to infection, since the neutrophils will produce an excess of hydrogen peroxide that compensates for the lack of the enzyme.

Miscellaneous Neutrophil Abnormalities

Job's syndrome is a disorder in neutrophil chemotaxis, especially in response to *Staphylococcus* spp. As a consequence, the affected people develop, like the biblical Job, large numbers of staphylococcal abscesses in

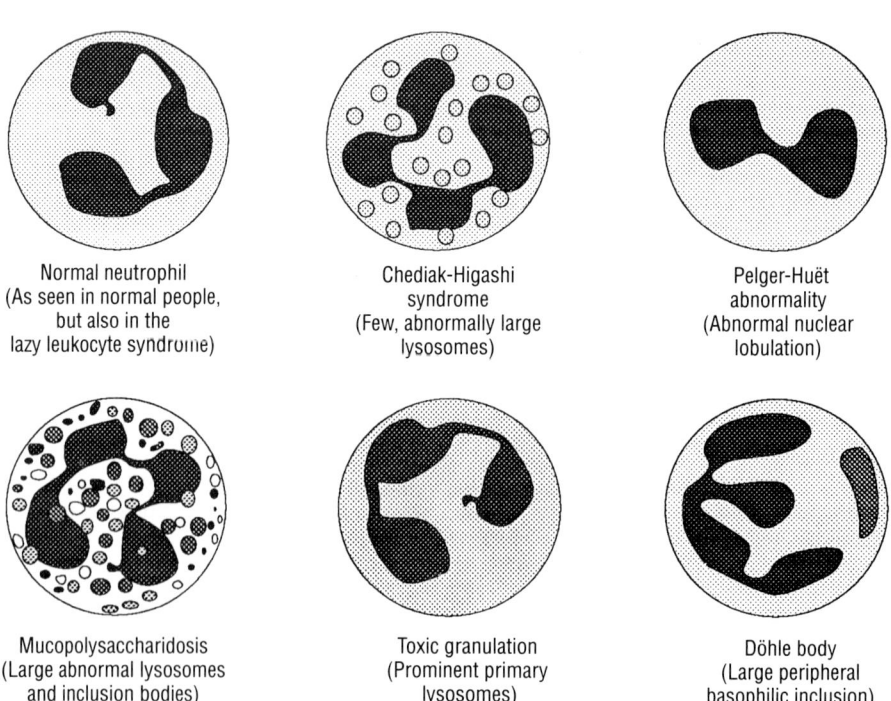

Normal neutrophil
(As seen in normal people,
but also in the
lazy leukocyte syndrome)

Chediak-Higashi
syndrome
(Few, abnormally large
lysosomes)

Pelger-Huët
abnormality
(Abnormal nuclear
lobulation)

Mucopolysaccharidosis
(Large abnormal lysosomes
and inclusion bodies)

Toxic granulation
(Prominent primary
lysosomes)

Döhle body
(Large peripheral
basophilic inclusion)

Figure 17.19   *Abnormalities in neutrophil morphology and function*

many organs of their body with carbuncles and furuncles on the skin. The IgE concentration in the blood is also raised.

Changes in neutrophil appearance may occur with a variety of infective and benign states. For example, **Döhle bodies**, which are peripheral, bright-blue-staining inclusions in neutrophils consisting of aggregates of granular endoplasmic reticulum and ribosomes, appear in benign reactive processes. **Toxic granules**, staining a dark purplish blue, may appear in the cytoplasm of neutrophils and consist of primary lysosomes that are deficient in alkaline phosphatase. Such cells appear in the blood of people with severe burns and infections. In **mucopolysaccharidosis** large inclusions are seen in the cytoplasm of neutrophils (see Figure 17.19).

The Leukocytoses

The characteristic feature of the leukocytoses is that there are increased numbers of leukocytes in the bloodstream, these leukocytes showing normal structure and function. Any white cell in the blood may be affected and the corresponding increase is given the suffix '-philia' or '-cytosis', implying increased numbers but normal function. The commonest of these states is associated with the neutrophils and is known as **neutrophilia**.

Neutrophilia (Neutrophil Leukocytosis)

Neutrophilia is the commonest type of leukocytosis and the number of neutrophils in the blood may increase, to anything from 20 000 per µL to 40 000 per µL. The PBS in these patients shows what the haematologist calls a '**shift to the left**', meaning that many immature neutrophils (**myelocytes** and **metamyelocytes**) are seen in the blood smear. These immature forms have been recruited from the bone marrow as there is an increased demand and an increased consumption of these cells in the tissues. The immature forms are still able to function as phagocytic cells.

There are no symptoms and signs associated with neutrophilia *per se* but rather the patient presents with the symptomatology of the primary disease that has caused the neutrophilia. Rises in neutrophil numbers are seen in bacterial infections with the pyogenic bacteria. A boil or acute appendicitis may induce a rise of 10 000 neutrophils per µL. A large abscess, pneumonia or peritonitis may give the higher numbers. Moderate rises in neutrophil numbers accompany tissue necrosis without infection such as myocardial infarction, burns or crush injuries. In some cases strenuous exercise, labour and haemorrhage will induce neutrophilia.

Increased production of neutrophils in such circumstances is a controlled response to a stimulus and may be regarded as a physiological reaction by the myelopoietic tissue. It is an example of a physiological hyperplasia in response to increased demand for these cells by the tissues in the face of infection or tissue necrosis. There is also a rare, primary hereditary form of neutrophilia which is present in association with splenomegaly. Neutrophil numbers as high as 40 000 per µL are present and the condition often persists for many years. Affected individuals are otherwise well.

Eosinophilia (Eosinophil Leukocytosis)

Several conditions give rise to increased numbers of eosinophils in tissues and in the blood. Eosinophilia occurs when the eosinophils reach numbers greater than 3000 per µL. The following may lead to eosinophilia:

- **Parasitic infestations** with many kinds of worms (e.g. *Trichinella*, ankylostomes schistosomes). Eosinophils are thought to be important in destroying these organisms.
- **Hypersensitivity reactions** such as hay fever, asthma, angio-oedema. It is thought that the eosinophils antagonize the effects of histamine in these situations.
- **Chronic skin diseases**, for example dermatitis, psoriasis, eczema, pemphigus and urticaria. The function of the eosinophil in such disorders is not known.
- **Malignant tumours** are often accompanied by an eosinophilia (e.g. Hodgkin's disease).
- **Primary hereditary eosinophilia**, which is an autosomal dominant disorder in which there are persistent increased numbers of eosinophils in the blood.

Basophilia (Basophil Leukocytosis)

Sometimes in chronic myeloid leukaemia or myxoedema there are accompanying rises in basophil numbers in the bloodstream. Occasionally in severe type I hypersensitivity reactions basophilia is observed. Otherwise, no conditions are known which regularly induce basophil leukocytosis.

Lymphocytosis (Lymphocyte Leukocytosis)

The lymphocyte count is normally higher in children

than adults. The number is higher just after birth, reaching numbers of 6000 per μL and then gradually falls to the adult levels of about 3000 per μL. In true lymphocytosis, there may be an increase of up to 100 000 lymphocytes per μL. Lymphocytosis usually accompanies specific infective fevers, for example whooping cough, typhoid fever, brucellosis, secondary syphilis, influenza, measles, mumps, rubella and other viral infections. Often what in an adult will induce neutrophilia will in the infant induce lymphocytosis.

Monocytosis

This is commonly seen in subacute bacterial endocarditis, undulant fever, TB, syphilis, sarcoidosis, regional enteritis and sometimes SLE. There may also be an increase of monocytes in typhus and other rickettsial infections. In malaria, increased numbers of monocytes are a striking feature with monocytes in numbers of 3000 per μL to 4000 per μL seen in such cases.

The Leukaemias

The leukaemias are conditions resulting from the **neoplastic proliferation of leukocytes**. In the more common varieties either lymphoid or myelogenous cells are involved. When the proliferation involves the immature, precursor cells, the disease is recognized as an **acute leukaemia** and tends to run a rapid course (the disease is also given the suffix '-blastic' leukaemia). In the more slowly progressive states, predominantly more mature cells have undergone the neoplastic transformation and are present in excess. These are the **chronic leukaemias** (given the suffix '-cytic' leukaemias). The age incidence of the leukaemias varies greatly, with the acute leukaemias generally having a high incidence is childhood (mainly the lymphoblastic type) and another peak in 40–60-year-old subjects (mainly myeloblastic). Chronic leukaemias are more common in the older age groups (refer to Figures 17.20 and 17.21).

In general the following predisposing factors are related to the development of the leukaemias:

- association with **congenital disorders** such as Down's syndrome;
- **chromosome abnormalities** such as the Philadelphia chromosome (see below);
- exposure to **ionizing radiation** (e.g. X-rays, nuclear fission products);
- **chemicals and drugs** (e.g. benzene, cytotoxic drugs);
- **virus infections** (e.g. HTLV I virus);
- **immune deficiencies**, as occurs in HIV infection or congenital immunodeficiencies;

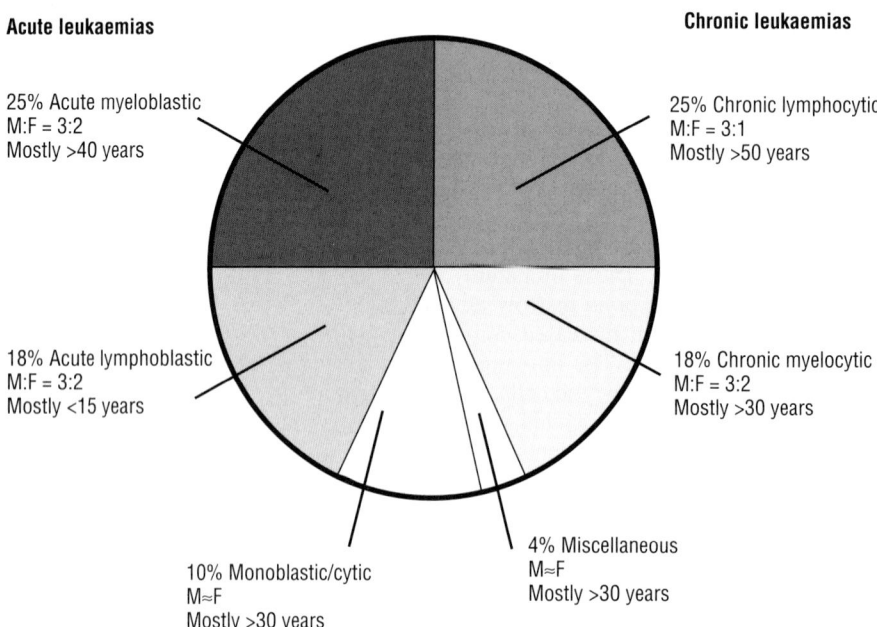

Acute leukaemias

25% Acute myeloblastic
M:F = 3:2
Mostly >40 years

18% Acute lymphoblastic
M:F = 3:2
Mostly <15 years

10% Monoblastic/cytic
M≈F
Mostly >30 years

Chronic leukaemias

25% Chronic lymphocytic
M:F = 3:1
Mostly >50 years

18% Chronic myelocytic
M:F = 3:2
Mostly >30 years

4% Miscellaneous
M≈F
Mostly >30 years

Figure 17.20 *The incidence of the various types of leukaemia*

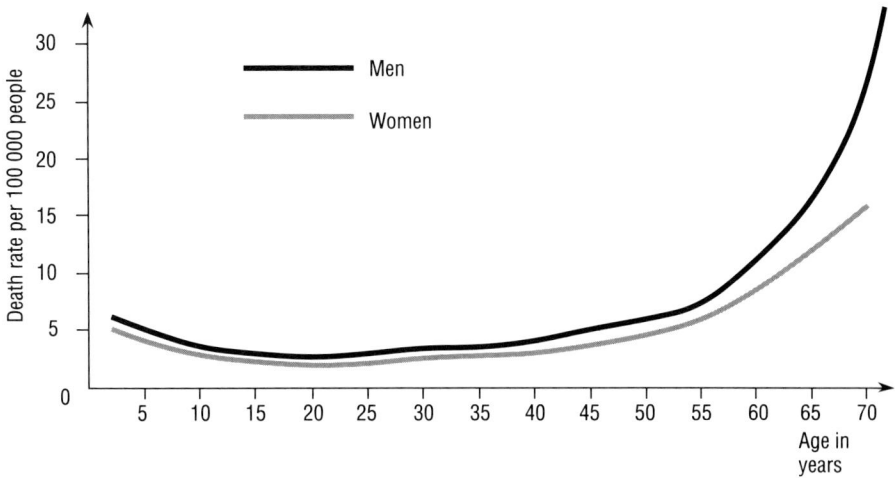

Figure 17.21 *The age and sex incidence of the leukaemias*

- **other disease states**, especially those involving the marrow, may be complicated by leukaemia (e.g. primary aplastic anaemia, polycythaemia rubra vera, paroxysmal nocturnal haemoglobinuria and myelofibrosis).

It should be noted, however, that many types of leukaemia are idiopathic and in many patients none of the aetiological factors above may be demonstrated.

In all forms of leukaemia the abnormal proliferating cells involve the bone marrow. Normal haemopoiesis is disorganized and therefore these conditions sooner or later produce:

- **anaemia** (with all of its attendant symptomatology);
- **neutropenia, lymphopenia** (leading to severe infections);
- **thrombocytopenia** (leading to haemorrhages); and
- **total failure of bone marrow** function in the later stages.

Acute Leukaemias

Acute Myeloblastic Leukaemia (Acute Myeloid Leukaemia, AML)

AML is a disease that causes one death per 100 000 of the population. The disease affects males more commonly than females (M:F = 3:2), and although a person struck with the disease may be of any age, most patients are over 40 years old. The proliferating cells in this type of leukaemia are the myeloblasts and the neoplastic cells may be derived from different stages of the development of these cells. The French–American–British (FAB) classification of leukaemias subdivides this type of leukaemia into four types, M1 to M4, but there are also three types of closely related leukaemias, M5 to M7 (see Table 17.3). It is often difficult to distinguish in a PBS between some of the different types of acute myeloid, acute monocytic leukaemia and erythroleukaemia, and some haematologists group all of these types of leukaemia into the 'acute, non-lymphoblastic leukaemia'.

The peripheral blood shows moderate increases in the white cell count, 20 000 to 50 000 leukocytes per μL being observed in about a quarter of patients. In about half of the cases of AML, the total white cell count is normal or even reduced and the clinical presentation is that of an acute marrow failure. These are the so-called **aleukaemic leukaemias**. Most of the circulating leukocytes are primitive-looking cells with large nuclei and nucleoli and little cytoplasm, resembling the myeloblasts of the bone marrow. In about a third of cases the myeloblasts have more than one nucleolus and show in their cytoplasm crystalline structures known as **Auer rods**. In bone marrow aspirates a marked increase in cellularity is usual and primitive leukoblasts constitute the majority of the cells present, the malignant cells replacing the fat spaces and extending into the shafts of the long bones. When the patients first present they are usually anaemic, with haemoglobin values around 5 g/dL. Thrombocytopenia is also present in most patients. Atypical erythrocytes, reticulocytes, erythroblasts and abnormal platelets are often noted in the PBS. 'Smudge' cells are disrupted,

Table 17.3 *The FAB classification of the acute non-lymphoblastic leukaemias*

FAB type of leukaemia	Morphological type	Common chromosomal anomalies
M1 (25% of cases of AML)	Undifferentiated leukaemia	Often trisomies are present (e.g. trisomy 7 or 8)
M2 (35% of cases of AML)	Differentiated myeloblastic leukaemia	Transposition between chromosomes 8 and 21
M3 (5% of cases of AML)	Promyelocytic leukaemia	Transposition between chromosomes 15 and 17
M4 (35% of cases of AML)	Myelomonocytic leukaemia	Pericentric inversion of chromosome 16
M5	Monocytic leukaemia	Transposition between chromosomes 9 and 11
M6	Erythroleukaemia (Di Guglielmo's disease)	Variable
M7	Megakaryocytic leukaemia (haemorrhagic thrombocythaemia)	Variable

fragile neoplastic cells that have been damaged during the preparation of the PBS.

In most young patients with AML the disease appears abruptly with fever, weakness, pallor, bleeding in the gums and petechial haemorrhages in the skin. In older people the disease may be more insidious but has similar clinical features (see Table 17.4). If untreated, the disease runs a very rapid course with death occurring in a few weeks or months; almost no patients live for a year.

In about half of the patients with AML, the spleen and liver are enlarged due to the accumulation of the malignant cells in the sinusoids. The same infiltration will be seen in the lymph nodes (causing lymphadenomegaly) and kidneys. The kidneys may be so infiltrated with the leukaemic cells that they double in weight and assume a creamy colour. Although renal function is not interfered with in most cases, some patients may develop the nephrotic syndrome. The skin may show purplish patches due to infiltration with neoplastic cells and in some patients other organs may also be affected. The sternum is tender in about 70% of patients because of the extensive marrow activity and hyperplasia. In children, the long bones will be tender and painful for the same reason.

Treatment of AML is essential for preserving patients' lives and also improving their quality of life.

Spontaneous remissions occur in a small proportion of patients and are short lived, the disease quickly re-establishing itself. Cytotoxic drugs such as vincristine, 6-mercaptopurine and cytarabine used in various combinations together with prednisone will be effective in about 50% of cases, causing a remission. The symptoms disappear and the PBS shows no leukoblastic cells. The 3-year survival with such treatments is rarely better than 10%. Only a handful of patients are cured with this drug therapy. The best chance for a cure is with bone marrow transplants after cytotoxic drug therapy. The proportion of patients alive after 2 years of such treatment is 50% and they may be cured. Most patients die as a result of infections and haemorrhages. The best prognosis is with leukaemias where the cells show a transposition between chromosomes 8 and 21 (i.e. FAB type M2), the worse in those with abnormalities of chromosome 5 (seen in any of the FAB types).

Erythroleukaemia (also termed **Di Guglielmo's disease**) is a rare disease in which malignant leukocytes coexist with neoplastic erythroblasts in the circulation. **Erythraemic myelosis** is used to name the disease if the erythroblast-like cells predominate in the circulating blood. These disorders resemble acute myeloblastic leukaemia in their behaviour, although uncommonly there are corresponding chronic forms that are more

Table 17.4 *Symptoms and signs associated with the acute leukaemias*

Frequency/nature	Symptoms	Signs
Common, non-specific	Fatigue, malaise, fever, loss of weight	Anaemia, fever, loss of weight
Less common and suggestive	Infection, recurrent skin, gum and uterine haemorrhages, splenic, sternal and periarticular pain	Ulcerative pharyngitis, gum hypertrophy, purpura, bruises, retinal haemorrhage, hepatosplenomegaly, sternal tenderness, lymphadenopathy

Table 17.5 *Types of acute lymphoblastic leukaemia*

Type	Marker on cell	FAB type	Age incidence
T cell leukaemia	T cell marker	—	10% of adults 15% of children
'Common' leukaemia	Common antigen	L1	15% of adults 75% of children
Unclassified leukaemia	None	L2	70% of adults 5% of children
B cell leukaemia	B cell marker	L3	5% of adults 5% of children

like chronic myelocytic leukaemia in presentation. The bone marrow in erythroleukaemia is infiltrated with malignant myeloblasts and erythroblasts. The malignant erythroblasts are demonstrated by the PAS stain (malignant erythroblasts are positive while the normal erythroblasts are negative).

Acute Lymphoblastic Leukaemia (ALL)

Acute lymphoblastic leukaemia is predominantly a disease of children, most cases occurring below the age of 15 years. About five children per 100 000 develop the disease per year compared with one adult per 100 000 per year. The leukaemia is more common in males than females and occurs in the ratio of 3:2. The neoplastic cells that are proliferating in ALL are lymphoblasts and depending on the surface markers on the cell membrane ALL may be subclassified into four types (refer to Table 17.5).

In about 60% of patients with ALL the PBS shows a dramatic increase in the number of circulating leukocytes, most of which are the neoplastic lymphoblasts. The white cell count ranges between 10 000 and 120 000 cells per μL, the neutrophils being greatly reduced in number, usually below 1000 per μL. Thrombocytopenia and anaemia are almost invariably present and the haemoglobin count is 8 g/dL or less. Hyperuricaemia is also present in many patients, the proportion of patients with high uric acid levels in their blood increasing after treatment. The cells in the blood and bone marrow resemble lymphoblasts but, depending on the subtype of ALL, there will be subtle variations in nuclear morphology, amount of cytoplasm and staining characteristics of the malignant cells. Generally, in all types the cells are large, with large nuclei and prominent nucleoli and a scanty, basophilic cytoplasm (except cells of ALL of FAB type L3, which have abundant cytoplasm).

Clinically, ALL presents rather similarly to acute myeloblastic leukaemia (see Table 17.4). Most children with the disease complain of fatigue and pains in the bones and joints. Fever and loss of weight are common. In some cases a mass may be palpated by the child's parents, this being an enlarged lymph node, liver or spleen (see Table 17.6). If the condition is left untreated infections and haemorrhages are life threat-

Table 17.6 *Clinicopathological features of the acute leukaemias*

Feature	Acute myeloblastic leukaemia	Acute lymphoblastic leukaemia
Splenomegaly	86% of cases	60% of cases
Hepatomegaly	74% of cases	54% of cases
Lymphadenomegaly	76% of cases	47% of cases

ening complications, usually causing death of the patient within a year of diagnosis. Leukaemic cell infiltration is seen in many organs, especially the kidneys, central nervous system, heart, testes and ovaries. Haemorrhages and infections become uncontrollable.

Treatment of this type of leukaemia is by combination chemotherapy as has been described already for acute myeloblastic leukaemia. In addition, irradiation of the brain may be necessary to control the neoplastic cell infiltrates. Children who undergo such treatments show complete remission within a few weeks and with maintenance chemotherapy the 5-year survival is 60% or better. Many of these children remain in remission after treatment stops and may be said to be cured. The prognosis tends to be better with the common or unclassified types of ALL. The higher the leukocyte count the worse the prognosis. Boys tend to have a worse prognosis than girls (recurrence of the leukaemia in the testes is common). T cell and B cell leukaemias have a poorer prognosis and the presence of a mediastinal mass indicates a T cell leukaemia and is an ominous sign. Maintenance therapy consists of administration of lower doses of drugs such as 6-mercaptopurine and methotrexate for 3 years or more. The longer the remission achieved, the less likely is the recurrence of the disease. About 20% of people on maintenance therapy have a recurrence of the disease and this is a bad sign as the disease cannot be controlled in such cases. Bone marrow transplantation has brought permanent remissions in some patients.

Complications that are seen during treatment are **temporary alopecia** (baldness, because of irradiation of the brain), **hyperuricaemia** and **hyperkalaemia** (because of breakdown of neoplastic cells; the patient may be prescribed allopurinol and given more fluids), **fever** (because of release of endogenous pyrogens or associated infection) and **temporary somnolence**. In some cases leukoencephalopathy develops, the brain being injured severely and brain damage causing neurological problems. A variety of viral, fungal and protozoal micro-organisms may cause life threatening **infections** in patients under treatment (immunosuppression due to the drugs).

Monoblastic Leukaemia (ML)

Monoblastic leukaemia (often referred to as a 'monocytic' or 'myelomonocytic' leukaemia) is relatively uncommon, typically being seen in adults over the age of 30 years, and may run an acute or subacute course. This leukaemia is of FAB type M5 and some haematologists consider it to be a subtype of acute myeloblastic leukaemia. In the PBS various mixtures of malignant monoblasts and myeloblasts will be seen, the leukocyte count on average being around 20 000 cells per µL, but may reach 250 000 leukocytes per µL in some patients. The circulating monoblasts are large and irregular in outline, with large, uneven, nuclei. If most of the circulating cells are monoblasts or monocytes, the leukaemia is the so-called **Schilling type** of ML. In addition, there is the **Naegeli type** in which the proliferating cells are a mixture of monoblasts and myeloid cells. Presumably, in the latter case the neoplastic cells retain the ability to differentiate into either type of cell line.

Patients with ML present with anaemia, fever associated with infections, and thrombocytopenic purpura. It is commoner in these patients to see leukaemic infiltration of various organs including lymph nodes, gums and skin than it is with acute myeloblastic leukaemias. There is pronounced hepatomegaly and moderate splenomegaly, the patient often feverish and complaining of lassitude and malaise.

Treatment of ML is by chemotherapy with 6-mercaptopurine, vincristine and methotrexate, but remissions are more difficult to induce than with the other types of acute leukaemia. Antibiotics are administered for the infections that develop and steroids may help in the control of haemorrhages. In some cases spontaneous remissions that last for a few months may be observed. The disease generally has a poor prognosis.

Chronic Leukaemias

Chronic Myelocytic Leukaemia (Chronic Myeloid Leukaemia, CML)

This type of leukaemia can occur in any age group but more commonly affects the middle aged and elderly, the disease seen more commonly in men in the ratio of 3:2. About two persons per 100 000 per year are affected by this disorder. CML is characterized by a very large number of circulating leukocytes which is usually around 300 000 cells per μL, but may reach levels of 1 000 000 cells per μL. Most of these cells are well-differentiated neutrophil-like cells, although about 30% of the cells are metamyelocytes and myelocytes. A small number of myeloblasts are also found. The haemoglobin content of the blood is around 9 g/dL and the erythrocytes show anisocytosis and reticulocytosis. Usually platelet numbers are increased to levels of more than 1 000 000 per μL, although as the disease progresses, thrombocytopenia supervenes. In the bone marrow there is a predominance of the myelogenous precursors, but erythropoiesis continues normally. In about 95% of cases of this type of leukaemia, the neoplastic marrow cells show the acquired chromosomal abnormality known as the **Philadelphia chromosome**. This is a reciprocal translocation, where the long arm of chromosome 9 is exchanged with the long arm of chromosome 22. The abnormal chromosome 22 is termed the Philadelphia chromosome because it was first described in that city. The breaks in the chromosomes and translocations involve abnormalities in the control of the proto-oncogenes c-sis and c-abl which are thought to bring about the neoplastic transformation.

In about a fifth of patients, CML is diagnosed as a consequence of a haematological examination that is performed routinely in the course of a medical check-up. In the other cases the patient presents with an insidious disease, eventually bringing about loss of weight, fever or fatigue. The person may have experienced night sweats and loss of appetite, or may have noticed abdominal distension due to a splenomegaly. Pain in the left hypochondrium may occur acutely in association with thrombotic episodes in the spleen or may be due to perisplenitis. Tenderness of the sternum may be elicited by pressure, but other bone tenderness or pain is rare.

In this type of leukaemia there is marked organ involvement, particularly of the liver and spleen, both of which can become grossly enlarged due to the infiltration of very large numbers of the neoplastic leukocytes which reach these organs via the bloodstream. The spleen may weigh anything between 1 to 3 kg. Other organs such as the kidney may show marked infiltration with abnormal cells. This infiltration may be regarded as a form of metastasis as the primary site of the tumours is the bone marrow and the secondary deposits after blood spread are seen to occur in the distant sites of the liver, spleen and kidney.

Treatment of CML is mainly through the use of cytotoxic drugs, especially busulphan. This treatment controls the symptoms but does not destroy the clone of neoplastic cells in the marrow and recurrences of the disease occur regularly. Most of the patients with treated CML survive for a period of 3 to 4 years. In a small number of cases survival is for a period of 15 to 20 years. Most patients with CML suffer from acute attacks named 'blast crises'. This occurs when the myelocyte and myeloblast numbers increase suddenly in the PBS. This change is often indicative of transformation of the chronic leukaemia to an acute terminal phase, an event called a **myeloblastic transformation**, which generally heralds the rapid demise of the afflicted person within a period of weeks to months. Death usually results from complications of haemorrhage, thrombosis or because of massive infection. A small number of long-term survivors and cures have been reported after bone marrow transplantation.

Other Types of Chronic Myelocytic Leukaemia

Although **chronic monocytic leukaemia** exists it is very rare. It is generally classified as a subtype of chronic myelocytic leukaemia. Most of the circulating neoplastic cells resemble normal monocytes, but there is also a smaller component of neutrophilic cells. The neoplasm is thought to arise in the myelomonocytic cell precursor which then differentiates into the two cell types seen in the PBS of patients with this disorder. The symptoms and signs are similar to those encountered in chronic myelocytic leukaemia.

Eosinophilic leukaemia is another uncommon variant of chronic myelocytic leukaemia in which the neoplastic cells are mostly eosinophils. Acute forms of this leukaemia are also known but are very rare. In the chronic form 'blast crises' may occur as in chronic myelocytic leukaemia. **Basophilic leukaemia** resembles eosinophilic leukaemia, except that the circulating neoplastic cells are basophils. It is a very rare disorder in both the acute and chronic form.

Chronic Lymphocytic Leukaemia (Chronic Lymphoid Leukaemia, CLL)

CLL is a disease of middle to old age, being very rare before the age of 35 years. It affect males more than females in the ratio of 7:3, with about three people per 100 000 being affected per year. This type of leukaemia is rare in Japan and China. The characteristic feature of the disorder is a marked increase in the peripheral lymphocyte count to around 100 000 cells per μL. In untreated cases the lymphocyte number increases gradually over the years to levels around 1 000 000 cells per μL. Although most of the neoplastic cells are well-differentiated small lymphocytes, some of the leukaemic cells are larger, more primitive looking, with cytoplasmic inclusions of IgM. In about 99% of cases of CLL the neoplastic lymphocytes are B cells, the remainder of cases being of the T cell type. Monoclonal IgM hypergammaglobulinaemia only occurs in about 5% of cases of the disease, and most cases show a hypogammaglobulinaemia. There may be mild anaemia, neutropenia and thrombocytopenia, the decreases in numbers of circulating erythrocytes, neutrophils and platelets becoming more marked as the disease progresses.

The disease originates in the haemopoietic marrow with subsequent involvement of the blood, lymphoid tissues and, later, the liver. In some patients, chromosomal abnormalities may be demonstrated in the leukaemic cells, including trisomy 12 and translocations involving chromosomes 11 and 14. There is a marked, generalized enlargement of lymph nodes and spleen which is quite conspicuous. The enlarged spleen and nodes may impinge on important structures such as the bile duct. The affected lymph nodes show on biopsy a diffuse involvement and replacement of normal cells by the neoplastic lymphocytes. Other organs may be infiltrated but not to the extent seen in myeloid leukaemia. Occasionally, a diffuse infiltration of the skin by neoplastic cells causes the patient to present with a reddened and thickened skin, a condition called *l'homme rouge* ('the red man').

CLL may cause little disability or symptoms for several years and in about a quarter of cases the disease is diagnosed incidentally during the course of other investigations because of the abnormally high lymphocyte count in a PBS or because of enlarged lymph nodes. The remainder of patients present because of weight loss, fatigue, malaise or because they have become aware of enlarged lymph nodes. Some patients present because of infections.

Treatment of the disease is by radiotherapy of the enlarged lymphoid tissues and chemotherapy with chlorambucil. Adjunctive treatment with steroids may also be administered, especially when anaemia and thrombocytopenia are a problem. Death of the patients usually results from anaemia and bacterial infections (especially bronchopneumonia). Viral and fungal infections are also problematic. In many elderly patients with CLL death occurs owing to unrelated disorders such as myocardial infarction, stroke or carcinomata. Most patients with the disease survive for about 5 years after diagnosis.

Chronic Lymphocytic Leukaemia Variants

A small number of cases of CLL (less than 5%) will be the so-called **hairy cell leukaemia**. The neoplastic cells in this subtype are characterized by numerous cytoplasmic projections from the periphery of the cell, best seen under the electron microscope. Many patients with this disorder are leukopenic, anaemic and thrombocytopenic when diagnosed. The spleen is grossly enlarged and the bone marrow shows massive infiltration by the neoplastic cells, or in some cases has a similar appearance to myelofibrosis. Treatment with recombinant α interferon brings about remission in most cases, and the 8-year survival is about 50%.

Prolymphocytic leukaemia is another very rare variant of CLL. The circulating lymphocyte numbers are grossly increased, most of these cells being large and resembling prolymphocytes. The spleen and liver are grossly enlarged while infiltration of lymph nodes is absent or not marked. This is a variant with a very poor prognosis, chemotherapy being almost useless in its treatment. Most patients die within a year of diagnosis.

Leukaemoid Reactions

The leukaemoid reactions are conditions that may mimic the leukaemias through the appearance of large numbers of white blood cells in the circulation. Two types are known, the myeloid and lymphoid leukaemoid reactions, the names indicating the types of cells affected. Often the total leukocyte count in these disorders is as high as 40 000 per μL. The leukaemoid states are thought to be reactive hyperplasias that are seen in the bone marrow in response to some other disease process or state that is occurring in the body concurrently. The leukaemoid reactions are different from the leukocytoses in that the cells are considerably more primitive in appearance. The causes of these reactions are summarized in Table 17.7.

Table 17.7   *States associated with the leukaemoid reactions*

Myeloid leukaemoid reaction	Lymphoid leukaemoid reaction
Bacterial infections (e.g. pyelonephritis, TB)	Infections (e.g. whooping cough, mumps)
Anaemias (e.g. leukoerythroblastic, haemolytic)	Infectious mononucleosis
Autoimmune disease (e.g. polyarteritis nodosa)	Some cases of carcinoma (e.g. colonic)

Malignant Lymphomata (Lymphosarcomata)

The malignant lymphomata are all neoplastic proliferations of the peripheral lymphoid tissue, the primary site of origin usually being the lymph nodes, occasionally the spleen, thymus, Peyer's patches or lymphoid tissue in other organs. The cells undergoing neoplastic transformation are most commonly the lymphocytes and less commonly the macrophages present in these sites. In some cases, although the cell may be demonstrated to be lymphoblastic, the precise stage in the differentiation ladder may not be able to be determined. Systemic spread outside the primary sites usually occurs later in the course of these disorders. Two major groups of lymphomata are known, the **Hodgkin's disease group** and the **non-Hodgkin's group**. Further subdivisions within the groups have been effected by various international medical organizations and specialist committees. There is a degree of overlap between the lymphoid leukaemias and the non-Hodgkin's lymphomata, especially in the poorly differentiated members of both groups.

Hodgkin's Disease (HD)

This is the most common form of malignant lymphoma arising in the lymphoreticular tissues, accounting for 40% of all types of lymphomata. Approximately four people in every 100 000 develop HD per year, the disorder being commoner in males in the ratio of 3:2. Although HD may occur at any age two peaks exist, one in early adult life (20–35 years, being the commonest presentation) and the second in the older age groups (over 50 years). The aetiology of HD is idiopathic although there are various suggestions as to links with viral infection (the Epstein-Barr virus and a putative virus similar to the murine leukaemia virus have been suggested) and genetic/familial causes. Hodgkin's disease is classified into four histological types, as is shown in Table 17.8.

Progressive and painless enlargement of lymph nodes is the commonest early feature of the disease, constitutional symptoms not seen until the later stages of the disease. The supraclavicular lymph nodes are very commonly affected, the left side of the neck being slightly more often involved than the right side. Cervical, abdominal and mediastinal lymph nodes show primary involvement in some patients, while the disease rarely starts in the spleen, thymus or other lymphoid organs. If the disease is untreated, it tends to spread from one group of lymph nodes to the next, eventually occurring in many lymphoid organs throughout the body. The nodular sclerotic type of HD differs from the other types in that it arises in the mediastinal and supraclavicular nodes and tends to remain confined to these situations. If patients complain of fever, it is rarely above 38°C, and it tends to occur with

Table 17.8   *Histological types of Hodgkin's disease*

Type	Proportion	Behaviour
Lymphocyte predominant	15% of cases	Slow growth (years), best prognosis
Nodular sclerosing	40% of cases	Slow growth (years–months), good prognosis
Mixed cellularity	30% of cases	Progressive growth (months), poorer prognosis
Lymphocyte depleted	15% of cases	Rapid growth (months–weeks), worst prognosis

weight loss and night sweats. Pruritus may be present and about a fifth of patients complain of painful affected nodes after they consume alcohol. Other symptoms include respiratory distress or a cough, jaundice or abdominal pain.

The microscopic feature, common to all types of HD and on the basis of which diagnosis is made, is the **Reed-Sternberg** giant cell (refer to Figures 17.22 and 17.23). This is present in the affected lymphoid tissues in varying numbers and is a large cell, 40 µm in diameter, with a double nucleus and prominent nucleoli ('owl-eyed cell'). Various pleomorphic variants of the Reed-Sternberg cell may be seen also. The various histological types of HD have differing cell populations and characteristic features:

- The **lymphocyte predominant** type contains many small lymphocytes that involve the lymphoid tissue diffusely. The classic Reed-Sternberg cells are present in small numbers, there are few background inflammatory cells and necrosis is rare.
- The **nodular sclerosing** type involves the lymphoid tissue in a nodular pattern with bands of fibrous

tissue separating the nodules of neoplasm. There are many lymphocytes in the neoplasm and characteristic **lacunar cells** are present, which may be considered to be variants of Reed-Sternberg cells. Focal

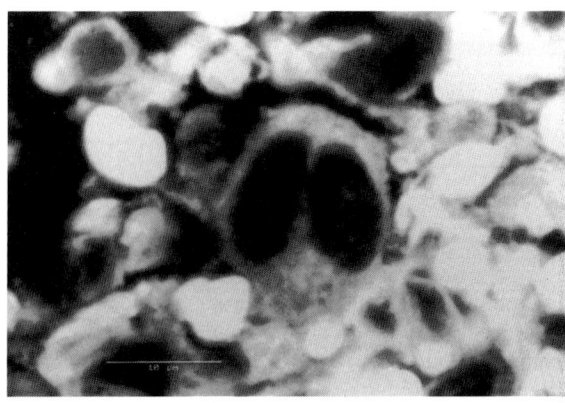

Figure 17.23   *A Reed-Sternberg giant cell in the spleen of a patient with Hodgkin's disease (scale bar is 10 µm)*

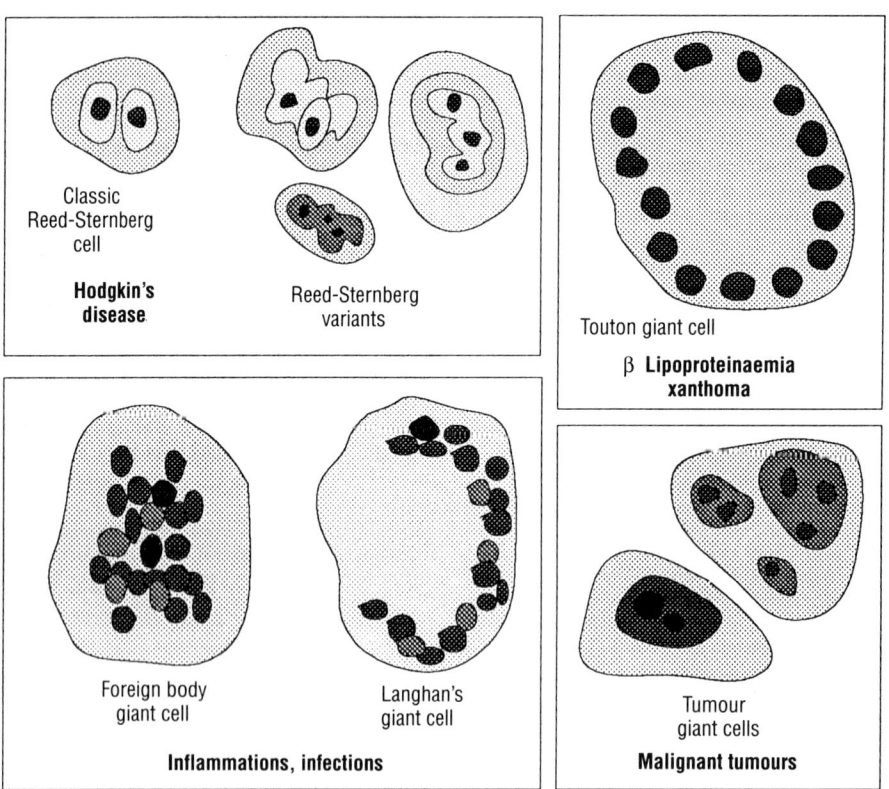

Figure 17.22   *Reed-Sternberg giant cells compared to other types of giant cells*

regions of necrosis may be seen and some eosinophils and other inflammatory cells may occur in the background.

- The **mixed cellularity** type contains a large variety of cells with lymphocytes, Reed-Sternberg cells and many of their variants, eosinophils, macrophages and plasma cells in the background. Focal regions of necrosis may be present.

- The **lymphocyte depleted** type contains scanty lymphocytes, Reed-Sternberg cells and their variants, and few inflammatory cells in the background. Occasionally, extensive loose fibrous tissue may be seen between the neoplastic cells. Focal regions of necrosis may be present.

The origin of the neoplastic cells is still undetermined. They may be derived from lymphoid cells or from cells of the mononuclear phagocyte system. The Reed-Sternberg cells are thought to be derived from macrophages. Depressed T cell function is notable in most cases of HD and may predispose patients to infection. B cell function and antibody production are normal. In many patients the lymphocyte count is decreased to levels of 1500 cells per µL or less. Anaemia may often be seen, but it is not severe until the late stages of the disease.

The staging of HD is complex and a common system in use is shown in Table 17.9 (Ann Arbor Conference, 1971). Each stage is subdivided into groups A and B, depending on whether constitutional symptoms such as unexplained weight loss (more than 10% of the body weight), unexplained fever ($\geq$ 38°C) or night sweats are absent (A) or present (B). Subscripts may be used to further clarify the extent of involvement (e.g. subscript E implies extralymphatic organ; S = spleen, H = liver, L = lung, N = nodes, M = marrow, D = skin, O = bone, P = pleura). In addition, a prefix may be used to indicate whether the stage is clinical (prefix CS = based on physical findings) or pathological (prefix PS = based on biopsy or surgical findings). It should be noted that this staging scheme is also used for non-Hodgkin's lymphomata.

If HD is left untreated half of the patients will die within 2 years and only 10% will survive for 5 years. Treatment of the disease will cure most patients. Patients in stages I or II are treated by radiotherapy of the affected fields or extended fields. Adjuvant chemotherapy may also be given. The 5-year survival of such patients ranges between 95% and 70%, depending on the type of HD and the stage. Patients in stage IIIA are treated by a combination of radiotherapy and chemotherapy, the drugs used being nitrogen mustard, vincristine, procarbazine and prednisone (MOPP treatment). Five-year survival figures in this case vary between 45 and 60%. In HD of stages IIIB and IV, combination chemotherapy is used, usually the MOPP treatment. Five-year survivals for these patients range between 20 and 40%. The histological type of HD influences the prognosis and generally the younger the patient the better the prognosis.

Non-Hodgkin's Lymphomata (NHL)

This is a mixed group of tumours derived from mononuclear cells which have been classified by at least five different systems, each of which is in widespread use. The **Rappaport** classification proposed in 1956, the **Lukes-Collins** classification introduced in 1974, the **Kiel** classification published in 1981 and the **USA Cancer Institute's working formulation** of 1982 have all attempted to deal with the problems of no-

Table 17.9 *Staging of Hodgkin's disease*

Stage	Features
I	Involvement of a single lymph node region (I) or of a single extralymphatic organ or site (I_E)
II	Involvement of two or more lymph node regions on the same side of the diaphragm (II) or localized involvement of an extralymphatic organ or site and of one or more lymph node regions on the same side of the diaphragm (II_E)
III	Involvement of lymph node regions on both sides of the diaphragm (III) which may also be accompanied by localized involvement of an extralymphatic organ or site (III_E) or by involvement of the spleen (III_S) or of both (III_{SE})
IV	Diffuse or disseminated involvement of one or more extralymphocytic organs or tissues with or without associated lymph node enlargement. Sites of involvement are specified by symbols (e.g. IVB_{SHM})

menclature and categorization of this very diverse group of tumours. The basic premise upon which the Rappaport system is based is whether the tumour is follicular or diffuse in growth pattern; subsequently, further subdivisions are created, depending on the histology of the tumour. The Lukes-Collins classification subdivides the lymphomata on the basis of their histogenetic origin into three basic groups, B cell tumours, T cell tumours and histiocytic tumours; further classification is based on histological types. The Kiel classification uses clinical behaviour of tumours as its basic criterion and thus divides the lymphomata into two major groups, tumours of low-grade malignancy and tumours of high-grade malignancy, further subdivisions being created by the use of histological and histogenetic criteria. The USA Cancer Institute's working formulation attempted to bring the three classifications together into what was hoped to be a generally accepted system, but unfortunately this failed to gain wide acceptance. This classification subdivides tumours into three clinical groups of low-, intermediate- and high-grade malignancy, each group then being subdivided on histological grounds. No consideration of the histogenesis of the tumour is taken into account (Table 17.10 attempts to correlate the four classifications).

The NHL represent approximately 60% of all lymphomata and as a group they have certain features in common. In about two-thirds of patients, lymph node enlargement is the feature of the disease that prompts the patient to seek medical advice. The cervical or supraclavicular area nodes are most commonly involved, unilaterally, followed by the axillary nodes, inguinal nodes and others. In a small proportion of patients many lymph nodes around the body are involved at the time of diagnosis. The age incidence is usually 10 to 20 years older than patients with Hodgkin's disease, making the NHL disorders of middle to old age. Males are affected more commonly than females in the ratio of 2:1 to 3:2, the proportion of males increasing as the age increases. Approximately six people in every 100 000 are affected by NHL per year.

Certain types of NHL are common in children or in certain geographical areas associated with certain aetiological agents. In particular, Burkitt's lymphoma is the commonest paediatric malignant tumour in Uganda and Nigeria, and only occurs commonly in Africa and New Guinea. This tumour is caused by the Epstein-Barr virus. The adult T cell lymphoma/leukaemia is caused by the human T cell leukaemia virus type I (HTLV I, a C-type retrovirus related to HIV) and is particularly prevalent in southern Japan and the Caribbean. The aetiology of some other NHL may be related to chromosomal abnormalities that are present in

the neoplastic cells; for example, trisomy 12 is common in the B cell tumours, while in others chromosome 14 shows derangement. Many of the NHL are associated with disruptions to proto-oncogenes, for example c-myc, bcl-1 and tcl-1 genes. Irradiation predisposes to the development of these tumours as also do immunodeficiency states (both congenital and acquired, e.g. Di-George syndrome, AIDS and immunosuppressive drug treatment). Certain autoimmune diseases such as rheumatoid arthritis and SLE increase the risk of developing NHL by a factor of 2.5. Coeliac disease also increases the risk of developing these tumours.

As can be gauged from Table 17.10, the histological appearance of the various NHL is a specialist area and only a few general features will be pointed out here. The term '**follicular**' is used to describe those tumours that form follicle-like groups of neoplastic cells in the affected nodes. '**Diffuse**' implies that the neoplastic cells replace the whole of the lymph node in sheets. '**Lymphocytic**' tumours have cells that are well differentiated and resemble mature lymphocytes with small, dark, round nuclei. '**Lymphoblastic**' is the term used to describe tumour cells that are large, with large, paler convoluted nuclei, and that resemble the lymphoblast in lymph nodes. '**Plasmacytic**' and '**plasmacytoid**' tumours possess cells that more or less resemble plasma cells. '**Cleaved**' tumour cells are those that possess a round to oval nucleus with an indentation (the 'cleaving' that gives the cells their name); small and large variants of these types of cells are found. '**Non-cleaved**' cells are larger cells with abundant cytoplasm and round to oval nuclei with one or more prominent nucleoli. '**Histiocytic**' tumour cells resemble macrophages in that they have abundant foamy cytoplasm and large nuclei (occasionally more than one nucleus) with several prominent nucleoli (see the tumour giant cells in Figure 17.22).

In **Burkitt's lymphoma** the tumour cells are closely packed in the affected lymph nodes (usually in the jaw area). They are B cells with little cytoplasm and a large ovoid nucleus that stains irregularly. Scattered throughout the tumour are normal macrophages in large numbers, some of them containing whole tumour cells or their fragments. In the **Sézary syndrome** and **mycosis fungoides** the tumour cells are T cells that cause forms of cutaneous lymphoma. Mycosis fungoides presents as reddened, scaly plaques on the skin in many regions that often cause severe pruritus and may be mistaken for eczema, psoriasis or other non-neoplastic conditions. The plaques show an essentially pleomorphic chronic inflammatory infiltrate with large, pleomorphic 'mycosis' cells that are scattered in moderate numbers among the normal cells. The lesions grow, thicken,

Table 17.10 *The various schemata of classification of the non-Hodgkin's lymphomata*
(L indicates low-grade, I indicates intermediate-grade, H indicates high-grade malignancy)

General type	Rappaport	Lukes-Collins	Kiel	Working formulation
Well-differentiated B cell tumours (≈ 7% of all cases)	• Diffuse, well-differentiated lymphocytic	• B small lymphocytic	• B chronic lymphoid leukaemia (L)	• Small lymphocytic consistent with chronic lymphoid leukaemia (L)
	• Diffuse well-differentiated lymphocytic with plasmacytoid features	• Plasmacytoid lymphocytic	• Immunocytoma, plasmacytoid or plasmacytic (L)	• Small lymphocytic, plasmacytoid (L)
	—	—	• Plasmacytic (L)	—
Follicular type of B cell tumours (≈ 65% of all cases, ≈ 40% are follicular, ≈ 25% are diffuse)	• Nodular well/poorly differentiated lymphocytic	• Small cleaved cell tumours		• Follicular, mainly small cleaved cell tumours (I)
	• Nodular mixed lymphocytic and histiocytic		• Centroblastic–centrocytic (L)	• Follicular, mixed small and large cleaved cell tumours (I)
	• Nodular histiocytic			
	• Diffuse poorly differentiated lymphocytic	• Large cleaved cell tumours	• Centrocytic (L)	• Follicular, mainly large cell tumours (I)
				• Diffuse, small cleaved cell (I)
	• Diffuse mixed lymphocytic and histiocytic		• Immunocytoma, mixed (L)	• Diffuse small and large cell (I)
		• Non-cleaved cell tumours	• Centroblastic–centrocytic (L)	
			• Centrocytic (L)	
	• Diffuse histiocytic		• Centroblastic (H)	• Diffuse large cell (I)
Poorly differentiated B cell tumours (≈ 7% of all cases)	• Diffuse histiocytic	• B immunoblastic sarcoma	• B cell immunoblastic (H)	• Large cell immunoblastic (H)
	• Burkitt's lymphoma	• Burkitt's lymphoma	• Burkitt's lymphoma (H)	• Burkitt's lymphoma (H)
T cell tumours (≈ 10% of all cases)	• Diffuse well-differentiated lymphocytic	• T small lymphocytic	• T chronic lymphoid leukaemia (L)	• Large cell immunoblastic (H)
	• Diffuse histiocytic	• T immunoblastic sarcoma	• T cell immunoblastic (H)	
	• Lymphoblastic, convoluted, non-convoluted cell	• Convoluted lymphocytic	• Lymphoblastic convoluted cell (H)	• Lymphoblastic, convoluted, non-convoluted cell (H)
	—	• Sézary syndrome	• Sézary syndrome (L)	—
	—	• Mycosis fungoides	• Mycosis fungoides (L)	• Mycosis fungoides (I)
Macrophage tumours (< 1% of all cases)	• Diffuse histiocytic	• Histiocytic	—	• Histiocytic (I)
Unknown cell origin tumours (≈ 10% of all cases)	• Diffuse histiocytic	• U cell	• Unclassified lymphoblastic (H)	• Lymphoblastic, non-convoluted cell (H)

multiply and ulcerate and the lymph nodes are also involved. The Sézary syndrome is a variant of mycosis fungoides, with hyperkeratotic, scaling, pruritic plaques on most of the skin. Unlike mycosis fungoides, the pleomorphic Sézary tumour cells, as well as being found in the lesions, will also circulate in the blood, the leukocyte count being about 20 000 cells per μL, with a fifth of these cells being Sézary cells.

Patients with NHL usually present with enlarged lymph nodes and, uncommonly, with constitutional symptoms such as malaise, fever, weight loss or night sweats. A few patients present with abdominal pain and gastrointestinal symptoms because of abdominal lymph node or GALT involvement. If the extranodal tissues are involved, the organ becomes enlarged through the formation of a well-defined tumour mass or masses. For example, the tonsils, stomach, intestine, spleen and bone may be affected in this way. Macroscopically the tumours may show a nodularity associated with the follicular forms or a greyish to yellowish, uniform, 'fish-flesh' appearance that may be difficult to distinguish from Hodgkin's disease macroscopically. Burkitt's lymphoma will cause dramatic distortion of the face with massive enlargement of the mandible or maxilla. Mycosis fungoides and the Sézary syndrome will produce characteristic skin lesions. Staging of NHL is carried out through the utilization of the criteria used for Hodgkin's disease, as set out in Table 17.9, although it should be noted that over two-thirds of patients with NHL are at stage IV at the time of diagnosis.

Treatment of NHL is through the use of radiotherapy, chemotherapy or a combination of both. In the low-malignancy variants of the disorder the disease may progress so slowly that treatment makes no difference to the prognosis of the patient, which is usually good. Radiotherapy of isolated lesions in stage I or II is sufficient in most patients to cause remissions that persist for 10 years or more, although eventually the disease does recur. If more extensive disease is present, chemotherapy with cyclophosphamide and/or chlorambucil may bring about remissions. High dosages of chemotherapeutic agents are needed for treating the more malignant forms of NHL. Surgical adjuncts may be required in some cases (e.g. Burkitt's lymphoma or lymphoma involving the gut) as well as radiation of the brain or mediastinum. Chemotherapy is effective in bringing about remissions in approximately 75% of patients, cures being said to occur in about half of these cases. The cure rates for Burkitt's lymphoma are 50% or better with chemotherapy and surgery. With all types of NHL, the younger the patient, the fewer the sites affected and the earlier the disease is treated the better the prognosis. Histiocytic reticulosis,

histiocytic sarcoma and adult T cell lymphoma have a very bad prognosis, as do any of the tumours that do not respond to chemotherapy. Most patients with such tumours die within a year, usually of infections, haemorrhages, impingement of important structures by the tumour or because of other malignancies developing (many patients with NHL progress to leukaemia).

Paraproteinaemias (Gammopathies)

In the group of diseases known as paraproteinaemias (PPAs), the common factor is the circulation in the blood of abnormal immunoglobulins or parts of immunoglobulins. Multiple myeloma is by the far the most important cause of PPAs, and this disorder has already been discussed with tumours of the bone. Another important cause of PPAs is B cell lymphoma of the non-Hodgkin's lymphoma group. The other diseases that may cause PPAs are Waldenström's macroglobulinaemia, heavy-chain disease, light-chain disease and various other benign gammopathies. A typical plasma protein electrophoretic pattern from a patient with a typical PPA is shown in Figure 17.24. Similar electrophoretic patterns will be seen in the other PPAs, but on the basis of the site and magnitude of the peak on the electrophoretic record, the various abnormal immunoglobulins may be identified.

Waldenström's macroglobulinaemia is an uncommon condition affecting more commonly middle-aged and elderly males (usually 50 years old or older, M:F = 7:3). It is a low-grade neoplasm of lymphoid cells accompanied by secretion of excessive levels of IgM antibody, thus giving rise to an IgM gammopathy. The bone marrow of the patients is excessively cellular, a single clone of B cells that produce IgM being the major abnormal component. As the disease progresses, the liver, spleen and lymph nodes may also be populated by these cells. The blood remains clear of the abnormal B cells but the plasma protein levels are markedly elevated, in particular the γ-globulins, with levels of 80 g/L or more of protein. A light-chain proteinuria, similar to the Bence-Jones proteinuria seen in multiple myeloma, will develop in a third of cases of the disease but there is little renal damage associated with this presentation. Deposition of IgM in the gut may cause malabsorption in some patients. Anaemia is usually severe in the last stages of the disease.

The disease is very slowly progressive and most patients remain symptomless for many years. When clinical disease manifests itself, the patient complains of weakness, tiredness, spontaneous haemorrhages and enlargement of the liver, spleen and lymph nodes. There is increased plasma viscosity with blurring of

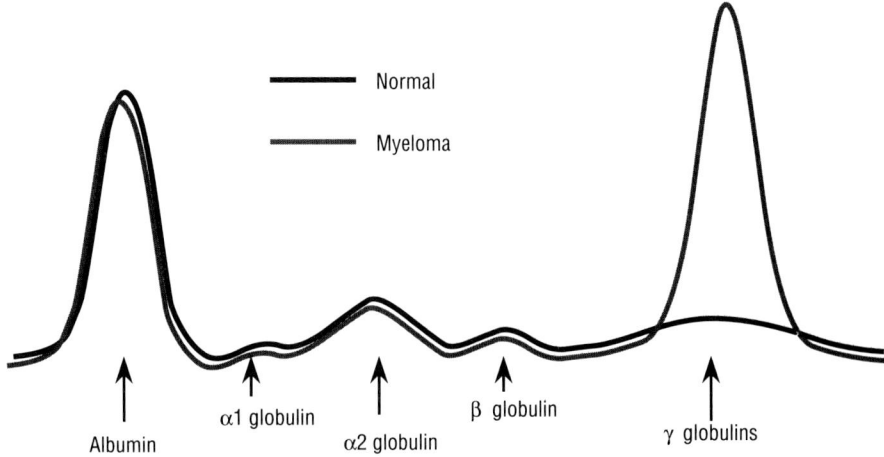

Figure 17.24 *Serum protein electrophoretic pattern of a normal person and of one showing serum myeloma gammaglobulins*

vision, neurological disturbances and haemorrhages. Once symptoms are apparent the disease is treated with chemotherapy as a B cell lymphoma. Remissions are usually temporary and the onset of symptoms generally indicates that the disease is becoming terminal. Few patients survive for about 5 years after diagnosis.

Heavy-chain diseases of several kinds are known and these are neoplastic proliferations of B cells characterized by production of excessive levels of one of the different kinds of heavy chains of immunoglobulins. The major features of these disorders are summarized in Table 17.11. Similarly, **light-chain diseases** are due to monoclonal proliferations of plasma cells that produce excessive levels of either κ or λ light chains. The proliferation of the cells tends to be less aggressive and extensive than in the heavy-chain diseases.

Some **benign gammopathies** will also cause monoclonal increases in the gamma globulin levels in the plasma in the absence of multiple myeloma, lymphoma or leukaemia. These become commoner as people age and may be associated with the collagen diseases or other autoimmune diseases, an unrelated malignancy or chronic infections. The quantity of the abnormal plasma protein is rarely more than 30 g/L and IgG is the most common immunoglobulin class produced. An abnormal clone of plasma cells in the body of these patients is presumably the source of the globulin. The diseases tend to be mostly benign with only about 3% of patients progressing to multiple myeloma or some type of lymphoma.

Cryoglobulinaemia is a condition where there are circulating globulins that precipitate when the plasma

Table 17.11 *The heavy-chain diseases*

Type	Incidence	Age and sex	Nature	Prognosis
α Heavy chain	Commonest (often in Middle Eastern people)	10–30 years, M = F	Anaplastic B cell lymphoma-like, gut involvement with malabsorption	Poor
γ Heavy chain	Less common	> 50 years, M > F	Similar to plasmacytoid lymphoma with lymphadenopathy, splenomegaly	Very poor
μ Heavy chain	Rarest	> 60 years, M > F	B cell lymphoma-like or leukaemia-like or like a plasmacytoid lymphoma	Poor

is cooled and then redissolve when the plasma is warmed. This disorder may be associated with multiple myeloma, Waldenström's macroglobulinaemia or a B cell lymphoma. In a few patients a primary cryoglobulinaemia is seen, not associated with malignancy; such people may have autoimmune disorders or chronic infections. The major pathological features of the disease in all types of presentations develop in skin which is cooled, causing the precipitation of the cryoglobulins with subsequent vascular occlusive manifestations. Raynaud's disease may develop, arthralgia and stiffening of the knees, ankles or hands is common and ulcers of the extremities are another manifestation. Keeping warm is one of the ways to prevent the complications of the condition.

Haematological Tests

The Complete Blood Count (CBC)

When normal functioning of the blood is investigated it is necessary to examine a multitude of variables to see how they differ from the normal and, therefore, how they may contribute to the disease process that has prompted the examination. Within the bloodstream are many hundreds of different substances which vary in concentration almost constantly, since blood is a dynamic living system. It must also be kept in mind

that there is immense individual variation in the normal range of these values and there will be a 'normal range of values' rather than a 'normal value' for each variable. In a complete blood examination some of these important variables relating to blood are examined and the following routine examinations are performed (refer also to Figure 17.25):

Red blood cell (RBC) count. The number of erythrocytes is of importance as there are a very large number of conditions in which this is reduced. A reduction of the red blood cell number below normal levels results in **anaemia**, which is a state where there is a compromise in the respiratory function of the blood, less oxygen than is needed being delivered by the blood to the tissues. Less often there may also be an increase in the red blood cell number (**polycythaemias**) which has the effect of making the blood more viscous, sometimes seriously hampering circulation.

White blood cell (WBC) count. This is subdivided into the **absolute count** and the **differential count**. Very important disease processes involve increases in WBC count. These include the **leukaemias**, where the increased number of white blood cells are due to a cancer in the bone marrow, the excess white blood cells being malignant. There may be increases in the number of normal white cells in some other disease process. **Neutrophilia** is an increase in the number of neutrophils

NAME: Norman Average AGE: 26 years SEX: Male CLINICAL DETAILS: No symptoms of disease, subject healthy; routine check-up MEDICATIONS PATIENT IS TAKING: Nil	
Haemoglobin: 15.7 g/dL	LEUKOCYTES WBC: 7100/µL
ERYTHROCYTES RBC: 5.1 million/µL PCV: 46% MCV: 90 µ³ MCHC: 34 g/dL MCH: 30 pg	Neutrophils: 64% (4551/µL) Eosinophils: 2% (140/µL) Basophils: <0.5% (29/µL) Monocytes: 7% (490/µL) Lymphocytes: 27% (1890/µL)
RETICULOCYTES 1.3%	FILM APPEARANCE: Normochromia, normocytosis
PLATELETS 350 000/µL	REMARKS: Nil

Figure 17.25 *A typical laboratory report of the CBC examination in a healthy person*

and is the change most commonly seen (e.g. with many infections).

Inspection of the peripheral blood smear (PBS). As must be obvious even to a lay person, it is not only quantitative differences that are of interest in the examination of the blood cells but also qualitative differences. A drop of the blood sampled is spread as a thin film on a slide, fixed, stained and examined under the microscope to detect abnormalities in the shape, size, nuclear morphology, etc. of the blood cells. The most common staining procedures utilize the dyes **haematoxylin**, which is a blue, basic dye, and **eosin**, which is a red, acidic dye (hence the name eosinophil, meaning having an affinity for the acid dye eosin). Common stains for blood that utilize these dyes are **Wright's stain**, **Leishman's stain** and **Giemsa stain**. A haematologist can diagnose a large variety of blood disorders simply by looking at the PBS of a patient. Many of the anaemias and leukaemias are diagnosed in this way (refer to Table 17.12).

Haematocrit. The haematocrit is the packed cell volume of red blood cells found in 100 mL of blood. For example, a normal value obtained is 46%, which implies that there are 46 mL of packed red bood cells in 100 mL of blood. The haematocrit is obtained after centrifugation of a blood sample in a graduated tube or, more commonly nowadays, by multiplying the **mean corpuscular volume (MCV)** of erythrocytes by the number of erythrocytes, both in standard units. The haematocrit is an important measurement since it gives an idea of size, capacity and number of cells in the blood. Together with the haemoglobin count it is very important in determining the severity of anaemia that is present.

Haemoglobin. Haemoglobin is the respiratory pigment and measurement of the amount of haemoglobin in the blood gives an idea of the oxygen-carrying capacity of the blood. Values for haemoglobin are quoted as grams of the pigment per dL. Haemoglobin measurement is important in evaluating the severity of anaemic states and establishing the effectiveness of a given treatment.

Erythrocyte indices. Erythrocyte indices refer to three variables of the red blood cells which may nowadays be very readily measured thanks to complex, automatic, electronic equipment. The first variable is **mean corpuscular volume (MCV)**, which measures the average volume of the erythrocytes. The second is **mean corpuscular haemoglobin concentration (MCHC)**, indicating the amount of haemoglobin present in all red blood cells, on average. The last variable is **mean corpuscular haemoglobin (MCH)**, which gives an indication of the amount of haemoglobin in a red blood cell, on average. These erythrocyte indices give an indication of the subtle interrelationships between volume, haemoglobin content and size of cells. Such investigation of erythrocyte indices may diagnose some disorders with a higher level of accuracy than other tests. For example, they may help identify an anaemia as **normocytic** (where the cells are of normal size) or **microcytic** (where the cells are smaller than normal).

Table 17.12 *Special morphological types of erythrocytes and the disorders in which they occur*

Cell type	Conditions where it occurs
Acanthocyte	Cirrhosis, alcoholic hepatitis, abetalipoproteinaemia, post-splenectomy
Codocyte	Thalassaemia, haemoglobinopathies, iron deficiency, post-splenectomy
Dacryocyte	Myelofibrosis, leukoerythroblastic anaemia, thalassaemia
Drepanocyte	Sickle cell disease
Echinocyte	Pyruvate kinase deficiency, chronic peptic ulcer, carcinoma of stomach, uraemia
Elliptocyte	Hereditary elliptocytosis, thalassaemia, iron deficiency
Leptocyte	Thalassaemia, liver disease
Macrocyte	Pernicious anaemia, pyruvate kinase deficiency, autoimmune anaemia
Microcyte	Iron deficiency, thalassaemia, hereditary spherocytosis
Reticulocyte	Haemolytic anaemias, pernicious anaemia, sickle cell disease, spherocytosis
Schizocyte	Post-valve prosthesis operations, severe burns, march haemoglobinuria
Siderocyte	Lead poisoning, haemolytic anaemias, myeloproliferative diseases
Spherocyte	Hereditary spherocytosis, haemolytic anaemias, water dilution anaemia
Stomatocyte	Hereditary stomatocytosis, liver disease

Reticulocyte count. Reticulocytes are immature erythrocytes, being slightly larger than the mature red blood cells and containing in their cytoplasm a small network (= reticulum) of basophilic staining material representing the last fragments of the degenerating nucleus. Their numbers are reported as a percentage of the mature erythrocytes. This figure is used as an indicator of bone marrow activity.

Red cell distribution width (RDW). Automated blood counts often provide this value as a histogram and its examination is a useful adjunct to MCV. The graphical representation gives an indication of the number of large, normal or small erythrocytes.

Other Routine Screening Tests

A variety of other blood tests are available and may be indicated when the CBC does not give a definite diagnosis or where it does not measure the variable under investigation.

Erythrocyte sedimentation rate (ESR). This value is the speed at which red blood cells settle to the bottom of the vessel holding a sample of well-mixed venous blood. The rate is increased in conditions where the negative charge on the RBC membrane decreases, allowing cells to aggregate together forming **rouleaux** (stacks of aggregated erythrocytes, see Figure 17.26). Such would be the case when there are elevated fibrinogen and globulin levels. The test is often used as a monitor of inflammatory or malignant disease and also in the diagnosis of many connective tissue diseases (e.g. rheumatoid arthritis).

Platelet count. The number of platelets in the bloodstream may increase or decrease giving rise to a number of important disorders. The platelet count measures the number of platelets per microlitre of blood when the CBC indicates some abnormality in the platelet numbers. This test is vital in the diagnosis of many haemorrhagic diseases.

Routine blood chemistry. This detects a number of substances in the bloodstream. They may be mineral ions (e.g. Na^+, K^+, Mg^{2+}, Cl^-), enzymes (e.g. acid phosphatase, lactate dehydrogenase), carbohydrates (e.g. glucose), proteins (e.g. albumin), or other organic compounds (e.g. uric acid, urea, bilirubin, cholesterol). Each of these tests is carried out in a variety of clinical situations where the symptoms would indicate an abnormality in the levels of these substances, as part of the major pathological processes.

Indications for the Patient about to have a CBC

1. Patients may eat or drink prior to collection of the blood sample.
2. Approximately 10 mL of venous blood is collected and placed in a lavender topped tube which contains anticoagulant. The tube is completely filled with blood and then inverted repeatedly to mix the blood with the anticoagulant.
3. A limb receiving intravenous fluid is not used to withdraw blood as this causes the sampled blood to be diluted. Similarly the tourniquet is not left on for more than a minute as this causes haemoconcentration.
4. For infants, capillary blood may be taken and a capillary tube used; however, the adjacent tissue should not be compressed as this will cause dilution of the blood with tissue fluid.
5. Drugs taken by the patient may affect the blood. All drugs taken should be listed on the slip accompanying the sample.
6. The specimen is handled gently to prevent haemolysis. The specimen should be sent immediately to the laboratory. If a delay is anticipated refrigeration of the specimen is imperative.

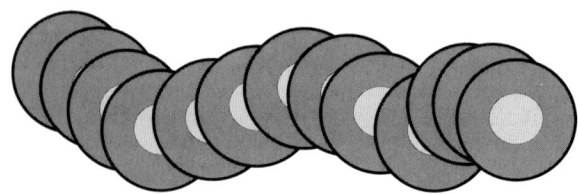

Figure 17.26 *A red blood cell rouleau indicating membrane changes which cause the aggregation of erythrocytes*

7. Both specimen and request form accompanying it are labelled with all of the patient's details.

8. The patient is informed about what is being done and why it is being done. Something like the following should be said: 'We have taken a blood sample from you and this will be sent to the laboratory for various tests to be done. The report from the laboratory will tell us the number and condition of your red blood cells, whether or not you are anaemic, and whether your body is able to fight infections'.

Guide for Infection Control (Blood Related)

The following guideline for blood-related infection control is from *Infection Control Guidelines — AIDS and Related Conditions*, published by the AIDS Task Force in March 1985, Canberra, AGPS.

1. No eating, drinking or smoking in the place where blood is to be collected or handled.

2. No pipetting of blood samples by mouth.

3. Laboratory coats or gowns must be worn at all times in the laboratory or clinic where the blood is collected or handled.

4. Gloves must be worn by the collector or handler of the blood at all times during the collection or handling of the blood if he or she has cuts, abrasions or wounds on his or her hands.

5. Gloves must be worn by all handlers of blood when handling specimens known to be HBsAg (hepatitis B) or HIV (AIDS) positive.

6. All glassware and non-disposable equipment that have been in contact with the blood should be soaked for 30 minutes in 1% sodium hypochlorite solution before routine washing.

7. Disposable items that have been in contact with blood should be collected into biohazard bags that are then autoclaved (121°C for 50 minutes) or alternatively incinerated.

8. All blood spills must be wiped up with 1% sodium hypochlorite solution. This solution should be in contact with the contaminated area for at least 30 minutes.

9. If blood is spilt on an item of clothing, remove the article contaminated and thoroughly soak the affected area with 1% sodium hypochlorite solution. Leave to dry before laundering in the usual manner.

10. Use 0.2% sodium hypochlorite solution for general cleaning of benches and equipment not affected by any definite blood spill.

Iron Studies and Anaemia

The average diet contains 10 to 20 mg of iron which is sufficient for children, men and non-pregnant women. Additional requirements are needed during pregnancy. Iron is absorbed in the duodenum where absorption is regulated by the mucosal cellular content of iron. Iron is transported by transferrin to red blood cells and excess iron is stored by the reticuloendothelial system. Iron is stored as ferritin molecules and small amounts of ferritin circulate in serum (reflecting the amount of iron stored). The presence of iron stimulates the formation of the protein apoferritin with subsequent ferritin formation. Circulating ferritin is thought to control transferrin synthesis by the hepatic parenchymal cells, so that iron deficiency is associated with increased transferrin production and iron overload with reduced transferrin production. Haemosiderin is thought to be composed of denatured ferritin molecules. The total body iron content of the normal adult is 2 to 3 g.

Measurements

Serum iron (SI). This measures the amount of iron bound to the protein transferrin. This bound iron is available for the formation of haemoglobin in the red blood cells. There is a physiological diurnal variation in levels, the lowest being in the afternoon. In women serum iron is low at the time of menstruation because of the loss of blood in the menstruum. As a consequence of these variations, a single measured SI value may not indicate whether the iron transport to erythrocytes is normal or abnormal. Several measurements may be needed. Serum iron estimations will also measure unbound iron after iron has been administered parenterally. In this situation the measurement does not indicate the amount of iron available for haemoglobin synthesis.

Total iron binding capacity (TIBC). This measures the amount of circulating transferrin which is usually inversely proportional to the amount of serum ferritin or iron stores.

Serum ferritin (SF). This measures the amount of circulating ferritin which in most instances reflects the amount of iron stores. Liver disease and the leukaemias increase serum ferritin levels, such that high levels may not indicate increased iron stores.

Iron saturation (IS). This is expressed as a percentage of iron bound to transferrin, with normal values being 25 to 50%.

Iron Metabolism in Common Anaemic States

Iron deficiency. With reduced iron from either poor diet, blood loss or both, iron stores are first depleted, which results in a low serum ferritin which stimulates transferrin production, giving a high transferrin. Later, serum iron falls and saturation is low; red blood cells become hypochromic and microcytic.

SI ↓   TIBC ↑   % Saturation < 16%   Ferritin ↓
Haemoglobin normal to ↓ MCH normal to ↓   MCV normal to ↓

Haemoglobinopathy. With anoxia there is increased intestinal uptake of iron and this may result in an increase in serum iron as well as increased stores.

SI normal or ↑   TIBC normal or ↓   % Saturation, normal or ↓
Ferritin ↑

Acute or chronic inflammation or malignancy. There is impaired flow of iron from the iron stores to the red blood cells, that is, 'iron starvation in the face of plenty'.

SI ↑   % Saturation, normal or ↓
Red cells,   Ferritin ↑
70% normochromic   TIBC normal or ↓
normocytic, 20% normocytic
hypochromic, i.e. MCH ↓ and
MCV normal

Anaemia due to liver disease. The anaemia may be due to the disease process itself or be secondary to blood loss, nutritional disturbances, haemolysis or hypersplenism. Because the liver is a site of iron storage, the breakdown of liver tissue associated with liver disease (acute or chronic) liberates ferritin into the bloodstream so that serum ferritin levels suggest that iron stores are greater than they actually are. Thus, a normal ferritin level may be associated with reduced iron stores.

SI normal or ↑   TIBC ↓   % Saturation, normal or ↑
Ferritin ↑

Haemolytic anaemia. Haemolysis results in increased serum iron and increased ferritin levels. These levels depend on the rate of haemolysis and normal iron and ferritin levels may occur when iron stores are diminished.

SI normal or ↑   TIBC normal or ↓   % Saturation, normal or ↑
Ferritin normal or ↑

Leukaemia. The highest levels of ferritin occur with **acute myeloblastic leukaemia** but high levels may also occur with other leukaemias due to the increased apoferritin production by the cells. This also occurs with some lymphomata, for example Hodgkin's disease.

SI ↓ or ↑   TIBC ↓   % Saturation, normal or ↑
Ferritin ↑↑

Renal disease. Serum ferritin levels reflect the amount of iron stores and iron stores are usually normal and transferrin normal.

SI normal   TIBC normal   % Saturation, normal
Ferritin normal

Summary

Iron studies including serum iron and ferritin are of great assistance in the diagnosis of normochromic, normocytic anaemias and hypochromic anaemias. A summary of the findings of iron investigations in various disease states is given in Table 17.13.

Table 17.13 *Summary of findings of iron investigations in various conditions (N = normal value)*

Condition	Serum iron	Ferritin
Iron deficiencies	↓	↓
Haemoglobinopathy	N or ↑	N or ↑
Inflammation and malignancy	↓	↑
Liver disease	N or ↑	↑↑
Haemolytic anaemia	N or ↑	N or ↑
Leukaemia	N or ↑	↑↑
Renal disease	Normal	Normal

Revision Questions and Case Studies

1. Define the term 'anaemia' and indicate all of the possible symptoms and signs that patients with anaemia may be expected to present with. How are the anaemias classified?
2. What are the characterizing features of the haemorrhagic anaemias?
3. Explain the clinical features observed in an iron deficiency anaemia and relate these to the pathological features of this disorder.
4. Define the following terms:
   (a) Hypochromia
   (b) Microcytosis
   (c) Anisocytosis
   (d) Poikilocytosis
   (e) Reticulocytosis
5. Discuss briefly the following conditions:
   (a) Toxic dyshaemopoietic anaemia
   (b) Leukoerythroblastic anaemia
   (c) Aplastic anaemia
   (d) β thalassaemia
6. Discuss the pathology of pernicious (Addisonian) anaemia.
7. Write brief notes on the following:
   (a) Sickle cell anaemia
   (b) Acquired haemolytic disease
   (c) Folate deficiency
   (d) Megaloblastic anaemias
8. Discuss the pathology of neutropenia and inherited abnormalities of neutrophil function.
9. Define the terms:
   (a) Di-George syndrome
   (b) Agranulocytosis
   (c) Eosinophil leukocytosis
   (d) Polycythaemia
   (e) Polycythaemia rubra vera
10. What are the general characteristics of the leukaemias?
11. Discuss the pathology of acute lymphoblastic leukaemia.
12. Discuss the pathology of the chronic leukaemias.
13. What are the characteristic features of the acute leukaemias?
14. Write brief notes on the following disorders:
    (a) Acute myeloid leukaemia
    (b) Chronic lymphocytic leukaemia
    (c) Burkitt's lymphoma
    (d) Mycosis fungoides
15. Discuss the pathology of thrombocytopenia and thrombocythaemia.
16. Discuss briefly the primary leukopenias.

17. Write a short account of the lazy leukocyte syndrome and chronic granulomatous disease of childhood.
18. Define the following terms:
    (a) Myelogenous precursor cells
    (b) 'Shift to the left'
    (c) Secondary leukopenia
    (d) Thalassaemia
19. Discuss the pathology of Hodgkin's disease.
20. Describe the characteristic findings of the group of disorders known as the 'lymphomata'.
21. Discuss the clinical findings observed in patients with leukaemia and relate these to the pathological changes occurring in the body of such patients.
22. Discuss briefly the pathology of primary and secondary immunodeficiency states.
23. Describe fully the changes in the immune system that are observed in a patient with HIV infection during the course of the disease.
24. Discuss briefly the pathology of Chediak-Higashi syndrome.
25. Define the following terms:
    (a) Haemoperitoneum
    (b) Haemorrhagic anaemia
    (c) Haemosiderosis
    (d) Haemolysis
    (e) Haemochromatosis
    (f) Haematoma
    (g) Codocytosis
    (h) Myeloblastic transformation
    (i) Quartan fever
    (j) Malignant malaria
    (k) Heinz bodies
    (l) Pappenheimer inclusions
    (m) Siderocytes
    (n) Naegeli type leukaemia
    (o) Auer rods
    (p) Aleukaemic leukaemia
    (q) Dacryocyte
26. What characteristic abnormalities in neutrophil morphology may be seen in a PBS? Describe the changes that may be seen in three different disorders.
27. What are the characteristics of cryoglobulinaemia?
28. Of what use is plasma protein electrophoresis in the diagnosis of haematological disorders?
29. What are the haematological implications of a positive Coombs' test?
30. What is the Philadelphia chromosome?

Case study 1. Mr Robert D., a 67-year-old Caucasian male, presents with disease of a very insidious onset, the main presenting symptom being a painless enlargement of his cervical and other superficial lymph nodes. The affected nodes are firm, freely mobile and of a rubbery consistency. There is moderate splenomegaly and hepatomegaly. A maculopapular rash is observed by the examining physician on Mr D.'s ab-

NAME: Robert D.	AGE: 67 years	SEX: Male

CLINICAL DETAILS:
Painless enlargement of superficial lymph nodes, extensive maculopapular rash, herpes zoster
MEDICATIONS PATIENT IS TAKING:
Labetalol 100 mg/four times daily (antihypertensive); aspirin 600 mg daily (antiarthritic)

Haemoglobin: 11.0 g/dL (N = 12–18 g/dL)	LEUKOCYTES WBC: 198 000/µL (N = 4000–10 000/µL)
ERYTHROCYTES RBC: 3.9 million/µL (N = 4.5–6.5 million/µL) PCV: 36% (N = 39–54%) MCV: 92 µ³ (N = 76–96 µ³) MCHC: 31 g/dL (N = 32–36 g/dL) MCH: 29 pg (N = 27–32 pg)	Neutrophils: 3% (6365/µL) (N = 60–70%) Eosinophils: <0.2% (315/µL) (N = 1–4%) Basophils: <0.05% (50/µL) (N = 0–1%) Monocytes: 0.5% (990/µL) (N = 5–10%) Lymphocytes: 96% (190 280/µL) (N = 25–30%)
RETICULOCYTES 1.9% (N = 0.5–2.2%)	FILM APPEARANCE: Normochromia, some prolymphocytes seen, many smudge cells
PLATELETS 93 000/µL (N = 150 000–400 000/µL)	REMARKS: Massive increase in the WBC caused by almost normal looking lymphocytes

For *Case Study 1*

domen and limbs, and there are also active herpes zoster lesions present on the midriff. There is no fever, malaise or excessive feelings of fatigue. Results of the blood examination ordered during the investigation of his condition are shown above.

(a) What is the differential diagnosis for the man's condition?
(b) What is the most likely diagnosis and what features of the case point towards this?
(c) How is this disorder treated?
(d) What is the prognosis?
(e) What are the common causes of death in this condition?

Case study 2. A 3-year-old male infant is admitted into hospital after his parents (Vietnamese illegal immigrants) are detained by the Immigration Department. The child looks quite sick and his growth is retarded, the conjunctivae and mucosae very pale, the skin yellow. There is abdominal distension and the spleen is markedly enlarged, the liver less so. Ulcers are found around the malleoli. A blood sample is taken and aliquots sent to haematology and biochemistry. Some rapid blood examinations in the hospital ward reveal

the following findings: haemoglobin, 4.6 g/dL (N = 12–18 g/dL); serum bilirubin, 2.1 mg/dL (N = 0.1–1.0 mg/dL); urine urobilinogen, increased.

(a) What is the presumptive diagnosis?
(b) What features of the case indicate this diagnosis?
(c) What are the main features of the PBS in this condition?
(d) What is the prognosis for the child?

Case study 3. Mrs Muriel F, a 43-year-old Caucasian woman, presents with an acute disease characterized by fever, rigors, fatigue and pallor. Lately she has noticed that she bleeds rather easily and examination shows evidence of purpura and other haemorrhagic manifestations on her skin and mucous membranes. The woman also shows evidence of skin infection, with two large boils seen on the nape of her neck and also stomatitis with ulceration. There is associated enlargement of the cervical lymph nodes, although there is no evidence of generalized lymphadenopathy. The spleen is moderately enlarged and there is bone tenderness, especially of the sternum. Results of the blood examination ordered during the investigation of her condition are shown overleaf.

NAME: Mrs Muriel F.	AGE: 43 years	SEX: Female

CLINICAL DETAILS:
Acute disease, fever, rigors, pallor. Purpura, ulcers, stomatitis, cervical lymphadenomegaly
MEDICATIONS PATIENT IS TAKING:
Self-administration of paracetamol 0.5–2 g daily, for 2–3 weeks (for bone aches and pains)

Haemoglobin: 5.0 g/dL (N = 12–18 g/dL)	LEUKOCYTES WBC: 25 000/μL (N = 4000–10 000/μL)
ERYTHROCYTES RBC: 1.9 million/μL (N = 4.5–6.5 million/μL) PCV: 18% (N = 39–54%) MCV: 95 μ³ (N = 76–96 μ³) MCHC: 31 g/dL (N = 32–36 g/dL) MCH: 29 pg (N = 27–32 pg)	Neutrophils: 14% (3500/μL) (N = 60–70%) Eosinophils: 11% (2750/μL) (N = 1–4%) Myeloblasts: 65% (16 250/μL) Monocytes: 3.5% (875/μL) (N = 5–10%) Lymphocytes: 6.5% (1625/μL) (N = 25–30%)
RETICULOCYTES 5.5% (N = 0.5–2.2%)	FILM APPEARANCE: Normochromia, 5 nucleated erythrocytes per 100 white cells
PLATELETS 19 000/μL (N = 150 000–400 000/μL)	REMARKS: Pleomorphic myeloblasts and promyelocytes with many smudge cells

For *Case Study 3*

A bone marrow biopsy is also performed and the bone marrow film examined.

MARROW EXAMINATION	Mrs M. F. Age 43

The marrow is markedly hypercellular and shows a vast majority of cells of the myeloblastic series. There is depressed haemopoiesis, although there is extension of active marrow at the expense of fatty marrow. The erythroid tissue and megakaryocytes are greatly reduced in quantity. There is thinning of the trabeculae and destruction of the cancellous bone.

For *Case Study 3*

(a) What is the diagnosis?
(b) What is known about the aetiology of this condition?
(c) What is the prognosis for untreated patients?
(d) How is this disorder treated?
(e) What is the prognosis for treated patients?
(f) What are the complications seen in the disease and what are the common causes of death?

Case study 4. Mrs Wilma S., a 39-year-old Caucasian female, presents with disease of a very acute onset, the main presenting symptoms being haematuria, rigors and pyrexia. There are also gastrointestinal upsets with abdominal discomfort and nausea. The patient is considerably weakened and fatigued and is seen to be very pale and thin on examination. There is no lymphadenopathy or splenomegaly. It was initially suspected that her presenting condition is attributable to a generalized infection that she had suffered from about 2 weeks earlier. However, there was no evidence of infection when she was examined, the infection having been successfully treated with chloramphenicol.

On questioning the woman it is revealed that her father suffers from allergic asthma and her elder brother (45 years old) suffers from hives. The woman herself is allergic to strawberries and fish, which she avoids eating. She has not had any of these foods for many years now. Blood samples were taken for bacterial culture, which was negative. Results of the haematological examination ordered during the investigation of her condition are shown overleaf.

NAME: Mrs Wilma S. AGE: 39 years SEX: Female CLINICAL DETAILS: Acute disease, haematuria, rigors and pyrexia. Abdominal discomfort, nausea MEDICATIONS PATIENT IS TAKING: Self-administration of antacids; oral contraceptive pill	
Haemoglobin: 7.5 g/dL (N = 12–18 g/dL)	LEUKOCYTES WBC: 16 800/µL (N = 4000–10 000/µL)
ERYTHROCYTES RBC: 2.0 million/µL (N = 4.5–6.5 million/µL) PCV: 24% (N = 39–54%) MCV: 120 µ³ (N = 76–96 µ³) MCHC: 35 g/dL (N = 32–36 g/dL) MCH: 28 pg (N = 27–32 pg)	Neutrophils: 60% (10 080/µL) (N = 60–70%) Eosinophils: 2% (336/µL) (N = 1–4%) Basophils: <0.05% (8/µL) (N = 0–1%) Monocytes: 8% (1344/µL) (N = 5–10%) Lymphocytes: 30% (5040/µL) (N = 25–30%)
RETICULOCYTES 25% (N = 0.5–2.2%)	FILM APPEARANCE: Polychromasia, anisocytosis, spherocytosis, macrocytosis
PLATELETS 160 000/µL (N = 150 000–400 000/µL)	REMARKS: Direct Coombs' test is positive, Ham's test is negative.

For *Case Study 4*

Other laboratory tests ordered are shown below.

OTHER EXAMINATION   Mrs W. S. Age 39 Serum bilirubin: 2.8 mg/dL (N = up to 1.0 mg/dL) Serum haemoglobin: Raised (N = < 2–3 mg/dL) Serum iron: 205 µg/dL (N = 50–150 µg/dL)

For *Case Study 4*

(a) What is the diagnosis?
(b) What is known about the aetiology of this condition?
(c) How is this disorder treated?
(d) What is the prognosis?

Case study 5. Mr Hans P., a 74-year-old Caucasian male, presents complaining of malaise, fatigue and weight loss. A PBS shows a reduction in erythrocyte number and there are many nucleated erythrocytes present. Other features are reticulocytosis, anisocytosis, and marked poikilocytosis with many dacryocytes. Haemoglobin is 10.2 g/dL, haematocrit 40%. Leukocyte and platelet numbers are normal, but the differential white cell count shows increased numbers of granulocytes with 8% metamyelocytes and myelocytes. A hepatosplenomegaly is present while the lymph nodes are normal.

(a) What type of anaemia is the patient suffering from?
(b) Discuss the various causes of this type of anaemia.

(c) Given the patient's age what are the most likely causes?
(d) What is the prognosis of this disorder?

Case study 6. Mrs Debbie L., a 22-year-old Caucasian, brings her 3-year old male infant for examination as the boy has suffered from sudden onset of fever, chills and generalized aches and pains. In the past week she had noticed that the boy had developed several bruises on his arms and legs and Mrs L. suspected child abuse at the crêche where she leaves her boy while she is at work. Examination shows evidence of pallor, purpura and haematomata on the infant's skin and mucous membranes. The boy has had bouts of diarrhoea for the past 2 weeks and there is infection of the skin in the perineum. There is enlargement of the cervical and other superficial lymph nodes, with evidence of generalized lymphadenopathy. The spleen is markedly enlarged. There is bone tenderness, especially in the joints and the sternum.

NAME: William Brett L. AGE: 3 years SEX: Male	
CLINICAL DETAILS: Acute disease, pyrexia, aches, pains. Haemorrhage, generalized lymphadenopathy MEDICATIONS PATIENT IS TAKING: Nil	
Haemoglobin: 8.2 g/dL (N = 12–18 g/dL)	LEUKOCYTES WBC: 118 800/μL (N = 4000–10 000/μL)
ERYTHROCYTES RBC: 2.6 million/μL (N = 4.5–6.5 million/μL) PCV: 25% (N = 39–54%) MCV: 96 μ³ (N = 76–96 μ³) MCHC: 31 g/dL (N = 32–36 g/dL) MCH: 26 pg (N = 27–32 pg)	Neutrophils: 1.5% (1747/μL) (N = 60–70%) Eosinophils: <0.5% (583/μL) (N = 1–4%) Basophils: 1% (1165/μL) (N = 0–1%) Monocytes: 1% (1300/μL) (N = 5–10%) Lymphocytes: 26% (31 455/μL) (N = 25–30%) Prolymphocytes: 35% (40 700/μL) Lymphoblasts: 35% (41 850/μL)
RETICULOCYTES 3% (N = 0.5–2.2%)	FILM APPEARANCE: Polychromasia, anisocytosis, spherocytosis, macrocytosis
PLATELETS 13 500/μL (N = 150 000–400 000/μL)	REMARKS: Massive increase in the WBC caused by large numbers of immature lymphocytes.

For *Case Study 6*

Results of the blood examination ordered during the investigation of the condition of the woman's child are shown above.

(a) What is the diagnosis?
(b) Do you think the woman's fears about child abuse are justified? How can the lesions of the child be explained in view of your diagnosis?
(c) How is the child treated?
(d) What are the complications associated with the treatment?
(e) What is the treatment that has the best chance of a cure for the condition?

Further Reading

Alderson M. 'The Epidemiology of Leukemia.' *Adv Cancer Res* 1980; **31**: 2.

Antin JH, Rosenthal DS. 'Acute Leukemias, Myelodysplasia and Lymphomas.' *Clin Geriatr Med* 1985; **1**: 795.

Bagby GC (ed.). 'Hematological Aspects of Systemic Disease.' *Hematol Oncol Clin North Am* 1987; **1**: 167.

Bank A. 'Genetic Disorders of Hemoglobin Synthesis.' *Hosp Pract* 1985; **20**(9): 109.

Bastian I. 'HTLV-I.' *Today's Life Sci* 1992: **4**(7): 16.

Bennett JM, *et al.* 'Proposals for the Classification of the Acute Leukaemias.' *Br J Haematol* 1976; **33**: 451.

Berlin NI (ed.). 'Polycythemia Vera.' *Semin Hematol* 1986; **23**: 131.

Bonham L, Symonds G. 'Murine Bone marrow Repopulation: A Model for Leukohaemogenesis.' *Today's Life Sci* 1992: **4**(1): 24.

Boxer LA, Morganroth ML. 'Neutrophil Function Disorders.' *Dis Mon* 1987; **32**(12): 681.

Cacciola E (ed.). 'Hemato-oncology and Hemato-immunology.' *Acta Haematologica* 1987; **78**(Suppl 1): 1.

'CDC Criteria for Anaemia in Children and Childbearing Age Women.' *Morbidity and Mortality Weekly Report* 1989; **38**: 400.

Chaplin H Jr. 'Immune Hemolytic Anaemias.' *Meth Hematol* 1985; **12**: 1.

Colvin BT. 'Thrombocytopenia.' *Clin Haematol* 1986; **14**: 661.

Dinsmore R, O'Reilly RJ. 'Bone Marrow Transplantation.' *Pathobiol Annu* 1982; **12**: 213.

Doll DC, Weiss RB. 'Neoplasia and the Erythron.' *J Clin Oncol* 1986; **23**: 131.

Elwood N, Begley G. 'Chromosomal Translocations and Lymphoid Tumours.' *Today's Life Sci* 1991: **3**(11): 16.

Fucharoen S, Winichagoon P. 'Hemoglobinopathies in Southeast Asia.' *Hemoglobin* 1987; **11**: 65.

Gale RP (ed.). 'Acute Leukemias.' *Semin Hematol* 1987; **24**: 1.

Gaston MH. 'Sickle Cell Disease.' *Semin Roentgenol* 1987; **22**: 150.

Golde DW. 'The Stem Cell.' *Sci Am* 1991; December: 36.

Golde DW, Gasson JC. 'Hormones that Stimulate the Growth of Blood Cells.' *Sci Am* 1988; July: 34.

Harker LA. 'Acquired Disorders of Platelet Function.' *Ann N Y Acad Sci* 1987; **509**: 188.

Herbert V. 'Megaloblastic Anemia.' *Lab Invest* 1985; **52**: 3.

Marcus DL, Freedman ML. 'Folic Acid Deficiency in the Elderly.' *J Am Geriat Soc* 1985; **33**: 552.

Myint-Oo, Yuthavong Y, O'Sullivan W. 'Malaria in South-East Asia.' *Today's Life Sci* 1991; **3**(7): 42.

Pearson TC, Messinezy M. 'Polycythaemia and Thrombocythaemia in the Elderly.' *Baillière's Clin Haematol* 1987; **1**: 355.

Peschle C (ed.). 'Normal and Neoplastic Blood Cells.' *Ann N Y Acad Sci* 1987; **511**: 1.

Rao AK, Holmsen H. 'Congenital Thrombocytic Disorders.' *Semin Hematol* 1986; **23**: 102.

Rifkind JM. 'Hemoglobin.' *Adv Inorg Biochem* 1988; **7:** 155.

Rosse WF. 'Autoimmune Hemolytic Anemia.' *Hosp Pract* 1985; **20**(8): 105.

Scrimshaw NS. 'Iron Deficiency.' *Sci Am* 1991; October: 24.

Silver RT, Gale RP. 'Chronic Myeloid Leukemia.' *Am J Med* 1986; **80**: 1137.

Steinberg MH, Embury SH. 'Alpha-thalassemia in Blacks.' *Blood* 1986; **68**: 985.

Worwood M. 'Serum Ferritin.' *Clin Sci* 1986; **70**: 215.

Zucker S. 'Anemia in Cancer.' *Cancer Invest* 1985; **3**: 249.

Zucker-Franklin D, *et al. Atlas of Blood Cells*, second edition, 1988; Lea & Febiger, Philadelphia.

18

Endocrine System Disorders

The Normal Endocrine System

The function of the endocrine system is regulation and homeostasis. This is achieved through the secretion, directly into the bloodstream, of specialized messenger compounds, the **hormones**, by the many organs of this system, the **endocrine** (or ductless) **glands**. The glands considered below have a very important role in the endocrine system, but it must be remembered that the gonads and the placenta also function in an endocrine role. In addition, some endocrine tissue is distributed so diffusely that it is not regarded as a distinct organ. An example of this tissue is the endocrine cells of the lining of the duodenum or the pancreatic islets within the exocrine pancreas. The disorders of some of these tissues not arranged in distinct organs (e.g. the pancreatic endocrine tissue) have been considered elsewhere (refer also to Figure 18.1).

The Adrenal Gland (Suprarenal Gland)

The adrenal glands are situated on the upper pole of each kidney and are yellowish, triangular organs, richly supplied with blood. When sectioned, the adrenals show three differently coloured layers immediately subjacent to the stout connective tissue capsule: the outer cortex, which is a yellowish colour, the inner cortex, which is a brownish red, and the medulla, which is a dark greyish colour. The cortex and medulla function as though they were distinct organs.

The cortex is essential to life, although even one-tenth of the tissue is sufficient to produce adequate hormone levels. Cortical hormones include **glucocorticoids**, **mineralocorticoids** and **sex hormones** and these have important functions in carbohydrate metabolism, water and electrolyte balance, and assist the gonads in maintaining normal sexual functions. The medulla is not essential to life and it is said to be an organ functioning only in emergencies, mediating 'fight or flight' responses through secretion of **adrenaline** and **noradrenaline**. These hormones are important in control of blood pressure and cardiovascular system function.

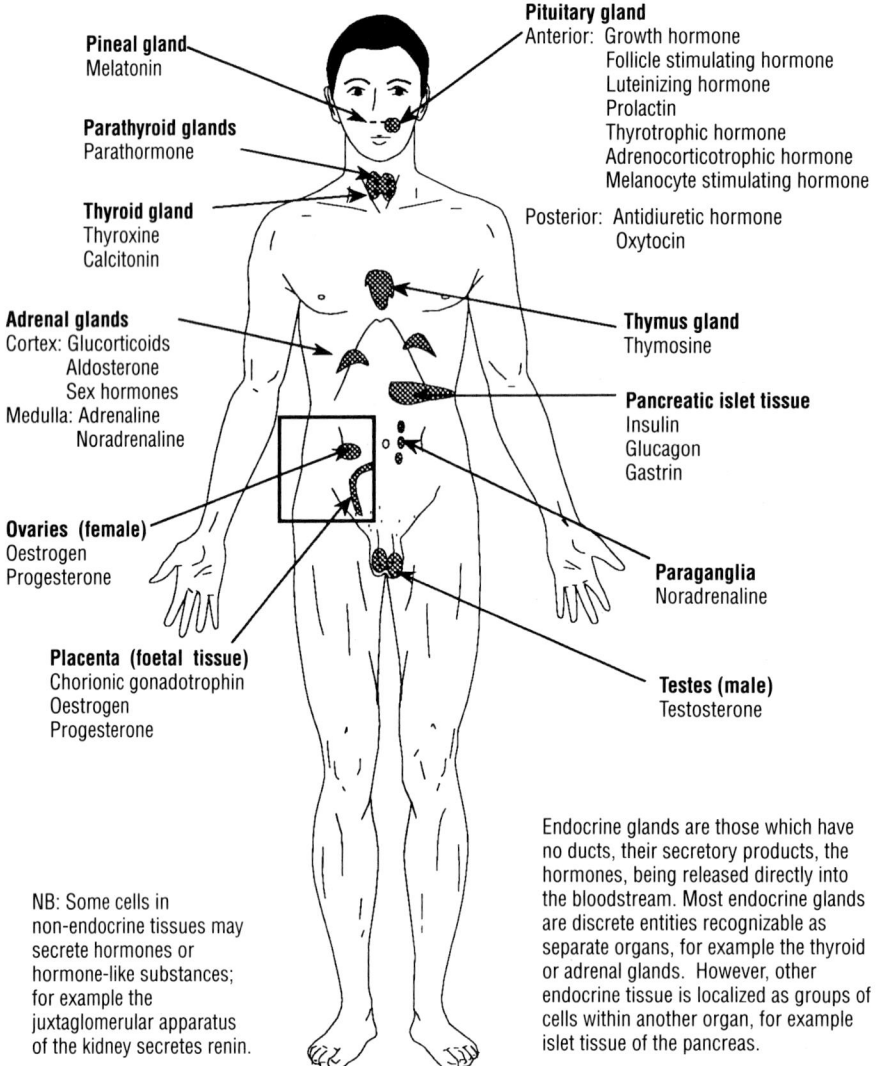

Pineal gland
Melatonin

Parathyroid glands
Parathormone

Thyroid gland
Thyroxine
Calcitonin

Adrenal glands
Cortex: Glucorticoids
Aldosterone
Sex hormones
Medulla: Adrenaline
Noradrenaline

Ovaries (female)
Oestrogen
Progesterone

Placenta (foetal tissue)
Chorionic gonadotrophin
Oestrogen
Progesterone

Pituitary gland
Anterior: Growth hormone
Follicle stimulating hormone
Luteinizing hormone
Prolactin
Thyrotrophic hormone
Adrenocorticotrophic hormone
Melanocyte stimulating hormone

Posterior: Antidiuretic hormone
Oxytocin

Thymus gland
Thymosine

Pancreatic islet tissue
Insulin
Glucagon
Gastrin

Paraganglia
Noradrenaline

Testes (male)
Testosterone

NB: Some cells in non-endocrine tissues may secrete hormones or hormone-like substances; for example the juxtaglomerular apparatus of the kidney secretes renin.

Endocrine glands are those which have no ducts, their secretory products, the hormones, being released directly into the bloodstream. Most endocrine glands are discrete entities recognizable as separate organs, for example the thyroid or adrenal glands. However, other endocrine tissue is localized as groups of cells within another organ, for example islet tissue of the pancreas.

Figure 18.1 *Endocrine glands*

Thyroid Gland

This gland is situated in front of the trachea in the neck, just below the cricoid cartilage, and is in two lobes, connected by a thin isthmus (a pyramidal lobe may also be present just above the isthmus in 50% of people) and weighs 15 g to 25 g. Each main lobe is normally the size of half a golf ball. A capsule surrounds the gland and when sectioned the bulk of the tissue within is seen to be of a mucoid, translucent nature in which numerous small follicles may be discerned. The gland normally contains much hormone stored within the follicles.

The thyroid secretes **thyroxine**, a hormone that controls growth, metabolism and heat production. Thyroxine is an iodine-containing hormone and normal dietary intake of iodine is essential to its formation. The hormone produced by the gland is **tetra-iodothyronine** (T_4), which in the tissues is deiodized to form **triiodothyronine** (T_3), which has a greater biological activity. Another hormone secreted is **calcitonin**, lowering plasma calcium and phosphate levels and inhibiting bone resorption, thus it is a hormone having the opposite effect of parathormone.

Parathyroid Glands

These are four, brownish, small glands (120 mg to 140 mg total weight, about the size of an apple seed) embedded superficially and symmetrically within the tissue of the posterior aspect of the thyroid. In about a third of normal people other accessory glands also occur. Each gland is covered by a capsule and within this the parenchyma consists of plates of cells richly supplied with vessels. The parathyroid glands produce **parathormone**, a hormone regulating calcium resorption and phosphate excretion. Its effects are opposite to calcitonin, in that parathormone causes bone resorption, raising plasma calcium and phosphate levels.

Pituitary Gland (Hypophysis)

This small gland (600 mg to 800 mg, the size of a large pea) is situated on the base of the brain, embedded in the bony ridge of the sella turcica, a fossa of the sphenoid bone. It comprises two distinct regions of different embryological origin: the **adenohypophysis**, arising from glandular tissue derived from the oral epithelium and secreting **growth hormone (GH)**, **prolactin (PL)**, **adrenocorticotrophic hormone (ACTH)**, **thyroid stimulating hormone (TSH)**, **follicle stimulating hormone (FSH)**, **luteinizing hormone (LTH)**, **melanocyte stimulating hormone (MSH)**, and the **neurohypophysis**, derived as a downgrowth from the base of the brain, which secretes **oxytocin (OT)** and **antidiuretic hormone (ADH)**. The pituitary is the central controlling gland with many of its hormones affecting the function of other endocrine glands.

Hormones secreted by the pituitary have the following functions: they affect growth and metabolism, initiate lactation, stimulate other endocrine tissue to produce hormones, maintain normal gonadal function, stimulate melanocytes and contraction of smooth muscle of the uterus and breast and regulate fluid balance and water reabsorption. This gland may be regarded as the master controller of many body activities and regulates the function of other endocrine tissue, thereby coordinating many different bodily actions.

Pineal Gland (Epiphysis)

This is a tiny (7 mm long) gland situated above the posterior part of the third ventricle. It is surrounded by a capsule and its lobulated interior may contain calcified concretions (**acervuli**). This gland reaches its full development in middle childhood and from puberty onwards begins to undergo involution, with increasing fibrous elements and more marked lobulation being demonstrable. It secretes **melatonin**, which is thought to have an important function in melanocyte function and regulation of body rhythms. The gland is also thought to inhibit the development of the gonads. The normal function of the pineal has not been well established, however, the organ is not a vestigial one and is required for normal body functions.

Thymus Gland

This is not strictly speaking a purely endocrine gland as it is mainly lymphoid tissue in its nature. It consists of two fused halves and is situated beneath the upper sternum, in the upper mediastinum. It attains its full size (5 cm by 3 cm) at the age of 2 years and then subsequently dwindles in size having shrunken to insignificance by puberty. Each lobe consists of numerous lobules, varying in size from 0.5 mm to 2 mm. The cortex of the gland has a population of mainly lymphocytes, whereas the medulla has a predominant population of reticuloepithelial cells.

There is active lymphopoiesis in the thymus and the T cells of the cell-mediated immune response differentiate here. **Thymosine** is a humoral factor (interleukin) produced in the gland that is important in lymphocyte maturation and function. The thymus illustrates several endocrine characteristics that are inherent in immune system function, namely production of humoral factors that travel via the bloodstream in order to exert control functions on cells and sites distant from their point of origin.

Adrenal Gland Diseases

Cortical Hypofunction

Acute Cortical Hypofunction

Acute cortical hypofunction of the adrenal results when the gland suddenly is no longer capable of maintaining an adequate production of cortical hormones. Glucocorticoids and mineralocorticoids are both involved and the condition may be brought about by any disease that involves destruction of the adrenal cortical substance. Various causes of this condition include:

- **infections**; for example the Waterhouse-Friedrichsen syndrome seen in association with meningococcal septicaemia;
- **haemorrhage** within the gland, as is seen in various coagulopathies;
- **surgical extirpation** as may occur after the excision of an adrenal tumour;
- **hypopituitarism** with no ACTH being secreted;
- **after other disorders**, as occurs after trauma to the adrenals, in association with severe burns, after long-standing Addison's disease, etc.

Following acute hypofunction of the gland, the patient rapidly goes into an adrenal crisis. There is shock with hypotension and oliguria, epigastric pain, apathy, vomiting and finally coma and death if left untreated. The patient shows severe dehydration and haemoconcentration, increased plasma potassium, decreased sodium and azotaemia. The condition is largely due to the effects of glucocorticoid deficiency and unless hormone substitution therapy is initiated immediately, death will result within approximately 48 hours.

Chronic Cortical Hypofunction (Addison's Disease)

Addison's disease is a condition resulting from partial destruction of the adrenal cortex, which leads to hormonal deficiency of varying degree, ranging from subclinical mild deficiencies to severe, life threatening disorders. The condition may lie dormant until the patient is placed in a stressful situation such as a surgical operation or a serious infection. The disease is uncommon, affecting only one person in every 100 000. Most cases of the disorder are brought about by an idiopathic autoimmune destruction of the cortex and manifestations of the disease usually result only if 90% or more of the gland is destroyed. Various other, less common causes are:

- **tuberculosis** of the adrenals;
- **amyloidosis**;
- **neoplasia**, either primary or secondary, causing cortical destruction;
- **pituitary hypofunction**;
- **iatrogenic**, after prolonged steroid administration which causes adrenal cortical atrophy.

The prime features of this disorder are weakness, fatigue, languor and a gradual failing of health. The plasma sugar is low and attacks of hypoglycaemia may be easily induced by stress. A characteristic feature is increased pigmentation of the skin like an uneven suntan. Some patients show a bluish or greyish tinge on their skin and there may be dark freckles and patches of dark pigmentation on the lips and mucous membranes. Hypotension is found in most patients, the blood pressure often falling to values as low as 80/50 mmHg, and the patient in these cases will often suffer from giddiness or syncope. Severe nausea, diarrhoea, vomiting and anorexia are very common symptoms, and in women loss of axillary and pubic hair is also a frequent finding.

More than half of the patients with Addison's disease show an atrophy of the adrenal cortex consistent with an autoimmune destruction of tissue. In others,

infection, haemorrhage or tumour is the cause of the destruction. In the early stages of the disease the unaffected adrenal tissue copes with the demands placed upon it, but as more and more tissue is destroyed the hormones produced decrease dramatically. The lack of cortisol causes the fatigue, languor and decreased levels of plasma glucose. Lack of aldosterone causes hyperkalaemia and reduction in plasma sodium with raised plasma potassium levels. Lack of water and sodium causes the hypotension. Decreased levels of androgens causes the loss of body hair in women, testicular androgens being sufficient to prevent this in men. In children, there is a stunting of growth due to the decreased hormone levels.

Addison's disease is treated by replacement of hormones normally produced by the adrenal cortex. Cortisol or prednisolone are administered to replace the cortisol and fludrocortisone replaces the aldosterone. Careful monitoring of the dosage is essential, but also any other incidental disorders must be treated accordingly.

Medullary Hypofunction

Removal or destruction of the adrenal medulla produces no functional disturbance in the body. The medulla normally produces adrenaline and noradrenaline in the ratio of 3:1, but these hormones are not essential as the sympathetic system in which they act as stimulators operates normally since the direct neural pathways still perform all of their necessary duties even in the absence of the adrenal gland.

Cortical Hyperfunction

Adrenal cortical hyperfunction may result if there is an abnormality in the pituitary gland where excessive levels of ACTH are secreted; alternatively, adrenal causes (most commonly hyperplasia and tumours) may lead to spontaneous oversecretion of the adrenocortical hormones. In some situations where excessive levels of steroids are administered therapeutically for prolonged time intervals, syndromes mimicking cortical hyperfunction may be seen.

Glucocorticoid Excess (Cushing's Syndrome)

Excessive levels of cortisol secreted by the adrenal gland due to any cause result in Cushing's syndrome. The term **Cushing's disease** is used when the cause of the adrenal hyperfunction is excessive ACTH production by the pituitary gland. Primary Cushing's syndrome is not a common disease, accounting for only one hospital admission in every 4000. If iatrogenic causes (secondary cause) are included, the disorder then increases in incidence. The disease is commoner in women, in the ratio of 7:3, and is seen most frequently between the ages of 20 and 40 years. The severity varies considerably from patient to patient and ranges from the almost subclinical to the grave disease.

Patients with Cushing's syndrome present with central obesity affecting the trunk, their limbs looking thin and spindly. The face is rounded and oedematous, justifying the name 'moon-face'. A pad of fat across the shoulder blades is often termed 'buffalo-hump'. The muscles are wasted, atrophic and weak due to the depletion of protein caused by the excess cortisol. Children show stunted growth. The skin becomes thin, atrophic and easily injured. Purple striae are seen in the protuberant abdomen as the weak skin stretches over the growing obesity. Osteoporosis and collapse of vertebrae are other common findings, as are pathological fractures in other bones. Hypercalciuria and renal calculus formation may be seen in association with the bone rarefaction. Most patients are hypertensive as water and sodium are retained because of the excessive glucocorticoid levels. Diabetes mellitus will develop in about a quarter of cases and another third of cases show abnormal glucose tolerance. There is an increased incidence of infection associated with depression of immunity and inflammation. Abnormalities in menstruation, infertility and impotence are commonly observed and in women, hirsutism develops in most cases (see Figure 18.2).

The majority of clinically observed cases of Cushing's syndrome are seen in association with the therapeutic administration of glucocorticoids. In other cases, by far the most important cause is a small pituitary adenoma that secretes an excessive level of ACTH, which cannot be easily detected radiologically. In a few cases, Cushing's syndrome is caused by adrenal cortical tumours or hyperplasia. Rarely, neoplasms in extra-adrenal sites may produce adrenal or adrenocorticotrophic hormones, most often the tumours being **oat cell carcinoma of the bronchus**, or **thymomata**.

Diagnosis of the disease depends on various laboratory investigations as well as on the clinical findings. It may be demonstrated in patients that there is diurnal variation in the levels of plasma cortisol as occurs in healthy people. Urinary excretion of cortisol is greater than 1000 nmol/day as compared to less than 400 nmol/day in healthy subjects. The dexamethasone test involves the use of this compound in order to suppress ACTH secretion by the pituitary and hence suppress glucocorticoid secretion by the adrenal. Its results are interpreted according to Table 18.1.

Treatment of Cushing's syndrome depends very much on its cause. If tumours of the adrenal gland or of the pituitary are the cause, surgical resection of the tumour or radiotherapy in the case of pituitary tumours will cause control of the hypersecretion of adrenal hormones and the clinical effects of the glucocorticoid excess will gradually regress. Drugs that interfere with the synthesis of cortisol (e.g. metyrapone) may be administered or the adrenal cortices may be destroyed by administration of mitotane (o,p-DDD). Bilateral adrenalectomy controls the syndrome in all cases but this is an operation of relatively high mortality, 5% of patients dying post-operatively. In addition, in about a sixth of the survivors **Nelson's syndrome** will occur, which is due to an ACTH-secreting adenoma of the pituitary developing, with hyperpigmentation due to MSH secretion which is secreted at the same time as ACTH. If Cushing's syndrome has followed therapeu-

Table 18.1 *The dexamethasone test*

Dexamethasone	Normal subject	Cushing's due to small tumours	Cushing's due to large tumours
Low dose for 2 days	Plasma cortisol < 140 nmol/L Urine cortisol < 80 nmol/L	Cortisol levels in plasma and urine stay well above that of normal subject	No change in high cortisol levels that were present before the test
High dose for 2 days	As above	Suppression, cortisol levels fall to less than 50% of previous levels	Rarely causes fall in cortisol levels (if yes, hyperplasia is more likely as a cause)

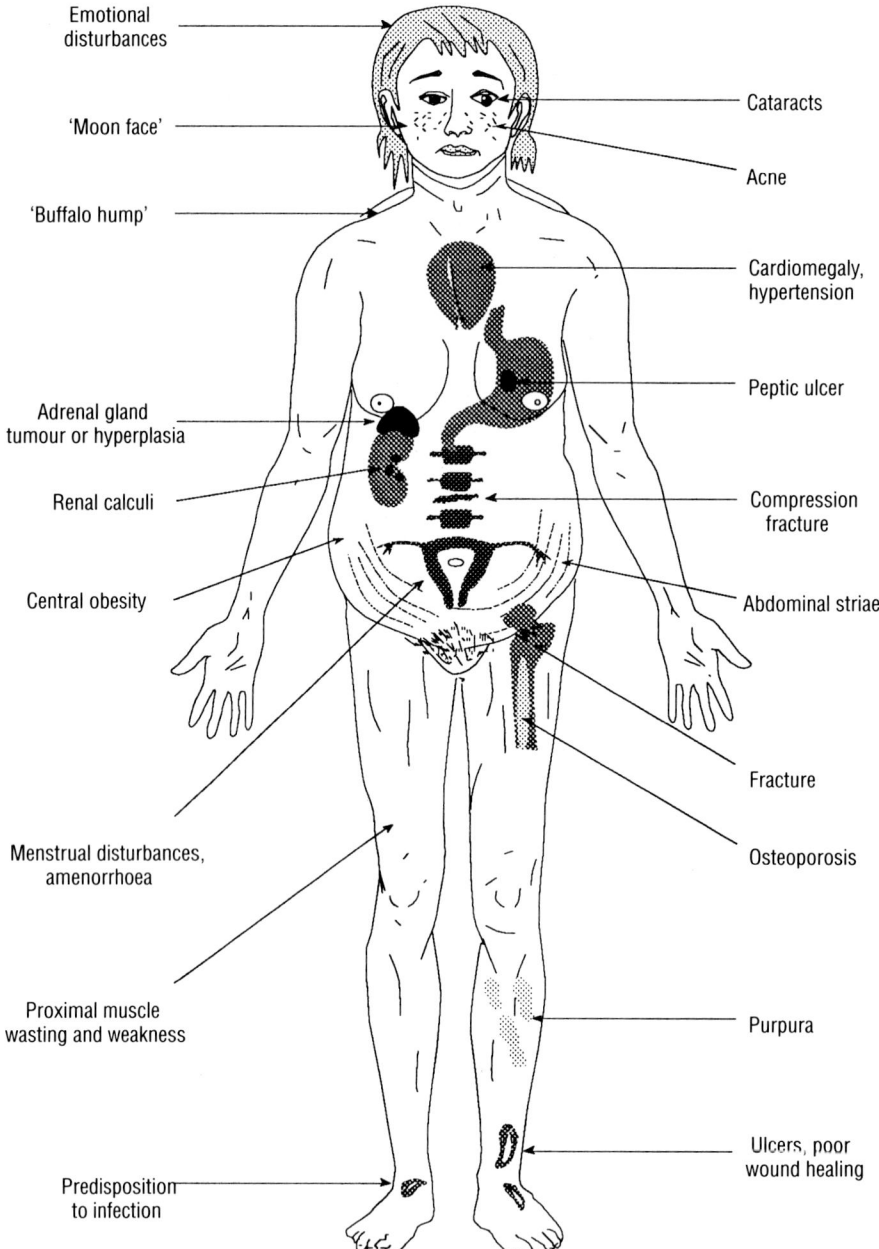

Figure 18.2   *Clinical features of Cushing's syndrome*

tic steroid administration, sudden cessation of administration will be followed by Addison's disease, so the patient must be slowly weaned off the steroids.

Mineralocorticoid Excess (Conn's Syndrome)

Conn's syndrome is an uncommon disease that is seen more frequently in women (7:3 sex ratio) and typically occurs in adults between 30 and 50 years of age. The disease occurs in primary and secondary forms, the former due to disease of the adrenals (mainly adenomata or occasionally hyperplasia), while the latter occurs when the kidney is secreting excess quantities of renin, causing the adrenals to secrete more aldosterone. In both cases, oversecretion of aldosterone causes electrolyte disturbances: there is hypokalaemia with muscle weakness, cramps and cardiac arrhythmias; there is slightly raised plasma sodium causing raised systemic blood pressure, the hypertension sometimes very severe and of the malignant form; and metabolic alkalosis and polydipsia with polyuria will also be apparent. If the disease is untreated for many years, renal failure may result, the patient showing uraemia.

Examination of the gland will show evidence of an adenoma in about three-quarters of cases while hyperplasia of the zona glomerulosa will be found in a quarter of cases. In a small number of patients with adenoma, the tumour may undergo malignant change and a hormone-secreting carcinoma will be the cause of the syndrome. Diagnosis of the condition depends on examination of renin levels and other tests. In the primary form of the disease, the renin levels in the plasma are decreased while in the secondary form the renin levels are greatly increased. Another test is the administration of two litres of normal saline intravenously. In normal people this salt loading will suppress the production of aldosterone within 4 hours, but in Conn's syndrome aldosterone will continue to be secreted.

Treatment of Conn's syndrome will depend on the aetiology. If an adenoma or carcinoma is the cause, surgical excision of the mass may be followed by a cure. If a hyperplasia is responsible, a salt-restricted diet and administration of aldosterone antagonists (e.g. spironolactone) will control the condition. In cases of secondary Conn's syndrome control of the primary disease that has brought about the adrenal disorder may be enough to control the overproduction of aldosterone. Excessive renin production may be seen in such states as renal disease, heart failure and cirrhosis of the liver, and obviously, some of these diseases may not be controlled easily.

Sex Hormone Excess (Adrenogenital Syndromes)

The adrenogenital syndromes are caused by oversecretion of sex hormones by the adrenal cortices. The most usual type of syndrome is that which is caused by an oversecretion of androgenic hormones. The patient presentation depends on the sex and age of the patient at the time of the androgen excess. In adults, the excessive secretion of androgens is most commonly caused by adrenal gland hyperplasia, while in children the condition is most often brought about by benign or malignant tumours of the adrenal cortex.

In adult males, excess androgens secreted by the adrenal will cause no clinical effects. Adult women with an adrenally caused androgen excess will undergo **virilization**: they will develop hair loss from the scalp, while hirsutism of the facial and truncal areas will be seen (i.e. a typical male distribution of body hair), their breasts will undergo atrophy as will their external genitalia and the clitoris will enlarge. There is deepening of the voice, which is often interpreted as 'hoarseness' and there will be disturbances in the menstrual cycle with oligomenorrhoea or amenorrhoea. The woman may also develop acne.

Children with androgen excess will show a growth spurt with well-developed muscles. At the same time, there will be premature fusion of the epiphyses and growth will be prematurely stunted. There will be premature development of body hair and the skin may show acne or excessive greasiness. In boys there will be precocious puberty with development of the secondary sexual characteristics at an early age. The testes, however, will remain infantile due to suppression of secretion of pituitary gonadotrophins. In girls, the excess androgens will cause masculinization with abnormal development of the external genitalia, clitorimegaly and male distribution of body hair. Puberty will not be attained as the pituitary gonadotrophin production is suppressed.

A rare form of oestrogenic excess also exists where the hormones are always produced by a tumour (mostly a carcinoma). The effects of this state are most marked in men and boys with **feminization** being the result. Gynaecomastia (development of breasts) and loss of body hair usually cause the male to present early for treatment. In women, there may be menstrual irregularity (refer to Table 18.2 for a summary of the hormonopathies of the adrenal glands).

Diagnosis of the adrenogenital syndromes depends very much on clinical findings and the results of the physical examination; however, laboratory investigations of hormone levels in blood and urine may be used to confirm the diagnosis. For example, high plasma

Table 18.2 *Hormonopathies of the adrenal gland*

Syndrome	Cause	Incidence	Characteristics
Addison's disease	Decreased glucocorticosteroids	1:100 000 30–50 yrs, F>M	Azotaemia, hyperkalaemia, hyponatraemia, loss of body hair, stunted growth in children, hypotension
Cushing's syndrome	Increased glucocorticosteroids	1:4000 + iatrogenic causes 20–40 yrs, 7:3 (F:M)	Obesity, 'moon face', 'buffalo hump', striae, muscle wasting, diabetes, osteoporosis, hirsutism, hypertension, weakness
Conn's syndrome	Increased mineralocorticosteroids	Uncommon 30–50 yrs, 7:3 (F:M)	Severe hypertension, alkalosis, hypernatraemia, hypokalaemia, muscle cramps, weakness
Androgenic adrenogenital syndrome	Increased male sex hormones	Rare Children, adults, F≈M	*Boys:* Precocious 2° sex characters, stunted growth *Men:* No clinical effects *Girls:* Masculinization, no puberty, clitorimegaly *Women:* Virilization, amenorrhoea, atrophy of breasts, clitorimegaly
Oestrogenic adrenogenital syndrome	Increased female sex hormones	Very rare Children, adults, F≈M	Gynaecomastia in men and boys, menstrual disorders in women

concentration of androgens or increased excretion of 17-ketosteroids in the urine suggests the adrenogenital syndrome. It should be noted that virilization may also be due to ovarian disorders and the dexamethasone suppression tests will help to distinguish between ovarian and adrenal causes of the disorder. In any case, virilization is invariably associated with increased plasma androgen levels.

Medullary Hyperfunction

Phaeochromocytoma

Phaeochromocytoma is a tumour that secretes hormones, most such neoplasms of the adrenal secreting both adrenaline and noradrenaline. Some of the neoplasms will secrete only noradrenaline, especially those that are found in extra-adrenal sites. About two-thirds of patients with the tumour will present with symp-

toms arising out of the excessive hormone production. The clinical presentation is one of elevated blood pressure. In some patients the rise in pressure resembles primary benign hypertension with moderate increases that remain constant over the weeks, progressively worsening with the passage of time. In other patients, the blood pressure is elevated but shows immense variations in the reading taken over time, different pressures being recorded from day to day. Spells of extremely high pressure in the region of 260/160 mmHg may be recorded and during these attacks the patient may experience palpitations, pounding headaches, abdominal discomfort, may feel anxious or apprehensive or may have attacks of angina pectoris. The attacks of extremely high blood pressure may occur at weekly or monthly intervals and may last for minutes to hours, but as the disease progresses the attacks become more frequent and last longer. Anything that compresses the tumour may trigger off an attack, for example exercise or tight clothing. Other symptoms and signs associated with the tumour include profuse sweating, loss of weight, cardiac arrhythmias, tachycardia, bradycardia and flushed or pale skin.

Paroxysmal hypertension with great variation in the readings over a period of time in a young adult and associated with cardiac anomalies should be viewed with suspicion and the patient should be investigated for the presence of a phaeochromocytoma (see below).

Tumours of the Cortex

Cortical Adenoma

These tumours of the adrenal are the commonest and are routinely discovered in as many as a tenth of all autopsies performed. Functionally, they are often indistinguishable from hyperplasia of the adrenals although hyperplastic nodules tend to be smaller than true adenomata, and multiple rather than the single masses of the adenomata. A typical adenoma is usually 2 cm in diameter or greater and consists of an encapsulated, yellow nodule that resembles adrenal tissue. Microscopically the tumour is seen to contain regions that resemble normal adrenal cortex, although the general arrangement is quite disorderly.

The effects of an adenoma may be minimal, many persons with these tumours never showing clinical evidence of the presence of the tumour during their life and the tumour being discovered as an incidental finding at autopsy. Alternatively, the tumour may give rise to Cushing's syndrome, Conn's syndrome or the adrenogenital syndromes. If symptomatic, the neoplasms are surgically excised and a cure results.

Cortical Carcinoma

This is a very rare tumour and only a handful of new cases are diagnosed in Australia per year. It is more common in young adults and occasionally seen in children. The neoplasms are large, segmented masses, yellowish in colour and often showing regions of necrosis and haemorrhage. Often, malignant tumours are not easily distinguished from benign ones, even microscopically, for the malignant masses may be very well differentiated and will even secrete hormones. The larger an adrenal mass is the more likely it is to be malignant. In addition, the carcinoma will also invade adjacent tissues such as the kidney and will metastasize to distant sites such as the lymph nodes, the other adrenal gland, brain, lungs and bone.

The tumour may be functionally inactive or alternatively may secrete hormones, leading to Cushing's or the adrenogenital syndromes. It may be difficult or impossible to predict the clinical effects of the tumour simply by examining it under the microscope. Treatment of the tumour by surgical means is nearly always impossible as the tumour is well advanced at the time of diagnosis. The drug mitotane (o,p-DDD) will lead to temporary remission of the tumour in some cases, but few patients survive for more than 2 years after diagnosis.

Secondary Tumours

Secondary tumours in the adrenal gland are much commoner than primary ones. The commonest primary tumours that are likely to metastasize to the adrenals are carcinomata of the bronchus, breast and stomach as is involvement by leukaemias and lymphomata. The presence of a secondary tumour in the adrenals is unlikely to compromise the hormonal function of the glands, although commonly the tumour deposits are bilateral.

Tumours of the Medulla

Phaeochromocytoma

Phaeochromocytoma is a rare tumour with an incidence of one in 1 000 000 population per year. It is a tumour that may occur in any age group although it is typically seen between the ages of 20 and 55 years, affecting men and women equally. It is a neoplasm which is most commonly benign, only about 5% of such tumours being malignant. It may be bilateral and may also arise in extra-adrenal sites, such as in a chromaffin ganglion or the organs of Zuckerkandl (these are a retroperitoneal group of paraganglia located along the abdominal aorta, and which undergo involution during childhood).

The tumour may vary greatly in size and in some patients a large abdominal mass may be palpated, but most tumours are about 4 to 5 cm in diameter. The tumour is pink to grey in section, with regions of necrosis, haemorrhage, cystic degeneration and calcification, and surrounded by a capsule. Under the microscope the tumour consists of columns or sheets of tumour cells. It is impossible to distinguish between benign and malignant tumours microscopically, as both may show pleomorphism, mitotic activity and even invasion; the only reliable indicator of malignancy is the development of metastases. The symptoms and signs of the tumour have been considered above.

The tumour is diagnosed by taking a 24-hour sample of urine and measuring the content of cate-cholamines and their metabolites. Free catecholamines in the urine of normal people are rarely above 150 µg/day, while in the patient with phaeochromocytoma the urine contains over 250 µg/day. If a 24 hour sample of urine contains more than 50 µg of adrenaline, the tumour is likely to be in the adrenal gland because non-adrenal tumours very rarely secrete adrenaline. The tumour may be treated by surgical means in most cases and this will lead to cures. However, the operation carries a considerable risk and the patient may suffer from excessive hypertension and cardiac arrhythmias caused by handling of the tumour and anaesthesia. If the patient is given α-adrenergic blocking agents before the operation, the risk of surgical complications is somewhat decreased. The tumour recurs in only a small number of patients. The prognosis is much poorer in the case of malignant tumours that have metastasized and the only treatment option is the control of symptoms through administration of adrenergic blocking agents.

Neuroblastoma

This is a tumour derived from the neuroblasts, which develop into the sympathetic nervous system cells. Although the tumour most commonly arises in the adrenal medulla, it may also be seen as a primary in the posterior sympathetic chain of the mediastinum, the coeliac plexus, within and around the brain and in the neck. Neuroblastoma is a tumour of infancy and childhood, very rarely seen in adults, and is one of the commoner childhood tumours, more than three-quarters of them arising in the first year of life.

The left adrenal is more commonly affected than the right and the tumour is a lobulated, pale, soft mass that may attain a large size and thus be palpated as an abdominal swelling. Foci of necrosis, haemorrhages and fine, microscopic regions of calcification may also occur. Under the microscope, neuroblastomata are composed of masses of small dark cells that resemble lymphocytes. The cells are arranged in sheets or rosettes and they are supported by a fine collagenous tissue stroma and many blood vessels. If cells resembling ganglion cells are present within the tumour, it is termed a **ganglioneuroblastoma**. The tumour may superficially resemble Ewing's tumour of bone, something to be considered as neuroblastomata do metastasize to bone.

The tumour is clearly malignant in its behaviour and will invade the surrounding tissues early in its growth and will metastasize via the lymphatics and blood-stream, forming secondary deposits most commonly in the other adrenal, liver, bone and lungs. Two syndromes are recognized in association with this tumour: **Hutchinson's syndrome**, when the tumour (usually a primary of the left adrenal) has metastasized extensively to bone with resultant anaemia, involvement of the skull, orbital masses and haemorrhages around the eyes; and **Pepper's syndrome**, when the tumour (usually a right adrenal primary) has prominent secondaries in the liver with marked hepatomegaly.

Symptoms and signs associated with the tumour are the presence of an abdominal mass, hepatomegaly, masses protruding from the skull or causing proptosis of the eye, weight loss, anaemia or pathological fractures. Rarely the patient may develop the carcinoid syndrome, hypertension or even Cushing's syndrome. Dopamine, catecholamines and their metabolites (e.g. vanillylmandelic acid, VMA, and homovanillic acid, HVA) are secreted by most tumours and these substances may be detected in the urine and may help in diagnosing the tumour.

Treatment of the neoplasms involves a complex regime of surgery, radiotherapy and chemotherapy; however, more than two-thirds of children will die within 18 months of diagnosis. The prognosis of the tumour is better if ganglion cells are present within the mass and in the cases where the tumour spontaneously and inexplicably 'matures' into the benign ganglioneuroma. If the tumour has not metastasized, the combined treatment will generally affect a cure. Large doses of vitamin B_{12} have been reported to be helpful in treating some forms of the tumour.

Multiple Endocrine Neoplasia (MEN) Syndrome

The MEN syndrome is a familial disorder in which neoplasms develop in many endocrine glands during life either at the same time (synchronously) or in succession, over a number of years (asynchronously). Depending on the glands involved, the syndrome is subdivided into type I (**Wermer's syndrome**) or type II (**Sipple's syndrome**). The major characteristics of these syndromes are considered in Table 18.3.

Congenital Dyshormonogeneses of the Adrenal

The enzymes that are needed for the biosynthesis of the adrenocortical hormones are shown in Figure 18.3. Deficiencies of these enzymes may occur as a number of Mendelian autosomal recessive defects. The defi-

Table 18.3 *Multiple endocrine neoplasia syndrome*

Type	Synonym	Tumours	Glands affected
MEN I	Wermer's syndrome	Adenomata	Pituitary, thyroid, adrenal cortex, parathyroid, islet tissue
MEN IIa (II)	Sipple's syndrome	Carcinomata	Thyroid, parathyroid, adrenal medulla (phaechromocytoma)
MEN IIb (III)	—	Adenomata, carcinomata	Mucosae (lips, tongue neuromata), adrenal medulla (phaechromocytoma)

ciencies may result in adrenal hyperplasia or they may have no effect on the size of the gland. The hyperplastic disorders are seen primarily in girls, the sex ratio being 4:1, and their incidence is one in every 10 000 population. The non-hyperplastic disorders are rarer and they affect the synthesis of the mineralocorticoids only.

The precise effects of the various deficiencies depend on the particular enzymes that are lacking and on the hormones whose synthesis is affected. Various anatomical malformations of the genitalia may be seen in the young infant because of aberrations of sex hormone levels.

Hyperplastic Deficiencies

20,22-Desmolase deficiency is rare and in this condition gonad hormonal synthesis is affected as well as adrenal hormonal synthesis. All adrenal cortical hormone synthetic activity is blocked and large quantities of cholesterol accumulate in the adrenal cortex. Affected infants do not survive for very long after birth.

3β-Hydroxysteroid dehydrogenase deficiency results in a lack of both glucocorticosteroids and mineralocorticoids, as well as of some sex hormones. An accumulation of dehydroepiandrosterone (DHEA)

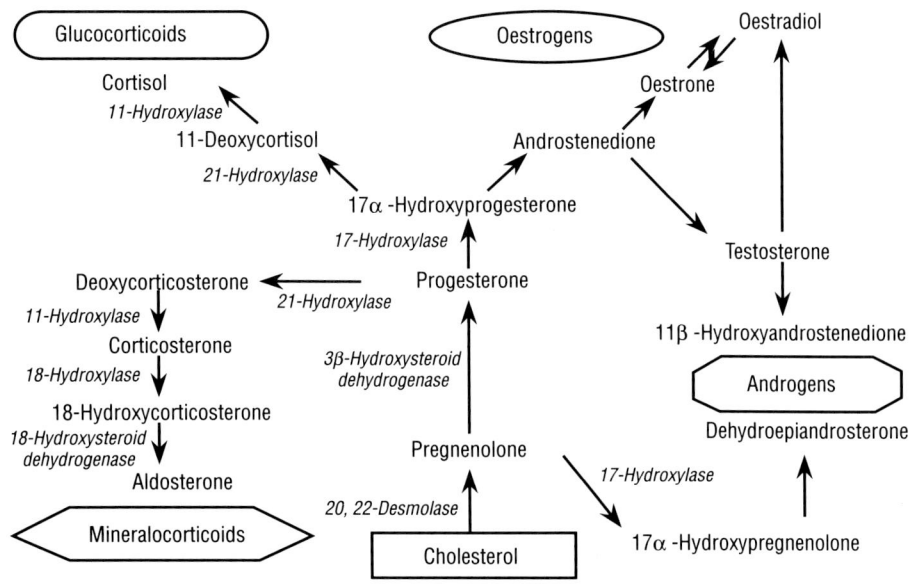

Figure 18.3 *Biosynthetic pathways of the adrenal cortical hormones*

occurs, as production of this weak androgen is not blocked. Affected children of both sexes have malformed genitalia: girls because of the masculinizing effects of excess DHEA and boys because of the lack of potent androgens. Loss of excessive salt and water will cause diarrhoea, feeding difficulties, vomiting, apathy and weakness during the first weeks of life and death may occur due to circulatory collapse.

17-Hydroxylase deficiency is rare and it causes impairment of cortisol, androgen and usually aldosterone production. Progesterone (and pregnanetriol, its metabolite), deoxycorticosterone and corticosterone are present in excess amounts. In boys the genitalia are hypoplastic and in girls there is reduction in normal sexual development and amenorrhoea at puberty. Hypertension and hypokalaemia occur in both sexes.

21-Hydroxylase deficiency is the commonest form of congenital adrenal hyperplastic dyshormonogenesis. There is impairment of glucocorticoid and mineralocorticoid synthesis, which results in excessive ACTH synthesis by the pituitary and subsequently, the adrenal gland undergoes hyperplasia. There are two variants of the disorder, possibly reflecting different genetic defects. In one of the variants there is excessive loss of salt from the body and the metabolic block in the adrenal is complete; in the other variant there is no excessive salt loss and this form is thought to represent an incomplete metabolic block. Excessive accumulation of androgens occurs in both forms but is more marked and has earlier results in the salt-losing form. Masculinization occurs in girls and there is growth of the penis with the testes remaining small in boys. These changes occur a few weeks after birth in the severe deficiency but in the milder form they may take between 2 to 12 years to manifest themselves. There is potassium retention, and hyponatraemia with perhaps a metabolic acidosis. Similar clinical effects are seen as in 3β-hydroxysteroid dehydrogenase deficiency. Diagnosis of the condition is made by demonstrating high levels of 17-hydroxyprogesterone in the plasma: a normal 36-hour-old infant has <6 nmol/L of the compound in its plasma, whereas an affected infant has >200 nmol/L of the compound in its plasma.

11-Hydroxylase deficiency impairs the production of aldosterone and cortisol, with an increased ACTH production by the pituitary causing hyperplasia of the adrenal and overproduction of androgens. Virilization

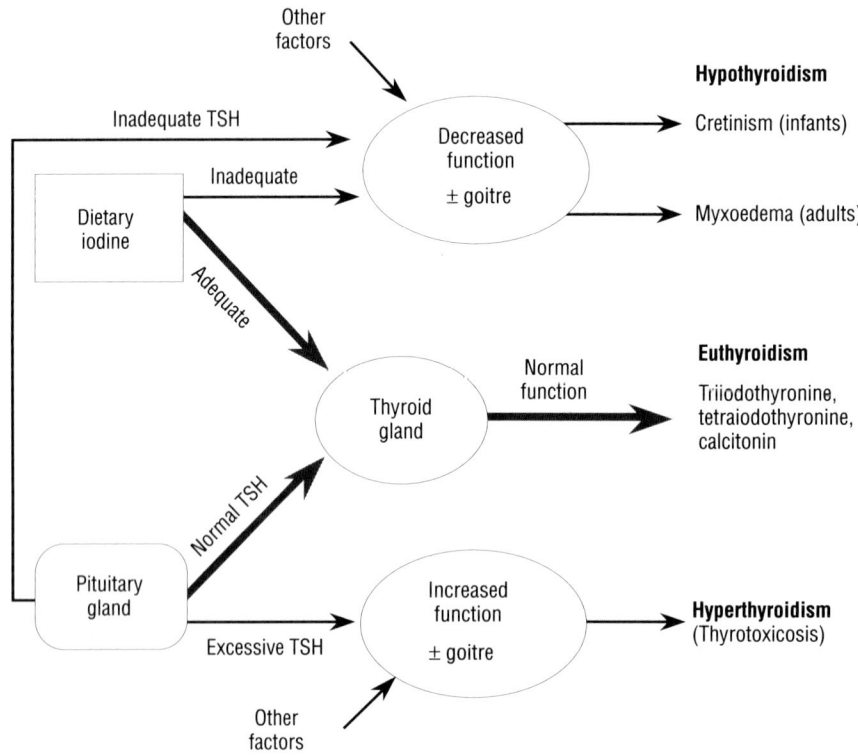

Figure 18.4 *Euthyroidism, hypothyroidism and hyperthyroidism*

occurs in the affected patients but the excess 11-deoxycortisol and 11-deoxycorticosterone overcome to a large extent the effects of lack of cortisol and aldosterone. Salt loss does not occur and hypertension is produced in much the same way as in Conn's syndrome.

Non-hyperplastic Deficiencies

18-Hydroxylase deficiency causes decreased production of 18-hydroxycorticosterone and aldosterone. The affected infants suffer from salt loss, dehydration and fever; the plasma renin levels are increased. Allotetrahydrocorticosterone, the metabolite of corticosterone, is found in excessive amounts in the urine. The condition is treated by administration of the mineralocorticoid that is lacking. **18-Hydroxysteroid dehydrogenase deficiency** prevents the formation of aldosterone through lack of the last dehydrogenation step. There is loss of sodium and water, hypotension and hypovolaemia, as well as hyperkalaemia and increased renin production. The condition is treated with mineralocorticoid supplements.

Thyroid Gland Diseases

Goitre

The word goitre is derived from the Latin word *guttur*, meaning throat, and is used to describe any swelling in the throat region caused by an enlargement of the thyroid gland. In certain cases the word **struma** is used synonymously for goitre. Goitre may be caused by a variety of disorders, and it must be remembered that an enlarged thyroid gland is not always accompanied by hyperthyroidism. In some cases of goitre, the patient may indeed be hypothyroid, as occurs, for example, in Hashimoto's disease, or he or she may show normal thyroid function (i.e. be **euthyroid**). The enlargement of the gland may be due to infiltration by inflammatory or neoplastic cells, but is more commonly due to an increase in the number of thyroid cells. The thyroid will undergo hyperplasia in response to TSH secretion by the pituitary but functional euthyroidism will also depend on the presence of adequate levels of dietary iodine; therefore, a hyperplastic stimulated gland may be associated with clinical evidence of hypothyroidism due to dietary deficiencies. In many cases the goitre may resolve by a process of involution if the primary disorder causing the hyperplasia is treated. Toxic goitre is a special case of thyroid enlargement that occurs independently of in-

creased TSH levels and need of thyroxine by the body as it is a case of a stimulatory, type V hypersensitivity reaction involving the gland (see Figure 18.4).

Inflammations

Acute Thyroiditis

Acute thyroiditis is one of the seven or so types of inflammations that are seen in the thyroid gland and is nowadays one of the most uncommon. It results after acute infection with bacteria which reach the gland via the bloodstream or via direct extension from surrounding infected sites. Usually it is the pyogenic bacteria, such as *Staphylococcus* spp., that are involved and they cause a typical acute inflammatory presentation which usually resolves with little, if any, damage to the gland. Occasionally, viral infections may involve the thyroid but the disorders seldom cause any clinical symptomatology or any permanent damage to the gland.

Granulomatous Thyroiditis

Chronic granulomatous thyroiditis due to tuberculosis, syphilis or other specific causes have all been described but are very rare. In most such cases, typical chronic inflammatory granulomata will form. Congenital syphilis affecting the thyroid may lead to extensive scarring and a diffuse inflammation with lymphocytes and plasma cells. Sarcoidosis may also rarely affect the thyroid and, although it is a nonspecific disease, it is usually included in this group as its lesions and clinical presentation are well characterized as a typical granulomatous inflammation. In all of these disorders, the chronic inflammatory reaction may cause extensive destruction and fibrosis of the gland with resultant hypothyroidism

Chronic Thyroiditis

Chronic non-specific thyroiditis may occur, in which case there is a diffuse infiltration of the gland by chronic inflammatory cells. This disease is most often seen in older women but it usually does not cause functional aberration and the patient remains euthyroid. Another variant of the disorder is **chronic lymphocytic thyroiditis**, a disease more common in the young, causing about 40% of cases of goitre in children. The gland shows diffuse infiltration by lymphocytes and these cells may also form germinal centres within the substance of the gland. Although most patients show normal levels of thyroxine in the serum, some may become hyperthyroid, usually mildly so. In both cases, the disease generally requires no major form of treatment, a monitoring of thyroid function typically being carried out and hypothyroidism or hyperthyroidism being treated supportively. The disorders may subside spontaneously within a period of a few months. A small number of patients may suffer relapses.

Hashimoto's Disease (Struma Lymphomatosa, Autoimmune Thyroiditis)

Hashimoto's disease is an autoimmune disease affecting one person in every 1600 and it appears to be becoming more common. The patients are most usually women, the sex ratio being 9:1, and persons between the ages of 30 to 50 years are most commonly afflicted, although the disorder may also be seen in children. There is a definite association of the disease with antigen HLA DR5 in Caucasians and antigen HLA BW35 in Japanese. About a third of the blood relatives of patients with Hashimoto's disease have some form of thyroid disorder. Autoimmune disorders such as rheumatoid arthritis, Sjögren's syndrome, pernicious anaemia and others are frequently found in association with Hashimoto's disease and contribute to the evidence that the disease is an autoimmune one.

The characteristic feature of Hashimoto's disease of the thyroid is an enlargement of the gland so that it becomes goitrous, often weighing ten times its normal weight. The enlargement is caused by a uniform expansion with retention of the shape and encapsulation of the gland. The cut surface has been likened to that of a bisected, raw potato and the consistency is hard, often with a lobulated structure. The microscopical appearance of the gland is essentially one which resembles lymphoid tissue, in that the thyroid follicles have been almost totally replaced by infiltrating lymphocytes and plasma cells that are grouped into follicular structures that even contain germinal centres. Only vestigial remnants of the thyroid tissue remain. As the disease progresses, no thyroid follicles may be seen at all in the gland. Some of the remaining follicles are lined by cuboidal, very sharply defined eosinophilic cells that are termed **Hürthle cells**. Antigen–antibody complexes are found enmeshed in the basement membrane of such acini. Fibrosis of the gland increases as the years pass. Electron micrographs often show lymphocytes in close contact with epithelial cells or with their fragments.

The morphological findings and the clinical features that point towards an autoimmune pathogenesis are supported by laboratory data in patients with the disease. Although the disease is thought to be caused by a cell-mediated reaction primarily, autoantibodies to thyroglobulin are found in over 90% of cases of the disease. Other autoantibodies against thyroid cell components or thyroid products are also commonly found in Hashimoto's thyroiditis. The disease can be induced experimentally in animals by injecting thyroid gland antigens in association with Freund's adjuvant and the lymphocytes from such animals, when transferred to healthy animals, will transmit the disease.

Hashimoto's disease is treated by giving the patients thyroxine in order to make them euthyroid; this treatment causes a decrease in the titre of TSH and a shrinkage in the gland. Radiation or surgical ablation of the thyroid may be necessary in grossly enlarged glands, but these forms of treatment are followed by a marked hypothyroidism and thyroxine administration has to be maintained throughout the individual's life.

De Quervain's Disease (Subacute or Granulomatous Thyroiditis)

De Quervain's disease of the thyroid is an idiopathic disorder that is seen in the frequency of one in 10 000 people, the patients being usually in their 50s and female (the sex ratio being 4:1). It is suspected that the disease may be due to a viral infection as in some patients with the disease the mumps virus has been demonstrated in the thyroid cells and in other patients the disorder often follows a viral respiratory infection. However, the evidence is not conclusive. Autoantibodies against the thyroid are absent or present in low titre and the disease is not considered to be an autoimmune one. It should be noted that low titres of autoantibodies against the thyroid are often present in normal, euthyroid people.

In de Quervain's disease the thyroid is usually doubled in weight and may be enlarged symmetrically or only one lobe of the gland may be affected. The gland is hard and a pale yellowish colour on section, the affected portions becoming adherent to the surrounding muscles. Microscopically there is evidence of chronic inflammation in the affected regions of the gland and granulomata may form with collections of macrophages, giant cells, lymphocytes and plasma cells. It appears that disruption of the thyroid follicles and spillage of the colloid in the substance of the gland stimulates the formation of granulomata and giant cells, the macrophages often containing phagocytosed colloid. Neutrophils are also present in the affected areas and they may form small, abscess-like collections. Fibrosis is quite marked as is the loss of follicular tissue.

Clinically, the patient with de Quervain's disease presents with hyperthyroidism in the early stages of the disease and hypothyroidism in the later stages. This presentation is caused by disruption of the follicles and spillage of stored hormone in the early phases with reduction in the functional endocrine tissue in the later, inflammatory–fibrotic phases of the disease. The patient very often presents with pain in the thyroid region (usually very severe) that is brought about by swallowing, turning the head or anything that compresses the gland. The pain may also be referred to the lower jaw or ear and may become worse for a period of weeks. Fever, malaise, leukocytosis and an increased ESR are also seen commonly in patients. If the disease remains untreated, it will resolve within a period of a few months, but may persist for a year or so. Treatment is through the administration of anti-inflammatory steroids such as prednisone, which causes the resolution of the condition within 3 to 4 weeks. Thyroid function returns to normal even though the gland may show microscopic evidence of focal non-specific chronic inflammation.

Riedel's Disease (Ligneous Thyroiditis)

Riedel's disease is a very rare, idiopathic disorder of the thyroid usually seen in adults of around 40 to 50 years, and is more common in females, the sex ratio being 3:1. The disease is characterized by extensive fibrosis of the gland, which gives it an extremely hard consistency (ligneous = woody). The thyroid becomes firmly attached to surrounding structures, often causing compression of the trachea. The substance of the gland is replaced by great tracts of fibrocollagenous tissue in which a few functioning follicles remain (these being sufficient to keep the patient euthyroid). A few lymphocytes and plasma cells infiltrate the scarred gland.

Patients with the condition generally present with symptoms and signs relating to the compression of structures by the sclerotic gland. They may complain of a choking feeling, dyspnoea and cough because of tracheal involvement, dysphagia because of oesophageal compression, hoarseness because of recurrent laryngeal nerve compression and paralysis of the vocal cords. The treatment is surgical and is designed to relieve these symptoms arising out of compression. In rare cases where hypothyroidism also occurs, thyroxine treatment is instituted in addition to surgery.

Hypothyroidism

Hypothyroidism occurs when inadequate levels of hormones are secreted by the thyroid gland. The condition may occur in adults, in which case it is termed **myxoedema**, or it may occur in infants, in which case it is termed **cretinism**. Hypothyroidism in older children resembles the adult form of the disease and is known as **juvenile hypothyroidism**. Endemic hypothyroidism in children and infants used to be much commoner in the past in regions where dietary intake of iodine was low.

Cretinism

Cretinism usually manifests as a congenital disorder, although the infant may not show signs of the disease until the maternal levels of circulating thyroid hormone fall below active levels. The disorder occurs in two major forms, the **endemic** and the **sporadic**. This is a distinction of aetiological and morphological considerations, as in the endemic form the disorder is seen in association with iodine deficiency and a goitre is present, whereas the sporadic form is caused by congenital anomalies of the thyroid and goitre may or may not be present.

Sporadic cretinism occurs in one in every 5000 children in areas where endemic cretinism is not a problem. Most often, the condition is caused by aplasia or hypoplasia of the thyroid and in these cases a goitre may not be present. Rarely, the disease is due to genetic enzymatic defects in the thyroid that are inherited as an autosomal recessive trait. The gland becomes goitrous due to excessive TSH production, but the hyperplastic thyroid tissue is unable to form active thyroid hormone and hence hypothyroidism results.

The child suffering from sporadic cretinism will show signs of the disease a few weeks or months after birth when the maternal levels of thyroid hormones are exhausted in the child's circulation. The child develops a dry, coarse skin and thick and dry hair, the face becomes puffy and dull, the abdomen becomes protuberant often with an umbilical hernia being present, and macroglossia, enlarged heart (which may show congestive heart failure), constipation and slow reflexes occur. If the child is not treated, mental retardation develops and there is failure of normal development, resulting in dwarfism, delayed or absent sexual maturation and bone and muscular disorders.

Such cases of hypothyroidism may be diagnosed at birth by estimating levels of TSH and thyroxine in the plasma, in some hospitals this being a routine procedure. Treatment is initiated immediately the condition

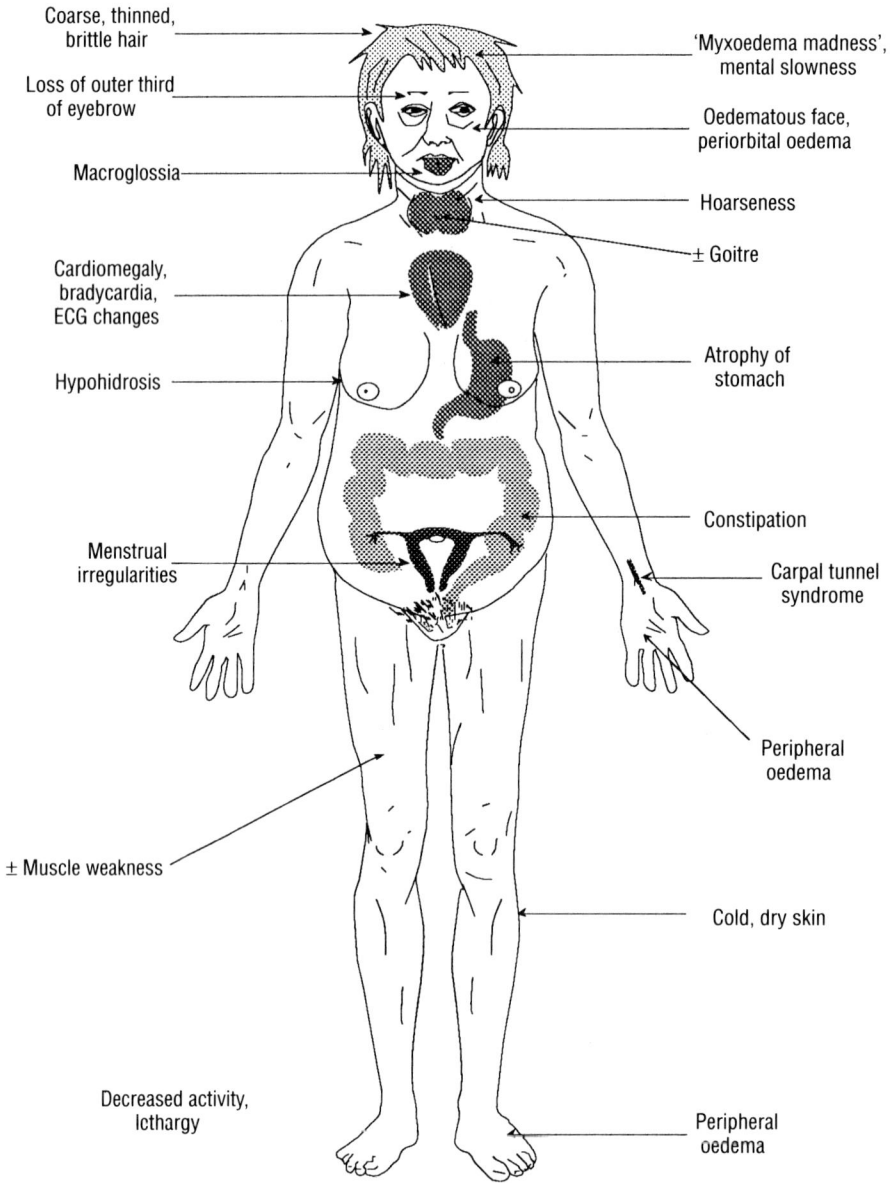

Figure 18.5 *Effects of myxoedema*

is diagnosed by administration of thyroid hormone in order to prevent maldevelopment and mental deterioration.

Endemic cretinism is still prevalent in the populations of some developing countries where iodine intake is low. Usually the areas are mountainous and remote with poor medical care and social welfare. Regions in the Himalayas and Andes, for example, still have a high incidence of the condition. Endemic

cretinism is subdivided into two types, the **myxoedematous form** and the **neurological form**. Both of these forms may coexist in a population or either type may predominate. In some remote villages of the Andes as many as 10% of inhabitants show mental deficiency due to endemic cretinism. The iodine deficiency in the diet in these populations may be complicated by other hypothyroid and goitrogenic factors, such as infections and intake of toxic thyrotropic plants.

In the **myxoedematous form**, the affected children show all the features of adult myxoedema (see below) with mental and growth retardation. However, the patients are not deaf and mute and the thyroid may be of normal size. In the **neurological form**, growth retardation is not as marked but the mental deficiency still develops. In addition, the affected children are usually deaf-mutes that may also show muscular disorders such as spasticity and incoordination.

In both cases of endemic goitre, supplementation of the diet with iodine will prevent the development of the condition even if other factors contribute to the development of goitre and hypothyroidism (i.e. infections and goitrogens in the diet). In a small number of cases thyroid hormone may need to be administered in order to prevent the condition and the individuals in these cases are thought to be cases of sporadic cretinism in an endemic area.

Myxoedema (Gull's Disease)

Myxoedema is hypothyroidism seen in adults and is a fairly common disorder with approximately three in every 2000 people being affected. It is most often seen in females in middle to old age. A juvenile form may also affect older children. The condition is associated with a variety of aetiologies, but dietary iodine deficiency is not a common cause, the iodine intake needing to be completely abolished if the disease is to develop. Various causes of myxoedema are:

- **thyroiditis**, especially Hashimoto's disease, occasionally Riedel's thyroiditis, etc.;
- **radiation** used for therapeutic purposes, or exposure to radioactive iodine (a common problem in scientific laboratories);
- **drugs**, administration of such antithyroid substances as lithium, phenylbutazone, thiocyanate, etc.;
- **iatrogenic**, caused by excessive antithyroid treatment of a toxic goitre, including surgical resection of the thyroid;
- **hypopituitarism** with inadequate levels of TSH secreted;
- **congenital**, caused by a relative deficiency in synthetic enzymes needed for thyroxine production;
- **dietary**, with complete removal of iodine from the diet or interference with dietary iodine absorption by high-fat diets, high calcium, fluoride and chloride consumption and high consumption of members of the *Brassica* (cabbage) group of vegetables;
- **'burnt out' thyroid** following thyrotoxicosis (see below);
- **idiopathic**.

In most cases of myxoedema, the disease develops slowly over a number of years. The patient may first complain of feeling cold and is noted to be listless and slow or sleepy. There may be weight gain, constipation or hair loss. The fall in circulating thyroid hormone levels causes a decrease in the metabolic rate, which makes the patient increasingly dull and sluggish. Neurological symptoms and signs begin to develop and these include vertigo, tinnitus, deafness, hallucinations and psychosis. The skin becomes dry, scaly, rough and cold with hypohidrosis (diminished sweating). The hair becomes brittle and coarse, tending to fall out; the lateral third of the eyebrows may be lost and the patient often does not need to shave or have hair cuts. The face is oedematous, pale and expressionless, and the eyelids are quite puffy. The tongue is swollen and this, together with the oedema of the vocal cords, makes the patient speak slowly and the words are slurred. The swelling of tissues is caused by the deposition of ground substance in the connective tissue, hyaluronic acid being especially plentiful; this substance binding water causes the oedema (increased ground substance = 'myx-', and increased water = '-oedema').

The muscles and joints are also affected in myxoedema. The muscles often show slowing of the contraction and relaxation processes and the duration of the reflexes is prolonged. The joints become thickened and there may be an increased volume of joint fluid in the joint spaces. The remodelling of bone is slowed down and although occasionally there may be hypercalcaemia, parathyroid function remains normal. The patient often shows gastrointestinal abnormalities with anorexia and constipation being mainly due to the slowed movements of the intestinal muscles. The heart also is involved, with a decreased cardiac output and stroke volume, effects of decreased heart muscle contractility. There is cardiomegaly due to dilatation of the ventricles. Angina pectoris may be present and digitalis administered to such patients does not relieve the cardiac condition. Anaemia is common in patients with myxoedema and often the absorption of vitamin B_{12} will be reduced due to autoantibody formation to gastric mucosa and to intrinsic factor. Dysfunction of the reproductive system may manifest itself as amenorrhoea or menorrhagia in women, and decreased libido or impotence in men (refer to Figure 18.5).

Myxoedema is treated by administration of thyroid hormone, which causes most of the symptoms and signs of the disease to disappear within a period of weeks. Basal metabolic rate increases, the puffiness of the face is reduced, cardiac function returns to normal and a diuresis signals the excretion of excess water and mucopolysaccharides. The patient regains alertness and normal activity and begins to display interest and initiative again. The skin and hair returns to normal within a period of months.

Hyperthyroidism

Toxic Goitre (Graves' Disease, Thyrotoxicosis)

Graves' disease is an autoimmune disorder affecting one person in 5000 each year, the patients usually being female (sex ratio 7:1) and between 20 and 40 years of age. The aetiology of the disease is unknown but several hypotheses have been proposed. Genetic factors in the development of the disease are indicated as the frequency of HLA DR3 and HLA B8 is increased in Caucasians with the disorder, while Japanese with Graves' disease are more likely to have HLA BW36 and Chinese HLA BW46. Some researchers suggest that a virus may be the triggering factor for the autoimmunity while other investigators suspect that the autoimmunity is a manifestation of the failure of self-tolerance mechanisms due to suppressor T cell dysfunction.

The pathogenesis of Graves' disease has been dealt with previously in Chapter 5, but the major features will be summarized here. In the plasma of patients with the disease there is present an autoantibody called long acting thyroid stimulating (LATS) antibody. This is an antibody that attaches to the membrane receptors of thyroid gland cells that are normally reserved for TSH. Other autoantibodies are also present and react with other surface proteins of the thyrocytes, either blocking the binding of TSH or alternatively having no effect on thyrocyte function. The LATS antibodies will cause excessive and continuous activity of the thyroid cells with hyperplasia of the gland and hypersecretion of thyroid hormone.

The thyroid gland in Graves' disease becomes enlarged with a noticeable goitre visible in most patients. On section the organ is firm, vascular and fleshy with no prominent colloid-filled follicles. The glandular epithelium is hyperplastic and microscopically the follicles are lined by tall cells that often form groups that project as papillae into the lumen of the follicles. There is a remarkably scalloped margin around the border of the colloid of the follicles, indicating active resorption of colloid. The vessels in the thyroid are prominent and congested, and variable lymphocytic infiltration of the tissue will be seen.

The dysfunction of Graves' disease is related to the overproduction of thyroid hormone and the symptoms and signs associated with the disorder include the following. Ophthalmopathy, which is seen in about three-quarters of patients, comprises retraction of the eyelids and proptosis of the eye, giving rise to **exophthalmos**, a bulging outwards of the eyeball. These changes are the result of increased secretion of catecholamines caused by the hyperthyroidism and also by oedema of the periorbital tissues. Dermopathy affects the skin and many patients show pretibial oedema, with large 20 cm long plaques developing over the tibiae. In the fingers and toes there is oedema and osteoarthropathy causing **acropachy**, a clubbing of the fingers and toes. The patient will also show systemic effects of hyperthyroidism such as **increased metabolic rate**, loss of weight, hyperactivity and anxiety, **hyperhidrosis** (excessive sweating), **tachycardia** (often progressing to arrhythmias, cardiac failure and atrial fibrillation) and **myopathy** with muscle wasting and tremor (refer to Figure 18.6).

Treatment of Graves' disease may be carried out through surgical means with the diseased thyroid being partially removed. The remaining thyroid tissue is sufficient to carry out the functions of the gland. If surgical treatment is not advisable, antithyroid drug treatment may be administered (e.g. propylthiouracil) or alternatively radioactive iodine administration will be followed by sequestration of the radionuclide by the thyroid and its antithyroid effects will last for many years, in some cases to the extent of causing hypothyroidism many years later.

Tumours

Adenoma

The term adenoma of the thyroid gland is often used interchangeably with the term 'thyroid nodule', even when the gland appears to be uniformly nodular as occurs in the case of hyperplasia. It is better to reserve the term 'adenoma' for a true benign tumour that develops in an otherwise non-nodular thyroid. If such a definition of adenoma is adhered to, less than about 5% of nodular thyroids contain these neoplasms. Most patients with these adenomata are over 30 years of age and the sex ratio shows a female predominance to the extent of 4:1.

An adenoma of the thyroid gland is an encapsulated, usually single lesion that is 1 to 5 cm in diameter. When sectioned, the tumour is brownish in colour and appears gelatinous if much colloid is present. If the tumour is more cellular it appears firmer, paler and not gelatinous. Often, cysts, regions of fibrosis, calcification or haemorrhage may be seen within the tumour

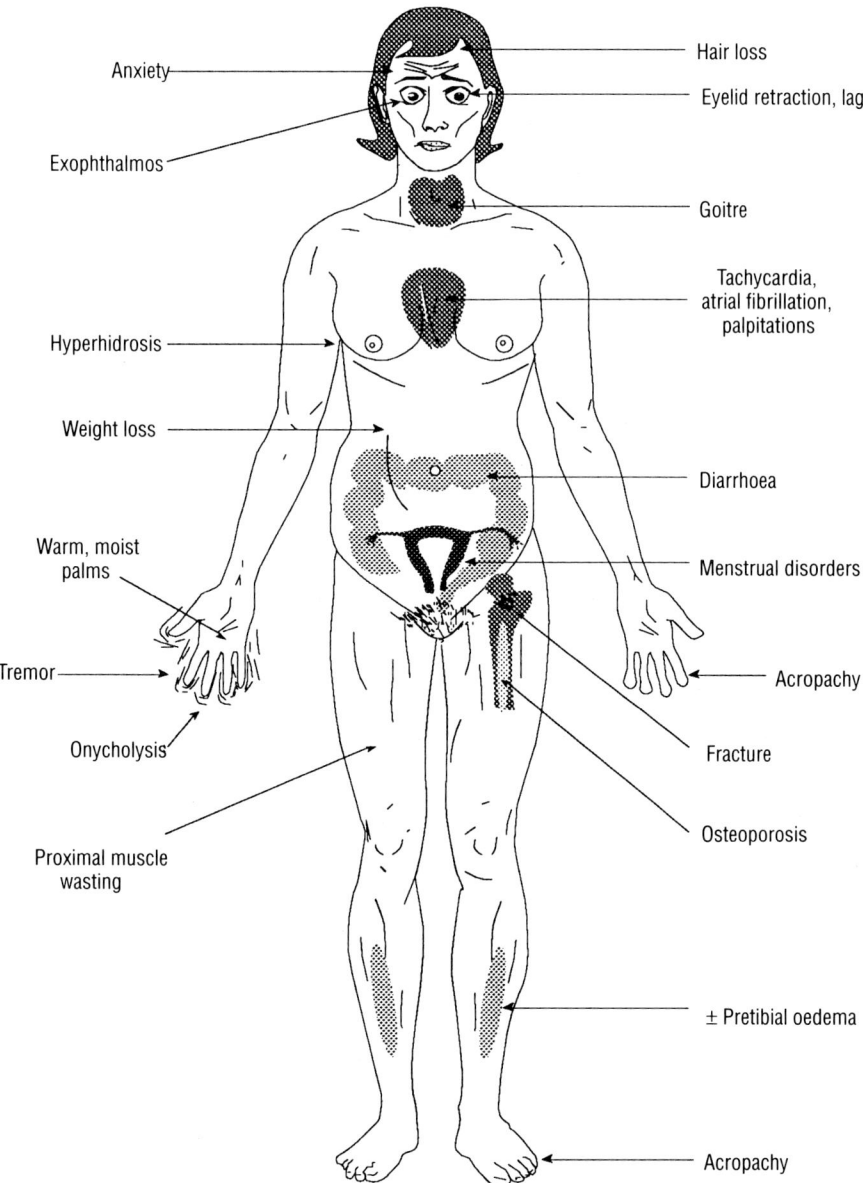

Figure 18.6 *Clinical features of Graves' disease*

mass. A number of different histological types of thyroid adenomata are distinguished:

- **Simple adenoma**: this contains tissue very similar in appearance to normal thyroid tissue, however, a great variation in the size of thyroid follicles may be observed. This is a common type of adenoma.
- **Colloid adenoma**: this type of tumour resembles the simple adenoma, but the follicles are very large

in size and distended with large quantities of colloid. Such types of adenomata are commonly seen.
- **Embryonal adenoma**: the tumour shows a resemblance to embryonic thyroid tissue, with columns of epithelial cells in a loose stroma. There are few or no follicles in this tumour.
- **Foetal adenoma**: a resemblance to foetal thyroid tissue is seen in these tumours, and the follicles which are present are small, have little colloid within

them and are lined by low cuboidal cells. They are separated by stroma and the tumour may often show cyst formation and haemorrhage. Such a tumour is the commonest of the adenomata.

- **Hürthle cell adenoma**: this is an uncommon variant of thyroid adenoma, consisting of a solid nodular aggregate of large, eosinophilic cells that are packed in cords and show little stroma and no follicle formation. The cells on electron microscopy show large, pale nuclei or sometimes small pyknotic nuclei and an abundant cytoplasm with many mitochondria.
- **Papillary adenoma**: this type of tumour is often cystic and the cysts are lined by epithelium that projects into the lumen with many small, papillary projections. In many cases, it is impossible to differentiate this type of adenoma from papillary carcinoma.

Most types of thyroid adenomata follow a typical, benign course in which the tumours grow slowly, are encapsulated, do not invade and do not metastasize. Some adenomata may show malignant change, particularly the Hürthle cell tumours and papillary tumours. Only approximately one in ten adenomata secrete high enough quantities of thyroid hormone to cause hyperthyroidism. In this case, the tumour is termed a **toxic adenoma**. If radioactive iodine is given to patients with adenomata, some tumours will accumulate the radioactive iodine selectively and these are termed 'hot nodules'.

Diagnosis of adenoma of the thyroid is difficult because, clinically, it is difficult to differentiate between non-neoplastic nodules, adenomata and carcinomata. A needle biopsy or an open excisional biopsy may be needed to diagnose the condition definitively. Many cases of adenoma of the thyroid require no treatment, especially if the lesion is small and produces no symptoms and signs other than goitre. If the lesion is large, administration of thyroid hormone may cause a reduction in the size of the adenoma due to suppression of secretion of TSH. Surgical excision is sometimes performed, especially if the tumour is a toxic adenoma. Radioactive iodine sometimes may be used in the treatment of 'hot adenomata' as these lesions accumulate the most radioactive iodine and are most damaged by the radiation.

An **adenoma of parafollicular cells** may rarely occur in the thyroid and this is a tumour of the C cells that normally secrete calcitonin. The lesion is solid, pinkish brown and encapsulated. Under the microscope the lesion is seen to consist of small, closely packed cuboidal cells that by immunohistochemical methods may be seen to contain calcitonin.

Carcinoma

Carcinoma of the thyroid gland is not a common tumour, accounting for only about 1% of all malignant tumours. The tumour occurs typically in middle to old age and affects women more than men in the ratio of 3:1. The tumour may be associated with benign lesions of the thyroid but it is also seen more frequently in some countries where endemic goitre is common, for example Switzerland, where one in 8000 people develop the tumour per year compared to Australia where one in 25 000 people develop the tumour per year. Predisposing factors to the development of carcinoma of the thyroid include irradiation of the thyroid region during childhood, the presence of adenomata of the thyroid, and possibly conditions of long-standing oversecretion of TSH. Irradiation of the thyroid in adulthood does not predispose to any great extent to thyroid carcinoma.

About 90% of tumours are of follicular cell origin and the rest are derived from the parafollicular cells; this latter type of tumour is termed **medullary carcinoma**. Carcinoma of the follicular cells is subdivided into many types and each of them has different macroscopic and microscopic appearance. The types of tumour that are found in the thyroid are:

- **Papillary carcinoma**: such a carcinoma is a well-differentiated tumour of a low-grade malignancy, which will nevertheless metastasize to the draining regional lymph nodes, often the affected lymph nodes being larger than the primary tumour mass in the thyroid. However, more distant metastases are rare and will be seen only in untreated cases after many years. This type of tumour is often found in children and young adults. The tumour cells are grouped in branching, frond-like arrangements, with occasionally some follicles also present.
- **Follicular carcinoma**: this tumour is also a slowly growing one and, as is the case with the papillary carcinoma, it may grow for many years and give rise to no symptoms. The tumour tissue consists of cuboidal to columnar cells arranged in acinar structures. Metastasis to the lymph nodes will occur and also to the lungs, liver and bone.
- **Anaplastic carcinoma**: this tumour forms a hard, irregular enlargement of the thyroid and consists of irregular clumps or cords of pleomorphic cells with no follicles formed and no resemblance to thyroid tissue. The tumour may resemble fibrosarcoma or lymphosarcoma microscopically. These carcinomata are very aggressive and will metastasize widely and quickly.

- **Medullary carcinoma**: this is a rare type of thyroid carcinoma and arises from the parafollicular cells. The tumour usually grows slowly and at presentation the patient will only show spread to involve the local lymph nodes. This tumour secretes calcitonin and the level in the plasma may be up to about 40 times the normal level, but usually there are no ill effects associated with this, hypocalcaemia seen in only a few patients. Other hormones may also be secreted, including ACTH, prolactin and VIP.

Usually only carcinomata that contain well-differentiated follicles are likely to be able to secrete thyroid hormone. Therefore, if radioactive iodine is administered only a small proportion of patients will show a 'hot nodule' in the region of the carcinoma. Uncommonly, a patient may show hyperthyroidism in association with a well-differentiated carcinoma that secretes excessive quantities of thyroid hormones. Most patients have either euthyroid or hypothyroid status, the quantity of thyroid hormones that they are secreting reflecting the quantity of normal thyroid tissue which is remaining undamaged by the tumour.

Treatment of thyroid carcinoma is in most cases by surgical means, a partial or total thyroidectomy being performed with dissection of the regional lymph nodes. Radioactive iodine may be given as an adjunctive treatment to surgery, or when there is widespread metastatic disease. The patient is also given supplements of thyroid hormones as they are required. Most patients with papillary carcinoma have a very good prognosis with treatment, only a small proportion of them dying as a result of their tumour. On the other hand, patients with anaplastic carcinoma have a very poor prognosis, almost all patients dying within a year of diagnosis. With follicular and medullary carcinoma the 10-year prognosis for the tumours is 50% with treatment.

Parathyroid Gland Diseases

Hypoparathyroidism

The cause of hypoparathyroidism is almost always due to the inadvertent removal of the glands during surgical procedures involving ablation of the thyroid. Other causes are neck surgery that may damage the blood supply to the parathyroids, or in some rare cases infection of the thyroid and parathyroids. Primary hypoparathyroidism may also occur very rarely, and in this case there is idiopathic hypofunction of the glands.

The primary features of hypoparathyroidism are hypocalcaemia and hyperphosphataemia. There is a reduction in the amount of calcium resorbed by the kidneys and the amount of phosphate retained is increased. Bone resorption is reduced and gut absorption of calcium is impaired. If the condition develops acutely, the plasma levels of calcium will decrease dramatically over a short period of time and the disease manifests itself as **tetany** and hyperexcitability of the nerves. Muscle spasm, abdominal cramps, bronchospasm, biliary colic or spasm of the glottis occur. There may paraesthesiae of the hands, feet or of the mouth. The patient becomes depressed, confused and irritable, occasionally suffering from hallucinations. If the condition occurs in children and it persists untreated it may cause mental retardation.

Hypoparathyroidism developing over a more prolonged time period will manifest itself as skin changes that are reminiscent of myxoedema. The skin becomes dry, coarse and prone to developing eczematous and psoriatic lesions. Thinning and falling out of the hair also occur and the nails become brittle and split easily. The eyes may show cataracts if the hypoparathyroidism becomes chronic. *Candida albicans* infections of the skin and its appendages are common in these individuals.

The treatment for hypoparathyroidism is initially by intravenous calcium preparations to restore normal plasma levels and relieve the muscle and neurological manifestations. Longer term treatment involves increased oral calcium and vitamin D supplements, but this is a treatment that must be carefully monitored as vitamin D intoxication may develop. In most patients this form of treatment is adequate to maintain normal levels of plasma calcium, and thus a lifetime of parathormone injections is avoided (parathormone cannot be administered orally).

Hyperparathyroidism

Primary Hyperparathyroidism

Approximately one person in every 1000 will secrete excessive quantities of parathormone, although this excess is in most cases a slight one and will not adversely affect the individual. As the age of the person increases, the hyperparathyroidism is more likely to become clinically significant and most patients suffering from adverse effects of hyperparathyroidism are over 40 years of age. About 70% of patients are female. The causes of primary hyperparathyroidism reside within the gland itself and are idiopathic. The disease arises because of:

- **adenoma** of the parathyroid in one or more glands (84% of cases);

- **hyperplasia** of the parathyroids in about 15% of cases;
- **carcinoma** of the parathyroids in less than about 1% of cases.

Rarely, hyperparathyroidism may develop if a carcinoma elsewhere in the body (e.g. carcinoma of the bronchus) secretes a parathormone-like substance.

If adenoma is the cause of the condition, the glands show a single nodule of tumour (multiple adenomata are only present in 5% of cases) which is usually in the lower glands. The adenoma is an encapsulated lesion, of a reddish brown colour, varying greatly in size from case to case but rarely larger than 1 cm in diameter. The microscopical appearance is variable with about half of the tumours composed of mainly chief cells, the remaining half being composed of mixtures of cell types. The carcinomata resemble the adenomata, except that invasion is seen and the encapsulation of the mass is incomplete or absent. Hyperplastic glands are uniformly enlarged, sometimes attaining a combined weight of 20 g or more. Increased quantities of adipose tissue in the parathyroids with diffuse nodularity and enlargement suggest that hyperplasia is present rather than an adenoma.

Primary hyperparathyroidism manifests itself through effects caused by hypersecretion of parathormone. The most important effect is rise in plasma calcium, which will cause depression, constipation and polyuria. Most commonly, patients with primary hyperparathyroidism present with renal calculi and metastatic calcification lesions in the blood vessels, stomach and kidney. As the elevated calcium in the blood is due to excessive resorption of bone, the condition may be detected radiologically as subperiosteal erosions in the phalanges. Von Reckinghausen's disease of bone will result in long-term untreated cases of the disease.

Diagnosis of the condition depends on demonstration of elevated levels of plasma calcium and PTH and a variety of other biochemical findings, including:

- decreased plasma phosphate and decreased renal tubular reabsorption of phosphate;
- increased renal tubular reabsorption of calcium;
- increased serum alkaline phosphatase;
- increased urinary hydroxyproline excretion.

Treatment of primary hyperparathyroidism is surgical in most cases, the adenomata, carcinomata or hyperplastic tissue being removed. The carcinomata tend to grow slowly and tend to spread locally rather than metastasizing to distant sites, and hence are associated with a good prognosis. In some cases the surgeon may not be able to localize all of the affected glandular tissue and the disease may recur after surgery.

Secondary Hyperparathyroidism

Secondary hyperparathyroidism will occur whenever there is lowering of the plasma calcium levels or raising of the plasma phosphate concentration. The condition may be seen in pregnancy and lactation where there is a drain of body calcium, it may be seen in association with renal diseases (especially chronic renal failure, or renal tubular disorders such as Fanconi's syndrome), or it may be associated with the malabsorption syndrome and steatorrhoea.

The glands are enlarged but not as markedly as in the primary condition. The microscopic appearance shows a loss of adipocytes and increased numbers of parenchymal cells, mainly chief cells. Diagnosis depends on demonstration of raised PTH levels, raised alkaline phosphatase and raised plasma phosphate. Serum calcium is low to normal and there are the characteristic radiological spinal changes known as 'rugger jersey spine'. Most often, patients with secondary hyperparathyroidism will present with whatever symptoms and signs are due to the primary disease. The patient will only develop renal osteodystrophy and metastatic calcification in very severe cases that remain untreated.

Secondary hyperparathyroidism may be regarded in most cases as a response by the body to dropping calcium levels in the bloodstream and is an attempt to re-establish a new equilibrium; thus in most cases, hyperactivity of the glands is beneficial for the patient, the calcium and phosphate levels stabilizing to normal concentrations in the plasma as a new equilibrium is attained. In severe, long-standing, untreated cases of secondary hyperparathyroidism, complications will develop. This is especially true where renal disease is the cause of the hyperparathyroidism. The increased secretion of parathormone in such patients will not be sufficient and hypocalcaemia with hyperphosphataemia will occur. Renal osteodystrophy will supervene and osteoporosis and osteomalacia or osteitis fibrosa cystica will develop in the bones. Metastatic calcification will be seen in the kidneys, arteries, skin and conjunctivae.

The treatment of secondary hyperparathyroidism varies greatly depending on the patient presentation. Mild forms of the disease may require no treatment. If the primary disease which is causing the hyperparathyroidism is treated, the condition of excess parathormone production will be controlled also and the parathyroid function will return to normal. If the condition is severe, restriction of dietary intake of phosphorus or increased calcium and vitamin D in the diet will help to control the bone changes. Severe bone disease is less likely to occur with secondary hyperparathyroidism than it is with primary hyperparathyroidism.

Tertiary hyperparathyroidism is sometimes seen to supervene in severe cases of secondary hyperparathyroidism, and in this condition an adenoma of the parathyroids will complicate the disease, making the patient present with symptoms and signs similar to primary hyperparathyroidism. Even if the cause of secondary hyperparathyroidism is treated, the hyperfunction of the parathyroids will continue as the adenoma will continue to secrete large quantities of parathormone.

Pituitary Gland Diseases

Hypofunction

Adenohypophyseal Hypofunction

Growth Hormone Deficiency — Dwarfism
The deficiency of growth hormone production in children is a congenital defect that may be inherited as a Mendelian character with a variety of patterns of transmission, most commonly as an autosomal recessive trait. Occasionally it may be caused by congenital malformations in the region, tumours, trauma or infarction of the pituitary. Adult growth hormone deficiency may be caused by tumours in the pituitary or adjacent tissues, surgical removal or radiotherapy of the gland, infections, infarction or non-specific inflammations of the gland. A special variety of necrosis of the anterior pituitary is known as **Sheehan's syndrome** and develops as a complication of childbirth in the obstetric patient who has suffered from circulatory collapse. In this case the hyperplastic anterior pituitary gland, which is under increased tension (an effect of pregnancy), is more likely to undergo ischaemia either because of spasm of the arteries supplying this part of the gland or because of disseminated intravascular coagulation. The necrotic part of the pituitary in all of these cases undergoes fibrosis but the neurohypophysis usually remains intact.

The most serious effects of growth hormone deficiency occur in children, in adults the deficiency causing no symptoms or dysfunction and therefore needing no treatment. A child who has a deficiency of growth hormone at birth will appear to grow normally for a few months, but after this, growth is retarded and the epiphyseal growth plates mature slowly, making the bone look as though it is that of a much younger infant. The growth of the teeth is delayed and the child is of small stature, plump, with small hands and feet and small, underdeveloped genitalia. Puberty occurs late and although growth continues for longer than normal, stature is greatly reduced. Intelligence is usually normal and the body proportions are normal, although the affected person never attains full height, a pituitary dwarf being 100 to 140 cm high (see Figure 18.7).

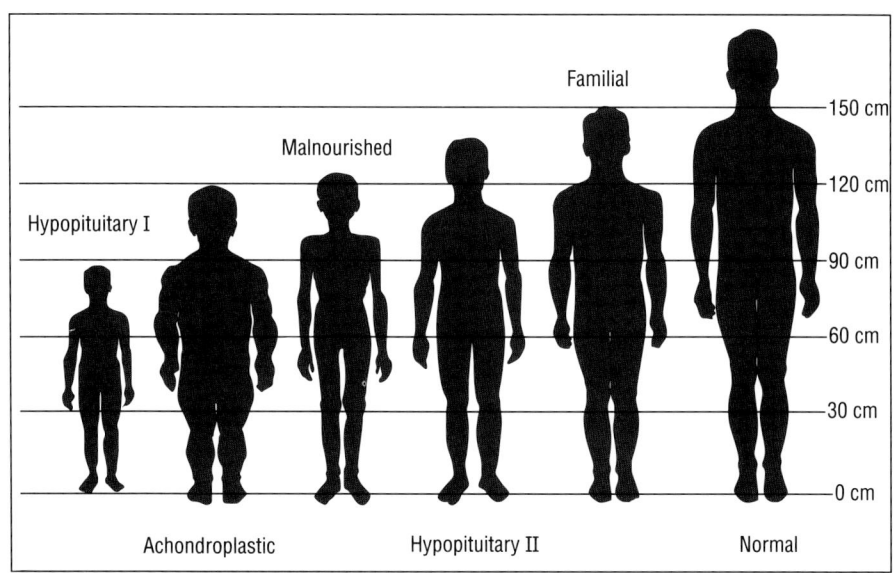

Figure 18.7 *Hypopituitary dwarfs compared to other types of dwarfs*

In most cases, the decreased stature is not due to a deficiency of growth hormone but rather a decreased sensitivity of the body tissues to the effects of the hormone, these individuals showing pituitary dwarfism type II. Only one in 1000 children of short stature have a demonstrable defect in growth hormone production, and these are said to show pituitary dwarfism type I. If the defect in the production of growth hormone is linked with defects in the production of other hormones, most commonly gonadotrophins, the child shows abnormal growth together with genital hypoplasia and is said to suffer from the **Peter Pan type of hypopituitarism** (or **Lorain type**). These patients are of normal intelligence, have childlike features, poor muscular development, poor reproductive system development but show normal bodily proportions. Often the height of these pituitary dwarfs is less than 100 cm and later in life they may show obesity due to the absence of the lipolytic effects of growth hormone.

Familial dwarfs have normal pituitary function but have inherited fewer genes regulating height from their (short) parents. Height is a trait regulated by a number of codominant alleles and the more dominant genes that are present in an individual, the taller that person is. A familial dwarf has fewer of these dominant genes than a tall person. If the familial dwarf has a child with a partner who is tall, the offspring will have a height intermediate to that of the parents. Achondroplastic dwarfs have a Mendelian genetic abnormality in the growth of the long bones and this condition has already been covered in detail in the chapter on disorders of bone. Dwarfism may also be seen in cases of extreme malnutrition where the food intake is insufficient for the normal build-up of body tissues. Hence the affected individual is much shorter than normal, greatly emaciated and usually shows other effects of poor nutrition, for example generalized oedema, ascites and skin lesions.

Diagnosis of growth hormone deficiency can be demonstrated by the insulin challenge test, where a dose of insulin sufficient to lower blood sugar levels to below 2 mmol/L is given to a fasting person. In a normal person there is a rise in the plasma growth hormone levels to more than 8 µg/L, while in the person with growth hormone deficiency the plasma levels of the hormone remain lower than 2 µg/L. The condition in children is treated by intramuscular injections of growth hormone, which has the effect of re-establishing normal growth. The treatment is continued until the epiphyses fuse and normal adult height is reached.

Progeria

Progeria is a rare, idiopathic disorder which develops in children that appear normal as babies. However, after a variable period of normal growth that may last between a few months to a few years, growth slows and stops, the epiphyseal plates fuse and the child begins to show signs of premature ageing. The skin becomes thin and atrophic, hair whitens and falls out and diseases of old age such as atherosclerosis, neoplasms and dementia, with all of their complications, will cause the death of the child in the early teens from 'old age'.

TSH Deficiency

Deficiency of TSH is usually always associated with deficiency of growth hormone and gonadotrophins, although, rarely, isolated TSH deficiency occurs as a congenital defect. The defect causes mild hypothyroidism, the symptoms, signs and clinical history all suggesting pituitary disease rather than thyroid gland disease as the cause of decreased thyroid hormone levels. The levels of TSH in the plasma are low or absent, in contrast to other forms of hypothyroidism where TSH levels are elevated. Thyroid hormone replacement therapy is given to these patients.

ACTH Deficiency

The deficiency of ACTH is usually associated with other adenohypophyseal hormone deficiencies, although rarely a pure ACTH deficiency occurs congenitally. The result is an adrenocortical hormone insufficiency, the affected individuals responding abnormally to stressful situations with nausea, vomiting or collapse. The skin is pale and the nipples are not highly pigmented as MSH levels are also low, this hormone being synthesized in association with ACTH. Individuals with ACTH deficiency do not show hypoaldosteronism because the secretion of aldosterone is maintained by the renin system. Various tests are used to confirm ACTH deficiency, namely, the insulin administration test or metyrapone administration test. The deficiency of adrenocortical hormones is treated by administering prednisone or hydrocortisone.

Gonadotrophin Deficiency

Gonadotrophin deficiency is often a congenital disorder that is seen in children, but it may also develop in adults when there is destruction of the pituitary due to any cause. In the affected children the absence of gonadotrophins will interfere with normal development of the reproductive system and development of normal secondary sexual characteristics.

Affected boys show poorly developed testes with

marked reduction in the circulating androgen levels. This causes failure of epiphyseal plate fusion, which if combined with normal growth hormone secretion will lead to very elongated limbs that are osteoporotic. The penis and testes remain small and the prostate does not grow to its adult size. The beard fails to grow, axillary and chest hair is scant, pubic hair is fine and the larynx remains small and the voice high pitched. Girls with gonadotrophin deficiency show amenorrhoea and the failure of breast development. The arms and legs become abnormally long because of failure of epiphyseal plate fusion and the hair in the pubic and axillary regions may be very fine and scant or completely absent.

Adults with gonadotrophin deficiency will show reduction in body hair, development of wrinkled skin in association with loss of dermal collagen, and in women there is amenorrhoea. If the deficiency is severe, there will be shrinkage of the breasts, atrophy of the uterus in women, and in men shrinkage of the testes, impotence and loss of libido. The circulating LH and FSH levels are low, although several samples of the patients' blood must be analysed in order to demonstrate the low levels because of episodic secretion of gonadotrophins in some cases of the disorder.

Treatment of the condition in females is through the administration of the contraceptive pill, which will cause an induction of menstruation and maintain normal breast size. Males are given dosages of testosterone sufficient to induce or maintain secondary sexual characteristics. If a person of either sex who is on this therapy wishes to become fertile, human gonadotrophins must be administered in order to stimulate normal ovarian and testicular function.

Panhypopituitarism — Simmonds' Disease

Panhypopituitarism develops when all of the hormones produced by the adenohypophysis are produced in very low quantities or not at all. Clinically, the signs and symptoms will depend on the severity of the hormone deficiencies, but usually in adults the hypogonadism is the most prominent feature while in children the growth hormone deficiency effects are the most conspicuous. Patients with severe panhypopituitarism show a pale skin with loss of capillary flushing, depigmentation, loss of body hair, genital hypoplasia and infertility, somnolence, weight gain, mental slowness and apathy, sensitivity to cold, puffy face and progression to coma. All of these are effects of the pituitary hormone deficiency or deficiency of the hormones produced by endocrine glands on which trophic hormones have an effect. Treatment of the condition involves correction of the multiple hormonal deficiencies that are demonstrated in the diagnosis of the condition.

Neurohypophyseal Hypofunction

Diabetes Insipidus

Diabetes insipidus is a condition caused by a deficiency in the production of ADH by the neurohypophysis. Diabetes is a term which implies production of an increased volume of urine, leading to polyuria, while insipidus refers to the insipid taste of the extremely dilute urine produced by these patients, in contrast to diabetes mellitus where the urine has a sweet taste. This condition is not related to diabetes mellitus, the only common factors being the polyuria that is seen in both disorders and the fact that both are due to hormonal dysfunction. Although diabetes insipidus is caused usually by posterior pituitary disorders, it may also be caused by renal tubular dysfunction, where the responsiveness of the renal tubules to ADH is reduced. This renal lesion may be congenital or acquired, as occurs after administration of drugs such as lithium salts or demeclocycline.

Pituitary-caused diabetes insipidus usually affects young adults, the sex ratio being equal. The condition may result if there is damage to the fibres of the hypothalamohypophyseal tract, which will cause a retrograde degeneration of the cell bodies. About a third of patients have demonstrable tumours that cause this damage; adenomata, craniopharyngiomata, pinealomata or metastatic tumours may be the cause. In about a third of cases diabetes insipidus is caused by surgical procedures, radiotherapy, meningitis, cerebral trauma or systemic disease (e.g. sarcoidosis). The remaining third of the cases have 'idiopathic' causes, although there is evidence that such cases may be of an inherited nature, several inheritance patterns being apparently involved, with usually an autosomal dominant or sex-linked recessive trait being demonstrated.

Patients with diabetes insipidus of a pituitary aetiology will present with a sudden onset of polyuria and polydipsia, with between 5 L and 20 L of urine passed daily, the specific gravity of the urine being less than 1.010, its osmolality less than 290 mmol/kg. The patient will usually drink enough cold drinks to maintain hydration. Various tests may be performed in order to diagnose diabetes insipidus and differentiate it from compulsive water drinking that may mimic the condition. The **water deprivation test** involves depriving the patient of water until the urine osmolality becomes constant (usually around about 10 to 12 hours) with a loss of 1 kg in weight. ADH is then administered subcutaneously. If this causes a 9% or more increase in urine osmolality, the diabetes insipidus is due to posterior pituitary causes. Normal people will have an increase in urine osmolality that is less than 9%, while people with renal causes of diabetes insipidus will show no change in urine osmolality. Another test performed is that of **hypertonic saline infusion** involving intravenous injection of hypertonic saline determining if there is a threshold where ADH production begins. In diabetes insipidus caused by pituitary aetiologies, no threshold will be found, even if the plasma osmolality is raised to over 300 mmol/kg. It should be noted that these tests are performed under the strictest controls, since inadequate fluid intake may cause dehydration with disorientation, weakness, fever, collapse or death.

Treatment of pituitary-caused diabetes insipidus is with drugs such as desmopressin or other synthetic hormones given intranasally or parenterally. If some hormone is being secreted by the pituitary, drugs such as clofibrate or chlorpropamide can increase secretion of ADH and increase sensitivity of renal tubules to ADH. Adequate hydration of the patient must be maintained.

Other Syndromes

Fröhlich's syndrome or dystrophia adiposogenitalis is a rare condition that affects children and causes obesity, genital hypoplasia, growth inhibition and pronounced mental retardation. Diabetes insipidus, visual disturbances and somnolence may also be seen in some cases. Boys are affected more than girls in Frölich's syndrome and the condition is caused by any lesion that damages the hypothalamus, thus causing interference with the production of gonadotrophins and disturbance to the eating centre.

The **Laurence-Moon-Biedl syndrome** is a genetic disorder inherited as an autosomal recessive character, presumably causing hypothalamic dysfunction although no lesions are demonstrable in the region. Affected children show similar features to those observed in Frölich's syndrome, but in addition have retinitis pigmentosa causing night blindness, polydactyly and syndactyly, and occasionally other congenital malformations.

The **diencephalic syndrome** is a disease caused by the involvement of the hypothalamus by astrocytoma in infants. The child eats well but becomes emaciated and has nystagmus, and is of an extremely affectionate disposition. Usually, most children die within a year of diagnosis but if they survive they may become obese.

Hyperfunction

Adenohypophyseal Hyperfunction

Growth Hormone Excess in Children — Gigantism
Growth hormone excess is usually caused by an adenoma of the pituitary. If this adenoma occurs before puberty, the excessive growth hormone produced by the tumour will cause abnormal growth of the whole body, especially marked during puberty, the affected person showing gigantism. The final height of these individuals may be as much as 2.8 m and their weight above 200 kg. Both the skeleton and soft tissues show proportional growth, but as the individual ages there is a predisposition to skeletal deformities, for example kyphosis and scoliosis. In later life, the adenoma may cause hypopituitarism with amenorrhoea and hypogonadism due to the deficiency of gonadotrophins. The growth may continue after epiphyseal fusion, leading to an acromegalic giant. Treatment of the condition is as for adenoma of the pituitary (see the section on tumours of the pituitary below).

Growth Hormone Excess in Adults — Acromegaly
Growth hormone excess due to an adenoma developing after epiphyseal plate fusion will cause the condition of acromegaly. The condition is usually seen between the ages of 20 and 40 years and one person per 300 000 will develop the condition every year, males and females affected equally. The effects of the excessive growth hormone will be seen mainly in bones that are still able to grow after epiphyseal fusion (i.e. the costochondral junctions, mandibular condyles, subperiosteally in most bones), in the soft tissues and viscera. The patients usually suffer from the disease for many years before presentation but the change is so subtle that they and the people in their immediate environment are not able to detect the changes in the appearance of the sufferer until the disease is quite advanced.

The affected person shows generally thickened bones and an enlarged, protruding lower jaw, prominent supraorbital ridges, and enlarged bones and cartilages of the chest leading to a thorax of enlarged diameter. The long bones are bowed, osteoarthritis develops and later in the disease osteoporosis will be evident, with collapse of the vertebrae, neuritis and myopathy. The hands and feet enlarge greatly mainly because of increased soft tissue deposition, often leading to a change in shoe size. The tongue, lips and ears grow larger and coarser and the skin thickens and shows exaggerated wrinkling, pigmentation, hair growth and sweating. The viscera also enlarge, sometimes attaining a weight of three times the normal. The voice deepens because of laryngeal enlargement and the endocrine glands become hyperplastic and nodular (see Figure 18.8).

Insulin resistance caused by excessive growth hormone levels occurs in about 80% of cases and about 15% will develop diabetes mellitus, this occurring especially in people genetically predisposed to the condition. Systemic hypertension develops in a quarter of cases and cardiomegaly with congestive heart failure is a common finding in such cases. Hyperparathyroidism will cause hypercalcaemia in many cases and renal calculi will be found in about 20% of patients. Increased levels of prolactin will be found in about half the patients and in some cases these increases are enough to cause amenorrhoea, galactorrhoea or reduction in libido. Other endocrine system dysfunction such as hyperthyroidism will be found in a smaller number of cases. Clinically, many patients will present with headache, ocular disturbances, arthralgia, muscular weakness and paraesthesiae.

As over 90% of cases of acromegaly are caused by

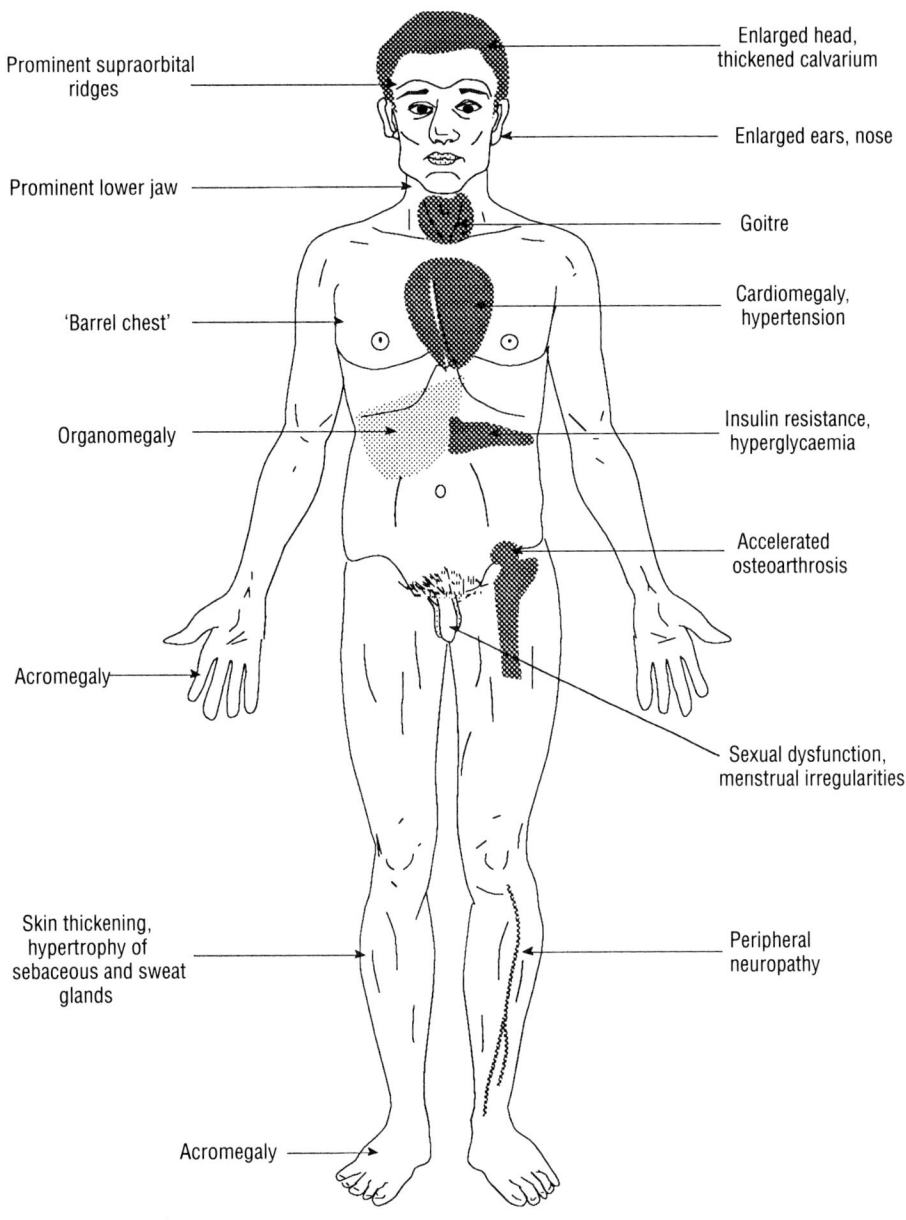

Prominent supraorbital ridges

Prominent lower jaw

'Barrel chest'

Organomegaly

Acromegaly

Skin thickening, hypertrophy of sebaceous and sweat glands

Acromegaly

Enlarged head, thickened calvarium

Enlarged ears, nose

Goitre

Cardiomegaly, hypertension

Insulin resistance, hyperglycaemia

Accelerated osteoarthrosis

Sexual dysfunction, menstrual irregularities

Peripheral neuropathy

Figure 18.8 *Systemic manifestations of acromegaly*

an adenoma, surgical treatment and/or radiotherapy is the major form of management of the disorder (see the section on adenoma below). In a small number of cases, no adenoma will be found in the pituitary, but rather a diffuse hyperplasia of the growth hormone cells of the adenohypophysis will cause the acromegaly. Bromocriptine treatment will lower the growth hormone levels in the plasma, but alone will not control the disorder. The prognosis of patients is excellent following surgical ablation of a localized tumour.

Other Hormone Excesses

Rarely, other hormone excesses of the adenohypophysis will occur and these will cause dysfunction associated with the target organs on which they have a trophic effect. **Cushing's disease** will be caused by excessive secretion of ACTH, usually by a corticotroph adenoma. **Hyperprolactinaemia** will cause amenorrhoea, galactorrhoea and infertility in women, reduction in libido, impotence, rarely gynaecomastia and galactorrhoea in men. The cause is usually an adenoma of the pituitary and approximately three-quarters of all women presenting with amenorrhoea and galactorrhoea suffer from this condition. About 10% of impotent men suffer from hyperprolactinaemia. Rarely, adenomata of the pituitary will cause **hyperthyroidism** due to excessive TSH production, and **increased gonadotrophin** production that is occasionally associated with gynaecomastia in men and precocious puberty in children.

Neurohypophyseal Hyperfunction

Primary hypersecretion of the hormones of the neurohypophysis does not occur. Secondary hypersecretion may be seen in association with some pathological states, most commonly cardiac failure and other conditions precipitating generalized oedema. In some cases, lung lesions such as tuberculosis, COAD, pneumonitis or lung abscesses will cause an excess of ADH production by the pituitary because of a reduced blood volume being returned to the left atrium. Injury to the pituitary or hypothalamus will sometimes be associated with excessive ADH production. Some extracranial tumours may produce ADH, the most common neoplasms that do so being oat cell carcinoma of the lungs, carcinoma of the pancreas or lymphoma.

An excess of ADH in the body will cause retention of water in the body, loss of sodium in the urine and generalized oedema with hypotonic interstitial fluid. The plasma concentration of sodium is less than 120 mmol/L and the urinary concentration of sodium is more than 20 mmol/L. The concentrations of chloride, creatinine, albumin and uric acid in the plasma are also low. Treatment of the condition involves replacement of sodium and chloride with restriction of water intake. Treatment of the primary condition (if possible) relieves the secondary hypersecretion of ADH.

Tumours

Adenoma

Adenoma of the pituitary gland is the commonest tumour in this organ, accounting for approximately 11% of primary intracranial neoplasms. Each of the specialized secretory cells in the gland may undergo neoplastic transformation and the resulting tumour usually shows hormone production associated with the particular cell type from which the tumour arose (see Table 18.4). The hormone produced by the cells may be demonstrated by immunoelectron microscopy of the tumour, or occasionally the amount of hormone production may be enough to cause dysfunction.

The adenomata are usually spheroidal in shape and range in size from microscopic to a few centimetres in diameter. They may be extremely slow growing tumours, thus producing no symptoms or signs at all during the individual's life and approximately 10% of autopsied people will show such a small, asymptomatic pituitary adenoma. These tumours will produce little or no hormone and will cause no wholesale destruction of the pituitary or adjacent structures during the patient's life, hence they are clinically silent. Pituitary adenomata that are symptomatic constitute less than 5% of intracranial tumours. Adenomata of this gland usually arise in adulthood, most patients being between 30 and 50 years of age, with an equal sex incidence. The only exception is the prolactin cell adenoma that usually affects women between 20 and 40 years of age.

If the tumour is visible with the naked eye, it forms a spheroidal or lobulated structure that is surrounded by a thin fibrous capsule. The neoplasm is a brownish red colour reflecting its very good blood supply. Microscopically, adenomata of the pituitary are composed of sheets of regular cells with much cytoplasm and small, spherical, dense, regular nuclei. Acidophilic adenomata have a red granular cytoplasm, basophilic adenomata a blue granular cytoplasm while chromophobe tumours have no granules in the pale cytoplasm. The staining character of the neoplasm depends on the number of secretory granules in the tumour cells and may be correlated with the amount of hormone pro-

Table 18.4 *The pituitary adenomata*

Adenoma type	Staining features	Percentage incidence	Clinical effects due to hormones
Growth hormone cell	Acidophilic or chromophobe	≈ 20	Acromegaly in adults or gigantism in children
Prolactin cell	Acidophilic or chromophobe	≈ 30	Amenorrhoea, infertility, galactorrhoea in women. Delayed puberty and hypogonadism in males
Mixed growth/ prolactin cell	Acidophilic or chromophobe	9	Mixtures of the above clinical effects
Corticotroph cell	Basophilic or chromophobe	15	Cushing's disease
Gonadotroph cell	Basophilic or chromophobe	3	Usually no clinical effects, although in men high levels of FSH and LH demonstrable
Thyrotroph cell	Basophilic or chromophobe	< 1	Mild hyperthyroidism
Null cell	Chromophobe, acidophilic or basophilic	≈ 25	No hormone is secreted by these tumours

duced by the cells, tumours with markedly granular cells being likely to produce clinical effects due to excessive hormone production.

The symptoms and signs attributable to pituitary adenomata are largely due to the space-occupying effects of the tumour and are independent of hormone production by the neoplasm. In about half of the patients with symptomatic tumours, the first symptom is visual disturbance taking the form of unilateral blindness, bitemporal hemianopia or scotomata, all effects of the tumour compressing the optic nerves. Eventually as many as three-quarters of all patients with pituitary adenomata will develop a headache, and about a sixth of patients will complain of headache as the first symptom. A third of patients will have symptoms attributable to excessive hormone production (see Table 18.4) or symptoms due to hypopituitarism caused by destruction of the gland by the tumour. In some patients, adenomata of the pituitary will develop in association with the multiple endocrine neoplasia (MEN) syndrome.

Treatment of pituitary adenomata is usually surgical, although if the treatment is only by excision, recurrence of the tumour within 10 years of the operation will occur in half of the patients. If radiotherapy is given after surgery, only 15% patients will have a recurrence of the tumour. Radiotherapy alone will control the growth of pituitary neoplasms, but if the tumour is hormonally active, the concentration of hormone in the blood falls very slowly, as opposed to the immediate reduction of hormone levels that is seen following surgery. Radiotherapy of the pituitary may cause hypopituitarism in some patients. Drug treatment may control small prolactin-secreting tumours, the dopamine agonist, bromocriptine, being used. The prognosis of pituitary adenomata is relatively good if the tumour is treated.

Craniopharyngioma

Craniopharyngioma is a tumour derived from the remnants of Rathke's pouch, embryologically derived from the pharyngeal epithelium. It constitutes approximately 5% of all intracranial tumours, typically arising in children or young adults. Most tumours arise above the diaphragm of the sella turcica and when diagnosed the tumour has invaded locally, to erode the base of the brain, optic and other cranial nerves, extending into the anterior, middle or posterior cranial fossa. Craniopharyngiomata may grow into the third ventricle, destroy the pituitary stalk or invade the sella.

With the naked eye, the tumour appears as a solid, well demarcated, brownish grey mass that frequently contains cysts, foci of cholesterol crystal accumulation, calcification and necrosis. Microscopically, craniopharyngiomata consist of masses of squamous epithelial cells arranged in clumps or cords, sometimes showing keratin pearl formation. The groups of tumour cells are sometimes lined by an outer region of columnar cells arranged in a palisade fashion, making the tumour resemble a basal cell carcinoma or an adamantinoma.

The tumours are of low-grade malignancy and although they invade locally they will not metastasize. As the tumour grows it compresses the adjacent structures and pressure atrophy of the pituitary gland in about a third of patients will result in hypopituitarism; the tumour itself is not hormonally active. Extension of the tumour to involve the hypothalamus will interfere with regulation of pituitary function and an excess secretion of prolactin may result. Compression of the cranial nerves may lead to the same symptoms and signs as a pituitary adenoma. Because of the delicate situation in which the tumour develops surgical resection is very difficult, but if it can be effected, it is curative.

Malignant Tumours

Carcinoma of the pituitary gland is rarely seen and in most cases arises *de novo*, although a few patients with a pre-existing adenoma may progress to a carcinoma. The tumour is most often of the chromophobe type and is not hormonally active. Because of local invasion and destruction of the adjacent tissues, the tumour may cause hypopituitarism. Occasionally, a carcinoma may show hormonal effects and in this case the cellular population is a mixed one.

Astrocytoma may rarely occur in the posterior pituitary, the infundibular stalk or hypothalamus. This tumour behaves in the same way that astrocytomata elsewhere in the brain behave, but in addition it may cause diabetes insipidus or malfunction of the anterior pituitary. Both this tumour and carcinoma of the pituitary tend to have a poor prognosis.

Secondary Tumours

Secondary tumours of the pituitary gland are not common, being found in about 3% of patients dying of malignant disease. They are most often derived from carcinomata of the breast, bronchus, colon and pros-

tate, usually affecting the posterior part of the gland. In most cases the tumours are not large enough to cause hormonal dysfunction, but occasionally hypopituitarism may be the result of metastatic tumour growth in the pituitary.

Pineal Gland Diseases

Pinealoma

The rare tumours of the pineal gland are often called collectively **pinealomata**, although they are a diverse group of neoplasms. Three-quarters of pineal tumours are germ cell tumours such as teratomata or germinomata (tumours that resemble a seminoma). Clinically, these tumours are seen most frequently in children and they may cause precocious puberty. Surgical removal of such masses is difficult and radiotherapy is the form of treatment given which ensures that the affected children have a 5-year survival of about 60%. Occasionally astrocytoma and ependymoma arise in the pineal gland from resident neuroglial cells and these tumours follow the same course as their counterparts in other CNS sites.

Some pathologists reserve the use of the term pinealoma for the tumours that arise out of the pinealocytes, tumours which constitute about a quarter of all neoplasms of the gland. Two types of such neoplasms are known: the **pinealocytoma**, occurring mainly in young adult males, and the **pinealoblastoma**, occurring mainly in children. Both tumours have a similar macroscopic appearance, forming soft, greyish masses that may contain regions of necrosis, haemorrhage and calcification. The pinealocytoma is better differentiated and has a population of both glial-type cells as well as regular, spheroidal, pinealocyte-type cells. Such tumours grow slowly, and although they impinge on surrounding tissues they do not invade them. Some tumours contain high concentrations of melatonin. The pinealoblastoma, on the other hand, is poorly differentiated, consisting of masses of pleomorphic large cells, that invade into the surrounding tissues. Because these tumours are faster in their growth, they will produce symptoms earlier than pinealocytomata.

Symptoms and signs associated with pinealomata are due to damage of surrounding structures. For example, the tumour will frequently damage the optic nerves, causing visual disturbances. Hydrocephalus and headache are common findings because of impingement on the third ventricle. Behavioural anomalies will result from destruction of nervous tissue, and precocious puberty may be seen in young boys with the tumour because of inadequate melatonin production (which suppresses gonadotrophin action). Pinealoblastomata may sometimes be found to metastasize to distant parts of the CNS, presumably an embolic spread by the CSF being the mode of metastasis.

Treatment of all forms of pinealomata is difficult because of the delicacy of the situation in which the gland is found. Even if surgery is decided upon, usually not all of the tumour will be removed. Pinealoblastomata have a very poor prognosis and few patients with these tumours live for more than 2 years after diagnosis. Pinealocytomata are more slowly growing tumours and are therefore associated with a better prognosis, most patients surviving for at least 5 years after diagnosis.

Thymus Gland Diseases

Hyperplasia

The thymus gland reaches its maximum size in childhood and from the time of puberty onwards begins to undergo involution. The size of the gland varies greatly from individual to individual within the same age groups. In the past, children who were unfortunate enough to be blessed with a large thymus gland were subjected to irradiation for its 'treatment', a procedure that in many cases was followed about 15 years later by carcinoma developing in the thyroid gland. Therefore, purely large size is not a good feature to use when judging whether or not a thymus gland is hyperplastic. Instead, the relative number of active germinal centres in the cortex of the gland is used as a means of identifying hyperplastic conditions of this organ. By far the most common cause of thymic hyperplasia is myasthenia gravis, hyperplasia also occurring in many other autoimmune diseases, such as SLE, rheumatoid arthritis, hyperthyroidism and scleroderma. It is suspected that thymic hyperplasia in these cases is reflecting the immune abnormalities that have led to the development of the autoimmune diseases.

Immunodeficiency States

The disorders of the thymus associated with primary immunodeficiency states have already been considered in Chapter 5. It should be noted that in almost all of these states, the thymus is smaller than normal or indeed completely absent and the number of lymphocytes within the shrunken gland are dramatically reduced. The concentration in the blood of the thymic hormones thymosine, thymine and thymopoietin are also decreased in these patients. The immunological incompetence that is seen in these conditions may be linked to the absence of sufficient quantities of the thymic hormones.

Tumours

Thymoma

Although primary tumours of the thymus gland are rare, they are one of the commonest causes of an anterior mediastinal mass. They are tumours of adults and the risk of developing the neoplasm increases with increasing age. Thymomata are mostly localized, non-invasive, encapsulated tumours that will grow locally, causing enlargement of the thymus (about 90% of cases). In a small number of cases the tumour will invade the adjacent tissues, growing into the pericardium or pleura, and even more rarely a thymoma will metastasize, usually only forming secondary deposits in the lungs.

The tumours form masses of 5 to 10 cm diameter in the anterior, superior mediastinum, and the tumour is usually encapsulated, with a soft, pinkish grey cut surface that may show lobulation and cyst formation. Microscopically both epithelial cells and lymphocytes comprise the tumour substance, but it is thought that the presence of lymphocytes is only incidental, the epithelial cells being the neoplastic component. A great variation in epithelial cell shape and size is found in different tumours, and variation is also seen in the proportion of epithelial cells to lymphocytes in any one tumour. In some thymomata, Hassal's corpuscles form.

In about half of the cases of thymoma, the tumour produces no symptoms and is only discovered incidentally in the course of other investigations. In about a third of cases the patient develops myasthenia gravis, red blood cell aplasia and/or hypogammaglobulinaemia with defects in cell-mediated immunity. In the remaining patients, symptoms such as chest pain, dyspnoea or cough may prompt investigations that lead to the diagnosis of the tumour.

Treatment of thymomata is by surgical excision if the tumour is encapsulated and has not metastasized. In these cases this form of treatment is curative. Removal of the thymoma may also benefit the patient in terms of the myasthenia gravis, if it is present (in about a quarter of cases of a patient having both conditions, surgical excision of the thymoma effectively treats both conditions). If excision of the neoplasm is impossible, irradiation is used and this will lead to shrinkage of the mass and possibly cure.

Other Tumours

Lymphomata may arise in or involve the thymus gland. Both Hodgkin's disease and the non-Hodgkin's lymphomata involve mediastinal structures such as the thymus and lymph nodes in the region. The morphology and clinical features of these tumours are similar to their counterparts in other body sites. **Neuroendocrine tumours** may arise in the gland and these are mostly encapsulated and follow a benign course; however, because of the hormones that they secrete, many patients with such tumours may develop Cushing's syndrome. Occasionally, neuroendocrine tumours of the thymus are malignant and will metastasize to distant sites, or be associated with neoplasms of other endocrine glands. **Germ cell tumours** may also occur in the thymus and any of the tumours normally found in the ovaries or testes may be seen as a primary in this situation. Germinoma (seminoma) is the commonest, but teratoma and choriocarcinoma may also occur. the prognosis is good for germinomata and teratomata but poor for choriocarcinomata.

Revision Questions and Case Studies

1. What is Addison's disease? How is this disease managed?
2. Discuss Cushing's syndrome, explaining the underlying pathogenesis of the clinically observed symptoms and signs.
3. What name is given to the disease which occurs as a result of excess mineralocorticoid production by the adrenal gland? What are the main features of this disorder?
4. What do you understand by the term 'adrenogenital syndromes'? Why are many sequelae seen in a disorder which primarily involves overproduction of only one type of sex hormone?
5. What are the most commonly occurring primary tumours of the adrenal gland? What do you know of their clinical effects?
6. Compare and contrast the pathology of:
   (a) Phaeochromocytoma
   (b) Neuroblastoma
7. Discuss the pathology of childhood hypopituitarism.
8. What is diabetes insipidus? Does this condition have any relation to diabetes mellitus? Comment.
9. Compare and contrast the results of hyperfunction of the adenohypophysis before and after fusion of the epiphyseal plates.
10. Enumerate the various tumours of the pituitary gland and indicate significance of these, especially in relation to their clinical effects on other endocrine glands.
11. What is meant by the term 'goitre'? Is a goitre always associated with hyperthyroidism?
12. Discuss the pathology of Hashimoto's thyroiditis.
13. Discuss the pathology of Graves' disease of the thyroid.
14. Distinguish between cretinism and myxoedema. Compare and contrast the major features of these two disorders.
15. Discuss the pathology of tumours of the thyroid gland.
16. What do you know of the pathology of hyperparathyroidism? Distinguish between primary and secondary forms of this condition in your discussion.
17. Is hypoparathyroidism of any clinical significance? Explain.
18. Discuss the pathology of tumours of the thymus gland.
19. Write short notes on the following topics:
    (a) Hyperpigmentation due to endocrine disease
    (b) Hypertension as a sign of endocrine disorders
    (c) Adrenal-caused hyperkalaemia
    (d) LATS antibody
    (e) De Quervain's disease
    (f) Craniopharyngioma
    (g) Congenital adrenal gland dyshormonogeneses
    (h) The dexamethasone test
20. What is the multiple endocrine neoplasia (MEN) syndrome?

Case study 1. A 65-year-old Caucasian woman presents because she is losing weight and because there has been hoarseness and hair growth which is embarrassing to her. When questioned about the weight loss she remarks that over the past 5 months she has lost about 10 kg. She says that her appetite is poor and even when her family try to tempt her with her favourite foods she cannot bring herself to eat much at all. When questioned about her bowel motions she admits that she is occasionally constipated but she has been self-administering laxatives on those occasions, the constipation not having been too problematic. There are no abdominal pains or discomfort and no obvious or occult blood in the faeces. The liver and spleen are normal on palpation. The woman has typical angina pectoris that is relieved by rest and glyceryl trinitrate. Her blood pressure is 120/80 and her heart rate is 80 beats per minute, although there is irregularity in this; no cardiac murmurs were auscultated. The respiratory system is normal except for a small region of calcification in the right upper lobe (she has a healed tuberculous Ghon focus in that region). There is no muscle wasting or abnormalities in sweating and the woman does not suffer from depression. The mouth and throat were normal although there was a noticeable goitre present, which was easily and freely movable. Her breasts showed atrophy and no masses were palpated. Examination of the pelvis showed findings consistent with the patient's advanced years, an atrophic vaginitis being present.

The patient had excessive facial and truncal hair while there was temporal hair loss. When asked about the hoarseness and hair changes, she replied that they had developed over the past 3 months. She also said that she avoided going out as she 'didn't look her best, but besides, she did not feel she had the energy'. Various laboratory investigations were ordered and the following results were obtained:

NAME: Edwina G. M. AGE: 65 years SEX: Female CLINICAL DETAILS: Weight loss, hoarseness, growth of facial, truncal hair, temporal hair loss, loss of appetite. MEDICATIONS PATIENT IS TAKING: Glyceryl trinitrate (symptomatically for angina); Coloxyl (laxative occasionally)	
Haemoglobin: 10.8 g/dL (N = 12–18 g/dL)	LEUKOCYTES WBC: 6910/μL (N = 4000–10 000/μL)
ERYTHROCYTES RBC: 3.9 million/μL (N = 4.5–6.5 million/μL) PCV: 37% (N = 39–54%) MCV: 95 μ^3 (N = 76–96 μ^3) MCHC: 31 g/dL (N = 32–36 g/dL) MCH: 29 pg (N = 27–32 pg)	Neutrophils: 63% (4347/μL) (N = 60–70%) Eosinophils: 2% (138/μL) (N = 1–4%) Basophils: <0.05% (10/μL) (N = 0–1%) Monocytes: 5% (345/μL) (N = 5–10%) Lymphocytes: 30% (2070/μL) (N = 25–30%)
RETICULOCYTES 1.9% (N = 0.5–2.2%)	FILM APPEARANCE: Mild hypochromia, occasional microcytes, some poikilocytes.
PLATELETS 245 000/μL (N = 150 000–400 000/μL)	REMARKS: Mild anaemia

For *Case Study 1*

The results of other laboratory tests ordered are shown below:

OTHER EXAMINATION	Mrs Edwina M. Age 65
Serum bilirubin	0.8 mg/dL (N = up to 1.0 mg/dL)
Serum albumin	32 g/L (N = 33–49 g/L)
Aspartate transaminase	18 IU/L (N = 7–27 IU/L)
Alkaline phosphatase	90 IU/L (N = 13–39 IU/L)
T4	125 nmol/L (N = 52–154 nmol/L)
T3	2.5 nmol/L (N = 1.16–3.00 nmol/L)
Serum testosterone	0.33 μg/dL (N = 25–90 ng/dL)
Urinary ketosteroids	58 mg/24 hrs (N = 5–15 mg/24 hrs)

For *Case Study 1*

(a) Consider as fully as possible the differential diagnosis and give reasons for your exclusions.

(b) What is the most likely diagnosis?

(c) Are any further tests to be considered?

(d) What is the treatment and what is the prognosis of the condition?

Case study 2. Mrs Dorothy P., an 82-year-old Caucasian woman, is admitted into hospital because the gradual deterioration in her health for the previous 10 months has led to headaches, hallucinations and somnolence. The woman had been becoming increasingly confused and alarmed over the past 3 months and complained to her niece (with whom she lived) that burglars were breaking into the house every night, chickens were parading on her bedspread and that legs of lamb were hanging from the ceiling of her bedroom (the woman does not drink alcohol and there is no liver disease in the history). The hallucinations were very distressing and the occipital headaches that she suffered from caused her great discomfort. On the second day in hospital the nurse attending Mrs P. could not rouse her, and the woman was found to be comatose.

Examination showed her to be obese and oedematous with pale and dry skin. She had considerable hair loss and was almost bald on the crown of the head. She responded to painful stimuli by eye blinking only and reflexes were present and equal in the upper limbs. There were no knee and ankle reflexes while plantar responses were flexor. Tone was reduced in the arms and legs and the relaxation stage of the biceps reflex was delayed. Her rectal temperature was 35°C, her blood pressure 112/60 mmHg and her pulse rate 60 beats per minute.

Results of laboratory investigations were as follows:

NAME: Dorothy Rae P.   AGE: 82 years   SEX: Female

CLINICAL DETAILS:
Comatose; has suffered from hallucinations, occipital headaches, was confused and agitated.

MEDICATIONS PATIENT IS TAKING:
Antacids (symptomatically for indigestion); Coloxyl (laxative, occasionally); multivitamins

Haemoglobin: 11.5 g/dL (N = 12–18 g/dL)	**LEUKOCYTES** WBC: 9980/μL (N = 4000–10 000/μL)
ERYTHROCYTES RBC: 4.1 million/μL (N = 4.5–6.5 million/μL) PCV: 40% (N = 39–54%) MCV: 98 μ^3 (N = 76–96 μ^3) MCHC: 32 g/dL (N = 32–36 g/dL) MCH: 29 pg (N = 27–32 pg)	Neutrophils: 68% (6770/μL) (N = 60–70%) Eosinophils: 2% (195/μL) (N = 1–4%) Basophils: <0.5% (38/μL) (N = 0–1%) Monocytes: 5% (490/μL) (N = 5–10%) Lymphocytes: 25% (2487/μL) (N = 25–30%)
RETICULOCYTES 0.8% (N = 0.5–2.2%)	FILM APPEARANCE: Microcytosis, some poikilocytes.
PLATELETS 190 000/μL (N = 150 000–400 000/μL)	REMARKS: Mild anaemia

For *Case Study 2*

Additional test results are shown below:

OTHER EXAMINATION   Mrs Dorothy R. P. Age 82

Serum bilirubin	0.7 mg/dL (N = up to 1.0 mg/dL)
Serum potassium	4.1 mmol/L (N = 3.6–5.2 mmol/L)
Serum sodium	132 mmol/L (N = 135–146 mmol/L)
Aspartate transaminase	90 IU/L (N = 7–27 IU/L)
Alkaline phosphatase	82 IU/L (N = 13–39 IU/L)
Creatine kinase	190 IU/L (N = 16–95 IU/L)
Cholesterol	12 mmol/L (N = 3.7–8.7 mmol/L)

For *Case Study 2*

(a) What is the most likely diagnosis?

(b) Justify the reasons for your diagnosis by pointing out relevant features in the clinical presentation or laboratory investigations.

(c) What do you know of the aetiology of this condition?

(d) What is the treatment for this disorder?

(e) What is the prognosis of the condition?

Case study 3. A 19-year-old man was referred to an endocrinologist by his family doctor, for delayed puberty. The man saw the doctor 3 months ago because repeated headaches had become a problem for him. The man was of short stature and slightly obese, but otherwise showed no abnormality. Although Klinefelter's syndrome was suspected at one stage, a karyotype showed the normal 46, XY genotype. Routine blood evaluation of sex hormones showed low basal gonadotrophins. A full evaluation of pituitary function was deemed necessary and a CT scan of the pituitary region was ordered.

(a) What is the differential diagnosis?

(b) What do the headaches and the request for the CT scan suggest as the most likely diagnosis?

(c) What do you expect the full evaluation of pituitary function to show?

Case study 4. A 39-year-old woman, Mrs Deborah H., presented at her doctor's surgery complaining of feelings of nausea, visual field disturbances, headaches and a persistent low back ache, all of which had been troubling her for the past 4 to 5 weeks. Physical examination showed a Caucasian female 1.65 m tall and weighing 89 kg. The woman was centrally obese and her face was rounded and oedematous. The leg muscles were wasted and atrophic; when the woman was questioned about her legs, she said that she did 'feel weak and needed to rest a lot lately'. The woman's skin was thin, atrophic and showed purple lines in the abdominal region. Around the chest and facial regions there were some bruises and wounds and questioned about these the woman admitted that she had been growing hairs in the facial region and chest, but she had been using a depilatory preparation which caused the damage to the skin. The blood pressure was recorded at 165/105 mmHg. A 24-hour sample of urine was collected and the dexamethasone test was performed.

(a) What is the diagnosis?

(b) Explain each symptom and sign in relation to the woman's disease.

(c) Why was the urine sample collected?

(d) What do you expect the dexamethasone test to show?

Further Reading

Bottazzo GF, Doniach D. 'Autoimmune Thyroid Disease.' *Annu Rev Med* 1986; **37**: 353.

Bush TL. 'The Adverse Effects of Hormone Therapy.' *Cardiol Clin* 1986; **4**: 145.

Burke CW. 'Adrenocortical Insufficiency.' *Clin Endocrinol Metabol* 1985; **14**: 947.

Carpenter PC. 'Cushing's Syndrome.' *Mayo Clin Proc* 1986; **61**: 49.

Chopra IJ, Solomon DH. 'Pathogenesis of Hyperthyroidism.' *Annu Rev Med* 1983; **34**: 267.

Ciric I. 'Pituitary Tumors.' *Neurol Clin* 1985; **3**: 751.

Cryer PE. 'Phaeochromocytoma.' *Clin Endocrinol Metabol* 1985; **14**: 203.

Cundy T, *et al.* 'Hyperparathyroid Bone Disease in Chronic Renal Failure.' *Ulster Med J* 1985; **54**(Suppl): S334.

DeLellis RA, Wolfe HJ. 'The Pathobiology of the Human Calcitonin (C)-Cell.' *Pathol Annu* 1981; **16**(2): 25.

Doniach I. 'Histopathology of the Pituitary.' *Clin Endocrinol Metabol* 1985; **14**: 765.

Fraser R. 'Disorders of the Adrenal Cortex: Their Effects on Electrolyte Metabolism.' *Clin Endocrinol Metabol* 1984; **13**: 413.

Gluck WL. 'Thyroid and Parathyroid Cancer.' *Clin Geriatr Med* 1987; **3**: 729.

Hoffman HJ. 'Pineal Region Tumors.' *Prog Exp Tumor Res* 1987; **30**: 281.

Hughes IA. 'Congenital and Acquired Disorders of the Adrenal Cortex.' *Clin Endocrinol Metabol* 1982; **11**: 89.

Kameya T, *et al.* 'Morphologic and Functional Aspects of Hormone-producing Tumors.' *Pathol Annu* 1980; **15**(1): 351.

Magyar DM. 'Amenorrhea, Galactorrhea and Hyperlactinemia.' *J Am Osteopath Assoc* 1985; **85**: 375.

McFarlane J. 'Congenital Adrenal Hyperplasia.' *Am J Nurs* 1976; **76**(8): 1290.

Moses M, Notman DD. 'Diabetes Insipidus and the Syndrome of Inappropriate antidiuretic Hormone Secretion.' *Adv Intern Med* 1982; **27**: 73.

Müller-Hermelink HK, Marino M, Palestro G. 'Pathology of the Thymic Epithelial Tumours.' *Curr Top Pathol* 1986; **75**: 207.

Neselof C. 'Pathology of the Thymus in Immunodeficiency States.' *Curr Top Pathol* 1986; **75**: 151.

Robuschi C, *et al.* 'Hypothyroidism in the Elderly.' *Endocrin Rev* 1987; **8**: 142.

Rosai J. 'The Pathology of Thymic Neoplasia.' *Monogr Pathol* 1986; **29**: 161.

Sasano N, Ojima M, Masuda T. 'Endocrinologic pathology of Functioning Adrenocortical Tumors.' *Pathol Annu* 1980; **15**(2): 105.

Seale JP, Compton MR. 'Side-effects of Corticosteroid Agents.' *Med J Aust* 1986; **144**: 139.

Sherwood LM. 'Diagnosis and Management of Primary Hyperparathyroidism.' *Hosp Pract* 1988; **23**(3A): 9.

Steinmann GG. 'Changes in the Human Thymus during Ageing.' *Curr Top Pathol* 1986; **75**: 43.

Stulberg BN, *et al.* 'Hyperparathyroidism, Hyperthyroidism and Cushing's Disease.' *Orthop Clin N Am* 1984; **15**: 697.

Tunbridge WMG. 'Acromegaly.' *Nurs Times* 1979; **75**(3): 110.

Volpé R. 'Autoimmune Thyroid Disease.' *Mol Biol Med* 1986; **3**: 25.

19

Eye and Ear Disorders

The Normal Eye

The ancients believed that the eye was the window to the soul. Iridologists gaze into their patients' eyes in an attempt to diagnose all manner of bodily disease. The medical practitioner looks at the eyes for evidence of systemic diseases that cause characteristic eye signs. The ophthalmologist examines the eyes for evidence of ocular disease. The organ of sight is one of the major receptors in the body that conveys to the brain information about the immediate environment. In many cases the eye will show evidence of numerous disorders, not only ocular but also systemic.

The eyeball is contained within the osseous cavity of the orbit, thus being well protected from injury and allowing an extensive range of sight. It is acted upon by several muscles that may cause it to be moved in different directions. It is richly supplied by blood vessels and nerves and is further protected by the eyebrow and eyelid (see Figure 19.1). The eyeball consists of three investing layers and three refracting media. The first lamina is composed of the sclera and cornea, both of which are essentially fibrous in nature. The sclera is a tough, dense, opaque, fibrous membrane surrounding the eyeball and helping to retain its shape. The cornea is continuous with the sclera and constitutes approximately one-sixth of the first investing layer, being different to the sclera in that it is transparent. The cornea is almost circular in shape, being convex anteriorly. The exact degree of curvature of the cornea varies in different people, but also in the same individual at different stages of life (it tends to become flatter as one ages, hence the need for corrective lenses).

The second lamina of the eye is formed from behind forward, by the choroid, ciliary body and iris. The choroid is a pigmented, very vascular layer investing the posterior five-sixths of the eyeball, being pierced behind by the optic nerve. The ciliary body comprises the orbiculus ciliaris, the ciliary processes and the ciliary muscle. The ciliary processes are formed by folds of the choroid, received between corresponding folds of the suspensory ligament of the lens. The ciliary muscle is a circular band of smooth muscle fibres arranged radially and circularly and is the main muscle

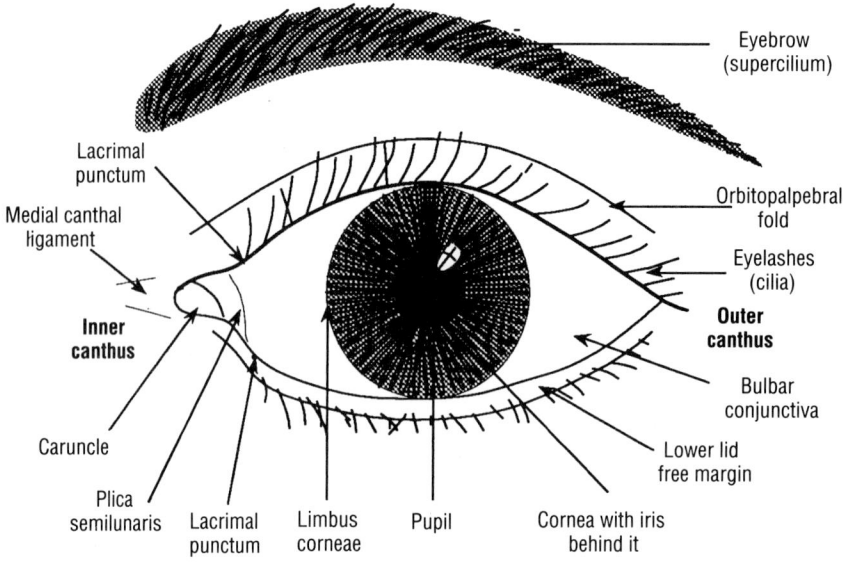

Eyebrow
(supercilium)

Lacrimal
punctum

Medial canthal
ligament

Orbitopalpebral
fold

Eyelashes
(cilia)

**Inner
canthus**

**Outer
canthus**

Bulbar
conjunctiva

Caruncle

Lower lid
free margin

Plica
semilunaris   Lacrimal   Limbus   Pupil   Cornea with iris
                punctum   corneae   behind it

Figure 19.1   *The external features of the normal eye*

involved in accommodation (i.e. adjusting the eye to vision of objects near to the eye). The iris is a thin, circular contractile membrane suspended in the aqueous humour. Its circumference is continuous with the ciliary body. Its inner edge forms the margin of the pupil, which is essentially an aperture that allows light to enter the eye. The anterior part of the iris is variously coloured in different individuals while the posterior aspect has a purplish tinge and is termed the uvea.

The third lamina of the eye is the retina, a delicate nervous membrane on which images of external objects are focused by the lens. Its outer surface is in contact with the choroid, while its inner surface is in contact with the vitreous humour. Behind, it is continuous with the optic nerve. The surface of the retina is purple in colour due to the presence of the pigment rhodopsin (visual purple). Exactly at the centre of the posterior part of the retina is an oval yellowish spot, called the macula lutea, and it is here that the sense of vision is most acute. Approximately 3 mm to the inner side of the macula is the point of entrance of the optic nerve, through the centre of which enters the central retinal artery. This is the only non-light-sensitive spot on the retina and is hence termed the 'blind spot'. The retina is very complex in structure and comprises ten layers, the rods and cones (specialized nerve cells for sensitivity to light) being found in the more superficial layers (refer to Figure 19.2).

There are three refracting media in the globe of the eye and these are the aqueous humour, vitreous hu-

mour and the crystalline lens. The aqueous humour is a slightly alkaline saline and this thin fluid fills the anterior and posterior chambers of the eye. The vitreous humour fills the concavity of the retina and has the consistency of thin jelly. It contains some salts and protein. The crystalline lens is enclosed by a capsule that is transparent and highly elastic. The anterior surface of the lens is covered by a layer of flattened, polygonal, nucleated cells that towards the circumference of the lens become elongated and fibre-like. No epithelium is present on the posterior aspect. The substance of the lens consists of concentric laminae. Each lamina is made up of closely fitting hexagonal fibres. The lens in the adult is colourless, transparent, avascular and firm in texture (see Figure 19.3).

The Normal Ear

The organ of hearing is divided into three parts (see Figure 19.4): the outer (external) ear, the middle ear and the inner ear. The outer ear comprises the pinna (auricle), whose function is to collect the vibrations of the air by which sound is produced and to direct these towards the auditory canal (meatus). The auditory canal ends at the tympanic membrane, which separates the outer ear from the middle ear.

The middle ear or tympanum is an irregular cavity within bone and placed above the jugular fossa. This cavity is filled with air and communicates with the

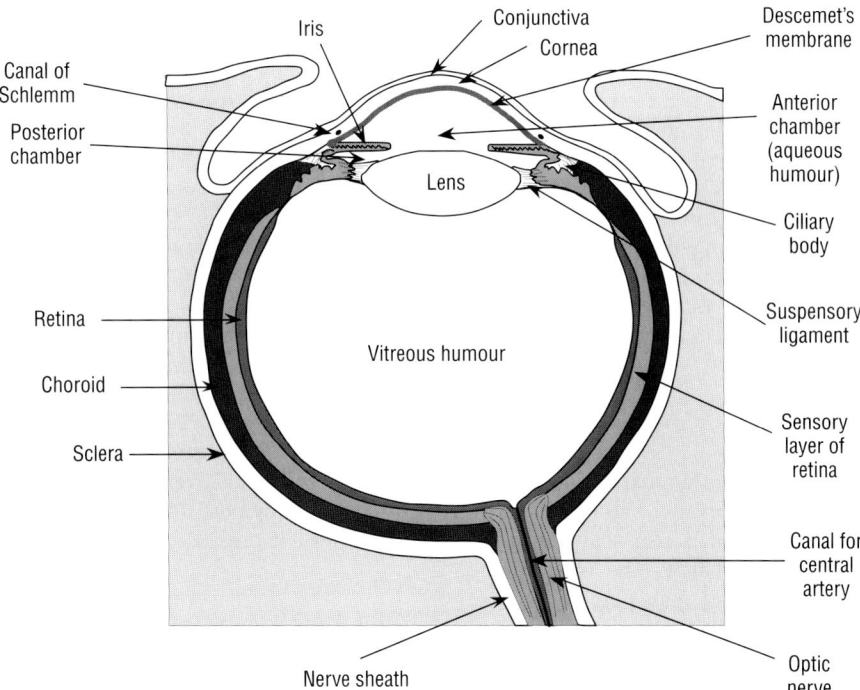

Figure 19.2 *Section through the normal eye*

nasopharynx via the Eustachian tube. A chain of three ear bones (auditory ossicles) crosses the tympanic cavity, connecting the tympanic membrane with the internal ear. These bones are the malleus, connected to the ear drum by its long limb, the incus in the centre, articulating with the other two ossicles, and the stapes, attached to the fenestra ovalis of the vestibule of the inner ear labyrinth.

The third part is the inner ear where the receptive apparatus for sound is located. The inner ear is very irregular in shape and is thus called the labyrinth. It is surrounded by bone and within the bony cavity is the membranous labyrinth, a system of interconnecting sacs and ducts filled with fluid and surrounded by fluid. The utricle and saccule are small sacs within a bony vestibule. Three semicircular ducts are positioned within bony semicircular canals. Finally a bony, snail-shaped cochlea encases the similarly shaped cochlear duct.

Within the internal ear, the membranous labyrinth serves two functions. The first is that of the auditory sense, residing in the cochlear duct where specialized nerve cells, the hair cells, are present within the organ of Corti. The second is that of the static and kinetic sense ('balance'), which resides in the semicircular canals and utricle.

Eye Diseases

Eyelid

Hordeolum (Stye)

Hordeolum is a typical pyogenic infection occurring in association with an eyelash follicle and its gland of Zeis. The commonest infecting organism is *Staphylococcus aureus* although occasionally other pyogenic bacteria are isolated. The affected lid becomes swollen, painful and red as the pus accumulates within the abscess. The application of hot compresses may provide relief and expedite the process of pointing and spontaneous discharge of pus at the lid margin. Usually no treatment is required and there are few complications, with minimal or no scarring seen.

Chalazion (Meibomian Cyst)

Chalazion is a chronic inflammatory lesion developing within an obstructed Meibomian gland, causing a firm and irritating lump to form, usually in the upper eyelid. Patients often complain that the lesion feels like a hailstone embedded in their eye (from which is derived the term for the disease). The lesion consists of inflamed granulation tissue which lays down a fibrous capsule around the reactive region. Often, a cystic cavity develops and this contains a mucous secretion, tissue debris and typical granulomata of chronic inflammation with giant cells and epithelioid cells. An infective organism is not isolated and confusion with tuberculosis is easily discounted because of the absence of caseation. The condition is treated by a vertical incision through the conjunctival surface, followed by evacuation of the contents of the cyst.

Blepharitis

Blepharitis is a generalized inflammation of the whole of the lid margin, involving many or all of the eyelash follicles. The affected eyelid is red, scaly, itchy and there is an occasional discharge. The inflammation tends to be non-specific and may persist for many years, causing the lashes to fall out or become grossly distorted. Ingrowing eyelashes cause the condition of **trichiasis**, where the eyelashes irritate and even ulcerate the cornea whenever the patient blinks. There are other variants of this condition, a **squamous blepharitis** being found in people with seborrhoea (dandruff), the eyelid disorder being an extension of the scalp condi-

tion. The other variant is an **ulcerative blepharitis** where there is widespread infection of the eyelids with *Staphylococcus aureus*, this causing a severe inflammation, with destruction of the lid margin and scarring.

Non-specific blepharitis is difficult to eradicate and the treatment used is one of the topical corticosteroid ointment applications, with topical antibiotic preparations often used to prevent secondary bacterial infection. Squamous blepharitis is treated in association with the scalp condition by frequent shampooing with anti-dandruff preparations. Trimming of long lashes may be useful as is also the washing of the eyelids with an alkaline solution and a topical antibiotic preparation. Ulcerative blepharitis requires long-term treatment with a cortisone and antibiotic ointment preparation, applied every 2 to 3 hours over the course of a few weeks until the infection is controlled and again after each relapse.

Entropion

Entropion is a displacement of the lower eyelid such that the lashes turn inward, together with inversion of the lid margin. It is often seen in the elderly where there is frequent rubbing of irritable eyes and constant squinting or 'screwing up' of the eyes associated with

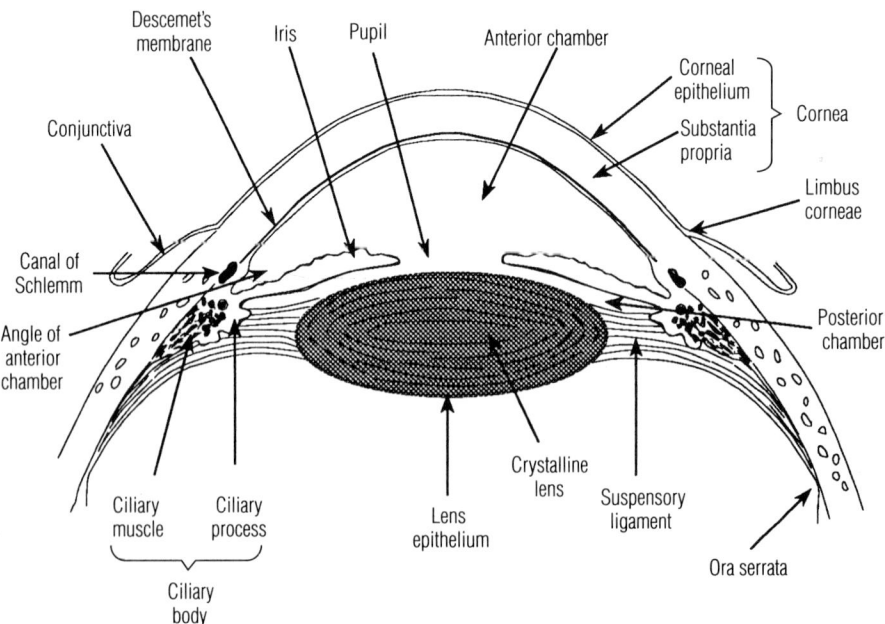

Figure 19.3   *The normal cornea, lens and related structures*

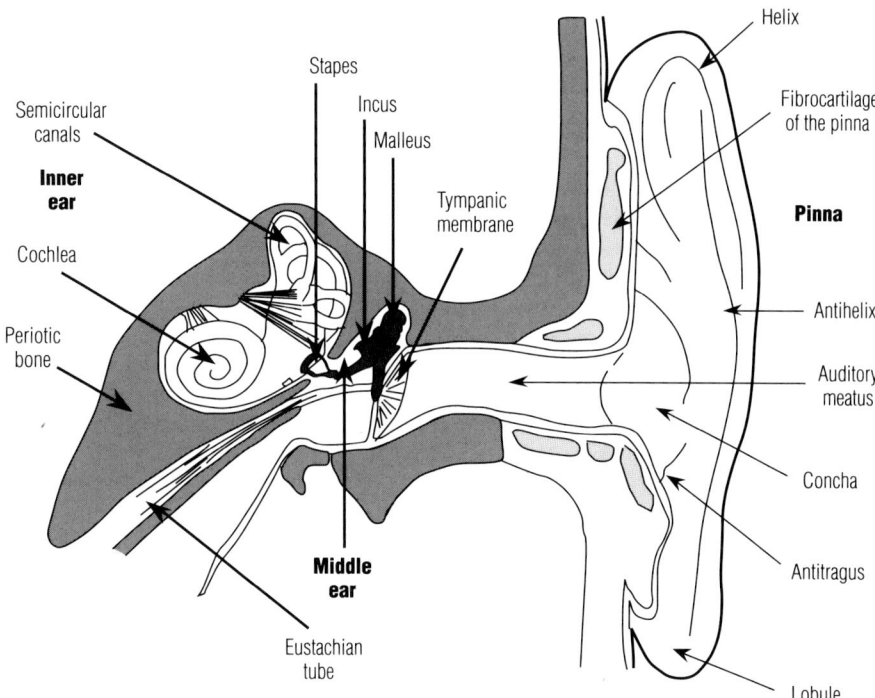

Figure 19.4 *The normal ear*

poor vision. The condition usually initiates a vicious cycle, the ingrowing eyelashes causing more irritation to the cornea, initiating another round of rubbing the eyes. Lubricating preparations and sedatives may help in the early stages of the condition, as will also correction of any treatable vision disturbances and treatment of any underlying blepharitis. In the more involved or severe cases, the treatment is surgical with removal of a small strip of skin and the underlying muscle from the lower lid. The scar resulting from the procedure and the weakening of the orbicularis muscle will prevent recurrence of the condition.

Ptosis

Ptosis is a droop of the eyelid, usually due to a bilateral congenital defect in the eyelid and external eye muscles. If the condition is severe enough it may cause interference with vision and the child will often tilt the head backwards in order to see. Surgical correction of the defect involves resection of some of the levator palpebrae superioris muscle and of the upper tarsal plate. Ptosis may also arise secondarily as a result of injury of the lid muscles or their motor nerves. Occasionally it is seen in association with senile atony of

muscles or in association with myasthenia gravis.

A variant of the condition is **atonic ectropion** where the lower eyelid will become everted, making the eye appear like that of a rabbit, justifying the synonymous term for the condition, **lagophthalmos**. This is due to a flaccid orbicularis muscle caused by facial palsy or to senile atonic changes of the lower lid muscles. A stagnant pool of tears forms in the lower fornix and this predisposes to infection, which will then cause inflammation and thickening of the lower lid, mechanically pushing the lid further down and increasing the secretion of tears. **Epiphora** (inappropriate and constant secretion of tears) is one of the prime symptoms of the condition. The disorder is treated with antibiotics to control the infection, astringents to reduce the epiphora, a surgical procedure to improve lacrimal drainage and a plastic operation to correct the ectropion.

Xanthelasma

Xanthelasma is seen either as a manifestation of hypercholesterolaemia, or more commonly not related to any systemic disorder of lipid metabolism, typically in middle-aged women who also suffer from cholelithiasis. The lesions of the disorder are elevated, yellowish, intradermal plaques several millimetres in length, situated near the inner canthus. Several xanthelasmata are usually present and are situated in the medial upper and lower aspects of the lids. Microscopically the plaques are seen to consist of deposits of many macrophages containing intracellular cholesterol and phospholipid granules ('foam cells'), within a fibrous stroma. The lesions do not cause any discomfort nor do they have any dire sequelae, but they may be excised for cosmetic reasons.

Carcinomata

Both basal cell carcinoma and squamous cell carcinoma (already considered in Chapter 16) are commonly observed to arise in the eyelid. Basal cell carcinoma, in particular, favours this site, giving rise to a small nodule that will ulcerate rapidly, forming the typical 'rodent ulcer' with the characteristic everted margins. The tumour is locally invasive and has a good prognosis if treated by excision. Left untreated, a basal cell carcinoma may invade deeply, causing extensive destruction and blindness of the affected eye.

Conjunctiva

Conjunctivitis

Conjunctivitis is an inflammatory condition, occurring in acute and chronic forms, affecting the conjunctivae and usually due to infective or allergic causes. In most cases, the condition will resolve with suitable treatment and no serious complications will be seen. In diagnosing conjunctivitis, microbiological examination of conjunctival scrapings and swabs of the secretion should be undertaken, but also a histological examination of the scrapings should be performed. Giemsa-stained material will provide a clue in identifying the cause of conjunctivitis (see Table 19.1).

Acute bacterial conjunctivitis is rather common in incidence and is due to a large variety of pyogenic organisms, including *Staphylococcus, Streptococcus, Haemophilus, Pseudomonas* spp. and *Neisseria gonorrhoeae*. The patient usually is responsible for the infection, having autoinoculated the bacteria in the eye with the fingers. Conjunctivitis may complicate the wearing of contact lenses or it may follow an allergic conjunctivitis if the patient persists in rubbing the irritated eyes and introducing bacteria. **Ophthalmia neonatorum** refers to a bacterial conjunctivitis contracted by newborn babies during the passage through an infected birth canal where *Neisseria gonorrhoeae* or *Chlamydia* spp. are present in a genital infection. Instillation of antibiotic eye drops into the eyes of all newborn babies routinely prevents this type of conjunctivitis.

The eyes in acute bacterial conjunctivitis show a diffuse redness, lacrimation and discharge (which may be purulent) that often has sealed together the eyelids on awakening. The patient experiences a gritty sensation in the eyes and will often rub the eyes in order to relieve the foreign body sensation. **Photophobia** (aversion to light) will often force the patient to wear dark glasses, but vision remains clear and the cornea is bright.

Diagnosis involves isolation of the causative organism, testing of antibiotic sensitivity and administration of the appropriate antibiotic in the form of eye drops instilled into the affected eye(s). Often, antibiotic ad-

Table 19.1 *Types of conjunctivitis*

	Acute bacterial	Chronic bacterial	Viral	Trachoma	Allergy
Examples	Staphylococcal, streptococcal	*Moraxella* spp., tuberculous	Herpetic, adenoviral	*Chlamydia trachomatis*	Pollen allergy, cosmetic allergy
Incidence	Common	Uncommon	Very common	Uncommon	Very common
Appearance	Suppuration, diffuse redness	Extreme redness, little secretion	Redness, lacrimation, chemosis	Papillation, follicle formation	Redness, lacrimation, chemosis
Histology	Neutrophils, purulent exudate	Lymphocytes, macrophages	Giant cells, lymphocytes	Plasma cells, inclusions	Eosinophils, basophils

ministration begins empirically immediately the microbiological specimen is collected and the treatment may be modified once the laboratory results are available. Antibiotic ointment may be also prescribed and this has a longer action and is especially useful during the night as it also prevents the sealing of the lid margins by discharge. The patient is educated regarding the infection and risk of spreading the infection to others, and is encouraged to maintain a good personal hygiene. Acute bacterial conjunctivitis usually resolves with treatment and no complications are seen.

Chronic bacterial conjunctivitis may sometimes follow an acute infection of the conjunctiva that has been left untreated or has been treated inadequately. It may also complicate persisting viral infections, unremoved foreign bodies in the eyes, or a chronic infection in the lacrimal passages. It is treated in the same manner as acute conjunctivitis; however, if a primary condition is present in addition to the secondary bacterial infection this must be addressed also in order for treatment to be effective.

Viral conjunctivitis is a very common infection of the eye and often occurs in an epidemic form. The commonest causative agents associated with the infection are the adenoviruses, types 1 to 28. Adenoviruses types 4, 8, 12 and 18 are especially involved with epidemic outbreaks of the disease. Other viruses involved are herpes viruses, measles, mumps and rubella viruses. Viral conjunctivitis is usually bilateral and causes **chemosis** (oedema of the conjunctiva and subconjunctival tissues), redness, follicular inflammation with many lymphocytes (and giant cells commonly), epiphora and a serous secretion (not often purulent). The cornea is likely to be involved and the condition presents often as a **keratoconjunctivitis** with **corneal ulcers** developing (see below).

The condition is treated by good hygiene and instillation of anti-inflammatory agents as eye drops. Antibiotics are also administered prophylactically in order to prevent secondary bacterial infection. The infection with adenovirus will persist for about 2 to 3 weeks and will usually subside with resolution. Antiherpetic drugs may be given in the case of herpes virus infections and if the pain associated with the condition is severe, analgesics may also be needed.

Allergic conjunctivitis is one of the commonest forms of conjunctivitis and is seen in association with exposure to various allergens such as house dust, pollens, cosmetics and drugs administered intraocularly. The condition is common during the flowering seasons when large quantities of pollen are in the air. The patient presents with a very inflamed conjunctiva, itching of the eyes (especially around the medial canthi) and epiphora; there may be an eczematous-type reaction around the eyelids. All of these symptoms and signs are often exacerbated by the rubbing of the eyes that the irritation experienced invariably compels the patient to do. Often allergic conjunctivitis is accompanied by allergic rhinitis ('hay fever'). In treating the allergic conjunctiva, the allergen is first identified and contact with it is limited or prevented altogether, if possible. Symptomatic relief may be provided by vasoconstrictors and antihistamines applied as eye drops or given orally. Desensitization in some cases has cured the condition.

Vernal conjunctivitis (**spring catarrh**) is a form of allergic conjunctivitis more often seen in warmer climates, affecting boys more commonly than girls and beginning in prepubertal years. It is commoner in springtime and is due to an allergic reaction to, usually, pollens and moulds. The patient complains of intense itching which is worse if the weather is warm. The palpebral, tarsal conjunctiva is severely affected by the inflammation and the thickened, red mucosa shows irregular thickening often described as having a 'cobblestone' appearance. The perilimbal conjunctiva is also thickened and inflamed, especially in the region of the palpebral aperture. There is a mucoid discharge produced by the inflamed mucosa and this contains large numbers of eosinophils. As the inflamed tarsal region rubs over the cornea, corneal ulcers may develop. Treatment of the condition is by instillation of weak solutions of corticosteroids and limitation of exposure to the allergen if this is known.

Phlyctenular conjunctivitis appears as small yellowish grey or pinkish lesions at the limbus, conjunctival epithelium and even on the cornea. The lesions of the disorder arise as hypersensitivity to a protein substance develops and most commonly they have been reported in association with hypersensitivity to tuberculoprotein.

Scleritis and **episcleritis** are conditions that involve the superficial vascular layers of the sclera and are associated with rheumatoid arthritis and some other autoimmune states. The main difference between scleritis and episcleritis is that in the latter, corneal or uveal tissue may be involved in the inflammation, whereas the former is a more superficial type of inflammatory change. Fibrinoid necrosis of collagen may be found in both types of lesion and an intense vascular reaction makes the tissue of the sclera look very red and congested.

Trachoma

This is a chronic, bilateral, cicatrizing keratoconjunctivitis which develops after infection with *Chlamydia trachomatis*, especially serotypes A, B, Ba and C (TRIC agents — trachoma, inclusion conjunctivitis agents). Trachoma is not a common disease in developed, Western-type countries and therefore it does not receive the attention that it deserves as one of the great scourges of humanity. Approximately 400 000 000 people worldwide are affected by the disease and it is estimated that 20 000 000 in the world are blinded by trachoma, making this disorder the single most important cause of blindness. Most cases of the disease occur in the Middle East, Africa, India, South East Asia, China, Russia and other Eastern European countries. In Australia, the Aboriginal population is still commonly affected, especially in northern states and the Territory. Conditions that predispose to trachoma are poor living conditions, poor hygiene, overcrowding, little washing, dirt and flies. The infection is transmitted by contact, often from mother to child or by fingers, fomites or flies. In the areas where trachoma is a problem, childhood infections are the rule and multiple reinfections will recur during life.

Trachoma begins insidiously with an acute stage, simple conjunctivitis seen about 5 days after the infection. There is watering of the eyes, perhaps a purulent discharge and the eyes feel gritty, being red and inflamed. The conjunctiva of the upper lids is affected particularly severely and on examination it appears red and granular. In a small number of people the infection will subside after this acute stage without further damage. In most cases, however, in the following weeks the inflammation will progress so that the granularity of the conjunctiva becomes even more marked, with small follicles on the tarsal conjunctiva developing into granulomatous lesions. Microscopically, the chlamydiae growing in the enlarged conjunctival cells will be seen as inclusion bodies in Giemsa-stained smears prepared from infected eyes a few days after infection. Some cells become necrotic and slough off, but the epithelium gradually becomes hyperplastic and the submucosa is infiltrated by lymphocytes and plasma cells, with large macrophages containing ingested debris.

With the passage of time the infiltrate becomes nodular and granulomatous with necrotic regions often seen in the centre of the granulomata. Fibrosis then begins and continues, to become more marked as the disease progresses. Growth of the chlamydiae in the corneal epithelium excites an inflammatory response and a pannus of inflammatory tissue grows into the cornea from the limbus. The pannus extends slowly across the cornea, making it opaque and bringing blindness. Scarring in the conjunctiva and eyelids causes entropion. Blockage of the tear ducts dries the eye and makes secondary infections particularly common. The disease is a slowly progressive one, taking months to years in order for it to develop fully. Approximately 80% of untreated patients will progress to serious complications such as conjunctival and corneal scarring, deformity, shrinkage, xerosis, ptosis, entropion of the lids and blindness.

Diagnosis of the infection is by identification of the characteristic inclusion bodies in conjunctival scrapings stained by the Giemsa method, serological tests (complement fixation test, fluorescent antibody techniques) and by culture of the causative agent in cell culture or embryonated hens' eggs. The infection is treated both medically and socially. Education of the populations at risk is an important factor in the control of the infection and improvement of living standards and hygiene must be a high priority. Antibiotic treatment brings a marked improvement in the condition but this is a slow process that may take 2 to 3 months. Antibiotics such as sulphonamides, tetracyclines and chloramphenicol orally are recommended for treating the infection and rendering the patient non-infectious. Tetracycline eye ointments may also be used.

Sarcoidosis

Sarcoidosis affects the eyes in about a quarter of cases of the systemic disease. The uveal tract is most commonly involved but the conjunctivae are also affected in a large number of cases. Typical sarcoid granulomata will form, about 1 to 2 mm in diameter, and these will be found in the fornix, the fold between the bulbar and palpebral conjunctiva. The lesions will show all the microscopical features of sarcoidosis and the absence of caseation and acid-fast bacilli easily differentiates these lesions from those of tuberculosis.

Age-related Changes

The conjunctiva will thicken slightly and become less white and less clear with increasing age. The epithelium tends to keratinize, thus roughening the surface of the mucous membrane. The submucosal tissues become thinner and microscopically will show hyalinization. Several distinct degenerative changes associated with ageing are described but it should be kept in mind that these are more likely to occur in people who expose their eyes to excessive wind, dust and ultraviolet radiation.

Pinguecula is an opaque, raised, yellowish, triangular nodule developing close to the limbus, especially common on the nasal side. Microscopic examination shows focal atrophy and hyperplasia of the epithelium over the lesion, while in the subconjunctival tissue there is hyalinization and proliferation of elastic tissue with subsequent degeneration and fragmentation. The condition is rarely treated and the patient is given advice regarding eye protection.

Pterygium is a trapezoidal lesion consisting of vascular connective tissue covered by epithelium that is found to extend from the conjunctiva to the cornea, usually on the nasal side and always present in the part of the eye exposed between the lids when the eye is open (palpebral aperture). The condition is associated with exposure to sunlight, wind and dust. The patient presents because of the obvious lesion, recurrent irritation and pain, and impairment of vision due to corneal opacity or astigmatism. The patient is advised to wear sunglasses and a hat when outdoors and this may stop further growth of the lesion. If the pterygium encroaches upon the pupillary area or if vision is otherwise impaired, the lesion is removed surgically.

Concretions may form on the tarsal conjunctiva of elderly or debilitated people and these present as yellow or white spots on the surface of the conjunctiva. They are due to obstructed serous gland openings which cause a retention and inspissation of secretions. The concretions are laminated and may attract calcium, forming calculus-like lesions. Concretions may cause irritation to the conjunctiva or damage the corneal epithelium as they move over it. They may be removed surgically if they are causing any problems.

Tumours

Both benign and malignant tumours may occur in the conjunctiva, but these are rather rare. The benign ones are: **papilloma**, a sessile or pedunculated mass that arises around the caruncle; **haemangioma**, resembling the lesion occurring elsewhere in the body; and **benign naevus**, appearing as a yellowish pink, occasionally pigmented nodule usually on the bulbar conjunctiva. The latter tumour may appear as a cystic lesion which is lined by the naevus cells and will appear as a smooth mobile nodule of variable pigmentation. **Conjunctival dermoid** is not uncommon and presents as a pale nodule at the limbus or the sclera. It is due to the persistence of germ cells at these sites, and skin, fat and hair follicles will be contained within the tumour. Such lesions cause disfigurement and are an irritant because of the production of keratin and the presence of hair. Corneal astigmatism due to the lesion will impair vision. Such lesions may be surgically removed.

The malignant tumours include **Bowen's disease**, a lesion similar to that already described on the skin

appearing on the limbus or the lid margin. This tumour will progress to a typical squamous cell carcinoma if left untreated. **Malignant melanoma**, **squamous cell carcinoma** and **basal cell carcinoma** may also occur on the conjunctiva, but they are all rare and behave in the same manner as their counterparts on the skin. Prompt removal of the tumour or enucleation of the affected eye are the treatments for these tumours.

Cornea

Keratitis, Corneal Ulcers

Keratitis is an infection or inflammation of the cornea. The infection may be derived from the outside, in which case it is called **exogenous keratitis** and is most commonly infectious in nature. Alternatively, if it starts deep in the corneal tissue it is called **endogenous keratitis**, with allergic-type reactions or toxic states being the cause. A common manifestation of keratitis is ulceration of the cornea, and these ulcers, which take several characteristic forms, may be associated with specific aetiologies (see Figure 19.5).

Corneal ulcers may be marginal or central and they may be associated with bacterial or viral infections or may be secondary to long-standing inflammation due to trauma or other aetiologies. In most cases the ulcer will resolve but in certain cases the severe inflammation and necrosis of tissue within the cornea will leave a scar or have the following serious complications:

- **scarring** of the cornea leading to opacities and impairment of vision;
- **corneal perforation** followed by prolapse of the iris or even the lens through the break (see Figure 19.6);
- **descemetocoele**, which is an outpouching of Descemet's membrane (lying anteriorly to the inner corneal epithelial layer) through the ulcerated outer layers of the cornea;
- **hypopyon**, a collection of pus within the anterior chamber (see Figure 19.7);
- **staphyloma**, which is a nodule of darkly coloured tissue caused by a bulging of the cornea or sclera lined by uveal tissue and covered anteriorly by epithelial cells;
- **uveitis**, **endophthalmitis**, **cataract**, **secondary glaucoma**.

Dendritic ulcers are a very common form of ulcerative keratitis and are due to herpes virus infection of the cornea. Such ulcers are usually demonstrated by instillation into the eye of a solution of rose Bengal 1% (showing the dead epithelial cells) or fluorescein 1%

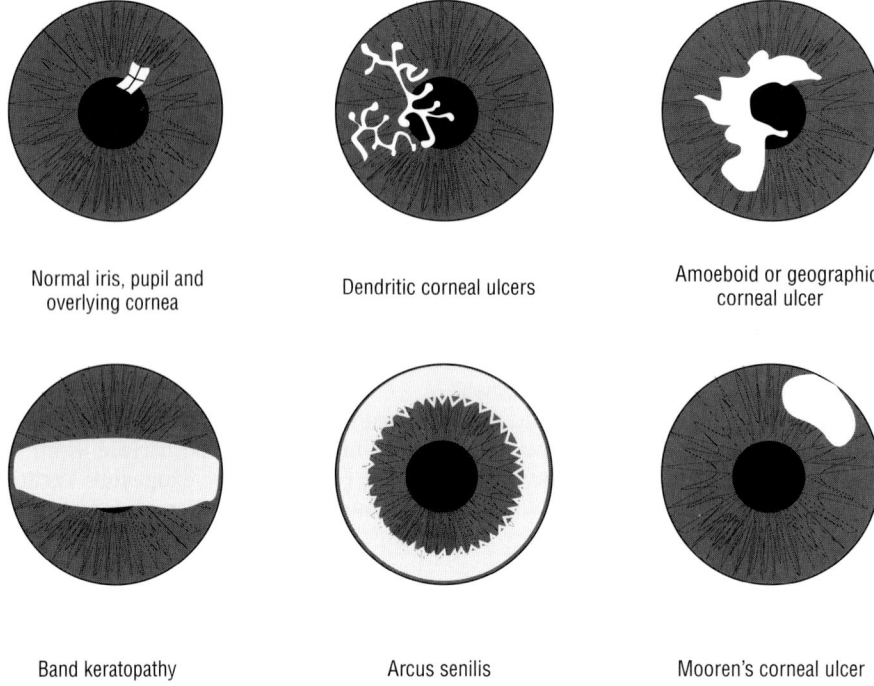

Normal iris, pupil and overlying cornea   Dendritic corneal ulcers   Amoeboid or geographic corneal ulcer

Band keratopathy   Arcus senilis   Mooren's corneal ulcer

Figure 19.5   *Corneal disorders (I)*

(staining breaks in the epithelium). They are termed dendritic ulcers as they show a tree-like pattern of destroyed corneal epithelium (refer to Figure 19.5). The symptoms of the condition are lacrimation, irritation, photophobia and blurred vision if the ulcer is placed centrally on the cornea. If the infection excites an excessive immune response the ulcer may become a **disciform herpetic keratitis** where the infection and inflammation spread to the deeper interstitial layers of the cornea and a large, disc-shaped opacity develops in the central cornea.

Herpetic infections in the cornea are treated by debridement of the ulcer under local anaesthesia, which removes the necrotic epithelium, much virus and debris. Following this, specific antivirals are instilled into the eye (e.g. iododeoxyuridine, adenosine arabinoside) and a broad spectrum antibiotic may also be administered to prevent secondary bacterial infections. Cycloplegic drugs (that paralyze the ciliary muscle temporarily, dilating the pupil and preventing accommodation) are given in order to prevent posterior synechiae (adhesions of the iris to the lens, see Figure 19.7). Dark glasses are worn to diminish the photophobia.

Other viral corneal infections are caused by herpes zoster virus (**herpes zoster ophthalmicus**) and by adenovirus. In herpes zoster ophthalmicus, the virus localizes in the ophthalmic division of the trigeminal nerve and periodically crops of typical herpetic vesicles will appear, limited to half the forehead and spreading downward towards the tip of the nose. The rash may be preceded by pain for 24 to 48 hours. The eyes look red, swollen, the cornea is oedematous with keratitis developing and the conjunctiva is inflamed. Various complications develop, including uveitis, secondary glaucoma, secondary bacteria infections, optic neuritis and ocular muscle paralysis. The condition is treated by topical antibiotic administration, mydriatic eye drops and steroid preparations in the case of uveitis or keratitis developing.

Adenoviral infections cause epidemic outbreaks due to their contagious nature. Adenoviral keratoconjunctivitis is heralded by swollen, tender, hard preauricular lymph nodes and then the typical signs and symptoms of keratitis and conjunctivitis are seen for 3 to 4 weeks. Punctate keratitis may persist for months to years. Such infections are treated by local antibiotic treatment to prevent secondary bacterial infections and topical corticosteroids if the corneal irritation is intense.

Mooren's ulcer is a rare, painful, progressive ulcer of the cornea that develops in the elderly and is idiopathic. It may be bilateral and usually develops in the limbus of the cornea, spreading over a period of months to a year to involve the whole of the cornea. Although the cornea is thinned under the ulcer, perforation is rare and inflammation with necrosis impairs the vision of the patient. Such ulcers are very difficult to treat.

Bacterial infections of the cornea with subsequent ulceration may occur when any one of several species of bacteria colonize this tissue. Organisms usually isolated from such infections are: *Staphylococcus* spp., *Streptococcus* spp., *Pseudomonas aeruginosa*, *Klebsiella pneumoniae* and Morax-Axenfeld bacillus (*Moraxella lacunata* and other species of *Moraxella*).

Bacterially caused ulcers of the cornea are usually central ulcers that involve the corneal tissue extensively, often perforating the cornea, leading to an abscess and **hypopyon**, a collection of pus or cloudy exudate in the anterior chamber of the eye (refer to Figure 19.7). The microscopic appearance of the ulcerated region is characterized by necrotic debris, acute and chronic inflammatory cells and much exudate. There is also infiltration of the iris, ciliary body and anterior chamber by many inflammatory cells and much exudate and the inflammation may cause anterior and posterior **synechiae** (where the iris margin adheres to the cornea anteriorly or to the lens posteriorly). *Pseudomonas aeruginosa* infection is a particularly dangerous one as the organism is very virulent and produces many enzymes that have a destructive effect on the tissue; perforation of the cornea can occur in as little as 48 hours, with loss of the eye if the infection remains untreated. Treatment of bacterial infections of the cornea and hypopyon is by topical administration of the appropriate antibiotics (garamycin, chloramphenicol and polymyxin B are often used), intravenous and subconjunctival injections of antibiotics being used in very severe infections.

Age-related Changes and Degenerations

Arcus senilis is a degenerative change of the cornea appearing in middle to old age and is generally associated with high lipid levels (especially if present in patients less than 55 years of age). The lesion causes no impairment of vision as the corneal periphery shows a diffuse infiltrate of lipid either as an arc or as a complete ring in the stroma of the cornea (refer to Figure 19.5). Although this condition is of no ophthalmological consequence it is advisable to investigate patients who present with the disorder for hyperlipidaemia.

Band keratopathy of the cornea presents as a band of opacity across the central region of the cornea (refer to Figure 19.5). It is associated with long-standing inflammation of the eyes (e.g. as observed in juvenile rheumatoid arthritis) and there is scarring and calcium deposition. The condition will cause vision impairment or blindness. Instillation of EDTA preparations into the eye may ameliorate the condition in the early stages by removing the deposits of calcium. Excessive scar tissue formed in the cornea in this condition may need excision.

Keratoconus is a deformation of the cornea, causing it to be conical in section, with a thinned central portion, instead of the normal, near-spherical cross-section and uniform thickness. If the eye is viewed from the side, the central part of the cornea bulges outwards (refer to Figure 19.6). The condition may be seen in both congenital and degenerative forms, and is usually bilateral, although the eyes may show different degrees of conical malformation in the corneae. The patient is grossly myopic and astigmatism may also be present. Treatment is by the use of corrective lenses (eyeglasses or contact lenses) in mild cases, but corneal grafting may be necessary in severe cases. Even after the corneal graft, patients may need to wear corrective lenses.

Pterygium and **pinguecula**, already considered in association with conjunctival diseases, may also involve the cornea. Reduction of visual acuity due to corneal opacity or astigmatism due to corneal deformity may complicate these conditions.

Tumours of the cornea are extremely rare and they may be benign or malignant. Dermoids of the cornea are the commonest benign tumours, while Bowen's disease and carcinoma of the limbus are the commonest malignant ones. Treatment and prognosis are similar to the conjunctival tumours.

Crystalline Lens

Cataract

A cataract is any opacity, partial or complete, of the crystalline lens. The disorder is either congenital (as may occur in congenital rubella) or occurs in an acquired form, following a variety of causes, but typically the disease is most often an age-related degeneration of the lens. The disease occurs because the lens fibres either are formed abnormally or may be formed normally but degenerate later. Acquired forms of cataract are:

- due to **trauma** caused by radiation, intraocular foreign bodies, severe contusions;

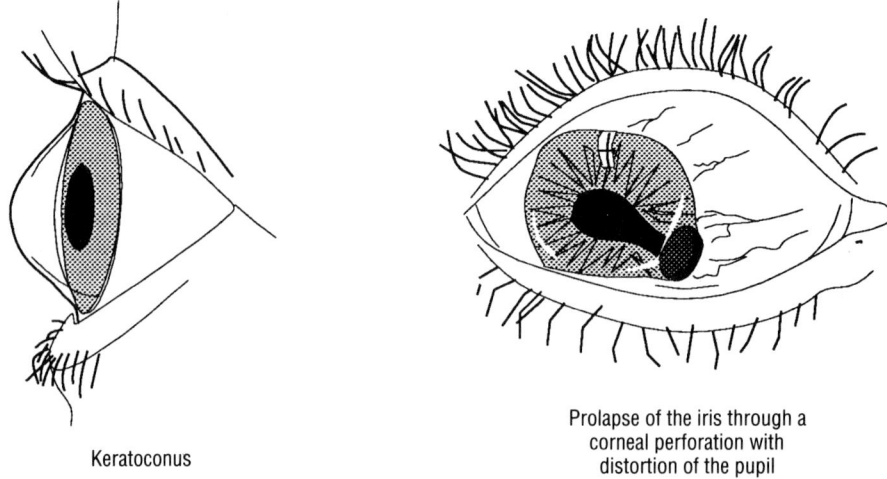

Keratoconus

Prolapse of the iris through a
corneal perforation with
distortion of the pupil

Figure 19.6   *Corneal disorders (II)*

- due to **systemic disease**, such as diabetes, galacto-saemia, myotonia dystrophica;
- **iatrogenic**, caused by the prolonged administration of some drugs (e.g. corticosteroids, powerful miotics) or after irradiation of the eye;
- **secondary**, as seen in association with other intra-ocular diseases (e.g. prolonged uveitis);
- **degenerative (senile)**, associated with age-related degenerative opacity.

A cataract may be seen primarily in the nucleus of the lens, in which case the opacity will develop in the central part of the lens, this being a **nuclear type** of cataract. Alternatively the cataract may be of the **cortical type** in which case there are multiple opacities scattered throughout the cortical region of the lens, associated with fluid accumulation and degeneration of the lens fibres. People with cataracts present with diminished vision which may be quite marked if most of the lens is involved. If the opacities in the lens are central (i.e. commonly with nuclear cataracts), vision usually improves when the patient is in a darkened room or at night as the pupil dilates and exposes the clearer lens on the periphery (i.e. vision will improve with mydriatics — drugs causing pupil dilatation). The cortical type of cataract will scatter light onto the retina, producing blurred vision and much discomfort with glare. Children with cataracts often present with **strabismus** ('squint'). An advanced ('ripe' or 'mature') cataract will appear as a grey or white pupil and the opacities in the lens will be seen quite clearly with the slit lamp during eye examination.

Treatment for cataract is undertaken when the condition has progressed to such an extent that the vision of the patient is seriously compromised. There are various forms of surgery for cataract, but the common factor in all methods is removal of the opaque crystalline lens. Once the lens is surgically extracted, the vision of the patient must be improved as an eye without a lens (**aphakia**) will not focus light on the retina. Three methods of vision improvement for cataract patients are:

- **Spectacles** of high refractive power (+11D to +14D may be needed) in order to correct the highly hypermetropic eye. Retinal images are enlarged by 30% with these glasses and the patient may find objects appearing very large and with curved outlines. Giddiness may be experienced with rapid head movements. Spectacles are not tolerated well if the patient has one good eye and an aphakic eye, as the difference in the size of the retinal image in the two eyes prevents fusion and the patient experiences double vision.
- **Contact lenses** correct the vision but magnify only about 9%, so that objects appear more normal and fusion of the images can occur with monocular aphakia. No giddiness occurs, but many elderly patients find the use of contact lenses very inconvenient.
- **Intraocular lens implants (IOL)** are the most promising and best method of correcting aphakia but the surgery is more difficult and carries increased risks, especially in the elderly. In this surgical operation a plastic lens is implanted into the eye, various such IOL implants being available. This type of prosthesis magnifies the image on the retina by about 5% of normal and successful procedures lead the best ap-

proximation to normal vision for patients with cataract. Generally, IOL implants are not carried out in the very young as the long-term effects of the implants are not known.

Complications of cataract surgery are haemorrhage, vitreous humour loss, general collapse or cardiac arrest. Iris prolapse may occur any time within the first 3 weeks after the surgery, and may be caused by sudden head movements or trauma to the eye. Infection, hyphaema and secondary glaucoma may also complicate cataract surgery, but even in the absence of serious complications the patient feels weak and tired.

Uveal Tract, Retina

Uveitis

The uveal tract comprises the iris, ciliary body and choroid, which although structurally continuous have different functions. The iris forms the anterior part of the uveal tract and it forms a pigmented, circular disc perforated by a round central aperture known as the pupil. The pupil size will be regulated by reflex mechanisms depending on the amount of ambient light. Strong light will cause a reduction of the pupil size, this being known as **miosis**. Miotic drugs such as pilocarpine, carbachol and prostigmine have the same effect. Little light will cause the pupil to dilate, a change known as **mydriasis**. Mydriatic drugs such as atropine, cocaine and phenylephrine have the same effect (see also Figure 19.7).

The ciliary body is a structure extending forward from the anterior termination of the choroid at the ora serrata, to the scleral spur close to the canal of Schlemm (refer to Figure 19.3). The ciliary processes secrete aqueous humour and also provide attachment to the crystalline lens. The ciliary muscles are responsible for the slight alteration in the shape of the lens, essential for accommodation and also serve to increase the aqueous outflow by contraction of the longitudinal muscle which causes a widening of the trabecular spaces. The insertion of the iris to the anterior portion of the ciliary body forms the angle of the anterior chamber and it is here that resorption of aqueous humour occurs. The choroid is the posterior part of the uveal tract extending from the ora serrata to the optic nerve. It consists of an outer brown, pigmented layer and an inner, very vascular layer. Bruch's membrane separates the choroidal vessels from the retinal pigment epithelium (refer to Figure 19.8). The function of the choroid is to provide nourishment to the external layers of the retina (neuroepithelium).

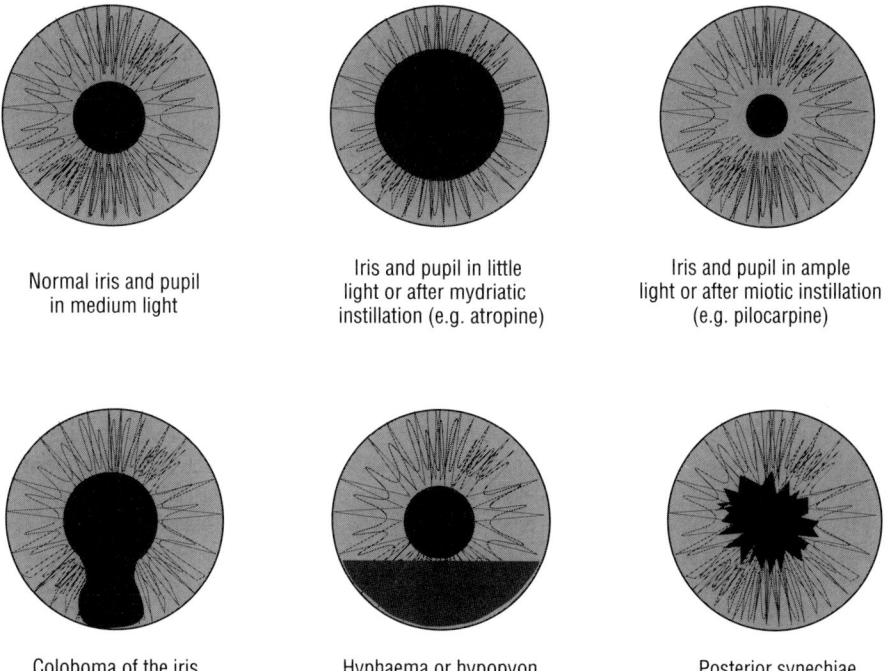

Normal iris and pupil in medium light

Iris and pupil in little light or after mydriatic instillation (e.g. atropine)

Iris and pupil in ample light or after miotic instillation (e.g. pilocarpine)

Coloboma of the iris

Hyphaema or hypopyon

Posterior synechiae

Figure 19.7 *The iris and pupil in various states*

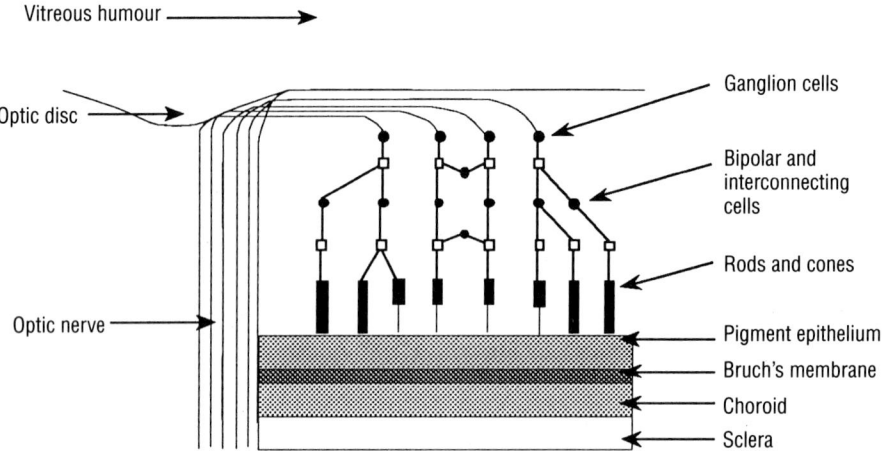

Figure 19.8 *The structure of the retina and associated structures*

Anterior uveitis may manifest itself as **acute iritis**, an inflammation of the iris, or as **acute cyclitis**, an inflammation of the ciliary body. Frequently both tissues are affected together giving rise to an **iridocyclitis**. Causes of acute anterior uveitis are:

- **traumatic**, especially with penetrating injuries to the eye;
- **infectious**, associated with systemic or local infections, viral or bacterial;
- **post-surgical**, associated especially with cataract surgery;
- **autoimmune disease**, with no other evidence of aetiological or predisposing factors;
- **systemic disease**, such as ankylosing spondylitis and rheumatoid arthritis (especially juvenile rheumatoid arthritis — Still's disease).

Symptoms of acute anterior uveitis are blurred vision and pain, the severity of which depends on the severity of the inflammation. Blepharospasm, photophobia, tenderness on palpation and lacrimation are also common complaints. Signs will be apparent upon close examination of the eye and include ciliary injection due to congestion of the ciliary vessels, a small pupil which is often unresponsive to light, and keratitic precipitates (inflammatory cells and debris that adhere to the cornea). In the anterior chamber there may be observed a 'flare' caused by leakage of protein from inflamed iridal or ciliary vessels, fibrinous networks associated with more severe inflammation and inflammatory cellular deposits. Secondary glaucoma may be caused by impedance of the outflow of aqueous humour from the inflamed region.

Posterior uveitis affects the choroid in the posterior regions of the eye and occurs without ciliary injection or pain. Vision is blurred to various degrees and this depends on the amount of tissue involved in the inflammation and also on the presence of more or less vitreous opacities. Various disorders may give rise to posterior uveitis, although toxoplasmosis is by far one of the commonest causes (see below). A number of autoimmune and systemic disorders may affect the posterior part of the choroid and chorioretinitis may be the consequence (see Table 19.2).

The treatment regimes for anterior and posterior uveitis are essentially similar and the principles of such treatments are first to treat the symptoms and provide relief for the patient. Then the inflammatory process is treated, with the aim being the prevention of complications. The underlying disorder which has led to the uveitis is then treated if it has been identified and if it is amenable to treatment. The local treatment of the condition involves mydriatic drugs that will dilate the pupil and prevent the adhesion of the iris to the lens or the cornea (i.e. prevention of posterior and anterior synechiae). Corticosteroids may be given locally to diminish the inflammation. Systemic therapy includes aspirin for its analgesic and anti-inflammatory effects, antibiotics and chemotherapeutic agents for any underlying infections (as needed) and whatever treatment is required for the underlying cause if this has been determined.

Complications of uveitis are:

- **cataract formation**, which usually begins posteriorly and is most often associated with chronic cyclitis. Prolonged corticosteroid treatment will also cause cataracts;

- **synechiae** — posterior adhesions of the iris to the lens form if the inflamed iris heals by scarring;
- **glaucoma**, if the pupil margin forms synechiae over 360° which prevent the flow of aqueous humour from the posterior to the anterior chamber; this may lead to **iris bombé**, which is a bulging of the peripheral iris towards the cornea, caused by high intraocular pressure; **anterior synechiae** may then form between the iris and cornea;
- **occlusion of the pupil** if the inflammatory exudate covers the pupillary aperture and thus occludes vision;
- **band keratopathy**, caused by involvement of the cornea by the chronic inflammation (see Figure 19.5);
- **retinal detachment** if the inflammation of the choroid is extensive, with the subretinal exudate lifting the retina off Bruch's membrane;
- **macular degeneration**, associated with oedema due to inflammation;
- **panophthalmitis**, which implies that the inflammation spreads to involve all of the eye with possibly retinal necrosis and loss of the affected eye.

Toxoplasmosis

Toxoplasmosis is an infection caused by an intracellular protozoon, *Toxoplasma gondii*. This is a crescent-shaped organism, approximately 5 μm by 2.5 μm, with a prominent nucleus. The organism has a worldwide distribution and is harboured by many domestic animals such as dogs, cats, rodents and pigeons. The disease may be contracted by eating undercooked or uncooked pork, beef or mutton (about 25% of pork and 10% of beef sold for human consumption contain cysts of *Toxoplasma gondii.*). Often, the disease may be contracted by contacting faeces of cats, or by congenital transmission. Immunocompromised patients and infants present with the most severe form of the disease, while normal adults are only mildly affected.

Toxoplasmosis of the eyes is most often seen to occur complicating congenital infections but it may also occur in adult infections. About a third of cases of chorioretinitis are caused by this infection. The patient suffers from blurred vision, strabismus, photophobia or scotoma. The eye may be painful and sometimes glaucoma or blindness are associated with the condition. The disease is episodic in nature and there are exacerbations and remissions. There are foci of necrosis in the retina, choroid and sclera, around which are areas of chronic granulomatous inflammation. In the early stages of the disease the organisms will be demonstrable, but in later stages the organisms are progressively harder to find. Untreated chorioretinitis will progress over many years, bringing blindness in its wake.

In congenital toxoplasmosis and in adults with immune dysfunction the disease is severe with widespread toxoplasmosis affecting many organs. The brain is particularly severely affected with encephalitis and meningitis resulting in brain damage and serious central nervous system malformations in the infant. Treatment is by administration of pyrimethamine and sulphonamides with folinic acid to prevent depression of the bone marrow. Adrenocortical steroids are usually given if the eye injury is particularly severe.

Retinopathies

A retinopathy is defined as any pathological condition of the retina that is not associated with inflammation. The major disorders that are associated with retinopathy are vascular diseases such as atherosclerosis, arteriolosclerosis, hypertension, and diabetes mellitus. Retrolental fibroplasia, involutionary changes associated with senility and some idiopathic and congenital disorders are also included in the group.

Atherosclerotic retinopathy is associated with the rather uncommon situation of atheromatous plaques developing in the retinal artery. If this occurs, the partial ischaemia associated with the condition will cause atrophy of the retina, especially the outer layers of the neuroepithelium. The inner layers are fairly well preserved because they are supplied with oxygen and nutrients from the choroidal vessels. The chronic ischaemia and atrophic changes in the retina will be associated with vision impairment as the cells undergo degeneration and necrosis. Through the ophthalmoscope, the retina will appear pale to milky white, the visible arteries being reduced to narrow threads. If most of the retina is involved, blindness will be the result.

Hypertensive retinopathy is seen in benign and malignant hypertension and is often given the name **arteriolosclerotic retinopathy** as the major changes in this disorder occur in the arterioles of the retina, which are damaged by the high blood pressure. The retinal disease in benign hypertension follows a characteristic progression and may evolve over a period of many years. The following steps are involved:

- **Spasm** of the arterioles occurs in localized areas rather intermittently and the blood columns in the vessels appear narrowed and there may be oedema in the retina making it appear opalescent (the normal retina is almost transparent, the fundus background observed being due to the choroidal epithelium and the blood in its blood vessels).

- **Sclerosis** is the next step that occurs in the retinal vessels and this is a thickening and opacity of the arteriolosclerotic vessel walls. This is seen through the ophthalmoscope as a 'copper and silver wire' appearance of vessels due to the high reflectivity of the thickened, sclerotic wall. Constrictions in the column of blood may be observed if the arteriolosclerotic plaques interfere with the flow of blood through the vessels.
- **Retinopathy** is fully developed when there are retinal haemorrhages (usually flame-shaped and superficial) and also some small, compact, whitish exudates. Small scars also appear where the haemorrhages are removed. Oedema of the optic disc (papilloedema) and of the perimacular areas are also features associated with the disorder.

Malignant hypertension will cause a rapidly developing retinopathy over a period of months. The appearance is similar to that of the retinopathy caused by benign hypertension, with the difference being that the spasm of the arterioles is more generalized and thus the whole of the retina may be affected, leading to ischaemia and gross retinal oedema which may be complicated by fluffy, whitish exudates ('cotton wool exudates') with a high fibrin content. Characteristically, the optic disc is involved in the oedema, with **papilloedema** being a prime feature of the disorder. Small vessels will show regions of fibrinoid necrosis and haemorrhages associated with these vessels may be observed (see Table 19.2).

Diabetic retinopathy is generally observed in the eyes of diabetics 10 to 20 years after onset of the disease, most patients thus affected being middle aged to elderly. The disease of the retina is complicated by senile and hypertensive changes. Both retinae are affected, the first sign of the disorder being microaneurysms developing in the small retinal vessels with many small haemorrhages developing subsequently as the aneurysms rupture (the so-called 'dot-and-blot-haemorrhages'). Small regions of exudation develop over the years and these are of small size and of an irregular margin, becoming gradually larger and more extensive, with progres-

Table 19.2 *Systemic diseases that cause eye changes*

Disease	Nature	Eye changes
Marfan's syndrome	Genetic	Subluxation of crystalline lens
Kinnier-Wilson's disease	Genetic	Kayser-Fleischer ring of copper pigment in Descemet's membrane of cornea
Arcus senilis	Genetic/metabolic	Pale ring of fat infiltration seen in the peripheral cornea
Diabetes mellitus	Genetic/metabolic	Cataracts, diabetic retinopathy, small haemorrhages, microaneurysms
Rheumatoid arthritis; Still's disease	Autoimmune	Scleritis and episcleritis; iridocyclitis
Ankylosing spondylitis	Autoimmune	Iridocyclitis
Reiter's syndrome	Infectious/autoimmune	Conjunctivitis, rarely uveitis and blindness
Syphilis	Infectious/autoimmune	Iridocyclitis, choroiditis, choroidoretinitis
Sarcoidosis	Autoimmune/idiopathic	Iridocyclitis, choroiditis
Thyrotoxicosis	Endocrine/autoimmune	Exophthalmos
Hypertension	Idiopathic	Papilloedema, retinal haemorrhages
Avitaminosis A	Dietary deficiency	Night blindness, keratomalacia

sively increasing vision impairment. A large haemorrhage into the vitreous humour may sometimes occur and this may bring on blindness, or alternatively retinal detachment, retinal degeneration and scarring that will cause blindness.

Central retinal vein occlusion may occur due to pressure effects from the adjacent artery in the region of the optic disc, occurring with atherosclerosis, hypertension, oedema in the region or with effects of infection and thrombosis. There is anoxia of the retina as the blood pools due to inadequate drainage and retinal degeneration causes sudden blindness of the affected eye. Haemorrhages appear to be scattered throughout the retina and these are superficial and irregular, lying parallel to the congested, tortuous retinal veins. In the period that follows, new vessels grow into the surface of the iris and into the filtration angles for unknown reasons, and this complication causes glaucoma. If the venous occlusion is resolved, the patient may regain some vision, but the developing glaucoma may cause rapid deterioration of sight. Treatment is difficult and ineffective in the majority of cases.

Retrolental fibroplasia occurs in premature babies after they are removed from the incubator where they have been breathing air with a high partial pressure of oxygen (usually greater than 30%). It is a bilateral condition affecting the retina with detachment and fibrosis. The high oxygen tension in the inspired air while the baby is in the incubator causes the retinal vessels to constrict and some of them may close off. When the baby is taken out of the incubator, the reduced oxygen tension in the air (and hence the blood) causes angiogenesis, especially in the peripheral retina within the inner retinal layer and the vitreous. Haemorrhages develop in these newly formed vessels and there is contracture of the retina causing detachment and degeneration. The fibrous tissue formed and the detached retina will cause marked deterioration in vision. New vessels in the iris can close off the filtration angle with secondary glaucoma supervening and complicating the condition. Prevention of the condition is achieved by avoiding high oxygen tension in incubators.

Senile retinopathy occurs in the retinae of the elderly even in the absence of hypertension and in this case the arterioles of the retina will be narrowed, pale and of variable diameter. Patchy fibrosis will cause a degree of visual impairment. **Senile macular degeneration** will occur if the choroidal vessels which normally supply the macula with blood undergo any degenerative changes associated with diseases of old age. Arteriolosclerosis of such vessels will result in damage to the retina and a central **scotoma** (an area of depressed vision in the visual field, surrounded by a region of less depressed or normal vision) will develop.

Retinal Detachment

Any lesion which causes the retina to separate from its bed of Bruch's membrane, which lies on the choroid, will manifest itself as retinal detachment. There are various forms of this condition and the classification is mainly an aetiological one.

- **Rhegmatogenous** or perforated detachment is one where there is a tear in the retina allowing vitreous and fluid to enter between the pigment epithelium and the layer of rods and cones.
- **Exudative** detachments are caused by inflammatory lesions or other disease (e.g. eclampsia) causing accumulation of fluid in the subretinal spaces.
- **Traction** detachments are caused by forces pulling on strands of the vitreous humour caused by trauma, inflammation, degenerations or neoplasms.
- **Neoplastic** detachment is caused by a neoplastic growth (retinoblastoma, malignant melanoma) beneath or on the retina, causing its detachment.
- **Retinoschisis** is any splitting caused by accumulation of fluid within the retina which is not associated with any of the above aetiologies.

The symptoms of retinal detachment are **photopsiae** (visions of flashing lights caused by the stimulation of visual receptors due to movement from their positions), '**floaters**' (black specks or lines in the vision caused by debris in the vitreous), and **scotoma** (a localized defect in the visual field). In addition, there may be a marked distortion or loss of vision if the macula is affected or if a retinal vessel is torn.

Treatment of the condition is surgical and involves sealing any defects that are present in the retina and creating apposition of pigment epithelium to neuroepithelium. Various techniques are used, including laser therapy, cryotherapy or diathermy, injection of air or gas into the vitreous to press back the detached retina, or various forms of scleral buckling with synthetic or biological implants. Post-operatively, the pupil is kept dilated with mydriatics to prevent synechiae from forming and to reduce movement of the choroid. Eye pads may be worn and the patients are advised not to bend and not to pick up heavy weights or exert themselves until the healing is complete.

Retinitis Pigmentosa

This is a congenital disease of various inheritance

patterns. There is an autosomal recessive severe form, an autosomal dominant, milder form and a sex-linked severe form limited to males. The disorder is brought about by premature degeneration of the retinal neuro-epithelium, commencing in early adult life and bringing about blindness by 55 years of age. The retinal rods are affected first and the patient initially experiences **nyctalopia** (night blindness), which progresses to loss of vision. The pigment accumulates as star-shaped aggregates in the retina, progressively affecting more one side of the optic fundus. The arteries are thinned and atrophic and the optic discs are pale and waxy.

Microscopically, in advanced cases of the disease, the rods and cones are almost totally absent, the pigmented epithelium is disorganized and the outer nuclear and plexiform layers of the retina are atrophic. The star-shaped pigmented areas are seen to be proliferating clumps of pigment epithelial cells. The optic disc may show atrophy. Macular degeneration or cataract may accelerate blindness, while in some pedigrees there is also a predisposition to deafness.

Coloboma

Coloboma is any defect or apparent absence of some ocular tissue. This is usually caused by a congenital failure of a part of the foetal fissure to close. It may affect the iris, lens, retina, optic nerve, choroid, eyelid or ciliary body (see Figure 19.7). If the defect is complete, it extends from the optic disc downwards and inwards to the pupillary margin of the iris. Along the region of the cleft, the sclera and choroid are thin, Bruch's membrane is absent and the retinal tissues overlying the lesion are atypical and atrophic. Varying degrees of vision impairment are observed.

Glaucoma

Glaucoma is the condition where there is an increased intraocular pressure, the normal intraocular pressure being 15 to 22 mmHg. A device known as a **tonometer** measures intraocular pressure when it is placed on the anaesthetized cornea. Changes in intraocular pressure that remain untreated will cause damage to the eye. Glaucoma may be acute, subacute or chronic and its development may be associated with the following factors:

- **genetic predisposition**, which may be a very important factor in some patients;
- **increased resistance** to the outflow of aqueous humour from the eye;
- **obstruction** to the circulation of aqueous humour within the eye;
- **increased secretion** of aqueous humour, a very rare cause;
- **idiopathic factors**, although the circulation may be involved in these.

Normally, the ciliary processes secrete the aqueous humour into the posterior chamber. The aqueous is a fluid similar to blood plasma except that its protein content is very low. It fills the anterior chamber and some of the posterior chamber and serves to nourish the cornea, the lens and the vitreous humour, these structures having no blood vessels of their own. If the composition of the aqueous humour changes (e.g. in diabetes, uveitis, effects of drugs) the lens may become damaged and cataracts will develop. The aqueous passes through the pupil into the anterior chamber and there it is resorbed by the trabecular processes to enter the canal of Schlemm, a modified vein which returns the aqueous to the blood (refer to Figure 19.3).

A high intraocular pressure will cause the following effects on the eye:

- **Distension** of the eyeball, which will occur in its weakest part, which may be a region damaged or inflamed. In the infant, the whole of the eyeball becomes enlarged such that it is readily apparent as an 'ox-eye' or **buphthalmos**.
- **Loss of visual field**, due to cupping of the optic disc by the high pressure, this being the weakest spot in the adult eye. Visual impairment occurs if nerve fibres are damaged in this process.
- **Corneal oedema**, caused by the high pressure forcing fluid into the cornea. The cornea becomes thickened and the patient sees hazily, often with rainbow-coloured rings seen around lights.

The classification of glaucoma depends on the aetiology and pathogenesis of the condition. Using such criteria, we may divide glaucoma into **primary** and **secondary**, **acute** and **chronic**, **closed angle** and **open angle**. Clinically, glaucoma may be divided into the following groups.

Infantile glaucoma (buphthalmos). This is seen as a congenital condition where the increased intraocular pressure causes enlargement of the affected eye, making it resemble the eye of a bullock. There is maldevelopment of the filtration angle of the anterior chamber with persistence of mesodermal remnants and impedance in the outflow of aqueous humour. The condition may be bilateral or unilateral and if untreated the raised intraocular pressure will cause splits in Descemet's membrane, oedema in the cornea with opacification, atrophy of the optic disc with cupping and myopia, photophobia and eventually blindness. Treatment of the condition is surgical and **goniotomy** is the procedure where the mesodermal remnants in the filtration angle are excised, allowing drainage of the aqueous.

Chronic simple glaucoma (open angle). The changes that cause this condition are thought to reside primarily in the trabeculae of the filtration spaces, causing obstruction to the outflow of the aqueous. The condition is idiopathic although some genetic factors appear to be operating. Patients present with the disorder after the age of 40 years (some cases are observed in youth). In the early stages there are few to no symptoms, although a small number of patients will experience pain in the eye or complain of vision impairment. As the condition progresses, loss of field of vision is demonstrable with the nasal quadrants first affected and gradually a definite scotoma will appear within the field of vision. The optic nerve fibres will progressively degenerate as the elevated pressure inside the eye increases, the optic disc being pale and atrophic, the optic cup growing larger, until it extends into the disc margin (**glaucomatous cupping**; see Figure 19.9).

Diagnosis of chronic glaucoma may be carried out by measuring the intraocular pressure on several occasions (usually at 4-hourly intervals) with a tonometer and in addition the water drinking test may be used. In this test, the patient presents in the morning before eating or drinking anything. The ocular tension is measured and a litre of water is given to the patient to consume within 5 minutes. Ocular tension is measured again at 15-minute intervals for the next 2 hours. In a normal subject there is little or no rise in intraocular tension, whereas the glaucomatous patient shows a rise of 4 mmHg or more in intraocular tension.

Treatment of simple chronic glaucoma is carried out by the local application of several drugs (e.g. anticholinesterase drugs, pilocarpine and laevoepinephrine) or by the systemic administration of drugs (e.g. carbonic anhydrase inhibitors or short-term treatment with mannitol or urea). Surgical management involves the creation of passages for the adequate drainage of the aqueous humour. Several such operations are carried out and they include anterior sclerotomy, cyclodialysis and cyclodiathermy procedures. The prognosis for this type of glaucoma is good, providing treatment is initiated rapidly after the onset of the disease.

Acute congestive glaucoma (closed angle). Closed-angle glaucoma implies that the filtration angle is obstructed by contact between the iris and cornea. The iris may be pushed forward from behind, it may be the result of long-term mydriasis where the iridal tissue occludes the angle or it may be the result of anterior synechiae. The condition develops over a short period of time and generally the patient presents with aching in the affected eye, blurred vision or the seeing of haloes around bright lights. These tend to be transient features and the eye then progresses into the congestive phase where it looks red, is painful, lacrimates excessively and vision is markedly impaired. The cornea is generally hazy because of corneal oedema, the anterior chamber is obstructed and shallow and the pupil appears oval and is dilated. Pupillary reactions in this stage are diminished or may be totally absent. The optic disc may not be seen because of the opacity of the cornea, but cupping does not occur until later in the

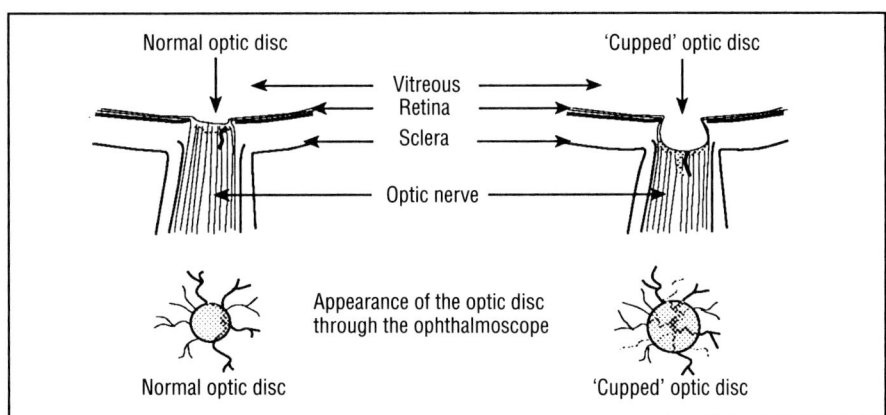

Figure 19.9 *Glaucomatous 'cupping' of the optic disc seen in section and through the ophthalmoscope*

course of the untreated disease. The intraocular tension is raised when measured with the tonometer.

Treatment of this type of glaucoma is through the instillation into the eyes of eserine or pilocarpine drops together with intravenous or intramuscular acetazolamide. If the condition persists after the drug treatment surgical intervention is necessary. Various forms of surgical procedures are carried out, all of them having the feature of opening up the obstructed filtration angle and allowing the outflow of aqueous. Although the choice of operation depends on the individual case and the surgeon, one of the common procedures that is carried out is peripheral iridectomy.

Secondary glaucoma. As the name for this condition implies, it is a disorder that complicates some other eye disease and it arises because the filtration angle becomes obstructed in the course of that disorder. Some common causes of secondary glaucoma have already been mentioned above but they are listed here for convenience:

- **Trabecular obstruction** may occur with a variety of diseases, such as inflammations, tumours, disintegrating damaged crystalline lens or iridal tissue.
- **Anterior synechiae** may block the filtration angle in association with a variety of disorders that cause fibrosis and synechiae to form. This may be a common aftermath of inflammations in the eye, as occurs, for example, with iridocyclitis. New vessels formed in the periphery of the iris (**rubeosis iridis**) may also cause anterior synechiae and glaucoma and various states in which this is seen are diabetic retinopathy, retrolental fibroplasia, central retinal vein thrombosis and choroidal tumours.
- **Trauma** may cause obstruction of the filtration angle.
- The cause may be **iatrogenic**, as is seen in association with topical steroid instillation into the eyes of people predisposed to glaucoma (familial) and is more likely to occur with some steroid preparations (e.g. prednisolone, dexamethasone). The glaucoma subsides after the steroid administration ceases.
- **Obstruction** of aqueous flow from the posterior to the anterior chamber through the pupil may be caused by ring synechiae of the pupil, pupil block between the iris and the lens or be the result of various inflammations of the iris.
- **Ciliary block** glaucoma occurs when the anterior chamber is flat and may occur after eye operations (e.g. cataract, glaucoma). The aqueous in this case becomes trapped around or in the vitreous and pushes the lens and iris against the cornea, closing off the filtration angle.

Treatment of secondary glaucoma depends on the early treatment of underlying primary disease which has brought about the glaucoma secondarily. The glaucoma may be treated concurrently by the administration of oral acetazolamide. Some cases are very refractory to such treatments and surgical methods must be employed.

Retinoblastoma

Retinoblastoma is a malignant tumour which is transmitted as an autosomal dominant characteristic and is therefore most often seen in infants less than 3 years old. A deletion of the long arm of chromosome 13 is often demonstrable in the tumour cells. In about a third of cases the tumour is bilateral, each eye showing an independently arising primary tumour. The children of survivors of the tumour will develop the condition in about 60% of cases. In the past, when the tumour was commonly fatal because of inadequate treatment, retinoblastoma was a rather uncommon tumour. Nowadays, with effective treatment of the tumour, the patients survive to adulthood and will contribute their genes to the next generation, making this tumour a more commonly occurring one.

Retinoblastoma forms a pale mass, often lobulated, arising from the retina and spreading in several directions. Depending on the growth pattern of the mass, the tumour is given the following names:

- **planum**, spreading flatly within the retina;
- **exophytum**, spreading posteriorly into the subretinal spaces;
- **endophytum**, growing within the eye into the vitreous humour;
- **diffuse infiltrating**, spreading along the retinal wall and involving the ciliary body and iris.

All forms of retinoblastoma, if left untreated, will eventually spread to involve the whole globe and will cause glaucoma in the affected eye. The tumour often grows along the optic nerve spreading directly to involve the brain. Blood-borne metastases are common and will most often involve the bones. Early signs of the tumour are strabismus and a pale pupil. Any whitish reflex seen through the pupil is known as **leukokoria** and this sign may be caused by a variety of aetiologies (in adults, cataract and retinal detachment are the most common; in childhood, as well as retinoblastoma the following conditions may cause leukokoria and thus must be considered as differential diagnoses for the tumour: congenital cataract, primary hyperplastic vitreous and retrolental fibroplasia). The cells of retinoblastoma appear as elongated or round, arranged in sheets or rosette-shaped masses. There is no pigmentation associated with the tumour cells. Necrosis and calcification are frequent findings and in a few cases extensive necrosis may cause a spontaneous remission.

Treatment of the tumour is by enucleation of the affected eye if the condition is unilateral. If the condition occurs bilaterally, treatment consists of enucleation of the most severely affected eye and radiotherapy of the less severely affected eye in order to treat the condition, preserve the life of the patient and at the same time conserve vision. The 5-year survival is 85% although recurrence of the tumour may occur in the radiotherapy-treated eyes. If recurrence does not occur within 5 years, it is unlikely to occur later in life.

Malignant Melanoma

Malignant melanoma in the eye most often occurs in the choroid, less frequently in the ciliary body and rarely in the iris. It is by far the commonest intraocular tumour, and typically arises in adults.

Tumours of the choroid begin as a small mass of malignant cells confined to the sclera, but soon grow in the subretinal space, lifting the retina and destroying it. The entire globe may soon be filled by the malignancy and eventually the tumour will invade past the sclera into the orbit. Pigmentation of the tumour is variable and amelanotic melanomata may also occur. Glaucoma is frequently present as the tumour grows because of blockage of the filtration angles by the growing mass or by necrotic debris from the neoplasm. In the ciliary body and iris the tumour will typically cause glaucoma early and the crystalline lens may become subluxated or may show cataract. The lesion may be seen on the iris, often causing its enlargement and in some cases altering its pigmentation.

Microscopically the melanoma may show several forms. **Spindle cell** tumours show elongated cells arranged in groups, resembling the naevus cells present in blue naevi. Mitotic figures in such tumours are scanty and the tumours are not highly malignant in behaviour. **Epithelioid cell** tumours consist of groups of large polyhedral cells with giant cells. There is pleomorphism with many mitotic figures readily observable. Pigmentation may be so heavy that the section must be bleached in order to be interpreted histologically; generally, highly pigmented tumours carry the poorest prognosis. **Mixed tumours** show populations of cells that resemble the two previous types and their behaviour is intermediate.

The tumour spreads locally around the orbit and may involve the brain if left untreated. Metastasis via the bloodstream to involve distant sites will also occur, but most often the liver will be affected. Although the primary tumour may have been removed, death from metastasis may occur as long as 20 years after treatment (the 'big liver and glass eye' syndrome). Treatment of malignant melanoma is by enucleation of the affected eye. The prognosis is much better than with melanoma in other parts of the body, the 5-year survival for the ocular tumour being 50% or better.

Lacrimal Apparatus

Inflammations

The function of the lacrimal system is to secrete tears in order to lubricate the surface of the cornea, thus preventing it from drying and maintaining a smooth surface for optical purposes. The tears will also wash away foreign bodies from the conjunctival surfaces and they contain lysozyme, which has an antibacterial effect. The lacrimal glands are situated in the fossa beneath the lateral part of the upper eyelid. They are oval-shaped bodies covered by the orbital septa, orbicularis muscles and skin. The collecting system of the lacrimal system comprises the lacrimal puncta, the upper and lower canaliculi, the lacrimal sac and the nasolacrimal duct.

Inflammations of the lacrimal apparatus may be acute or chronic, and if they affect the lacrimal glands are termed **dacryoadenitis**; if they affect the lacrimal passages of the collecting system they are termed **dacryocystitis**. Acute dacryoadenitis is often associated with viral infections such as mumps. Bacterial infections of the lacrimal gland are less commonly observed but will cause a typical suppurative response and may progress to abscess formation. Acute dacryocystitis is almost always associated with obstruction of the lacrimal passages and secondary bacterial infection. A low-grade infection may produce mucocoele of the lacrimal sac, whereas a pyogenic infection will cause an abscess to form in the sac, which in poorly managed cases may form a discharging fistula through the overlying skin.

Chronic dacryoadenitis is in most cases due to **Mikulicz's syndrome**, a chronic inflammation of the lacrimal and salivary glands (especially the parotids) due to many disorders, the commonest of which is sarcoidosis. Other conditions in which Mikulicz's syndrome is seen are tuberculosis, autoimmune disorders, Hodgkin's disease and other lymphomasarcomatous and leukaemic conditions. There is a chronic, bilateral involvement of the glands and there is an associated dysfunction seen together with chronic inflammation in the parenchyma of the affected tissue.

Sjögren's Syndrome

Sjögren's syndrome is an autoimmune disease that primarily affects post-menopausal women and leads to a defective secretion of the lacrimal and salivary glands and the mucous glands of the nose, trachea and bronchi. There appears to be an increased incidence of antigens HLA DR2, HLA DR3, HLA DR4 and HLA B8 in patients with Sjögren's syndrome. Autoantibodies may also be demonstrated in a large proportion of patients, and rheumatoid factor is frequently one of these autoantibodies. Many patients with Sjögren's syndrome will also suffer from rheumatoid arthritis, SLE, dermatomyositis, scleroderma, primary biliary cirrhosis or Hashimoto's disease.

The patient presents with dry conjunctivae, atrophic rhinitis and pharyngitis. Frequently, the patient complains of feelings of grittiness or soreness in the eyes, blurred vision and pain if the corneal epithelium is damaged. There is an increased secretion of mucus that may form flakes or stringy ropes in the fornices. Both salivary and lacrimal glands are slightly enlarged and firm. Microscopically a lymphocytic and plasma cell infiltrate is seen between the atrophic acini of the secretory tissue. Increasing fibrosis will be observed in the tissue. The severity of involvement of tissue will vary not only from gland to gland in the same patient, but also, different parts of the same gland may show different degrees of involvement. Lymphocytes in the tissue may aggregate to form germinal centres.

Clinical presentation of the patient is characteristic of the syndrome, but diagnosis may be confirmed by Schirmer's test which measures tear production and also by biopsy of one of the minor salivary glands. Treatment of the condition is by replacement of the absent secretions, for example artificial tear solutions such as lacril, which are frequently instilled into the eyes. Complications such as an increased risk of infections occur even in treated patients and about 10% of patients will develop a non-Hodgkin's, B cell lymphoma in either the affected glands or in adjacent lymph nodes.

Tumours

Tumours of the lacrimal glands and sacs are rare. A 'mixed parotid' tumour identical in appearance to that developing in salivary glands will occasionally be seen in the lacrimal glands. Usually, these tumours develop before the age of 50 years and are firm, encapsulated and lobulated masses. They are tumours of mucus-secreting cells and large quantities of mucus in the tumour give a false impression that cartilage is present between the cells (hence the name 'mixed'). Although these are slow-growing tumours that enlarge by expansion, they will recur unless they are completely excised with a sleeve of normal tissue around them. Occasionally, such a tumour will undergo malignant transformation and behave like a typical adenocarcinoma. Malignant lymphoma of the lacrimal gland is most often associated with Sjögren's syndrome and behaves in exactly the same manner as lymphomata in other sites.

Optic Nerve

Inflammations

Inflammations of the optic nerve may be an **optic perineuritis** or an **optic neuritis**. In the former case the nerve sheath is involved, usually as a result of adjacent infection, such as meningitis caused by pyogenic organisms. In this instance if the primary infection is treated, the optic perineuritis will resolve and there will be no permanent damage to the optic nerve. In the case of optic neuritis the infection and inflammation involves the neural tissue itself and may be secondary to optic perineuritis or it may have resulted from spread directly to the nerve tissue either through local spread or blood spread. In some cases the inflammation of the optic nerve is associated with non-infectious causes (e.g. multiple sclerosis, lead, arsenic or drug effects). Nerve fibres within the optic nerve are destroyed by the inflammation.

Optic atrophy is the result of optic neuritis, the symptoms of the disorder being varying degrees of visual impairment, pallor of the optic nerve head and absent or reduced pupil response to direct illumination. If the condition remains untreated it may lead to blindness (e.g. toxic causes), or in some cases vision may return to normal, although pallor of the temporal parts of the optic disc will in most cases persist (e.g. with multiple sclerosis). Other factors that may bring about optic atrophy are glaucoma, papilloedema, vascular disorders in the region (aneurysms, central retinal artery thrombosis, etc.) and trauma.

Papilloedema

Papilloedema is the condition of oedema within the optic disc (papilla) that may often be associated with non-inflammatory causes. Common causes of papill-oedema are:

- **raised intracranial pressure**, as may occur with space-occupying lesions in the cranium, hydrocephalus and inflammations;
- **ocular diseases**, such as optic neuritis, low intra-ocular pressure, leaking incisions, uveitis and thyroid exophthalmos;
- **vascular diseases**, most commonly malignant hypertension, atherosclerosis, but also central retinal vein occlusion, temporal arteritis and cavernous sinus thrombosis;
- **other diseases**, as may be seen in toxaemia of pregnancy.

The disorder occurs in well-defined stages, with congestion of the retinal veins and blurring of the margins of the optic disc being the first signs observed. The oedema in the region of the optic disc will cause it to swell and protrude into the vitreous humour and, gradually, haemorrhage will be seen in and around the disc. Optic atrophy and pallor of the optic disc will occur in untreated cases. The patient experiences visual disturbances and in long-term untreated cases blindness may result.

Tumours

The primary tumours affecting the optic nerve are very similar to those affecting the central nervous tissue, the commonest tumours in this site being gliomata and meningiomata. Glioma usually affects children and is unilateral in most cases, astrocytomata or oligodendrogliomata being the tumours most often observed in this site. Any part of the optic nerve may be involved by the tumour although most gliomata of this nerve arise within the orbit. If the tumour grows anteriorly towards the optic disc, blindness will be unilateral whereas if the optic chiasma is involved by posterior spread, the resulting blindness will be bilateral. The effects of the tumour are due to direct spread and, as with equivalent brain tumours, no metastasis will occur. Surgical excision of the tumour before cerebral invasion occurs is curative.

Meningioma of the optic nerve arises from the arachnoid of the nerve and is usually seen in older patients. Most of these tumours arise in the region of the optic foramen and they will spread along the nerve sheath to give rise to a tumour that bulges anteriorly into the orbit and posteriorly into the cranium, resembling a dumb-bell. In behaviour these tumours resemble those of the brain and excision before spread to involve the cerebrum may be curative although the patient loses sight in the affected eye.

Refraction Errors

The shape of the normal eye is such that near parallel rays of light from distant objects pass through the convex corneal and crystalline lens areas and are brought to focus on the retina. Light rays from objects that are closer to the eye can be brought to focus by the reflex mechanism of **accommodation** where the ciliary muscles contract and cause the lens to become more spherical, thus focusing the rays from the object onto the retina. There are four basic types of refractive errors in the eye and in all of these the light rays fail to be focused sharply on the retina, giving rise to a blurry or hazy image. All such errors of refraction may be corrected by the wearing of corrective lenses in the form of spectacles or contact lenses that compensate for the errors and allow focusing of the light rays on the retina (see Figure 19.10).

Presbyopia

The range of accommodation of the eye decreases steadily throughout life so that in middle age, when the lens has become firmer and less able to be deformed through the action of the ciliary muscles, the nearest point that can be effectively focused on the retina recedes beyond the normal reading range. The affected person usually presents at the age of about 45 years and requests 'reading glasses' as there has been considerable difficulty reading and doing close work with the hands (needlework, etc.). The condition can be compensated for by the prescription of weak convex lenses that generally require strengthening every few years as the lens becomes even firmer with advancing years and the accommodation reflex becomes weaker.

Myopia ('Short-sightedness')

The condition of myopia occurs when the eyeball is too long, such that distant objects are brought into focus on a plane lying in the vitreous in front of the retina, the retinal image being out of focus. Prevention of the normal accommodation reflex when viewing near objects will allow focusing of light rays on the retina (thus myopes are 'short-sighted' — refer to Figure 19.10). In some cases of myopia, termed **pro-**

gressive myopia the eyeball continues to lengthen throughout life and the condition becomes more marked, leading to retinal detachment and degeneration. However, in most cases the myopia stabilizes after the growing years and may even be slightly reduced in late middle age. The myopic eye requires a concave spectacle lens in order to correct the distance vision defect.

Hypermetropia ('Far-sightedness')

Hypermetropia will occur when the eyeball is too short and the focal plane for distant objects will lie beyond the retina, somewhere to its posterior. In the young hypermetrope, distant objects are brought into focus by accommodation of the lens spontaneously, such that these people will have normal distance vision ('far-sighted'). However, this process will leave less reserve for accommodation to occur when viewing near objects and fatigue will develop when too much near work is done requiring a concentrated viewing of near objects. This usually occurs around adolescence and the individual will require convex spectacles to correct the defect. Thus the patient with hypermetropia is similar to the presbyopic patient but presents during adolescence rather than after the age of 45 years (see Figure 19.10).

Astigmatism

Astigmatism occurs when the eyeball is flattened causing blurry vision for both near and distant vision. The

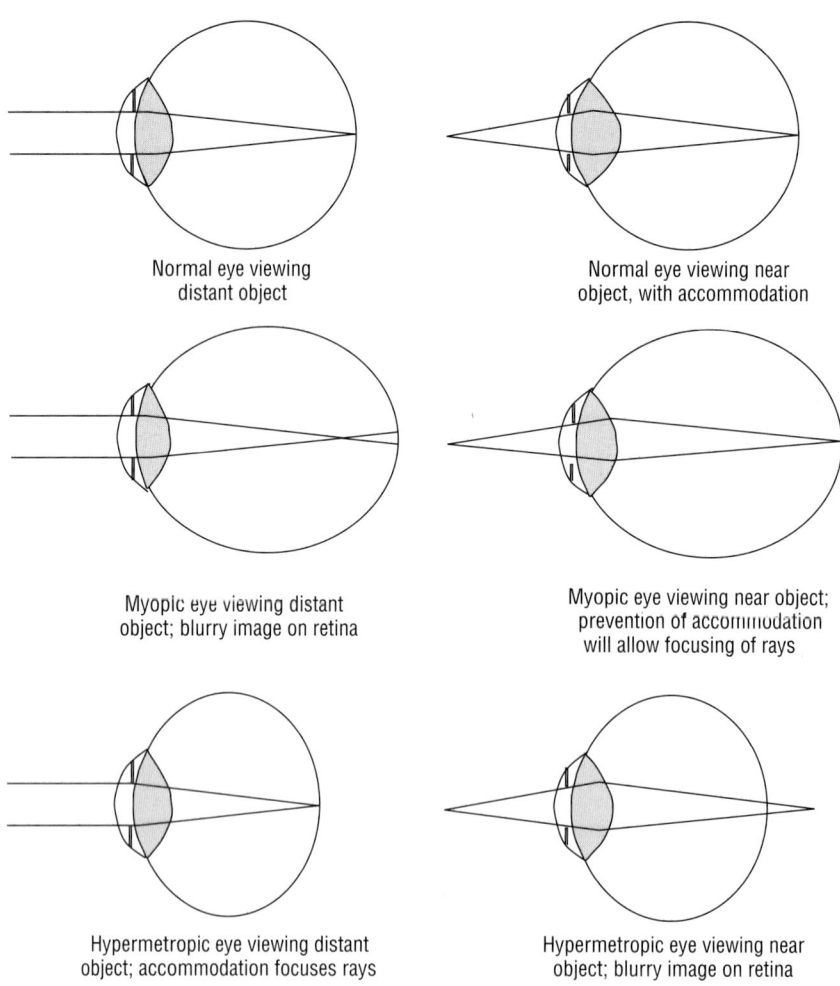

Normal eye viewing
distant object

Normal eye viewing near
object, with accommodation

Myopic eye viewing distant
object; blurry image on retina

Myopic eye viewing near object;
prevention of accommodation
will allow focusing of rays

Hypermetropic eye viewing distant
object; accommodation focuses rays

Hypermetropic eye viewing near
object; blurry image on retina

Figure 19.10   *Refractive errors of the eye*

most usual defect is a downward flattening, although sideways or oblique deformations of the eyeball may also occur. The effect is one of variation of the cornea curvature in different meridians, causing 'straying' of the refracted light rays away from the point of focus on the retina. Accommodation cannot correct such a defect. Visual fatigue and headaches may accompany the vision impairment. The condition is corrected by the appropriate astigmatic lenses that have a different curvature in the two meridians (in severe cases only spectacles will effectively correct the defect, contact lenses only correcting the milder cases of astigmatism).

Testing the eye for refractive errors is carried out by optometrists and the test may be subjective (trying out a variety of lenses to find the combinations giving best vision by trial and error, the patient telling the optometrist which is the best lens combination), or testing may be objective by **retinoscopy**. This is the more accurate procedure and may be the only appropriate one in the very old or the very young. On retinoscopy, the appropriate lens is used to neutralize the movement of a beam of light reflected from the fundus. A mydriatic is used to keep the ciliary muscle at rest and make the measurements reliable. It is a technique requiring much practice and experience but gives highly reliable results.

Recent advances in the correction of refractive errors involve **keratomileusis**, which involves removing a thin slice of the cornea, shaping it to the appropriate curvature to correct the error of refraction and then stitching it back onto the remaining cornea. This is a new technique and although in successful cases obviates the need for corrective lenses, in the unsuccessful cases it may lead to permanent vision impairment which is much worse than the refractive error it attempted to correct.

Keratoplasty is a surgical operation where defective corneae are excised and replaced with a corneal graft taken from a cadaveric donor. **Optic keratoplasty** is where the grafted cornea replaces a damaged or scarred cornea and thus is essential for correcting serious visual impairment or blindness. **Refractive keratoplasty** is used to correct refractive errors in a similar manner to keratomileusis, or in the variant of **keratophakia**, a part of the donor cornea is shaped appropriately and inserted between layers of the patient's own cornea. **Tectonic keratoplasty** is where a donor cornea is used to replace part of the patient's cornea that has been lost through injury.

Ear Diseases

External Ear

Inflammations

Inflammations of the external ear involving the skin and meatus due to infectious causes are quite common. The conditions are termed **otitis externa**. If they are severe, the infections will progress down to the level of the cartilage and may even destroy it. This occurs with **furunculosis** of the ear, the presence of a boil on the auricle, a condition also called otitis externa circumscripta. Most cases of otitis externa involve the external auditory canal and from this site the infection spreads to involve the auricle and periauricular skin, a condition often described as otitis externa diffusa. This presentation is often termed 'swimmer's ear' because of the regularity with which swimmers present with this type of infection, having contracted it in poorly disinfected swimming pools. Improper drying of the ear following bathing or washing greatly predisposes to such infections. Otitis externa is commoner in teenagers and adults than in young children.

The organisms causing such infections are usually bacterial or fungal and rarely viral. More than one organism may be involved in any one infection and the microbes most commonly isolated are:

- *Pseudomonas* spp., *Proteus* spp., *Staphylococcus* spp. and diphtheroids, in various combinations;
- *Streptococcus* spp.;
- *Aspergillus niger* and *Candida albicans* (Otomycoses);
- herpes viruses (viral cause).

The symptoms and signs of these infections are exquisite pain of the affected ear, redness, swelling and the production of a moderate volume of foul-smelling discharge from the ear. The patient often develops fever and may experience a degree of hearing loss on the affected side. The pain is exacerbated by moving the jaw, as occurs in chewing. If the disease is left untreated, the fever and pain will diminish and disappear, but the discharge persists. Itching of the ear becomes the prominent feature of the chronic disorder and introduction of a fingertip or foreign body into the auditory canal may further aggravate the condition.

Treatment of the condition is firstly by removing all traces of debris from the auditory canal. During this aural toilet procedure a swab is taken for microbiological investigation. The infection is then treated by dressing the ear with medicated gauze or cotton wool. The medications include topical antibiotics, steroid preparations (especially where there is marked oedema) and analgesics. Antibiotic sensitivity tests that have been performed on the microbe isolated by the microbiology laboratory are taken into account when the dressing is changed in 24 hours. Dressing the ear should continue until the meatal skin has returned to normal. Systemic antibiosis in otitis externa is only indicated if the patient presents in an acute febrile state with signs of widespread involvement or cellulitis. Fungal infections benefit from application of baby oil as well as specific antifungals such as nystatin.

Once treated, patients should be instructed not to scratch their ears, prevent water from entering the ear and after bathing or swimming to dry the ears carefully with clean cotton wool. Application of baby oil or petroleum jelly to the ear and external auditory canal before swimming or bathing may be helpful in preventing infection. Recurrence of otitis externa is common and is thought to be more common in patients who do not produce adequate quantities of cerumen (wax).

In some cases, otitis externa is not due to an infectious cause but rather is a manifestation of systemic or localized allergic reactions. For example, ingestion of beer or chocolate in some individuals will cause otitis externa. Neurodermatitis of the external ear also commonly occurs, a typical eczematous appearance seen in relation to emotional crises or other psychological stimuli.

Tumours and Tumour-like Lesions

The ear is a frequent site for the development of **gouty tophi**. These are circumscribed, pale, hard nodules developing on the pinna of the ear and involving the cartilage. They consist of chalky, crystalline deposits of sodium biurate surrounded by variable amounts of chronic inflammatory infiltrate with giant cells, encapsulated by fibrous connective tissue.

Exostoses are likely to develop around the region of the external auditory meatus fairly commonly and these lesions are often bilateral. They have been associated with exposure to cold water and swimmers or surfers are likely to present with them. The lesions are hard, sessile and smooth, covered with thin skin and when touched are exquisitely sensitive to pressure. They are very slowly growing benign masses, often giving rise to no symptoms. In some cases, cerumen will accumulate between the exostosis and the tympanic membrane, interfering with normal hearing. Such lesions may be removed surgically with an operating microscope and a dental burr.

Cauliflower ear is a term applied to a haematoma occurring beneath the skin or perichondrium of the pinna of the ear and refers to the irregular and thickened nodule that forms in the affected region, deforming the ear. The lesion is totally benign and consists of initially a typical haematoma that later becomes organized into irregular bands of fibrous tissue or occasionally into cartilage.

A **ceruminoma** (adenoma of the ceruminous glands) occurs rarely and this is a tumour resembling an adenoma of the salivary glands or a pleomorphic adenoma of the salivary glands. In most cases although the tumour is microscopically benign it will grow slowly and invade the surrounding tissues. Even if such tumours are surgically removed they tend to recur. In some cases, a typical malignant variant will be found and such ceruminocarcinomata will metastasize to the lungs or kidneys.

The commonest tumours of the external ear are **squamous cell carcinomata**. A **basal cell carcinoma** may also arise very frequently in this site. Both of these tumours have been already considered in Chapter 16, and such tumours developing on the ear behave in exactly the same manner as these tumours in other situations.

Myringitis

Myringitis is an inflammation of the tympanic membrane and may be seen in association with middle or external ear inflammations as the tympanic membrane separates the external from the middle ear. The membrane becomes thickened and inflamed. In some cases haemorrhagic myringitis (bullous myringitis) will be associated with viral infections, especially influenzal infections. If the condition that precipitates myringitis is left untreated, the ear drum may rupture.

Tympanic Membrane Injury

Injury to the ear drum may have many causes, but in all cases early diagnosis and treatment is vital. The causes of tympanic rupture are:

- **direct trauma**, as may occur when the patient tries to clean out the ears too vigorously, or attempts to remove wax or foreign bodies from the ear;
- **infection**, especially long-standing otitis media;
- **indirect trauma**, as occurs with gunfire, blasts, fireworks, rapid descent in an aircraft or a slap on the ear (rock concerts?);
- **fracture** of the temporal bone.

The patient will usually experience pain at the time of the rupture, but this is a transient feature. Later, hearing loss, tinnitus and vertigo, together with haemorrhage and haematoma formation, are observed and upon examination a tear may be visible on the ear drum. The major features of treatment are non-interference and observation for signs of superinfection. Infection should be treated with systemic antibiotics but the ear should not be syringed, nor the clot removed. The edges of the tear will unite rapidly and no permanent hearing loss will be seen.

Middle Ear

Inflammations — Acute Otitis Media

Acute otitis media is a common infection occurring mainly in infants and children, about 10% of children under 10 years suffering from one or more attacks in any one year and about 30% of all children having at least one attack of otitis media. The route of the infection is in almost all cases via the Eustachian tube. The Eustachian tube in children lies horizontally and is quite short, making access of nasopharyngeal organisms to the middle ear very easy. As the individual ages, the Eustachian tube lengthens and the pharyngeal orifice moves downwards as the tube assumes a more vertical pitch. These changes in the anatomy of the tube with increasing age tend to reduce the incidence of middle ear infections as bacteria find it in-

creasingly difficult to gain access to the ear from the throat.

The bacteria involved in the causation of otitis media are mainly commensal organisms that are found in the throat and are β-haemolytic *Streptococcus*, *Streptococcus pneumoniae*, *Haemophilus influenzae* and *Staphylococcus* spp.

Any infection of the upper respiratory tract will predispose to a middle ear infection. Otitis media is a common complication of acute tonsillitis, pharyngitis, scarlet fever, the common cold, influenza, measles, mumps, whooping cough, sinusitis, and less commonly is a result of injury and perforation of the ear drum. Acute otitis media is an infection of the mucous membrane lining of the middle ear, the Eustachian tube, tympanic cavity, attic, aditus, mastoid antrum and mastoid cells. It should be noted that **mastoiditis** is involvement of the mastoid cells by inflammation which causes necrosis of the bone lining the cells (see Figure 19.12).

The pathogenesis of otitis media is complex and depends firstly upon the organisms accessing the middle ear via the Eustachian tube. Their presence excites an acute inflammatory response in the mucosa with oedema, hyperaemia and exudate formation, followed later by suppuration. The oedema involves the lining of the Eustachian tube, which has the effect of decreasing the lumen of the tube until the tube finally closes. This causes an increase in pressure within the tympanic cavity with bulging of the ear drum outwards, until the membrane ruptures. A purulent exu-

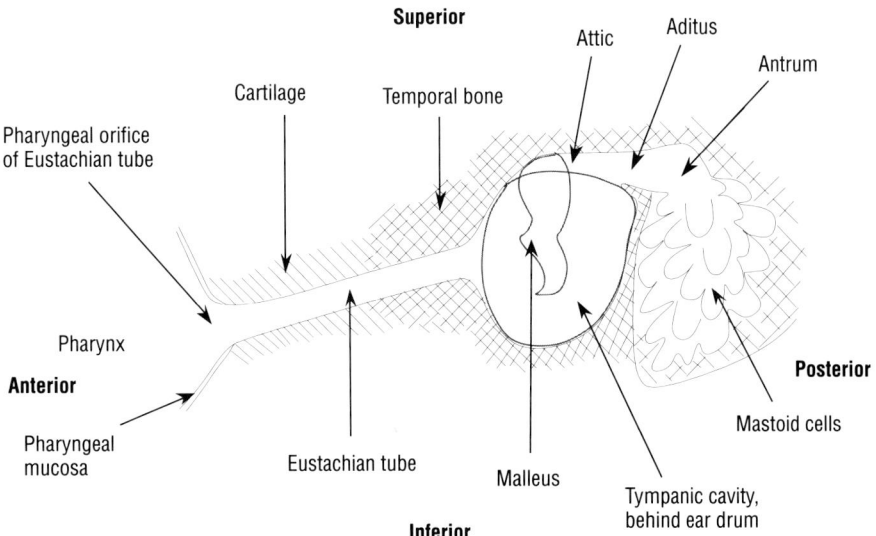

Figure 19.12 *The relationship between the Eustachian tube and the middle ear*

date begins to discharge through the ruptured tympanic membrane until the infection resolves.

Symptoms and signs associated with acute otitis media are a severe and throbbing **otalgia** (earache, often causing the child to weep and cry out in pain), fever (often as high as 40°C), loss of hearing (of the conductive type), tinnitus, tenderness, and a purulent discharge from the ear. A differential diagnosis of otalgia must be carried out as both aural conditions and disorders of the head and neck will produce earache (Table 19.3 outlines the various causes of earache). A radiograph will often show some opacity of the mastoid cells in otitis media. Examination of the tympanic membrane will show it to be very inflamed with the handle of the malleus vertical; later the membrane will bulge outwards and appear plum-coloured, and in the last stages it will perforate and discharge a purulent exudate.

Treatment of the condition will depend on the stage at which the patient presents: early, 'bulging' (when the ear drum bulges out but is not perforated) and discharging (after perforation of ear drum). In the early stage, analgesics and antibiotics given systemically will control the symptoms and the infection. Penicillin is usually given and if an improvement is not seen, a broad spectrum antibacterial is prescribed. Nasal vasoconstrictors such as ephedrine may be administered. The coexistent infection of the upper respiratory tract or pharynx is also controlled. In the bulging stage, the procedure followed is a surgical one, **myringotomy** (incision of the tympanic membrane) being performed under general anaesthesia. Following this procedure, the condition is treated as for the discharging type of otitis media. Discharging otitis media is managed by aural toilet and isolation of the causative organism (upon which the appropriate antibiotic sensitivity tests may be carried out), and antibiotics and analgesics are given.

If otitis media is treated in the manner outlined above, most cases will resolve and hearing will return to normal. Complications of otitis media occur in untreated or poorly managed cases and these include the following:

- **chronic otitis media**;
- **perforation of the tympanic membrane**, which may cause problems with hearing later;
- **organization of exudate**, with fibrous adhesions of the ossicles causing deafness;
- **mastoiditis**, with necrosis of the bone and suppuration;
- **inner ear infection** (e.g. labyrinthitis);
- **central nervous system infection** (e.g. meningitis).

Inflammations — Chronic Otitis Media

Chronic otitis media is in most cases a sequela of untreated or poorly treated acute otitis media. In some cases chronic otitis media will appear to arise spontaneously, but supervening on serous otitis media or being associated with chronic nasopharyngeal inflammations. The infecting organisms most often associated with chronic otitis media are: β-haemolytic *Streptococcus*, *Streptococcus pneumoniae*, *Staphylococcus* spp., *Haemophilus influenzae*, *Escherichia coli* and *Pseudomonas* spp., in any combination.

The most common sign indicating chronic otitis media is a perforated ear drum, through which drainage of exudate constantly occurs, and the patient will at the same time complain of hearing loss on the affected side. The perforation of the tympanic membrane seen with chronic otitis media may be of two

Table 19.3 *Differential diagnosis of otalgia*

Aural otalgia	Referred otalgia, via			
(Auriculotemporal nerve (V), but also C2, 3, VII and X)	Greater auricular nerve (C2, 3)	Auriculotemporal branch of trigeminal nerve (V)	Facial nerve (VII)	Glossopharyngeal and vagus nerves (IX & X)
Furunculosis	Wounds of the neck	Dental disease (e.g. caries, abscesses)	Geniculate herpes	Tonsillitis
Otitis externa	Lymphadenopathy of neck glands	Sphenoidal sinusitis		Tonsillectomy
Otitis media	Cervical disc lesion	Temporomandibular joint disorders		Quinsy
Mastoiditis	Osteoarthrosis	Arthritis		Glossopharyngeal neuralgia
Otitis interna				Neoplasm (pharynx, tongue, larynx, tonsil)
Neoplasms				

types (see Figure 19.13): the less dangerous **central perforation** in the tense part of the drum and the more dangerous **marginal perforation** in the more peripheral part of the membrane, involving the annulus tympanicus. Any perforation of the pars flaccida of the membrane (Schrapnell's membrane) is considered to be a marginal perforation. Marginal perforations are more likely to be associated with many sequelae, some of which may prove life threatening.

Two subtypes of chronic otitis media are recognized, the so-called **mucosal type** and the **osseous type**. Central perforations of the tympanic membrane are the usual feature of the mucosal type and peripheral perforations occur with the osseous type. In the mucosal type, the mucosa of the middle ear and the mastoid air cells are thickened and fibrous, with infiltrates of chronic inflammatory cells such as lymphocytes, plasma cells and macrophages. The epithelium retains its ciliated cells but there is hyperplasia of the goblet cells with an increased secretion of mucus, making the mastoid air cells look like mucous glands. The discharge from the ear is definitely mucous and the infection may be quiescent periodically. However, if the condition is not treated the tympanic perforation will enlarge and the hearing loss will become more profound. In the osseous form of the condition, the infection is extensive and involves all of the middle ear and its bony walls, and a purulent, foul-smelling exudate is seen draining from the perforated ear drum. Untreated osseous-type chronic otitis media will often progress to various complications, the main ones being:

- **organization** of exudate with destruction of the ossicles, causing hearing loss;
- **cholesteatoma**, see below;
- the development of **aural polypi** consisting of masses of inflamed granulation tissue, filling the meatus and becoming visible in the concha;
- **acute mastoiditis**, with bone necrosis as the infection involves the mastoid air cells;
- **meningitis**, with pyrexia, headache, neck rigidity, photophobia and positive Kernig's sign;
- **abscesses**, including extradural, subdural, cerebellar and cerebral, resulting from direct or haematogenous spread of the infection; symptoms and signs depend on the precise area involved, but any patient with middle ear infection complaining of headache, malaise or nausea should be suspected of suffering from a CNS abscess;
- **petrositis**, involving the apex of the petrous; this rarely occurs but involves the sixth cranial nerve with diplopia, trigeminal pain and headache (**Gradenigo's syndrome**);
- **facial nerve paralysis**, with a tendency to dribble on one side of the mouth;
- **lateral sinus thrombosis**, the pus tracking through from the mastoid air cells to form a perisinus abscess;
- **labyrinthitis**, where the infection reaches this area through a fistulous communication in the medial wall of the middle ear.

Treatment of chronic otitis media is complex and depends on the extent of the infection, whether a mar-

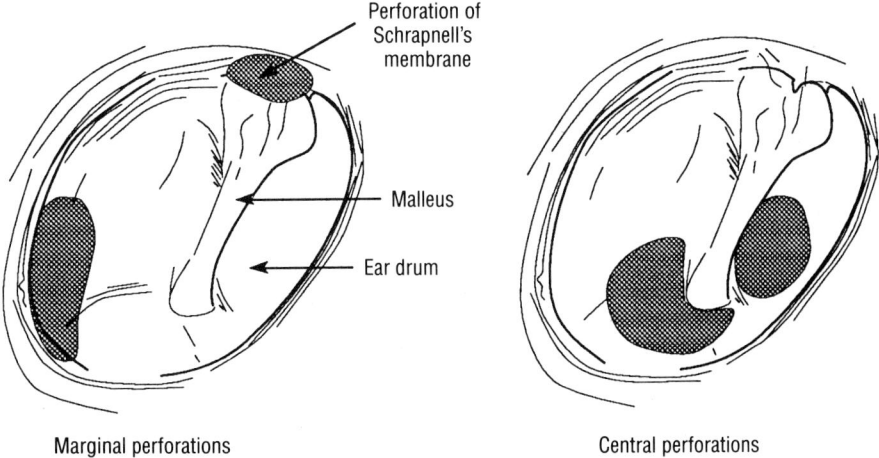

Marginal perforations   Central perforations

Figure 19.13 *Types of tympanic membrane perforation in chronic otitis media*

ginal or central perforation is present and whether any complications have developed. In uncomplicated, mucosal-type disease, sepsis is eradicated from the nasopharyngeal area, aural toilet is meticulously carried out daily and a simple antiseptic solution is instilled into the ear. The patient in which the infection and inflammation has been controlled is a candidate for **tympanoplasty**, a surgical manoeuvre where the pathways of sound conduction are reconstructed utilizing skin grafts and the undamaged ossicles. In the osseous-type disorder a conservative treatment similar to that initiated for the mucosal type should be tried first. In addition, aural polypi are resected and a careful watch is kept on the patient in case complications develop. If a rapid improvement is not evident shortly, or in the case of complications, the osseous type of chronic otitis media is treated surgically with **mastoidectomy** (removal of the mastoid air cells and associated debris), several variants of which are carried out, depending on the extent of the disease. Tympanoplasty may also be performed. Systemic antibiosis is not undertaken in chronic otitis media, any antibiotic treatment, if given, being topical.

Inflammations — Serous Otitis Media ('Glue Ear')

Serous otitis media is also termed catarrhal otitis media or secretory otitis media, while to the layperson it is known as 'glue ear'. The condition is important because non-treatment will result in deafness in most cases. Although in about half of the patients no bacteria are isolated, in the other half the commonest isolate is *Haemophilus influenzae*. The exact pathogenesis of the condition is obscure but it has been associated with nasopharyngeal infections and obstruction, frequently virally caused, as occurs with the common cold. Obstruction of the Eustachian tube with resorption of the air from the middle ear and serous effusion following this may be an important mechanism. Allergic factors are an important cause of Eustachian tube oedema and obstruction. A pharyngeal tumour at the orifice of the Eustachian tube may also cause obstruction and serous otitis media.

The mucosa of the middle ear in this condition is oedematous with a small number of chronic inflammatory cells infiltrating the tissue. The mucosal epithelium may become pseudostratified and the goblet cells undergo hyperplasia, contributing mucus to the serous fluid that fills the middle ear. The ear drum bulges outwards and is yellowish in colour, and on otoscopy the meniscus of fluid is seen behind the drum or air bubbles within the serous fluid will be detected (see Figure 19.14).

The patients with 'glue ear' will rarely complain of otalgia, but rather report a 'stuffy feeling' in the ear and also complain of hearing loss of the conductive type. If earache is present it usually implies that a bacterial infection is present. Sometimes the patient complains of a roaring or a ringing noise in the affected ear. If the patients tilt the head, some of them will report that they can feel the fluid within the ear. Most patients will also complain of nasopharyngeal symptoms such as a 'stuffed up nose', difficulty in normal breathing and 'congestion'. These findings are very characteristic of the condition and differential diagnosis is relatively easy, the other causes for hearing loss which need to be investigated being cerumen or foreign bodies in the external auditory canal.

Treatment of the condition begins by an evaluation of the patient in order to detect factors in the causation

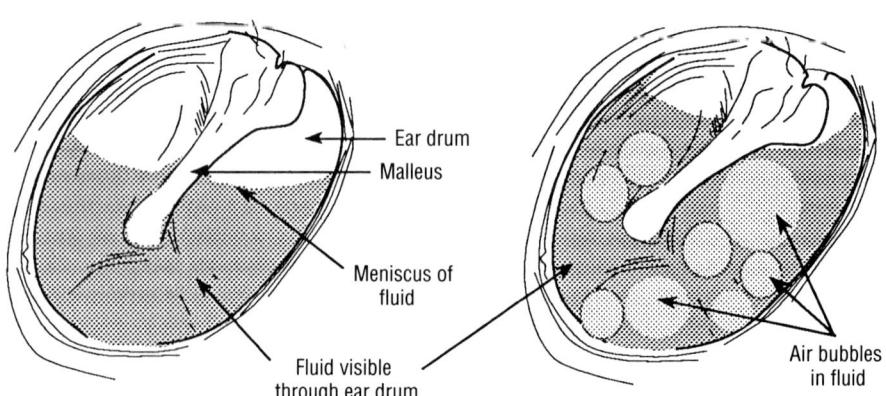

Figure 19.14 *The appearance of serous otitis media on otoscopy*

of the condition. Allergic causes are treated by prevention of exposure to the allergen, nasopharyngeal infections are treated, adenoids may be removed and obstructions to the orifice of the Eustachian tube treated. Decongestion of the nasal passages by nasal administration of ephedrine is useful and a procedure known as **politzerization** may be carried in order to promote drainage of fluid and open up the Eustachian tube. In this procedure, Politzer's bag (a rubber sac with a tube attached) is used and the nozzle at the end of the tube is inserted into one of the nostrils, the other end of the tube being compressed. The sac is squeezed and the patient swallows, raising the pressure within the nasopharynx, opening the Eustachian tubes and promoting drainage of fluid from the middle ear. This procedure is repeated daily until the condition resolves. A myringotomy may be performed in certain cases, in order to allow drainage of fluid. If the condition is left untreated it will be complicated by organization of the serous fluid and the formation of fibrous adhesions between the ossicles, retracting the ear drum and causing a conductive type of deafness. Such a complication is sometimes treated by tympanotomy but in most cases a hearing aid is needed.

Cholesteatoma

Cholesteatoma is a double misnomer as it neither involves metabolic disorders of cholesterol nor is a tumour. It is a condition that is almost always associated with chronic otitis media, rarely following trauma to the ear. It is essentially a hyperplasia of squamous epithelium within the confined space of the middle ear which may extend into the mastoid air cells. It forms a pale, firm nodule of tissue that grows slowly and erodes the bone underlying it. Within its centre there are whorled deposits of keratin, purulent debris and epithelial breakdown products. The nodular mass is often foul smelling and if left untreated it will lead to erosion of the tegmen, involvement of the cranial fossa and central nervous system complications such as extradural, subdural or temporal lobe abscesses and meningitis. Treatment of the condition involves removal of the lesion and management of the chronic otitis media.

Inner Ear

Inflammations — Labyrinthitis

Labyrinthitis is an inflammation of the inner ear involving the labyrinth and is also termed **otitis interna**.

The commonest cause of labyrinthitis is extension of infection and inflammation from a case of acute or chronic otitis media; less commonly it may occur as an extension of meningitis into the inner ear. In many patients with otitis interna, a cholesteatoma is also present if the condition arose in association with chronic otitis media. The organisms involved in infections of the inner ear include β-haemolytic *Streptococcus*, *Streptococcus pneumoniae*, *Staphylococcus* spp., *Haemophilus influenzae*, coliforms, *Pseudomonas* spp. and *Neisseria meningitidis*, in any combination.

The infection of the labyrinth may be circumscribed or diffuse and in most cases a purulent exudate will form in association with the infection. The clinical presentation involves loss of labyrinthine function and loss of hearing. Whether or not severe disease develops is determined by the extent of the infection, the most severe symptoms being experienced with the diffuse inflammation. The patient usually presents with vertigo (see below), vomiting, nausea and nystagmus (involuntary rapid movement of the eyeball).

Treatment of the disorder is highly specialized and depends very much on the individual case, cause of the labyrinthitis and degree of tissue involvement. Prompt antibiotic treatment is likely to control serous forms of labyrinthitis associated with otitis media. If the infection in the labyrinth is associated with cholesteatoma and severe otitis media mastoidectomy would be necessary. In some severe cases of otitis interna labyrinthectomy may be indicated.

Ménière's Disease

Ménière's disease is an idiopathic condition associated with increased endolymphatic system pressure within the inner ear. There is a distension of the membranous labyrinth by the raised endolymph pressure and the hair cells of the organ of Corti show a progressive degeneration. The disease usually first affects people between the ages of 40 and 60 years, one ear being affected initially and in a quarter of cases the other ear showing similar involvement later.

The clinical features of the disorder include **vertigo**, which is a sensation of rotation of the patient's own self (**subjective vertigo**) or of the patient's surroundings (**objective vertigo**) in any plane. The patient often describes vertigo as a feeling of 'giddiness' or 'dizziness'. Vertigo in Ménière's disease is intermittent, the attacks lasting between a few minutes to hours. Vertigo is often preceded by a feeling of pressure in the ear and is often followed by malaise for several days. **Nausea** and **vomiting** are almost always associated with the attacks and may be very difficult to control. The patient will complain of **hearing loss** which is of a sensorineural type and is particularly marked immediately before and after an attack. The hearing loss is progressive and associated with extreme distortion of any of the sound still perceived, this being the bane of the music lover. **Tinnitus** is also present and this is a complaint of ringing, buzzing, pulsating or hissing noises heard by the patient in the ears or the head region. This symptom is also worse before the attacks and often it may precede all other symptoms of the disease by a period of months or years. Differential diagnosis of Ménière's disease is very important, as many other common and less severe states may present with tinnitus and vertigo (refer to Table 19.4).

The attacks of Ménière's disease occur in bouts, becoming progressively more frequent and severe. In the early stages, the patient may experience three or four attacks in a period of 2 to 3 weeks and then remain symptom-free for a period of months. The recurring attacks finally cause deafness in the affected ear. The other ear then begins to suffer from the disease, or as is the case in bilateral disease, both ears may be involved in the attacks.

Diagnosis of the condition depends on **audiometry** (see below) which demonstrates a sensorineural hearing loss, the audiogram curve being fairly flat, the hearing loss involving high and low tones being similar. The **caloric test** is performed and involves the patient lying supine with the head flexed forward about 30° from the horizontal and looking at a small spot on the ceiling overhead. Using a special can and nozzle, each ear is irrigated with water first at 30°C and then at 44°C for 40 seconds. The period of time elapsing between the start of irrigation and the stopping of the nystagmus induced by the procedure is measured and

recorded on a calorigram. Normally, the period of time is about 120 seconds. Treatment of Ménière's disease during the attacks involves the use of agents to control the vertigo and nausea, and these may provide considerable symptomatic relief for the patient. During the quiescent stages numerous regimes have been advanced but they are of limited usefulness. The patient is often advised to stay on a low-fluid, low-salt diet, is prescribed vasodilators, and histamine desensitization may be tried. In severe unilateral cases labyrinthectomy is effective but is not advised when the patient can still hear in that ear or when the other ear is affected by hearing dysfunctions. Stellate ganglionectomy and selective destruction of the labyrinth by ultrasonic means may also be performed in an attempt to preserve hearing in the affected ear.

Otosclerosis

Otosclerosis is a rare disease involving the ossicles of the ear, appearing to have a genetic predisposition and being about twice as common in females as in males. The usual age of onset is between 15 and 30 years of age and the condition although first occurring in one ear will then progress to become bilateral. Characteristic of the condition is a conductive hearing loss with **paracusis** (ability to hear conversation more easily in noisy surroundings). Although air conduction is poor, the patient has good bone conduction (at least in the early stages of the disease) and will therefore speak quietly.

The hallmark of otosclerosis is the formation of new bone of a vascular, spongy nature around the region of the footplate of the stapes, at the oval window and the promontory, occasionally extending to involve the

Table 19.4 *Differential diagnosis of tinnitus and vertigo*

Condition	Tinnitus	Vertigo
Ménière's disease	✓	✓
Labyrinthitis (e.g. suppurative, traumatic, syphilitic, post-operative)	✓	✓
Excessive cerumen in the outer ear ('wax')	✓	✓
Alcohol abuse	✓	✓
Ototoxic drugs (e.g. streptomycin, quinine, salicylates)	✓	✓
Neoplasms (e.g. acoustic neuroma, glomus tumour, carcinoma)	✓	✓
Vascular disease (e.g. atherosclerosis, hypertension, haemorrhage)	✓	✓
Presbycusis (senile hearing loss)	✓	—
Otosclerosis	✓	—
Vestibular neuronitis	—	✓
Benign positional vertigo	—	✓

cochlear side of the oval window (refer to Figure 19.15). The new bone formed shows a similarity to the bone formed in Paget's disease with osteoclastic and osteoblastic activity leading to a vascular bone with prominent cement lines and an irregular structure. The bone causes ankylosis of the stapes and the conduction of vibrations from the tympanic membrane to the cochlea is thus seriously compromised. If otosclerosis is treated in the early stages, many cases are remediable; neglected disease is often untreatable and will progress to deafness.

The diagnosis of the disorder depends on the clinical presentation, a young person presenting with hearing loss, tinnitus, paracusis and family history of deafness. The patient may complain of increasing hearing loss, firstly unilateral and then bilateral. Pregnancy may result in increased hearing loss. The tympanic membranes are normal on examination and hearing tests (see below) will show good bone conduction in the early cases but poor conduction in advanced disease and a negative Rinne's test.

Treatment of the disorder is surgical and two types of operation are carried out in an attempt to mobilize the stapes or to bypass the ankylotic ossicle. **Stapedectomy** will in most cases partially or totally restore hearing. The ossicles are exposed via an incision in the posterior wall of the meatus and the stapes is removed and replaced by some form of prosthesis. In **fenestration**, the lateral semicircular canal is approached by an endaural incision and after excision of the incus a fenestra is made in the lateral wall of the semicircular canal and covered by a mobile membrane of thin meatal skin, thus bypassing the ankylotic stapes. In both cases, sound waves are able to be transmitted to the cochlea. Inoperable cases of otosclerosis may be helped to a certain extent by the use of a hearing aid.

Tumours — Chemodectomata

Chemodectomata are tumours derived from the chemoreceptive tissue of non-chromaffin paraganglia that is sensitive to changes in the chemical composition of blood. The tumours arise in the carotid body, aortic bodies and the glomus jugulare. These are all rare tumours and they should not be confused with the chromaffin tumours such as the adrenal phaeo-chromocytoma. The tumour likely to be encountered in association with the ear is the **glomus jugulare tumour**. This arises from the wall of the jugular bulb and frequently first presents as a vascular polypoid mass within the auditory meatus. It typically arises in middle-aged females and is associated with some hearing loss. The neoplasm consists of clumps of large, polyhedral cells within a fibrous stroma that contains many blood vessels. The tumour is a locally invasive one, growing from the site of origin to involve the petrous portion of the temporal bone, destroying the structures of the ear and presenting in the external ear. As the tumour is excessively vascular, any surgical

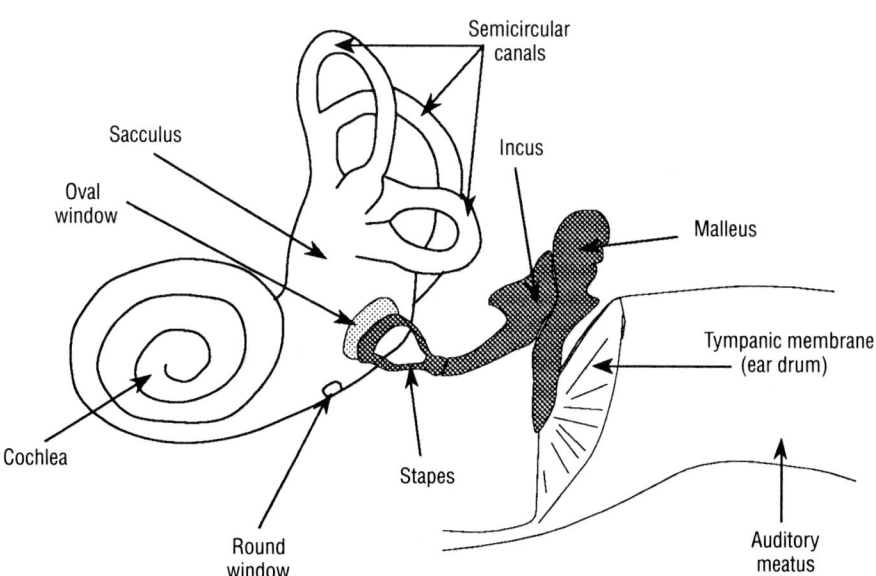

Figure 19.15 *The ossicles of the middle ear in relation to the ear drum and sacculus*

manipulation is likely to precipitate a massive haemorrhage, making the preferred treatment for this tumour radiotherapy.

Carotid body tumours do not involve the ear but are considered here for the sake of convenience. They are rare tumours but by far the most common type of chemodectoma. They are seen in adults between 30 and 60 years of age and affect males and females equally. The neoplasms arise from the carotid body at the bifurcation of the common carotid artery and present as small solid, firm masses that envelop the artery. The cells are large, polyhedral and show all the features of a benign tumour. There is abundant fibrous tissue stroma in which are found large vascular spaces. The tumours are typical benign neoplasms in that they grow slowly and expansively, causing compression of the arteries around which they grow. Surgical intervention may be required to relieve the pressure effects on the vessel. Rarely, a carotid body tumour is malignant and will invade widely into the surrounding tissues and metastasize to distant sites.

Hearing Loss

The term **deafness** is often loosely used to describe any form of hearing loss, when such a term should be reserved for conditions which involve a total inability to hear any sound. Therefore hearing loss is a preferable term as it allows degrees of hearing dysfunctions, ranging from minor hearing defects, through marked inability to hear or understand, to profound and total hearing loss implicit in the correct usage of the word deafness. There are two major forms of hearing loss, **conductive** and **sensorineural (perceptive) hearing loss**, the causation of these two types varying greatly, with almost any pathological process in the general region of the ears being responsible; however, the mechanism underlying the two forms of hearing loss is different.

Conductive Hearing Loss

Conductive hearing loss is present if no lesions can be demonstrated in the cochlea, eighth nerve or brain, the cause of the hearing loss being demonstrable in the external or middle ear. The lesion in these regions will cause an interference with the normal conduction of sound to the cochlea, the energy of the sound waves reaching the hair cells being too low to allow normal sound perception. Treatment of the lesion or surgical operations involving the ossicles or tympanic membrane, may be sufficient to treat the hearing loss effec-

tively. If this fails, hearing aids that amplify the sound waves restore a normal hearing range.

Sensorineural (Perceptive) Hearing Loss

In this type of hearing loss a lesion of the cochlea, eighth nerve or brain is responsible for the condition. Generally, sensorineural hearing loss implies a permanent loss of hearing as the conditions that cause this type of hearing loss are not treatable. It must be noted that in some patients both types of hearing loss may be present and treatment of the conductive hearing loss may produce a striking improvement in the aural acuity of the patient, even if a sensorineural component has been demonstrated (e.g. in an elderly patient who is showing signs of **presbycusis**, senile deafness, a treated superimposed middle ear infection may produce an improvement in hearing).

Testing Hearing

Hearing may be tested in a variety of ways, the standard 'office-type test' involving tuning forks and the more specialized **audiometry** where hearing is tested through the use of electronic equipment by an audiometrist. A term which often leads to confusion is **good bone conduction**. This term implies that the patient hears sound waves conducted by bone well and hence implies that the cochlea, eighth nerve and brain are functioning in detecting the sound (i.e. not a sensorineural hearing loss). **Poor bone conduction** implies that the patient hears poorly sounds that are conducted by bone and therefore the cochlea, eighth nerve or brain are not functioning in detecting the sound (i.e. a sensorineural hearing loss).

Rinne's test involves the use of tuning forks of 256, 512 and 1024 cycle frequency, comparing the duration of sound perception when conducted by air and by bone. The tuning fork is struck and held close to the auditory meatus until the patient signals that the sound is no longer heard. The fork's vibrating base is then immediately applied to the mastoid process. If the patient cannot hear any sound a positive or normal Rinne is recorded. Sound is heard better by air conduction than by bone conduction, therefore if hearing loss is present it will be of the sensorineural type. If the patient signals that sound is still heard when the fork is applied to the mastoid process, the test result is negative, implying that bone conduction is better than air conduction and therefore the patient is likely to have a conductive hearing loss. The principle underpinning Rinne's test is that in normal hearing more sound is conducted through to the cochlea after it has passed through the 'amplifier' of the middle ear, compared to sound which passes through bone and thus reaches the cochlea through bone conduction (refer to Figure 19.16).

A **false negative Rinne's test** will be seen in a patient with severe unilateral sensorineural hearing loss. In this case, the patient will appear to hear better by bone conduction than by air conduction in the deaf ear. This is because the bone conduction transfers the sound to the opposite cochlea where the patient does not have sensorineural hearing loss.

Weber's test involves the use of a tuning fork and is performed in association with Rinne's test. The tuning fork is struck and its vibrating stem is placed on the vertex or midline of the forehead. The patient is then asked in which ear the sound is heard better. If the patient has conductive hearing loss, the sound seems to be better heard by the affected ear. If the sound is better heard by the normal ear, the hearing loss is probably of the sensorineural type.

Absolute bone conduction is a test comparing the sensorineural hearing of the examiner and the patient. The ear of the patient being tested is occluded by pressure being put on the tragus and the vibrating tuning fork base is placed on the mastoid process on the same side as the occluded ear, until the patient signals that the sound disappears. The examiner occludes his own ear and immediately the patient signals applies the base of the fork to his or her own mastoid process. If the examiner hears a sound, it may be deduced that the patient has a degree of sensorineural hearing loss (provided that the examiner does not suffer from sensorineural hearing loss, in which case the test is useless).

Schwabach's test is a test performed with the ear opposite to the one tested stopped for both the examiner and the patient. The vibrating tuning fork base is placed on the mastoid process of the patient and examiner alternately. The results are expressed as: **Schwabach prolonged** if the patient hears the sound longer than the examiner does, indicating in this case a conductive type of hearing loss for the patient; **Schwabach diminished** if the examiner perceives the sound for longer than the patient, indicating a sensorineural hearing loss for the patient; and **Schwabach normal** if both the examiner and patient hear the sound for the same time (once again assuming the examiner has good hearing).

Audiometry involves the use of an electronic instrument, termed an audiometer, which generates pure tones between 120 and 12 000 Hertz. The patient

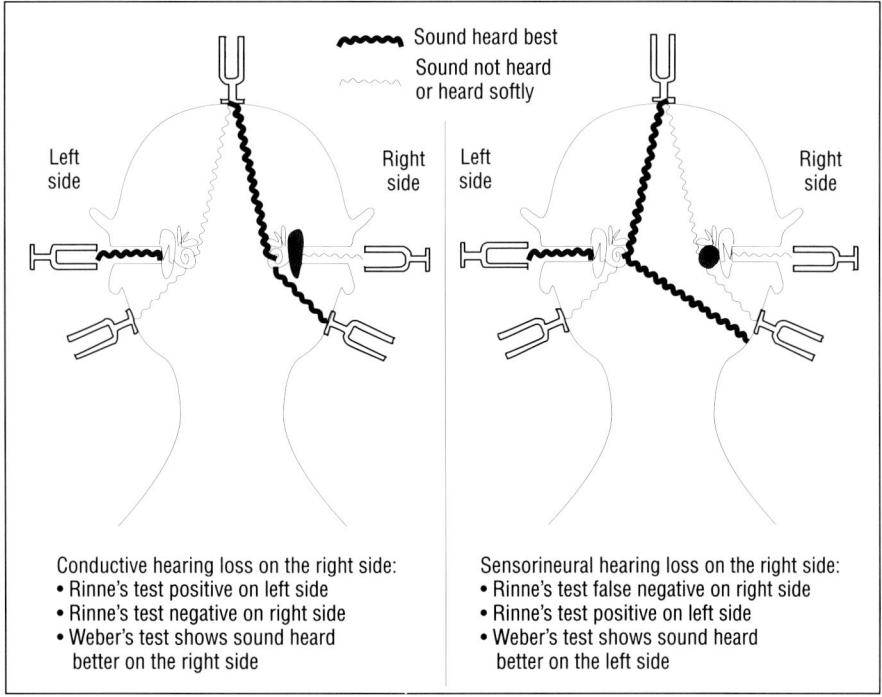

Figure 19.16 *The testing of hearing loss by the Rinne and Weber tests*

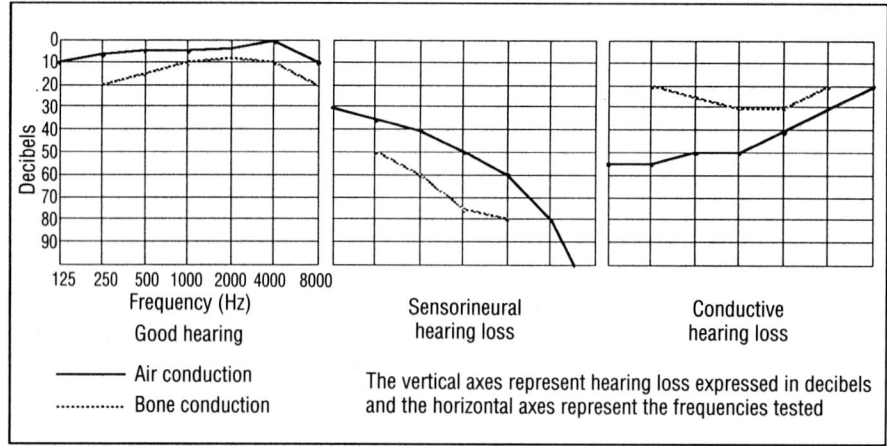

Figure 19.17   *Three audiograms, comparing a person showing good hearing with two people showing different types of hearing loss*

wears headphones through which a selected tone at a selected volume is generated by the audiometrist. The volume of the tone is increased until the patient signals that it can be heard. Volume thresholds for hearing a spectrum of tones are recorded and a graphic representation of this is made and is known as an audiogram. Hearing loss is recorded as decibels (logarithmic units of relative sound intensity) over a range of frequencies (see Figure 19.17).

Revision Questions and Case Studies

1. Discuss the pathology of conjunctivitis.
2. Define the term trachoma and discuss in full the microbiology and pathology of this disease.
3. What is the significance of the discovery of a corneal ulcer?
4. Define the following terms:
   (a) Arcus senilis   (f) Chalazion
   (b) Pterygium   (g) Hypopyon
   (c) Pinguecula   (h) Xanthelasma
   (d) Cataract   (i) Glaucoma
   (e) Ophthalmia neonatorum (j) Coloboma
5. Discuss the pathology of cataract.
6. What are the causes of glaucoma and what are the sequelae of the untreated condition?
7. What are the most important features of retinoblastoma?
8. Discuss the significance of pigmented lesions of the retina.

9. What systemic diseases commonly affect the eye and what are their manifestations in this organ?
10. Define the term papilloedema and discuss the pathological features of the condition.
11. What is epiphora and what may cause this condition?
12. Discuss in full the microbiology and pathology of acute otitis media.
13. What is otosclerosis?
14. What do you know of the pathology of the inner ear tumours?
15. Discuss the pathology of Ménière's disease.
16. Define the following terms:
    (a) Petrositis   (f) Otalgia
    (b) Cholesteatoma   (g) Vertigo
    (c) Chemodectoma   (h) Mastoiditis
    (d) Myringitis   (i) Tinnitus
    (e) Cerumen   (j) Myringotomy
17. What disease may be responsible for earache in a 6-year-old child?
18. How is deafness investigated?
19. What are the complications of acute otitis media?
20. Discuss in full the pathology of chronic otitis media, outlining aetiology, pathogenesis, macroscopic and microscopic appearance, symptoms and signs, complications and treatment.

Case study 1. Mrs Jane G., a 68-year-old Caucasian woman, was referred to an audiologist because she complained to her family doctor of 'ringing in her ears' and 'difficulty in hearing'. The woman had insisted that her ears be syringed but her problems were not resolved upon cleaning of the external ear. No

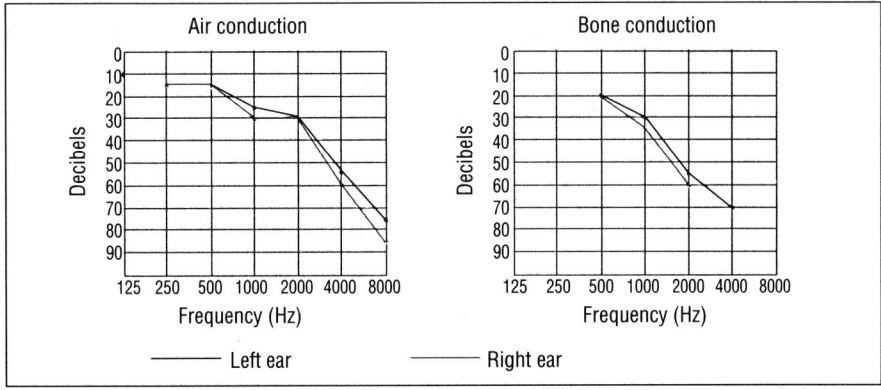

For *Case Study 1*

abnormalities were visible through the otoscope and no evidence of throat infection was found. The Rinne test was positive for both ears and the Schwabach test showed that the patient was experiencing hearing loss on both sides. Audiometric examination elicited the audiograms above.

The patient says that she has difficulty in hearing conversation in noisy places or when many people are talking in a group and the sounds shift from one direction to another.

(a) What is the diagnosis?
(b) Explain the findings of the Rinne and Schwabach tests.
(c) What do the findings of the audiograms illustrate?

Case study 2. An Aboriginal boy aged 5 years is brought to an Aboriginal Community Health Centre near Alice Springs because of itchy red eyes that water excessively. Upon examination, both eyes are seen to be affected with periorbital oedema, chemosis of the bulbar conjunctiva, hyperaemia, exudation, photophobia and pain. The upper tarsi show papillary hyperplasia and numerous follicles, each about 1 to 2 mm in diameter. The preauricular nodes are small but tender. A conjunctival scraping is taken and stained by the Giemsa method. Plasma cells, neutrophils, numerous macrophages containing debris and some epithelial cells containing dark blue inclusions around the nuclei are seen. Upon questioning the child's parents, it is revealed that the child had spent some days with his grandparents about 3 weeks ago.

(a) What is the diagnosis?
(b) What laboratory tests will confirm this diagnosis?
(c) How is the disorder treated?
(d) What are the complications of the untreated disease?

Case study 3. A 3-year-old Caucasian child is experiencing problems in the day care centre where she is left by her working parents. Over the past 3 weeks there have been behavioural changes, agression and uncharacteristic tantrums. One of the centre workers has suggested that the child be taken to a doctor to have her hearing tested as a hearing problem is suspected. Hearing assessment shows a moderate hearing loss and inspection of the ears shows the ear drum bulging outwards and of a yellowish colour, and air bubbles are seen within fluid behind the tympanic membrane. There is no earache and the child's kindergarten performance and speech are normal.

(a) What is the diagnosis?
(b) How is the condition treated?
(c) What are the complications of the untreated condition?

Case study 4. A 28-year-old Caucasian male presents at his doctor's surgery with both of his eyes red, tearing and painful, and swollen, tender preauricular nodes. These symptoms first appeared a week ago and they affected the right eye first, the left eye becoming affected 2 days later. The eyes are itchy, painful and the patient experiences photophobia. Examination of the eyes shows a follicular conjunctivitis with chemosis and oedema of the eyelids. The upper right conjunctiva shows two small haemorrhages and the left lower palpebral conjunctiva a small region occupied by a pale whitish pseudomembrane. Conjunctival scrapings show few neutrophils and mainly a mononuclear infiltrate with epithelial debris. No epithelial cell inclusions are demonstrable upon Giemsa staining. The man works as a clerk in a city office and says that one of his fellow workers had a similar eye problem about 2 weeks ago. The man does not wear contact lenses or spectacles and his vision is normal and the corneae clear.

(a) What is the diagnosis?

(b) How is the condition treated?

(c) What are the complications of the untreated condition?

Case study 5. A 46-year-old female presents because of feelings of intermittent 'giddiness' in attacks lasting for a few minutes each. The patient also says that she feels 'very poorly' after the attacks and often she is 'sick' during the attack. When questioned about her hearing she says that she has noticed some hearing loss especially immediately before and after an attack. She says that she enjoyed listening to music before these attacks started to plague her about 6 months previously, but now she cannot stand listening to even her favourite songs because they 'sound terrible', a 'buzzing' in her head contributing to this aversion to music. Tuning fork tests show a sensorineural hearing impairment that is worse on the left side. There is no earache and the ear drum looks normal upon otoscopy, and there is no cerumen blocking the ear canals.

(a) What is the most likely diagnosis?

(b) What findings of the Rinne and Weber tests would confirm this?

(c) What will occur in untreated cases of the disorder?

(d) How is the disorder treated?

Case study 6. A 28-month-old male Caucasian infant is brought to the doctor's surgery because of a squint. The right eye is esotropic (looks towards the nose) and also shows leukokoria. Ophthalmoscopic examination reveals a normal left eye but the right eye shows the presence of several small, pale yellowish white, nodular masses on the posterior retina which are growing into the vitreous. Immediate enucleation of the right eye is recommended.

(a) What is the differential diagnosis for leukokoria?

(b) What is the diagnosis?

(c) What questions are asked of the parents in connection with the infant's disease?

(d) Is the other eye likely to be spared by this disease?

(e) Why was enucleation of the right eye performed?

(f) What is the treatment if the left eye is affected by this disease at a later stage?

(g) If the infant survives to adulthood, what advice needs to be given in later life?

Further Reading

Ash JE, Beck MR, Wilkes JD. *Tumors of the Upper Respiratory Tract and Ear*, 1964; Armed Forces Institute of Pathology, Washington DC.

Batsakis JG. 'The Lymphoepithelial Lesion and Sjögren's Syndrome.' *Head Neck Surg* 1983; **5**: 150.

Bell TA. '*Chlamydia trachomatis, Mycoplasma hominis* and *Ureaplasma urealyticum* Infections of Infants.' *Semin Perinat* 1985; **9**: 29.

Bernstein JM. 'Recent Advances in Otitis Media with Effusion.' *Ann Allergy* 1985; **55**: 544.

Beverley JKA. 'Toxoplasmosis.' *Br Med Bull* 1973; **29**: 475.

Black N. 'Causes of Glue Ear.' *J Laryngol Otol* 1985; **99**: 953.

Bryan PA, Fagan PA. 'The Role of CT Scanning in Ear Disease.' *Mod Med Aust* 1992; **33**(7): 71.

Capon M, Jacobs M. 'Lasers in Ophthalmology.' *Curr Ther* 1990; **31**(3): 11.

Coster DJ, Mills RAD. 'Treatment of Tear Film Dysfunction.' *Curr Ther* 1990; **33**(1): 47.

Coster DJ. 'Common Corneal Conditions.' *Mod Med Aust* 1991; **34**(3): 97.

Darougar S. (ed.), 'Chlamydial Disease.' *Br Med Bull* 1983; **39**: 107.

Ellingham TR. 'The Dry Eye: Modern Management.' *Curr Ther* 1987; **28**(9): 99.

Emerick LL. *A Workbook in Clinical Audiometry*, 1971; Charles C. Thomas, Springfield, Illinois.

Frenkel JK. 'Toxoplasmosis.' *Pediatr Clin N Am* 1985; **32**: 917.

Giebink GS, Quie PG. 'Otitis Media.' *Annu Rev Med* 1978; **29**: 285.

Goldberg I. 'Current Treatment of Glaucoma.' *Curr Ther* 1991; **32**(8): 49.

Grieg MH. 'Otolaryngology.' *Curr Ther* 1990; **31**(4): 11.

Hipwell GC, Lawless M. 'The Ocular Complications of Connective Tissue Disease.' *Mod Med Aust* 1991; **34**(5): 47.

Huang MY, Schacht J. 'Drug-Induced Ototoxicity.' *Curr Ther* 1991; **32**(10): 71.

Hunter RM, Davis BW, Gray GF Jr, Rosenfeld L. 'Primary Malignant Tumours of Salivary Gland Origin.' *Am Surg* 1983; **49**: 82.

King J. 'Loss of Vision.' *Mod Med Aust* 1990; **33**(5): 52.

Kirkness CM. *Ophthalmology*, 1985; Gower Medical Publishing, London.

Leflar RB, Lillie H. *Cataracts*, 1981; Facts on File Inc., New York.

Long J, Buckley C. 'Eye Problems in the Elderly.' *Mod Med Aust* 1991; **34**(6): 55.

Maclean H. 'Infections. Part VI: Common Eye Infections.' *Curr Ther* 1991; **32**(3): 41.

Meyerhoff WL, Giebink GS. 'Pathology and Microbiology of Otitis Media.' *Laryngoscope* 1982; **92**: 273.

Naumann GOH, Apple D. *Pathology of the Eye*, 1986; Springer Verlag, Berlin.

Prince JH. *You and your Eyes*, 1970; AH & AW Reed, Sydney.

Schachter J. 'Chlamydial Infections.' *N Engl J Med* 1978; **298**: 428.

Smith PH. 'Advances in Lens Replacement.' *Mod Med Aust* 1991; **34**(7): 52.

Strand V, Tala N. 'Advances in the Diagnosis and Treatment of Sjögren's Syndrome.' *Bull Rheum Dis* 1980; **30**: 1046.

Tonkin JP. 'Management of Ménière's Disease.' *Curr Ther* 1987; **28**(10): 153.

Wiet RJ, Raslan W, Schambaugh GE Jr. 'Otosclerosis 1981 to 1985.' *Am J Otol* 1986; **7**: 221.

Unger H. 'Eye Problems in General Practice.' *Mod Med Aust* 1990; **33**(7): 113.

Vorrath J. 'Glue Ear: Treatment and Management in Childhood.' *Mod Med Aust* 1991; **31**(3): 69.

Yermankov V, *et al.* 'Disseminated Toxoplasmosis.' *Arch Pathol Lab Med* 1982; **106**: 534.

Systemic Pathology Test

Allow 3 hours for this test.

Part A: Multiple Choice Questions

The following questions or statements have only **one correct response**. Read carefully all choices and indicate the **best** response by marking the letter corresponding to it (allow 60 minutes for this section).

1. Which of the following is not a sequela of acute appendicitis?
   (a) Peritonitis
   (b) Regional enteritis
   (c) Septicaemia
   (d) Localized abscess formation
   (e) Gangrenous appendicitis
2. Males are affected more than females by:
   (a) Rheumatoid arthritis
   (b) The seronegative arthropathies
   (c) Viral hepatitis (type A)
   (d) Rheumatic fever
   (e) Meningitis
3. The following are malignant skin tumours:
   (a) Squamous cell carcinoma, anaplastic tumour of the dermis
   (b) Malignant melanoma, keratoacanthoma
   (c) Keratoacanthoma, acanthosis
   (d) Papilloma, squamous cell carcinoma
   (e) Squamous cell carcinoma, junctional naevus
4. The commonest cause of death in people suffering from benign hypertension is:
   (a) Massive gastrointestinal haemorrhage
   (b) Myocardial insufficiency
   (c) Cerebral infarction
   (d) Atherosclerosis
   (d) Renal failure
5. Centrilobular necrosis of the liver is seen in all of the following, *except:*
   (a) Yellow fever virus infection
   (b) Chronic venous congestion
   (c) Hepatitis
   (d) Cardiac failure
   (e) None of the above

6. The nephrotic syndrome would be seen in an individual with:
   (a) Hypolipidaemia
   (b) Diabetes insipidus
   (c) Renal amyloidosis
   (d) Perirenal abscess
   (e) Renal vein thrombosis

7. The *commonest* site for ectopic pregnancies is the:
   (a) Fallopian tube
   (b) Peritoneal cavity
   (c) Vagina
   (d) Ovary
   (e) Cervix

8. Spongiosis of the epidermis is a marked feature of:
   (a) Xeroderma pigmentosum
   (b) Basal cell carcinoma
   (c) Keratoacanthoma
   (d) Pigmentary incontinence
   (e) Contact dermatitis

9. An encapsulated, rubbery, freely mobile breast lump is most likely to be a:
   (a) Scirrhous carcinoma
   (b) Medullary carcinoma
   (c) Fibroadenoma
   (d) Non-neoplastic lesion

10. A tumour found more frequently in men than in women is:
    (a) Meningioma
    (b) Carcinoma of the bladder
    (c) Carcinoma of the breast
    (d) Carcinoma of the colon
    (e) Reticulosarcoma

11. Prophylaxis of rheumatic fever is best accomplished by:
    (a) Steroid therapy
    (b) Salicylate therapy
    (c) Antiserum therapy
    (d) Early antibiotic therapy of streptococcal infections
    (e) Early antibiotic therapy of staphylococcal infections

12. Average 5-year survival figures generally quoted for malignant melanomata are:
    (a) 15%
    (b) 30%
    (c) 50%
    (d) 75%

13. Mitral valve stenosis is most often the result of:
    (a) Rheumatic endocarditis
    (b) Arteriosclerosis
    (c) Syphilis
    (d) Congenital heart disease

(e) Healed subacute bacterial endocarditis

14. Cardiac failure is the result of:
    (a) Inadequate myocardial oxygenation
    (b) Inability of the heart to maintain an adequate circulation
    (c) Myocardial hypertrophy
    (d) Increased venous pressure
    (e) None of the above

15. Acute pancreatitis:
    (a) Is due to the digestive enzymes of the pancreas acting on itself
    (b) Is due to acute poisoning
    (c) Is most commonly due to alcoholism
    (d) Is a congenital disease due to excessive mucus accumulation
    (e) Is due to islet cell tumours of the pancreas

16. Myocardial hypertrophy is the result of:
    (a) Dilatation of the chambers of the heart
    (b) Increased numbers of muscle fibres
    (c) Proliferation of myocardial caveolae
    (d) An excessive work load being placed on the heart
    (e) Endocardial thickening due to proliferation of cells

17. Anaphylactic reactions, such as bronchial asthma, are caused by the release of histamine and histamine-like substances from:
    (a) Kupffer cells
    (b) Monocytes
    (c) Mast cells
    (d) Killer T cells
    (e) B lymphocytes

18. Pylephlebitis with resulting liver abscesses is often due to:
    (a) Chronic non-specific ulcerative colitis
    (b) Appendicitis
    (c) Amoebiasis
    (d) Meckel's diverticulum
    (e) Rheumatic fever

19. Production of a peptic ulcer requires:
    (a) Gastric hypermotility
    (b) Increased nervous activity
    (c) An acid environment
    (d) Intrinsic factor
    (e) Histamine

20. Average 5-year survival in carcinoma of the colon is about:
    (a) 25%
    (b) 35%
    (c) 45%
    (d) 65%
    (e) 85%

21. In amyloidosis the following is *not* true:
    (a) Amyloidosis often occurs as a sequela of

rheumatoid arthritis
- (b) The body reacts weakly to the presence of amyloid
- (c) Renal involvement occurs in both primary and secondary amyloidosis
- (d) Secondary amyloidosis may develop in people with tuberculosis
- (e) Amyloid material is composed of immunoglobulin heavy chains

22. Activated macrophages will be found in a lesion of eczema.
    - (a) True
    - (b) False

23. The main factors in the development of bronchiectasis are:
    - (a) Congenital diseases
    - (b) Bronchial adenomata and carcinomata
    - (c) Hyperdistention and infection
    - (d) Smoking and lack of α-antitrypsinase activity
    - (e) Silicosis and asbestosis

24. In carcinoma of the lungs the overall 5-year survival rate is:
    - (a) 0–20%
    - (b) 21–40%
    - (c) 41–60%
    - (d) 61–80%
    - (e) Better than 81%

25. Bronchogenic carcinomata tend to *metastasize* early:
    - (a) By local invasion only
    - (b) Via the lymphatics
    - (c) By haematogenous routes
    - (d) By bronchial dissemination
    - (e) Within the thorax only

26. Multiple sclerosis is characterized by:
    - (a) Focal axonal degeneration followed by demyelination
    - (b) Flattened, brownish skin lesions
    - (c) Focal cerebral necrosis
    - (d) Demyelination without destruction of the axons

27. The origin of the commonest type of brain tumours is:
    - (a) Glial
    - (b) Meningeal
    - (c) Vascular
    - (d) Osseous
    - (e) Neuronal

28. In familial polyposis coli the polyps tend to appear most frequently:
    - (a) At birth
    - (b) During childhood and youth
    - (c) After the age of 40 years
    - (d) During the fourth decade of life
    - (e) Following gastrointestinal haemorrhage

29. A malignant melanoma is most likely to arise in a:
    - (a) Neurofibroma
    - (b) Basal cell carcinoma
    - (c) Junctional naevus
    - (d) Wart
    - (e) Freckle

30. Predisposing factors to the development of carcinoma of the stomach are:
    - (a) Gout, amyloidosis and/or sarcoidosis
    - (b) Spicy diets, ingestion of hot liquids, eating of meat, benign tumours
    - (c) Gastritis, oesophagitis and enteritis
    - (d) Peptic ulcer, gastritis, pernicious anaemia, benign tumours
    - (e) Benign tumours, sarcoidosis, gout

31. The commonest sequelae of Crohn's disease are:
    - (a) Haemorrhage, perforation, ulceration
    - (b) Suppuration, ulceration, fistula formation
    - (c) Intestinal obstruction, fistula formation, malabsorption
    - (d) Obstruction, haemorrhage, suppuration
    - (e) Malabsorption syndrome, suppuration, ulceration

32. The progress of pulmonary tuberculosis is enhanced by the inhalation of which of the following particles?
    - (a) Talc
    - (b) Silica
    - (c) Iron oxide
    - (d) Carbon
    - (e) Beryllium oxide

33. The majority of peptic ulcers heal with bed rest and only approximately 15% fail to do so.
    - (a) True
    - (b) False

34. Chronic pyelonephritis is only rarely fatal.
    - (a) True
    - (b) False

35. The kidney is a common site for cysts to occur.
    - (a) True
    - (b) False

36. Hydronephrosis is often associated with urolithiasis.
    - (a) True
    - (b) False

37. Which of the following statements about diverticular disease is *not* correct:
    - (a) It is characterized by patchy hypertrophy of the colonic muscle
    - (b) Perforation of the bowel may occur
    - (c) Up to two-thirds of people aged 60 years or

over are affected to some degree

(d)   It is an important cause of fibrous colonic narrowing

(e)   Most diverticula are found in the sigmoid colon

38.   Fibroleiomyomata of the uterus are uncommon tumours.
(a)   True
(b)   False

39.   Leukoplakia is a premalignant condition.
(a)   True
(b)   False

40.   The incidence of ectopic pregnancy is:
(a)   Once in every 50 pregnancies
(b)   Once in every 125 pregnancies
(c)   Once in every 500 pregnancies
(d)   Once in every 1000 pregnancies
(e)   Once in every 2000 pregnancies

41.   Obstruction in the large bowel is most commonly due to:
(a)   Herniation through the abdominal wall
(b)   Intestinal bands and adhesions
(c)   Neoplasms
(d)   Volvulus
(e)   Mesenteric vessel thrombosis

42.   Breast carcinoma is commoner in women whose menarche was before the age of 13 years.
(a)   True
(b)   False

43.   Carcinoma of the gall bladder is *not:*
(a)   Seen more often in women than men
(b)   Associated with cholelithiasis
(c)   Usually an adenocarcinoma
(d)   A tumour with a good prognosis
(e)   Seen to spread early via the bloodstream and lymphatics

44.   The most *important* effects of cirrhosis are:
(a)   Ascites, haemorrhage, blood in the faeces
(b)   Jaundice, hepatoma, haemorrhage
(c)   Hepatoma, liver failure, ascites
(d)   Renal failure, portal hypertension
(e)   Portal hypertension, liver failure, hepatoma

45.   Glomerulonephritis is most often due to:
(a)   An inflammation of the kidney
(b)   An infection of the glomeruli
(c)   Diseases of the kidney medulla
(d)   Injury to the glomeruli caused by the presence of antigen–antibody complexes in the glomerular capillary walls
(e)   An autoimmune disease in which antibodies are produced and which destroy the renal parenchyma

46.   A *malignant* skin tumour which rarely, if ever, metastasizes is the:

(a)   Basal cell carcinoma
(b)   Squamous cell carcinoma
(c)   Malignant melanoma
(d)   Keratoacanthoma

47.   A common feature seen in sarcoidosis is:
(a)   Onset after the age of 55 years
(b)   Hyperparathyroidism
(c)   Raised serum level of angiotensin-converting enzyme
(d)   Erythema multiforme
(e)   None of the above

48.   Inflammatory cells in the alveolar *walls* are characteristic of:
(a)   *Pneumocystis carinii* pneumonia
(b)   Bronchopneumonia
(c)   Lobar pneumonia
(d)   Interstitial pneumonitis
(e)   Organizing pneumonia

49.   All of the following are thought to be autoimmune diseases *except:*
(a)   Thyroiditis
(b)   Ulcerative colitis
(c)   Gas gangrene
(d)   Rheumatoid arthritis
(e)   Amyloidosis

50.   Exposure of the skin to ionizing radiation most often gives rise to a basal cell carcinoma.
(a)   True
(b)   False

51.   Abscess formation tends to occur more commonly in the right lung.
(a)   True
(b)   False

52.   Malignant hepatomata are liver tumours, and about 50% of them arise in relation to cirrhosis.
(a)   True
(b)   False

53.   The commonest joint disease is rheumatoid arthritis.
(a)   True
(b)   False

54.   Post-streptococcal glomerulonephritis is an:
(a)   Endergonic reaction
(b)   Anaphylactic reaction
(c)   Arthroid-type reaction
(d)   Immune complex-mediated hypersensitivity
(e)   Autoimmune disease

55.   Glioblastoma multiforme is a tumour that has a good prognosis ($\approx 65\%$ 5-year survival).
(a)   True
(b)   False

56.   Well-differentiated tissues of many different kinds are seen in:
(a)   Anaplasia

(b) Hamartoma
(c) Seminoma
(d) Teratoma of the ovary
(e) Teratoma of the testis

57. Carcinoma of the pancreas:
(a) Occurs more commonly in females than in males
(b) Is very uncommon (<1% of cancers)
(c) Most usually involves the tail and body of the organ
(d) May cause biliary obstruction and jaundice
(e) Has a good prognosis (>50% 5-year survival)

58. All of the following are associated with chronic lymphocytic leukaemia *except:*
(a) It is the commonest type of leukaemia in children < 10 years of age
(b) It involves a neoplastic proliferation of lymphocytes
(c) There is infiltration of lymph nodes with the malignant cells
(d) It is more common in males
(e) It is associated with anaemia

59. Anaemia may be commonly brought about by, or be the result of:
(a) Benign tumours
(b) Haemochromatosis
(c) Sarcoidosis
(d) Lobar pneumonia
(e) Autoimmune disorders

60. A primary carcinoma of the breast is most likely to give rise to metastatic deposits in the:
(a) Intestines, bone or brain
(b) Lymph nodes, lungs or bone
(c) Viscera, brain, ovaries or lymph nodes
(d) Lymph nodes, muscles and skin
(e) Liver, lungs, genitalia

61. In chronic cholecystitis:
(a) Infecting organisms are often isolated
(b) No association with cholelithiasis is observed
(c) Marked fibrosis is seen in the organ wall
(d) The mucosa is grossly thickened and hyperplastic
(e) Pain is unusual

63. Syndesmophytes are lesions associated with Reiter's disease.
(a) True
(b) False

64. Carcinoma of the kidney (Grawitz tumour) is:
(a) Most commonly seen in elderly women
(b) A tumour of infancy
(c) Most commonly seen in elderly men
(d) Associated with ingestion of large quanti-

ties of sugar
(e) Caused by diabetes mellitus

65. Tertiary syphilis affects which systems of the body most commonly?
(a) Musculoskeletal and cutaneous
(b) Alimentary tract and liver
(c) Cardiovascular and central nervous
(d) Haemopoietic (including spleen)
(e) Genitourinary

66. Myocardial infarction is often associated with coronary artery atherosclerosis.
(a) True
(b) False

67. Seminoma is commoner in males with undescended testes than in normal males.
(a) True
(b) False

68. Osteoporosis may be seen in many bones of the skeleton in scurvy.
(a) True
(b) False

69. Alzheimer's disease is characterized by:
(a) Delirium tremens
(b) Primary hydrocephalus
(c) Tabes dorsalis
(d) Involuntary choreiform movements
(e) Extensive cortical atrophy of the cerebrum

70. Ulcerative colitis:
(a) Is a diffuse granulomatous inflammation
(b) Involves the entire thickness of the bowel wall
(c) Is the result of peptic ulcers
(d) Predisposes to the development of amyloidosis
(e) Results in pseudopolyp formation

71. Sterile fibrinous pericarditis may be seen in:
(a) Uraemia
(b) Tuberculosis
(c) Viral infections
(d) Hypertrophy of the heart due to hypertension
(e) Hepatitis

72. Emphysema:
(a) Is a permanent dilatation of the alveoli
(b) Results in a constriction of the bronchial airways
(c) May result in carcinoma of the lungs
(d) Is associated with increased surface area of the alveoli
(e) Results in accumulation of mucus in the airways

73. Which is the tumour associated with the best prognosis?
(a) Ewing's sarcoma

(b) Chondrosarcoma
(c) Giant cell tumour of the bone
(d) Osteosarcoma
(e) Fibrosarcoma

75. Obstruction in the small bowel is most commonly due to:
(a) Herniation through the abdominal wall
(b) Intestinal bands and adhesions
(c) Neoplasms
(d) Volvulus
(e) Mesenteric vessel thrombosis

74. Leukopenia is indicated by a circulating leukocyte number of less than:
(a) 4000 per µL
(b) 5000 per µL
(c) 8000 per µL
(d) 10 000 per µL
(e) 20 000 per µL

75. The administration of specific gamma globulin is a recognized form of prophylactic treatment in which disease?
(a) Rubella
(b) Influenza
(c) Hepatitis A
(d) Hepatitis B
(e) Hepatitis C

76. A 59-year-old woman, who smokes about five cigarettes a day presents at her local community health centre 5 years after a modified radical mastectomy. She complains of respiratory difficulties, shortness of breath and a persistent, dry, non-productive cough. She is most likely suffering from:
(a) Pneumonia
(b) A primary lung carcinoma
(c) Bronchiectasis and emphysema
(d) Secondary lung tumours
(e) Tuberculosis

77. An 82-year-old woman presents with loss of weight and anaemia, bowel disturbances (bouts of constipation and diarrhoea) and excessive mucus in the faeces. There is slight ascites and pain in the right upper quadrant of the abdomen. There is jaundice present. The most likely diagnosis is:
(a) Alcoholic liver disease
(b) Diverticular disease
(c) Crohn's disease
(d) Ulcerative colitis
(e) Carcinoma of the colon

78. A man of 68 years with left costovertebral angle sharp pain complains of blood-stained urine. There is dysuria and dribbling with poor urine flow. The urine is acid to litmus and there is excessive oxalate present. The most likely diagnosis is:
(a) Prostatitis and prostatomegaly
(b) Kidney tumour
(c) Urinary calculi
(d) Pyelonephritis
(e) Urinary calculi and prostatomegaly

79. Which of the following is *not* a primary immune deficiency disease?
(a) Congenital thymic aplasia
(b) Swiss-type immunodeficiency
(c) Di-George syndrome
(d) AIDS
(e) Bruton agammaglobulinaemia

80. Hydatid disease:
(a) Does not occur in rural Australia
(b) Causes eosinophilia in peripheral blood
(c) Is routinely diagnosed by biopsy of suspected lesions
(d) More commonly causes lesions in the lung than in the liver
(e) Commonly involves rupture of a cyst into a bronchus

Part B: Multiple Choice Questions

The following 20 questions or statements **may have more than one correct response** out of (i) to (v). Read carefully all responses and mark the letter **a, b, c, d**, or **e** of **the one correct choice** on your paper (allow 15 minutes for this section).

81. Tumours of the large intestine:
(i) Are most commonly found in the rectum and the sigmoid colon
(ii) May cause obstruction
(iii) Are most frequently sarcomata
(iv) Rarely metastasize to the liver
(v) Are often adenocarcinomata, if malignant

(a) Responses (i), (ii) and (iii) are correct
(b) Responses (i), (ii) and (iv) are correct
(c) Responses (i), (ii) and (v) are correct
(d) Responses (ii), (iii) and (iv) are correct
(e) Responses (ii), (iv) and (v) are correct

82. Cholecystitis:
(i) Is often associated with cholelithiasis
(ii) May be associated with obstruction of the gall bladder
(iii) Is more commonly seen in women
(iv) Is due to a fatty diet
(v) May cause cholelithiasis

(a) Responses (i), (ii) and (iii) are correct

(b) Responses (i), (ii) and (iv) are correct
(c) Responses (i), (ii) and (v) are correct
(d) Responses (ii), (iii) and (iv) are correct
(e) Responses (ii), (iv) and (v) are correct

83. Obstruction of the urethra may:
(i) Cause hydronephrosis
(ii) Be caused by coeliac disease
(iii) Be seen frequently in elderly men
(iv) Predispose to infection
(v) Lead to glomerulonephritis

(a) Responses (i), (ii) and (iii) are correct
(b) Responses (i), (iii) and (iv) are correct
(c) Responses (i), (iii) and (v) are correct
(d) Responses (ii), (iii) and (iv) are correct
(e) Responses (ii), (iv) and (v) are correct

84. Chronic obstructive airways disease is often associated with:
(i) Bronchitis
(ii) Congenital chymotrypsin deficiency
(iii) Sarcoidosis
(iv) Infarction
(v) Interstitial fibrosis

(a) Responses (i), (ii) and (iii) are correct
(b) Responses (i), (ii) and (iv) are correct
(c) Responses (i), (ii) and (v) are correct
(d) Responses (ii), (iii) and (iv) are correct
(e) All responses are correct

85. Pulmonary hypertension may:
(i) Accelerate atherosclerosis
(ii) Cause right ventricular failure
(iii) Cause generalized oedema
(iv) Activate the renin–angiotensin system
(v) Cause chronic venous congestion of the liver

(a) Responses (i), (ii) and (iii) are correct
(b) Responses (i), (ii) and (iv) are correct
(c) Responses (i), (ii) and (v) are correct
(d) Responses (ii), (iii) and (iv) are correct
(e) All responses are correct

86. Conditions with a very poor 5-year survival rate are:
(i) Hodgkin's disease
(ii) Acute myeloid leukaemia
(iii) Chronic lymphocytic leukaemia
(iv) Hypochromic anaemia
(v) Acute lymphoid leukaemia

(a) Responses (i), (ii) and (iii) are correct
(b) Responses (i), (ii) and (iv) are correct
(c) Responses (i), (ii) and (v) are correct
(d) Responses (ii), (iii) and (v) are correct
(e) Responses (ii), (iv) and (v) are correct

87. The following are characteristic of carcinoma of the cervix:

(i) The highest incidence is in the age group 60 to 75 years
(ii) The Pap smear is used in diagnosis
(iii) It has an average 5-year survival rate of 85%
(iv) It is associated with sexual promiscuity
(v) It is treated by conization, partial or radical hysterectomy

(a) Responses (i), (ii) and (iii) are correct
(b) Responses (i), (iii) and (iv) are correct
(c) Responses (i), (iii) and (v) are correct
(d) Responses (ii), (iii) and (iv) are correct
(e) Responses (ii), (iv) and (v) are correct

88. The following are malignant tumours:
(i) Ovarian teratoma
(ii) Testicular teratoma
(iii) Meningioma
(iv) Hepatoma
(v) Lymphosarcoma

(a) Responses (i), (ii) and (iii) are correct
(b) Responses (i), (ii) and (iv) are correct
(c) Responses (i), (iii) and (v) are correct
(d) Responses (ii), (iii) and (v) are correct
(e) Responses (ii), (iv) and (v) are correct

89. The following are characteristic of breast carcinoma:
(i) Paget's disease of the nipple
(ii) *Peau d'orange*
(iii) Spread to involve the ovaries
(iv) Most commonly metastasizes to the brain
(v) Seen usually in women between the ages of 40 to 75 years

(a) Responses (i), (ii) and (iii) are correct
(b) Responses (i), (iii) and (iv) are correct
(c) Responses (i), (ii) and (v) are correct
(d) Responses (ii), (iii) and (iv) are correct
(e) Responses (iii), (iv) and (v) are correct

90. Rheumatoid arthritis is characterized by:
(i) Pannus formation
(ii) Osteophyte formation
(iii) Autoimmunity
(iv) Degeneration of cartilage of weight-bearing joints primarily
(v) Deformation of joints in advanced cases

(a) Responses (i), (ii) and (iii) are correct
(b) Responses (i), (ii) and (iv) are correct
(c) Responses (i), (iii) and (v) are correct
(d) Responses (ii), (iii) and (iv) are correct
(e) Responses (iii), (iv) and (v) are correct

91. Osteosarcomata:
(i) Arise commonly in the vicinity of the knee joint

(ii) Are primarily a tumour of old age

(iii) Are associated with injuries, fractures, wounds, etc.

(iv) Are seen more commonly in young adults

(v) Have a poor prognosis

(a) Responses (i), (ii) and (iii) are correct

(b) Responses (i), (ii) and (v) are correct

(c) Responses (i), (iii) and (v) are correct

(d) Responses (i), (iii) and (iv) are correct

(e) Responses (i), (iv) and (v) are correct

92. Giant cell tumours of bone, on average:

(i) Have a better prognosis than osteosarcomata

(ii) May arise in elderly patients in association with Paget's disease

(iii) May not give rise to symptoms for years

(iv) May spread via the bloodstream and lymphatics, killing the patient quickly

(v) May arise in pre-existing benign tumours

(a) Responses (i), (ii) and (iii) are correct

(b) Responses (i), (ii) and (iv) are correct

(c) Responses (i), (ii) and (v) are correct

(d) Responses (ii), (iii) and (iv) are correct

(e) All responses are correct

93. The following may be autoimmune diseases:

(i) Dermatitis

(ii) Pernicious anaemia

(iii) Pick's disease of the pericardium

(iv) Thrombocytopenia

(v) Atherosclerosis

(a) Responses (i), (ii) and (iii) are correct

(b) Responses (i), (ii) and (iv) are correct

(c) Responses (i), (iii) and (v) are correct

(d) Responses (ii), (iii) and (iv) are correct

(e) All responses are correct

94. Amyloidosis:

(i) Is an autoimmune disorder

(ii) May be seen in association with chronic infective states

(iii) Is an idiopathic granulomatous chronic inflammation

(iv) Is seen most frequently in the brain, skin and intestines

(v) Is seen most frequently in the heart, liver, spleen

(a) Responses (i), (ii) and (iii) are correct

(b) Responses (i), (ii) and (iv) are correct

(c) Responses (i), (ii) and (v) are correct

(d) Responses (ii), (iii) and (iv) are correct

(e) Responses (ii), (iii) and (v) are correct

95. Malignancies of the colon are very common. Such tumours are often:

(i) Associated with *Clostridium paraputrificum*

and bile acids in the faeces

(ii) Staged by Duke's system, A–D

(iii) Grouped by the Lancefield system A–E

(iv) Involved with a high animal fat intake

(v) Seen in patients 20 to 50 years of age

(a) Responses (i), (ii) and (iv) are correct

(b) Responses (i), (ii) and (v) are correct

(c) Responses (i), (iii) and (iv) are correct

(d) Responses (i), (iii) and (v) are correct

(e) Responses (ii), (iv) and (v) are correct

96. Sarcoidosis:

(i) Is an atypical mycobacterial infection

(ii) Is commoner in women than it is in men

(iii) Is an idiopathic granulomatous chronic inflammation

(iv) Is seen most frequently in the brain, skin and intestines

(v) Is seen most frequently in the lungs, liver, spleen

(a) Responses (i), (ii) and (iii) are correct

(b) Responses (i), (ii) and (iv) are correct

(c) Responses (i), (ii) and (v) are correct

(d) Responses (ii), (iii) and (iv) are correct

(e) Responses (ii), (iii) and (v) are correct

97. Cerebral infarction:

(i) Is the leading cause of death after cancer in Australian men aged 60 years or more

(ii) Is often preceded by TIA

(iii) Is associated with atherosclerosis of the carotid, vertebral and basilar arteries

(iv) Results in an apoplectic cyst within the brain

(v) Causes headache as a typical symptom in most patients

(a) Responses (i), (ii) and (iii) are correct

(b) Responses (i), (ii) and (iv) are correct

(c) Responses (i), (ii) and (v) are correct

(d) Responses (ii), (iii) and (iv) are correct

(e) All responses are correct

98. Subarachnoid haemorrhage:

(i) Is associated with berry aneurysms

(ii) Is often seen in people with polycystic disease of the kidneys

(iii) Has a relatively good prognosis, with approximately 50% of patients surviving

(iv) Is associated with Kernig's sign, Budzhinki's sign, and neck stiffness

(v) May be seen in association with chronic infective states

(a) Responses (i), (ii) and (iii) are correct

(b) Responses (i), (ii) and (iv) are correct

(c) Responses (i), (ii) and (v) are correct

(d) Responses (ii), (iii) and (iv) are correct

(e) All responses are correct

99. Disorders arising from the actions of a type II hypersensitivity are:
    (i) Dermatitis
    (ii) Hyperacute graft rejection reactions
    (iii) Serum sickness
    (iv) Hashimoto's thyroiditis
    (v) Agranulocytosis associated with administration of quinidine

    (a) Responses (i), (ii) and (iii) are correct
    (b) Responses (i), (ii) and (iv) are correct
    (c) Responses (i), (iii) and (v) are correct
    (d) Responses (ii), (iii) and (iv) are correct
    (e) Responses (ii), (iv) and (v) are correct

100. Spina bifida:
    (i) Occurs in approximately 1.5% of births
    (ii) May remain undiagnosed during an individual's life
    (iii) In its most severe form is termed rachischisis
    (iv) Is a Mendelian genetic disorder
    (v) Leads to hydrocephalus in many patients

    (a) Responses (i), (ii) and (iii) are correct
    (b) Responses (i), (ii) and (iv) are correct
    (c) Responses (i), (ii) and (v) are correct
    (d) Responses (ii), (iii) and (iv) are correct
    (e) Responses (ii), (iii) and (v) are correct

Part C: Case Study

Read the following information carefully and then complete the questions below.

A 28-year-old Caucasian male was admitted to the Fairfield Infectious Diseases Hospital because fatigue, considerable weight loss over a short period of time, swollen cervical and axillary lymph nodes and a chronic watery diarrhoea were becoming increasingly problematic. The patient is an intravenous drug user. On examination he is seen to be 1.85 m tall, 67 kg in weight, pale, slightly jaundiced. He is very irritable and anxious about being examined and not very co-operative. Laboratory findings showed a pancytopenia in the blood film and a depressed T4 to T8 ratio.

For the following questions there is one correct choice; mark each correct choice, **a**, **b**, **c**, **d** or **e** on your paper (allow 15 minutes for this section).

1. The differential diagnosis for the man's condition is:
    (i) Hepatitis B or hepatitis C

    (ii) HIV infection
    (iii) Hepatitis A
    (iv) Infectious mononucleosis
    (v) Septicaemia

    (a) Responses (i), (ii) and (iii) are correct
    (b) Responses (i), (ii) and (v) are correct
    (c) Responses (i), (iii) and (iv) are correct
    (d) Responses (ii), (iii) and (v) are correct
    (e) Responses (ii), (iv) and (v) are correct

2. Based on the clinical findings the most likely diagnosis is:
    (a) Hepatitis (due to a hepatitis virus)
    (b) Septicaemia and subacute bacterial endocarditis
    (c) Infectious mononucleosis
    (d) HIV infection
    (e) Gay bowel syndrome

3. The aetiological agent of this disease may be transmitted by:
    (i) The respiratory route (droplet spread)
    (ii) Reused, shared syringes
    (iii) Mosquitoes and other biting insects
    (iv) Sexual intercourse
    (v) Congenital infection

    (a) Responses (i), (ii) and (iii) are correct
    (b) Responses (ii), (iii) and (iv) are correct
    (c) Responses (ii), (iii) and (v) are correct
    (d) Responses (ii), (iv) and (v) are correct
    (e) Responses (i), (ii) and (v) are correct

4. Frequently, this aetiological agent contributes to the causation of:
    (a) Primary hepatocarcinoma
    (b) Cervical carcinoma
    (c) Leukaemia and lymphoma
    (d) Bronchogenic carcinoma
    (e) Carcinoma of the colon

5. The aetiological agent may be *easily* isolated from the patient's:
    (i) Blood
    (ii) Urine
    (iii) Saliva
    (iv) Semen
    (v) Lymph nodes

    (a) Responses (i), (ii) and (iii) are correct
    (b) Responses (i), (ii) and (v) are correct
    (c) Responses (i), (iii) and (iv) are correct
    (d) Responses (i), (iv) and (v) are correct
    (e) Responses (ii), (iii) and (v) are correct

6. Another three, secondary infectious agents were isolated from the patient subsequently. These are most likely to have been:
    (i) *Mycobacterium avium*

(ii)   Cytomegalovirus
(iii) *Candida albicans*
(iv)   *Bacteroides fragilis*
(v)   Echovirus, serotypes 9 and 11

(a)   Responses (i), (ii) and (iii) are correct
(b)   Responses (i), (ii) and (v) are correct
(c)   Responses (i), (iii) and (iv) are correct
(d)   Responses (i), (iv) and (v) are correct
(e)   Responses (ii), (iii) and (v) are correct

7. The following people that have contacted the patient should be examined for evidence of direct transmission of the primary infection:
(i)   The patient's girlfriend
(ii) The chiropractor who was treating the patient before he presented at Fairfield
(iii) Drug user friends
(iv) The patient's brother who received a kidney transplant from the patient 4 years ago
(v)   The patient's mother

(a)   Responses (i), (ii) and (iii) are correct
(b)   Responses (i), (ii) and (v) are correct
(c)   Responses (i), (iii) and (iv) are correct
(d)   Responses (i), (iv) and (v) are correct
(e)   Responses (ii), (iii) and (v) are correct

8. The man was treated with:
(i)   Antibiotics and antifungal drugs
(ii) Interferon and CD_4
(iii) Iododeoxyuridine and related compounds
(iv) Vaccination and passive immunization against hepatitis
(v)   Azidothymidine (Zidovudine) and other anti-AIDS drugs

(a)   Responses (i), (ii) and (iii) are correct
(b)   Responses (i), (ii) and (v) are correct
(c)   Responses (i), (iii) and (iv) are correct
(d)   Responses (i), (iv) and (v) are correct
(e)   Responses (ii), (iii) and (v) are correct

The man died 5 months after he first presented at Fairfield and an autopsy is performed. It is seen that he is extremely wasted and markedly jaundiced. Throughout his skin and mucous membranes there are multiple dark purplish blotches that formed, large, irregular, slightly raised plaques, that in some cases were ulcerated.

9. These plaques are a manifestation of:
(a)   Septicaemia
(b)   Hodgkin's disease
(c)   Leukaemia and lymphoma
(d)   Kaposi's sarcoma
(e)   Liver failure and jaundice

The lungs were examined and were seen to be heavy, consolidated and non-crepitant. Both lungs were involved diffusely and looked as though they were made of coarse sponge. When the lung was squeezed, the cut surface exuded considerable, thick, non-purulent exudate. Histological samples were taken and it was observed that a foamy, eosinophilic and generally acellular alveolar exudate filled the air spaces and the alveolar cells in many cases had undergone cuboidal metaplasia. A silver stain on the sections shows the foamy exudate to be teeming with round, ovoid and semilunar dark bodies that have a diameter of 3.5 to 6 µm. The organisms are found in large clusters throughout the lung but in no other organ of the body.

10. The lung disease is:
(i)   Due to *Legionella pneumophila*
(ii) A typical massive pneumonia
(iii) Due to *Pneumocystis carinii*
(iv) Due to *Bacteroides fragilis* (i.e. a mixed infection with another organism)
(v)   The commonest opportunistic infection in these patients

(a)   Responses (i), (ii) and (iv) are correct
(b)   Responses (i), (ii) and (v) are correct
(c)   Responses (i), (iii) and (iv) are correct
(d)   Responses (i), (iv) and (v) are correct
(e)   Responses (ii), (iii) and (v) are correct

11. During life, the patient would have presented with the following symptoms and signs due to the respiratory disease:
(i)   Acute onset of disease
(ii) Cyanosis
(iii) Low fever, dry cough and tachypnoea
(iv) Insidious onset of disease
(v)   Productive cough with purulent sputum

(a)   Responses (i), (ii) and (iii) are correct
(b)   Responses (i), (ii) and (v) are correct
(c)   Responses (i), (iii) and (v) are correct
(d)   Responses (ii), (iii) and (iv) are correct
(e)   Responses (ii), (iii) and (v) are correct

12. The respiratory disease is treated by:
(a)   Ethambutol, isoniazid, para-amino salicylic acid for many months
(b)   Tetracyclines, erythromycin or chloramphenicol
(c)   Penicillin in massive doses, preferably
(d)   Vancomycin or neomycin
(e)   Pentamidine or trimethoprim-sulfamethoxazole

The liver was found to be slightly enlarged and bile-stained on section, with some lighter regions scattered throughout it. Microscopically an active chronic hepatitis was evident with scarring and regenerative nodule formation. It was decided that this disease was of several years' duration.

13. The lesions in the liver may be attributed to:
    (i) The disease the man presented with at Fairfield
    (ii) An infection that occurred before he contracted the disease that caused his death
    (iii) Autoimmune reactions and hypersensitivity
    (iv) Immunodeficiency
    (v) A carrier state

    (a) Responses (i), (ii) and (iv) are correct
    (b) Responses (i), (ii) and (v) are correct
    (c) Responses (i), (iii) and (v) are correct
    (d) Responses (ii), (iv) and (v) are correct
    (e) Responses (ii), (iii) and (iv) are correct

14. Jaundice as seen in this case would be predominantly of which type?
    (a) Obstructive
    (b) Haemolytic
    (c) Hepatocellular
    (d) All of the above
    (e) None of the above

The liver was also found to contain several regions of gross focal scarring with some associated calcification.

15. These lesions are evidence of infection with:
    (a) *Mycobacterium avium*
    (b) *Candida albicans*
    (c) *Bacteroides fragilis*
    (d) Cytomegalovirus
    (e) Any of the above

An examination of the central nervous system was carried out as the patient exhibited neurological motor symptoms and progressive signs of encephalitis immediately prior to his death. The brain showed cerebral atrophy with bilateral widening of the sulci. Microscopically it was subsequently seen that extensive demyelination was present in the white matter with numerous, perivascular aggregates of inflammatory cells (mainly lymphocytes). Some multinucleated giant cells were found scattered in the cerebral lesions and there was some gliosis apparent. The meninges were relatively normal.

16. The lesions described in the brain may be attributed to:

    (i) The original disease the man presented with
    (ii) A new infection
    (iii) Autoimmune reactions
    (iv) Immunodeficiency
    (v) Hypersensitivity reactions

    (a) Responses (i), (ii) and (iv) are correct
    (b) Responses (i), (ii) and (v) are correct
    (c) Responses (i), (iii) and (v) are correct
    (d) Responses (ii), (iv) and (v) are correct
    (e) Responses (ii), (iii) and (iv) are correct

17. The autopsy attendant accidentally cuts himself while handling the corpse's viscera and some ascitic fluid from the corpse comes into contact with the wound. The attendant was vaccinated against hepatitis B 12 months previously. What treatment steps are open to him after thorough disinfection and dressing of the wound, in order to prevent further disease?
    (i) Antibiotics and antifungal drugs
    (ii) Interferon and CD_4
    (iii) Iododeoxyuridine and related compounds
    (iv) Passive immunization for hepatitis
    (v) Azidothymidine (Zidovudine) and other anti-AIDS drugs

    (a) Responses (i), (ii) and (iii) are correct
    (b) Responses (i), (ii) and (v) are correct
    (c) Responses (i), (iii) and (iv) are correct
    (d) Responses (i), (iv) and (v) are correct
    (e) Responses (ii), (iii) and (v) are correct

18. How long after death is the body considered to be no longer infectious, as far as this particular patient is concerned?
    (a) 24 hours
    (b) 48 hours
    (c) 3 days
    (d) 5 days
    (e) The body must be cremated immediately after death to prevent risk of infection

19. What way of decontaminating surfaces in the autopsy room should be used after this autopsy?
    (a) Bleach (hypochlorite) solutions
    (b) Phenolic agents
    (c) Alcoholic preparations
    (d) Soap and hot water
    (e) Iodine preparations

20. The disease the patient died of is a notifiable disease (i.e. the Health Department must be notified)
    (a) True
    (b) False

Part D: Short Answer Questions

Answer the following questions lucidly and concisely, covering all of the important main points. You should spend about 50 minutes answering this section. The suggested time you should spend on each question is given after it.

1. What is the aetiology and pathogenesis of myasthenia gravis? (3 minutes)
2. What are the major complications of a chronic benign gastric ulcer? (2 minutes)
3. What are the symptoms and signs associated with untreated diabetes mellitus? (4 minutes).
4. Compare and contrast carcinoma of the bronchus and mesothelioma, using the following headings (a table may be used):

Cells of origin	Rate of growth
Age incidence	Routes of spread
Sites found	Sites of metastasis
Macroscopic appearance	Treatment
of cut surface of lung	Prognosis
	(6 minutes)

5. What are the predisposing factors in the development of carcinoma of the colon? What do you know of the pathogenesis of this condition? (4 minutes)
6. What is the incidence of primary intracranial tumours? What common complication do they give rise to and what is the prognosis of these tumours if they are treated in their early stages ? (5 minutes)
7. Differentiate prostatic nodular hyperplasia from carcinoma of the prostate as far as aetiology and sites of the gland in which each condition arises. Also differentiate the effects caused by each of these disorders. (4 minutes)
8. (a) What is meant by the term glomerulonephritis?
   (b) Give examples of four different types of glomerulonephritis.

(c) Which of these glomerulonephritides is the most benign (i.e. causes least pathology, has the best prognosis)?
(d) Which of these glomerulonephritides is the one associated with (in most cases) renal failure?
(e) Briefly describe the microscopic appearance of the nephron and kidney of an advanced case of any one of the glomerulonephritides that causes severe disease. (10 minutes)

9. What characterizes Conn's syndrome? (3 minutes)
10. What is Graves' disease? (1 minute)
11. What are the predisposing/aetiological factors leading to the development of leukaemia? (3 minutes)
12. Choose any common eye disorder and describe briefly its major characteristics. (5 minutes)

Part E: Essay Question

Choose *only one* of the following topics and write an essay, including all relevant information, concisely and thoroughly. (40 minutes)

1. Discuss cirrhosis of the liver, giving an indication of incidence in the community, characteristics of the disease (signs, symptoms; microscopic and macroscopic findings in the liver), predisposing factors in its development, complications; briefly mention prognosis and treatment.
2. Discuss three important commonly occurring malignant tumours of the skin, giving their salient features, presenting symptoms and signs, treatment, prognosis, etc.
3. Compare and contrast osteoporosis and osteomalacia.
4. Discuss in detail the pathology of ischaemic heart disease

Appendix I

Etymology of Pathological Terms

Many of the terms used in pathology, as in most of the sciences in general, have been derived from classical Greek and Latin roots. A knowledge of these languages is therefore a boon to anyone beginning to study pathology. However, since most people are no longer formally taught these languages at school it is sufficient for the serious students to familiarize themselves with a few commonly occurring prefixes and suffixes of Greek and Latin origin.

Once this basic vocabulary has been mastered the students' (and teachers'!) task has been considerably lightened and the study of the subject becomes much less tedious and infinitely more enjoyable. In the pages that follow there is a list of some of the most important of these terminological roots that are used in the nomenclature of things biological, physiological and of course pathological.

It is not advised that the students lock themselves in a room for days on end until they have memorized these lists; although such an undertaking would no doubt be beneficial, it would be of little enjoyment and of little attractiveness to the individual concerned. It is

suggested instead that these lists are kept in mind and are used constantly as a reference when the student is studying from this text, reading through lecture notes or doing any other form of study connected with the subject. When a term with which the student is unfamiliar is encountered in such study, the lists should be consulted and the student should attempt to break down the unknown word to its component parts and derive a possible meaning. The term's exact definition can then be looked up in the glossary at the back of this text, a medical dictionary, or other reliable sources.

In such a way the students' awareness of the language of pathology is slowly built up and with increasing familiarity it will become easier to use it meaningfully and to derive the maximum information from it whenever and where it is encountered.

The lists are arranged in alphabetical order, prefixes given in Table 1 and suffixes and combining forms given in Table 2. An example is given with each of the roots so that the student is immediately aware of the functional significance of each of these combining forms.

In parentheses following each of the terms is an etymological note giving the source language of the word.

Key: G = Greek
       L = Latin

In addition, a large number of terms used in pathology are based on proper names, commemorating the person who first described a particular disorder or who first successfully treated a condition with a novel procedure, etc. This is the so-called **eponymic** nomenclature, an example of which is Crohn's disease. Many of these terms are firmly entrenched, although the use of most of these names in pathology and other branches of medical science is rapidly disappearing, for example Crohn's disease is now being referred to as regional enteritis.

Table 1 *Prefixes in common use in pathology*

Prefix	Meaning	Examples
a- (G)	Without	Asepsis, acrania
ab- (L)	From, away, apart	Abduction
acro- (G)	Extremity, limb	Acromegaly
ad- (L)	To, toward	Adduction
aden/o- (G)	Gland	Adenitis, adenoma
adipos- (L)	Fat	Adipose, adipocyte
ambi- (L)	Both sides	Ambidextrous
an- (G)	Without	Anaemia, anuria
andr/o- (G)	Man	Andrology, androgen
angi/o- (G)	Vessel	Angiitis, angiotensin
aniso- (G)	Unequal, dissimilar	Anisocytosis
ante- (L)	Before, in front of	Ante mortem
anthrac/o- (G)	Carbon, coal	Anthracosis
anti- (G)	Against, inhibiting	Antitoxin, antibody
append/o- (L)	Appendix	Appendicitis
arthr/o- (G)	Joint	Arthritis, arthralgia
auto- (G)	Self, independent	Autolysis, automatic
bi- (L)	Two, double	Bilateral, bisexual
bio- (G)	Life	Biology, biochemistry
brachi/o- (G)	Relating to arm	Brachial
brachy- (G)	Short	Brachycephalic
brady- (G)	Slow	Bradycardia
bronch/o- (G)	Airway	Bronchitis, bronchogenic
carcin/o- (G)	Epithelial cancer	Carcinoma, carcinogenic
cardia/o- (G)	Heart	Cardiomegaly, cardiac
cary/o- (G)	Nucleus	Caryotype, caryolysis
cervic- (L)	Cervix, neck	Cervical
chlor/o- (G)	Green	Chlorophyll, chloasma
chol/e- (G)	Bile	Cholic acid, cholangitis
chondr/o- (G)	Cartilage	Chondroma, chondrocyte
chrom/o/a- (G)	Colour	Chromophobic
circum- (L)	Around	Circumcision
col/o- (G)	Large intestine	Colitis, colostomy
colp/o- (G)	Vagina	Colposcopy
con- (L)	Together, with	Congenital
contra- (L)	Against	Contraception

Table 1 *Continued*

Prefix	Meaning	Examples
crani/o- (G)	Skull	Cranial
crypt/o- (G)	Hidden	Cryptorchidism
cyan/o- (G)	Blue	Cyanosis
cyst/o- (G)	Bladder, cavity	Cystitis, cystoscopy
cyt/o- (G)	Cell	Cytology, cytolysis
dacry/o- (G)	Tears	Dacryoadenitis
de- (L)	From, removal	Deamination, denature
derma/to- (G)	Skin	Dermatitis, dermis
dia- (G)	Through	Diarrhoea, diapedesis
di/plo- (G)	Two, double	Diatomic, diploid
dys- (G)	Bad, ill, difficult	Dyspnoea, dysfunction
ecto- (G)	Outside	Ectoderm, ectopic
em-/en- (G)	In, into	Encyst, empyema
encephal/o- (G)	Brain	Encephalomyelitis
endo- (G)	Within	Endocytosis, endometrium
entero- (G)	Gut, intestine	Enteritis, enterotoxin
epinephr/o- (G)	Adrenal gland	Epinephrine
erythro- (G)	Red	Erythrocyte, erythrasma
eu- (G)	Good, well	Euphoria, eugenics
ex/o- (G)	Outside, out from/of	Exostosis, exocytosis
extra- (L)	Outside, beyond	Extraembryonic
febr- (L)	Fever	Febrile
fibro- (L)	Connective tissue	Fibrosis, fibrosarcoma
gastr/o- (G)	Stomach	Gastritis, gastric
gli/a/o- (G)	Supporting cells of brain	Glial, gliosis
gloss/o- (G)	Tongue	Glossitis
glott- (G)	Tongue	Glottal, glottic
gon/o- (G)	Semen, seed	Gonad, gonorrhoea
gynaec/o- (G)	Woman	Gynaecology, gynaecomastia
haem/a/o- (G)	Blood	Haemolysis, haemorrhage
hemi- (G)	Half	Hemisphere
hepat/o- (G)	Liver	Hepatitis, hepatoma
hetero- (G)	Dissimilar, different	Heterocellular
hist/o- (G)	Tissue	Histopathology, histology
holo- (G)	Whole, complete	Holoenzyme
homo/eo- (G)	Same, similar	Homozygous, homograft
hydro/hygro- (G)	Water, fluid	Hydronephrosis, hygropic
hyp/o (G)	Deficiency, lack	Hypoplasia, hypoacidity
hyper- (G)	Excessive, above	Hyperplasia, hyperacidity
hyster/o- (G)	Uterus, womb	Hysterectomy
infra- (L)	Below, under	Infra-orbital, infrared
inter- (L)	Between, amongst	Intercellular
intra- (L)	Within, into	Intracellular
iso- (G)	Equal, same	Isotonic
kary/o- (G)	Nucleus	Karyotype, karyolysis

Table 1 *Continued*

Prefix	Meaning	Examples
laryng/o- (G)	Vocal cords, throat	Laryngitis
leiomyo- (G)	Smooth muscle	Leiomyoma
leuc/o- (G)	White	Leucocyte, leucocytosis
leuk/o- (G)	White	Leukocyte, leukaemia
lip/o- (G)	Fat	Lipoma, lipocyte
lith/o- (G)	Stone	Lithotomy, lithiasis
lymph/o- (G)	Lymph	Lymphocyte, lymphadenitis
macro- (G)	Large	Macrophage, macroscopic
mal- (L)	Bad, ill, abnormal	Malnutrition
mamm/o- (L)	Breast	Mammary, mammotrophic
mast/o- (G)	Breast	Mastectomy, mastitis
mega- (G)	Great	Megacolon
melan/o- (G)	Black	Melanocyte, melanosis
men/o/s- (G)	Month	Menarche, menopause
meso- (G)	Middle	Mesoderm, mesosome
meta- (G)	After, beyond	Metaphase, metastasis
micro- (G)	Small	Microscope, microcephaly
mono- (G)	One, single	Monoclonal, monocyte
multi- (L)	Many	Multicellular
myco- (G)	Fungus	Mycosis, mycodermatitis
my/o- (G)	Muscle	Myositis, myocardium
myx/o- (G)	Mucus	Myxoedema, myxoma
necr/o- (G)	Death, dead	Necrosis, necropsy
neo- (G)	New	Neoplasm, neomycin
nephr/o- (G)	Kidney	Nephritis, nephrotic
neur/o- (G)	Nerve	Neuritis
noso- (G)	Disease	Nosocomial
nucle/o- (L)	Nucleus, nuclear	Nucleic acid, nucleoid
odont/o- (G)	Tooth	Odontoma
olig/o- (G)	Few, scanty, scarce	Oliguria, oligodendroglia
oö- (G)	Egg, ovum	Oöcyte, oöphoritis
ophthalm/o- (G)	Eye	Ophthalmoscope
orchid/o- (G)	Testis	Orchidectomy
orth/o- (G)	Straight, correct	Orthodontist, orthopaedic
oste/o (G)	Bone	Osteitis, osteopath
osteomyel/o- (G)	Bone and bone marrow	Osteomyelitis
ot/o- (G)	Ear	Otolaryngologist, otitis
oxy- (G)	Acid, acidic	Oxyphilic
paed/o- (G)	Child	Paediatrics
pan- (G)	All, many	Pancarditis, pandemic
para- (G)	Beside	Para-aortic, parenteral
path/o- (G)	Disease, suffering	Pathology, pathetic
ped- (L)	Foot	Pedometer, pedal
peri- (G)	Around, about	Peribronchial, peristalsis
periton/eo- (G)	Coelomic cavity	Peritonitis
phago- (G)	Eat, devour	Phagocytosis
phleb/o- (G)	Vein	Phlebitis, phlebotomy

Table 1 *Continued*

Prefix	Meaning	Examples
phren/o- (G)	Diaphragm	Phrenocolic
pneumo- (G)	Lungs, air	Pneumonia, pneumothorax
poly- (G)	Many, much, diverse	Polyarthritis, polydipsia
post- (L)	After, behind	Post-prandial, post mortem
pre- (L)	Before	Pre-clinical
proct/o- (G)	Terminal colon, anus	Proctitis, proctoscopy
pseud/o- (G)	False	Pseudoarthrosis
psych/o- (G)	Mind, spirit	Psychology, psychiatrist
pyel/o-	Pelvis of kidney	Pyelitis, pyelonephritis
pyle- (G)	Portal	Pylephlebitis
pyo- (G)	Pus	Pyogenic, pyonephrosis
rachi- (G)	Back, spine	Rachischisis, rachitic
re- (L)	Again, once more	Reversal, retraction
retro- (L)	Behind, backward	Retrovirus, retrograde
rhabdomy/o- (G)	Striated muscle	Rhabdomyosarcoma
rhin/o- (G)	Nose	Rhinitis, rhinophyma
sacchar/o- (G)	Sugar, sweet	Saccharolytic, saccharine
salping/o- (G)	Uterine tube	Salpingitis
sarc/o- (G)	Flesh, non-epithelial	Sarcoma, sarcoidosis
sclero- (G)	Hard, firm	Scleroderma, sclerosis
semi- (L)	Half	Semilunar
sesqui- (L)	One and a half	Sesquihydrate
somat/o- (G)	Body	Somatic, somatostatin
splen/o- (G)	Spleen	Splenectomy
spondyl/o- (G)	Vertebra	Spondyloarthropathy
ster/eo- (G)	Solid, three dimensional	Sterol, stereotactic
sterc- (L)	Dung, faeces	Stercobilin
stomat/o- (G)	Mouth	Stomatitis
sub- (L)	Under, beneath	Subcutaneous
super- (L)	Above	Superinfection
supra- (L)	Above	Supra-orbital
sym-/syn- (G)	With, together	Symbiosis, synchronous
tachy- (G)	Quick, rapid	Tachycardia
tele- (G)	At a distance, far	Telekinesis, telereceptor
thromb- (G)	Clot, lump	Thrombosis, thrombocyte
tox/o- (L)	Poison	Toxin, toxic
trache/o- (G)	Windpipe	Tracheostomy, tracheitis
trans- (L)	Through, across	Transmural, transplant
troph- (G)	Feed, nurture	Trophic
visc- (L)	Internal organ, cavity	Visceral, viscus
vesic- (L)	Urinary bladder	Vesical, vesicovaginal
xanth/o- (G)	Yellow	Xanthoma, xanthine
zygo- (G)	Double, even	Zygote, homozygous
zym/o (G)	Fermentation	Zymogen, enzyme

Table 2 *Suffixes and combining forms in common use in pathology*

Suffix	Meaning	Examples
-ac (G)	Pertaining to	Cardiac, iliac
-aden- (G)	Gland	Lymphadenitis
-aem/ia (G)	Blood	Anaemia, pyaemia
-aesthe/s/t- (G)	Sense, feeling	Anaesthesia, anaesthetic
-algia (G)	Pain, suffering	Arthralgia, neuralgia
-ang/io- (G)	Vessel	Lymphangiitis
-ase (G)	Enzyme	Coagulase, kinase
-asia (G)	Condition or state	Aphasia
-asis (G)	Condition or state	Amoebiasis, haemostasis
-blast/o- (G)	Primitive cell	Haemocytoblast
-blastoma (G)	Malignant mass of primitive cell origin	Retinoblastoma
-carcinoma (G)	Malignant epithelial mass	Adenocarcinoma
-centesis (G)	Puncture	Amniocentesis
-cephal/e/o- (G)	Head	Hydrocephaly
-chrom/at/o- (G)	Colour	Polychromatophil
-chol/e (G)	Bile	Acholic, dyscholic
-cide (L)	Killing, destroying	Biocide, homicide
-clon/o- (G)	Branch, relation	Monoclonal
-coel/e- (G)	Herniation, swelling	Meningocoele
-cyt/e (G)	Cell, mature cell	Adipocyte, fibrocyte
-dipsia (G)	Thirst	Polydipsia
-ectasis (G)	Stretching, dilating	Bronchiectasis
-ectomy (G)	Surgical removal	Appendectomy
-emesis (G)	Vomit	Haematemesis
-encephal/o/y (G)	Brain	Anencephaly
-gen (G)	Produced, generated	Pathogen, antigen
-genesis (G)	Origin, production	Angiogenesis
-gram (G)	Written record	Electrocardiogram
-graph- (G)	Write, record	Radiography
-hidrosis (G)	Sweating	Anhidrosis
-ic (G)	Pertaining to	Gastric, toxic
-icter/o- (G)	Jaundice	Kernicterus
-ism (G)	Condition or state	Alcoholism
-ist (G)	One who practises	Pathologist
-itis (G)	Inflammation	Gastritis, neuritis
-kin/i/o- (G)	Movement	Bradykinin
-lith/o- (G)	Stone, calculus	Cholelithiasis
-logous (G)	Relating to	Homologous
-logy (G)	Study of	Pathology
-lysis (G)	Dissolution	Haemolysis
-malacia (G)	Softening	Osteomalacia
-mast/o- (G)	Breast	Gynaecomastia

Table 2 *Continued*

Suffix	Meaning	Examples
-megal/o/y (G)	Large, enlargement	Splenomegaly
-men/o- (G)	Month, menses	Amenorrhoea
-metr/o- (G)	Uterus	Endometritis, myometrium
-oid (G)	In the form of, like	Adenoid, epithelioid
-oma (G)	Mass, tumour, cancer	Granuloma, adenoma
-onych/o- (G)	Nails	Paronychia
-osis (G)	State, disorder	Psychosis, necrosis
-ose (L)	Characterized by	Comatose, scabiose
-ost/e/o- (G)	Bone	Exostosis
-ous (L)	Full of	Poisonous
-path/ia/y (G)	Disease, suffering	Adenopathy, sympathy
-penia (G)	Poverty, lack of	Thrombocytopenia
-petr/o- (G)	Stone, increased density	Osteopetrosis
-phag/o/e/y (G)	Eating, devouring	Dysphagia, lipophage
-phil/o/e (G)	Loving, liking	Acidophilic, neutrophil
-phob/o/ia (G)	Fear, non-affinity	Acrophobia, hydrophobic
-plasia (G)	Formation, growth	Hyperplasia, aplasia
-plasty (G)	Reconstruction	Rhinoplasty
-plegia (G)	Paralysis	Paraplegia
-pnoea (G)	Breath	Apnoea, dyspnoea
-pod (G)	Foot	Arthropod
-poiesis (G)	Formation, creation	Haemopoiesis
-por/e/o (G)	Hole, passage, pore	Osteoporosis, pore
-ptosis (G)	Falling, degeneration	Apoptosis, nephroptosis
-ptysis (G)	Spitting	Haemoptysis
-py/e/o- (G)	Pus	Empyema, haemopyoarthrosis
-pyr/o/exia (G)	Heat, fever	Hyperpyrexia, pyrogen
-rrhag/e/ia (G)	Discharge	Haemorrhage, metrorrhagia
-rrhexis (G)	Disintegration	Karyorrhexis
-rrhoea (G)	Flow	Diarrhoea, dysmenorrhoea
-scope (G)	Instrument for viewing	Microscope, otoscope
-stasis (G)	Stopping, standing	Haemostasis
-stomy (G)	Artificial opening	Colostomy, tracheostomy
-taxi/a (G)	Order, arrangement	Ataxia
-taxis (G)	Ordered movement	Chemotaxis
-thromb/o- (G)	Blood clot	Prothrombin
-thrombocyt/o- (G)	Blood platelet	Dysthrombocytogenesis
-top/o/y (G)	Place	Ectopic
-troph/o/y (G)	Nutrition, growth	Hypertrophy, atrophy
-ur/o/ia (G)	Urine	Proteinuria

On the Formation of the Plural

As so many of the terms encountered in medicine and pathology have Greek or Latin roots, or are often complete, unchanged Greek or Latin words, the plural of these terms is formed by following the accidence of these classical languages. A short list of the commonest such plural formations is given below, but it must be remembered that often there are many exceptions to the general rules and that there are many irregular plurals in both Latin and Greek.

Singular ending	Plural ending	Examples
-a	-ae	Fistula, fistulae
-axis	-axes	Epistaxis, epistaxes
-ex	-ices	Cortex, cortices
-is	-ides	Ephelis, ephelides; iris, irides
-itis	-itides	Nephritis, nephritides
-ix	-ices	Varix, varices
-ma	-mata	Carcinoma, carcinomata
-o	-ones	Comedo, comedones
-sis	-ses	Prosthesis, prostheses
-um	-a	Bacterium, bacteria
-us	-i	Calculus, calculi

Some common irregular plural formations are given below:

Singular form	Plural form
corpus	corpora
faex	faeces
femur	femora
lumen	lumina
meninx	meninges
os (mouth, opening)	ora
os (bone)	ossa
phalanx	phalanges
thorax	thoraces
viscus	viscera

Other Grammatical Trivia

In some diseases or processes or names of body parts that retain the original Latin or Greek terminology there is agreement between the adjectives and nouns in both gender and number. In Greek and Latin there are three genders (masculine, feminine and neuter) and two numbers (singular and plural). Often the words are further modified because of accidence relating to case (i.e. nominative, accusative, genitive, etc). Examples are:

- Corpus albicans (singular), corpora albicantia (plural).
- Corpus amylaceum (singular), corpora amylacea (plural).
- Zona pellucida (*pellucida* agreeing in gender and number with the feminine *zona*).
- Xeroderma pigmentosum (not the feminine *pigmentosa* as the noun xeroderma is neuter and requires the neuter adjective).
- Carcinoma corpus uteri (*uteri* being in the genitive case implying 'of the uterus').
- Falx cerebri (*cerebri* being in the genitive case implying 'of the cerebrum').
- *Escherichia coli* (*coli* = genitive, 'of the colon').

Appendix II

Anthropometric Measurements and Common Abbreviations

Height and Weight Ratios

Measurements relating to body parameters are used widely to assess body composition, especially with respect to fat stores and muscle mass. The measurements are used to determine growth patterns in children and appropriate body weight for adults of a given height. **Relative weight** is the actual weight divided by the desirable weight multiplied by 100. A relative weight greater than 120% indicates obesity. Recent **changes in weight** are probably a better indication of undernutrition than a low relative weight. A weight loss of 10% of body weight or more within a 1 to 2 month period is usually considered predictive of a poor clinical outcome in many diseases.

The **body mass index (BMI)** uses both height and weight to determine obesity. It is calculated by dividing the weight in kilograms by the height, in metres, squared.

$$BMI = \frac{weight\ (kg)}{height \times height\ (m^2)}$$

The **normal BMI** is 19 to 27 and persons with a BMI of 30 or greater are considered to be **obese**. Those with a BMI of 40 or greater are considered to be pathologically obese. '**Overweight**' implies that there is a slight disruption to height/weight ratio and for a male to be considered overweight the BMI exceeds 24, while for a female it exceeds 26.

Obesity is defined as an excess of body fat, frequently resulting in a significant impairment of health. The excess body fat is generated when the calories consumed exceed those expended in exercise and activity. Factors contributing to this imbalance are numerous and probably exist in differing combinations among obese people. Heredity, socioeconomical factors, culture, environment, diet, psychological influences and activity levels are implicated. Hormonal factors are a very rare cause.

Body weight reflects both lean body mass and adipose tissue and cannot be used as a method for describing body composition or the percentage of fat tissue present. The proper **body-fat ratio** is age and sex specific. For young adults under 30 years the recommended range for males is 12–15%, and for females is 19–23%. The upper limit for a 50-year-old male is 19% and for a female about 27%. During physical exercise, the body fat decreases and lean body mass increases.

The tables that follow are based on health and life insurance statistics and these usually relate height and weight to survival. The upper and lower frame sizes appear to be based on the upper and lower quartiles of the population, with the medium frame representing the two middle quartiles. Using such tables obesity is defined as the condition in which body weight is greater than 30% of the weight for the specific height and frame.

There are some problems associated with such tables: the weight ranges define lowest mortality and not necessarily ideal body weight; they are based on an ill-defined concept of **frame size**; they may not be representative of the population as there may be sampling biases; and finally they do not differentiate between weight gain due to increased muscle mass and weight gain due to increased fat content.

Table 1 *Women's height to weight table*
(25–60 years, in indoor clothes weighing ≈1.5 kg, and shoes with 2 cm heels)

| Height (cm) | Weight (kg) | | |
	Small frame	Medium frame	Large frame
147	46–50	49–55	54–59
150	47–51	50–56	54–61
152	47–52	51–57	55–62
155	48–54	52–59	57–64
158	49–55	54–60	58–65
160	50–56	55–61	59–67
162	52–58	56–63	61–69
165	53–59	58–64	62–70
168	54–60	59–65	64–72
170	56–62	60–67	65–74
173	57–63	62–68	66–76
175	59–64	63–69	68–77
178	60–66	64–71	69–79
180	61–67	66–72	70–80
183	63–69	67–74	72–81

Table 2 *Men's height to weight table*
(25–60 years, in indoor clothes weighing ≈2.5 kg, and shoes with 1 cm heels)

| Height (cm) | Weight (kg) | | |
	Small frame	Medium frame	Large frame
158	58–61	59–64	63–68
160	59–62	60–65	64–69
162	60–63	61–66	64–71
165	61–64	62–67	65–73
168	62–64	63–69	66–74
170	63–66	64–70	68–76
173	64–67	65–71	69–78
175	64–69	67–73	70–80
178	65–70	69–74	72–82
180	66–71	70–75	73–84
183	68–73	71–77	74–85
185	69–74	73–79	76–87
188	70–76	74–81	78–89
191	72–78	76–83	80–92
193	74–80	78–85	82–94

Abbreviations Used in Tables

<	=	less than	ImU	=	international milliunit
>	=	greater than	mOsm	=	milliosmole
dL	=	decilitre (100 mL)	mμ	=	millimicron (= nanometre, nm)
g	=	gram	mU	=	milliunit
IU	=	international unit	ng	=	nanogram
kg	=	kilogram	pg	=	picogram
L	=	litre	μEq	=	microequivalent
mEq	=	milliequivalent	μg	=	microgram
mg	=	milligram	IμU	=	international microunit
mL	=	millilitre	μL	=	microlitre
mM	=	millimole	μU	=	microunit
mmHg	=	millimetres of mercury	U	=	unit

Commonly Used Abbreviations

a/aa	=	artery/ies	CMV	=	cytomegalovirus
Ab	=	antibody	CoA	=	coenzyme A
ACh	=	acetylcholine	COPD	=	chronic obstructive pulmonary disease
AChE	=	acetylcholinesterase			
ACTH	=	adrenocorticotrophic hormone	CT	=	computed tomography
ADH	=	antidiuretic hormone	CV	=	cardiovascular
ADP	=	adenosine diphosphate	CVA	=	cerebrovascular accident
AFP	=	α-foetoprotein	CVP	=	central venous pressure
Ag	=	antigen			
AIDS	=	acquired immunodeficiency syndrome	D&C	=	dilatation of cervix and curettage of uterus
ALT	=	alanine aminotransferase			
AMI	=	acute myocardial infarction	DLE	=	discoid lupus erythematosus
AMP	=	adenosine monophosphate	DNA	=	deoxyribonucleic acid
ANA	=	antinuclear antibody	DOA	=	dead on arrival
Å	=	Ångstrom unit = 10^{-10} m	DPT	=	diphtheria, pertussis, tetanus (vaccine)
AP	=	angina pectoris			
APUD	=	amine precursor uptake and decarboxylation	EBV	=	Epstein-Barr virus
aq	=	water, aqueous	ECF-A	=	eosinophil chemotactic factor A
AR	=	aortic regurgitation	ECG	=	electrocardiogram
ASA	=	acetylsalicylic acid	ECT	=	electroconvulsive therapy
AST	=	aspartate aminotransferase	EDTA	=	ethylenediaminetetraacetic acid
ATP	=	adenosine triphosphate	EEG	=	electroencephalogram
AV	=	atrioventricular; arteriovenous	EKG	=	electrocardiogram
			EKY	=	electrokymogram
BCG	=	*bacille Calmette-Guérin*	Em	=	emmetropia
BP	=	blood pressure	ENG	=	electronystagmography
BSA	=	body surface area	ENT	=	ear, nose and throat
BUN	=	blood urea nitrogen	ERV	=	expiratory reserve volume
			ESR	=	erythrocyte sedimentation rate
CA	=	cardiac arrest			
cAMP	=	cyclic adenosine monophosphate	Fab	=	fragment, antigen binding (of an antibody)
CDC	=	Center for Disease Control, Atlanta			
CF	=	cardiac failure; Christmas factor	Fc	=	fragment, cell binding (of an antibody)
ChE	=	cholinesterase			
CMI	=	cell-mediated immunity	FFA	=	free fatty acids

FSH	=	follicle stimulating hormone
GALT	=	gut-associated lymphoid tissue
GFR	=	glomerular filtration rate
GH	=	growth hormone
G6PD	=	glucose-6-phosphate dehydrogenase
H	=	hyperopia
H&E	=	haematoxylin and eosin (stain)
HAV	=	hepatitis A virus
Hb	=	haemoglobin
HBV	=	hepatitis B virus
HCV	=	hepatitis C virus
HDL	=	high-density lipoprotein
HDV	=	hepatitis delta virus
HEV	=	hepatitis E virus
Hg	=	mercury
HGH	=	human growth hormone
5-HIAA	=	5-hydroxyindoleacetic acid
HIV	=	human immunodeficiency virus
Hl	=	latent hyperopia
HLA	=	human leukocyte antigen (histocompatibility antigen)
Hm	=	manifest hyperopia
HSV	=	Herpes simplex virus
5-HT	=	5-hydroxytryptamine (serotonin)
IC	=	inspiratory capacity; irritable colon
ICSH	=	interstitial cell stimulating hormone
ICU	=	intensive care unit
IE	=	immunoelectrophoresis
Ig	=	immunoglobulin (antibody)
IHD	=	ischaemic heart disease
IM	=	intramuscularly
IP	=	intraperitoneally
IPPB	=	intermittent positive pressure breathing
IQ	=	intelligence quotient
IR	=	infrared
IRV	=	inspiratory reserve volume
IUD	=	intrauterine contraceptive device
IV	=	intravenously
IVT	=	intravenous transfusion
L&A	=	light and accommodation (reaction of pupils)
LATS	=	long acting thyroid stimulator
LD	=	light difference; lethal dose
LDH	=	lactic dehydrogenase
LDL	=	low-density lipoprotein
LH	=	luteinizing hormone
LIF	=	leukocyte inhibitor factor; left iliac fossa

LT	=	lymphotoxin
LTH	=	luteotrophic hormone
Ly	=	T cell antigen type
M	=	myopia; mixture; macerate
mϕ	=	macrophage
MCH	=	mean corpuscular haemoglobin
MCHC	=	mean corpuscular haemoglobin concentration
MCV	=	mean corpuscular volume
MHC	=	major histocompatibility complex
mm	=	millimetre; muscles
MOPP	=	drug combination used in cancer treatment; mechlorethamine, Oncovin (vincristine), procarbazine, prednisone
MS	=	multiple sclerosis
MSH	=	melanocyte stimulating hormone
n	=	refractive index
NAD$^+$	=	oxidized nicotinamide-adenine dinucleotide
NADH	=	reduced nicotinamide-adenine dinucleotide
NADP$^+$	=	oxidized nicotinamide-adenine dinucleotide phosphate
NADPH	=	reduced nicotinamide-adenine dinucleotide phosphate
NPN	=	non-protein nitrogen
NREM	=	non-rapid eye movements (sleep)
OB	=	obstetrics
OD	=	*oculus dexter* (right eye)
OL	=	*oculus laevus* (left eye)
OR	=	operating room
OS	=	*oculus sinister* (left eye)
OT	=	occupational therapy
OTC	=	over the counter (drugs)
OU	=	*oculi uterque* (each eye)
P	=	presbyopia; pupil; pulse
p	=	short arm of a chromosome
PABA	=	para-aminobenzoic acid
PAF	=	platelet activating factor
PAHA	=	para-aminohippuric acid
PASA	=	para-aminosalicylic acid
pc	=	*post cibum* (after meals)
PCB	=	polychlorinated biphenyl
PCG	=	phonocardiogram
pCO$_2$	=	carbon dioxide partial pressure
PCV	=	packed cell volume
pd	=	prism dioptre
PG	=	prostaglandin
PGA	=	pteroylglutamic (folic) acid

pH	=	negative logarithm of the hydrogen ion concentration
PLT	=	psittacosis, lymphogranuloma venereum, trachoma (group)
PMI	=	point of maximal impulse (of heart)
PO	=	*per os* (by mouth, orally)
pO_2	=	oxygen partial pressure
POR	=	problem oriented record
PPD	=	purified protein derivative
PPLO	=	pleuropneumonia-like organisms
ppm	=	parts per million
prn	=	*pro re nata* (according to circumstances)
PSP	=	phenolsulfonphthalein
PTT	=	partial thromboplastin time
PUO	=	pyrexia of unknown origin
PVP-I	=	povidone iodine
PZI	=	protamine zinc insulin
q	=	long arm of a chromosome
qd	=	*quaque die* (every day)
qh	=	*quaque hora* (every hour)
qid	=	*quater in die* (four times daily)
qs	=	*quantum satis* (a sufficient amount)
R	=	an organic radical; Roentgen
℞	=	*recipe* (take): prescription; treatment
r	=	ring chromosome
RAST	=	radioallergosorbent test
RBC	=	red blood cell; red blood cell count
RBE	=	relative biological effectiveness
REM	=	rapid eye movements (sleep)
rem	=	Roentgen equivalent man (= 1 rad × RBE)
rep	=	Roentgen equivalent physical (= absorption of 93 erg/g H_2O)
RES	=	reticuloendothelial system
Rh	=	Rhesus factor
RIA	=	radioimmunoassay
RNA	=	ribonucleic acid
RNase	=	ribonuclease
rpm	=	revolutions per minute
RQ	=	respiratory quotient
rRNA	=	ribosomal RNA
RUL	=	right upper lobe (of lung)
RV	=	residual volume
Rx	=	*recipe* (take): prescription; treatment
S	=	*semis* (half); sight
SCID	=	severe combined immunodeficiency disease
SD	=	skin dose; standard deviation
SE	=	standard error
SED	=	skin erythema dose

SI	=	*système international d'unitès*
SIDS	=	sudden infant death syndrome
sig	=	*signa* (mark)
SISI	=	short increment sensitivity index
SK	=	streptokinase
SLE	=	systemic lupus erythematosus
SOS	=	*si opus sit* (if necessary)
SR	=	sedimentation rate
SRH	=	somatotropin releasing hormone
SRS-A	=	slow reacting substance of anaphylaxis
ss	=	*semis* (half)
stat	=	*statim* (at once)
STD	=	sexually transmitted disease
STH	=	somatotrophic hormone
STS	=	serological test for syphilis
T_m	=	tubular maximum (in renal function tests)
T_3	=	triiodothyronine
T_4	=	thyroxine
t	=	translocation
TB	=	tuberculosis
TD_{50}	=	median toxic dose
THC	=	tetrahydrocannabinol
tid	=	*ter in die* (three times daily)
TLC	=	thin layer chromatography
TNM	=	tumour, node, metastasis (staging system)
TNT	=	trinitrotoluene
TPA	=	total parenteral alimentation
TPN	=	total parenteral nutrition
TRH	=	thyrotrophic releasing hormone
TRIC	=	trachoma inclusion conjunctivitis (group of organisms — *Chlamydia*)
tRNA	=	transfer RNA
TSH	=	thyroid stimulating hormone
TU	=	tuberculin unit
U	=	unit
UDP	=	uridine diphosphate
UMP	=	uridine monophosphate
ung	=	*unguentum* (ointment)
USP	=	United States Pharmacopoeia
UTP	=	uridine triphosphate
v/vv	=	vein/s
VC	=	acuity of colour vision
VCG	=	vector cardiogram
VD	=	venereal disease
VDG	=	venereal disease — gonorrhoea
VDH	=	valvular disease of the heart
VDRL	=	venereal disease research laboratory
VDS	=	venereal disease — syphilis

VF	=	vocal fremitus
Vf	=	visual field
VLDL	=	very low density lipoproteins
VR	=	vocal resonance
VS	=	volumetric solution
v/v	=	volume of solute per volume of solvent

WBC	=	white blood cell; white blood cell count
WHO	=	World Health Organization
WR	=	Wassermann reaction
wt	=	weight
w/v	=	weight of solute per volume of solute
Z	=	atomic number

Appendix III

Some Normal Parameters and Measurements of Normal Values

Table 1 *Normal parameters of important organs (healthy adult, 20–25 years)*

Adrenal glands: weight together	10–15 g
Brain: weight	1200–1350 g
Gastrointestinal tract:	
Oesophagus, length (cricoid to cardia)	25 cm
Stomach, length	25–30 cm
Duodenum, length	25 cm
Small intestine, length	550–660 cm
Large intestine, length	150–170 cm
Heart:	
Weight	275–350 g
Left ventricle, thickness	8–14 mm
Right ventricle, thickness	2–4 mm
Kidney:	
Weight	110–160 g
Cortex, thickness	5–8 mm
Medulla, thickness	12–16 mm
Liver: weight	1350–1600 g

Lungs:
Right lobes (3), weight	350–450 g
Left lobes (2), weight	275–375 g

Ovaries: weight together — 15–25 g

Pancreas: weight — 80–120 g

Parathyroids (4): weight — 100–150 mg

Pituitary gland: weight — 600–750 mg

Prostate gland: weight — 14–20 g

Spleen: weight — 125–175 g

Testis and epididymis: weight — 17–27 g

Thyroid gland: weight — 20–40 g

Uterus:
Nulliparous weight	40–60 g
Weight after pregnancy	75–125 g

Normal parameters vary considerably depending on the individual and this table takes some account of the normal variation, but it should be kept in mind that extreme values on either side of those quoted may be seen in some normal, healthy individuals because of their physique.

Table 2 *Normal values for some laboratory tests (healthy adult subject)*

Enzymes:
Serum acid phosphatase	0.01–0.63 IU/L
Serum alkaline phosphatase	13–39 IU/L
Serum cholinesterase	700–1500 IU/L
Serum creatine kinase	30–170 IU/L
Serum lactic dehydrogenase	45–90 IU/L

Glucose:
Blood, random	3.6–9.3 mmol/L
Cerebrospinal fluid	2.7–4.4 mmol/L
Urine	0

Lipids:
Total faecal lipids	0–5 g/day
Serum cholesterol	2.5–7.0 mmol/L
Serum triglycerides	0.17–2.00 mmol/L

Metals:
Serum calcium	2.13–2.62 mmol/L
Urine calcium	3.7–6.2 mmol/day
Serum iron	7–35 μmol/L
Serum magnesium	0.7–1.3 mmol/L
Serum potassium	3.5–5.5 mmol/L
Urine potassium	10–90 mmol/day
Serum sodium	137–147 mmol/L
Urine sodium	150–250 mmol/day

Non-metals:

Serum hydrogen carbonate ion	20–30 mmol/L
Serum chloride	92–107 mmol/L
Cerebrospinal fluid chloride	120–130 mmol/L
Serum phosphorus	0.73–1.37 mmol/L

Proteins:

Total serum proteins	61–83 g/L
Total serum albumin	35–48 g/L
Total serum globulin	20–32 g/L
Total plasma fibrinogen	20–45 g/L
Total cerebrospinal fluid proteins	0–0.4 g/L
Total urine proteins	0–0.2 g/day

Serum B_{12}	150–900 ng/L
Serum bilirubin	2–9 μmol/L
Serum folate	3–20 μg/L
Serum insulin	0–25 mU/L
Serum ketones	0–10 U

Urea:

Serum urea	0.17–2.00 mmol/L
Urine urea	41–50 mmol/day

Uric acid:

Serum uric acid	0.18–0.47 mmol/L
Urine uric acid	1.2–3.0 mmol/day

Urine pH	5–8 pH units
Urine specific gravity	1.003–1.030

Table 3 *Normal haematological values*

Bleeding time (Duke's method)	1–3 minutes
Blood cells:	
Erythrocytes	4.2–6.4 million/μL
Leukocytes:	5000–10 000/μL
Granulars — Neutrophil polymorphs	2500—7000/μL
— Eosinophils	40–400/μL
— Basophils	15–100/μL
Agranulars — Lymphocytes	1500–3500/μL
— Monocytes	100–800/μL
Platelets:	200 000–400 000/μL
Reticulocytes	0.5–1.5%
Blood pressure:	
Systolic	120 mm Hg
Diastolic	80 mm Hg
Blood volume	6–8% of body weight
Clot retraction time:	
Begins	< 2 hours
Is completed	< 24 hours
Coagulation time (capillary tube)	2–5 minutes
Erythrocyte life span	80–120 days
Erythrocyte sedimentation rate (ESR), Wintrobe:	
Males	9–15 mm/hour
Females	20 mm/hour
Haemoglobin:	
Males	14–18 g/dL
Females	12–16 g/dL
Children	11–17 g/dL
Haematocrit:	
Males	40–50% (0.4–0.5 L/L)
Females	37–47% (0.37–0.47 L/L)
Children	35–49% (0.35–0.49 L/L)
Partial pressures of blood gases:	
pCO_2	35–45 mmHg
pO_2	95–100 mmHg
pH of arterial blood	7.35–7.45 pH units

NB: 'Abnormal' laboratory test values are those measurements of body parameters or constituents that fall outside of the normal range. It should be remembered, however, that the tests and measurements of approximately 5% of all normal, healthy individuals fall outside of the 'normal' range. This simply means that these individuals are different not sick. There is always the possibility that an abnormal value may be the result of a laboratory error.

Glossary of Terms

NB. The terms in SMALL CAPITALS within the body of the definitions refer to related items that may be cross-referenced within this glossary of terms. The mark '=' signifies synonymous terms. Terms in quotation marks are 'common' or 'students' slang' terms.

Abetalipoprotcinacmia: An hereditary condition in which the levels of β lipoproteins in the bloodstream are greatly reduced, with hypercholesterolaemia. In severe cases ATAXIA, NYSTAGMUS, motor incoordination and retinitis occur.

Abscess: A localized collection of pus within a cavity that is formed by the destruction of tissue. It is usually the result of pyogenic infection, quite commonly *Staphylococcus aureus* being the organism responsible.

Acantholysis: A disruption to the prickle cell layer in the epidermis resulting from the breakdown of the cytoplasmic bridges between the cells. Spaces are apparent between the cells and many prickle cells appear shrunken and degenerate.

Acanthosis: A great thickening of the stratum spinosum of the epidermis, leading to thickening of the skin (hyperplasia of the prickle cell layer).

Achalasia: Failure of relaxation of smooth muscular rings, which form valves and sphincters, along the length of the gastrointestinal tract (e.g. achalasia of the cardia in the stomach).

Acholia: Failure of secretion of bile.

Achlorhydria: A condition characterized by the greatly reduced or totally absent secretion of hydrochloric acid by the gastric mucosa.

Acholuric jaundice: Yellowing of the skin and sclerae of the eyes (see JAUNDICE), coexistent with lack of excretion of bile pigments in the urine.

Achondroplasia: An hereditary disorder of aberrant cartilage formation leading to defective growth in the long bones and the formation of achondroplastic dwarfs.

Acidosis: A state marked by the lowering of the blood pH due to excessive levels of hydrogen ions or lowered levels of bicarbonate.

Acne vulgaris: A skin condition characterized by infection (*Staphylococcus aureus*, *Propionibacterium acnes* and *Corynebacterium* spp.), severe inflammation and scarring.

Acquired disease: A disease which develops as a result of factors from the external environment; not an hereditary or genetic disease.

Acquired immune deficiency syndrome (AIDS): An infection (usually sexually transmitted, but may also be acquired through body fluid to body fluid exchange, or congenitally) with the human immunodeficiency virus (HIV) causing a marked reduction in the level of the helper T subclass of lymphocytes, resulting in greatly reduced efficiency of the immune system. Patients invariably die of massive infection or cancer.

Acromegaly: Gross enlargement of the fingers, toes, jaws and nose caused by overproduction of pituitary hormone in a mature person (cf. GIGANTISM).

Actinic keratosis: A premalignant skin lesion developing in the elderly as a result of excessive exposure to ultraviolet light and resembling a localized horny or warty growth.

Active immunity: A type of immune response in which the body's immune cells are actively taking part in recognizing and reacting to the antigen (cf. PASSIVE IMMUNITY).

Acute: Short lasting, being over within hours to days (cf. CHRONIC).

Acute abdomen: A characteristic clinical presentation of acute abdominal pain of a severe nature that may be seen with a variety of diseases, for example DIVERTICULITIS, ovarian cyst rupture.

Acute inflammation: The reaction of tissue beginning with sublethal injury and ending with complete healing. Primarily a vascular response, the function of which is to increase blood flow to the injured area, flood it with plasma and plasma proteins, convey neutrophils to the area for phagocytosis of debris and, if necessary, initiate scarring to heal the tissue.

Adamantinoma: See **Ameloblastoma**.

Addisonian anaemia (= pernicious anaemia): A type of anaemia due to either congenital causes (lack of intrinsic factor secretion) or a complex aetiology associated with genetic factors or autoimmunity (= 'classical' form). In the congenital form there is severe anaemia with the stomach being normal, while in the classical form there is pallor, jaundice, weakness, paraesthesia, stiffness of limbs, glossitis, weight loss, anorexia and achlorhydria with atrophy of the mucosa of the stomach. The prognosis is poor and in untreated cases the disease is fatal.

Addison's disease: Severe hypofunction of the adrenal glands resulting from haemorrhage, infection or autoimmune disease, leading to bronzed skin pigmentation, prostration, anaemia, hypotension and digestive disorders. It is a potentially fatal disorder.

Adenocarcinoma: A malignant neoplasm arising in glandular tissue and characterized by the aggregation of the tumour cells into masses resembling the acini of glands, mimicking to an extent the tissue in which the tumour arose.

Adenoids: Hyperplasia of the pharyngeal tonsils causing partial respiratory obstruction, seen predominantly in children. The condition causes anomalies in breathing and speaking, and may lead to ear infections, hypoventilation and pulmonary hypertension. Treatment is by surgical removal of the excessive lymphoid tissue.

Adenoma: A benign tumour arising in glandular tissue and resembling normal tissue to the extent that acinar structures are seen within the tumour cell masses.

Adenomatosis coli: See **Polyposis coli**.

Adenomyosis of the uterus: An example of ECTOPIA, where normal tissue is found in an abnormal location. In this condition endometrium is found deep in the wall of the uterus. The myometrium is thickened and contains haemorrhagic or cystic foci, as normal menstrual cyclical changes occur in this endometrial tissue. The condition may cause menorrhagia, dyspareunia or premenstrual pain (see also ENDOMETRIOSIS).

Adenosis of the breast: A hyperplastic/dysplastic condition of the female breast where there is increased epithelial cellularity at the acinar level. Increased numbers of lobules will be seen in the breast tissue and there may be associated hyperplasia of connective tissue around the lobules producing distortion of the epithelium with, eventually, sclerosis (sclerosing adenosis).

Adhesion: Abnormal union of two surfaces, usually the result of ORGANIZATION, as a sequela of inflammation.

Adipose: Of a fatty nature, in reference to tissue.

Adjuvant: A substance which when administered together with an ANTIGEN will improve the body's immune response to that antigen. A common adjuvant is Freund's which contains *Mycobacterium* extracts and mineral oil.

Adrenogenital disorders: Disorders of the adrenal gland characterized by excessive secretion of adrenocortical androgens, resulting in virilization in females and precocious development of secondary sex characteristics in young boys. The disorder may be caused by neoplasms in the gland, hyperplastic conditions or a genetic enzymatic defect.

Aetiology: Referring to cause, especially of a disease or disorder.

Afferent: Conveying towards a centre.

Afibrinogenaemia: A rare congenital disorder where there is no synthesis of fibrinogen by the liver. The blood is virtually incoagulable and widespread haemorrhages occur in the affected infants. Occasionally, with severe liver disease (e.g. CIRRHOSIS), an acquired form of afibrinogenaemia is seen.

Agammaglobulinaemia: The condition where no gamma globulins (ANTIBODY) is found within the body. This is a rare congenital disorder arising from a complete lack of B lymphocytes in the body, also known as Bruton's disease.

Agenesis: The failure of an organ or tissue to develop from its primordia, leading to the complete absence of that organ or tissue in the body. The condition may be fatal (e.g. agenesis of the brain = ANENCEPHALY) or may not manifest itself at all (e.g. unilateral kidney agenesis).

Agglutinin: An ANTIBODY that clumps a particular ANTIGEN.

Agglutinogen: An antigen stimulating the production of an AGGLUTININ.

Agnosia: Total or partial loss of the ability to recognize familiar objects or people through any of the sensory pathways. It usually reflects organic brain damage.

Agranulocytosis: A condition in which there is marked reduction in the circulating number of all granular white cells (but especially the neutrophils, cf. NEUTROPENIA). It may be caused by primary or secondary tumours in bone, radiotherapy or chemotherapy in association with neoplasm treatments or it may be an autoimmune or idiopathic disorder. Patients present with fever, infections, prostration and ulceration of mucous membranes.

AIDS: See **Acquired immune deficiency syndrome**.

Albers-Schönberg disease: See **Osteopetrosis**.

Albinism: An autosomal recessive condition in which there is partial or total lack of melanin in the body. Total albinos have a very pale skin, white hair, pink eyes, NYSTAGMUS, photophobia and ASTIGMATISM. They are more prone to developing actinic cancers of the skin, sunburn and dermatitis.

Albright's syndrome (= fibrous dysplasia of bone): An uncommon syndrome, which in its complete form has a complex of changes: fibrous dysplasia of bone, skin pigmentation ('café au lait spots') and precocious puberty. The disease is idiopathic and in the monostotic form the mandible and maxilla are affected commonly. In the polyostotic form there is bilateral jaw involvement with other bones also affected. In the long bones the lesions are unilateral but multiple. Fibrous tissue replaces bone and pathological fracture is very common. Fibrosarcomata may rarely arise in the affected sites.

Aleukaemic leukaemia: A form of leukaemia in which the total leukocyte number is not raised above the upper limit of normal (10 800 per µL or 10.8×10^9 per L). Any type of leukaemia may present as such but the bone marrow will always show the cells typical of the leukaemia and therefore bone marrow smears are mandatory in diagnosis.

Alkalosis: A condition in which the blood is abnormally alkaline.

Alkaptonuria: Rare, autosomal recessive disorder in which tyrosine is not metabolized normally due to an enzymatic defect. Glycosuric acid is excreted in large amounts in the urine, staining it dark. The symptoms of the disease do not usually develop until middle age where OCHRONOSIS may be seen as a presenting feature.

Alkylating agents: Mutagenic substances or CARCINOGENS which exert their effect by adding alkyl groups to cell components, for example, vinyl chloride.

Allergen: An ANTIGEN which initiates an ALLERGIC RESPONSE.

Allergic response (= allergy, hypersensitivity): An abnormality of the immune response in which destruction of tissue and other harmful effects are seen in response to an antigen, instead of the normal protective effects and inactivation of the antigen by the body's immune system. The immune system in allergy destroys body tissue or perverts the normal functioning of the tissue. Five main types of allergy are described (see ANAPHYLAXIS, ARTHUS REACTION, CYTOTOXIC HYPERSENSITIVITY, DELAYED HYPERSENSITIVITY, STIMULATORY HYPERSENSITIVITY).

Allograft (= homograft): The transplantation of tissue between two genetically dissimilar individuals of the same species. For example, a kidney transplantation from parent to offspring.

Alopecia: An abnormal loss of hair caused by the cessation of growth in the follicle.

Alzheimer's disease: The commonest form of DEMENTIA, characterized by rapid loss of neurones over a relatively short period of time (4 to 8 years). There is progressive loss of the higher intellectual functions of the brain, with confusion, loss of memory, restlessness, nocturnal wandering, AGNOSIA, disturbances of speech and behaviour.

Amaurosis: Blindness due to any cause, but especially when it develops without any apparent lesions within the eye.

Amaurosis fugax: Transient episode of monocular or partial blindness, as may be seen, for example, in TRANSIENT ISCHAEMIC ATTACKS.

Amaurotic familial idiocy: See **Tay-Sachs disease**.

Ameloblastoma (= Adamantinoma): A neoplasm of the tissue of the enamel organ of teeth, not well differentiated enough to form enamel. It is a rare, locally malignant, highly destructive tumour of youth that most commonly arises in the lower jaw and is treated adequately by local excision.

Amenorrhoea: Absence or abnormal stoppage of the menses.

Ametropia: Failure of images to be focused sharply on the retina as a result of discrepancies between the size and refractive powers of the eye.

Amniocentesis: Removal of ≈25 mL of amniotic fluid by transabdominal puncture into the amniotic cavity, performed between the 16th and 20th weeks of gestation in order to detect congenital foetal abnormalities such as DOWN'S SYNDROME or TAY-SACHS DISEASE.

Amoebic colitis (dysentery): See **Ulcerative colitis (specific)**.

Amyloid: A proteinaceous substance deposited extracellularly in many tissues of the body in the condition of AMYLOIDOSIS. There are two major biochemical classes of amyloid. Amyloid light-chain protein, derived from immunoglobulin molecule fragments, and amyloid-associated protein, which is derived from an apoprotein of a high-density lipoprotein.

Amyloidosis: A systemic disorder which may be primary (unknown aetiology, may be hereditary) or secondary (seen after, or in association with, chronic infections or inflammations such as rheumatoid arthritis; also seen in malignancies, especially multiple myeloma). A characteristic proteinaceous substance, AMYLOID, is deposited intercellularly in various tissues throughout the body and represents immune dysfunction.

Anaemia: A state in which there is reduction of haemoglobin in the blood below the normal for the patient's age and sex. WHO defines as anaemic anyone whose haemoglobin is below 13 g/dL (males) and 12 g/dL (females). Anaemia is due to many aetiologies, ranging from genetic diseases which affect the haemoglobin molecule itself, to acquired diseases, and also it may be the consequence of diseases in non-related body systems (e.g. as an effect of malignancy or chronic systemic diseases).

Anaesthesia: Any loss of sensation, but especially on a systemic level as induced prior to major surgery, with loss of consciousness.

Analgesia: Loss of sensitivity to pain, without loss of consciousness.

Analgesic nephropathy: A condition associated with excessive intake of phenacetin and other analgesics which induce renal papillary necrosis. The tips of the renal pyramids projecting into the minor calyces become necrotic and eventually become detached from the rest of the pyramid. The condition is usually bilateral, involving several papillae.

Anamnestic antibody response (secondary antibody response): The immune response seen on the second and subsequent times the same ANTIGEN is encountered by the immune system. It is characterized by a rapid rise in specific ANTIBODY and, generally, a protective immunity, with no clinical evidence of the disease.

Anaphylactic shock: A very marked type of ANAPHYLAXIS seen on a systemic level, characterized by profound systemic vasodilatation, bronchoconstriction and a typical SHOCK presentation, as is seen after bee stings in some hypersensitive individuals. The condition may be fatal. It is an example of a type I hypersensitivity.

Anaphylaxis (= Type I hypersensitivity): A hypersensitivity (allergic) response in which an ALLERGEN enters the tissues and stimulates IgE antibody formation instead of IgG or IgA. The IgE antibody (= REAGIN) attaches to mast cells and sensitizes them such that the next time the allergen is encountered it binds to the IgE-coated mast cells, causing their degranulation with release of histamine and serotonin causing widespread inflammation, vasodilatation and bronchoconstriction. A typical reaction of this kind occurs in ASTHMA.

Anaplasia: A characteristic of some malignant neoplasms in which the 'de-differentiation' of the cells is so complete that they lose all resemblance to the parent tissue from which they have arisen. It may not be possible to classify or identify the origin of such anaplastic tumours.

Anasarca: Marked generalized OEDEMA.

Anastomosis (plural, **anastomoses**): A surgical connection between two tubular or hollow organs such that their lumina are directly connected.

Andersen's disease: A rare glycogen storage disease (type IV), in which there is a congenital enzyme defect leading to the deposition of abnormal glycogen in the liver and striated muscle predominantly. The babies look normal at birth but there is failure to thrive with development of hepatomegaly, hypotonia of muscles, CIRRHOSIS and liver failure or cardiac failure. It is not treatable and most children die within the first few years of life.

Anencephaly: Congenital absence of the brain, not compatible with life. It may be detected early in the pregnancy by ultrasonography or AMNIOCENTESIS.

Aneuploidy: Any variation in chromosome number which is not in the normal, exact multiple of the haploid number (23 in humans). There may be fewer chromosomes (e.g. Turner's syndrome: 45, X0) or more (as in DOWN'S SYNDROME: 47, XY+21 or 47, XX+21).

Aneurysm: A localized, abnormal dilatation of any vessel or the heart. It may develop in any part of the vascular system, but is most commonly seen in the arteries. Most aneurysms occur in the aorta, arteries of the brain and head, iliac arteries and renal arteries.

Angina: Any disorder characterized by SPASMODIC, choking or suffocating pain.

Angina pectoris: A severe, crushing, left-sided chest pain, which often radiates down the left arm. The pain of angina is felt upon exertion, emotional stress, overeating, extremes of temperature or any other cause of increased myocardial activity. It is caused by severe coronary artery atherosclerosis which compromises cardiac blood flow.

Angioma: A benign tumour-like mass of blood vascular elements. It may be a HAEMANGIOMA or a lymphangioma.

Anhidrosis: The abnormal absence of perspiration.

Anisocytosis: A condition in which the red blood cells are of abnormal and varying size.

Anitschkow myocytes: Cells seen in ASCHOFF BODIES of RHEUMATIC FEVER. They are altered myocytes with a bar-shaped nucleus which has little projecting fibres of chromatin, making the nucleus look like a caterpillar, hence the name 'caterpillar cells'.

Ankylosing spondylitis: An autoimmune disease affecting the spine more prevalent in young men. It often begins in the sacroiliac joints and may later involve the vertebral column and more rarely, adjacent major joints (e.g. hip and shoulder). Initially there is an inflammatory reaction in the sacroiliac joints and ligaments of the vertebral column, which ossify, progressing to complete bony fusion of these joints and the spine. The patients have a characteristic bowed, rigid posture.

Ankylosis: The fixation of a joint with loss of normal movement due to the destruction of the joint tissue and repair by fibrosis, for example as occurs in severe RHEUMATOID ARTHRITIS.

Anosmia: Loss of the sense of smell, either temporarily as occurs in upper respiratory tract infections or permanently as occurs after destruction of olfactory epithelium or the olfactory nerve.

Anorexia nervosa: A psychoneurotic disorder in which the patient persistently refuses to eat leading to gross emaciation. Usually seen in young women or adolescents.

Anoxia: Reduction of oxygen in the tissues of the body below the physiological levels (see also ISCHAEMIA).

Anthracosis: Deposition of carbon particles within the body. Most commonly this occurs as a PNEUMOCONIOSIS where carbon particles in the form of smoke or smog are inhaled and are ingested by alveolar macrophages, which convey the particles to the lymph nodes. Generally not a severe disease unless there is massive deposition of carbon as occurs in coal workers' pneumoconiosis.

Antibody: A protein manufactured by PLASMA CELLS of the body in response to the presence of an abnormal component in the tissues (the ANTIGEN). Antibody and antigen react very specifically together with a lock and key structure, the purpose of this being the inactivation of the noxious antigen.

Antigen: A substance which when in the tissues will generate an immune response. Most commonly antigens are derived from components of infecting microorganisms.

Antrum: A cavity or chamber.

Anuria: Absence of excretion of urine.

Aphthous stomatitis: A painful condition of the oral cavity in which shallow ulcers or erosions form in the mucosa. It may be associated with stress or immune dysfunction, but usually is self-limiting and most commonly resolves spontaneously.

Aplasia: A sudden cessation of growth with the affected tissue never reaching its full size or extent, usually as a result of failure of normal differentiation and growth. The term aplasia has now become confined to the condition of aplastic anaemia in which the bone marrow fails to produce the blood cells which it does normally.

Apoplectic cyst: A cystic glial structure in the brain representing a healed cerebral infarct.

Apoplectic haemorrhage: Extravasated blood in the brain causing a sudden loss of consciousness.

Apoplexy: See **Stroke**.

Apoptosis (= '**shrinkage necrosis**'): A mechanism of cellular death which occurs in such situations as INVOLUTION or within certain tumours. The cells that undergo this process are isolated cells within the tissue and they begin to lose water, their organelles group together and become membrane-bound packets, the nucleus undergoes PYKNOSIS and KARYORRHEXIS and eventually the whole cell breaks down into small, dense, membrane-bound fragments which are then phagocytosed by surrounding, normally non-phagocytic cells.

Appendicitis: Infection or inflammation of the vermiform appendix.

Apraxia: Impairment in the performance of purposeful acts (learned movements) or manipulation of objects. It is primarily a neurological condition and is seen to occur in the absence of motor paralysis, ATAXIA or sensory loss.

Arachnodactyly: A congenital condition seen usually in association with MARFAN'S SYNDROME in which there are long, spindly, spider-like fingers and toes.

Arnold-Chiari malformation: A congenital defect of the central nervous system often associated with SPINA BIFIDA or MENINGOCOELE, in which there is herniation of the brainstem and lower cerebellum through the foramen magnum into the cervical vertebral canal.

Arrhenoblastoma: A rare tumour of the ovary in which there is proliferation of cells similar to those in testicular tissue in that they secrete male sex hormones causing VIRILIZATION of the woman.

Arrhythmia: Any abnormal variation from the normal rhythm of the heartbeat.

Arteriosclerosis: A group of arterial diseases characterized by a loss of elasticity, thickening and hardening of the vessels of the arterial system. The most important of the group is ATHEROSCLEROSIS.

Arteritis: Infection or inflammation of the wall of an artery.

Arthritis: Infection or inflammation of a joint.

Arthus reaction: A type III hypersensitivity reaction in which there is local formation of antigen–antibody complexes with stimulation of acute inflammation, complement fixation and platelet adhesion with severe, necrotic and haemorrhagic lesions resulting.

Artificial immunity: A resistance to infection that is acquired by artificial means, as occurs, for example, in immunization (active artificial immunity) or after the injection of pooled human immunoglobulins (passive artificial immunity).

Asbestosis: A PNEUMOCONIOSIS resulting after inhalation of asbestos fibres, causing a diffuse fibrosis of the lungs with pleural thickening, especially in the lower lobes. It greatly predisposes to pulmonary tuberculosis, bronchial carcinoma and pleural MESOTHELIOMA.

Aschoff body: A characteristic lesion found in RHEUMATIC FEVER. It consists of a central degenerating region of collagen and fibrinoid necrosis, surrounded by a granulomatous reaction with macrophages, fibroblasts, plasma cells and lymphocytes, and multinucleate giant cells being present. The Aschoff giant cells contain two to five nuclei. ANITSCHKOW MYOCYTES may also be seen in association with the lesion.

Ascites: The collection of oedema fluid within the peritoneal cavity, seen commonly in association with liver failure and as an adjunct of generalized OEDEMA.

Asphyxia: A condition brought about by drowning, electrocution, blockage of the trachea or major airways, inhalation of toxic gases or smoke. It is characterized by a severe hypoxaemia and hypercapnia, loss of consciousness and, if untreated, death.

Asterixis (= 'flapping tremor'): A hand flapping tremor that often accompanies metabolic disease which affects the central nervous system. It commonly accompanies CIRRHOSIS of the liver and can be induced in a patient by extending the arm and dorsiflexing the wrist.

Asteroid bodies: Star-shaped eosinophilic inclusions composed of lipoproteins found in the cytoplasm of giant cells in sarcoidosis (see also SCHAUMANN BODIES).

Asthma: A condition characterized by widespread bronchial obstruction due to muscular spasm, producing expiratory wheezing with prolongation of expiration. Typically, a thick, white mucus is produced by the respiratory epithelium of the bronchi and this leads to plugging and distension of the airways, the patient experiencing considerable difficulty in breathing. It may be an extrinsic or intrinsic type according to whether the aetiology is environmental in origin or whether the patient's own idiosyncrasy is more important in the causation of the disorder.

Astimatism: A type of AMETROPIA caused by a flattened eyeball causing a proportionate blurring both for near and distance vision, irrespective of accommodation, with visual fatigue and headaches occurring. The condition is corrected by astigmatic lenses with an appropriately different curvature in the two meridians.

Astrocytoma: The commonest of the primary intracranial tumours, accounting for approximately 34% of them. It is a grossly infiltrative tumour usually in the cerebral hemispheres of adults or in the cerebellum of children. Astrocytomata of the cerebrum in adults are very invasive and kill within a few months to years, while astrocytomata of the cerebellum in children behave much less aggressively. Divided into grades according to their behaviour: Grade I less aggressive to Grade IV, very aggressive.

Ataxia: Loss of voluntary muscle co-ordination.

Atelectasis (= **atelectasia**): Failure of the lungs to aerate at birth. It may result from brain damage causing respiration failure or may occur due to bronchial obstruction by mucus or aspirated amniotic fluid. The baby may die of ASPHYXIA.

Atheroma (plural, **atheromata**): The characteristic fibrofatty, intimal lesion of ATHEROSCLEROSIS, also commonly used synonymously with the disease.

Atherosclerosis (= **atheroma**): The commonest of the arteriosclerotic group of diseases, found in some degree in all people over the age of 45 years. It affects males more commonly below 45 years but the incidence in post-menopausal women increases. Large elastic arteries are affected, such as the aorta (especially the abdominal portion), the coronary and cerebral arteries, the carotids, the renal and iliac arteries. The disease is associated with several well-defined risk factors: genetic predisposition, hormonal effects and age, all of which affect the degree of HYPERLIPIDAEMIA which is seen in the disorder, with HYPERTENSION, DIABETES MELLITUS and cigarette smoking also being major risk factors. The characteristic lesions or ATHEROMATA develop over many years and cause important complications such as ISCHAEMIA, THROMBOSIS, ANEURYSMS and myocardial and cerebral INFARCTS.

Athetosis: Involuntary and repetitive, slow, writhing movements that are most noticeable in the hands or arms.

Atresia: The congenital absence or closure of any part of the body which would normally have an opening, or the congenital obstruction of a tubular structure; for example, atresia of the oesophagus.

Atrial fibrillation: An involuntary, recurrent contraction of an isolated group of muscle fibres in the atrium leading to inefficient or random contraction of the chamber with disruption to the normal sinus rhythm of the heart.

Atrium: A chamber or cavity, the term usually applied to the upper chambers of the heart.

Atrophy: A wasting away or diminution in the size of a cell, a tissue or an organ. It is a decrease in the size of a part due to the decrease in the numbers or size (or both) of its constituent specialized cells.

Australia antigen: This is equivalent to the hepatitis B virus surface antigen (HBsAg), found in the serum of acute cases of the disease or the serum of carriers of the virus. It was originally discovered in the serum of Australian Aborigines.

Autoantibody: An antibody which reacts with tissues of the same body that has produced it, i.e. an antibody forming in response to an AUTOANTIGEN.

Autoantigen: A body component functioning as an antigen and stimulating an AUTOIMMUNE DISEASE, usually with the formation of AUTOANTIBODIES.

Autograft: Transplantation of tissue from one body site to another body site in the same individual, commonly carried out with skin grafts or vascular grafts.

Autoimmune disease: A disorder of the immune system resulting in immune reactions which cause destruction of the body's own tissues. There are organ-specific autoimmune diseases such as chronic autoimmune thyroiditis, where only one tissue is affected, and generalized autoimmune diseases, such as SYSTEMIC LUPUS ERYTHEMATOSUS (SLE), where many tissues are affected throughout the body.

Autolysis: The destruction of body cells through the activity of their own lytic enzymes derived from their lysosomes. Autolysis is seen in necrosis and in some tissues may progress almost to completion resulting in complete lysis of the cells (e.g. brain tissue after infarction).

Autophagy: A reactive change to sublethal injury in parenchymal tissues where isolated lysosomes within the cell release their lytic enzymes, causing limited lysis and damage within the cytoplasm of the cell. Such a reactive change may progress to NECROSIS and AUTOLYSIS.

Axonopathy: Any disease of peripheral nerves mainly, where the lesions are seen to affect primarily the axons.

Azoöspermia: Lack of spermatozoa in the semen caused by testicular disorders, blockages in the ducts of the epididymis or vasectomy. Sexual potency is maintained but the man is sterile.

Azotaemia: An abnormally high concentration of nitrogenous wastes in the blood.

Bacteraemia: The presence of bacteria in the bloodstream. This may be a transient event and not give rise to symptoms and signs.

Bacteraemic shock: See **Endotoxic (septic) shock**.

Bacterial endocarditis: An infection of the heart valves with *Staphylococcus aureus* or *Streptococcus pneumoniae* (the acute form, usually occurring in healthy valves), or with *Streptococcus viridans* (the subacute form, usually occurring in damaged valves). Septic VEGETATIONS form on the heart valves and septic emboli arise from the valves. Patients present with heart murmurs, fever, bacteraemia and manifestations of EMBOLISM.

Bacteriuria: The presence of significant numbers of bacteria in the urine indicating a urinary tract infection. Bladder urine is sterile normally and if it is sampled aseptically and shows bacteria within it, this may be taken to be indicative of a urinary tract infection.

Bagassosis: An organic PNEUMOCONIOSIS caused by inhalation of dusty, mouldy, sugar cane refuse (bagasse). It is essentially a hypersensitivity reaction in the lungs causing dyspnoea, fever and malaise mediated by inflammatory reactions and oedema in the lung tissue. It is treated by corticosteroids and avoidance of the allergens. Generally it does not cause fibrosis or permanent damage to the lung tissue.

Balanitis: Infection or inflammation of the glans penis.

Balanoposthitis: Infection or inflammation of the glans penis and prepuce, commonly associated with sexually transmitted disease or poor hygiene.

Basal cell carcinoma: A slow growing, malignant tumour of the basal cells of the epidermis, presenting as a pearly, flattened nodule. The centre breaks down with an ulcer and a scab developing ('rodent ulcer'). The periphery forms a smooth, slightly raised margin which as it spreads forms characteristically a 'rolled edge'. Generally it does not metastasize but can cause extensive damage locally through direct invasion and spread. It is common on the face of elderly people and excision is curative.

'Battered baby syndrome': SCURVY seen in babies and young children leading to multiple haemorrhages and bruises on the skin. This may be misdiagnosed as child abuse.

Bence-Jones protein: A characteristic protein found in the urine of patients with MULTIPLE MYELOMA. It is derived from the light-chain portion of the immunoglobulins secreted by the malignant plasma cells of the tumour. When the urine is heated to ≈50°C the protein coagulates and then redissolves when the urine is boiled.

'Bends': See **Caisson disease**.

Benign: Not MALIGNANT, not serious or life threatening in the majority of cases.

Beri beri: A disease brought about by thiamine deficiency endemic in areas of poor diet and countries where rice is the staple food. Peripheral neuropathy is associated with the disease, with paralysis, wasting of limbs, weight loss, heart failure and oedema.

Berry aneurysm: A type of ANEURYSM, shaped like a berry, which commonly occurs in the arteries of the circle of Willis in the brain. It is due to congenital weaknesses in the wall of the arteries. It may rupture, leading to a brain haemorrhage.

Berylliosis: A type of PNEUMOCONIOSIS due to inhalation of beryllium-containing dusts. Granulomata form in the lungs and diffuse pulmonary fibrosis occurs leading to DYSPNOEA, dry cough and chest pain, symptoms which may not be apparent until many years after exposure to the beryllium.

Bilirubin: An orange-yellow pigment found in bile, formed mainly from the breakdown of haemoglobin of erythrocytes. In a normal person ≈250 mg of bilirubin are produced daily, the majority of which is excreted in the faeces.

Biliverdin: A greenish bile pigment formed from haemoglobin and converted to BILIRUBIN.

Biopsy: Removal of a small piece of tissue from the living body for microscopic examination in order to diagnose a disorder.

'Birthmark': See **Haemangioma**.

'Blackhead': See **Comedo.**

-Blast: An immature or primitive stage in the development of a cell or alternatively a young, very active cell.

Blastoma: A usually malignant neoplasm arising from embryonic tissues, for example NEPHROBLASTOMA, RETINOBLASTOMA.

Bleeding time: A test of the clotting cascade of blood, where the time required for bleeding to stop from a small puncture wound is recorded. The Duke method involves wounding the free hanging ear lobe, whereas the Ivy method involves wounding the volar aspect of the forearm. Bleeding time is normally 2–6 minutes and prolongation of the bleeding time implies disorders of platelet function, ingestion of anticoagulants or uraemia.

Blood groups: Classification of the blood into specific types depending on the presence or absence of specific proteins (antigens) on the surface of erythrocytes and the presence or absence of specific antibodies to these antigens in the serum. Many different blood group types occur and include the ABO, Rh, MNS, Xg, Kidd and Lutheran groups.

B lymphocytes: A small (8 μm) agranular blood cell arising from stem cells in the bone marrow which together with T LYMPHOCYTES (from which they are indistinguishable microscopically) make up 25% of the white cells in the circulation. B lymphocytes are important in HUMORAL IMMUNITY, giving rise to the PLASMA CELLS which synthesize antibodies.

Boil: See **Furuncle**.

Bowen's disease: An intraepidermal malignancy of the skin arising from the squamous cells, which, if left untreated, will progress to SQUAMOUS CELL CARCINOMA.

Bradycardia: A disorder of heartbeat where the myocardium contracts steadily at a rate of less than 60 contractions a minute. It may indicate a brain tumour, digitalis poisoning or vagotonus. The patient presents with faintness or dizziness, chest pain and eventually SYNCOPE, all a result of diminished cardiac output.

Bradykinin: A nonapeptide produced from plasma α2 globulin by kallikrein and which is a potent vasodilator important in acute inflammatory reactions.

'Brittle bone syndrome': See **Osteogenesis imperfecta**.

Bronchiectasis: A permanent, abnormal dilatation of the bronchi and bronchioles (enlargement of airways above the level of the terminal bronchioles). It is often associated with chronic infectious/inflammatory states, for example as a sequel to a whooping cough, adenovirus infection and measles, or seen in association with obstruction, scarring, tumours, strictures, EMPHYSEMA, pressure anomalies, etc.

Bronchiolitis: Infection or inflammation of the bronchioles, commonly caused by infection with respiratory syncytial virus, parainfluenza viruses, *Mycoplasma pneumoniae* and rhinoviruses.

Bronchitis: Infection or inflammation of the bronchi, acute or chronic in nature, commonly caused by viral infection (e.g. measles) or bacterial infection (e.g. whooping cough). Chronic bronchitis is very debilitating and destructive and may be linked with BRONCHIECTASIS and COAD; it is commonly caused by bacteria of low virulence, for example *Haemophilus influenzae*.

Bronchopneumonia: Inflammation of the bronchi, bronchioles and immediately adjacent alveoli. It tends to occur throughout the lung lobes, but it is a patchy lesion, the inflamed and consolidated areas being observed adjacent to relatively normal areas. It is caused by a large variety of bacteria, e.g. *Streptococcus pneumoniae, Staphylococcus aureus* and *Haemophilus influenzae*. It does not follow a well-characterized clinical course and repair by scarring is usual in the affected lung tissue.

'Bronzed diabetes': See **Haemochromatosis**.

Brown atrophy of the heart: In this condition there is a wasting of the heart so that its size and weight is much lower than normal. The condition is seen in extreme old age and with wasting diseases such as advanced malignancies, the myocardium atrophying and becoming brown in colour due to the accumulation of a brown pigment known as LIPOFUSCIN. In most cases the atrophy does not interfere with the function of the heart, the damaged areas being replaced by scar tissue. In some cases, especially in diphtheria, the conducting system of the heart is damaged with heart block, arrhythmias and acute cardiac failure leading to the sudden death of the patient.

Bruton-type agammaglobulinaemia: A sex-linked disorder in which there are no circulating gamma globulins in the bloodstream, making the sufferers very susceptible to bacterial infections.

Bubo: A swelling of the inguinal lymph nodes as is characteristically seen with the bubonic plague.

Bulla (plural, **bullae**): A thin-walled blister in the skin or mucous membranes, greater than 1 cm in diameter and filled with a serous fluid. Alternatively, the term may be applied to a greatly dilated emphysematous space in the lungs, especially one of those found subpleurally.

Burkitt's lymphoma: A malignant tumour derived from lymphoreticular cells which commonly forms a large, osteolytic mass in the jaw of children. The tumour is found chiefly in central Africa and is associated with exposure to the Epstein-Barr virus. Chemotherapy is very effective in the treatment of the condition.

Bursa (plural, **bursae**): Sac or sac-like cavity filled with a viscous fluid situated in areas where friction would otherwise develop.

Bursa of Fabricius: An organ in fowl which is an outpouching of the gastrointestinal tract and in which the differentiation of B LYMPHOCYTES occurs. There is no such organ in mammals and the bursa-equivalent organ is believed to be the bone marrow.

Cachexia: A profound and marked state of constitutional disorder, usually associated with a loss of fat stores, wasting away of muscle tissue and generalized debilitation. It may be seen in chronic serious diseases and advanced malignancy.

Caisson disease: A type of gas EMBOLISM due to the formation of nitrogen bubbles in the bloodstream. It is seen in deep sea divers who surface too quickly. It is also known as 'the bends' as it causes excruciating pains in the joints forcing the sufferer to double up in pain. Brain damage may result from nitrogen bubbles lodging in brain vessels.

Calcification: The deposition of insoluble calcium salts in tissues; it may be physiological, such as occurs in bone, or pathological, such as occurs in METASTATIC CALCIFICATION.

Calcinosis: A condition in which there is abnormal deposition of calcium salts in the soft tissues (cf. MYOSITIS OSSIFICANS).

Calculus (plural, **calculi**): An abnormal concretion or 'stone' composed of mineral salts or hardened organic residues, occurring within the animal body, for example urinary or biliary calculi.

Callus: **(1)** Localized hyperplasia of the horny layer of the epidermis due to pressure or friction. **(2)** An unorganized network of woven bone formed between the ends of a broken bone, eventually resorbed as new normal bone is regenerated. Its function is to immobilize the broken bone and also to act as a scaffold on which the true bone is to form.

Canaliculus: A small canal or channel.

Cancer: A malignant tumour (see also CARCINOMA and SARCOMA).

Cancer-en-cuirasse (French: cancer in the form of a breastplate): A term commonly applied to a specific form of carcinoma of the breast in which the tumour cells infiltrate the dermal lymphatics, producing multiple tumour nodules, thickening of the skin and a dense dermal fibrosis.

Cancrum oris: A rare, gangrenous condition of the mouth usually seen in children. It is most often preceded by severe malnutrition or debilitating illnesses and is usually due to an opportunistic infection by normal flora bacteria including anaerobes. It may prove fatal in untreated cases.

Caput medusae: A case of TELANGIECTASIA of the umbilical veins associated with CIRRHOSIS of the liver, caused by portal hypertension and leading to an appearance similar to the head of the snake-headed goddess of Greek mythology, Medusa.

Carbuncle: A large, multilocular ABSCESS in which there are several interconnecting chambers of pus. It is commonly caused by infections with *Staphylococcus aureus*. It is often seen in the back of the neck and the buttocks of diabetics and people with agammaglobulinaemia.

Carcinogen: Any agent or substance which produces a cancer or acts on a population to change its total frequency of cancer in terms of numbers of tumours or distribution by site and age. Terms that are used synonymously for carcinogen are: cancerogen, tumourigen and oncogen.

Carcinogenesis: The origin or causation of cancer; the factors that contribute to the development of cancer.

Carcinoid syndrome: The systemic effects manifested by the secretion of serotonin and other catecholamines from CARCINOID TUMOURS. The patient presents with flushing, diarrhoea, cramps, cyanosis, bronchospasm, laboured breathing, palpitations, ascites, oedema and signs of pulmonary stenosis.

Carcinoid tumour: Small, yellowish, malignant, rare tumours of the intestinal crypts derived from the argentaffin cells secreting catecholamines. The tumours tend to grow slowly at first with only local invasion but they may later spread widely.

Carcinoma: A malignant mass composed of neoplastic cells that tend to invade and infiltrate into the surrounding tissues. It is derived from epithelial tissues, for example breast, colonic, skin, liver cells.

Carcinoma-in-situ (Latin: cancer at the site in which it arose): A carcinoma where the tumour is still confined to the epithelial layer in which it arose, not yet having invaded beyond the basement membrane of that epithelium.

Carcinosarcoma: Very rare tumours found in the uterus, lungs, oesophagus, genital tract, etc. where both the epithelial component and the connective tissue stroma are recognizably malignant.

'Cardiac cirrhosis': A consequence of long-standing chronic venous congestion of the liver in which the liver tissue undergoes reactive changes and necrosis as a consequence of anoxia. Fibrosis of the liver occurs diffusely, prompting some pathologists to dub it a type of cirrhosis; however, regenerative nodule formation is not a prominent feature (see CIRRHOSIS).

Cardiogenic shock: A state of SHOCK caused by abnormalities in the heart, very commonly associated with myocardial infarction or cardiac failure. Usually it is seen in association with a reduced cardiac output. It is fatal in approximately 80% of cases.

Cardiomyopathies: A broad group of cardiac disorders which are usually not inflammatory but present as myocardial dysfunction, which is not associated with hypertension, coronary heart disease or rheumatic heart disease. There may be both primary and secondary cardiomyopathies.

Carrier: A person who appears healthy but may pass on a disease to offspring or other people. There may be carriers of genetic disease (e.g. carrier of HAEMOPHILIA) or carriers of microbial disease (e.g. *Salmonella typhi*, typhoid carrier).

Caseous necrosis (= caseation): A type of necrosis associated with infection with *Mycobacterium tuberculosis*. Macroscopically it resembles white, crumbly, cottage cheese. Microscopically there is no definition of cellular outlines, an amorphous eosinophilic mass being all that is discernible.

Cast: An amorphous material composed of a variety of compounds usually found within a duct or epithelial cavity, for example protein or red blood cell casts found in the kidney tubules in renal disease.

Cataract: A loss of transparency of the lens of the eye which is slowly progressive and usually seen in the elderly. A grey-white opacity may be seen in the lens behind the pupil. Uncomplicated cataracts of old age are usually treated surgically and the patient is prescribed special eyeglasses.

Catarrhal inflammation: An inflammation of the mucous membranes characterized by the production of excessive mucus, such as is seen, for example, with the common cold where there is catarrhal inflammation in the upper respiratory tract and excessive nasal discharge.

Catecholamine: A group of related compounds composed of a catechol molecule joined to the aliphatic portion of an amine. Some catecholamines are formed naturally by the body, for example serotonin, and have various functions in the CNS or in inflammation.

Cell-mediated immunity: A type of immune response reliant on the activity of macrophages and T LYMPHOCYTES and the secretion of specific messenger substances, the INTERLEUKINS, by these cells, facilitating the mounting of immune responses. Cell-mediated immunity is effective against viral, fungal and protozoal infections and some bacterial infections (e.g. TB, leprosy, brucellosis) and also is effective in protecting the body against malignant cells and is important in graft rejection.

Cellulitis: A diffuse infection throughout loose tissue, usually caused by *Streptococcus* spp. and occurring in the subcutaneous tissues.

Cerebral infarction: Ischaemic necrosis of the brain associated with atherosclerosis of the carotid, cerebral and basilar arteries. Often thromboembolism will be the cause of the infarction. Haemorrhagic infarcts are common in the brain and, together with cerebral haemorrhages, infarcts of the brain are given the term 'stroke' or cerebrovascular accidents (CVAs). COLLIQUATIVE NECROSIS is the aftermath of a cerebral infarction and the lost brain tissue is replaced by GLIOSIS.

Ceruloplasmin: A plasma glycoprotein of the α globulin group by which most of the plasma copper is transported.

Chalone: A hormone-like compound which is a polypeptide and which is elaborated by a variety of tissues, the function of which is to inhibit the functioning of target organs.

Chancre: A skin lesion, the first manifestation of syphilis, found most commonly in the genital areas. It is a painless, bloodless, clean ulcer with a hard base which heals spontaneously in about 2 months with little or no scarring. The lesion is teeming with *Treponema pallidum* and is highly infectious.

Chancroid: A sexually transmitted disease caused by infection with *Haemophilus ducreyi*, a Gram-negative coccobacillus. The lesion that develops on the genitals begins as a papule which then ulcerates to form a soft ragged ulcer with a deep, suppurating base, enlarging to 2 to 3 cm in diameter. Inguinal lymphadenopathy follows with formation of BUBOES.

Charcot arthropathy (= neuropathic arthropathy): A progressive degenerative disease of joints, especially affecting the stress-bearing regions, due to neurological disorders involving loss of sensation in the joint. Hypertrophic changes occur in the periphery of the joint. It may be seen commonly at the knee, hip and shoulder and a typical cause is leprosy.

Chediak-Higashi syndrome: This is a rare, congenital, lysosomal defect in polymorphs leading to an impaired capacity of the phagocyte to destroy bacteria intracellularly. Patients present at a young age with pyogenic infections.

Cheilitis: Inflammation or infection of the lips.

Chemotaxis: The ordered movement of cells in response to a chemical gradient (e.g. neutrophils actively moving towards a clump of bacteria).

Chickenpox (= varicella): A mild, very common and highly contagious disease of childhood caused by the varicella virus. It has an incubation period of about 2 weeks and is manifested by a characteristic skin eruption beginning on the trunk and spreading outwards. Only rarely does the disease lead to complications such as pneumonia or encephalitis which may prove fatal.

'Childbed fever': See **Puerperal sepsis**.

Chimaera: An organism carrying cell populations derived from two or more genetically distinct individuals. A chimaera may be produced artificially by introducing foreign cells into a zygote developing *in vitro* or it may be a consequence of medical treatment, for example a bone marrow graft.

Chloasma (= melasma): A tan or brownish pigmentation seen in the facial area and commonly associated with pregnancy or the use of oral contraceptives. It is due to increased production of melanin and may be permanent or transient.

Chloroma: A malignant, greenish coloured tumour arising from the myeloid tissue. The greenish pigment is mainly myeloperoxidase.

Cholangiocarcinoma: A rather uncommon, malignant tumour of the bile duct epithelium, growing and spreading early, associated with a very poor prognosis.

Cholangitis: An infection or inflammation of the intrahepatic bile ducts, leading to the formation of multiple abscesses in the liver.

Cholecystitis: An infection or inflammation of the gall bladder, commonly associated with CHOLELITHIASIS.

Cholelithiasis: The condition in which gall stones form in the gall bladder.

Cholestasis: Interruption to the normal flow of bile in any part of the biliary system from the liver to the duodenum.

Cholesterosis of the gall bladder (= 'strawberry gall bladder'): An idiopathic condition where there are multiple yellow deposits of cholesterol on the surface of the gall bladder epithelium associated with a reddened, inflamed mucosa. There is no systemic cholesterol metabolism anomaly and the condition is normally symptomless, although a large number of cases coexist with cholecystitis.

Chondroma: A rare benign tumour of cartilage.

Chondrosarcoma: A rare malignant tumour of cartilage, occurring later in life (average age 45 years) and affecting proximal ends of the long bones, limb girdles and ribs. Males are affected twice as often as females and 10% of cases arise from pre-existing benign chondromata. Patients often have a long history of symptoms when they first come for treatment. The tumours are slow growing and it may be 20 years or more before a patient dies from the tumour. Following amputation there is a moderately good prognosis.

Chordoma: A rather rare, malignant tumour arising from the embryonic remnants of the notochord.

Chorea: A clinical presentation arising out of cerebral irritability or damage with sudden, involuntary, irregular, rapid 'dance-like' movements with muscular incoordination and weakness. It may be seen in association with RHEUMATIC FEVER in which case it is termed Sydenham's chorea or it may develop as the result of a Mendelian dominant inherited disorder producing symptoms in middle life, the so-called HUNTINGTON'S CHOREA.

Choriocarcinoma: A malignancy derived from the chorionic trophoblast. It is extremely rare, affecting one in 50 000 Caucasians, but one in 1000 Asians. There is raised HCG in blood and urine which is diagnostic. The tumour is bulky, haemorrhagic and invasive. It may present as haemorrhage from the vagina. There is very early blood spread of metastases to lungs and brain most commonly. This tumour is very aggressive in its behaviour. Therapy with suitable cytotoxic drugs (e.g. methotrexate) is very effective, the mortality being 40% or even less.

Choristoma: A focal mass of normal cells in a tissue most commonly arising during development but it differs in that these cells are present in a tissue or organ that normally does not contain them. An alternative name for the condition is ECTOPIA or ectopic tissue. An example of the condition is normal functional glandular cells of the mucosa of the stomach being present in the lower intestinal wall.

Christmas disease (= haemophilia B): A sex-linked Mendelian defect in clotting factor IX, manifesting as a bleeding tendency. The prognosis is similar to HAEMOPHILIA A and the disease is treated by injection of factor derived from donated blood.

Chronic: Prolonged, persistent or of long duration; i.e. weeks to months to years.

Chronic granulomatous disease of childhood: This is due to an undefined enzyme defect which prevents the neutrophils destroying phagocytosed bacteria. It is an X-linked genetic disorder.

Chronic inflammation: The prolonged inflammatory state in which tissue injury and attempts at healing are proceeding at the same time. Usually this is due to the persistence of the injurious agent.

Chronic obstructive airways (or **pulmonary**) **disease** (= **COAD**; **COPD**): A group of respiratory disorders in which there is the common factor of long-term obstruction of the respiratory passages. The causes of the obstruction may be inflammatory, infectious, neoplastic, associated with pneumoconiosis, emphysema and bronchiectasis or congenital diseases. There may be regions of lung collapse, fibrosis, infection, abscess formation and extreme fibrosis (see also HONEYCOMB LUNG).

Chyle: The milky fluid absorbed by the lacteals from food in the intestine during digestion, consisting of lymph and triglycerides.

Chylothorax: The presence of effused CHYLE in the thorax.

Chyluria: The presence of chyle in the urine, leading to its milky appearance.

Cicatrix: See **Scar**.

Cirrhosis: A condition of the liver in which there is diffuse fibrosis and necrosis of the organ, making it appear tawny in colour. Cirrhosis is a diffuse disease of the liver with gross disruption to liver architecture, the parenchyma changed to a large number of lobules separated by fibrous tissue tracts. The anatomical criteria for diagnosis of cirrhosis are: diffuse involvement of the liver; disorganization of lobular architecture; necrosis of liver cells at some stage; the presence of regenerative nodules of hepatocytes; diffuse fibrosis (NB: little collagen is normally present in liver); and bile duct hyperplasia with or without aberrant bile ducts.

Claudication: A weakness of the legs which manifests itself as cramps or pains in the calves, usually seen in association with some activity. It is mostly caused by ATHEROSCLEROSIS of the leg arteries and the resultant poor blood supply to the legs seen with the condition. The patient may show limping or lameness when walking.

Clear cell carcinoma: Carcinoma of the kidney which is the commonest renal tumour (80% of kidney malignancies), and arises from tubular epithelium. It commonly arises in the cortex, and the tumour shows a propensity to grow along veins. It is composed of large, pale clear cells. Metastasis occurs to lung, liver, bone and the other kidney.

Clone: A population of identical cells.

Clonus: Rapidly successive, involuntary episodes of muscular contraction and relaxation.

Clubbing: A deforming enlargement of the terminal phalanges, usually acquired, associated with disorders of the cardiovascular, respiratory and gastrointestinal systems (usually indicative of anaemia).

COAD: See **Chronic obstructive airways disease** (= COPD).

Coagulase: An enzyme produced by some bacteria (e.g. *Staphylococcus aureus*) which acts on fibrinogen converting it into fibrin.

Coagulative necrosis: The commonest type of cellular death in the living body characterized by its macroscopic appearance about 7–8 hours after the cells have died. The affected tissue looks pale, slightly shrunken and is firm to the touch. It is seen in most solid organs in the body, for example heart, kidney, spleen, liver, pancreas, skin, lungs.

Co-carcinogen: A substance which on its own is not CARCINOGENIC and will not transform a normal cell into a neoplastic one when it contacts it. However, a co-carcinogen will aid the carcinogenic effects of another agent which is itself an ultimate or active carcinogen.

Coeliac disease (= **gluten enteropathy**): A genetic disease in which there is a deficiency in enzymes required for the hydrolysis of peptides contained in gluten. The patients present with abdominal distension, vomiting, diarrhoea, steatorrhoea, muscle wasting and lethargy. Elimination of gluten products from the diet usually leads to complete recovery.

Cold abscess: A collection of caseous necrotic material as occurs in tuberculosis. The caseous material may collect in myofascial planes and may induce an inflammatory response. However, the tissue swelling that is seen is not characteristically red and hot as would be seen with a typical acute inflammatory abscess (see also POTT'S DISEASE).

Colitis: An infection or inflammation of the colon.

Colliquative necrosis (= **liquefactive necrosis**): A type of NECROSIS in which the cells undergo almost complete lysis resulting in a collection of fluid in the affected tissue. Typically, autolytic colliquative necrosis occurs in the brain and is the result of the action of the cells' own enzymes digesting the cells' own substance. Alternatively heterolytic colliquative necrosis may occur when any tissue is subjected to the action of neutrophilic enzymes which lyse the necrotic cells around the area (as occurs typically in an abscess, PUS being the manifestation of this latter process).

Coma: A profound loss of consciousness from which a patient cannot be roused. There are no spontaneous eye movements and no response to painful stimuli. It may be due to brain damage, poisoning, intoxication, diabetic acidosis or infection.

Comedo (plural, **comedones**): A blackhead. A skin lesion arising out of sebaceous gland dysfunction where the sebum plugs the duct of the gland with accumulation of fatty material within the duct and its protrusion from the surface. The upper region of the secretion becomes oxidised and black. Comedones may become infected and lead to the formation of ABSCESSES.

Complement: A complex of 11 enzymatic serum proteins which interact in a cascade series of reactions similar to the blood clotting cascade. Complement activation is stimulated by antigen–antibody reactions, bacteria and inflammatory stimuli. Its function is to aid phagocytosis, increase effectiveness of the inflammatory response, and ultimately cause lysis of cell membranes.

Condyloma acuminatum (plural, **condylomata acuminata**): A genital wart usually seen as a sexually transmitted disease and caused by infection with the human papilloma virus (HPV). It arises as a soft, papillomatous growth on moist skin and mucous membranes of the genitalia.

Congenital disorder: A disorder which is present at the time of birth. It may have a genetic basis or be a congenital malformation. Although some genetic diseases are present at birth they may not be apparent until later on in life (e.g. HAEMOCHROMATOSIS).

Congestion: The dilatation of blood vessels such that they carry much more blood than they do normally. The condition may be an active process such as occurs in inflammatory conditions or a passive process caused by failure of the right ventricle to pump away the blood from the venous system at an adequately fast rate.

Congestive heart failure: A circulatory system aberration caused by a variety of heart diseases, especially myocardial infarction. There is congestion of the circulation which stimulates sodium and water retention by the kidneys, further aggravating the condition. Pulmonary congestion and oedema is also seen with the condition thus impairing the ventilatory function of the lungs. Dyspnoea, high venous pressure, increased circulation time, oedema and decreased vital capacity also occur.

Conn's syndrome (= primary aldosternonism): A condition where there is hypersecretion of aldosterone occurring as a primary disease of the adrenal cortex. Usually it is a hyperplasia or a tumour of the adrenal cortex that causes the syndrome. It results in sodium and water retention, potassium excretion, increased blood volume and pressure, alkalosis, cardiac anomalies, muscle weakness and tetany. Electrolyte imbalances lead to polydipsia and polyuria.

Contact dermatitis: A type IV hypersensitivity in which an allergy develops to objects or substances contacting the surface of the skin (e.g. cosmetics, jewellery, plant components, substances encountered in an occupational setting). Inflammation and irritation of the skin develop with many lymphocytes and macrophages accumulating in the affected area, causing tissue damage.

Convulsion: A violent involuntary contraction or group of contractions of skeletal muscles.

COPD: See **Chronic obstructive airways disease** (= COAD).

Cor bovinum (Latin: heart of an ox): Very marked left ventricular hypertrophy most often caused by systemic hypertension. Heart valve disease may also result in myocardial hypertrophy.

Cor pulmonale (Latin: heart state resulting from a pulmonary condition): Right ventricular hypertrophy commonly arising from pulmonary hypertension. Heart valve disease may also result in myocardial hypertrophy.

Corpus (Latin: body; plural, **corpora**): The body as a whole, or the main part of an organ.

Corpus amylaceum (Latin: starch-like body; plural, **corpora amylacea**): Small hyaline mass of degenerate cells and/or inspissated secretion found in the prostate gland.

Coryza (= rhinitis): An acute inflammation of the nasal cavity with increased nasal discharge. It may be caused by bacterial or more commonly by viral infection or by allergic reactions.

Cretinism: A severe congenital hypothyroidism seen in areas where there is an endemic iodine deficiency (from which the pregnant mother suffers) or associated with congenital thyroid anomalies. The baby is small in size, shows mental deficiency, oedematous face, dry skin, macroglossia, umbilical hernia and muscular incoordination. If the condition is due to iodine deficiency, iodine supplements in the diet will prevent the condition from causing permanent damage (see also MYXOEDEMA).

Creutzfeld-Jakob disease: A CNS infection caused by a member of the polyoma subgroup of papovaviruses, which are oncogenic in experimental animals. The disease occurs in middle age and produces DEMENTIA and myoclonus, leading to death within a year.

Crohn's disease (= regional enteritis): A relapsing granulomatous inflammatory disorder of unknown aetiology which commonly affects the terminal ileum or colon (regional colitis) but may occur anywhere in the gastrointestinal tract. In some patients the intestinal involvement is associated with inflammation of the joints, eyes, skin and liver. The disease is similar to idiopathic ulcerative colitis and it is sometimes difficult to differentiate the two. It is most prevalent in the Western world. There is chronic inflammation with adhesions forming, and with occasional cases of perforation and FISTULA formation. There may also be obstruction, rarely haemorrhage and in the late stages, MALABSORPTION SYNDROME.

Curling's ulcer: A type of peptic ulcer developing in the duodenum of people with extensive burns on their body surface.

Cyanocobalamin: A dietary requirement with activity similar to vitamin B_{12}. It contains cobalt and is a water soluble, reddish crystalline substance found in liver, kidney, fish and dairy products.

Cyanosis: A bluish appearance of the skin and nails secondary to deficient oxygenation of the blood.

Cyst: A true cyst is a cavity lined by epithelium and filled with a clear fluid, usually some secretion, for example renal cysts or cysts in the female breast. A false cyst is any cavity filled with fluid, for example hydatid cyst.

Cystadenocarcinoma: A malignant tumour arising from glandular epithelium and in which large CYSTS form.

Cystadenoma: A benign tumour arising from glandular epithelium and in which large CYSTS form, commonly found in the ovaries.

Cytotoxic drugs: Chemotherapeutic agents which have a toxic effect on rapidly dividing cells in the body. Such agents are frequently used in the treatment of cancer but one of their undesirable side effects is the death of other dividing cells in the body (e.g. hair follicular cells, causing temporary baldness, intestinal cells, causing diarrhoea and malabsorption, and bone marrow cells, causing anaemia).

Cytotoxic hypersensitivity (type II): This type of allergic reaction involves direct damage to cells caused by antibodies, usually of the classes IgG or IgM. The antibody is directed against some cell surface component or against a small molecule that may have attached itself to the cell surface. The cells commonly affected in this hypersensitivity are erythrocytes and platelets.

Dacryoadenitis: Inflammation or infection of the tear glands.

Dacryocystitis: Inflammation or infection of the lacrimal apparatus.

Degeneration: Departure from a former state of health and normal appearance, in which tissues and cells deteriorate, showing a corresponding degree of functional aberration, as well as changes in biochemistry and morphology.

Degenerative joint disease: See **Osteoarthrosis**.

Delayed hypersensitivity (type IV) reaction: An example of an allergic response in which the perverted immune response responsible for the damage to the tissues is mediated by T cells, macrophages and interleukins. Examples of this type of hypersensitivity include CONTACT DERMATITIS (e.g. to occupationally contacted chemicals, cosmetics or to items of jewellery) and also the extreme tissue damage seen in some individuals with severe tuberculosis.

Dementia: A severe and ineluctable disorder in which the higher intellectual functions of the brain deteriorate, owing to a progressive loss of neurones. The patient presents with confusion, disorientation, loss of memory which becomes progressively worse, personality disorders and deterioration of the intellectual capacity. It may be caused by a variety of agents: drugs, hyperthyroidism, brain tumours, infections with viruses, alcohol. The majority of cases are idiopathic and untreatable and are due to ALZHEIMER'S DISEASE.

Dementia paralytica: A nervous system disorder seen in some patients with tertiary syphilis, many years (sometimes decades) after initial infection. There is degeneration of cortical neurones with progressive DEMENTIA, tremor, speech disturbances, muscular weakness and ultimately generalized paralysis.

Demyelinating disorders: A group of disorders whose common feature is a progressive demyelination of the nerve sheath, for example MULTIPLE SCLEROSIS.

Dermatitis: Infection or inflammation of the skin; commonly due to autoimmune or allergic causes, for example contact dermatitis due to organic dyes.

Dermatofibroma: A painless skin nodule that is elevated, firm and rounded, most commonly found in the extremities and sometimes associated with SLE. It is a benign mass and requires no treatment unless it is disfiguring or interferes with normal function.

Dermatomyositis: A group of disorders affecting muscles and skin which in many cases is due to autoimmune disease, idiopathic causes or associated with malignancies. There is involvement of connective tissues, joints and muscular tissues, the skin showing a typical rash and a pruritic, eczematous inflammation. Destruction of muscular tissue may be very severe, leading to inability to walk or perform even the simplest of tasks.

Dermoid cyst: TERATOMA of the ovary.

Desensitization: A procedure whereby an attempt is made to cure a hypersensitivity response by introducing the ALLERGEN in a form or by a route which is not its normal way of entering the body and causing the allergy. For example, for an inhaled or ingested food allergen, very dilute preparations of allergen may be injected subcutaneously. These subcutaneous injections are continued over a period of time, the concentration of the allergen being slightly increased with each injection. Desensitization is a very unreliable process and there is immense variation in the individual response to it. Some people are not cured of their hypersensitivity, others are.

Diabetes insipidus: Diabetes insipidus is a condition

caused by a deficiency in the production of ADH by the neurohypophysis. 'Insipidus' refers to the insipid taste of the extremely dilute urine produced by these patients, in contrast to DIABETES MELLITUS where the urine has a sweet taste. The condition is not related to diabetes mellitus, the only common factors being the polyuria that is seen in both disorders and the fact that both are due to hormonal dysfunction.

Diabetes mellitus: A metabolic disorder, in many cases with a genetic basis, characterized by an absolute or relative lack of insulin, which results in impaired metabolism of carbohydrates, fat and protein. Diabetes may have a primary, idiopathic form (97%) or a secondary fom (3%) due to pancreatic islet destruction by inflammation, surgery, tumour or HAEMOCHROMATOSIS. It may occur as a result of excessive production of insulin antagonists. Diabetes may also be seen accompanying other endocrine disorders such as Cushing's syndrome, acromegaly or phaeochromocytoma. 'Diabetes' unqualified generally implies diabetes mellitus.

Diapedesis: The passage of blood cells through the junctions of the endothelial cells in small vessels as seen in acute inflammatory processes.

Diarrhoea: The frequent passage of loose and watery stools because of increased mobility of the large intestine. The faecal material may also contain large amounts of mucus, traces of blood and pus, or fat. It may be due to infection, inflammatory conditions of the bowel, allergic reactions to foodstuffs or reactions to ingested toxins.

Differential diagnosis: A diagnosis made by closely comparing a case of a disease with several diseases producing a range of similar symptoms and signs, so as to exclude as many alternatives as possible, arriving at what is hoped to be the correct and definitive diagnosis.

Differentiation: The process whereby unspecialized, primitive cells undergo a process of specialization, becoming modified in their structure and function such that they are able to perform specific, different, complex tasks that are required in various body sites.

Di-George syndrome: A congenital disorder in which there is agenesis or aplasia of the thymus and parathyroid glands. The affected babies have no T cell function and are very susceptible to viral, fungal, protozoal and tuberculous infections. Death usually occurs before the age of 2 years.

Diphtheria: A serious throat infection with *Corynebacterium diphtheriae* that was very common before the 1920s, nowadays seen only rarely because of widespread immunization programmes that prevent it effectively. The disease causes a pseudomembrane to form in the laryngeal region, which may be extensive enough to cause asphyxia. The organism also produces a potent exotoxin that may cause myocarditis, polyneuritis, adrenal, liver and kidney focal necrosis and ultimately death.

Disease: Any abnormality in the structure and/or function of any tissue in the body.

Dissecting aneurysm: A type of ANEURYSM, commonly seen in the aorta, where the vessel wall splits along the damaged media and blood courses within the split wall, separating inner and outer layers and forming a false lumen while at the same time obliterating the true lumen. This condition is usually rapidly fatal.

Disseminated intavascular coagulation (DIC): Generalized formation of thrombi in the body using up very large numbers of platelets which leads to a THROMBOCYTOPENIA. This occurs after the release into the bloodstream of various thromboplastic substances such as occurs after severe tissue trauma, intrauterine death and amniotic fluid embolism.

Disseminated sclerosis: See **multiple sclerosis**.

Diuresis: Increased formation of usually dilute urine with an increased volume of urine voided. It may be an effect of disease (e.g. DIABETES) or it may be an effect of increased fluid consumption, or an effect of diuretic compounds ingested.

Diurnal: Occurring during the day.

Diverticulitis: Infection or inflammation associated with DIVERTICULA.

Diverticulosis: The condition which is characterized by the presence of (usually multiple) DIVERTICULA.

Diverticulum (plural, **diverticula**): Pouch or sac formed by the herniation of the lining mucous membrane through a tear or weakness of the muscular coat in any tubular organ.

DOPA reaction: A reaction used in the laboratory to identify cells that possess the enzyme tyrosinase (DOPA positive cells). Melanocytes are DOPA positive cells and they are able to carry out the DOPA reaction:

Dihydroxyphenylalanine (DOPA) → tyrosinase oxidation → blackened DOPA

Down's syndome (= Mongolism): A congenital disorder arising as a cytogenetic defect, which usually occurs as a result of non-disjunction of chromosomes, for example trisomy 21. The affected children are mentally retarded and have a characteristic 'Mongoloid' facies, usually dying in puberty or early adulthood.

Duchenne muscular dystrophy: An X-linked recessive disorder, affecting primarily males where there is progressive degeneration of leg and pelvic muscles. It accounts for about half of all muscular dystrophies. The disease appears insidiously between 3 and 5 years of age and the affected children have a waddling gait and marked lordosis. Calf muscles appear large because as the muscle is destroyed it is replaced by fat.

By about 12 years of age, the patients are confined to wheelchairs and as the disease progresses it involves involuntary and cardiac muscles. Death results 10 to 15 years after the onset of symptoms.

Dysarthria: Any difficulty with articulation of speech caused by damage to nervous tissue.

Dysfunction: Partial disturbance, impairment or abnormality in the functioning of an organ.

Dysmenorrhoea: Painful or irregular menstruation.

Dyspareunia: Painful sexual intercourse.

Dyspepsia: An uncomfortable fullness after meals, with nausea, heartburn, belching and often abdominal distension.

Dysphagia: A difficulty in swallowing.

Dysphasia: A disorder in the use of symbols for communication (written, read, spoken, heard) arising because of a cortical disorder.

Dysplasia: A disorderly epithelial cell proliferation which is reversible. It comprises a loss in cellular uniformity together with a loss in architectural orientation of individual cells. This leads to a disordered, defective and atypical growth pattern with an associated compromise in function.

Dystonia: Involuntary, twisting movements over a period of time, usually affecting the proximal muscles.

Dystrophic calcification: An abnormal deposition of calcium in tissue occurring despite normal levels of plasma calcium and in the absence of derangements in calcium metabolism. The calcium is deposited in regions of coagulative, caseous and fat necrosis especially. The larger the area of necrosis and the longer it persists in the body, the more chance there is of calcification occurring (cf. METASTATIC CALCIFICATION; CALCINOSIS).

Dystrophy: A loosely used term to describe pathological changes in tissues occurring as a result of nutritional or metabolic disturbances which may in a large number of cases be related to genetic disease. Such disturbances in the metabolism of the cell will lead to changes in appearance and architecture of the tissue. The condition may also occur in combination with other variations in growth, such as atrophy. The term is now almost exclusively used to describe conditions of skeletal muscle.

Ecchondroma: A cartilaginous nodule, frequently occurring multiply, directed away from the epiphyseal line of origin, most commonly found adjacent to the knee joint. Some familial factors seem to be involved in the development of the lesions. They produce protuberances, pain and deformity and may give rise to malignant lesions. They are treated by surgical excision.

Ecchymosis: A very large HAEMATOMA.

Echinococcosis (= hydatid disease): An infestation by the parasitic tapeworm *Echinococcus granulosus,* usually involving the liver or lungs, but which may occur anywhere in the body. The principal host is the dog, and cattle, sheep, rodents and deer are the intermediate hosts. Humans can become interposed accidentally in the cycle (and act as terminal hosts) by ingesting ova on material contaminated by dog faeces or hair. Hydatid cysts form in the affected organ and may cause jaundice if in the liver, respiratory problems if in the lungs. The only treatment is surgical excision of the cyst. If the cyst ruptures, spontaneously or at surgery, there is the risk of an anaphylactic reaction occurring, which is often fatal.

Eclampsia (= toxaemia of pregnancy): A condition developing in pregnancy and affecting approximately 0.2% of pregnant women, characterized by: epileptiform convulsions, coma and disseminated intravascular coagulation. There may be no preliminary signs, onset can be sudden. If the condition is untreated, there is high foetal (25%) and maternal (10%) mortality. Eclampsia may occur following delivery, usually immediately post-partum. It is more common in first pregnancies and is associated with large placenta, hydatidiform mole, Rh incompatibility, diabetes mellitus and multiple pregnancy. It is also more common in patients with existing hypertension and renal disease.

Ectasia: Dilatation, enlargement (usually applied to ducts or acini of glands).

Ectopia: The presence of normal tissue in an abnormal site (see also CHORISTOMA, HAMARTOMA).

Eczematous disorders: Inflammatory reactions in the skin usually due to hypersensitivities to a large variety of substances. The ALLERGENS may be externally or locally applied or be more distant in origin as manifestations of a generalized hypersensitivity reaction (systemic allergy), producing many and varied skin lesions which may be acute or chronic. Acute eczema is a common condition, a typical example of which is contact dermatitis, in which there is a variable rash of macules, papules and vesicles, later coalescing to produce a diffuse red rash. Chronic eczema is a more severe, long-standing inflammation (for example, neurodermatitis) in which the skin thickens, with mixtures of scaling, oozing, crusting and fissure formation.

Efferent: Conveying away from a centre.

Effusion: The escape of fluid into a part or tissue.

Ehlers-Danlos syndrome: A connective tissue disorder developing congenitally leading to hypermobility of joints, hyperelasticity of skin and tissue fragility ('India rubber man'). Minor trauma may cause severe wounding and bleeding. Joint problems are very common with dislocations, effusions and inflammations being often seen. Life expectancy is usually normal if the patient takes adequate precautions against injury.

Elephantiasis: A condition of long-standing OEDEMA in (usually) the legs where the skin swells and thickens so much that it resembles the skin of elephants. The deformed oedematous and thickened limbs of such people are shaped like those of elephants hence the term to describe this condition.

ELISA: Enzyme-linked immunosorbent assay; a commonly used procedure for carrying out serological tests.

Embolism: The transfer of abnormal material by the bloodstream and its subsequent impaction in the vascular system. The solid or insoluble material is called an embolus and the commonest type of embolus is a thromboembolus which is derived from a dislodged THROMBUS elsewhere in the vascular system.

Embryo: The stage of human development beginning 2 weeks after conception (time of implantation) and ending in the 7th or 8th week of gestation (see also FOETUS).

Emesis: Vomiting.

Emphysema: Permanent increase, beyond the normal, in the size of air spaces distal to the terminal bronchiole, either from dilatation or destruction of their walls. Sometimes both destruction and dilatation of the alveolar walls may be seen. Classification of emphysema depends on the distribution of dilated air spaces within the lung lobule, but severity of the disease is more important in the clinical presentation.

Empyema: Accumulation of pus within a natural cavity in the body, as for example, within the chest or gall bladder.

Encephalitis: An inflammation or infection of the brain caused commonly by viruses such as arboviruses, poliovirus and rabies virus. Herpes simplex can produce encephalitis in the neonate and the elderly. There is progressive degeneration and destruction of nerve cells, with inclusion bodies in some cases. There is proliferation of microglial cells and blood vessels are surrounded by lymphocytes and plasma cells. The disease may be mild or severe with serious residual effects. Encephalitis may also be due to bacterial infections and allergic/autoimmune reactions (e.g. post-measles encephalitis).

Encephaloid cacinoma: A type of malignant tumour which on palpation has a soft, 'brain-like' consistency, for example encephaloid carcinoma of the breast.

Encephalomyelitis: An inflammation or infection of the brain and spinal cord, usually an autoimmune reaction to a viral infection (e.g. rubella, chickenpox or influenza).

Enchondroma: A benign tumour of cartilage which may develop anywhere in the skeleton where cartilage is present. Most occur in the small bones of the hands and feet, deep in the bone (in the spongiosa). Young adults are principally affected. These tumours erode bone and cause pain, swelling and pathological fractures.

Endometriosis externa: Ectopic endometrial tissue outside the uterine wall, the most common sites of occurrence being the ovaries, Fallopian tubes, the rectovaginal septum, pelvic peritoneum, intestinal wall, abdominal wall, umbilicus, laparotomy scars and more rarely lymph nodes, lung, pleura, etc. Endometriosis may be asymptomatic or may produce a painful, swollen mass in the area. Adhesions are common due to fibrosis at the site of endometriosis, and may produce complications such as intestinal obstruction.

Endometriosis interna: See **Adenomyosis of the uterus**.

Endometritis: An inflammation or infection of the endometrium, being in most cases of an acute nature and most commonly due to PUERPERAL SEPSIS. The condition may be very serious or fatal.

Endorphin: One of a group of neuropeptides made by the pituitary gland and acting on the central and peripheral nervous systems to reduce pain by a similar pharmacological action to morphine. Beta-endorphin is a powerful analgesic in humans and animals and is released into the CNS under certain circumstances.

Endotoxic shock (= toxic or **septic shock)**: A type of SHOCK which is brought about by invasion of Gram-negative bacteria into the bloodstream. Inflammatory cells break down the bacterial cell wall and release lipid-rich endotoxin into the circulation. This brings about fever, chills, shock, leukopenia and a host of other symptoms and signs depending on the organism and individual factors. Toxic shock usually has a poor prognosis.

Endotoxin: A product of mostly Gram-negative bacteria which is an integral component of the bacterium and is not released outside the bacterial cell unless the cell is destroyed and degraded. It is a rather weakly toxic compound and relatively large amounts are needed to cause death if released in the body, mainly by mediating ENDOTOXIC SHOCK. Examples include: Pseudomonas endotoxin elaborated by *Pseudomonas aeruginosa* and Proteus endotoxin produced by *Proteus vulgaris.*

Enkephalin: One of two analgesic pentapeptides produced in the brain, pituitary and gastrointestinal tract. Depression of neuronal function is mediated by the compounds and they reduce both physical and emotional perceptions of pain (see also ENDORPHIN).

Enteritis: Infection or inflammation of the small intestine.

Enterocolitis: Infection or inflammation of the small and large intestines.

Ependymona: Tumour of the central nervous system, arising from the cells lining the ventricles of the brain, and the central canal of the spinal cord. Peak incidence is in early childhood. They comprise over half of intraspinal gliomata. They are invasive tumours with a poor prognosis. Only tumours of the conus or filum terminale are sufficiently accessible to allow surgical curative resection.

Epididymitis: Infection or inflammation of the epididymis, such as may occur with gonorrhoea or tuberculosis.

Epiglottitis: Inflammation or infection of the epiglottis, for example by bacteria such as *Haemophilus influenzae*.

Epilepsy: A disturbance in the electrical activity of the brain causing paroxysmal, transient disturbances in brain function. Manifestations include loss of consciousness, abnormal motor function, psychic and sensory disturbances, or perturbation of the autonomic nervous system.

Epiphora: Excessive flow of tears, usually due to an obstruction in the lacrimal duct.

Epispadias: A congenital anomaly of the urethra, where its opening is on the dorsal aspect of the penis, proximal to the glans. There may be urinary incontinence and sexual dysfunction (see also HYPOSPADIAS).

Epistaxis: Bleeding from the nose caused by local irritation, sneezing, fragility of the nasal mucosa, infection, trauma, hypertension, leukaemia or haemorrhagic diatheses.

Epithelioid cell: A derivative of the macrophage seen in chronic inflammatory granulomata. It has a secretory role and is not actively phagocytic. It is an elongated cell resembling an epithelial cell.

Erosion: A superficial destruction of the topmost cells in an epithelial surface, generally confined to the layers above the basement membrane or the muscularis mucosae (see also ULCER).

Erythema (= rubor): A reddened area, usually applied to a reddened area of skin or mucous membrane. It is mostly caused by an active hyperaemia to the site as may be seen with acute inflammation.

Erythroblastosis foetalis: A type II hypersensitivity reaction developing in cases of Rh factor incompatibility between an Rh negative pregnant mother and an Rh positive unborn foetus. The condition develops in the second and subsequent pregnancies, the first pregnancy having sensitized the mother to produce IgG antibody against the baby's Rh positive erythrocytes. As the IgG crosses the placenta there is destruction of the foetal red blood cells with severe anaemia, jaundice and hepatosplenomegaly developing in the foetus. Passive immunization of all Rh negative mothers just before delivery in all of their pregnancies with pooled human anti-Rh IgG prevents the condition in all cases.

Ewing's tumour (= 'round cell tumour'): A rare bone tumour, the exact cells of origin not being known but arising from cells of the reticuloendothelial system in bone marrow, generally seen most often in children. It is a fleshy, non-bony tumour with reactive bone formation around it causing the radiological 'onion skin' appearance. Radical operative procedures early on have yielded a few long-term survivors but generally there is a very poor prognosis for this tumour with an average 5-year survival of < 5%.

Exophthalmos: A bulging outwards of the eyeball, commonly associated with THYROTOXICOSIS or with lesions inside the bony orbit.

Exostosis cartilaginea (= osteochondroma): A common neoplasm due to localized overgrowth of bone. It gives a knobbly, bony projection of varying size, on the distal part of which is a small cap of cartilage. The neoplasm mostly occurs at the metaphyseal surface of long bones, mostly around the knee. It is not usually significant although it may impede joint movement or have pressure effects. There is an hereditary form where multiple cartilaginous exostoses occur, the condition having potential for malignant transformation to CHONDROSARCOMA or OSTEOSARCOMA.

Exotoxin: A product of mostly Gram-positive bacteria which is released to the exterior of the bacterial cell. It is a very potently toxic compound and only minimal amounts may be enough to cause death if released in the body. Examples include: tetanus toxin elaborated by *Clostridium tetani*, diphtheria toxin produced by *Corynebacterium diphtheriae*, enterotoxin produced by *Staphylococcus aureus*, botulinum toxin produced by *Clostridium botulinum* (see also ENDOTOXIN).

Exudate: The fluid portion of the acute inflammatory response formed as a consequence of increased vascular permeability, seen in the early stages of the reaction (cf. INFILTRATE).

Faecolith: An inspissated, hardened mass of faecal material that is seen in the lumen of the large intestine. It may cause obstruction, especially when it occurs in the lumen of the appendix, where it is often associated with appendicitis.

Fat necrosis: A type of necrosis seen in adipose tissue. It may be traumatic, in which the adipocytes degenerate following trauma (e.g. after a blow to the breast), or it may be enzymatic, in which lipases break down the triglycerides in the cells, forming calcium salts with the free fats (this subtype is only seen in the vicinity of the pancreas).

Fatty change: A reactive change of cells to injury in which fat droplets accumulate in the cell cytoplasm as a result of impaired lipid metabolism. Very commonly seen in the liver, myocardium and kidney tubules.

Fatty streak: A lesion found in the intima of large arteries which consists of a shallow, yellow intimal plaque, beginning as a lesion less than 1 mm in diameter, soon growing to streaks 2 mm in width and 1–2 cm long. They are flattened or slightly raised lesions, lifting the endothelium slightly, and are often hard to distinguish macroscopically unless they have been stained with a lipophilic stain. They occur in childhood and young adulthood and some workers consider them to be precursors to the ATHEROMA.

Fibrin: Insoluble, polymerized form of FIBRINOGEN.

Fibrinogen: A soluble plasma protein that may be converted to its insoluble form, fibrin, by thrombin when the coagulation cascade is activated. It is important in haemostasis and THROMBOSIS.

Fibroadenoma: A benign tumour composed of dense collagenous stromal tissue in which are interspersed glandular nests, most commonly seen in the female breast. It is an encapsulated, freely mobile lump, non-tender and round, seen in the breast of women under 25 years and is associated with oestrogen excess. The lesion does not have a high potential for malignant transformation but is nevertheless excised for histological examination.

'Fibroid': See **Leiomyoma**.

Fibroma: A rather uncommon, benign tumour of connective tissue derived from the fibroblast. It forms a circumscribed, hard mass which is freely mobile and easily excised.

Fibrosarcoma: A rather uncommon, malignant tumour of connective tissue derived from the fibroblast. It is very aggressive and is associated with a poor prognosis.

Fibrosis: The process of repair by connective tissue or scarring is known as fibrosis and is the sequela of many injuries to the body where tissue has been irreversibly damaged and has undergone necrosis. It is a reaction of fibroblasts in connective tissues and much collagen is laid down by these cells to give rise to the scar.

Fibrous dysplasia of bone: See **Albright's syndrome**.

Fistula (plural, **fistulae**): An abnormal communication between two organs with a lumen or between one such organ and the exterior of the body. Fistulae form commonly in association with inflammatory/infectious processes or in association with tumours, for example a vesicovaginal fistula in association with carcinoma of the bladder.

Foetus: The stage in the development of the human beginning with the 8th week of gestation and ending with birth (see also EMBRYO).

Fomites (singular, **fomes**): Contaminated inanimate objects that may spread infection.

Fracture: Any discontinuity of bone caused by trauma. It includes bone breaks, cracks and crushing injuries. Fracture may occur after direct application of force to the bone or after force is transmitted indirectly along the line of the bone (e.g. fracture of the radius due to falling on an outstretched hand).

Furuncle (= '**boil**'): A large ABSCESS of the skin, often caused by *Staphylococcus aureus.*

Gammopathy: Any disorder characterized by increased levels of gamma globulins in the blood.

Ganglioneuroma: A tumour of the ganglionic nerve cells.

Gangrene: A condition where necrotic lesions affecting skin or mucosal surfaces, for example the bowel, are infected by bacteria which cause putrefaction (the production of foul-smelling gas with brown, green or black tissue discolouration). This putrefactive form of necrosis is called gangrene (or gas-gangrene if gas is produced in the tissues). The main causative bacterium is *Clostridium perfringens.*

Gardner's disease: An inherited disease transmitted as an autosomal dominant in which multiple polyps form in the large intestine but there are other associated disorders such as fibrous dysplasia of the skull, extra teeth, osteomata, fibromata and epidermal cysts. The patients have an increased risk of developing malignancies in the bowel, bone and connective tissues (cf. POLYPOSIS COLI).

Gastritis: An inflammation of the stomach mucosa which may be acute or chronic. Often the term is used vaguely and is applied to any clinical syndrome which presents with pain or discomfort in the left upper abdominal quadrant, whether or not there is any indication of pathological changes in the gastric mucosa.

Ghon focus: The first site (and the resultant lesion) at which *Mycobacterium tuberculosis* lodges in the lung in a case of TB, usually subpleurally in the midzone of the lung. Over 2–3 weeks a tubercle develops at this primary site and is 1–2 cm in size. Caseation is present and the tubercle enlarges gradually. The mycobacteria, in macrophages, spread to the local hilar lymph nodes in which tubercles and caseation also form. The combination of the Ghon focus and caseous lymph nodes is known as the Ghon complex or primary complex. The Ghon complex will usually heal by fibrosis and often calcify, becoming easily visible on chest X-ray.

Giant cell: Any cell formed (usually) from fusion of macrophages or other cells of the monocyte line and possessing more than two nuclei. Examples are Aschoff giant cells (approximately two to five nuclei, found in rheumatic heart disease), Langhan's giant cells ($\approx$50 to 150 nuclei, found in tubercles), Reed-Sternberg giant cells (two to three nuclei, found in HODGKIN'S DISEASE).

Gigantism: A disorder of growth hormone secretion by the pituitary occurring before fusion of the metaphyseal growth plates and leading to excessive lengthening of the long bones of the body causing an excessive increase in size and stature of the patient.

Glaucoma: A condition of raised intraocular pressure due to obstruction of the normal outflow of aqueous humour. There is pain, impaired vision, red eye and a dilated pupil with nausea and vomiting.

Glioblastoma multiforme: A highly malignant form of ASTROCYTOMA (Grade III, IV), which is rapidly fatal.

Gliosis: The process of glial cell proliferation in the central nervous system, occurring after destruction of nervous tissue. It is a repair process and is equivalent to FIBROSIS in other tissues.

Glomerulonephritis (plural, **glomerulonephritides**): A general term embracing a wide group of disorders. The renal lesions in these disorders are primarily glomerular, usually some form of injury to the glomeruli initiating the disease. All other lesions seen in glomerulonephritis are secondary to the disease process in the glomeruli. Many cases of glomerulonephritis are due to an immunological mechanism operating, especially related to deposition of immune complexes on the glomerulus. There is destruction of glomerular tissue and inflammation contributing to the damage.

Glossitis: An infection or inflammation of the tongue.

Gluten enteropathy: See **Coeliac disease**.

Glycosuria: The presence of glucose in the urine.

Goitre: Any enlargement of the thyroid gland, whether associated with hyperthyroidism or hypothyroidism.

Gout: An inherited autosomal dominant metabolic disease affecting males more commonly than females. Due to defects in the metabolism of nitrogen (protein) excessive uric acid is formed and may be deposited in the soft tissues where the sodium biurate crystals set up a chronic inflammatory granulomatous reaction, leading to TOPHUS formation. There are long-term complications in gout. The production of excessive uric acid leads to its increased excretion via the kidneys, leading to kidney stone formation (urate stones). There is also associated vascular disease and renal failure due to nephritis.

Granulation tissue: A tissue found wherever repair and ORGANIZATION processes are operating, consisting of fibroblasts producing collagen and 'budding' (proliferating) capillaries. The fibroblasts divide and migrate into the area, along with the budding capillary loops. Granulation tissue migrates inwards towards the centre of an injured area from the undamaged margins and its function is to repair the tissue by laying down collagenous scar.

Granuloma: A characteristic lesion of chronic inflammatory states in which a grain-like lump 1 mm to 1 cm forms in the inflamed tissue. It consists of an aggregation of chronic inflammatory cells such as macrophages, their derivatives (EPITHELIOID CELLS, GIANT CELLS), lymphocytes, plasma cells and few granulocytes. There may be a central region of necrosis (e.g. caseous in the TUBERCLE, gummatous in the GUMMA) and a surrounding capsule of collagen and fibroblasts.

Granulomatosis: A condition where multiple granulomata develop in tissues as in berylliosis or Wegener's granulomatosis.

Granulomatous disease of childhood: An inherited disease transmitted as an X-linked genetic disorder in which an undefined enzyme defect prevents neutrophils destroying phagocytosed bacteria. Patients present in infancy suffering from multiple pyogenic infections.

Granulosa-theca cell tumour: A usually benign tumour of the ovary, often oestrogen secreting, occurring more often post-menopausally. These tumours may result in hyperoestrinism, and can lead to menstrual irregularity, endometrial hyperplasia, endometrial carcinoma and fibrocystic disease of the breast.

Graves' disease: See **Thyrotoxicosis**.

Guillain-Barré syndrome: This is an ascending paralysis that occurs days to weeks after a non-specific viral illness or viral immunization. It starts in the feet, ascends to the leg, affects the upper limbs and finally the muscles of respiration within hours or a day or two. The disease reaches a peak in a week, remains static for a fortnight then gradually subsides, usually leaving no sequelae. Artificial respiration for the duration of the illness is essential if respiration is affected. Widespread segmental demyelination and lymphocytic infiltration is seen in the cord and CSF protein is raised.

Gumma (plural, **gummata**): The lesion of tertiary syphilis, a GRANULOMA 1 mm to 1 cm in diameter. There is a central region of gummatous necrosis surrounded by chronic inflammatory cells and a fibrous capsule. Many gummata may coalesce to form large lesions, or they may rupture onto a surface and give rise to ulcers.

Gynaecomastia: Breast enlargement in a male.

Haemangioma (= 'birthmark', 'port wine stain'): An example of a HAMARTOMA, which is an excessive focal overgrowth of blood vessels in a tissue, most obvious in the skin. It consists of normal blood vessels in continuity with the rest of the circulation. It appears as a red area in the skin and may be unsightly but usually causes no other problems. If subjected to trauma it may bleed very easily as it is composed of vessels with very thin walls.

Haematite lung (= **silicosiderosis**): A PNEUMOCONIOSIS caused by the inhalation of iron oxide (haematite) dust usually seen in miners and quarry workers. It gives the lungs a rusty red colour and there is diffuse fibrosis and emphysema. The patients have a higher incidence of tuberculosis and lung carcinoma than normal individuals.

Haematemesis: The vomiting of blood.

Haematoma (= 'bruise'): A localized mass of extravasated blood in tissue.

Haematuria: The presence of blood in the urine.

Haemochromatosis (= 'bronzed diabetes'): An autosomal dominant disorder causing increased absorption of iron in the body. Affected individuals have ten or more times the normal level of iron in their tissues (2–3 g normal, up to 35–40 g in the condition). Males are affected more commonly, females being protected by menstruation. Patients present at ≈40 years with liver damage, pancreatic damage (with diabetes mellitus), testicular atrophy and skin pigmentation, all effects of iron deposition in tissues.

Haemolytic anaemia: A type of anaemia resulting after excessive destruction of erythrocytes, as seen, for example, after some inherited diseases or after autoimmune reactions.

Haemopericardium: An accumulation of blood within the pericardial sac, usually due to haemorrhage into the pericardium. It occurs as a result of rupture of the heart, either as a result of a stab wound or more commonly associated with a myocardial infarct.

Haemophilia A: An X-linked recessive genetic disorder affecting primarily males, in which there is a deficiency in clotting factor VIII. There is tendency for haemorrhage from even trivial trauma and the disorder must be treated by injections of the missing factor (see also CHRISTMAS DISEASE).

Haemoptysis: The expectoration of blood by coughing from the larynx or lower respiratory tract (cf. HAEMATEMESIS).

Haemorrhage: The loss of blood from the vascular system into the exterior of the body or into body cavities. Usually caused by trauma to blood vessels and/or HAEMORRHAGIC DIATHESES.

Haemorrhagic diathesis (plural, ~ **diatheses**): Any abnormality or defect in the blood coagulation mechanism which leads to a predisposition to HAEMORRHAGE.

Haemorrhagic pancreatitis: An acute inflammatory condition of the pancreas characterized by the release of pancreatic enzymes into the substance of the pancreas, leading to autodigestion of the tissue, damage to blood vessels, haemorrhage and FAT NECROSIS. It may be caused by excessive alcohol consumption, atherosclerosis or idiopathic disease. It may be fatal or lead to chronic disease and uncommonly to DIABETES MELLITUS.

Haemorrhoid: A varicose dilatation of the superior or inferior haemorrhoidal plexus of veins.

Haemosiderosis (= **siderosis**): The accumulation of haemosiderin in tissues, usually seen to be inside macrophages. It occurs whenever there is a transient excess of iron in a localized area of tissue, as may occur after a haemorrhage or prolonged congestion.

Hamartoma: A focal developmental anomaly which may be seen in any tissue of the body and usually arises because of excessive proliferation of a group of normal cells when the tissue is differentiating or growing. It may be defined as an excessive, focal overgrowth of normal, mature cells in an organ that contains identical cellular elements normally found in that organ. A typical example is a naevus ('mole' or 'birthmark') which consists of large nests of normal melanocytes situated in the skin.

Hashimoto's thyroiditis: An autoimmune disorder of the thyroid gland seen more frequently in women between the ages of 30 and 50 years. The thyroid substance is replaced by a lymphocytic cell infiltrate until the tissue resembles a lymph node rather than a gland. There is goitre and hypothyroidism which may in severe cases progress to MYXOEDEMA. Treatment is by thyroid hormone replacement therapy.

Heberden's nodes: Small bony projections which occur on the terminal joints of the fingers in the elderly in association with OSTEOARTHROSIS.

Helper T cells: A subgroup of lymphocytes also called T4 cells that are involved in 'turning on' the immune response. They are important in the cell-mediated response but also assist in the formation of antibody by secreting factors that stimulate B cells and plasma cells.

Hemiplegia: Paralysis of one side of the body. A common aftermath of CEREBRAL INFARCTION.

Hepatitis: Any infection or inflammation of the liver which is diffuse in its nature, affecting the whole liver. There may be acute and chronic forms of hepatitis. Most commonly the term hepatitis refers to viral hepatitis caused by the hepatitis B virus.

Hepatitis B: See **Serum hepatitis**.

Hepatization: A consolidation of lung tissue in which the normally air-containing alveoli become filled with exudate, blood and inflammatory cells in the course of pneumonia. The term is descriptive and draws attention to the resemblance of the consolidated lung tissue to liver tissue.

Hepatoblastoma: A very rare, primary malignant tumour of the hepatocytes occurring in neonates and composed of embryonic liver cells.

Hepatocarcinoma (= **malignant hepatoma**): A rather uncommon primary malignancy of the hepatocytes. It is often associated with cirrhosis of the liver (alcoholic, chronic hepatitis B), and is often multiple. There are infrequent metastases but the prognosis is very poor. There is only a 5% 5-year survival. It is usually rapidly fatal, within months of diagnosis. In some countries this is the commonest malignancy (e.g. in China, Indonesia, some parts of Africa). The high incidence of HEPATITIS and dietary factors are thought to be important in these cases.

Hernia: A protrusion of a body viscus outside its natural cavity. It may be internal (within the body) or external (into the exterior environment).

Heterograft: See **Xenograft**.

Hiatus hernia: An internal HERNIA where part of the stomach herniates into the thoracic cavity through the oesophageal hiatus.

Hidradenoma: A tumour of the sweat gland acini, usually well differentiated and slow growing, forming papillary, cystic or solid lesions.

Hirschsprung's disease: A disease arising out of the congenital absence of autonomic ganglia in the smooth muscle coat of the colon resulting in poor or absent peristalsis in the involved region of the colon. There is subsequent accumulation of faeces and MEGACOLON develops. There may be intermittent vomiting diarrhoea alternating with constipation and abdominal distension. The condition develops in childhood and the procedure is to remove surgically the abnormal portion of bowel.

'Hives': See **Urticaria**.

Hodgkin's disease: The most common form of LYMPHOMA arising in the lymphoreticular tissues. The origin of the neoplastic cells is still undetermined (may be derived from lymphoid cells or from cells of the mononuclear phagocyte systems). There is progressive, painless enlargement of lymph nodes (especially the cervical) and spleen, anorexia, weight loss, night sweats, generalized pruritus, anaemia and low-grade fever. It is more common in males and generally has a good prognosis with treatment.

Homograft: See **Allograft**.

Honeycomb lung: A descriptive term indicating that extensive and severe EMPHYSEMA is present in a lung. It may be seen in a variety of conditions such as congenital disorders, pneumoconioses or long-standing cases of COAD.

Hordeolum (= 'stye'): A pyogenic infection of one of the glands at the base of an eyelash, equivalent to a FURUNCLE elsewhere in the skin.

Horseshoe kidney: A developmental anomaly of the kidneys in which the two kidneys are fused at their lower pole (usually). There is no associated abnormality in function. The condition often remains undiagnosed during life.

Human immunodeficiency virus (HIV): A RETROVIRUS, the cause of AIDS.

Human T cell lymphotropic virus (HTLV): A group of RETROVIRUSES, the cause of amongst other diseases a type of leukaemia.

Human papilloma virus (HPV): A Papovavirus, the cause of the common and genital warts. Many different serotypes exist.

Humoral immune response: The type of immunity relying on the activity of B cells and PLASMA CELLS, the secretors of ANTIBODY.

Huntington's chorea: An autosomal dominant disorder in which symptoms usually become manifest at middle age (although a juvenile form, the Westphal variant, is known). Degeneration of the head of the caudate nucleus and putamen occurs with neurone loss followed by gliosis. Changes may be so marked that almost total atrophy of the head of the caudate nucleus occurs. The disease is characterized by abnormal involuntary movements of the limbs and fingers. Choreiform movements are followed by dementia and both progress until over a period of 10–15 years the patient is totally incapacitated and bedridden.

Hydatid disease: See **Echinococcosis**.

Hydatidiform mole: A rather rare disorder of the chorionic tissue of the placenta. There is conversion of some or all of the chorionic villi into clear grape-like vesicular masses. In affected villi, blood vessels are absent, and stroma is oedematous. A foetus is usually not present (= complete mole), but rarely there is a foetus present (= incomplete mole). Usually there is spontaneous abortion of the mole by the 18th to the 20th week. There will be haemorrhage and passage of grape-like masses in some cases. In 5% of cases, the mole may undergo malignant change to CHORIO-CARCINOMA. The hydatidiform mole secretes HCG.

Hydrocephalus: Hydrocephalus results from obstruction of cerebrospinal fluid outflow either at the aqueduct of Sylvius or the foramen of Magendie or of Luschka. Associated with the condition is an increase in CSF pressure in some part of the CNS. There may be ventricular distension, which may convert the cerebral cortex into an atrophic shell surrounding an enormous bag of fluid. Causes of hydrocephalus include compensatory (increased CSF, due to decreased brain volume) congenital malformations (e.g. ARNOLD-CHIARI MALFORMATION), obstructing tumours, infectious scars (usually from tuberculous meningitis) or idiopathic.

Hydrocoele: Accumulation of serous fluid in any cavity or sac-like organ or duct. The term is most commonly used to describe such fluid accumulations in the tunica vaginalis of the testis or in the spermatic duct. It is caused by inflammatory, obstructive or lymphatic drainage disorders of the tissue. Persisting hydrocoele has to be treated by surgery and treatment of the underlying cause.

Hydronephrosis: A condition of the kidneys which may be unilateral or bilateral. There is progressive pressure atrophy of the renal parenchyma due to retention of urine in the renal pelvis caused by some obstruction in the urinary flow. In advanced hydronephrosis there is less urine excretion and renal failure supervenes, with hypertension and uraemia.

Hydropericardium: An accumulation of TRANSUDATE within the pericardial cavity. It may be seen with conditions causing generalized oedema.

Hypercapnia: An excessively high partial pressure of carbon dioxide in arterial blood.

Hyperemesis gravidarum: An abnormal, idiopathic condition of pregnancy in which there is vomiting, weight loss and fluid and electrolyte imbalances. If the condition persists there may be brain, liver and kidney damage with a fatal outcome.

Hyperlipidaemia: The presence of abnormally high levels of lipids in the blood.

Hypermetropia (= hyperopia): The eyeball is shorter than normal in this condition and the retina lies in front of the focal point, with vision better for far objects than for near objects ('farsightedness'). A convex lens is used in spectacles to correct this disorder.

Hyperopia: See **Hypermetropia**.

Hyperostosis frontalis interna: An idiopathic disorder, the characteristic of which is thickening of the frontal bones of the cranium while the posterior of the skull presents a normal appearance. Foci of hyperostosis in the skull may sometimes be associated with slowly growing tumours of the cranial cavity, for example meningioma.

Hyperparathyroidism: A disorder in the activity of any or all of the four parathyroid glands associated with an increased secretion of parathormone. This causes an increased resorption of calcium from bones, increased absorption of calcium from the gut and by the kidney and a consequent hypercalcaemia and META-STATIC CALCIFICATION. There may be CALCULUS formation in the kidneys, OSTEOPOROSIS in bones, pancreatitis and peptic ulceration. In long-standing cases CNS changes will develop.

Hyperplasia: The increase in the size of a tissue or organ due to an increase in the number of its specialized, parenchymal cells. It is usually caused by excessive action of a normal stimulus and may be physiological (e.g. breast tissue in lactation), pathological (e.g. breast tissue in adenosis) or compensatory (kidney tubules in the remaining kidney after a unilateral nephrectomy).

Hypersensitivity: See **Allergic response**.

Hypertension: A persistent elevation of blood pressure. It may be associated with the systemic circulation in which case values above 140/90 mmHg are considered to be hypertensive or it may be associated with the portal circulation as is commonly seen in CIRRHOSIS of the liver.

Hyperthermia: An excessively high body temperature.

Hypertrophy: The increase in the size of a tissue or organ due to an increase in the size of its individual, specialized, parenchymal cells. It is usually caused by a mechanical stimulus, i.e. increased work load, and pure hypertrophy without accompanying hyperplasia is seen only in striated muscles. It may be physiological (e.g. skeletal muscles of an athlete) or pathological (e.g. left ventricle of the heart in systemic hypertension).

Hypoplasia: The condition whereby an organ has failed to attain full size. Such a tissue or organ is much smaller than normal and may be dysfunctional, for example microcephaly in which the foetus has a brain much smaller than normal. Although this condition is not fatal there is usually some mental retardation.

Hypospadias: A congenital anomaly of the urethra, where its opening is on the ventral aspect of the penis, proximal to the glans. Urinary incontinence does not occur as the sphincters are unaffected. Any sexual or urinary dysfunction is treated surgically (see also EPISPADIAS).

Icterus: See **Jaundice**.

Ileitis: Inflammation or infection of the ileum. A common form is regional ileitis or CROHN'S DISEASE.

Ileus: Any obstruction of the intestines, whether mechanical as may be caused by tumour growth or intraluminal masses, or adynamic, caused by failure of normal peristalsis.

Infarct: A region of tissue which has undergone anoxic necrosis due to an acute interruption to its normal blood flow. A pale infarct is seen usually when end-arteries in organs with a single blood supply are obstructed (usually by a THROMBOEMBOLUS), whereas red infarcts are seen when venous channels are obstructed, preventing outflow (and ultimately inflow) of blood.

Infiltrate: The cellular component of the inflammatory response (cf. EXUDATE).

Inflammation: The reaction of connective tissue elements to sublethal injury.

Insulinoma: A benign neoplasm of the insulin-secreting cells of the islets of Langerhans of the pancreas. The tumour secretes excessive quantities of insulin which may bring about hypoglycaemia.

Interleukin: A soluble, chemical messenger secreted by white cells (mainly lymphocytes and macrophages), capable of transmitting information to other white cells. Interleukins are important compounds of the immune system.

Intertrigo: An inflammatory condition of opposing skin surfaces caused by friction (e.g. the axillae or the inner aspect of the thighs).

Intussusception: The invagination of one portion of the intestine into the lumen of the bowel immediately distal (like a telescope). The apex passes down the lumen, dragging mesentery and its vessels with it, thus strangulating vessels and causing the trapped portion of bowel to undergo necrosis.

Involucrum (plural, **involucra**): A coating or a sheath.

Involution: The process of physiological atrophy (e.g. seen in the uterus after parturition).

Ischaemia: The acute interruption of blood supply to an organ or tissue, as occurs with EMBOLISM in a nutritive artery. The tissue suffers from ANOXIA and dies unless the vessel is made patent again rapidly.

Isograft: A transplanted tissue between two genetically identical individuals, for example between identical twins or between highly inbred laboratory animals.

Jaundice (= **icterus**): A yellow colouration due to deposition of bilirubin (conjugated or unconjugated) in the skin and sclerae. It becomes visible when the serum bilirubin concentration exceeds 34 mmol/L (normally less than 12 mmol/L). Jaundice can be prehepatic, hepatic or post-hepatic. Most bilirubin comes from the splenic breakdown of red blood cells (85%); the rest comes from bone marrow and metabolism of cytochromes and myoglobin.

Karyolysis: Dissolution of the nucleus in a moribund cell.

Karyorrhexis: Fragmentation of the nucleus in an injured cell.

Keloid: The laying down of excessive amounts of collagen which occurs in some individuals, forming a protruding, tumour-like growth of scar tissue. This tends to occur more commonly in people with dark skin pigmentation, being rare in Nordic-type Caucasians and redheads. Instead of contracting and settling down, as most scars do, keloid scars may continue growing, producing large protruding masses. This bulging scar is disfiguring and unsightly but often removal of the keloid simply leads to further keloid scar formation. Laser therapy may be employed in this case.

Keratosis: A reaction occurring in keratinized epithelium in response to an irritant or injurious stimulus, resulting in overgrowth and thickening of the keratinized layer of the epithelium.

Kernicterus: An abnormal toxic accumulation of bilirubin in the CNS especially seen in neonates (= hyperbilirubinaemia of the newborn). In this case the disease develops because of congenital liver diseases (especially enzyme defects), haemolytic disease (e.g. ERYTHROBLASTOSIS FOETALIS) or immaturity of the liver (in premature babies). The bilirubin in the brain may cause damage and mental deficiency if untreated.

Koilonychia: The condition where the nails become concave, having a spoon-shaped depression on their surface. It may be seen in anaemia.

Krukenberg tumour: A secondary, mucoid, adenocarcinoma of the ovary, most frequently seen in association with carcinoma of the stomach. The tumour metastasizes from the stomach to the ovary by transcoelomic spread.

Kyphosis: Abnormal convexity in the curvature of the thoracic spine when viewed from the side.

Lazy leukocyte syndrome: A defect in the motility of leukocytes, leading to poor chemotaxis and a failure of the cells to localize in sites where they are needed. Hence, bacteria and other microbes proliferate unchecked causing serious or even fatal infections.

'Leather bottle stomach': See **Linitis plastica**.

Leiomyoma (= **fibroleiomyoma** = **'fibroid'**): A benign tumour of smooth muscle. Very commonly seen in the uterus.

Leiomyosarcoma: A rare malignant tumour arising from smooth muscle cells occurring in any situation of the body which possesses these cells, for example the uterus.

Leukaemias: Conditions resulting from neoplastic proliferation of leukocytes. Lymphoid or myelogenous cells are most commonly involved. When the proliferation involves the early immature cells the disease is recognized as an acute leukaemia and tends to run a rapid course (sometimes also called a '-blastic' leukaemia). In more slowly progressive states, predominantly mature cells are present in excess. These are the chronic leukaemias ('-cytic' leukaemias).

Leukocytosis: An increased number of normal white cells in the circulation, as may be seen after a serious infection.

Leukopenia: A decrease in the numbers of circulating white cells to below 4000 per μL. May be primary due to a decreased production of white cells in the bone marrow or may be secondary to other diseases. Any or all types of the white cells may be affected and depending on the cell component affected there is a more or less severe disease.

Leukoplakia: A raised, whitish plaque seen on mucous membranes or thin skin, which on microscopy shows typical dysplastic changes of the epithelium. Due to chronic irritation or injury, this condition is premalignant and will usually progress to a SQUAMOUS CELL CARCINOMA.

Lichen planus: An idiopathic skin disease in which there is chronic dermatitis leading to the formation of reddish purple, flat-topped papules on the skin over the extensor surfaces and around the mouth. The disease is episodic in nature and may involve the mucous membranes. Often the nails of the affected people have longitudinal ridges.

Linitis plastica (= 'leather bottle stomach'): An infiltrating form of carcinoma of the stomach in which the tumour rapidly grows along the stomach wall, invading and infiltrating it, causing gross thickening and contraction of the stomach and making it appear like a 'leather bottle'.

Lipofuscin: A non-toxic, yellow-brown, insoluble pigment seen to accumulate intracellularly, especially within permanent cells such as cardiocytes and neurones. It represents the remains of indigestible debris that the cell cannot dispose of.

Lipoma: A benign tumour of the adipocytes, commonly occurring in the subcutaneous tissues.

Liposarcoma: very rare, malignant tumour of the adipocytes, associated with a poor prognosis.

Liquefactive necrosis: See **Colliquative necrosis**.

Lobar pneumonia: Pneumonia in which the inflammation is sharply confined to one or two lobes which are diffusely affected. Rarely, larger areas of the lungs may be involved. More than 90% of cases of lobar pneumonia are caused by *Streptococcus pneumoniae* ('pneumococci'). Follows a well-characterized clinical course over 8 days, the patient either dying on the eighth day or surviving, with the pneumonia resolving in the next 2 to 3 weeks (cf. BRONCHOPNEUMONIA).

Lymphadenitis: An inflammation or infection of the lymph nodes generally causing their enlargement and prominence with pain or discomfort.

Lymphadenopathy: Any disorder of the lymph nodes which causes them to become enlarged and more prominent. For example, lymphadenopathy may be seen when a tumour is invading lymph nodes or when there is hyperplasia of the lymph node due to an infection.

Lymphangitis: An inflammation of the lymphatic vessels generally caused by infection with *Streptococcus* spp. The lymphatic vessels are seen as red streaks beneath the skin and there is associated fever, leukocytosis, myalgia and headache.

Lymphocyte: A mononuclear, agranular blood cell, making up approximately 30% of the white cell count. Lymphocytes are subdivided into functional groups, B LYMPHOCYTES and T LYMPHOCYTES being the two types. Lymphocytes are the effector cells of the immune response.

Lymphoma (= **lymphosarcoma** in most cases): The malignant lymphomata are all neoplastic proliferations of the peripheral lymphoid tissue, the primary site of involvement usually being the lymph nodes or the spleen. The systemic tumour spread, outside the primary sites, usually occurs later in the course of these disorders. Many variants are known and the course of the disease may be very long and follow an almost benign progression or, at the other extreme, there may be a typical malignant rapid progression with extremely poor prognosis (see also HODGKIN'S DISEASE, RETICULOSARCOMA, PLASMACYTOMA, LEUKAEMIA).

Macroglobulinaemia: See **Waldenström's macroglobulinaemia**.

Macronodular cirrhosis: A type of CIRRHOSIS in which the regenerative nodules are uniform in size and rather large.

Macrophage: The cell in tissues derived from the monocyte of the blood. It is a long-lived phagocytic cell that also has important functions in cell-mediated immunity.

Macule (Latin: a spot): A colour change in the skin without elevation or depression.

Malabsorption syndrome: A collection of symptoms and signs arising in any condition where there is impaired intestinal absorption of nutrients. Depending on the substance malabsorbed, different presentations will be observed for example STEATORROEA when fats are malabsorbed.

Malaria: A protozoal infection of the blood caused by members of the genus *Plasmodium* transmitted by mosquitoes which act as the VECTOR of the infection. It is a disease characterized by high fever, debilitation and fatigue and may be fatal.

Malformation: An abnormality in the structure of a body part, usually implying a gross, congenital anomaly.

Malignant: 'Evil', tending to go from bad to worse, life threatening and eventually causing the death of the patient if left untreated; for example malignant tumour, malignant hypertension (cf. BENIGN).

Malignant hepatoma: See **Hepatocarcinoma**.

Malignant melanoma: A very aggressive malignant tumour of the melanocytes which tends to spread early. It is most commonly seen in the skin but may also occur as a primary in the brain, squamous mucosae (e.g. vagina) or eye. Australia has the highest incidence of this tumour in the world.

Mallory-Weiss syndrome: Massive haemorrhage from a tear in the oesophagogastric junction, usually caused by protracted vomiting seen in alcoholics or in patients with pyloric obstruction. Excellent prognosis after surgery.

Malnutrition: Any abnormality in nutrition, resulting from an unbalanced, inadequate or excessive diet, or alternatively due to MALABSORPTION of nutrients by the intestine.

Marfan's syndrome: An autosomal dominant disorder of connective tissues causing musculoskeletal system abnormalities. Patients show muscular underdevelopment, ligament laxity, joint hypermobility and bone elongation. Connective tissues in the cardiovascular system and the eyes may also lead to severe disease in these regions (e.g. aortic ANEURYSMS, dislocation of the lens).

Margination: The phase of acute inflammation in which neutrophils stick firmly to the internal aspect of the endothelium of vessels prior to DIAPEDESIS and emigration out into the intercellular spaces to form the INFILTRATE.

Mast cells: Cells found in loose connective tissue throughout the body and derived from the basophils of the blood. They contain numerous granules full of histamine, serotonin and other pharmacologically active compounds important in inflammatory reactions. They play an important role in ANAPHYLACTIC RE-ACTIONS and ASTHMA.

Mastitis: Infection or inflammation of the breast.

Meckel's diverticulum: This is a congenital anomaly found in 2 to 3% of the population, arising from persistence of the omphalomesenteric duct. It is a solitary DIVERTICULUM usually within 60 cm of the ileocaecal valve. It varies in appearance from a fibrotic cord to a pouch with a lumen larger than the ileum and is up to 5 or 6 cm in length. The wall of the diverticulum is like the small bowel, but there may be nests of gastric mucosa or, rarely, even pancreatic rests. Sometimes there may be peptic ulceration in the diverticulum with perforation, adhesions, haemorrhage, etc. Otherwise there are no symptoms.

Meconium ileus: An obstructive disease of the small intestine of neonates caused by the impaction of a plug of thick and tenacious meconium (mucus, amniotic fluid, epithelial cells, bile pigment and debris), usually close to the ileocaecal valve. There is abdominal distension, vomiting, failure to pass faeces in the first 24–48 hours after birth, and rapid dehydration. Enemas or, in complicated cases, surgery is needed to treat the condition. Frequently this condition is an indication of cystic fibrosis in the neonate.

Medial calcification (Mönckeberg's): A common idiopathic disease affecting men and women equally over the age of 50 years. It affects small and medium-sized muscular arteries. The media only is involved by this process. Calcium deposits are seen in a hyalinized media, as plate-like or ring-like patches. It causes few clinical symptoms as the affected vessels remain patent.

Medulloblastoma: A malignant tumour, the peak incidence of which occurs at about the age of 10 years, but which also may arise in adults. It is believed to be derived from embryonic cerebellar cells. In children the tumours are usually midline in location and rapidly obstruct the fourth ventricle, causing massive hydrocephalus. Primitive cells may differentiate along both glial and neuronal lines. Survival beyond 2 years is a rarity.

Megacolon: Extreme dilatation of the colon, usually due to retention of faeces.

Melaena: The passage of black, tarry-looking faeces containing digested blood. It is usually a sign of upper gastrointestinal tract haemorrhage often associated with peptic ulceration or small intestinal disease.

Melanin: A dark-brown pigment derived from tyrosine, occurring naturally in the body and synthesized by melanocytes. This pigment is found in the skin, adrenal cortex, choroid of the eye, substantia nigra in the brain, the meninges and some mucous membranes.

Melanoma: See **Malignant melanoma**.

Melanosis coli: An asymptomatic brownish or black discolouration of the large bowel associated with constipation, due to a local conversion of proteins to a melanin-like pigment. Sometimes it is due to anthracene purgatives. The pigment is not true melanin and is found accumulating in macrophages within the colonic mucosa.

Melasma: See **Chloasma**.

Menarche: The commencement of menstruation.

Meningioma: A benign tumour arising from cells at the junction of the arachnoid and dura mater. These tumours are uncommon in children. They do not invade the brain substance but by pressure may indent the brain and erode into the skull bones. Most can be surgically removed. A spectrum of differentiation is seen and controversy exists as to the presence of malignant behaviour; some experts recognise a malignant form, the so-called meningosarcoma, which is anaplastic and recurs after excision.

Meningitis: An infection or inflammation of the meninges of the brain or spinal cord. Usually due to a bacterial or viral infection.

Meningocoele: A fairly common type of SPINA BIFIDA in which there is a simple herniation of the meninges through a defect in the neural arches, usually in the thoracolumbar region. Although the spinal cord is normal there is often an associated deformity such as the ARNOLD-CHIARI MALFORMATION. The condition carries with it the risk of infection and also there may be some neurological disability.

Meningoencephalitis: An infection or inflammation of the meninges and neural parenchyma of the brain or spinal cord. Usually due to a bacterial or viral infection.

Meningomyelocoele: A variant of SPINA BIFIDA in which there is herniation of the meninges and spinal cord through defects in the neural arches into a skin-covered sac, usually in the thoracolumbar region. The nerve roots are abnormal and there is commonly paralysis below the level of the defect.

Menopause: The cessation of menstruation.

Menorrhagia: Heavy menstrual bleeding.

Mesothelioma: A malignant tumour of mesothelium

seen in the peritoneum, pericardium or more commonly in the pleura and until the 1960s a rare tumour. There is a strong correlation with asbestos exposure. As little as 3 months exposure has been shown to be sufficient, but the tumour may take 20 to 40 years to develop. Prognosis is very poor, with death usually occurring within a year of appearance of symptoms.

Metaplasia: The conversion of one fully differentiated, adult-type cell to another type of similar differentiated cell, usually as the result of chronic inflammation or irritation, for example the conversion of respiratory epithelium to stratified squamous epithelium in the airways of smokers.

Metastasis: The spread of malignant neoplastic cells from their site of origin such that they involve distant organs and tissues, forming deposits and growing there. Malignant cells achieve this by growing, invading and destroying normal tissue. Mechanisms of spread frequently involve embolic spread via blood and lymphatic vessels.

Metastatic calcification: A type of pathological calcification in which the deposition of calcium occurs even in normal, living tissues and it is always the result of some derangement of calcium metabolism, which is reflected by raised plasma calcium levels. There are many causes of hypercalcaemia. It should be noted that if necrotic tissue is present in an individual with hypercalcaemia, the calcium deposition is greatly enhanced and accelerated (see also DYSTROPHIC CALCIFICATION).

Micronodular cirrhosis: A type of CIRRHOSIS in which the regenerative nodules are uniform in size and rather small, also called Laennec's cirrhosis. It is commonly seen in alcoholics.

Miliary tuberculosis: Spread of tubercle bacilli occurring via the bloodsteam by erosion of a tubercle as it enlarges into a blood vessel, discharging bacilli directly into the bloodstream, or by lymphatic spread into the thoracic duct and into the venous blood. The disease is so named because of the appearance of numerous tiny tubercles (which result from such widespread dissemination simultaneously) resembling tiny 'millet seeds' scattered throughout the tissues. Miliary TB is 100% fatal without antibiotics, most deaths being from tuberculous meningitis.

'Mole': See **Naevus**.

Mongolism: See **Down's syndrome**.

Mucocoele: The collection of mucus within a saccular organ, usually associated with obstruction. It very commonly occurs in the appendix or the gall bladder in association with appendicitis or cholecystitis respectively.

Multiple myeloma: A malignant tumour derived from the PLASMA CELL arising in many situations of the skeleton and usually seen in old age. The neoplastic cells secrete excessive quantities of antibody and there may be BENCE-JONES PROTEIN present in the urine. The tumour has a poor prognosis.

Multiple sclerosis (= **disseminated sclerosis**): A rather common, idiopathic progressive disease characterized by 'plaques' or foci of demyelination throughout the CNS, affecting young adults, and being more common in women. Clinically, it is characterized by long chronicity, and periods of remissions and of relapses, with new neurological signs which partially resolve for long periods but which ultimately lead to progressive disability. Some patients live a normal life span, albeit with increasing disability; in others the disease may be fatal in a few years.

Mutagen: A factor or substance that may cause a heritable change in genetic material. The term is often used synonymously with CARCINOGEN.

Myasthenia gravis: A relapsing–remitting neuromuscular disorder producing a generalized weakness of muscles which is exacerbated by fatigue. The disease is due to an autoimmune process (type V hypersensitivity) in which antibody is formed against the acetylcholine receptors. Antibody attaches to these receptors at the neuromuscular junction and destroys them. Most muscles throughout the body show disease and atrophy in the later stages. Initially there may be little obvious change.

Mycosis fungoides: A rare malignant lymphomatous disorder manifesting itself in the skin, causing cutaneous tissues to assume an appearance suggestive of eczema or a skin tumour. The skin lesions are followed by microabscess formation in the epidermis and lesions resembling those of HODGKIN'S DISEASE in the spleen and lymph nodes.

Myelitis: An infection or inflammation of the spinal cord, being due to autoimmune reactions, viral or bacterial infections (see also POLIOMYELITIS).

Myelocoele: A form of SPINA BIFIDA that involves protrusion of the spinal cord through a focal defect in the vertebrae.

Myocarditis: Myocardial disorder marked by inflammatory changes. Myocarditis mostly involves microbial infections but also may be caused by hypersensitivities and physical or chemical agents and drugs which cause myocardial necrosis and inflammation.

Myopia (= **'nearsightedness'**): The eyeball is longer than normal, such that parallel light rays are focused at a point in front of the retina, vision being better for near objects than for distant objects as the eye inhibits the normal reflex of accommodation when viewing near objects. A concave spectacle lens is used to correct the disorder.

Myositis ossificans: An example of DYSTROPHIC CALCI-

FICATION, this condition is likely to develop if there has been haematoma formation in traumatized muscle near bone, and consists of calcification of necrotic muscle followed by ossification in the organizing lesion. The new bony mass formed in the muscle can be easily palpated or seen on X-rays.

Myxoedema: A state of hypothyroidism arising in adults, more commonly in elderly women, and characterized by a deficiency of thyroxine, obesity, decreased metabolic rate, oedema, listlessness and apathy, dry skin and brittle hair. It may be due to autoimmune disorders or iodine deficiency (cf. CRETINISM).

Myxoma: A benign tumour of fibroblasts associated with nerves. The tumour is composed of stellate cells embedded in a mucoid matrix. Myxomata are encapsulated and have a soft, gelatinous texture. They develop in fascial planes, subcutaneous tissues, the heart, gastrointestinal tract and intermuscular septa.

Naevus (plural, **naevi**): A benign proliferation of melanocytes in the skin to give rise to nests of normal cells which may be present in the junction of dermis and epidermis (= junctional naevus), within the dermis (= intradermal naevus) or both of the above situations (= compound naevus). A naevus is an example of a HAMARTOMA.

Necrosis: The death of cells while still part of the living body. Usually due to an injurious agent and the appearance of the necrotic tissue may give a clue as to the aetiology; for example caseous necrosis caused by *Mycobacterium tuberculosis*, gummatous necrosis caused by *Treponema pallidum*, liquefactive necrosis with suppuration caused by PYOGENIC BACTERIA.

Necrotizing enterocolitis: See **Pseudomembranous colitis**.

Neoplasm: An abnormal mass of tissue, the growth of which exceeds and is uncoordinated with that of the normal tissues, and persists in the same excessive manner after the cessation of the stimuli which evoked the change. The term is often used synonymously with 'tumour'.

Nephritic syndrome: A collection of symptoms and signs which is seen in association with various forms of glomerular injury. Often seen with the various forms of glomerulonephritis. The patient presents with haematuria, glomerular lesions, inflammation of glomeruli, mild PROTEINURIA, erythrocyte and protein casts in tubules, hypertension, OLIGURIA, AZOTAEMIA and OEDEMA.

Nephroblastoma (= Wilm's tumour): This tumour of the kidneys is almost exclusively found in children under 8 years of age. It accounts for 20% of solid tumours of childhood. It is a large tumour and may be found to fill the abdomen at laparotomy. A variety of mesodermal tissues occur in the tumour. Sarcomatous spindle cells with abortive tubules and glands are found together with a variety of other tissues such as fat, cartilage and bone. The patient presents with hypertension, a palpable mass, HAEMATURIA and pain. Metastases, especially to lung, are common. The tumour is highly sensitive to radio- and chemotherapy, and 75% of patients are cured with early detection.

Nephrotic syndrome: A clinical state characterized by heavy PROTEINURIA (1 to 10 g/day) hypoalbuminaemia, generalized oedema (osmotic effects) and hyperlipidaemia. It follows a severe prolonged increase in glomerular permeability to protein and is caused by glomerular lesions with the tubules usually intact. A whole variety of aetiologies are responsible for the syndrome but it is commonly associated with GLOMERULONEPHRITIS.

Nephrosclerosis: The degeneration and hyalinization of a renal corpuscle leading to its non-function, often seen in association with diabetes mellitus, hypertension, glomerulonephritis and SLE.

Neuroblastoma: A highly malignant tumour of primitive neurones occurring exclusively in young children. The tumour metastasizes widely early and has a poor prognosis unless diagnosed at an early stage, and is treated by radical surgery, irradiation and chemotherapy.

Neurofibroma: A benign fibrous-like tumour derived from Schwann cells in peripheral nerve sheaths.

Neurofibromatosis (= Von Recklinghausen's disease): An autosomal dominant disorder resulting in the formation of multiple neurofibromata in the nerves and skin, spotty café-au-lait skin pigmentation and in some cases developmental anomalies in the musculoskeletal system. Multiple soft tissue tumours may also occur leading to gross deformity ('elephant man').

Neutropenia: The reduction in the number of circulating neutrophils to numbers as low as 500 per μL. It is the commonest form of AGRANULOCYTOSIS and is associated with severe bacterial infections throughout the body.

'Nutmeg liver': A disorder of the liver associated with right-sided heart failure (e.g. mitral stenosis, pulmonary hypertension or tricuspid incompetence), which results in a pooling of blood in the liver whereby the central vein of the liver lobules becomes congested. The liver cells surrounding the central vein become anoxic and undergo fatty change. If chronic venous congestion is severe and prolonged these liver cells may undergo necrosis, and eventually CARDIAC CIRRHOSIS of the liver may ensue.

Nystagmus: An involuntary and rhythmic movement of the eyes where the movements may be vertical, horizontal, rotary or mixed. It may be a sign of barbiturate intoxication, neurological disease, MULTIPLE SCLEROSIS and ALBINISM.

Obstructive jaundice: A condition that results whenever there is obstruction of the biliary tree, the most common precipitating disease being CHOLELITHIASIS. Other causes include tumours of the liver, bladder, pancreas and of other surrounding organs. Cirrhosis may also give rise to this condition and therefore jaundice may be seen in alcoholics, hepatitis patients and in some cases of congenital disease.

Ochronosis: Deposition of a brownish or black pigment in connective tissue and cartilage, often associated with ALKAPTONURIA or phenol poisoning. The urine is also dark coloured and there may be bluish discolouration of fingers, sclerae, ears, nose and buccal mucosa.

Oedema: An excessive accumulation of extracellular fluid in the tissues or the body cavities. It may be localized, remaining confined to a small region, or generalized, involving the whole body (see also ASCITES, HYDROPERICARDIUM).

Oesophageal varices: Varicose dilatations of the veins of the lower oesophagus associated with portal hypertension and cirrhosis of the liver.

Oesophagitis: An infection or inflammation of the oesophagus, for example reflux oesophagitis caused by regurgitation of stomach acid into the lower oesophagus.

Oliguria: The production of a reduced volume of urine. It may be seen physiologically as, for example, occurs when the body is conserving water on a hot day, or pathologically as, for example, occurs in RENAL FAILURE or in SHOCK.

Ollier's disease: Multiple ENCHONDROMATA occurring in childhood and often undergoing malignant transformation to chondrosarcoma or osteosarcoma.

Oncogene: A normal cellular gene important in division and differentiation of cells (c-onc). Such normal cellular genes have been taken up by viruses and many viruses now possess viral oncogenes (v-onc). Cellular oncogenes and viral oncogenes may be involved in the process of neoplasia through various abnormalities of gene expression.

Oncovirus: Any virus that is associated with the formation of human or animal neoplasms.

Orchitis: An infection or inflammation of the testis, often spreading to the epididymis, being converted into an epididymoörchitis.

Organization: A sequela of acute inflammation in which the inflammatory exudate and fibrin are replaced by strands of collagen, laid down by activated fibroblasts. The result is a region of fibrosis, scarring.

Osteoarthrosis (= osteoarthritis, degenerative joint disease): A very common disease, usually beginning in late adult life with an insidious onset and taking a chronic course. This degenerative form of arthritis affects men more often than women, and the larger weight-bearing joints, such as the hip joint and knee, are more often involved, giving rise to pain and limited movement. The disease is considered to be a degenerative process of articular cartilage initially and then of bone in the joint area.

Osteochondroma: See **Exostosis cartilaginea**.

Osteoporosis: A condition of bone in which there is a reduction in the amount of bone, but the matrix mineralization remains normal. The bone is of normal texture but there is less of it. It may be due to decreased formation of bone, increased bone resorption or a combination of both. The commonest form of osteoporosis is so-called senile osteoporosis, seen mostly in women over the age of 45 years. It is also referred to as 'postmenopausal osteoporosis'. The bones become thin and there is a tendency towards vertebral collapse and fractures (particularly fracture at the hip). Thoracic humps known as 'dowager's hump' quite commonly occur with resultant KYPHOSIS. This produces a diminishing height and in advanced disease there is considerable pain. It is suspected that hormonal factors are important in its causation.

Osteogenesis imperfecta (= 'brittle bone syndrome'): This is a heterogeneous group of diseases of varying severity, in which there is failure of the skeleton to ossify properly. Bones are slender, with thin cortices, and very prone to fracture. In severe cases, multiple fractures occur *in utero*. During childhood, these patients run the risk of fracturing bones on trivial trauma.

Osteoma: This is a true, but rare, benign neoplasm of osteoid tissue. Most lesions are in the bones of the skull and nasal sinuses. The lesions are composed of normal bone and may project into the sinuses. There are usually no clinical effects except for pressure and these growths may only be removed for cosmetic purposes.

Osteomalacia: A condition of bone in which there is a normal amount of osteoid but, due to lack of calcium, it is defectively ossified. It is usually due to low dietary intake of vitamin D combined with little exposure to sunlight. It may occur in the malabsorption syndrome and also in people who are malnourished and housebound, such as elderly people. It may also develop during pregnancy when there may be lack of vitamin D and also loss of calcium to the foetus and later in breast milk. It may also arise following gastrectomy, various malabsorption syndromes and in obstructive jaundice. As the bones are deficient in calcium (demineralization) they are soft, leading to bowing, with incomplete fractures. The patient presents with muscular weakness, waddling 'penguin gait' and various aches and pains. They may have pathological fractures with no mineralized callus formation, which may cause pseudoarthrosis. Deformities of the bones may be present (see also RICKETS, OSTEOPOROSIS).

Osteomyelitis: Bone infection involving compact and cancellous bone occurring most often following bacteraemia or less commonly trauma, or infection of adjacent tissues (e.g. abscesses due to pyogenic organisms). *Staphylococcus aureus* may be responsible for acute or chronic osteomyelitis, characterized by suppuration within the bone and bone marrow, with destruction of bone. The affected region in the bone (most commonly in the long bones adjacent to the knee joint) causes great swelling and inflammation of overlying tissues, associated with severe pain.

Osteopetrosis (= Albers-Schönberg disease): A genetic disorder occurring in a severe form due to an autosomal recessive trait and a milder form due to an autosomal dominant trait. There is an increased density of all bones ossified from cartilage, especially vertebrae, pelvic bones and ribs. Bones are very hard, dense and yet brittle so that fractures are very common. Anaemia and neurological disease is seen in patients because of involvement of the bone marrow and skull.

Osteophyte: A bony outgrowth occurring around joint margin in a joint with OSTEOARTHROSIS. It is formed by reactive osteogenesis as the joint is destroyed in the disease process. Osteophytes commonly rub against one another, causing pain and may break off to form loose bodies within the joint space (joint 'mice').

Osteosarcoma: A primary malignant bone tumour which, although rare, is the most important and commonest of primary bone malignancies (19% of all primary bone malignancies). It affects young people primarily and males are affected slightly more than females. The majority of cases occur at the growing ends of long bones, particularly those around the knee. The tumours may be osteolytic or osteosclerotic. The periosteum is raised by the expanding tumour, and this periosteum lays down new bone. The tumour is highly malignant and metastases occur early via the bloodstream to the lungs, the prognosis being very poor.

Otitis: Infection or inflammation of the ear. Depending on the part of the ear affected the condition may be further differentiated into otitis externa, otitis media or otitis interna. These conditions are frequently seen in children because of the shortness and more horizontal arrangement of the Eustachian tube in childhood, allowing organisms to gain entry into the middle ear from the throat.

Paget's disease of bone: A fairly common, idiopathic disorder of bone, which may be widespread throughout the skeleton or localized to one bone. The affected bone is irregularly thickened, spongy, soft and vascular. The softening of bones results in bending of weight-bearing bones. Thickening of bones results in compression of nerves passing though foramina in the skull and vertebral column, causing pain and loss of function, for example deafness. The increased vascularity of the bones causes high cardiac output with subsequent cardiac failure. Pathological fracture is also common. Osteosarcoma develops in 1 to 10% of cases and represents 30% of all malignant primary bone tumours occurring in people over the age of 50 years.

Paget's disease of the nipple: A condition of the nipple associated with carcinoma of the breast. The nipple appears red and inflamed, with a scaly, eczematous, thickened appearance.

Pancarditis: Inflammation of all three layers of the heart as seen, for example, in RHEUMATIC FEVER.

Pancreatitis: An inflammation of the pancreas due to release of pancreatic enzymes into the parenchyma of the organ in association with arteriosclerosis, chronic alcoholism, obstruction or idiopathic disease (cf. HAEMORRHAGIC PANCREATITIS).

Pancytopenia: Failure of the bone marrow to produce enough blood cells to replace those lost in peripheral blood. Both red and white blood cells are involved.

Papilloma: A benign tumour of epithelium, usually arising from a surface and projecting into a lumen. It has an irregular surface and appears rather like a cauliflower. It commonly arises in the skin, squamous mucosae and gastrointestinal mucosae.

Papule: A small elevated lesion on the skin.

Paraesthesia: A spontaneous and abnormal sensation in any part of the body, such as tingling, tickling, itching, burning, pricking, etc.

Passive immunity: A method of immunity caused by the passive transfer of antibodies from an immune individual to a non-immune individual. The recipient's immune system takes no part in the immune response and the immunity transferred is only temporary, lasting for 2 to 3 months. Pooled human immunoglobulin is used, and this is a common procedure used in protecting travellers against hepatitis A.

Pathogenesis: The way in which an aetiological agent or factor interacts with tissue in order to bring about the disease and its effects.

Pathological fracture: A fracture occurring in a bone with pre-existing pathology (e.g. a tumour or osteoporosis). Minimal force is required to break such bones.

Peau d'orange (French = orange peel): An appearance of the skin overlying a breast in which a carcinoma is present occurring due to skin dimpling the lymphatics of the skin. It is due to lymphatics being infiltrated by cancer cells, which block the flow of lymph and cause localized oedema, leading to an exaggeration of the normal pore pattern of the skin, making the skin resemble orange peel.

Pelvic inflammatory disease (PID): A complication of untreated genital infections (especially gonorrhoeal and chlamydial) in females, with spread of the infection into the pelvic peritoneal cavity, leading to chronic inflammation and widespread scarring in all of the surrounding tissues. PID is associated with abortions, stillbirths, infant prematurity, ectopic pregnancy, puerperal infections and sterility.

Pemphigus vulgaris: A bullous eruption which affects any skin surface, but especially common at the groin, axilla and mouth. This is a very severe condition which was often fatal before cortisone therapy was available.

Peptic ulcer: A benign, localized defect consisting of a deep excavation of any part of the gastrointestinal tract mucosa that is in contact with acid and pepsin. The defect extends beyond the muscularis mucosae, which is contrary to the shallower and more superficial EROSIONS, the latter not extending beyond the muscularis mucosae.

Pericarditis: An infection or inflammation of the pericardium. It is most usually acute (e.g. as occurs in URAEMIA), although infrequently a chronic pericarditis may be seen (e.g. tuberculous).

Perinephric abscess: An abscess forming in the loose connective tissue and perirenal fat found around the kidney. Commonly, the pyogenic bacterium causing the infection arrives in that situation via the bloodstream, or alternatively the infection may spread outwards from a parenchymal kidney infection.

Peritonsillar abscess: See **Quinsy**.

Petechia (plural, **petechiae**): A tiny haemorrhage occurring from capillaries and seen especially in the mucosae and skin. It may indicate PURPURA or haemorrhagic infections.

Peutz-Jegher's syndrome: This is a congenital condition inherited as an autosomal dominant trait in which multiple benign polyps occur in the gastrointestinal tract associated with increased melanin deposition in the mouth and lips. The patients have an increased risk of developing colonic carcinoma when compared with the normal individual but less risk of developing carcinoma when compared with patients with familial polyposis coli (cf. POLYPOSIS COLI).

Phaeochromocytoma: A rather uncommon tumour of the chromaffin tissue of the adrenal medulla or sympathetic paraganglia which secretes large quantities of adrenaline or noradrenaline. It may give rise to persistent or intermittent hypertension.

Phlebothrombosis: Asymptomatic THROMBOSIS in the venous system (cf. THROMBOPHLEBITIS).

Phocomelia: A developmental anomaly in which the limbs are greatly reduced in size, resembling the flippers of seals. It was seen in the babies of women who had taken thalidomide during early pregnancy.

Pilonidal cyst: A cyst which contains hair, developing in the sacral region of the skin.

Pilonidal sinus: A lesion found most commonly over the tip of the coccyx and consisting of a PILONIDAL CYST which has become fistulous, communicating with the exterior. It may become infected and requires excision.

Plasma cell: A cell derived from the B cell of the blood. It is a large, oval cell with a basophilic cytoplasm and an eccentric, round, 'clock-face' nucleus. It is the active secretor of antibodies and thus important in HUMORAL IMMUNITY.

Plasmacytoma: See **Multiple myeloma**.

Pleomorphism: A greatly varying appearance in a cellular population, caused by either a great many different cells of a similar type (e.g. pleomorphic cellular infiltrate of chronic inflammation) or many cells of the same type which show a very greatly different morphology (pleomorphic cell population of a malignant tumour).

Plummer-Vinson syndrome (= sideropenic dysphagia): A rather rare, congenital condition of the oesophagus which is seen primarily in females. The patients present with DYSPHAGIA, GLOSSITIS, KOILONYCHIA, ACHLORHYDRIA and iron deficiency ANAEMIA.

Pneumaturia: The passage of gas during micturition. It may be seen in association with DIVERTICULITIS of the colon where there has been a fistulous communication between intestine and bladder.

Pneumoconiosis (plural, **pneumoconioses**): A group of disorders caused by inhalation of organic or inorganic fine dusts. These are usually diseases of occupational/industrial association. The dust particles inhaled must be less than 5 μm in diameter to reach the alveolar level.

Pneumonia: An acute inflammatory disorder of the lung, characterized by consolidation due to the presence of acute inflammatory exudate and infiltrate within the alveolar spaces. A large number of infective agents may cause pneumonia and these include protozoa, fungi, bacteria, mycoplasmata and viruses. Bacterial pneumonias are the most characteristic and common of these lesions and they have been divided into LOBAR PNEUMONIA and BRONCHOPNEUMONIA, depending on the distribution of affected tissue in the lungs.

Poliomyelitis: An infection with the polioviruses, which in most cases is an acute disease with fever, diarrhoea, sore throat, vomiting and headache and often stiffness of the neck and back. This minor disease is usually self-limited and presents few serious symptoms. In a small number of cases, there is central nervous system involvement, destruction of motor neurones in the anterior grey matter of the spinal cord with subsequent paralysis, atrophy of muscle groups, contraction and deformity. The disease is now prevented through immunization.

Polycystic disease: A congenital, hereditary disorder affecting the kidneys, pancreas and the liver. One-third of patients with polycystic disease have multiple cysts in the liver. There are two forms of the disease. The neonatal form is inherited as an autosomal recessive and is very severe, with death occurring very early. The adult form, inherited as an autosomal dominant, is compatible with life, until multiple cysts develop in adult years.

Polyp: A usually benign tumour resembling a mushroom in that it possesses a stalk and a head and projects from mucosal surfaces into a lumen.

Polyposis coli: This is an hereditary disorder which is usually transmitted as a Mendelian dominant by either sex, but in some families is of very poor penetrance or transmitted as a recessive character. Hundreds of adenomatous polyps form in the large intestine. The condition does not appear until late childhood or early adult life. This condition predisposes to cancer of the colon, the carcinoma being almost inevitable usually after 15 years of the onset of symptoms of polyposis. The entire colon must be excised, as soon as the condition is diagnosed.

Porphyria: A group of inherited disorders in which there is an increased production of porphyrins (iron-free pyrrole derivatives) in the body. As these substances are deposited in many tissues, including the skin, there is photosensitivity, abdominal pain and neuropathy. In some cases, porphyria may be acquired, especially after ingestion of some drugs or toxins (e.g. alcohol, barbiturates, arsenicals, phosphorus, sulphonamides). The urine may be coloured a deep red colour and the teeth may have a red-brown tinge.

Portal hypertension: A rise in the blood pressure within the portal vein, usually associated with CIRRHOSIS of the liver. It causes SPLENOMEGALY, ASCITES, CAPUT MEDUSAE, OESOPHAGEAL VARICES and HAEMORRHOIDS.

Pott's disease of the spine: Spinal tuberculosis involving one or more vertebrae, commonly seen in the thoracic vertebrae, especially T11. It arises when the microbe spreads haematogenously to these sites, usually from a primary lesion in the lungs. There is destruction of bone, vertebral collapse and angular KYPHOSIS. 'COLD ABSCESSES' may form in the adjacent region or track down muscle planes and consist of collections of caseous necrotic material. Pott's paraplegia may follow destruction of the cord and tubercu-

lous meningitis may be seen, especially after surgery.

Presbycusis: A progressive, bilateral and symmetric hearing loss occurring with advancing age.

Presbyopia: A condition caused by the decrease of the range of focusing ('accommodation') that occurs throughout life and is more marked in the elderly such that the nearest point that can be brought into focus on the retina recedes beyond the normal, necessitating the person holding their reading matter further and further away. The condition is corrected by the wearing of convex spectacles.

Primary: (1) Idiopathic in aetiology, of an unknown cause, for example primary hypertension. (2) The disease when or where it manifests itself first, for example primary tumour of the bronchus or primary syphilis (see also SECONDARY).

Procarcinogen: A substance that becomes a CARCINOGEN only after it is chemically altered by metabolic processes in the body.

Prolapse: The falling, sliding or any other downward displacement of an organ from its normal position in the body, for example a prolapsed uterus.

Prostatitis: An infection or inflammation of the prostate commonly associated with PROSTATOMEGALY.

Prostatomegaly: Enlargement of the prostate gland, commonly seen in elderly males. It may be due to prostatic hyperplasia (symptoms associated with urinary obstruction) or prostatic carcinoma (symptoms associated with metastatic disease, especially to the bones, e.g. pathological fractures).

Proteinuria: The presence of protein in urine.

Prothesis (plural, **prostheses**): An artificial part designed for replacement of a missing body part (e.g. an artificial heart valve or dentures). Alternatively it may be a device designed to improve the function of a diseased body part (e.g. contact lenses).

Pruritus: The subjective, cutaneous sensation of itching leading to the urge to scratch the affected site. It is the single most common presenting feature of many dermatological conditions and often may also accompany systemic diseases (e.g. ECZEMA may cause it, as may CIRRHOSIS of the liver).

Pseudoarthrosis: A 'false joint' which is formed in certain situations where a fractured bone is healing abnormally. When there is little or no immobilization, fibroblasts lay down collagen only, forming scar tissue between the broken bone ends. If scar joins the bone ends little or no further change occurs. The fracture is permanently unstable and healing is unsatisfactory.

Pseudomembranous colitis (= necrotizing enterocolitis): (1) An acute inflammatory disorder of the large and small intestine seen in neonates, especially premature ones, caused by infection with normal flora bacteria associated with a decreased immune response and defects in host defences. It may progress to ischaemic necrosis of the gut mucosa, perforation of the intestine and peritonitis. **(2)** An infection of the bowel with *Clostridium perfringens*. The patient presents with severe abdominal pain, diarrhoea and vomiting.

Psoriasis: A common, often familial, chronic progressive dermatitis with dry, sharply demarcated plaques of reddening covered by layers of silvery scales. On scraping, the scales are removed to expose fine, multiple bleeding points. Microabscesses may form. Psoriasis may also be drug-induced (iatrogenic). The disease is controlled by anti-inflammatory agents and phototherapy.

Ptosis: Drooping of an eyelid.

Puerperal sepsis (= 'childbed fever'): A condition developing after delivery, where normal flora bacteria from the vagina colonize the traumatized uterine tissues, causing a serious infection that often develops into a septicaemia. Anaerobic bacteria and streptococci are often involved in double infections. Puerperal sepsis was a common cause of death in the past as a complication of delivery but nowadays antibiotic therapy proves life saving.

Pumonary failure: See **Respiratory failure**.

Pulmonary hypertension: A persistent rise in the blood pressure within the pulmonary vascular system which can be rarely idiopathic or more commonly due to excessive pulmonary blood flow, chronic passive venous congestion and obstructive lung disease with obstruction of pulmonary vessels. Pulmonary hypertension results in thickening of the walls of pulmonary arteries and also in ATHEROMA of pulmonary arteries.

Purpura: Condition in which small haemorrhages occur from capillaries throughout the body resulting in small areas of haemorrhage called PETECHIAE, in the skin, mucous and serous membranes. Low platelet numbers cause an abnormal capillary fragility which may lead to persistent bleeding and purpura.

Purulent: Producing, containing or characterized by PUS.

Pus: A yellow, viscous fluid commonly found in sites that have been infected with pyogenic bacteria and composed of acute inflammatory exudate, large numbers of neutrophils, dead and living bacteria and liquefied tissue debris. It is a manifestation of heterolytic tissue necrosis.

Pustule: A small, focal, raised lesion in the skin that contains purulent fluid.

Pyaemia: The carriage of pyogenic organisms by the bloodstream.

Pyelitis: Inflammation or infection of the renal pelvis.

Pyelonephritis: Inflammation of the renal pelvis and renal parenchyma. Common in females as a result of ascending urinary tract infection most often caused by *Escherichia coli*. Acute and chronic forms are known, the latter an important cause of RENAL FAILURE.

Pyknosis: A reactive change to injury where the nuclear material condenses greatly to give rise to a small, dense, dark-staining nucleus; the nucleus may then show KARYORRHEXIS and KARYOLYSIS.

Pylephlebitis: A suppurative infection of the portal vein and its branches, spreading to the liver and forming multiple abscesses. It may be due to spread of bacteria from bowel infections, especially APPENDICITIS, ULCERATIVE COLITIS or DIVERTICULITIS.

Pyogenic micro-organisms: Those micro-organisms which when introduced into the tissues will cause an acute inflammatory reaction characterized by the formation of copious PUS.

Pyrogen: A fever-causing substance. Pyrogens may be endogenous (e.g. components released by neutrophils during acute inflammation) or exogenous (e.g. bacterial endotoxin components).

Pyrogenic: Causing fever, containing PYROGENS.

Q-fever: An acute febrile illness caused after infection with *Coxiella burnetii*. It is acquired by inhalation of the organism, and the lungs show a viral-like interstitial pneumonia which is patchy in distribution. The disease has a low mortality.

Quadriplegia: Paralysis of all four limbs.

Queyrat's erythroplasia: A condition seen on the prepuce and glans penis leading to the formation of multiple, flat, red, raised patches with marked keratosis and dysplasia of the epithelium. The condition is regarded as a severe dysplasia or carcinoma *in situ*.

Quinsy (= peritonsillar abscess): An infection of the tonsils and associated pharyngeal areas, the patients presenting with dysphagia, pain radiating to the ear and fever. A typical abscess develops and may be incised and drained if it does not spontaneously rupture. Penicillin and saline irrigation of the area are also indicated.

Rachischisis: A congenital condition in which there is fissuring in one or more vertebrae (see also SPINA BIFIDA).

Rales: Abnormal sounds originating from the trachea, bronchi or lungs. Very loud rales associated with terminal oedematous conditions of the lungs are known popularly as the 'death rattle'.

Raynaud's disease: A functional disorder of small arteries and arterioles of the extremities in which intense vasospasm is seen. Affects usually young, otherwise healthy, women. Seen in the peripheral tissues, mainly the fingers and hands, occasionally the toes and feet and sometimes the tip of the nose. The affected parts become very pale, almost white, then blue and then red.

Raynaud's phenomenon: A disorder characterized

by cold sensitivity in the fingers, pain and colour changes in the skin, and in which the patient may resemble a case of RAYNAUD'S DISEASE. In Raynaud's phenomenon all of the observed changes that develop in the tissue are secondary to some underlying, often serious disorder which is causing an organic lesion in the arterial wall, e.g. SCLERODERMA or SLE.

Reagin (= Reaginic antibody): Antibody of the IgE class formed in excessive amounts in ANAPHYLAXIS and which attaches to mast cells, thus sensitizing them.

Reed-Sternberg cell: A giant cell found in lesions of HODGKIN'S DISEASE. It is a large cell possessing two to five nuclei, centrally arranged. Most often such cells have two nuclei arranged symmetrically ('mirror image' or 'owl-eyed cells'). Diagnosis of Hodgkin's disease depends on the demonstration of Reed-Sternberg cells.

Regeneration: A sequela to injury in which parenchymal cells lost or destroyed in the injury are replaced by identical, fully functional, parenchymal cells. This process can only occur in labile and stable tissues and will occur only if the connective tissue matrix of the tissue remains intact.

Regional enteritis (= Crohn's disease): This is an idiopathic relapsing granulomatous inflammatory disorder which commonly affects the terminal ileum or colon (regional colitis) but may occur anywhere in the gastrointestinal tract. In some patients the intestinal involvement is associated with inflammation of joints, eyes, skin and liver. The disease is similar to idiopathic ulcerative colitis and is sometimes difficult to differentiate from it. It is most prevalent in the Western world. There is chronic inflammation with adhesions forming, and occasionally there may be perforation and fistula formation. There may also be obstruction, rarely haemorrhage, and in the late stages MALABSORPTION SYNDROME. Malnutrition may rarely cause death.

Renal failure (= kidney failure): The inability of the kidney to secrete urine, excrete wastes and conserve useful substances. Acute renal failure develops suddenly and the patient presents with anuria or oliguria. The condition develops with severe trauma, burns, incompatible blood transfusions, severe acute hypotension, toxic agents, drugs, septicaemia and some forms of glomerulonephritis. Chronic renal failure develops with progressive kidney diseases such as chronic glomerulonephritis, chronic pyelonephritis, hypertensive nephropathy, renal tubular syndromes and analgesic nephropathy. Haemodialysis and renal transplantation are the options when medical treatment of the conditions is no longer effective.

Repair: A sequela of a disease process after considerable damage has occurred in a tissue, resulting in the replacement of parenchymal cells of the tissue by fibrous scar tissue. It is a process of rapid healing of tissue in which the body is attempting to repair the damage sustained in the most rapid way, for example wound healing.

Resolution: A sequela of a disease process resulting in complete return to normality and usually occurring in association with conditions which cause little damage to the tissues, for example resolution following lobar pneumonia or mild thermal burns (cf. REGENERATION, REPAIR, ORGANIZATION).

Respiratory failure (= pulmonary failure): An inability of the cardiopulmonary systems to maintain an adequate exchange of carbon dioxide and oxygen in the lungs. Respiratory failure may be either hypoxaemic failure and characterized by hyperventilation (this is seen to occur with many lung diseases, e.g. emphysema and infections) or it may be ventilatory failure characterized by hypercarbia and due to obstructive lesions in the airways or depression of the respiratory function (e.g. brain trauma or administration of drugs). Respiratory failure may be brought about or exacerbated by cardiac conditions, surgery, anaesthesia, etc. It may result in COR PULMONALE, CONGESTIVE HEART FAILURE and respiratory acidosis.

Reticulosarcoma: This is a rare primary tumour of bone arising most frequently in the shaft of long bones. The tumour usually presents in young adults of about 30 years of age as a radiolucent, single lesion bearing no relationship to the lymphomata seen as a generalized disease. Patients with reticulosarcoma of bone remain in good health even when the tumour mass has reached a relatively large size. Surgery and radiotherapy bring about good results in localized tumours while chemotherapy is also given to patients with extraosseous metastases; the general prognosis of this tumour is relatively good.

Retinoblastoma: An hereditary malignant tumour transmitted as an autosomal dominant characteristic with poor penetrance and developing in the retina from germ cells. In many cases it is bilateral and, untreated, it will invade the brain and metastasize to distant sites. It is curable if detected early by removal of the affected eye(s). Genetic counselling is advisable.

Retrograde: Going backwards, in the reverse manner or usual mode, or against the current, for example retrograde spread of tumours in lymphatics whereby the tumour cells travel against the flow of the lymph.

Retroviruses (= Retroviridae): A family of RNA viruses of humans and animals, including the ONCOVIRUSES, the HUMAN IMMUNODEFICIENCY VIRUS causing AIDS and the HUMAN T CELL LYMPHOTROPIC VIRUS I causing certain types of human LEUKAEMIA.

Reverse transcriptase: A unique enzyme found only in the retroviruses and essential in the life cycle of the virus as it is used in the reverse transcription of RNA into DNA, prior to insertion of the viral genetic material into the genetic material of the cell.

Rhabdomyoma: A very rare, benign tumour of striated muscle, especially as it occurs in the heart.

Rhabdomyosarcoma: A very rare, malignant tumour of striated muscles, very aggressive and having a poor prognosis. Commonly presents as a large, rapidly developing mass in the muscles of the legs or occasionally of the trunk.

Rheumatic fever: An autoimmune/hypersensitivity-type reaction occurring as a sequela of streptococcal infection in certain individuals. As these people share some protein components with the streptococci, following infection, when antibody has been produced against the bacteria and after the infection subsides, tissues in the body cross-react with the antibodies produced leading to damage and disease. The heart, heart valves and joints are primarily involved. After each new infective episode with streptococci, the antibodies produced will cause more and more damage.

Rheumatoid arthritis: An autoimmune disorder, presenting as a generalized disease of connective tissues. Polyarthritis due to disease of synovial tissues is usually the dominant clinical and pathological feature. The disease is common, often familial and typically presents in females between the ages of 20 and the menopause, rather later in men. The sites affected are many of the small joints, particularly those of the feet, hands and wrists. The larger joints at ankle, hip and knee are also often affected. Inflammation and destruction of joints occur usually after an insidious, chronic course. The joints are painful, swollen and tender with limitation of joint movement.

Rheumatoid nodule: In RHEUMATOID ARTHRITIS subcutaneous nodules may form, mostly at the elbows. There may be similar nodules in the liver, lungs, heart and aorta. These nodules are composed of circular areas of denatured collagen surrounded by macrophages and lymphocytes.

Rhinitis: See **Coryza**.

Rhinophyma: A condition of the nose where there is erythema of the skin, sebaceous gland hyperplasia with nodular swelling and marked congestion of the nose.

Rhonchi: Continuous, coarse rattling sound arising from the trachea or bronchi.

Rickets: A disease of infants and early childhood in which the cartilage fails to ossify normally due to lack of vitamin. D. The softness of the bones leads to deformities such as bow legs. If severe and untreated it can cause deformities of the pelvis (important in females who will bear children). Growth will be stunted (cf. OSTEOMALACIA).

'Round cell tumour': See **Ewing's tumour**.

Rubor: See **Erythema**.

Salpingitis: Infection or inflammation of the Fallopian tube as may commonly be seen with *Mycoplasma* spp. infections, associated with PELVIC INFLAMMATORY DISEASE (PID).

Sarcoidosis: An idiopathic granulomatous inflammation which, although systemic, most commonly affects the lungs. Other sites in the body very frequently affected include the lymph nodes, skin, eyes, salivary glands, spleen, liver and bones. Microscopically the lesions of the disease are typical granulomata, each one appearing almost identical to the tubercle of tuberculosis, without the caseous necrosis of TB.

Sarcoma: A malignant tumour arising from non-epithelial tissue, for example FIBROSARCOMA.

Scar (= cicatrix): A deposit of fibrocollagenous tissue seen after REPAIR or ORGANIZATION processes have healed an injury to tissue. Examples are scarring after wounding or after removal of necrotic tissue in an infarct.

Schaumann bodies: Large (≤ 10 μm in diameter) basophilic inclusions composed of calcium and iron salts found within giant cells of the granulomata of SARCOIDOSIS (cf. ASTEROID BODIES).

Schick test: A skin test used to determine whether a person is immune to DIPHTHERIA. A small amount of diphtheria toxin is injected intradermally and a positive reaction (indicated by redness and swelling) demonstrates non-immunity and susceptibility to diphtheria.

Schmorl's node: A commonly seen, vertical herniation in the spinal column where there is protrusion of the nuclear tissue into the vertebral body above or below the disc. It is radiologically evident as there is reactive bone formation around the herniation.

Schwannoma: A benign tumour of nerve sheath cells, the commonest location of which is the acoustic nerve typically at the cerebellopontine angle. It is more frequent in patients with von Recklinghausen's disease. The tumours are almost always resectable. Acoustic nerve schwannomata produce tinnitus, deafness, and ataxia or dizziness if they impinge on the cerebellum. Large tumours impinge on the fifth and seventh nerve, producing palsies. Tumours arising outside the CNS tend to be invasive and metastasize.

Scirrhous carcinoma: A malignant tumour which on palpation is very hard, for example scirrhous carcinoma of the breast.

Scleroderma: A relatively rare autoimmune disease of skin and connective tissues where there is degeneration of connective tissue in skin, lungs, blood vessels, oesophagus, kidneys, etc. The patients may present with RAYNAUD'S PHENOMENON, oedema, thickening of the skin of the face and swelling of distal extremities. Severe renal disease develops and is usually the cause of death. No effective treatment exists and the disease is managed by administration of corticosteroids.

Scorbutic: Suffering from, showing signs of, or pertaining to SCURVY.

Scurvy: Severe vitamin C deficiency leading to capillary fragility and a haemorrhagic diathesis, poor wound and fracture healing and defective collagen formation. Patients usually present with many open bleeding sores in the gums and multiple bruises ('BATTERED BABY SYNDROME').

Seborrhoeic dermatitis: This is an extremely common condition in its mild form, seborrhoea or 'dandruff'. The scales of dandruff are composed of desquamated keratin matted together by sebaceous material. In the more florid form there is dermatitis present as well. Seborrhoeic dermatitis shows as raised, reddened, scaly plaques involving the scalp, eyebrows and eyelids, face, ears and sometimes the chest.

Secondary: Seen after another process or disease; caused directly or indirectly by a pre-existing process or disease, for example secondary hypertension seen after renal artery stenosis. A phase of a disease occurring some time after the initial (or PRIMARY) phase, for example secondary syphilis.

Secondary antibody response: See **Anamnestic antibody response**.

Seminoma: A malignant tumour of the seminiferous epithelium of the testis. There is a painless, uniform enlargement of the testis within the tunica albuginea, so that the tumour is usually well contained. Seminoma is most commonly seen in males between the ages of 30 and 40 years. Metastasis does not occur until late in the disease. Growth is slow and the tumour responds well to radiotherapy. Prognosis is very good if the tumour is treated early and the 10-year survival is 90%. GYNAECOMASTIA may occur in this disease if the tumour produces gonadotrophins. Seminoma is ten times more common in males with undescended testes rather than in the normal male.

Septicaemia: The presence of micro-organisms within the bloodstream.

Sequela: Any consequence of a disease process.

Sequestrum: A fragment of necrotic bone which is detached from the surrounding living bone and is often inaccessible to osteoclasts, blood vessels and inflammatory cells. It may act as a nidus of infection (chronic OSTEOMYELITIS).

Serotonin (= 5-hydroxytryptamine): A biological amine, a derivative of tryptophan found in platelets, brain and intestinal cells. It is a potent vasoconstrictor and constrictor of intestinal smooth muscle and acts as a neurotransmitter in the brain. Excess quantities are secreted by some tumours (in the small intestine, appendix and lungs) and may cause the CARCINOID SYNDROME.

Serum hepatitis (= hepatitis B): A liver infection caused by the hepatitis B virus (HBV) which is transmitted by transfer of body fluids between individuals and also by sexual intercourse. It is a serious disease, causing liver damage and inflammation. It may lead to CIRRHOSIS and HEPATOCARCINOMA (a carrier state is also possible).

Serum sickness: A type III, complex-mediated hypersensitivity occurring on a systemic level 2 to 3 weeks after administration of an antiserum (foreign protein). There is fever, splenomegaly, lymphadenopathy, joint pain, glomerulonephritis and a skin rash. It may be fatal and treatment is symptomatic. Corticosteroid administration may limit the inflammatory reactions seen.

Sexually transmitted diseases (= venereal diseases): A group of diseases that are transmitted mainly through the intimate contact of sexual intercourse. There are protozoal, fungal, bacterial and viral sexually transmitted diseases.

Shock: This is not a specific disease but rather a clinical syndrome with many presentations. The clinical state of shock results from reduction of the effective circulating blood volume. This circulatory insufficiency leads to an imbalance between the metabolic needs of the tissues and the blood available to them. There will be lowered amounts of oxygen and nutrients available to cells and an increased level of metabolites. This in turn may lead to cell damage, reactive changes and necrosis. Depending on the severity of the syndrome, shock may be either reversible or irreversible.

'Shrinkage necrosis': See **Apoptosis**.

Sideropenic dysphagia: See **Plummer-Vinson syndrome**.

Siderosis: See **Haemosiderosis**.

Silicosiderosis (= haematite lung, from haematite, iron oxide dust): A PNEUMOCONIOSIS seen in quarry workers and miners where the inhaled dusts are rich in iron oxides. A severe fibrotic damage to the lung tissue evolves. The condition is associated with a higher risk of development of lung cancers.

Silicosis: A PNEUMOCONIOSIS caused by inhalation of silica particles. It causes severe fibrosis in the lungs, with development of large fibrous nodules known as silicotic nodules. Patients show a predisposition to the development of tuberculosis.

Sinusitis: Inflammation or infection of the paranasal sinuses. It may be due to infections with bacteria or viruses, or due to allergies. Swelling and obstruction of nasal passages causes pain, discomfort, headaches, fever and local tenderness. Treatment of chronic sinusitis may be surgical.

Smallpox (= variola): A highly contagious serious viral disease caused by the variola virus, a poxvirus. The disease has been declared eradicated by WHO and no natural infections have been known to occur in recent years. This has been possible as the virus only infected human beings and worldwide vaccination succeeded in eradicating it.

'Small round cells': See **Lymphocytes**.

Somatic mutation: A heritable change in the DNA of the body cells (as opposed to mutation in the gametocytes) commonly caused by CARCINOGENS or MUTAGENS. A somatic mutation may lead to death of cells or to a NEOPLASM.

Spasmodic: Characterized by spasms or convulsions, usually of an involuntary nature.

Spider naevus: A type of TELANGIECTASIA in which there is a red spot on the skin the size of a pinhead from which radiate congested, small blood vessels. Seen in association with raised oestrogen levels as occurs during pregnancy or in cirrhosis of the liver.

Spina bifida: A congenital disorder occurring in 1 to 2% of births. It is a neural tube defect where there are varying degrees of failure of fusion of the neural tube and spinal canal. It may be a minor defect frequently remaining undiagnosed (spina bifida occulta) or it may be incompatible with life (RACHISCHISIS, MYELOCOELE). Various intermediate forms occur. Some types of spina bifida are associated with neurological deficits.

Splenomegaly: Enlargement of the spleen which may be gross, as occurs with a variety of disease processes, for example HODGKIN'S DISEASE or obstruction of the splenic vein.

Squamous cell carcinoma: A common, characteristic, malignant tumour of squamous epithelia and squamous mucosae. It may also arise in unexpected sites where squamous metaplasia of the epithelium precedes the neoplasia. It appears as a small raised papule or papillary lesion and forms an indolent ulcer with a central scab. Distant metastases may be seen. Overall prognosis is good as the majority of these tumours are discovered early and treated by excision (the exception is squamous carcinoma of the bronchus which has a poor prognosis).

Steatorrhoea: The presence of large amounts of undigested fat in the faeces.

Stimulatory hypersensitivity (cell receptor hypersensitivity or type V hypersensitivity): An antibody-mediated hypersensitivity in which antibodies form against a plasma membrane receptor molecule. This receptor may be destroyed by the autoantibody, making the cell less efficient in its function (as occurs in MYASTHENIA GRAVIS) or the antibody may stimulate the cell into hyperactivity (as occurs in THYROTOXICOSIS).

Stone: See **Calculus**.

Strabismus (= 'squint'): A deviation of the eyes such that their axes are not parallel, most commonly being a horizontal deviation (convergent or divergent).

'Strawberry gall bladder': See **Cholesterosis of the gall bladder**.

Stroke: See **Cerebral infarction/haemorrhage**.

Struma ovarii: A subtype of ovarian TERATOMA in which there is predominance of thyroid tissue in which are found follicles and hormone-secreting cells.

Suppressor T cell (= T8 cell): A subtype of the T lymphocyte group important in the control of the immune response. It dampens down the immune response after an infection and eliminates other types of activators of immunity. Normally there are fewer suppressor T cells in the bloodstream than HELPER T CELLS, but in some conditions (e.g. AIDS) the ratio may be reversed.

Syncope (= 'fainting'): A transient loss of consciousness associated with cerebral anoxia. It may be caused by extremes of temperature, vagal stimulation, stress, fear, anxiety and other factors. The person usually feels light-headed and nauseous before syncope and the condition may be prevented by placing the head between the knees or laying the person down.

Syndrome: A set of symptoms and signs that usually occur together and characterize a particular disorder.

Syringoma: A tumour of the sweat gland ducts, usually well differentiated and slow growing, forming papillary, cystic or solid lesions.

Syringomyelocoele: A type of SPINA BIFIDA anomaly in which the spinal cord is complete but there is dilatation of the central canal associated with a severe defect of the vertebral arches. There is associated neurological deficit and early death of the affected infants occurs.

Systemic lupus erythematosus (SLE): A systemic autoimmune disease with inflammatory changes in many tissues of the body but especially in the joints, kidneys, skin and nervous system. It is commoner in young females and the earliest manifestations are arthritis and a symmetrical skin rash over the nose and malar prominences. RENAL FAILURE may develop and is often the cause of death. The disease is controlled by systemic corticosteroid administration.

Tabes dorsalis: A manifestation of late or post-tertiary stage neurosyphilis in which there is atrophy of the posterior (sensory) roots in the lumbar region sometimes accompanied by atrophy of the optic nerves. Paroxysms of severe lightning pains occur, most commonly in the legs. There is loss of normal pain sensation, vibration sense and deep reflexes. The Argyll-Robertson pupil (accommodates but does not react) is nearly always present. ATAXIA is prominent, due to proprioceptive loss. ULCERS and CHARCOT TYPE JOINTS occur.

Taboparesis: A manifestation of tertiary syphilis seen in some patients 15 to 20 years after the primary infection characterized by nervous tissue involvement with

TABES DORSALIS and DEMENTIA PARALYTICA.

Tay-Sachs disease (=amaurotic familial idiocy): An autosomal recessive disorder more common in families of Eastern European Jewish origin, leading to a neurodegenerative disorder due to abnormal lipid metabolism caused by a defect of the enzyme hexosaminidase A. As a result sphingolipids accumulate in the brain causing progressive mental retardation and early death. Symptoms first appear at 6 months of age and most infants die between 2 and 4 years of age. There is no cure for the disease and therapeutic abortions are advised after the condition is diagnosed via AMNIOCENTESIS in a woman having a history of the disease in her or her husband's family.

T cell: A lymphocyte processed in the thymus gland, which takes part in the cell-mediated immune response. Many subclasses of T cells are known, each having specific functions, for example helper T4 cells, suppressor T8 cells, etc.

Telangiectasia: Permanent dilatation of superficial capillaries and venules causing them to become very prominent and the skin or mucosae to appear reddened. It may occur with high oestrogen levels, cirrhosis of the liver, dermatitides, actinic damage and so on (see also CAPUT MEDUSAE).

Tendonitis (= tendinitis): An inflammation of a tendon usually due to excessive stress or strain placed on it.

Tenesmus: Persistent but ineffectual contractions of the smooth muscle lining the rectum or bladder giving rise to desire to defaecate or to void urine. It may occur, for example, with irritable bowel disease.

Tenosynovitis: The inflammation or infection of a tendon sheath caused by trauma or other types of injury, calcification, various types of arthritis, or infections affecting joints such as gonorrhoea.

Teratogenesis: The production of developmental defects in the embryo, usually caused by exogenous, teratogenic agents (e.g. thalidomide causing PHOCOMELIA, rubella virus causing heart defects, blindness, etc.).

Teratoma: A tumour, either benign or malignant, most usually occurring in the testis (typically malignant) or the ovary (typically benign) and composed of a mass of cells derived from all three germ layers. In well-differentiated teratomata there may be tufts of hair, teeth, cartilage, epithelium, bone, nervous tissue and glandular tissue (especially thyroid, see STRUMA OVARII).

Tetanus: A potentially fatal infection and intoxication with the anaerobic bacterium *Clostridium tetani*. Once the bacterium enters the body it multiplies and produces a very potent neurotoxin which causes TETANY.

Tetany: A condition most often seen in abnormal calcium metabolism as occurs in hypoparathyroidism, vitamin D deficiency and alkalosis, in which there are convulsions, cramping and twitching of muscles.

Tetrad of Fallot: A congenital heart defect in which pulmonary stenosis is combined with a high ventricular septal defect, overriding of the septum by the aorta (which is supplied by both ventricles), and right ventricular hypertrophy (because the right heart pumps against the pressure of the left ventricle).

Thalassaemia beta: An inherited ANAEMIA, due to an autosomal dominant trait and more prevalent in certain geographical locations (Mediterranean basin, Burma, Iran, India and Africa). It presents as thalassaemia minor if the patient is heterozygous for the trait and there is only mild to moderate anaemia. Where the patient is homozygous for the trait it presents as thalassaemia major, and the patient suffers from severe anaemia and has a poor prognosis.

Thrombin: An enzyme in plasma and tissue fluids which is important in the blood coagulation cascade. It converts soluble FIBRINOGEN to insoluble FIBRIN, thus forming a haemostatic plug in association with platelets.

Thrombocythaemia: Essential or primary thrombocythaemia is a neoplastic condition of the megakaryocytes producing abnormal platelets in large numbers, which may be as high as 1×10^7 platelets per µL. It occurs in middle age or in the elderly with a recent history of spontaneous bleeding (NB: paradoxical; although increased platelets are present, often their function is not normal). In the bone marrow all cell elements are proliferating excessively but especially the megakaryocytes. Sometimes some of the platelets are normal in function, in which case the condition predisposes to thrombosis.

Thrombocytopenia: The reduction in the circulating platelet number below 100 000 per µL. If the count falls below 60 000 per µL there is the danger of spontaneous bleeding occurring. PURPURA is the condition in which small haemorrhages occur from capillaries throughout the body, resulting in small areas of haemorrhage called PETECHIAE in the skin, mucous and serous membranes.

Thrombocytosis: A transient increase in circulating platelets, usually self-limiting. Seen after injury, haemorrhage or removal of the spleen and accompanies some other disruptions in the blood cell numbers, for example neutrophil LEUKOCYTOSIS. The platelets are normal in structure and function and their increased numbers increase the risk of thrombosis.

Thrombophlebitis: A venous thrombosis, very often seen in the deep leg veins, associated with inflammation or infection at the site. The patient presents with pain and swelling in the region (cf. PHLEBOTHROMBOSIS).

Thrombosis: Process resulting in the formation of a

THROMBUS.

Thrombus: A solid or semi-solid mass composed of elements of the blood and forming within the intact bloodstream during life. Its colour and shape may reflect its composition and mechanism of formation. Important complications are EMBOLISM and INFARCTION.

Thymoma: Any of a variety of swellings of the thymus gland presenting as a mediastinal mass and being either a typically benign, non-metastasizing tumour (epithelial thymoma containing Hassal's corpuscles) or a malignant tumour which metastasizes and resembles the lymphomata (granulomatous and lymphomatous thymomata). Thymomata may be associated with MYASTENIA GRAVIS.

Thyroiditis: Any inflammation or infection of the thyroid gland which may be acute and due most commonly to bacteria such as staphylococci or streptococci, or chronic and due to mycobacterial infection or associated with autoimmunity such as in HASHIMOTO'S DISEASE.

Thyrotoxicosis (= Graves' disease): An autoimmune thyroid disease characterized by the presence of autoantibody (LATS antibody) which constantly stimulates the thyroid to produce thyroxine, thus leading to hyperthyroidism. This disease is an example of the type V, STIMULATORY HYPERSENSITIVITY.

Tinnitus: The perception of ringing, buzzing, hissing or pulsating noises in the ears or head.

T lymphocyte: See **T Cell**.

Tolerance (immunological): The ability to recognize a given antigen as privileged and hence not to mount an immune response against it. We are tolerant of the self-antigens of our tissues and hence do not normally mount immune responses against them. If this self-tolerance fails, AUTOIMMUNE DISEASE may result.

Tonsillitis: An infection or inflammation of the tonsils (palatine lymphoid tissue in the oropharynx) frequently caused in an acute form by streptococcal infection, resulting in a severe sore throat, fever, malaise, DYSPHAGIA and headache.

Tophus (plural, **tophi**): A calculus developing in the soft, fibrous periarticular tissues of patients suffering from GOUT. It consists of sodium urate deposits and is surrounded by inflammatory cells.

Toxaemia of pregnancy: See **Eclampsia**.

Toxic shock: See **Endotoxic shock**.

Transient ischaemic attack (TIA): A commonly observed clinical presentation in patients with mild, or transient embolic occlusions of the brain vessels, the manifestations of the disorder being over within 24 hours with complete recovery occurring, otherwise the patient is described as having sustained a cerebral infarct. Symptoms and signs associated with a TIA are variable depending on the site of the brain affected (see AMAUROSIS FUGAX).

Transplantation: The surgical transfer of tissue from one part of the body to another or from one individual to another in order to repair damage and restore function, to replace a diseased structure or to improve appearance. The tissues of recipient and donor must be closely matched according to the major histocompatibility antigens they possess, such that rejection of grafts is not as likely to occur. Often, immunosuppressive drugs are administered to prevent this rejection reaction. Identical twins possess identical MHC antigens and this problem does not arise. The same may be said of AUTOGRAFTS, where tissue from one part of the body is transplanted to another part.

Transudate: Intercellular non-inflammatory fluid.

Trauma: Injury due to a physical agent; for example, falling over and breaking a bone is a traumatic injury.

Triple response of Lewis: A series of reactions developing in the skin in mild acute inflammatory reactions such as those induced by release of histamine (after a scratch or after histamine injection in the skin). (1) Transient pallor of the region caused by transient vasoconstriction; (2) flare, caused by vasodilatation and active hyperaemia mediated by the histamine; (3) wheal, filled with oedema fluid caused by increased vascular permeability due to opening of interendothelial cell junctions in the venules. The response is short-lived and is over in less than 30 minutes.

Tubercle: The specific chronic inflammatory GRANULOMA associated with infection with *Mycobacterium tuberculosis*. It has a central region of CASEOUS NECROSIS and is surrounded by chronic inflammatory cells (LYMPHOCYTES, MACROPHAGES, EPITHELIOID CELLS and GIANT CELLS).

Ulcer: A local excavation or defect on the surface of a tissue, caused by necrosis and sloughing off of debris.

Ulcerative colitis (non-specific): A chronic, autoimmune, inflammatory disease of the large intestinal mucosa which is episodic in nature and generally presents in young adults. Symptoms and signs include a profuse, watery diarrhoea (may contain blood and pus), severe abdominal pain, TENESMUS, fever, chills, ANAEMIA and weight loss. The mucosa of the affected regions become ulcerated and acutely inflamed (often with secondary bacterial infections), the intervening intact mucosa undergoing hyperplasia to form pseudopolypi.

Ulcerative colitis (specific = amoebic colitis, amoebic dysentery): An inflammatory disease of the colonic mucosa, resembling the non-specific form in presentation and histopathological findings but caused by infection with *Entamoeba histolytica*.

Ultimate carcinogen: The substance which is directly involved in cellular changes leading to mutation in the cell undergoing CARCINOGENESIS. Most commonly the term is applied to a PROCARCINOGEN which has undergone chemical change through cellular metabolism, to give rise to the ultimate carcinogen, responsible for the carcinogenic effect.

Uraemia: Excessive amounts of urea in the bloodstream as occurs with RENAL FAILURE.

Urobilin: A brownish pigment formed by oxidation of UROBILINOGEN, and found in the faeces and urine.

Urobilinogen: A colourless compound formed in the intestine after bilirubin is degraded by normal flora bacteria. Some of the urobilinogen formed is excreted in the faeces, some is resorbed into the blood and excreted in the bile again or in the urine.

Urography: The X-ray examination of the urinary tract after a radio-opaque substance has been injected into the lumina of the structures under investigation; for example intravenous pyelography.

Urolithiasis: Urinary calculi which may form anywhere in the urinary tract (e.g. renal calculi, vesical calculi). They may cause obstruction, pressure atrophy, predisposition to infection, chronic inflammation and development of carcinoma.

Uroporphyria: A rare genetic disease in which excessive uroporphyrin is found in the urine. Patients present with photosensitivity, blistering dermatitis, haemolytic anaemia and SPLENOMEGALY.

Urticaria (= hives): A pruritic skin condition where acute inflammatory changes induce transient wheals of varying shapes and sizes, having a pale centre and red, raised margins. It may be due to allergic reactions or emotional factors, exposure to extremes of temperature or exercise.

Uveitis: Infection or inflammation of the uveal tract of the eye (iris, ciliary body and choroid). It may be caused by allergy, bacterial or viral infections, trauma, diabetes and systemic autoimmune diseases. An important complication is GLAUCOMA.

Vaccine: A suspension of living, attenuated or killed micro-organisms introduced into the tissues to induce ACTIVE, ARTIFICIAL IMMUNITY to disease.

Varicose veins: A condition in which the veins become enlarged and dilated, very tortuous and appear quite prominently below the surface of the skin if they are in a superficial situation. Varicose veins usually occur in the legs. Oesophageal varicose veins are seen in CIRRHOSIS of the liver.

Varicella: See **Chickenpox**.

Variola: See **Smallpox**.

Varix (plural, varices): An excessively dilated and tortuous vein.

Vector: A carrier which transmits disease from one organism to another. Vectors may be biological, in which case the infecting organism completes part of its life cycle in their tissues (e.g. mosquitoes in malaria), or may be mechanical, in which case they transmit the organism but they are not essential for the life cycle of the pathogen (e.g. flies carrying micro-organisms on their legs).

Vegetations: Thrombi forming on the heart valves which are often large and friable, consisting of large numbers of platelets, fibrin and inflammatory cells, sometimes also bacteria.

Venereal disease: See **Sexually transmitted disease**.

Ventricular fibrillation: The rapid and marked depolarization of the ventricular myocardium leading to cardiac ARRHYTHMIA. There is complete lack of electrical impulse, conduction and organized ventricular contraction resulting in a rapidly falling blood pressure and unconsciousness. Defibrillation and ventilation must be initiated immediately, otherwise patients may die within 5 minutes.

Verruca (plural, verrucae = 'warts'): A benign neoplasm of the skin caused by infection with the human papilloma virus (HPV). It may occur on dry skin, especially on the hands, or it may occur in moister areas of the perineum or genitals, in which case it is often transmitted by sexual contact.

VLDL (very low density lipoprotein): A plasma lipoprotein composed of triglycerides mainly, with small amounts of cholesterol and phospholipid. Its function is to transport lipids from the liver to peripheral sites. They may be converted to more soluble lipoproteins and eventually to low-density lipoproteins (LDL).

Vesicoureteric reflux: An abnormal backflow of urine from the bladder to the ureters. It may be caused by congenital anomalies, obstructions or infections and greatly increases the risk of ascending urinary tract infections and PYELONEPHRITIS.

Vincent's angina (= 'trench mouth'): An infection with spirilla in the periodontal tissues and gingivae, which recurs in predisposed individuals. It causes ulceration and necrosis with pain and offensive breath. It is treated with antibiotics.

Virilization (= virilism): The acquisition of male secondary sex characteristics by a female due to abnormalities of hormone levels, commonly seen in disorders of the adrenals.

Viscus (plural, viscera): A hollow organ.

Vitiligo: An idiopathic, acquired skin disorder where the patient has pale, irregular patches of non-pigmented skin on predominantly exposed areas of the skin.

Von Recklinghausen's disease: See **Neurofibromatosis**.

Von Willebrand's disease: An inherited blood clotting disorder characterized by a lack of factor VII. It is associated with EPISTAXIS, gingival bleeding, prolonged menstrual bleeding and bleeding after injury or surgery.

Waldenström's macroglobulinaemia: A monoclonal GAMMOPATHY in which plasma cells produce IgM antibody in inappropriately large quantities in response to an antigen. The blood becomes increasingly viscous with circulatory disturbances, fatigue and neurological symptoms. At the same time normal immune function is hampered and the patient is more prone to infections especially septicaemia and pneumonias.

Wallerian degeneration: The degeneration of a nerve fibre after it has been severed from its cell body.

Warts: See **Verrucae**.

Waterhouse-Friederichsen syndrome: A severe septicaemia with *Neisseria meningitidis* presenting with a sudden onset of fever, cyanosis, petechial haemorrhages and collapse from massive bilateral adrenal haemorrhages with adrenal failure. Emergency therapy centres around antibiosis, vasopressors, intravenous fluids, plasma and oxygen administration.

Wegener's granulomatosis: A relatively uncommon disease of a chronic inflammatory nature with formation of GRANULOMATA in the airways, necrotizing vasculitis and glomerulonephritis. The patient may present with a bloody, purulent nasal discharge, saddle nose deformity, chest discomfort and cough, weight loss and skin lesions.

Wernicke's encephalopathy: A degenerative disease of the brain affecting the hypothalamus, mamillary bodies and tissues around the ventricles and aqueducts. It is caused by thiamine deficiency and is seen in association with chronic alcoholism; it may also be seen in gastrointestinal disease such as HYPEREMESIS GRAVIDARUM. There is deterioration of mental function, double vision, muscular incoordination, and involuntary, rapid movements of the eyes.

Whipple's disease: A rare intestinal disease characterized by MALABSORPTION, STEATORRHOEA, anaemia, weight loss and arthritis. The symptoms may be alleviated by tetracycline and penicillin.

Whitlow: Inflammation of the end of a finger or toe resulting in suppuration around the nail region.

Wilm's tumour: See **Nephroblastoma**.

Wilson's disease: A rare congenital disorder in which there are abnormally high levels of copper in the body, especially in the liver, blood cells and brain. CIRRHOSIS may develop in the liver, HAEMOLYTIC ANAEMIA as the copper accumulates in the red blood cells, causing their destruction, and brain damage will cause neurological symptoms such as tremors, rigidity, DYSARTHRIA and DEMENTIA.

Xenograft (= heterograft): A tissue graft from a different species, usually rejected in the long term, but providing in the short term a protective or life saving function and used as an emergency treatment (cf. AUTOGRAFT, ISOGRAFT).

Xenobiotic: A substance that is not normally found in the body, a foreign (and often toxic) compound.

Xerophthalmia: Dryness of the cornea and conjunctiva due to vitamin A deficiency.

Yaws: A systemic, usually non-venereal infection of the tropics caused by *Treponema pertenue*. The initial lesion, called the mother yaw, is a GRANULOMA that ulcerates and then heals and scars. Weeks to months after the initial manifestation of the disease, successive granulomatous lesions form, all over the body including bone.

Yellow fever: A serious, often fatal, liver infection with a group B arbovirus of the family Flaviviridae, transmitted by mosquitoes of the genus *Aedes* and prevalent in the tropics. Characteristic necrosis of liver lobules develops and jaundice is what has given the disease its name. May nowadays be prevented by vaccination.

Zollinger-Ellison syndrome: A syndrome where a pancreatic tumour is secreting great quantities of gastrin which stimulate acid secretion by the stomach mucosa. Intractable peptic ulcers form in this condition.

Index

Page numbers appearing in *italics* allude to a major reference of the topic, while page numbers appearing in **bold** allude to a reference found in a diagram or a table. The symbol 'ff' after a page number implies that the pages after the quoted page also contain relevant information; the symbol '≈' indicates approximately equivalent terms. Refer also to the Glossary of Terms on page 766.

807